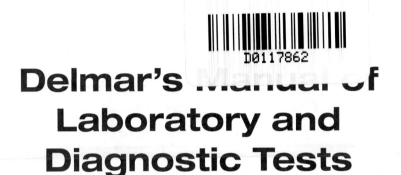

Delmar's Manual of Laboratory and Diagnostic Tests

Rick Daniels, RN, PhD
Oregon Health Sciences University
Ashland, Oregon

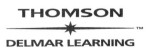

THOMSON
™
DELMAR LEARNING

Australia Canada Mexico Singapore Spain United Kingdom United States

THOMSON

DELMAR LEARNING

Delmar's Manual of Laboratory and Diagnostic Tests
by Rick Daniels, RN, PhD

Business Unit Director:
William Brottmiller
Executive Editor:
Cathy L. Esperti
Acquisitions Editor:
Matthew Filimonov
Developmental Editor:
Marah Bellegarde
Editorial Assistant:
Patricia Osborn
Executive Marketing Manager:
Dawn F. Gerrain

Channel Manager:
Jennifer McAvey
Project Editor:
Bryan Viggiani
Production Coordinator:
Nina Lontrato
Art/Design Coordinator:
Jay Purcell
Database Coordinator:
Linda Helfrich

ISBN-13: 978-0-7668-6235-7
ISBN-10: 0-7668-6235-6

NOTICE TO THE READER

Contents

Introduction

We are excited to announce the arrival of the trend-setting *Delmar's Manual of Laboratory and Diagnostic Tests.* This new reference book has a combination of features that make it a very unique laboratory and diagnostic book. It presents the most current knowledge, uses the latest in technological approaches, introduces an international perspective, and is in an extremely "user friendly" format. This must-have reference is organized by type of test, indexed, and fully cross referenced. Each test has an exceptionally straightforward and concise presentation of information. *Delmar's Manual of Laboratory and Diagnostic Tests* is designed to provide students and practitioners of nursing, medicine, and medical technology with the necessary information to provide comprehensive care for their clients who are having laboratory and diagnostic tests and procedures.

The reader will quickly see that the information provided for each test has been developed with careful attention to ease of use, concise explanations, and the most current up-to-date information. Overall, this manual is unique in its inclusion of international authors, information specific to the international aspects of laboratory and diagnostic testing, specific nursing considerations including home health care and rural nursing, and weblinks for each test. The book contains several comprehensive indices that allow the reader the ability to quickly locate what they need.

Organization

Section I: The first three chapters of the manual contain need-to-know information about laboratory and diagnostic testing. Chapter 1, A Guide to Understanding and Using *Delmar's Manual of Laboratory and Diagnostic Tests*, explains what information can be found for each test. Chapter 2, The Ever-

Expanding Role of Laboratory and Diagnostic Tests, provides a synopsis of the importance of these tests, their relationship to nursing, and the ethical considerations in their interpretation. Chapter 3, Standard Precautions, addresses the absolute priority that standard precautions and infection control have as related to laboratory and diagnostic testing. Chapter 4, Selected International Perspectives on Diagnostic Testing, "whets the appetite" for not limiting the focus of obtaining knowledge to any one culture. Chapter 5, Case Study Presentations, provides good examples for the reader to synthesize information and to integrate knowledge related to laboratory and diagnostic tests.

Section II of the manual presents information on more than 600 tests. It is organized by types of tests. Chapters in this section include blood studies; culture, tissue, and microscopic studies; electrodiagnostic studies; endoscopic studies; fluid analysis and sputum studies; physical examination, manometric, sensation, and breath studies; nuclear medicine studies; stool studies; ultrasound studies; urine studies; and radiologic (x-ray) studies. Within each of these typology chapters the reader will find the tests organized alphabetically. Each test has the necessary information, including, but not limited to, the normal findings, equipment needed to perform test, test description (including pathophysiology), a step-by-step procedure list, nursing care (before, during, and after) for each test, interfering factors, complications, contraindication, and nursing considerations for specific topics (e.g., geriatrics, pediatrics, pregnancy, home care, rural, and international).

The Appendices contain many useful references that the reader will find helpful in learning about and performing laboratory and diagnostic tests. The index section of this manual is unique. In fact, there are three different easy-to-use lists in the indices: Listing of Tests by Body System, Listing of Tests by Type, and a general index that includes test names as well as synonyms.

Features:

• Unique worldwide perspective provided by contributors from all over the United States, Mexico, Guatemala, and

Canada. This perspective provides a well-rounded knowledge base for our "shrinking world."

- Organized by type of tests and has several indices that promote ease of use and allow reader to quickly find what they need.
- Weblinks for every test provide the reader with web addresses to seek more information about the alteration that is being tested for.
- Phonetic pronunciations are provided for the more difficult-to-pronounce test names.
- Before, during, and after test nursing considerations are listed for every test reinforcing to the student and practicing nurse that care is needed beyond just the test procedure.
- Use of color and illustrative artwork adds a supportive environment for the information regarding the tests.

Also Available

Delmar's Guide to Laboratory and Diagnostic Tests Student CD-Rom, Order # 0766815099

Delmar's Guide to Laboratory and Diagnostic Tests WEB (academic license), Order #0766815080

Delmar's Guide to Laboratory and Diagnostic Tests WEB (corporate license), Order #0766831124

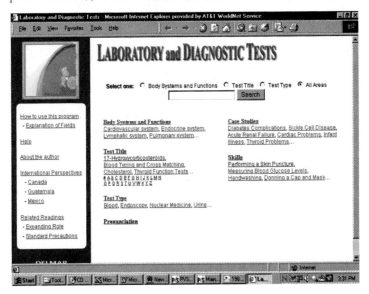

These exciting electronic versions of the *Delmar's Manual of Laboratory and Diagnostic Tests* bring interactivity to the quest for laboratory and diagnostic information. These electronic versions contain all of the information found in the book but have additional features including:

- Easy ability to search the entire database of information.
- Allow user to choose which information to view for a test.
- Audio pronunciation for selected tests that allows the user to hear the pronunciation.
- Ability to link to the weblink listed for each test.
- Ten additional case studies that enrich the reader's learning experience by showing how laboratory and diagnostic tests are used.
- The Web version will also feature quarterly updates that will reflect any new test or information available.

About The Author

Rick Daniels has been with the Oregon Health Sciences University, School of Nursing, since 1988. He received his Ph.D. from the University of Texas in Austin in 1994. Dr. Daniels teaches adult health and illness courses throughout the Bachelor of Science in Nursing curriculum. In addition, he teaches a distance learning course in pathophysioloy and administers clinical practicum electives in critical care and perioperative nursing settings. His clinical practice is kept current by practicing nursing as a lieutenant colonel in the Oregon Army National Guard. Dr. Daniels' research is primarily associated with the concept of health promotion (currently he is supervising a health promotion program in concert with the Department of Defense). In addition, Dr. Daniels publishes in nursing journals and authors nursing textbooks.

Acknowledgments

I would like to express my sincere appreciation to the contributors who bring a wealth of professionalism to this book. These contributors have applied their clinical practice, research efforts, and knowledge as they developed their respective sections of the book. I would also like to extend a thank-you to the reviewers of this book. Their comments and expertise were appreciated. Finally, appreciation and special thanks are also given to the editorial and production staff of Delmar Learning, who sustained our efforts from start to completion.

Contributors

Rosa Maria Cazares, RN, PG in
Neurology
Professor, Postgraduate Department
School of Nursing
National University of Mexico City
Mexico City, Mexico

Carol Craig, PhD, FNP-c, RN
Associate Professor
Oregon Health Sciences University
School of Nursing
Klamath Falls, Oregon

Heather Freiheit, RN, BSN, EMT-P
Associate Professor
Oregon Health Sciences University
Ashland, Oregon

Ellen M. Howe, RN, MS
Associate Professor of Nursing
Central Oregon Community College
Bend, Oregon

Josephine B. Jacavone, RN, MS,
CCRN
Clinical Nurse Specialist for Critical
Care Units
Rogue Valley Medical Center
Medford, Oregon

Katherine N. Moore, RN, PhD
Assistant Professor, Faculty of
Nursing
Adjunct Professor, Faculty of
Medicine
University of Alberta
Edmonton, Canada

Wendy Neander, BS, BSN, MN, RN
Assistant Professor
Oregon Health Sciences University
Ashland, Oregon

Linda M. Nisbet, FNP, MSN, CCRN
Cardiology Consultants, PC
Rogue Valley Medical Center
Emergency Department
Medford, Oregon

Jeanie Ouellette, RN, BScN, MN
Patient Care Manager, Pediatric
Medicine
Stollery Children's Health Centre,
University of Alberta Hospital
Associate Faculty, Faculty of Nursing,
University of Alberta
Edmonton, Canada

Marilyn Housel Poysky, RN, MSN
Assistant Professor
School of Health Sciences
Seattle Pacific University
Seattle, Washington

Milena Segatore, RN, MscN, MNI-PG,
CNRN
Clinical Nurse Specialist, Neurology
St. Joseph's Hospital
Milwaukee, Wisconsin

Valerie Lindquist Stalsbroten, RN, MN
Adjunct Faculty
Seattle Pacific University
Seattle, Washington

Debra L. Topham, PhD, RN, ACRN
Assistant Professor
Oregon Health Sciences University
Ashland, Oregon

Fred Wilkins, RN, BSN, CNOR
Nurse Manager, Operative Service
Roseburg Veterans Health Care
Adjunct Faculty Umpqua Community
College
Roseburg, Oregon

Reviewers

Jan Barrett, PhD, RN
Academic Dean
Deaconess College of Nursing
St. Louis, Missouri

Melanie King Gulliver, RN, MS
Coordinator/Adjunct Instructor
Broward Community College
Coconut Creek, Florida

Brenda Morris, RN, EdD
Clinical Associate Professor
Arizona State University
Tempe, Arizona

Ayda Gan Nambayan, DSN, RN
Assistant Professor
School of Nursing
University of Alabama
Birmingham, Alabama

Terrie Ortego, RN, CCM
Louisiana Technical College
T.H. Harris Campus
Opelousas, Louisiana

Kathy Simonsen, MT, AFCP
Medical Technologist
Southern Oregon Family Practice
Ashland, Oregon

Michele Woodbeck, RN, MS
Associate Professor, Nursing
Hudson Valley Community College
Troy, New York

Maryann Yzaguirre, RN, MS, MSN
Assistant Professor
Del Mar College
Corpus Christi, Texas

1

A Guide to Understanding and Using Delmar's Manual of Laboratory and Diagnostic Tests

A Wide Variety of Tests That Benefit the Client

This reference is an easy-to-use, concise summary of common laboratory and diagnostic tests and includes the physiological bases for the tests, clinical indications, and normal findings. Nursing care that precedes the examination and occurs during and after the examination is outlined. Absolute and relative contraindications, complications, and age-sensitive nursing considerations follow every description. Finally the reader is referred to related tests.

Every test reflects some facet of the structural or functional state of an organ or system. Some re-create the structure of an organ, a system, and even genes. For example, computerized tomography (CT) of the brain reconstructs for the viewer a two-dimensional image of the brain; an ultrasound of a pregnant uterus images a living, moving fetus; and densitometry of the hip joint in a geriatric patient identifies bone vulnerable to fracture because of its reduced density. These images can capture the normal, the pathological, and in the case of genetic mapping, the threat or inevitability of disease to come. Functional tests demonstrate, often in real time, biological processes. For example, positron emission tomography (PET) links data regarding cerebral blood flow, oxygenation, and glucose metabolism to illuminate metabolic activity in the brain. This technology is being used to better understand such phenomena as dementia, epilepsy, head injury, and even schizophrenia. Doppler ultrasound scanning of the peripheral arterial circulation equips the vascular surgeon with flow data that enrich surgical planning by differentiating critical stenosis from occlusion. A huge assortment of serological and blood tests sample organ function. Some monitor response to treatment or disease progression. Others search for disease or the tendency to develop disease in asymptomatic clients across all of the medical and surgical subspecialties. For example, ultrasound of the carotid arteries estimates the caliber of the carotid arteries in clients with bruits to identify those individuals who might reduce their risk of stroke by undergoing carotid endarterectomy. Serological evidence for the existence of carcinogenic embryonic antigen (CEA), a tumor-associated plasma marker, is an accurate marker in clients with curative resection of large bowel cancer for detecting liver metastases, though it lacks value for detecting the disease itself. Overall, the text includes the most pertinent and current laboratory and diagnostic tests designed to improve client outcomes.

Assumptions of the Text

There are basic assumptions for using this reference. The primary assumption is that the necessary information for each test is provided knowing that there are some practical limitations. In other words, every detail for every test cannot be presented, but the authors with their expertise have provided the information that they believe is cogent and accurate. For example, in the list of equipment for venipunctures "needle and syringe or vacutainer" and "alcohol swab" are listed. However, Band-Aids, cotton ball, gauze pad, tape, and gauge of needle are not included, but the color of the vacutainer is given. The assumption is that the readers know they need to apply a covering of their choosing after the venipuncture. However, the color of vacutainer is specific to tests and may not be known. Or, the reader may not know whether a plasma separator tube or serum separator tube can be correctly used. That information is provided when appropriate. Likewise, in nursing care after all venipunctures, the following statement is made: "Apply pressure to venipuncture site. Explain that some bruising, discomfort, and swelling may appear at the site and that warm, moist compresses can alleviate this. Monitor for signs of infection." However, phrases such as "resume normal activity" or "resume normal diet" are not written. The assumption is that the individual client care to be resumed is known by the health care provider and oversimplified statements might not be accurate from client to client. Therefore, the assumption is to present information that is necessary, but not to be so specific as to be inaccurate.

In addition, specific facilities may have their own procedures that vary slightly from region to region. The basic principles are the same, but slight differences may exist. This manual provides the most typical approaches to the information for each test but acknowledges the fact that the readers must be aware of the slight variations in their settings. For example, in urine testing, some facilities might have specific colors for containers that have different preservatives. These colors are not standardized, and therefore the list of equipment for urine specimen procurement is "sterile plastic container" without mention of a specific color. The assumption is that the readers will interpret their equipment list as they correlate that with their individual situations.

Last, this reference presents "just the right amount" of information as deemed necessary to perform laboratory and diagnostic testing on clients with health care needs. Interpreted, this means that the authors have chosen to select the appropriate knowledge from among the many interrelated disciplines that support each test. For example, this manual presents concise data on pathophysiology (in Test Description) and highlights the most necessary procedural steps to perform each test (in Test Procedure). However, this is not a nursing skills text or a pathophysiology text. The assumption is that the reader will access other materials for further knowledge specific to areas of interest, but the information provided is enough to provide comprehensive and quality client care.

Overviews of Types of Tests

Section II of the book is divided into chapters that are categorized by typology of testing. The test types are blood studies; culture, tissue, and microscopic studies; electrodiagnostic studies; endoscopic studies; fluid analysis and sputum studies; physical examination, manometric, sensation, and breath studies; nuclear medicine studies; stool studies; ultrasound studies; urine studies; and radiologic (x-ray) studies. Similar types of tests are grouped together to provide a more concise feel to the book. The reader will find at the beginning of the chapter an alphabetical listing of that chapter's tests. A general overview of the particular type of tests discussed follows. The purpose of these overviews is to provide background information. This information can include an introduction to the type of tests, the physiology of the body substance being discussed (e.g., blood, urine), methods of specimen collection, appropriate client care, and handling of the specimens. The remainder of the chapter is devoted to the actual tests. See below for an explanation of the fields of test information. It is understood that some tests may be done with more than one type of testing. For instance, a test could be performed using blood or urine. You will find the tests categorized under only the most prevalent method of testing. However, the test listings also include information on the alternative testing method, providing a comprehensive view of the test.

Explanation of Fields

The following is an item-by-item explanation for the information provided in the laboratory and diagnostic tests presented in this book. Each test will likely not have entries in all of these data entry fields but will have information as it is relevant to the specific test:

Title of test: The test title is provided as the primary identifier for each test. They are listed alphabetically, and then cross-referencing occurs throughout the text and in the appendix. There are over 600 tests covered in the body of this guide.

Pronunciation: Each test that may be considered difficult to pronounce has a phonetic pronunciation to allow the reader education on how to correctly state the names of the tests to other health care providers and clients (note: the accented syllables are in bold capital letters).

Synonym: As a test may have many synonyms for its usage, we have listed all the synonyms below the pronunciation. These synonyms are the most common ones and are listed in alphabetical order. This assists the reader in identifying other names for a given test. The synonyms can also be found in the test name index.

Type of test: Each test is identified as to its typology. This allows for groupings of tests that are similar in their inclusion. For example, Listing of Tests by Type of Test has the following categories, followed by the names and page numbers of specific tests for each division: blood, breath, culture, electrodiagnostic, endoscopic, fluid analysis, manometric, microscopic, nuclear medicine, physical examination, sensation, sputum, stool, tissue, ultrasound, urine, and x-ray. The reader immediately knows the specific category in which the specific test is enumerated.

Body systems and functions: Many pathologies are identified by the particular body system that is diseased. Therefore, each test has the primary body system identified. An example is seen in Listing of Tests by Body System. Each test is fitted into one of the following body systems: cardiovascular, endocrine, gastrointestinal, hematological, hepatobiliary, immunological, integumentary, lymphatic, neurological, pulmonary, metabolic, musculoskeletal, renal/urological, reproductive, or sensory. We have added two categories to the body system field that are not necessarily "systems" but are used to categorize (i.e., oncology and miscellaneous). There are obviously times when a test has more than one body system it could be correlated with, but for the purposes of this text, the primary body system is identified.

Normal findings: The normal findings for each test are identified. Norms for tests will vary according to different sources, so the normal findings presented are those that are used most frequently. In addition, there are tests that individual laboratories will have their norms for, and that is identified whenever appropriate.

Estimated time to complete test: The book includes the amount of time you can expect it will take to perform a given test. Look near the clock icon for the information. The reader must remember that these are estimates and that differences will exist, but generally speaking, the displayed amount of time is an accurate estimate.

Test results time frame: Each test has an estimated amount of time it takes to get the results back for the test. This is helpful for clients, as they naturally want to know how long they will have to wait before knowing the results of their test. And the health care providers can plan their care accordingly.

Clinical alert: Some tests have specific information that is "critical" for the health care provider to know. Some tests have conditions that can result in emergent complications and other tests have clinical manifestations that need to be observed. Therefore, this category depicts those concerns. For example, many contrast mediums used in tests can have anaphylactic reactions as a potential consequence. The health care providers need to know that emergency resuscitative equipment should be kept on hand during these tests.

Critical values: Some tests have values that indicate a medical and nursing concern of a critical nature. Thus, a number of tests will have this information as appropriate (e.g., blood glucose levels above or below the norm may require immediate attention).

List of equipment: A listing of the equipment necessary for performing the test is provided. When the test takes place in a specialized setting, this field may be blank. In addition, not every single item used for each test is given. For example, examination gloves are routinely worn with many types of physical contact and are therefore assumed but not listed. Also, when drawing a blood sample, the vacutainer tube, needle and syringe, and alcohol swab are listed, but a tourniquet, cotton ball, and Band-Aid are not. This encourages a concise approach to this data field without taking away important information.

Test description: A narrative paragraph explains what the test measures. If there is any appropriate anatomy/physiology or pathophysiology, it is presented in this category. The information is concise and pertinent in nature.

Test procedure: A step-by-step listing of how to do the test is provided in numerical sequence. Then, after some of the steps, the rationale for that step is provided in italics. For example: "Label the specimen tube. *Correctly identifies the client and the test to be performed.*" This italicizing allows the reader to quickly identify the information that is supporting the procedural activity. Again, only the necessary information is provided. For example, the fact that a test is performed by a medical technologist in the laboratory is not necessary to list. And the statement "send the specimen to the laboratory as soon as possible" is only used when time is of necessity. The reader will notice that consistency is advocated throughout the tests. For example, when a urine sample is collected for different tests, the same wording is used each time that method of collection exists.

Clinical implications and indications: This is a section for those things that cause the test values to be increased or decreased. It is also the area where specific reasons for why a certain test might be performed is provided. In addition, relevant clinical information is included that supports a particular test.

Nursing care: This section is for the nursing care for this test in its appropriate time frames (e.g., before test, during test, after test). Pertinent nursing assessments and nursing interventions are listed in narrative format for each of the categories (note: there may not always be information for each category for each test).

Before test: This section gives those items of nursing care needed prior to the test. To avoid duplication of another field, some things are not included, such as "obtain the informed consent." Also, "obtain a medication history and hold medications as ordered by physician" is not included but assumed.

During test: This section includes those items of nursing care performed during the test (e.g., "adhere to standard precautions").

After test: Those items of nursing care performed after the test are given here. To prevent duplication, "take specimen to laboratory" is not included here, as it is under test procedure.

See Tables 1-1, 1-2, and 1-3 for a complete discussion on before, during, and after test client care.

Potential complications: Some tests have potential complications that could develop as a result of performing the test (e.g., potential bleeding from a venipuncture on a client with a high prothrombin time).

Contraindications: Some tests should not be performed during certain conditions and these conditions are listed in this category. For example, a lumbar puncture should not be performed with clients suspected of having increased intracranial pressure.

Interfering factors: This category refers to factors that would interfere with the results of a test. For example, there are many tests where medications would alter the results. Those medications are listed in this category. However, the common interfering factor of hemolysis of a venipuncture sample that can occur with agitation is not included, but assumed.

Nursing considerations: This section includes additional information in any of several fields related to the nursing considerations for a specific test. These fields include pregnancy, pediatrics (including the fetus), gerontology, home care, rural, and international.

Listing of related tests: Many situations require multiple tests to be performed in conjunction with other tests. For example, hematocrit and hemoglobin are often evaluated at the same time.

Consent form: The importance of informed consent is recognized by this separate entry field and provides the reader with quick access to this knowledge. Occasionally, individual facilities will have their own requirements for consent. The assumption is that the reader will adhere to these individual practice requirements.

Weblinks: This field has website(s) for gathering more information about the test. This provides the reader with an additional method of accessing information. The assumption is that the reader is knowledgeable in respect to accessing the Internet. Note: URLs change frequently. The URLs listed under weblinks were current as of press date.

Table 1-1 Protocol: Preparing the client for diagnostic testing

Purpose	To increase the reliability of the test by providing client teaching on why the test is being performed, what the client can expect during the test, and the outcomes and side effects of the test. To decrease the client's anxiety about the test and the associated risk.
Level	Independent.
Supportive data	Increasing the client's knowledge promotes cooperation, enhances the quality of the testing, and decreases the time required to perform the study with an outcome of increased cost effectiveness. Proper physical preparation prevents delays.
Assessment	Check to be sure the client is wearing an identification band. Review the medical record for allergies and previous adverse reactions to dyes and other contrast media, a signed consent form, and the recorded findings of diagnostic tests relative to the procedure. Assess for presence, location, and characteristics of physical and communicative limitations or preexisting conditions. Monitor the client's knowledge of why the test is being performed and what to expect during and after testing. Monitor vital signs for clients scheduled for invasive testing to establish baseline data. Assess client outcome measures relative to the practitioner's preferences for preprocedure preparations. Monitor level of hydration and weakness for clients who are NPO (nothing by mouth), especially geriatric and pediatric populations.
Report to practitioner	Notify practitioner of allergy, previous adverse reactions, or suspected adverse reaction following administration of drugs. Notify practitioner of any client or family concerns you were not able to alleviate.
Interventions	Clarify with practitioner if regularly scheduled medications are to be administered. The NPO status is determined by the type of test. Administer cathartics or laxatives as denoted by the test's protocol; however, there must be a specific practitioner order to give children and infants a laxative. Instruct clients who are weak, especially geriatric clients, to call for assistance to bathroom.

Teach relaxation techniques, such as deep breathing and imagery.

Establish intravenous (IV) access if necessary for procedure.

Evaluation
Evaluate client's knowledge of what to expect.

Evaluate client's anxiety level.

Evaluate client's level of safety and comfort.

Monitor that someone will accompany a child to the department where the test is to be performed and remain with the child during the tests if not at risk of harmful exposure.

Client teaching
Discuss the following with the client and family as appropriate to the specific test:

- Reason for test and what to expect

- An estimation of how long the test will take

- NPO (if oral medication to be taken, how much water to drink)

- Cathartics or laxative: how much, how often

- Sputum: cough deeply, do not clear throat

- Urine: voided, clean-catch specimen, time to collect

- No objects (jewelry or hair clips) to obscure x-ray film

- Barium: taste, consistency, aftereffects (stools lightly colored for 24–72 hr, can cause obstruction/impaction)

- Iodine: metallic taste, delayed allergic reaction (itching, rashes, hives, wheezing, and breathing difficulties)

- Positioning during the test

- Positioning posttest (e.g., angiography—immobilize limb)

- Posttest, encourage fluids if not contraindicated

Documentation
Record the following in the client's medical record:

- Practitioner notification of allergies or suspected adverse reaction to contrast media

- Presence, location, and characteristics of symptoms

- Teaching and the client's response to teaching

- Response to interventions (client's outcomes)

Table 1-2 Protocol: Care of the client during diagnostic testing

Purpose	To increase cooperation and participation by allaying the client's anxiety and to provide the maximum level of safety and comfort during a procedure.
Level	Interdependent.
Supportive data	Increasing the client's participation and comfort encourages relaxation of muscles to facilitate instrumentation.
	Proper preparation of the client ensures efficient use of time during the test and reliable results.
Assessment	Check the client's identification band to ensure the correct client.
	Review the medical record for allergies.
	Assess the preprocedure sedatives administered to the client before the administration of anesthesia during the procedure.
	Assess airway maintenance and gag reflex if a local anesthetic is sprayed into the client's throat.
	Assess vital signs throughout the procedure and compare with baseline data.
	Assess the client's ability to maintain and tolerate the prescribed position.
	Assess the client's comfort level to ensure the effectiveness of the anesthetic agent.
	Assess for related symptoms indicating complications specific to the procedure (e.g., accidental perforation of an organ).
Report to practitioner	Notify the practitioner if the client has any concerns or questions that you were not able to resolve.
	Notify the practitioner if the client has family members present and where they are waiting during the procedure.
	Notify the practitioner when the client is positioned properly and the anesthetic agent has been administered to the client.
Interventions	Institute standard precautions or appropriate aseptic technique for the specific test.
	Report to all personnel involved with the test any known client allergies.
	Place client in the correct position, drape, and monitor to ensure that breathing is not compromised.
	Remain with the client during the administration of anesthesia.
	If the procedure requires the administration of a dye, ensure the client is not allergic to the dye; if the client has not received the dye before, perform the skin allergy test according to the drug manufacturer's instructions that accompany the medication.
	Maintain the client's airway and keep resuscitative equipment available.

Assist the client to relax during insertion of the instrument by telling the client to breathe through the mouth and to concentrate on relaxing the involved muscles.

Explain what the practitioner is doing so that the client will know what to expect.

Label and handle the specimen according to the type of materials obtained and the testing to be done.

Report to the practitioner any symptoms of complications.

Secure client transport from the diagnostic area.

Posttest in the diagnostic area:

• Assist client to a comfortable, safe position.

• Provide oral hygiene and water to clients who were NPO for the test if they are alert and able to swallow.

• Remain with the client awaiting transport to another area.

Evaluation   Evaluate client's ventilatory status and tolerance to the procedure.

Evaluate client's need for assistance.

Evaluate client's understanding of what was performed during the procedure.

Evaluate client's understanding of findings identified during the procedure.

Evaluate client's knowledge of what to expect after the procedure.

Client teaching   Discuss the following with the client and family as appropriate to the specific test:

• Explain what occurred during the procedure.

• Answer questions and concerns of the client or family member.

• Explain what to expect during the immediate recovery phase.

• Explain what to report to the nurse during the immediate recovery phase.

Documentation   Record in the client's medical record:

• Who performed the procedure

• Reason for the procedure

• Type of anesthesia, dye, or other medications administered

• Type of specimen obtained and where it was delivered

• Vital signs and other assessment data, such as client's tolerance of the procedure or pain/discomfort level

• Any symptoms of complications

• Who transported the client to another area (designate the names of persons who provided transport and place of destination)

Table 1-3 Protocol: Care of the client after diagnostic testing

---

Purpose	To restore the client's prediagnostic level of functioning by providing care and teaching relative to what the client can expect after a test and the outcomes or side effects of the test.
Level	Interdependent.
Supportive data	Increasing the client's participation and knowledge of expected outcome measures after a diagnostic test.
	Proper postprocedure care and client teaching alerts the client to what signs and symptoms need to be reported to the practitioner.
Assessment	Check the identification band and call the client by name.
	Assess the client closely for signs of airway distress, adverse reactions to anesthesia or other medications, and other signs that may indicate accidental perforation of an organ.
	Assess body area(s) where a biopsy was performed for bleeding.
	Assess the client's color and skin temperature.
	Assess vascular access lines or other invasive monitoring devices.
	Assess the client's ability to expel air if air was instilled during a gastrointestinal test.
	Assess the client's knowledge of what to expect during the recovery phase.
Report to practitioner	Notify the practitioner of any signs of respiratory distress, bleeding, or changes in vital signs; adverse reactions to anesthetic, sedative, or dye; and other signs of complications.
	Notify the practitioner regarding client or family concerns or questions that you are not able to answer.
	Notify the practitioner when any results are obtained from the diagnostic test.
	Notify the practitioner when the client is fully alert and recovered for an order to discharge.
Interventions	Implement the practitioner's orders regarding the postprocedure care of the client.
	Institute standard precautions or surgical asepsis as appropriate to the client's care needs.
	Position the client for comfort and accessibility to perform nursing measures.
	Monitor vital signs according to the frequency required for the specific test.
	Observe the insertion site for a hematoma or blood loss; replace pressure dressing as needed.

	Monitor the client's urinary output and drainage from other devices.
	Enforce activity restrictions appropriate to the test.
	Schedule client appointments as directed by the practitioner.
Evaluation	Evaluate the client's respiratory status to any anesthetic agents.
	Evaluate the client's tolerance of oral liquids.
	Evaluate the client's understanding of procedural findings or the time frame that written results should be reported to the practitioner.
	Evaluate the client's knowledge of what to expect after discharge.
Client teaching	Based on client assessment and evaluation of knowledge, teach the client or family about the following:
	• Dietary or activity restrictions
	• Signs and symptoms that should be reported immediately to the practitioner
	• Medications
Documentation	Record in the client's medical record on the appropriate forms:
	• Assessment data, nursing interventions, and achievement of client expected outcomes
	• Client or family teaching and demonstrated level of understanding
	• Written instructions given to the client or family members

Summary

Laboratory and diagnostic tests have a tremendous impact on the health of a wide variety of client populations. This reference provides the focused information for the health care provider to implement the precepts offered in a vital and necessary manner.

Bibliography

Barnett, H. J. M., & Meldrum, H. E. (2000). Carotid endarterectomy. *Archives of Neurology, 57*(1), 40–45.

Macdonald, J. S. (1999). Carcinoembryonic antigen screening: Pros & cons. *Seminars in Oncology, 26*(5), 556–560.

Small, G. W. (1999). Positron emission tomography screening for the early diagnosis of dementia. *Western Journal of Medicine, 171*(5–6), 294–295.

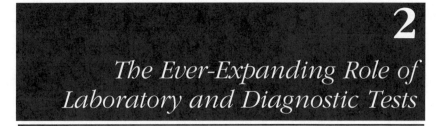

2

The Ever-Expanding Role of Laboratory and Diagnostic Tests

"The thinking activity—according to Plato, the soundless dialogue we carry on with ourselves—serves only to open the eyes of the mind."

Arendt, 1971, p. 6

Value of Laboratory and Diagnostic Tests

Perhaps the best way to come to an appreciation of the value of understanding the significance of laboratory and diagnostic tests is illustrated in the following example: A friend's husband recently experienced chest pain at home. He was rushed to the hospital by paramedics, triaged in the emergency room, and based on his clinical presentation and electrocardiogram, treated for the possibility of an acute myocardial infarction. In the emergency department, he received oxygen, aspirin, a beta blocker, and nitroglycerine. His laboratory values (i.e., myoglobin, tropinin) that are indicative of heart damage were assessed and found to be increased. Further blood was drawn to see if the more specific cardiac isoenzymes (e.g., creatine phosphokinase isoenzymes) would provide further information concerning his amount and location of heart damage. The laboratory tests and other diagnostic studies confirmed the need for immediate treatment. Within 50 min of symptom onset, he underwent surgical coronary treatment (i.e., angioplasty and stent placement). A transient arrhythmia (detected by the electrocardiogram) during the latter part of the surgery was successfully treated with lidocaine and magnesium. The family was ecstatic about the availability and competence of the health care team and very satisfied with the nursing care in the emergency department, surgical suite, and coronary care unit (CCU). They expressed appreciation for the kind, calm efficiency shown by the nurses and felt that they had been kept informed throughout the crisis. The value of laboratory and diagnostic tests is obvious in this client's healthy outcome.

Nurses' Role Associated with Laboratory and Diagnostic Testing

Nursing responsibilities related to clients undergoing diagnostic evaluation include education and advocacy; comforting, clinically monitoring and assisting clients prior to, during, and after the procedure. Postprocedure care can include monitoring recovery, managing complications, interpreting laboratory or procedural findings, taking corrective action for critical values, and organizing follow-up. The roles of nurses and physicians in the context of managing this acute coronary syndrome were convergent and complementary: Definitive action to correct the pathology was successfully undertaken. A variety of supportive activity also occurred, including monitoring and intervening to treat the arrhythmia and "just-in-time" instruction regarding procedural details and creating a calm and supportive environment. Nurses who attended this gentleman were able to support the client with timely rationales for every intervention along the way. Though nursing as a discipline lacks a systematic, coherent body of knowledge with boundaries, much of what nurses do is based on theoretical paradigms from a diversity of disciplines, including genetics, biology, biochemistry, microbiology, anthropology, epidemiology, ethics, psychology, and sociology. Thus, a compelling reason for mastering content related to the diagnostic process is that it augments, guides, and predicts events and processes relevant to the praxis of nursing. Nurses concern themselves with the nature and significance of laboratory and diagnostic findings because they directly influence the direction and scope of nursing interventions. Nursing has a broad base classically concerned with man, health, disease, and the environment—complex sets of variables with intricate and ever-changing interrelationships (Code of Ethics, 1998, p. 12):

> As part of the ever-changing relationship with society, nursing has an obligation to keep abreast of and contribute to those advancements in science and technology and in the arts and humanities that enhance nursing's goals.

The Future is Here

This reference of the proxy biochemical, structural, and functional markers of growth, development, and disease is especially timely given the fact that scientific knowledge is renewing itself every 18 months, if not sooner. The practice environment is ever more frantic, as the scientific, legislative, economic, and sociological contexts around it evolve. The American Nurses Association (ANA) Code of Ethics working draft is replete with nursing responsibility and obligation to remain up to date in this climate of accelerating knowledge growth and societal transformation. This reference is designed to provide the user with concise summaries of states of the sciences regarding a broad variety of specific tests. Using it will help avoid omissions or misinterpretations, thus improving the quality and efficiency of clinical problem solving. This reference facilitates the process of integrating diagnostic and clinical information to alter how nurses think about and intervene with clients (see Box 2-1 for a genetic testing example). The result is positively influenced client care outcomes.

Ethics of Interpreting Tests

With the continued mapping of the humane genome, the possibility of early identification of often lethal disease in asymptomatic individuals is raising ethical questions that few of us are equipped to address. Decisions flowing directly from a single laboratory test may have profound personal consequences for clients and their extended families. Today, the counseling and educational responsibilities demand that one acknowledges the scientific power, but more importantly the subtleties, limitations, and implications, inherent in the use of emerging technology. It is essential that clients be fully informed prior to exposing themselves or their families to the risks implicit in consenting to testing. Indeed, one can anticipate a growing need for nurses to support individuals who choose to avoid or defer diagnostic testing when financial, health, or personal consequences exceed any conceivable value in knowing the result. What issues ought to be raised by professional staff, if not by the client?

Box 2-1

A Genetic Testing Example

The following is an example of a case study involving genetic testing. It depicts the very nature of the complexity of genotyping: Adult children of a 70-year-old male had noted small problems with memory and felt that they should "do something" preemptively. Having recently heard in the popular press that there was an "Alzheimer's blood test," the family requested that the father be tested. Dementia of the Alzheimer type (AD), the most common of the dementias, is not a homogeneous disease. Three of the four confirmed genes—amyloid precursor protein, presenilin 1, and presenilin 2—contain rare mutations, are inherited as autosomal dominant traits, and tend to be associated with early-onset disease. This gentleman's family history excluded early-onset disease. But what of the fourth gene? Three alleles of the two apolipoprotein genes (Apo) we all inherit, ApoE 2, 3, and 4, are major determinants of the incidence and prevalence of AD. The 4/4 genotype may predispose one to AD with an earlier onset and higher relative risk of AD. Exactly how this happens is unclear. Although there is a commercially available ApoE marker, ApoE genotyping is not useful for predicting the development of AD in individuals who are cognitively intact. Current guidelines direct that testing should not be used for that purpose. If, on the other hand, patients have a nonfocal neurological exam and mental status findings supportive of dementia, then testing significantly improves the overall specificity for clients eventually confirmed at autopsy. At this time, this disease marker's value is limited to those who already carry a clinical diagnosis of AD. Then, and only then, testing is able to provide specificity for clients meeting clinical criteria for AD but is also the best predictor for younger memory-impaired individuals who will eventually develop full criteria for AD.

With this very specific indication, careful client selection and preparation are critical. The Alzheimer Association has emphasized that mere testing demands adequate pretest and posttest counseling, education, and psychosocial support and should include a full discussion of the implications of the test. For example, if positive, during the remaining time that the client is decisional, he faces financial, custodial, and medical decisions about such things as resuscitation, tube feeding, and nursing home placement. Conceivably, suffer the "many tortures" contemplating his fate. Consequences of error are obviously catastrophic in human terms. How does knowing the science help?

Given the limited utility of the test, the fact that AD has no cure and the good news that the client's neurological examination was normal, the family agreed to forego diagnostic testing. They felt a need to walk away from ambiguity, choosing to avoid the lack of control that might have arisen from "getting an answer." They prefer living with the uncertainty of not knowing and have made financial, housing, and other contingency arrangements for the future. The family shared the fact that their decision was based directly on the educational input and support they received from all caregivers. They felt affirmed by staff who trusted their judgment with complete and accurate information and appreciated not feeling pressured to consent to testing. This story, which continues to unfold, epitomizes the value of understanding laboratory and diagnostic tests. Judgments that can and do have immediate and long-term—even generational—consequences can be handled with compassion and humility and intelligence as we assist clients and their families in health-related decisions.

Ironically, the simplest questions may be the most difficult to answer: What does the result mean? Does a positive finding mean that disease is inevitable? Does a negative one exclude all risk? For every test, the answer will be rooted deeply in the biological sciences—whose mysteries are far from understood. Nurses are assuming personal responsibility for addressing the unknowable intelligently and with compassion. If one proceeds with testing, learns the results, and inaccurately understands the results, a deceptively "simple" yes or no may overwhelm, because every option flowing from either result implies life-altering choices. "Knowing" implies the necessity of confronting issues that the involved parties may be profoundly ill equipped to meet. Possessing easy access to state-of-the-art science information regarding the quality of diagnostic information in the management of disease and disease risk, particularly test sensitivity, specificity, and indications, will support that growing function. We encourage nurses to use resources like this reference as they find new ways in the millennium to meet their societal obligations. Nurses must use knowledge, skill, wisdom, and compassion as well as use the power that knowledge confers wisely.

Summary

We encourage you to take genuine pleasure in the use of *Delmar's Manual of Laboratory and Diagnostic Tests* and the practice that it supports. Indulge your curiosity, your capacity to explore, to digress, and to learn. May you enjoy privately the pleasure of your mastery of the subject matter, but for the public good. We are buttressed by the acceptance that nurses, doing and being with full comprehension and compassion and responsibility, are keeping faith with the public who have entrusted themselves into our care (Cicero, 1971, p. 90):

The third subdivision of intellectual activity is one which extends widely over all aspects of knowledge. This is the branch of learning that defines and classifies, draws logical consequences, formulates conclusions and distinguishes the true from the false. In other words, it is the art and science of reasoning: which is not only supremely useful for evaluating arguments of all kinds but also offers its devotees a noble satisfaction which merits the name of wisdom.

Bibliography

Adams, R. D., Victor, M., & Ropper, A. H. (1997). *Principles of Neurology* (6th ed.). New York: McGraw-Hill.

Arendt, H. (1971). *The life of the mind.* San Diego: Harcourt Brace Jovanovich.

Cicero. (1971). *On the good life.* (M. Grant, Trans.). London: Penguin.

Code of Ethics working draft #8 (rev. June 1998). [On-line]. Retrieved 4-17-2000: http://www.nursingworld.org/ethics/edraft.htm.

Fesmire, F. M. (Chair). (2000). Clinical policy: Critical issues in the evaluation and management of adult patients presenting with suspected acute myocardial infarction or unstable angina. *Annals of Emergency Medicine, 35*(5), 521–544.

Kaye, J. A. (1997). Oldest-old healthy brain function. *Archives of Neurology, 54,* 1217–1221.

Meleis, A. I. (1985). *Theoretical nursing development and progress.* Philadelphia: J. B. Lippincott.

Roses, A. D. (1997). Genetic testing for Alzheimer's disease. *Archives of Neurology, 54,* 1226–1229.

3

Standard Precautions

A reference on laboratory tests and diagnostics would not be complete without addressing standard precautions. The premise of standard precautions is relatively simple: to protect transmission of infectious agents from clients to health care workers (HCWs) or other clients. The human immunodeficiency virus (HIV) prompted serious concern about protecting HCWs from blood-borne pathogens. In addition, the Centers for Disease Control and Prevention (CDC) reports over 22,000 HCWs are infected with the hepatitis B virus (HBV) and over 200 die each year. This is despite the availability of hepatitis B vaccine (note: it is recommended that all HCWs receive the hepatitis B vaccine to reduce their risk of acquiring the infection). The newest blood-borne pathogen to become a prominent threat to HCW is the hepatitis C virus (HCV), which has no known cure or vaccine. Many other blood-borne pathogens necessitate health care workers following standard precautions (see Table 3-1).

Table 3-1 Examples of diseases caused by blood-borne pathogens

Cytomegalovirus	Rocky Mountain spotted fever
Creutzfeld-Jacob disease	Mononucleosis
Arboviral encephalitis	Syphillis
Brucellosis	Viral hemorrhagic fevers
Malaria	

Standard Precautions

Standard precautions that are to be used with all health care clients are listed in Table 3-2. The cornerstone of standard precautions is hand washing and the use of clean gloves when in contact with blood or any moist bodily fluids. The recommendation was for latex gloves, but with the growing number of HCWs with latex allergies, newer recommendations are for latex-free gloves. Other types of personal protective equipment, gowns, masks, and eye protection are only used when splashing of bodily substances is likely (Figure 3-1). The health care facility is legally responsible to provide for personal protective equipment in sizes that fit its workers. The final essential element of standard precautions is proper disposal of sharps, especially needles (Figure 3-2). Table 3-3 lists routes of transmission and the bodily fluids carrying blood-borne pathogens to HCWs.

Table 3-2 Standard precautions

1. Wash hands with soap and water after contact with blood, body fluids, secretions, excretions, and contaminated objects.
2. Wear clean gloves when touching broken skin, blood, body fluids, secretions, excretions, and contaminated objects.
3. Wear mask, goggles, or a face shield if splashing or spraying of blood, body fluids, secretions, or excretions is anticipated.
4. Wear a clean gown if splashing or spraying of blood, body fluids, secretions, or excretions is anticipated. The gown is to protect clothing and should be removed immediately after client care.
5. Soiled client equipment should be handled properly:
   - Dispose of single-use equipment correctly.
   - Clean reusable equipment and send for reprocessing, i.e., sterlization.
   - Dispose of scalpels, needles, and other sharps in a puncture-resistant sharps container.

Wash Hands (Plain soap)

Wash after touching **blood, body fluids, secretions, excretions,** and **contaminated items.**

Wash immediately **after gloves are removed** and **between patient contacts.**

Avoid transfer of microorganisms to other patients or environments.

Wear Gloves

Wear when touching **blood, body fluids, secretions, excretions,** and **contaminated items.**

Put on **clean** gloves just **before touching mucous membranes** and **nonintact skin.**

Change gloves between tasks and procedures on the same patient after contact with material that may contain high concentrations of microorganisms. Remove gloves promptly after use, before touching noncontaminated items and environmental surfaces, and before going to another patient, and wash hands immediately to avoid transfer of microorganisms to other patients or environments.

Wear Mask and Eye Protection or Face Shield

Protect mucous membranes of the eyes, nose, and mouth during procedures and patient-care activities that are likely to generate **splashes** or **sprays** of **blood, body fluids, secretions,** or **excretions.**

Wear Gown

Protect skin and prevent soiling of clothing during procedures that are likely to generate **splashes** or **sprays** of **blood, body fluids, secretions,** or **excretions.** Remove a soiled gown as promptly as possible and wash hands to avoid transfer of microorganisms to other patients or environments.

Patient-Care Equipment

Handle used patient-care equipment soiled with **blood, body fluids, secretions,** or **excretions** in a manner that prevents skin and mucous membrane exposures, contamination of clothing, and transfer of microorganisms to other patients and environments. Ensure that reusable equipment is not used for the care of another patient until it has been appropriately cleaned and reprocessed and single-use items are properly discarded.

Environmental Control

Follow hospital procedures for routine care, cleaning, and disinfection of environmental surfaces, beds, bedrails, bedside equipment, and other frequently touched surfaces.

Linen

Handle, transport, and process used linen soiled with **blood, body fluids, secretions,** or **excretions** in a manner that prevents exposures and contamination of clothing and avoids transfer of microorganisms to other patients and environments.

Occupational Health and Blood-Borne Pathogens

Prevent injuries when using needles, scalpels, and other sharp instruments or devices; when handling sharp instruments after procedures; when cleaning used instruments; and when disposing of used needles.

Never recap used needles using both hands or any other technique that involves directing the point of a needle toward any part of the body; rather, use either a one-handed "scoop" technique or a mechanical device designed for holding the needle sheath.

Do not remove used needles from disposable syringes by hand, and do not bend, break, or otherwise manipulate used needles by hand. Place used disposable syringes and needles, scalpel blades, and other sharp items in puncture-resistant sharps containers located as close as practical to the area in which the items were used, and place reusable syringes and needles in a puncture-resistant container for transport to the reprocessing area.

Use **resuscitation devices** as an alternative to mouth-to-mouth resuscitation.

Patient Placement

Use a **private room** for a patient who contaminates the environment or who does not (or cannot be expected to) assist in maintaining appropriate hygiene or environmental control. Consult Infection Control if a private room is not available.

The information on this sign is abbreviated from the HICPAC Recommendations for Isolation Precautions in Hospitals.

Figure 3-1 *Standard Precautions for Infection Control (Courtesy of Brevis Corporation).*

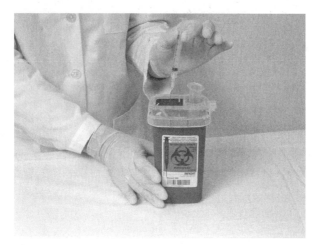

Figure 3-2 *Needle sticks are common among HCWs. Use proper technique and dispose of all sharp equipment in puncture-resistant containers.*

Table 3-3 Routes of transmission and bodily fluids carrying blood-borne pathogens to HCWs

Routes of transmission	Bodily fluids
Punctures—highest risk	Amniotic fluid
Mucous membranes	Blood
Open sores	Semen
Cuts	Vaginal secretions
Abrasions	Cerebrospinal fluid
Blisters	Pericardial fluid
Burns	Plural fluid
Acne	Synovial fluid
Chapped skin	Saliva in dental settings
	Unfixed human tissue

When clients have known or suspected infections that are passed via air, droplets, or contact, one of three transmission-based precautions is used *in addition* to standard precautions. To emphasize, transmission-based precautions are in addition to, not instead of, standard precautions.

Airborne precautions (Figure 3-3) are taken when clients infected with microorganisms smaller than 5 µm exhale the microbes into the air and potential hosts inhale the particles. An example of diseases transmitted by air include rubeola (measles), varicella (chicken pox and disseminated zoster), and tuberculosis.

Droplet precautions (Figure 3-4) are taken when clients infected with microorganisms greater than 5 µm exhale the microbes into the air and potential hosts inhale the particles. An example of diseases transmitted by air include diphtheria, meningitis, pertussis, mumps, rubella, pneumonia, and streptococcal pharyngitis.

Contact precautions (Figure 3-5) are taken when clients have a known or suspected microorganism that is transmitted by direct client contact or contact with items in the client's room. The CDC have identified several diseases that require contact isolation. Examples of these diseases include but are not limited to *Clostridium difficile*, enterohemorrhagic *Escherichia coli*, *Shigella*, hepatitis A, respiratory syncytial virus, parainfluenza virus, herpes simplex virus, impetigo, pediculosis, scabies, wound infections, or colonization with multi drug-resistant bacteria.

Obtaining Laboratory Specimens and Standard Precautions

In the process of obtaining specimens for the laboratory analysis or assisting with obtaining specimens for laboratory analysis, the nurse is obviously in contact with blood, body fluids, excretions, and secretions. Conscientious use of standard precautions is of highest priority while obtaining these specimens. After obtaining specimens, the rule of thumb is that while transporting specimens to the laboratory, two containers are used. The first container is a sealed, leakproof container with the specimen. The second container is usually a plastic biohazard bag. Additionally, biohazard symbols need to be prominently displayed on the outer container or bag. Laboratory requisitions or other paperwork should be kept on the outside of the bag. It should also be noted if the client is in isolation and the type of isolation. Specimens from clients in isolation should be placed in two plastic biohazard bags in addition to the original specimen container. In addition to the above, the nurse should take specific precautions with each type of specimen (Table 3-4).

Occupational Exposure

Even when using standard precautions, occupational exposure to bloodborne and other pathogens can still occur. Each health care facility is required by law [the Occupational Safety and Health Administration (OSHA)] to have an exposure control plan. This plan begins with standard precautions and moves to postexposure prophylaxis. With all exposure to pathogens, the area is to be cleaned thoroughly with soap and water and the incident reported to the occupational health nurse. Specific follow-up for blood-borne pathogens may include HIV antibody, HBV antigen, and HCV antigen testing of the client and the nurse; administration of prophylactic medication(s); and postexposure follow-up and counseling. The CDC recommends postexposure prophylaxis only in the cases of highest risk. This involves deep injury with bleeding from a hollow-bore contaminated needle or any exposure to blood or bodily fluids with a high HIV viral load. Postexposure prophylaxis is not recommended for percutaneous sticks or membrane contact with solid suture needles or splashes to eye or mouth in persons with low HIV viral loads.

VISITORS: Report to nurse before entering

Patient Placement

Private room that has:
Monitored negative air pressure
6 to 12 air changes per hour
Discharge of air outdoors of HEPA filtration if recirculated
Keep room door closed and patient in room.

Respiratory Protection

Wear an **N95 respirator** when entering the room of a patient with known or suspected infectious pulmonary **tuberculosis.** **Susceptible** persons should not enter the room of patients known or suspected to have **measles** (rubeola) or **varicella** (chickenpox) if other immune caregivers are available. If susceptible persons must enter, they should wear an **N95 respirator.** (Respirator or surgical mask not required if immune to measles and varicella.)

Patient Transport

Limit transport of patient from room to essential purposes only.
Use **surgical mask** on patient during transport.

Figure 3-3 Transmission-Based Precautions: Airborne Precautions. (Copyright 1996 by Brevis Corporation. Reprinted with permission.)

VISITORS: Report to nurse before entering

Patient Placement

Private room, if possible. Cohort or maintain spatial separation of **3 feet** from other patients or visitors if private room is not available.

Mask

Wear mask when working within **3 feet** of patient (or upon entering room).

Patient Transport

Limit transport of patient to essential purposes only.
Use **surgical mask** on patient during transport.

Figure 3-4 Transmission-Based Precautions: Droplet Precautions. (Copyright 1996 by Brevis Corporation. Reprinted with permission.)

VISITORS: Report to nurse before entering

Patient Placement
Private room, if possible. Cohort if private room is not available.

Gloves
Wear gloves when entering patient room.
Change gloves after having contact with infective material that may contain high concentrations of microorganisms (**fecal** material and **wound drainage**).
Remove gloves before leaving patient room.

Wash
Wash hands with an **antimicrobial** agent immediately after glove removal.
After glove removal and handwashing, ensure that hands do not touch potentially contaminated environmental surfaces or items in the patient's room to avoid transfer of microorganisms to other patients or environments.

Gown
Wear gown when **entering** patient room if you anticipate that your clothing will have substantial contact with the patient, environmental surfaces, or items in the patient's room or if the patient is **incontinent** or has **diarrhea,** an **ileostomy,** a **colostomy,** or **wound drainage** not contained by a dressing. **Remove** gown before leaving the patient's environment and ensure that clothing does not contact potentially contaminated environmental surfaces to avoid transfer of microorganisms to other patients or environments.

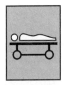

Patient Transport
Limit transport of patient to essential purposes only.
During transport, ensure that precautions are maintained to minimize the risk of transmission of microorganisms to other patients and contamination of environmental surfaces and equipment.

Patient-Care Equipment
Dedicate the use of noncritical patient-care equipment to a single patient.
If common equipment is used, clean and disinfect between patients.

Figure 3-5 Transmission-Based Precautions: Contact Precautions. (Copyright 1996 by Brevis Corporation. Reprinted with permission.)

Table 3-4 Specific precautions when handling various equipment

1. Capillary puncture: Blood is obtained in a microtube. The ends are sealed and the tube placed in a plastic biohazard bag for transport to the laboratory.

2. Venipuncture: Blood is obtained directly from the vein into vacuum tubes or by syringe and transferred to a vacuum tube. The vial is to be placed in a biohazard bag for transport to the laboratory. If a pneumonic tube system is used to transport tubes, they must be doubled bagged. Most institutions do not allow blood to be transported via pneumonic tube systems.

3. Biopsies:
   a. Laboratory transport: The tissue biopsy is placed in a sterile container with fixative. The container is closed. This container is placed in a plastic biohazard bag for transport to the laboratory. An example of this would be stereotactic breast biopsy tissue.
   b. Bedside slide preparation: Sometimes the biopsied material is placed on a slide, a slide smear is made, and fixative is added to the slide. The slide is then placed into a container for holding. The container is placed in a plastic biohazard bag for transport to the laboratory. An example of this would be bone marrow biopsies.

4. Urine specimens: Urine should be collected in a clean container. The container should be placed in a plastic biohazard bag for transport to the laboratory. For 24-hr specimens, a large container is kept on ice for collection of the urine. There is usually a preservative in this container, so if it spills, the laboratory should be notified immediately for proper instructions on cleanup.

5. Stool specimens: Feces should be collected in a dry, clean container such as a bedpan or commode. (A plastic "hat" that fits in the toilet to measure urine could also be used but it needs to be clean.) Unless otherwise specified, the entire specimen should be transferred to a container (clean denture holder works well) with a clean tongue blade. The specimen is covered and placed into a plastic biohazard bag. The bag is transported immediately to the laboratory.

6. Bodily fluids: For example, spinal fluid, pericardial fluid, synovial fluid, or pleural fluid is withdrawn from the corresponding body areas via needle and syringe. The sterile fluid is placed in sterile vial(s), which are sealed. The vials are placed in plastic biohazard bags and transported to the laboratory.

7. Cultures: The area to be culture, e.g., throat, conjunctiva, wound, is swabbed with a sterile swab. Moistening the swab with sterile normal saline can sometime increase the likelihood of obtaining microbes with the swabbing. The swab is placed in a vial and sealed. The sealed vial is placed in a plastic biohazard bag and transported to the laboratory.

Summary

Standard precautions are essential when considering laboratory and diagnostic testing. Therefore, every test described in this reference refers to "adhering to standard precautions." The desired outcome is for HCWs to function at the highest level of safety when their clients are having laboratory and diagnostic tests.

Bibliography

Annual number of occupational percutaneous injuries and mucocutaneous exposures to blood or potentially infective biological substances. (1998, June 15). Virginia: University of Virginia. [On-line]. Retrieved August 14, 2000: http://www.med.Virginia.EDU/medcntr/centers/epinet/estimates.html.

D'Souza, M., Carins, J., & Plaeger, S. (2000). Current evidence and future directions for targeting HIV entry. *Journal of the American Medical Association, 284*(2), 215–222.

McFarlane, M., Bull, S., & Rietmeijer, C. (2000). The internet as a newly emerging risk environment for sexually transmitted diseases. *Journal of the American Medical Association, 284*(4), 443–446.

Ross, R., Viazor, S., & Roggendor, F. (2000). Risk of hepatitis C transmission from infected medical staff to patients: Model based calculations for surgical settings. *Archives of Internal Medicine, 160*(15), 2313–2316.

Wong, J., McQuillan, G., McHutchinson, J., & Poynard, T. (2000). Estimating future hepatitis C mortality, morbidity, and costs in the United States. *American Journal of Public Health, 90*(10), 1562–1569.

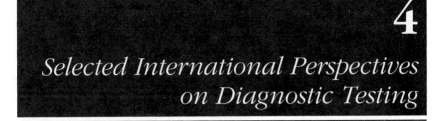

4

Selected International Perspectives on Diagnostic Testing

Diagnostic testing is quickly becoming extremely valuable to all health care systems in the world. While this reference does not attempt to provide a synopsis on a worldwide basis, the following is a presentation of three countries and their paradigm related to diagnostic testing. The information pertaining to each of the three countries is written from the perspective of nurse educators from each country, thereby providing unbiased information as to the most relevant content as determined by experts in their fields and their countries. The countries highlighted are Canada, Guatemala, and Mexico. A concise presentation is provided with the primary and important contributions of these authors related to their respective countries. An assumption is that the reader has some knowledge of health care systems in general and of diagnostic testing in specifics. The intended outcome goal for the reader is to have a broader perspective on how diagnostic tests are viewed from a more worldwide basis.

Diagnostic Testing in Canada

In Canada, as in any country, diagnostic tests are used to provide information that assists in diagnosis, provides a means of monitoring treatment and/or progress related to a pathological state, and assists in clarifying the status of specific states of wellness (e.g., pregnancy). What may cause diagnostic testing to look different when comparing Canada to other countries are issues related to coverage, access, monitoring of standards, measurement, and terminology.

Coverage

In 1966, Medical Care Insurance (Medicare), based on five identifiable principles, was introduced in Canada. In 1984, the Canada Health Act reaffirmed these principles and identified that health care fund transfers to provinces would be withheld if they were not respected. The principles apply to all aspects of the health care experience, including laboratory and other diagnostic testing. *Universality* implies that all Canadian residents, regardless of financial or social status, are entitled to health care services. *Comprehensiveness* ensures all necessary medical services will be covered. *Reasonable access* must exist and services must be provided on uniform terms and conditions. *Portability* requires that individuals remain covered when they are temporarily absent from their province of residence or out of country. Finally, *administration* of health plans must be assumed by *a nonprofit, public* authority that is regularly audited.

Listing these principles, however, should not lead the reader to assume that challenges did not exist in implementing this system or that these challenges do not continue to present themselves. Without delving further into the political history of Medicare, suffice it to say that health care in Canada remains universal, but there are provincial variations in the specific manner in which the principles are addressed and, as in many countries, continuing health care reform is a hotly debated topic. Any changes within the system are guaranteed to have direct or ripple effects in the area of diagnostic testing. Events such as the enactment of the North American Free Trade Agreement between Canada, Mexico, and the United States present new challenges for the Canadian system in maintaining a nonprofit health care environment. As well, further challenges have recently been introduced in the province of Alberta, where the provincial government has introduced changes that are largely viewed as the first step in a movement toward "for-profit" health care. At this point, however, all Canadians regardless of income or other status have access to medically required services (diagnostic tests included) and largely continue to access them through a national health care system.

Access

There are few situations in which a Canadian citizen would need (or be able) to access private services for diagnostic purposes. An exception currently receiving much attention is the establishment of private MRI (magnetic resonance imaging) clinics, a practice that began in 1993 in Calgary, Alberta. If an individual is unwilling to wait on a list in the regular system, they may purchase an MRI through a privately owned, for-profit clinic. Critics point out that this may then allow the individual to jump the line into their treatment, a topic that has received much attention, as this practice is not in keeping with the principles of universal health care. Since the same test could be accessed using universal coverage within the public system, many critics support the purchase of more publicly owned MRIs to reduce waiting lists, rather than indirectly causing jumping the line by allowing those who can afford it to purchase their tests. Needless to say, this remains a focus of much attention by citizens, health care providers, and politicians alike.

The use of diagnostic tests is largely physician driven since physicians bill for tests through the national health care plan. Some guidelines for specialized testing exist to control unnecessary use and resultant costs. Individual facilities also monitor use of tests and, in some cases, care maps have been helpful in providing guidelines for diagnostic testing needs in specific health care situations. Ultimately, however, physicians choose which diagnostic tests are needed to meet a client's specific needs. While some might wonder if this might lead to an increased use of tests and therefore health care costs, statistical information available regarding health care expenses indicates that a nationally insured system is no more expensive and, in most cases, is less expensive to provide than one that is not. The details and dynamics of why this is true are well covered in other publications and will not be addressed here.

Monitoring of Standards for Diagnostic testing within Canada

Within Canada, each province is responsible for the monitoring of diagnostic facilities, both in clinics and within hospitals. Bodies such as the Canadian Council on Health Services Accreditation, regional health authorities, and the Colleges of Physicians and Surgeons are utilized to act as proficiency monitors, but provinces do vary in the structure of their monitoring programs. Monitoring and accreditation for testing that occurs in the home setting done by clients themselves, as well as that done by pharmacists, are emerging issues likely to be of importance in any country where they are occurring with more frequency.

Measurement Differences for Diagnostic Testing within Canada

Some differences may be found in the reporting of diagnostic test results in Canada as compared to those in the United States. Conventional units are used more widely in the United States while Canadian test results are likely to be reported in SI (Système International d'Unites). Perhaps the best way to explain this is to give some examples of test results in their converted forms. In SI units, a few examples of reference ranges of normal values are:

Sodium	133–1466 mmol/L
Platelet	140–450 × 10^9 /L
Serum lipase	<190 U/L
Mucopolysaccharides	<41 U/mmol creatinine
Hemoglobin	115–155 g/L

This measurement format addresses quantity (where relative molecular mass is known) as "amount of substance" or mole rather than expressing it as mass. As well, many of the test results that might be reported as percentage in conventional units are reported as fractions. Note: This reference presents the norms for many of the tests in both the conventional and the SI units of measurement.

Terminology Used in Diagnostic Testing in Canada

Another area of difference between countries, and sometimes within countries, is that of terminology used by health care providers when referring to specific diagnostic tests. Traveling nurses who have worked in various countries and settings have noted specific terminology may vary. As an example, in Canada a fecal occult blood sample would usually be ordered as "stool for occult blood," while in many states in the United States this order would read "guaiac stool." Although differences are not usually so vast that there are difficulties in determining the purpose of the test, implications regarding clarification and verification do exist for the health care provider who is unfamiliar with the terminology to ensure that the client undergoes the expected diagnostic test. The majority of textbooks used by health care providers for interpreting diagnostic testing are those published in the United States. This reference has the advantage of international authors and specific implications for diagnostic tests as related to international implications.

Summary

Overall, the diagnostic testing in Canada has many similarities to the United States. The primary differences have been concisely discussed in this section, including coverage, access, monitoring of standards, measurement, and terminology.

Diagnostic Testing in Guatemala

In Guatemala, diagnostic testing is a method used to provide information with respect to the health status of an individual, family, community, or specific population. What may cause diagnostic testing to look different when comparing Guatemala to other countries are issues related to the historical, cultural, environmental, political, and economic context of the country. Coverage, accessibility, and the monitoring of standards of diagnostic testing in Guatemala are influenced by health care reform, the civil war of the past 30 years, and the present-day influence of peace.

Coverage

The Republic of Guatemala is located in Central America and has a land mass of 108,889 km. Guatemala shares borders with Mexico on the north and northeast, Belize on the northeast, and Honduras and El Salvador on the east and southeast. Guatemala has an estimated population of 11.562 million with 65% living in rural areas. The population is comprised predominately of indigenous people (approximately 60%) representing 21 different Mayan language groups.

Guatemala has a 30-year plus history of civil war. This humanitarian disaster caused by violent conflict has resulted in 75% of the population living in poverty. Peace accords were signed in 1996 to end the civil war in Guatemala. However, health services continue to struggle and the war has had a considerable impact on short- and long-term morbidity and mortality in the country. Additionally, government attention to health services was neglected during the civil war and left approximately 40% of the population without health care coverage.

Health care coverage in Guatemala is composed of private and public institutions, nongovernmental organizations, and traditional Mayan medicine (predominately in the rural areas). Institutional Health Services coverage of the Guatemalan population is as follows: Ministry of Health and Social Assistance (national health system open to all) covers 25%, the Guatemalan Institute of Social Security (IGSS) covers 17%, the Military Health Service covers 2.5%, nongovernmental organizations (NGOs) cover 4%, and the private sector covers 10% (PAHO, 1999).

Health Care Reform

As in many countries of the world, health care reform is occurring in Guatemala. The health sector reform has the following objectives: (1) to increase the coverage of basic health services focusing on the poorest segment of the population, (2) to increase the public spending and expand the sources of financing for the sector to ensure its sustainability, and (3) to rechannel the allocation of resources.

Many rural areas of the country have no access to diagnostic services; therefore the government is faced with the challenge of developing these services. People who require diagnostic services are often required to travel a day or more to reach a regional hospital or city in which diagnostic testing is offered. In some cases a person might walk 6 hr to reach bus transportation to a larger center. The poor economic situation, lack of infrastructure, and inaccessibility are present-day challenges for the rural population. The Guatemalan government is responding to these challenges with a new model for health care delivery called the Comprehensive Health Care System or Sistema Integral de Atencion en Salud (SIAS). This model (SIAS) intends to provide basic health care to the entire population that currently is without access to health services. The plans for implementation of the SIAS model include building on and utilizing existing resources, such as community organization and participation. SIAS implementation includes the delivery of specific, simplified, and ongoing health services provided by volunteers with the support and supervision of institutional personnel. Community participants in the SIAS model are expected to work closely with a health care team that provides them with technical, logistical, and decision-making support and whose members work in close contact with the community.

Monitoring the Diagnostic Services in Guatemala

With respect to diagnostic services, the challenge is to provide services that will help in the diagnosis, monitoring, and progress of pathological conditions that impinge upon the health of the population without coverage. The following focus areas are needed for the entire population before more specialized services can be developed: (1) women need prenatal screening, including basic services, such as hemoglobin, hematocrit, and Pap smears; (2) children need screening for iron deficiency anemia, parasitic infections, nutritional deficiencies, and respiratory infections; and (3) general screening is needed for parasitic infections, cholera, respiratory infections, malaria, dengue fever, tuberculosis, rabies, sexually transmitted diseases, and other local epidemiological problems.

In addition to the areas of focus for diagnostic testing, Guatemala is faced with the lack of surveillance systems that contain early-warning elements to identify elevated health risks. The Guatemalan government is strengthening its national epidemiological monitoring system and training epidemiologists to meet the need for a more responsible public health system, particularly at the local level. Malaria is a good example of a public health risk that needs improved surveillance. An effective local malaria surveillance system is influenced by collecting and analyzing blood smears to detect and type malaria parasites, beginning presumptive treatment, and returning laboratory results as quickly as possible to the community. It is effective to have the local technicians and health care providers provide treatment and prevention based on diagnostic results seen in their communities.

Present-Day Availability of Diagnostic Tests in Guatemala

In an attempt to meet the diagnostic testing needs of the Guatemalan population, a number of responses have been developed over the years. These responses include the following: (1) a large number of international nongovernmental (NGO) and governmental organizations have provided diagnostic screening on a short-term and often sporadic basis over the years in rural areas; (2) a number of nongovernmental Guatemalan organizations have also played a role in diagnostic services in rural areas; (3) some government health posts have provided screening for iron deficiency anemia, sexually transmitted diseases, tuberculosis, and stool specimen analysis for parasites, services contingent upon supplies, equipment (e.g., microscopes, centrifuges), and trained personnel; and (4) government hospitals are capable of a more comprehensive diagnostic screening but still lack equipment such as computerized axial tomography (CAT) scans and MRIs. When a person needs a CAT scan or MRI, it must be acquired privately at his expense. In certain cases, the government hospitals have negotiated a reduced cost for their clients.

Although these diagnostic services have been beneficial for the Guatemalan population, they have been somewhat disjointed and lack continuity in evaluation and monitoring. The Ministry of Public Health and Social Welfare needs to continue to develop its role as leader, regulator, financier, and executor of health services independently of the participation and the presence of international nongovernmental organizations.

Diagnostic Textbooks in Guatemala

Guatemala has severe limitations of standardization in diagnostic testing. Relatedly, health care providers use diagnostic textbooks that are developed from other countries and rely on the translation into the Spanish language. Unfortunately, there is not an adequate focus on the specific needs of the Guatemala system for diagnostic testing. Consequently, the inclusion of international implications for diagnostic testing is presented in this reference to attempt to bridge the knowledge gap for countries such as Guatemala.

Summary

Overall, Guatemala is more similar to Mexico than North American countries when comparing diagnostic testing. Guatemala continues to develop its health care services and technology, which is leading to better diagnostic testing.

Diagnostic Testing in Mexico

In Mexico, diagnostic tests are used to provide information that assists in diagnosis, provides a means of monitoring treatment and/or progress related to a pathological state, and assists in the prevention of disease processes. What may cause diagnostic testing in Mexico to vary from other North American countries are issues of access, availability of technological equipment, financial support, and textbooks written specifically for the Mexican culture and terminology.

Health Care Services in Mexico

Since 1990 and as a consequence of the economic globalization process (i.e., North American Free Trade Agreement, or NAFTA) (TLC in Mexico), important work has been exerted in health legislation in many North American and Latin American countries. The opening of commercial processes in the American countries provoked the review and elaboration of health norms in the interchange of benefits and services. In the Latin American countries, increasing economic resources are designated to the health assistance services. The majority of these medical services are established in the form of public social security services. However, there are also private services established throughout these countries.

In addition, the legislation and health coverage in the United States is primarily fee for service with about 58% having health services. In Mexico there are three different classes of health services, and they allow 51% of the people to have medical coverage. NAFTA gives financial support to Mexico, which allows for equipment and supplies for diagnostic services. Recently, Mexico had an agreement with NAFTA for South American countries to have a better interchange and interrelationships concerning health services.

Mexico Health Care Services and Access Issues

In Mexico, for the past 12 years, the monies designated for health care services have been progressively increased to provide better services. Unfortunately, many persons do not have access to any health care services. In Mexico, there is a General Health Care Law, which was reformulated during the 1995–2000 presidential period. During this time the health care structures were reformed by considering the demographic, social, and economic changes of the country. In addition, the various causes of illness and incidence of death were examined. Health care reform is continuing to focus more on prevention than on management of disease and more on health than on illness. The objectives of the General Health Care Law are primarily (1) to give health services to the people who do not have health care services, (2) to give better services to the people with services, and (3) to make better use of the materials and human resources that are currently available.

Health services are financed in a variety of methods. First, there is the structure of social security funding. The employers pay a specified amount of social security money for each employee. Then, the employees are provided with health services. Second, the government provides federal employees with health services coverage. Third, there is government support for limited health care services for unemployed persons. Fourth, and last, there are private hospitals and clinics where people pay for their services or the members pay for medical insurance that covers their health care services. Most of the above funding sources for health care cover diagnostic testing to some capacity.

Implementation of Diagnostic Testing in Mexico

Diagnostic testing has the same overall objectives in Mexico as in many other countries: to gather the most accurate information regarding a client's condition and to allow for the best treatments as a result of the diagnostic testing. The primary differences with Mexico's diagnostic testing when compared with other countries are the equipment available, the human resources and their level of training and education, and the financial resources for the diagnostic areas of implementation.

To provide an example of how diagnostic testing is implemented, Mexico City (population 20 million) is considered. Mexico City has private laboratories that are associated with both public and private hospitals. The private laboratories have different offices spread geographically throughout the city. The specimens are taken to one of three or four different laboratories by the different health care providers. In addition, the larger hospitals have their own laboratories, primarily used for clients housed within the acute care settings.

The nursing role is essential, due to their preparation of the clients prior to the diagnostic testing, checking the results of the tests, and techniques for performing the tests. Other technicians have important roles as related to diagnostic testing. However, such services as radiology are varied in their efforts. The maintenance and supply provisions may be lacking, which decreases the quality of the diagnostic testing. Therefore, even though there is access to free health care services, the quality of the individual services is varied and questionable. Another example is radiation protection. Many settings do not have adequate radiation protection supplies, which compromises the nursing staff involved as well as other health care providers associated with this type of testing.

Most of the laboratories in Mexico are private or associated with private hospitals. The laboratories work with an accreditation system established in each country, each having its own regulations. All of the techniques used in the laboratories are somewhat universal, but not all of the institutions are exactly the same. The primary focus in comparing one country to another is the interpretation of the diagnostic test results. This can involve something as simple as knowing which labels or values for a test are used. Or, there are laboratory tests that are potentially unique to a given country or region. The onus is with the health care providers to be able to identify the differences and similarities among the different countries.

Technology and Equipment for Diagnostic Testing

Some studies by the Pan American Health Organization (PAHO) (OPS in Mexico) have found that diagnostic testing is not as good in some countries in Latin America because they do not have an accurate understanding of the importance of having the right equipment to make a preventative diagnosis in cancer or cardiovascular disease. These countries are also not able to give viable economically affordable treatment that provides benefit to the client. The PAHO does not have the financial ability to purchase necessary equipment or hire properly trained personnel to have equitable diagnostic capabilities as other more developed countries. In addition, maintaining equipment is expensive and in Mexico is deficient, which compromises the diagnostic capabilities. Also, many of the supplies are imported from other countries, which is very expensive and adds to the difficulty of having technology necessary to compete with the health care delivered in other countries. Several countries (e.g., Argentina, Brazil, Bolivia, Chile, Peru, and Mexico) have an evaluation program of their technological services that is specifically related to diagnostic testing.

Diagnostic Textbooks in Mexico

Mexico does not have many laboratory and diagnostic textbooks developed specifically within Mexico. Health care providers rely on other countries for their texts and their translation to the Spanish language (see Box 4-1 for examples of common Spanish laboratory tests). Accordingly, there are diagnostic tests that are focused on in Mexico that may not be addressed by a text.

Summary

Overall, Mexico is more similar to the Latin American countries than the North American countries when comparing the use of diagnostic testing. Mexico is continuing to develop its resources and equipment to increase its diagnostic testing capabilities.

Box 4-1

Examples of Common Test Titles with Spanish Translations

English	Spanish
General Laboratory Tests	**Analisis de Laboratorioen General**
Biopsy	Biopsia
Blood test	Analisis de la sangre
Blood culture	Cultivo de sangre
Computed tomography (CT)	Tomografia computarizada
CAT scan	Tomografia axial computarizada
Endoscopy	Endosopia
Magnetic resonance imaging	Formacion de imagenes por resonancia magnetica
Ultrasound	Ultrasonido
Urinalysis	Analisis de orina
X-ray	Rayos X
Immune System and Blood Tests	
Differential blood cell count	Recuento diferencial de las celulas de sangre
Red blood cell count	Recuento de los globulos rojos de la sangre
White blood cell count	Recuento de los globulos blancos de la sangre
Clotting times	Tiempo de coagulacion
Hematocrit	Hematocrito
Hepatitis B	Hepatitis tipo B
Human immunodeficiency virus (HIV)	Virus de inmunodeficiencia humana
Platelets	Plaquetas
Bone marrow biopsy	Biopsia de la medula osea

Bibliography

Canada Health Act. [On-line]. Available: Canada.justice.gc.ca/FTP/EN/Cha/C/C-6.txt.

Cassels, A. (1992). *Implementing health sector reform.* Report prepared for the Health and Population Division, Overseas Development Administration, London.

Crichton, A., Hsu, D., & Tsang, S. (1994). *Canada's health care system: Its funding and organization.* Ottawa, Ontario: CHA Press.

Laurel, A. C., & Ortega, M. E. (1991). *El impacto del tratado de libre comercio en el sector salud.* Mexico City, Mexico: Mexico Fundacion Friedrich Ebert.

Mendoza, E. M., & Henderson, B. J. (1995). *International health care: A framework for comparing national health care systems.* Tampa, FL: American College of Physician Executives.

Organizacion Pan American de la Salud. (1998). *La salud en las Americas* (Vol. I.). Mexico Fundacion Friedrich Ebert, Mexico City.

Pan American Health Organization. [On-line]. Available: www.paho.org.

Secretaria de Salud. Programa Nacional de Salud Mexico, D. F. 1994–2000.

Secretaria de Salud. Reformas al programma Nacional de salud Mexico. D. F. 1995–2000.

Taft, K. & Steward, G. (2000). *Clear answers: The economics and politics of for-profit medicine.* Edmonton, Alberta: Duval House Publishing.

World Bank. (1993). *World development report 1993: Investing in health.* Oxford University Press, London, England: World Health Organization. [On-line]. Available: www.who.org.

5

Case Study Presentations

The knowledge of laboratory and diagnostic testing is invaluable information for nurses to possess. However, applying that knowledge during nursing practice is the true test for the professional nurse. The manner in which the nurse incorporates the laboratory and diagnostic testing data is essential for quality nursing care. Therefore, this chapter presents six case studies that realistically make the reader problem solve and work through the process of critical decision making as related to laboratory and diagnostic testing information. These scenarios are concise, yet portray accurate clinical situations where the nurse is given information about a client, including laboratory test results. Each case study asks the reader to (1) detect which laboratory values are abnormal, (2) present the normal limits of each laboratory test, (3) correlate the client's clinical manifestations with the correct laboratory values, and (4) describe the nursing care that needs implementing as related to the laboratory testing information. To enhance the learning process, there are correct responses provided with each of the six case studies. The outcome of this chapter is for the reader to incorporate problem-solving skills in the interpretation of laboratory and diagnostic test information for each of the case studies.

Case Scenario: Diabetes Complications

Mrs. Guadalupe Hernandez, age 65, has been hospitalized for complications of her diabetes. She was diagnosed with adult-onset diabetes mellitus (AODM) since age 51. She takes glyburide 10 mg q.d. She does not have a home glucose monitor. Last week she developed an ulcer on her left great toe, which she has been treating at home. She is unable to visualize her feet well, but she thinks it is getting worse. She noticed some red streaks on her ankle yesterday. The previous day at home she reports being very thirsty and needing to urinate frequently. Last evening she began feeling nauseated and vomited twice. When she came to the emergency room this morning she reported feeling very fatigued and had vomited once more. On physical examination, she has a fruity breath odor. Her vital signs are as follows: temperature (T) =100, pulse (P) = 102, respiration (R) = 28, and blood presure (BP) = 96/62. Her body mass index (BMI) is 32. Initial nursing assessment reveals a tired-looking woman with little ability to answer questions. She states that she has not eaten or taken her medication since yesterday morning. Her breakfast that morning was two corn tortillas with cheddar cheese and refried beans and two cups of coffee with milk and sugar. Her left great toe has a 5-cm round ulcer that involves the full depth of the skin and is bright red in color with a small amount of yellow-green exudate. The surrounding area is indurated and hot to the touch. Red streaks are present from her ankle to midcalf. She has little feeling in her feet and admits that the ulcer may have been present for some time.

Tests done in the emergency department indicate:
Blood glucose: 480 mg/dL
Blood pH: 7.0
Serum bicarbonate: 12 mEq/L
Serum positive for ketones
Potassium: 3.7 mEq/L
Sodium: 140 mEq/L
Calcium: 10 mg/dL
Leukocyte count: 22,000 U/L, with a shift to the left

Points to ponder:
1. Which laboratory values are abnormal?
2. Which values are within normal limits?
3. What clinical manifestations correspond to the abnormal values?
4. What nursing care needs to be implemented?

Discussion
   1. *Which laboratory values are abnormal?* Mrs. Hernandez's blood glucose
(480 mg/dL) is very high, reflecting hyperglycemia. Her blood pH (7.0) is acidic
and her bicarbonate (12 mEq/L) is too low, both of which indicate that Mrs.
Hernandez is acidotic. The presence of ketones in her serum suggests diabetic
ketoacidosis. Her white count (22,000 U/L) is high, and the shift to the left indicates increased neutrophils, reflecting infection. Infection is also indicated by
her low-grade fever. Adults with AODM who do not use insulin are most at risk
for diabetic acidosis when severe stress, such as infection, is present.
   2. *Which values are within normal limits?* Mrs. Hernandez's electrolytes (calcium, potassium, sodium) are within normal limits, even though vomiting and
acidosis can change electrolyte values.
   3. *What clinical manifestations correspond to the abnormal values?* The ulcerated toe and resulting infection are reflected in Mrs. Hernandez's high leukocyte
count and fever. Fatigue, nausea, and vomiting are common with hyperglycemia. The fruity breath odor is common with ketosis.
   4. *What nursing care needs to be implemented?* Diabetes is a disorder that
requires good self-management. Prevention of complications and the need for
hospitalization are essential. Mrs. Hernandez needs to learn the connection
between physical and emotional stressors and subsequent hyperglycemia. A
home glucose monitor is essential to track and maintain appropriate blood glucose levels. As Mrs. Hernandez has little feeling in her feet, she needs to be
taught how to examine her feet by using a mirror placed on the floor. Finally
her breakfast recall and her BMI may reflect a need for diabetic dietary education.

   While hospitalized, Mrs. Hernandez will need frequent blood glucose monitoring. Insulin will be needed to bring her sugar levels into normal range, and
she will need a diabetic diet to maintain an appropriate carbohydrate intake.
She should be monitored for hypoglycemic episodes and for appropriate therapeutic response. Her infected toe and subsequent sepsis require close monitoring for antibiotic effectiveness, as her ketoacidosis will not resolve until the
underlying cause has been successfully treated. Discharge education will
include the potential need for home health care visits.

Case Scenario: Sickle Cell Disease

Keesha Jones, an African-American boy age 8, has been hospitalized for complications of sickle cell disease. He is small for his age (20th percentile for height and weight) and complaining of severe pain in his abdomen. His conjunctiva and gingiva are pale. His abdominal pain is primarily in the left upper quadrant (LUQ). Keesha was adopted by the Joneses when he was 14 months of age. They have two other school-aged children and the parents take turns staying with Keesha in the hospital. Both parents are very caring and supportive in their relationship with Keesha. Keesha speaks well, asks age-appropriate questions, and responds politely to the nursing staff.

His CBC values are:

Hgb: 5 g/dL
MCV: 82
MCHC: 34%
RBCs: 3 million/μL
Reticulocytes: 8% of RBCs
Leukocytes: 8,000
PMNs: 60%
Lymphocytes: 31%
Monocytes: 7% μm^3

Points to ponder:

1. Which laboratory values are abnormal?
2. Which values are within normal limits?
3. What clinical manifestations correspond to the abnormal values?
4. What nursing care needs to be implemented?

Discussion

1. *Which laboratory values are abnormal?* Keesha has a normocytic (demonstrated by the MCV of 82), normochromic (MCHC of 34%) anemia. Combined with low RBCs (3 million/μL), low Hgb (5 g/dL), and a high reticulocyte count (8% of RBCs), the values are consistent with sickle cell crisis. During a crisis, RBCs are destroyed in high numbers and large numbers of reticulocytes are produced to replace destroyed cells.

2. *Which values are within normal limits?* All of the white cell counts are within normal limits (WNL) for Keesha; therefore, infection is not present. This is fortunate, as persons with sickle cell anemia are at risk of sepsis due to disruption of WBC formation in the engorged spleen.

3. *What clinical manifestations correspond to the abnormal values?* Keesha's fatigue is due to low oxygenation from his profound anemia, while his abdominal pain may reflect splenic engorgement due to sequestered RBCs. His pale conjunctiva and nail beds are due to his anemia. The chronic nature of his anemia has potentially resulted in poor height and weight gain. A more complete familial background is needed for further physiological evaluation.

4. *What nursing care needs to be implemented?* Keesha needs blood transfusion and adequate oxygenation and pain management during this acute episode of the sickle cell crisis. He is at risk for infection, and scrupulous hand washing and clean technique will be needed to prevent an iatrogenic infection.

Assessment of oxygen status and pain relief will take immediate precedence during the transfusion and early hospitalization. Long-term client and family support should include comprehensive psychosocial support as this disease is both chronic and difficult to manage. Keesha and his family need to be educated thoroughly as to the disease processes and management of sickle cell disease.

Case Scenario: Acute Renal Failure

Mrs. Jenny Lee, an Asian-American woman age 78, is hospitalized for acute renal failure. Her medical history includes osteoarthritis of the left knee and shoulder, cataract surgery in both eyes (OU) last year, and osteoporosis. She takes ibuprofen 400 mg q.i.d. for her arthritis pain, and recently she has added over-the-counter acetaminophen 325 mg q.i.d. for more effective pain control. She also has back pain, which her physician told her is due to osteoporotic spinal compression, and this is controlled with her current analgesics. Mrs. Lee noted that she only urinated once yesterday, and that was just a small amount. Today her hands and feet are swollen and her skin feels tight. The weather has been 100°F–105°F during the past week, and Mrs. Lee does not have air conditioning in her home. She knows she should drink extra fluids in the heat, but she was not feeling thirsty. Mrs. Lee lives alone and has two close friends that "look in every day to see how she is doing." Mrs. Lee is very cooperative and intelligent, as evidenced by the manner of conversation she maintains with the nursing staff.

Her laboratory values are:
Hgb: 14.2 g/dL
Blood urea nitrogen (BUN): 30 mg/dL
Creatinine: 1.8 mg/dL
Urine WBCs: 8 per high-powered field
Urine casts: moderate

Points to ponder:
1. Which laboratory values are abnormal?
2. Which values are within normal limits?
3. What clinical manifestations correspond to the abnormal values?
4. What nursing care needs to be implemented?

Discussion

1. *Which laboratory values are abnormal?* The BUN (30 mg/dL) has risen out of proportion to the creatinine level (1.8 mg/dL), an indicator of acute renal failure. The presence of WBCs (8 per high-powered field) and casts in the urine (moderate amount) is consistent with interstitial nephropathy, which could be precipitated by the additional nonsteroidal anti-inflammatory drug (NSAID) use and dehydration.

2. *Which values are within normal limits?* The Hgb (14.2 g/dL) is WNL, and Mrs. Lee has no other clinical manifestations related to anemia. Therefore, anemia is ruled out as an underlying factor in the acute renal failure.

3. *What clinical manifestations correspond to the abnormal values?* Mrs. Lee has both oliguria and tight skin, which reflect low renal perfusion and output.

These findings also correspond with the laboratory values indicating low renal perfusion in this client.

4. *What nursing care needs to be implemented?* Mrs. Lee's renal failure was potentially preventable, and client education could likely prevent another episode. The NSAIDs need to be discontinued with the assistance of Mrs. Lee. She needs to learn that NSAIDs can precipitate renal failure, especially in an older person. Adding over-the-counter medications should be discussed first with her primary health care provider and then with Mrs. Lee. In addition, perhaps Mrs. Lee's close friends could be advised as to the necessity of prevention of the same type of crisis and assist Mrs. Lee with her medication management. Also, older people are more prone to dehydration and decreased renal flow during hot weather, as sweat glands decrease and the thirst mechanism does not work as well as we age. Exploration of potential financial resources for adding cooling to Mrs. Lee's living environment could be examined. Last, if oliguria persists, dialysis will potentially be necessary until renal function is restored. Mrs. Lee would need to learn about dialysis and self-management of her care during treatment.

Case Scenario: Cardiac Problems

Mr. John Jamison, age 67, comes to his primary care provider complaining of dyspnea with mild exertion (walking up four stairs), fatigue, a dry, hacking cough, and sudden swelling in his feet. He had an 8-lb weight gain overnight. He has a history of hypertension with poor control, despite taking atenolol 10 mg q.d. Upon physical examination, Mr. Jamison is tachycardic with an S3 gallop and has expiratory crackles in the base of both lungs. His feet and ankles have 3+ pitting edema. His vital signs are T= 98.2, P = 112, R = 26, and BP = 154/108. Mr. Jamison lives with his wife at home and "takes care of her because she has had several mild strokes." He states that they have one adult child in the area who comes to visit them every week. And Mr. Jamison states that they have lived in the area for over 30 years and consequently have many friends nearby.

His laboratory and diagnostic results are:
Sodium: 142 mEq/L
Potassium: 3.9 mEq/L
Chloride: 100 mEq/L
Creatinine: 1.0 mg/dL
BUN: 15 mg/dL
Hgb: 15.0 g/dL
TSH: 2.5 μU/mL
Chest x-ray: left ventricular hypertrophy
ECG: normal sinus rhythm

Points to ponder:
1. Which laboratory values are abnormal?
2. Which values are within normal limits?
3. What clinical manifestations correspond to the abnormal values?
4. What nursing care needs to be implemented?

Discussion

1. *Which laboratory values are abnormal?* Mr. Jamison's chest x-ray shows left ventricular hypertrophy, a frequent compensatory mechanism to maintain sufficient cardiac output in a failing heart. This is suggestive of left-sided heart failure. In addition, the high blood pressure (154/108) is potentially dangerous, and uncontrolled hypertension can lead to cardiac failure.

2. *Which values are within normal limits?* Mr. Jamison has normal creatinine (1.0 mg/dL) and BUN (15 mg/dL) values, which rule out a renal cause for the congestive heart failure (CHF). Mr. Jamison's Hgb (15.0 g/dL) and TSH (2.5 μU/mL) are also normal, which rules out anemia and hyperthyroidism as precipitating causes. His electrolytes are within normal limits, which indicates that a sodium imbalance is not a problem at this time. The normal ECG rules out a myocardial infarction (MI) as an underlying cause of this episode.

3. *What clinical manifestations correspond to the abnormal values?* Mr. Jamison's fatigue and dyspnea likely have resulted from the failing heart's inability to provide sufficient oxygenation. The weight gain, swollen feet, and dry, hacking cough result from fluid pooling in the extremities and lungs. The S3 heart sound is vibration caused by blood distending a stiffened, hypertrophic left ventricular wall during diastole.

4. *What nursing care needs to be implemented?* Mr. Jamison needs diuretics and a moderate sodium restriction to rid his body of excess fluid. Once the acute episode has been treated, his blood pressure needs to decrease to normal levels to help reduce the strain on his heart. Mr. Jamison will need to learn about his medications and a sodium-reduced diet. He needs to be assessed for knowledge about his hypertension, the consequences of uncontrolled hypertension, and the potential prevention of disease through medication and life-style changes. In addition, exploration of assistance in caring for his spouse needs examination. Perhaps the adult child or friends could help in this matter, as well as determining the financial ramifications of a home health care provider.

Case Scenario: Infant Illness

Crystal Miller, age 4 months, has just come into the clinic with her mother. Crystal has had vomiting and diarrhea for 2 days. She has been fussy, felt very warm, and been refusing to bottle feed. Crystal's mother is worried because Crystal is listless and had only one wet diaper in the past 8 hr. Examination reveals an apathetic infant with decreased skin elasticity, a slightly depressed anterior fontanelle, slightly sunken eyes, and a dry diaper. Her vital signs are T = 103.2, P = 160, R = 30, and BP = 98/54. Crystal's mother states that this is a new condition for Crystal and that Crystal normally drinks well and urinates sufficient amounts. In addition, Crystal's mother states that Crystal recognizes her immediate family members with "smiles and cooing noises," moves her head toward sounds, and is normally "very aware of her surroundings." Crystal's mother is obviously very caring toward her child and appears very distressed over her daughter's condition.

Crystal's laboratory values are:

Stool culture: negative for ova and parasites and bacterial pathogens
Sodium: 130 mg/dL

Potassium: 3.2 mEq/L
Calcium: 8.2 mg/dL
Magnesium: 1.7 mg/dL

Points to ponder:
1. Which laboratory values are abnormal?
2. Which values are within normal limits?
3. What clinical manifestations correspond to the abnormal values?
4. What nursing care needs to be implemented?

Discussion
   1. *Which laboratory values are abnormal?* Crystal's electrolytes are all below normal levels (sodium, 130 mg/dL; potassium, 3.2 mEq/L; calcium, 8.2 mg/dL; magnesium, 1.7 mg/dL). This can potentially be expected in a dehydrated infant who has lost electrolytes through both vomiting and diarrhea.
   2. *Which values are within normal limits?* Crystal's stool culture is negative for pathogens, but the episode of diarrhea may be caused by a virus.
   3. *What clinical manifestations correspond to the abnormal values?* Crystal has been nauseated and vomiting, along with listlessness, sunken eyes, depressed fontanelle, and fatigue. These clinical manifestations can result from dehydration and electrolyte imbalance. The decreased urine output is likely due to dehydration.
   4. *What nursing care needs to be implemented?* Crystal needs rehydration. Since she is refusing to suck and drink from the bottle, it is necessary to replace both water and electrolytes parenterally. Crystal needs careful assessment of her response to rehydration, along with evaluation of her continuing fever, diarrhea, and vomiting. A continued monitoring of her urine output may necessitate an indwelling catheter. If not, then a careful examination of her diaper wetting will be required. A follow-up blood draw to monitor Crystal's electrolytes will likely be necessary. And continued assessment of her skin turgor, anterior fontanelle, and vital signs is necessary. In addition, emotional support of Crystal's mother during this acute hospitalization episode is needed. Assuming the rehydration is successful, a follow-up appointment with the primary health care provider needs scheduling.

Case Scenario: Thyroid Problems
   Mr. Thomas Brandon, age 39, comes to see his primary care provider because he has felt tired and listless for the past 4 months. Mr. Brandon is usually an active man, and he just "doesn't feel like himself." He noted an inability to concentrate at work as well as he usually does and stated he "feels colder." Mr. Brandon has gained 5 lb in the past few months, after being the same weight for 15 years. Upon questioning, Mr. Brandon states that his skin is drier and he has been having trouble with constipation. Upon physical examination, significant findings are coarse hair with dry skin and prolonged relaxation on DTRs; his vital signs are T = 98.6, P = 84, R = 16, and BP = 138/76. Mr. Brandon is an electrical engineer, has been married for 15 years, and has two children, ages 11 and 8.

His laboratory values are:
TSH: 7.8 μU/mL
T4: 3.8 μg/dL
Cholesterol: 240 mg/dL
Calcium: 9.3 mg/dL
Phosphorus: 4.0 mg/dL

Points to ponder:
1. Which laboratory values are abnormal?
2. Which values are within normal limits?
3. What clinical manifestations correspond to the abnormal values?
4. What nursing care needs to be implemented?

Discussion

1. *Which laboratory values are abnormal?* Mr. Brandon has a high TSH (7.8) level. His elevated TSH level in the presence of low T4 levels (3.8 μg/dL) confirms a diagnosis of hypothyroidism. Mr. Brandon's cholesterol (240) is high; hyperlipidemia is frequently found in people with low thyroid function.

2. *Which values are within normal limits?* Mr. Brandon's calcium (9.3 mg/dL) and phosphorus (4.0 mg/dL) are WNL. The calcium and phosphate levels may be low in hypothyroid states, but the disease process may take some time to cause their depletion.

3. *What clinical manifestations correspond to the abnormal values?* Mr. Brandon has several clinical manifestations that are indicative of hypothyroidism. As evidenced in Mr. Brandon, thyroid is a hormone that affects many body systems. Mr. Brandon's symptoms of hypothyroidism are the slowed metabolism, resulting in fatigue, constipation, difficulties with concentration, weight gain, and cold intolerance. In addition, coarse, dry hair and skin are also frequently found in people with hypothyroidism.

4. *What nursing care needs to be implemented?* Hypothyroidism is potentially a life-long condition, and Mr. Brandon will need to be evaluated for the potential of taking synthetic thyroid replacement therapy. If this treatment is prescribed, Mr. Brandon will need to understand the need to take the medication every day for the rest of his life. As people can sometimes develop hyperthyroidism from too much synthetic hormone, it will be important to include information on hyperthyroidism and to report symptoms to his health care provider. With daily medication, his signs and symptoms should be controlled or eliminated. In addition, quarterly laboratory testing of Mr. Brandon's thyroid levels will likely be ordered during his initial management. The importance of this follow-up will need to be emphasized and annual laboratory testing of his thyroid levels will likely be prescribed.

6

Blood Studies

45

EXAMINATION OF BLOOD

Blood is examined for many different purposes. The complete blood count with differential counts the numbers of red and white cells and the proportion of the different types of white cells. Blood may be drawn to examine substances within it, such as drugs and hormones.

PHYSIOLOGY OF THE BLOOD

Blood is composed of plasma and cells. The average person has 3 liters of plasma and 2 liters of cells. Plasma is formed from liquids absorbed by the intestines and transformed by body organs, while cells are manufactured primarily in the bone marrow. The primary physiological function of blood is the exchange of substances between cells and the external environment. Blood also provides defense against infection and assists in the regulation of pH and temperature.

Blood cells are composed of three basic types: red cells, white cells, and platelets. Red blood cells transport and exchange oxygen and carbon dioxide. White blood cells fight infection, and platelets maintain hemostasis. Blood cells have a limited lifespan and must be constantly manufactured by the body. All blood cells originate from a single type of cell found in the bone marrow called a stem cell. The stem cell differentiates to form red cells, white cells of several different types, and platelets.

METHODS OF OBTAINING BLOOD SPECIMENS

Three different procedures for obtaining blood are of importance to the nurse: capillary punctures, venipunctures, and samples taken from an indwelling apparatus. Gloves should always be worn when obtaining any blood sample. Ask the client about latex allergies before touching the skin with latex gloves. Skin punctures should always be made when the skin is dry because the sample can be diluted or contaminated by antiseptic.

Capillary Punctures
Capillary punctures may be taken from the earlobe, fingertip, or heel, although in adults the standard site is the fingertip. The fingers, heel, or earlobe can be warmed to dilate the capillaries and make collection easier. Never squeeze the extremity as it may dilute the blood sample with interstitial fluid. The skin is cleansed with an antiseptic and dried. The skin is punctured with a sterile lancet and the first drop of blood is wiped away with sterile gauze. The sample is collected in a capillary tube or dropped on a collection device for examination. Pressure is applied to the site to stop subsequent bleeding.

Venipuncture
Venipuncture is done on a peripheral vein in the arm, usually using a vacuum tube. Vacuum tubes come in several types which contain different reagents important to the specific test for which the blood is drawn. Do not draw blood on an arm that has an IV in place, as the IV fluid may dilute the sample. Have the client make a fist. A tourniquet is applied to the arm above the anticipated puncture site to identify a vein suitable for puncture. Warming the site or placing the arm in a dependent position may help to facilitate identification of a site. The skin is cleansed with an antiseptic and dried. A venipuncture needle is introduced into the vein and the tube is pushed onto the needle until the rubber stopper is punctured and blood flows into the tube. The tourniquet is released before the needle is withdrawn or after the first tube in a series of tubes is taken.

Collection from an Indwelling Device
Strict sterile technique is required when withdrawing blood from any indwelling device. Different devices have different procedures; follow the policy and procedure for each device separately.

HANDLING OF BLOOD SPECIMENS

Examination of Blood by the Nurse
Nurses frequently check hematocrit, hemoglobin, and blood glucose. All of these involve an examination of a capillary specimen. Each testing device will have

separate instructions. Blood must be refrigerated if it cannot be transported immediately to the lab.

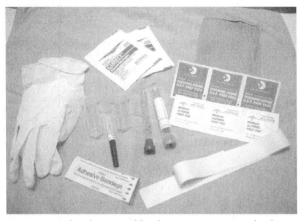

Equipment for obtaining blood specimen: nonsterile gloves, sponges, povidone-iodine, alcohol swabs, blood collection tubes, Vacutainer tube, Vacutainer needle, and rubber tourniquet.

Blood collecting tubes

Various vacuum tubes are used when collecting blood specimens (see table). When more than one type of tube is needed, the sequence is as follows: (1) blood culture tubes, (2) tubes with no additives, (3) tubes for coagulation studies, and (4) tubes with additives.

When all of the tubes are drawn, the needle is withdrawn and pressure applied at the puncture site. Pressure should be maintained for three minutes to prevent bleeding at the puncture site. Do not shake tubes. Label tubes and send them immediately to the laboratory.

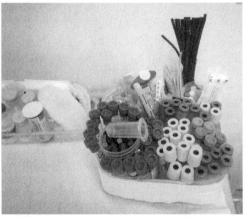

Vacutainer tubes used for collection of blood specimens

Examination of Blood by the Laboratory

Laboratory examination of blood provides valuable information about many disease processes and body systems. Blood examination is easily the most common method of diagnostic testing. Results are often obtained quickly and interventions are often employed based on the blood examination findings.

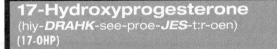

17-Hydroxyprogesterone
(hiy-*DRAHK*-see-proe-*JES*-t:r-oen)
(17-OHP)

5 min.

Type of Test: Blood

Body Systems and Functions: Endocrine system

Normal Findings:

Males:

Puberty stage 1	0.1–0.3 ng/mL
Adult	0.2–1.8 ng/mL

Females:

Puberty stage 1	0.2–0.5 ng/mL
Follicular	0.2–0.8 ng/mL
Luteal	0.8–3.0 ng/mL
Postmenopausal	0.4–0.5 ng/mL

Test Results Time Frame: Within 24 hr

Test Description: 17-Hydroxyprogesterone is one of the glucocorticoids produced in the synthesis of cortisol and estradiol. In women, levels are related to the ovulatory cycle. Newborns have a high level that rapidly decreases following birth. The test is done to detect congenital adrenal hyperplasia due to 21-beta-hydroxylase deficiency or other congenital enzyme deficiencies.

Consent Form: Not required

List of Equipment: Red-top tube or serum separator tube; needle and syringe or vacutainer; alcohol swab

Test Procedure:
1. Label the specimen tube. *Correctly identifies the client and the test to be performed.*
2. Obtain a 5-mL blood sample.
3. Do not agitate the tube. *Agitation may cause RBC hemolysis.*
4. Send tube to the laboratory.

Clinical Implications and Indications:
1. Increased levels are found with congenital adrenal hyperplasia due to 21-beta-hydroxylase deficiency and adrenal or ovarian tumors (note: levels have a marked variation in secretion, with the highest values in the morning).
2. Decreased levels are found with 17-alpha-hydroxylase and cholesterol desmolase congenital enzyme deficiency.
3. 17-OHP is occasionally used to detect adrenal or ovarian neoplasms.

Nursing Care:

Before Test: Explain the test procedure and the purpose of the test. Assess the client's knowledge of the test.

During Test: Adhere to standard precautions.

After Test: Apply pressure to venipuncture site. Explain that some bruising, discomfort, and swelling may appear at the site and that warm, moist compresses can alleviate this. Monitor for signs of infection.

Potential Complications: Bleeding and bruising at venipuncture site

Nursing Considerations:

Pediatric: Infants and children will need assistance in remaining still during the venipuncture and age-appropriate comfort measures following the test.

WEBLINKS

http://www.niddk.nih.gov

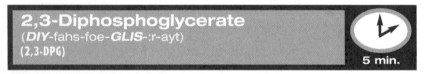

2,3-Diphosphoglycerate
(***DIY***-fahs-foe-***GLIS***-:r-ayt)
(2,3-DPG)

5 min.

Type of Test: Blood

Body Systems and Functions: Hematological system

Normal Findings:

Men   4.2–5.4 μmol/mL packed cells or 9.2–17.4 μmol/g of hemoglobin

Women   4.5–6.1 μmol/mL of packed cells or 8.4–18.4 μmol/g of hemoglobin

Test Results Time Frame: Within 24 hr

Test Description: 2,3-DPG is an organic phosphate in RBCs that alters the affinity of hemoglobin for oxygen. An increase in 2,3-DPG decreases oxygen binding capacity of hemoglobin so that increased amounts of oxygen are released and become available to tissues.

Consent Form: Not required

List of Equipment: Red-top tube or serum separator tube; needle and syringe or vacutainer; alcohol swab

Test Procedure:

1. Label the specimen tube. *Correctly identifies the client and the test to be performed.*
2. Obtain a 5-mL blood sample.
3. Do not agitate the tube. *Agitation may cause RBC hemolysis.*
4. Send tube to the laboratory.

Clinical Implications and Indications:

1. Elevated levels are found with hypoxia, thyrotoxicosis, pyruvate kinase deficiency, uremia, and anemia.

2. Decreased levels are found with alkalosis, polycythemia, hexokinase deficiency, phosphofructokinase deficiency, respiratory distress syndrome, and diphosphoglyceromutase deficiency.

Nursing Care:
Before Test: Assess the client's knowledge of the test. Explain the test procedure and the purpose of the test.
During Test: Adhere to standard precautions.
After Test: Apply pressure to venipuncture site. Explain that some bruising, discomfort, and swelling may appear at the site and that warm, moist compresses can alleviate this. Monitor for signs of infection.

Potential Complications: Bleeding and bruising at venipuncture site

Interfering Factors: Levels will be increased at high altitudes.

Nursing Considerations:
Pediatric: Infants and children will need assistance in remaining still during the venipuncture and age-appropriate comfort measures following the test.

Listing of Related Tests: CBC; iron binding; iron stores

WEBLINKS

http://www.methodisthealth.com

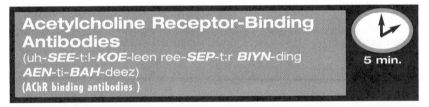

Acetylcholine Receptor-Binding Antibodies
(uh-*SEE*-t:l-*KOE*-leen ree-*SEP*-t:r *BIYN*-ding *AEN*-ti-*BAH*-deez)
(AChR binding antibodies)

5 min.

Type of Test: Blood

Body Systems and Functions: Musculoskeletal system

Normal Findings: Negative or <0.03 nmol/L

Test Results Time Frame: Within 24 hr

Test Description: Acetylcholine receptor-binding antibodies tests for the presence of elevated levels of serum AChRs. This test is considered diagnostic for myasthenia gravis. Myasthenia gravis (MG) is a neurological degenerative disease that destroys acetylcholine receptors bound by antibodies at the skeletal muscle end plate. The client with MG typically has clinical manifestations of fatigue, muscle weakness, particularly of the upper extremities, and often exacerbations/remissions throughout the disease process.

Consent Form: Not required

List of Equipment: Red-top tube or serum separator tube; needle and syringe or vacutainer; alcohol swab

Test Procedure:
1. Label the specimen tube. *Correctly identifies the client and the test to be performed.*
2. Obtain a 5-mL blood sample.
3. Do not agitate the tube. *Agitation may cause RBC hemolysis.*
4. Send tube to the laboratory.

Clinical Implications and Indications:
1. Detects AChR binding antibodies, which are increased in MG
2. Monitors the progression of MG after interventions

Nursing Care:
Before Test: Assess the client's knowledge of the test. Explain the test procedure and the purpose of the test.
During Test: Adhere to standard precautions.
After Test: Apply pressure to venipuncture site. Explain that some bruising, discomfort, and swelling may appear at the site and that warm, moist compresses can alleviate this. Monitor for signs of infection.

Potential Complications: Bleeding and bruising at venipuncture site

Interfering Factors: Clients with amyotrophic lateral sclerosis who have been treated with snake venom will have false-positive results.

Nursing Considerations:
Pregnancy: The physiological stress of the birthing process can stimulate a myasthenic crisis, which may cause severe respiratory complications and may require client to be placed in a critical care environment.
Pediatric: Infants and children will need assistance in remaining still during the venipuncture and age-appropriate comfort measures following the test (note: myasthenia gravis is relatively rare in this age group).

Listing of Related Tests: Glucose tolerance test; TSH; ESR; muscle biopsy; CBC

║WEBLINKS ║   ▣▨

http://www.nih.gov

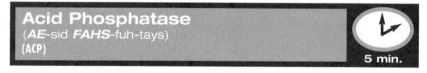

Acid Phosphatase
(*AE*-sid *FAHS*-fuh-tays)
(ACP)

5 min.

Type of Test: Blood

Body Systems and Functions: Oncology system

Normal Findings: (Note: values vary widely, depending on the laboratory).

Adults	0–0.8 U/L
Newborns	10.4–6.4 U/L
1 month–13 years	0.5–11.0 U/L

Test Results Time Frame: Within 24 hr

Test Description: Acid phosphatase is a group of enzymes that are widely distributed in the body and are active in an acid environment. The prostate, seminal fluid and RBCs have particularly high levels of these enzymes. Prostatic ACP is measured by adding tartaric acid to the sample, so that these samples are reported as atartaric inhibited levels. The test is done to assist in the diagnosis and course of prostatic cancer. ACP is also tested in the investigation of rape to establish the presence of seminal fluid.

Consent Form: Not required

List of Equipment: Red-top tube or serum separator tube; needle and syringe or vacutainer; alcohol swab

Test Procedure:
1. Label the specimen tube. *Correctly identifies the client and the test to be performed.*
2. Obtain a 5-mL blood sample.
3. Do not agitate the tube. *Agitation may cause RBC hemolysis.*
4. Send tube to the laboratory.

Clinical Implications and Indications:
1. Elevated levels of ACP are found with prostatic cancer, metastatic bone cancer, hyperparathyroidism, exacerbations of sickle-cell disease (from the destruction of RBCs) and other hemolytic anemias, and Paget's disease and disorders involving extensive destruction of kidney, liver, or bone tissue.
2. Decreased levels are found with alcohol ingestion and people with Down syndrome.

Nursing Care:
Before Test: Assess the client's knowledge of the test. Explain the test procedure and the purpose of the test.
During Test: Adhere to standard precautions.
After Test: Apply pressure to venipuncture site. Explain that some bruising, discomfort, and swelling may appear at the site and that warm, moist compresses can alleviate this. Monitor for signs of infection.

Potential Complications: Bleeding and bruising at venipuncture site

Interfering Factors: A number of drugs interfere with levels of ACP, including alcohol, flourides, oxalates, phosphates, androgens given to women, and clofibrate; vigorous prostatic massage within 48 hr can elevate levels.

Nursing Considerations:
Pediatric: Infants and children will need assistance in remaining still during the venipuncture and age-appropriate comfort measures following the test.

Listing of Related Tests: Alkaline phosphatase; bone scans; pelvic ultrasound

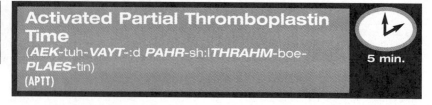

BLOOD

Activated Partial Thromboplastin Time
(*AEK*-tuh-*VAYT*-:d *PAHR*-sh:l*THRAHM*-boe-*PLAES*-tin)
(**APTT**)

5 min.

Type of Test: Blood

Body Systems and Functions: Hematological system

Normal Findings: 35–45 sec (times vary for clotting and widely depend on the laboratory and the substances used to activate the prothrombin)

CRITICAL VALUES:
Greater than 20 sec above the control time if client is not receiving heparin. Greater than 2.5 times the control time if the client is receiving heparin. Greater than 100 sec indicates a significant risk of severe bleeding.

Test Results Time Frame: Within 24 hr

Test Description: Blood clotting is a complex mechanism that requires a number of clotting factors to occur. Thromboplastin is one of those factors. The partial thromboplastin time (PTT) is a sensitive measure of blood-clotting ability. When this test is "activated," agents are added to the sample that "activate" or speed up the clotting of factor VII. The APTT test, therefore, measures the same functions as the PTT but is faster. This test is very useful to monitor anticoagulation therapy.

CLINICAL ALERT:
Normal findings vary so much between specific laboratories that misinterpretation of values can easily occur. It is vital to check the standard values of each laboratory. Do NOT use a tube with anticoagulant.

Consent Form: Not required

List of Equipment: Blue-top tube; needle and syringe or vacutainer; alcohol swab

Test Procedure:
1. Label the specimen tube. *Correctly identifies the client and the test to be performed.*
2. Obtain a 5-mL blood sample.
3. If client is receiving heparin, the blood is to be drawn 30–60 min before the next dose of heparin. *Ensures accurate results.*
4. Do not agitate the tube. *Agitation may cause RBC hemolysis.*
5. Send tube to the laboratory.

Clinical Implications and Indications:
1. Elevated levels are found with anticoagulant therapy, inherited deficiency of blood-clotting factors, liver disease, vitamin K deficiency, and disseminated intravascular clotting deficiency.

2. Decreased levels (hypercoagulable) are found with cancer, surgical procedures, pregnancy, heparin-induced thrombocytopenia, severe inflammation, and inherited causes.

Nursing Care:
Before Test: Explain the test procedure and the purpose of the test. Assess the client's knowledge of the test.
During Test: Adhere to standard precautions.
After Test: Apply pressure for at least 5 min to venipuncture site. Explain that some bruising, discomfort, and swelling may appear at the site and that warm, moist compresses can alleviate this. Monitor for signs of infection.

Potential Complications: Bleeding and bruising at venipuncture site

Interfering Factors: Traumatic venipuncture will alter times by inducing clotting; medications that alter results are salicylates, heparin, antihistamines, chlorpromazine, and ascorbic acid.

Nursing Considerations:
Pediatric: Infants and children will need assistance in remaining still during the venipuncture and age-appropriate comfort measures following the test.
International: About 20% of people of European descent who have a thromboembolism have an inherited problem with coagulation.

Listing of Related Tests: Prothrombin time

| WEBLINKS |

http://alice.ucdavis.edu

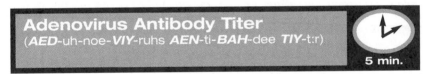

Adenovirus Antibody Titer
(*AED*-uh-noe-*VIY*-ruhs *AEN*-ti-*BAH*-dee *TIY*-t:r)

5 min.

Type of Test: Blood

Body Systems and Functions: Pulmonary system

Normal Findings: Negative titer

Test Results Time Frame: Within 24 hr

Test Description: Adenoviruses are a group of viruses that are the primary cause of upper respiratory infections. The infection tends to be self-limiting or inapparent. Groups most at risk for adenovirus infection are infants and young children and people on active duty in the military. An adenovirus titer is positive for people who are actively infected or who are convalescent with an infection. Asymptomatic infections will also have a positive titer. Serious infection is most likely to occur in the very young or those who are immunosuppressed. A titer is most useful in the diagnosis and management of serious disease.

Consent Form: Not required

List of Equipment: Red-top tube or serum separator tube; needle and syringe or vacutainer; alcohol swab

Test Procedure:
1. Label the specimen tube. *Correctly identifies the client and the test to be performed.*
2. Obtain a 5-mL blood sample.
3. Do not agitate the tube. *Agitation may cause RBC hemolysis.*
4. Send tube to the laboratory.
5. Repeat 10–14 days later for convalescent sample and label the tube as convalescent sample. *Allows for separate identification of the convalescent sample, which is compared in ratio to the acute sample.*

Clinical Implications and Indications:
1. The titer will increase from the onset of the infection to the convalescent state of the illness if infection with an adenovirus.
2. Monitors treatment for adenovirus.

Nursing Care:
Before Test: Explain the test procedure and the purpose of the test. Assess the client's knowledge of the test.
During Test: Adhere to standard precautions.
After Test: Apply pressure to venipuncture site. Explain that some bruising, discomfort and swelling may appear at the site and that warm, moist compresses can alleviate this. Monitor for signs of infection. Teach client to return in 10–14 days to repeat the test to see if the infection is subsiding.

Potential Complications: Bleeding and bruising at venipuncture site

Nursing Considerations:
Pediatric: Infants and children will need assistance in remaining still during the venipuncture and age-appropriate comfort measures following the test. Infants and small children may not have a positive titer, even though infection occurs.

WEBLINKS

http://www.rcjournal.com

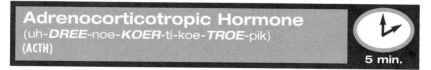

Adrenocorticotropic Hormone
(uh-*DREE*-noe-*KOER*-ti-koe-*TROE*-pik)
(ACTH)

5 min.

Type of Test: Blood

Body Systems and Functions: Endocrine system

Normal Findings: 4–22 pmol/L

Test Results Time Frame: Within 24 hr

Test Description: ACTH is a hormone secreted by the anterior lobe of the pituitary. The hormone maintains the functions of the renal adrenal glands by stimulating the adrenals to secrete glucocorticoids, androgens, and mineralocorticoids.

ACTH levels vary throughout the day and night cycle and rise in response to stress. The test is done to establish a diagnosis of Addison's disease, in which increased ACTH levels are found with low cortisol levels; Cushing's syndrome, where decreased ACTH is found with high cortisol levels; pituitary adenomas and malignant tumors that produce ACTH; and pituitary and hypothalamic disease.

BLOOD

Consent Form: Not required

List of Equipment: Lavender-top or green-top tube or plasma separator tube; needle and syringe or vacutainer; alcohol swab

Test Procedure:
1. Label the specimen tube. *Correctly identifies the client and the test to be performed.*
2. Obtain a 5-mL blood sample between 6 and 8 AM. *ACTH levels vary with diurnal rhythm, and levels are highest during this time.*
3. Do not agitate the tube. *Agitation may cause RBC hemolysis.*
4. Send tube to the laboratory.
5. Keep specimen cool. *High temperatures alter the results.*
6. A second sample may be drawn that evening to assess for diurnal variation.

Clinical Implications and Indications:
1. Elevated levels are found with Addison's disease, adrenal hyperplasia, and ACTH-producing tumors.
2. Decreased levels are found with Cushing's syndrome, adrenal carcinomas, and secondary adrenocortical insufficiency due to pituitary or hypothalamus disease.

Nursing Care:
Before Test: Explain the test procedure and the purpose of the test. Assess the client's knowledge of the test. Teach client to follow a low-carbohydrate diet 24 hr before the test and to be NPO for 12 hr before the test. Explain that glucose levels in the blood affect test results. Teach client not to do strenuous exercise 12 hr before collection. Assess client's stress level.
During Test: Adhere to standard precautions.
After Test: Apply pressure to venipuncture site. Explain that some bruising, discomfort, and swelling may appear at the site and that warm, moist compresses can alleviate this. Monitor for signs of infection.

Potential Complications: Bleeding and bruising at venipuncture site

Interfering Factors: Blood drawn at incorrect time; medications that alter results are adrenocorticosteroids (e.g., prednisone, dexamethasone), estrogens, androgens, calcium gluconate, amphetamines, alcohol, and spironolactone; exercise; stress; blood glucose levels

Nursing Considerations:
Pregnancy: Pregnancy will affect ACTH levels and may obscure interpretation of test results.
Pediatric: Infants and children will need assistance in remaining still during the venipuncture and age-appropriate comfort measures following the test.

WEBLINKS

http://www.niddk.nih.gov

BLOOD

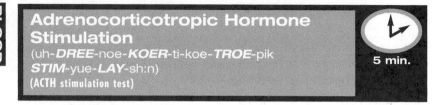

Adrenocorticotropic Hormone Stimulation
(uh-*DREE*-noe-*KOER*-ti-koe-*TROE*-pik
STIM-yue-*LAY*-sh:n)
(ACTH stimulation test)

5 min.

Type of Test: Blood

Body Systems and Functions: Endocrine system

Normal Findings: 4–22 pmol/L

Test Results Time Frame: Within 24 hr

Test Description: ACTH is a hormone secreted by the anterior lobe of the pituitary. The hormone maintains the functions of the renal adrenal glands by stimulating the adrenals to secrete glucocorticoids, androgens, and mineralocorticoids. ACTH levels vary throughout the day and night cycle and rise in response to stress. The test is done to establish whether the adrenals are responding to synthetic ACTH, to help differentiate adrenal disease from pituitary or hypothalamus disease. Normal adrenal function will produce a serum rise in cortisol of at least 20 μg/dL within 1 hr of stimulation with artificial ACTH.

Consent Form: Not required

List of Equipment: Lavender-top or green-top tube; needle and syringe or vacutainer; alcohol swab

Test Procedure:
1. Label the specimen tube. *Correctly identifies the client and the test to be performed.*
2. Give cosyntropin 0.25 mg IM or IV. *Stimulates the release of hormones by the adrenal glands.*
3. Obtain a 5-mL blood sample 30–60 min following cosyntropin. *Indicates adrenal response within a specified time period.*
4. Do not agitate the tube. *Agitation may cause RBC hemolysis.*
5. Send tube to the laboratory.
6. Keep specimen cool. *High temperatures alter the results.*

Clinical Implications and Indications:
1. Elevated levels are found when the adrenal glands are functioning normally, indicating problems in the pituitary-hypothalamus axis.
2. Decreased levels are found if adrenals are not functioning normally.

Nursing Care:
Before Test: Explain the test procedure and the purpose of the test. Assess the client's knowledge of the test. Instruct client to be NPO after midnight prior to test.
During Test: Adhere to standard precautions.
After Test: Apply pressure to venipuncture site. Explain that some bruising, discomfort, and swelling may appear at the site and that warm, moist compresses can alleviate this. Monitor for signs of infection.

Potential Complications: Bleeding and bruising at venipuncture site

Interfering Factors: Medications that alter results are adrenocorticosteroids (e.g., prednisone, dexamethasone, estrogens, androgens, calcium gluconate, amphetamines, alcohol, spironolactone); exercise; stress; blood glucose

Nursing Considerations:

Pregnancy: Pregnancy will affect ACTH levels and may obscure interpretation.
Pediatric: Infants and children will need assistance in remaining still during the venipuncture and age-appropriate comfort measures following the test.

Listing of Related Tests: ACTH

▌WEBLINKS ▣

http://www.ncbi.nlm.nih.gov/entrez/query.fcgi

African Trypanosomiasis
(*AEF*-ri-k:n tri-*PAN*-oe-soe-*MIY*-uh-sis)
(sleeping sickness; sleepy sickness)

5 min.

Type of Test: Blood

Body Systems and Functions: Immunological system

Normal Findings: No parasites present

Test Results Time Frame: Within 24 hr

Test Description: *Trypanosoma rhodesiense* (acute) and *T. gambiense* (chronic) are flagellates that cause forms of parasitic illnesses in the bloodstream of humans and transmitted by the tsetse fly. Finding *Trypanosoma* in blood provides a definitive diagnosis, but false negatives are high in chronic cases. Serologic assay is helpful in screening for trypanosomiasis. In the United States, bone marrow, lymph node aspirate, and cerebral spinal fluid may also be drawn for testing. Animal innoculation is also common in the United States. Since trypanasomes are found in the blood only 3 of 5 days, blood should be drawn and examined for 15 consecutive days. Drug treatment of the illness has a 10%–20% mortality rate; therefore treatment is never begun before a definitive diagnosis of the specific organism is made.

Consent Form: Not required

List of Equipment: Green-top tube or plasma separator tube; needle and syringe or vacutainer; alcohol swab

Test Procedure:
1. Label the specimen tube. *Correctly identifies the client and the test to be performed.*
2. Obtain a 5-mL blood sample.
3. Do not agitate the tube. *Agitation may cause RBC hemolysis.*
4. Send tube to the laboratory.
5. Repeat for ordered number of consecutive days

BLOOD

Clinical Implications and Indications:
1. Screens for trypanosomiasis
2. Diagnoses the parasitic illnesses caused by *T. rhodesiense* (acute) and *T. gambiense* (chronic)

Nursing Care:
Before Test: Explain the test procedure and the purpose of the test. Assess the client's knowledge of the test. Inform client that blood will need to be drawn for approximately 15 consecutive days
During Test: Adhere to standard precautions.
After Test: Apply pressure to venipuncture site. Explain that some bruising, discomfort, and swelling may appear at the site and that warm, moist compresses can alleviate this. Monitor for signs of infection. Instruct client regarding the potential continued serum blood draws for screening for the trypanosomiasis.

Potential Complications: Bleeding and bruising at venipuncture site

Nursing Considerations:
Pediatric: Infants and children will need assistance in remaining still during the venipuncture and age-appropriate comfort measures following the test.
International: Sustained screening programs in African countries at risk have been curtailed by cost, civil war, and low health budgets.

Listing of Related Tests: Sedimentation rate; WBC; bone marrow; CSF and lymph node aspirates; animal innoculation

║WEBLINKS   ▤▧

http://www.mic.ki.se/Diseases/c20.html

Alanine Aminotransferase
(*AEL*-uh-neen uh-*MEE*-noe-*TRAENZ*-f:r-ays)
(ALT; SGPT; GPT)

5 min.

Type of Test: Blood

Body Systems and Functions: Hepatobiliary system

Normal Findings: Normal laboratory findings vary among laboratory settings (note: different testing methods may have widely ranging normal findings).

Test Results Time Frame: Within 24 hr

Test Description: Alanine aminotransferase was once known as glutamic pyruvic transaminase (GPT), and the test was known as serum glutamic pyruvic transaminase (SGPT). References to the older names continue to be common. ALT is found in high concentration in liver cells, although smaller amounts are found in cardiac, renal, and skeletal tissues. The test is most useful in the evaluation and monitoring of hepatic disorders. The release of hepatocellular enzyme into the bloodstream occurs with injury or disease affecting the liver. This release will elevate the serum ALT. In viral hepatitis the ratio of ALT:AST is greater than 1.

BLOOD

CLINICAL ALERT:
Markedly high values (up to 20 times the reference range) are
considered to confirm liver damage.

Consent Form: Not required

List of Equipment: Red-top tube or serum separator tube; needle and
syringe or vacutainer; alcohol swab

Test Procedure:
1. Label the specimen tube. *Correctly identifies the client and the test to be performed.*
2. Obtain a 5-mL blood sample.
3. Do not agitate the tube. *Agitation may cause RBC hemolysis.*
4. Send tube to the laboratory.
5. Keep specimen cool. *High temperatures alter the results.*

Clinical Implications and Indications:
1. Elevated levels are found with drug toxicity, alcoholic hepatitis, cirrhosis,
   gallbladder obstruction, and hepatic cancer and are slightly increased with
   chronic cirrhosis and pancreatitis. Smaller rises can be noted with muscle tissue destruction, including cardiac tissue and renal failure.
2. The test may also be ordered in conjunction with AST to distinguish hepatic
   from cardiac damage. AST rises more consistently with cardiac damage than
   does ALT. However, AST may be more sensitive to alcoholic liver damage.

Nursing Care:
Before Test: Explain the test procedure and the purpose of the test. Assess the
client's knowledge of the test. Teach client to abstain from alcohol 24 hr before
blood is drawn.
During Test: Adhere to standard precautions.
After Test: Apply pressure to venipuncture site. Explain that some bruising, discomfort, and swelling may appear at the site and that warm, moist compresses
can alleviate this. Monitor for signs of infection.

Potential Complications: Bleeding and bruising at venipuncture site

Interfering Factors: Previous intramuscular injection elevates levels;
hepatotoxic medications; medications that alter results are acetaminophen,,
aminosalicylic acid, barbiturates, narcotics, phenytoin, phenothiazines, methyldopa, isoniazid, desipramine, oral contraceptives, gentamicin, allopurinol, and
antifungals (note: check with the pharmacist and the provider about other drugs
that might interfere with the ALT test).

Nursing Considerations:
*Pediatric: Infants and children will need assistance in remaining still during the
venipuncture and age-appropriate comfort measures following the test.*

Listing of Related Tests: AST

WEBLINKS

http://cpmcnet.columbia.edu

BLOOD

Aldolase
(**AEL**-doe-lays)
(ALS)

5 min.

Type of Test: Blood

Body Systems and Functions: Musculoskeletal system

Normal Findings:

Male	2.9–8.6 U/L
Female	2.0–6.5 U/L

Test Results Time Frame: Within 24 hr

Test Description: Aldolase is an enzyme found in skeletal muscle, the heart, and the liver, where it converts glycogen into lactic acid. The level is increased in some muscle diseases (e.g., muscular dystrophy) and in viral hepatitis. The level may also increase during an acute myocardial infarction.

Consent Form: Not required

List of Equipment: Red-top tube or serum separator tube; needle and syringe or vacutainer; alcohol swab

Test Procedure:
1. Label the specimen tube. *Correctly identifies the client and the test to be performed.*
2. Obtain a 5-mL blood sample.
3. Do not agitate the tube. *Agitation may cause RBC hemolysis.*
4. Send tube to the laboratory.

Clinical Implications and Indications:
1. Assists in the diagnosis of diseases involving cell destruction or increased membrane permeability. ALS is distributed throughout the body and elevated findings are possible with a large number of conditions.
2. The highest levels of ALS are found with muscular dystrophy, but levels are also increased with dermatomyositis, polymyositis, muscular dystrophy, myocardial infarction, and chronic viral hepatitis.
3. Elevated levels are also found with general body stress where cell destruction is involved (e.g., burns and gangrene will also cause moderately increased levels).

Nursing Care:
Before Test: Explain the test procedure and the purpose of the test. Assess the client's knowledge of the test. Fasting from midnight until the blood is drawn is required; water is allowed.
During Test: Adhere to standard precautions.
After Test: Apply pressure to venipuncture site. Explain that some bruising, discomfort, and swelling may appear at the site and that warm, moist compresses can alleviate this. Monitor for signs of infection.

Potential Complications: Bleeding and bruising at venipuncture site

Nursing Considerations:

Pediatric: *Infants and children will need assistance in remaining still during the venipuncture and age-appropriate comfort measures following the test.*

Listing of Related Tests: Creatinine phosphokinase; ANA; rheumatoid factor; electromyography; muscle biopsy

| WEBLINKS |

http://chorus.rad.mcw.edu

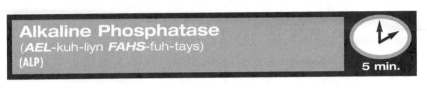

Alkaline Phosphatase
(**AEL**-kuh-liyn **FAHS**-fuh-tays)
(ALP)

5 min.

Type of Test: Blood

Body Systems and Functions: Hematological system

Normal Findings: Findings vary widely depending on the method of analysis. Check your laboratory for the reference values. Children generally have lower levels than adults.

Test Results Time Frame: Within 48 hr

Test Description: Alkaline phosphatase is a group of enzymes found primarily in the liver, gallbladder, and intestinal and bone tissues. They function best at an alkaline pH of 9. The test is done primarily to assist in the diagnosis of hepatic and bone disease. High levels are also found in the placenta, so that ALP levels rise during pregnancy.

Consent Form: Not required

List of Equipment: Red-top tube or serum separator tube; needle and syringe or vacutainer; alcohol swab

Test Procedure:
1. Label the specimen tube. *Correctly identifies the client and the test to be performed.*
2. Obtain a 5-mL blood sample.
3. Do not agitate the tube. *Agitation may cause RBC hemolysis.*
4. Send tube to the laboratory.

Clinical Implications and Indications:
1. Highly elevated levels are found with obstructive jaundice, liver cancer, cirrhosis, biliary obstruction, osteogenic sarcoma, metastatic bone disease, hyperparathyroidism, and Paget's disease.
2. Moderately elevated levels are found with infectious mononucleosis, pancreatitis, pregnancy, osteomalacia, rickets, bone infections, and extrahepatic duct obstruction.
3. Mildly elevated levels are found with viral hepatitis, chronic hepatitis, growing children, large doses of vitamin D, and leukemia.

4. Decreased levels are found with hypophosphatasia, malnutrition, cretinism, scurvy, hypothyroidism, pernicious anemia, placental insufficiency, and CHF.

Nursing Care:

Before Test: Explain the test procedure and the purpose of the test. Assess the client's knowledge of the test. Teach client to be NPO for 12 hr prior to the test. Assess medication history and specifically check for IV albumin administration within the past 10 days.

During Test: Adhere to standard precautions

After Test: Apply pressure to venipuncture site. Explain that some bruising, discomfort, and swelling may appear at the site and that warm, moist compresses can alleviate this. Monitor for signs of infection.

Potential Complications: Bleeding and bruising at venipuncture site

Interfering Factors: Postmenopausal women have higher levels of ALP; medications that cause false decreases are clofibrate, fluorides, and azathioprine; most of the drugs that cause an increase do so because they are toxic to the liver or cause cholestasis.

Nursing Considerations:

Pregnancy: Normal pregnancy will increase levels due to ALP in the placenta.
Pediatric: Infants and children will need assistance in remaining still during the venipuncture and age-appropriate comfort measures following the test. Rapid growth in children causes increases in ALP.

Listing of Related Tests: AST; ALT; albumin; GTT; bone studies

WEBLINKS

http://www.methodisthealth.com

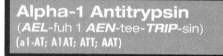

Alpha-1 Antitrypsin
(*AEL*-fuh 1 *AEN*-tee-*TRIP*-sin)
(a1-AT; A1AT; ATT; AAT)

5 min.

Type of Test: Blood

Body Systems and Functions: Immunological system

Normal Findings: 83–199 mg/dL

Test Results Time Frame: Within 24 hr

Test Description: Alpha-1 antitrypsin is an enzyme that is thought to inhibit protease release from dead or dying cells. This is one of three known protease inhibitors found in the blood. A congenital condition known as alpha-1 antitrypsin deficiency occurs in which early-onset emphysema and liver cirrhosis are common. In the general population, the test can be used as a nonspecific indicator of any tissue breakdown.

BLOOD

CLINICAL ALERT:
Persons with emphysema often have an acquired deficiency of alpha-1 antitrypsin.

Consent Form: Not required

List of Equipment: Red-top tube or serum separator tube; needle and syringe or vacutainer; alcohol swab

Test Procedure:
1. Label the specimen tube. *Correctly identifies the client and the test to be performed.*
2. Obtain a 5-mL blood sample.
3. Do not agitate the tube. *Agitation may cause RBC hemolysis.*
4. Send tube to the laboratory.
5. Keep specimen cool. *High temperatures alter the results.*

Clinical Implications and Indications:
1. Elevated levels are found with tissue damage and necrosis, as in any inflammation, cancer, thyroid infections, stress, pregnancy, and oral contraceptives.
2. Decreased levels are found with familial genetic disorders in which the enzyme is not produced, pulmonary disease, severe liver disease, and malnutrition.

Nursing Care:
Before Test: Explain the test procedure and the purpose of the test. Assess the client's knowledge of the test.
During Test: Adhere to standard precautions
After Test: Apply pressure to venipuncture site. Explain that some bruising, discomfort, and swelling may appear at the site and that warm, moist compresses can alleviate this. Monitor for signs of infection.

Potential Complications: Bleeding and bruising at venipuncture site

Interfering Factors: Pregnancy; oral contraceptives

Nursing Considerations:
Pregnancy: Elevations may be found with pregnancy and the use of oral contraceptives.
Pediatric: Infants and children will need assistance in remaining still during the venipuncture and age-appropriate comfort measures following the test.

WEBLINKS

http://www.nlm.nih.gov

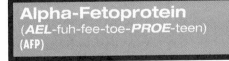

Alpha-Fetoprotein
(*AEL*-fuh-fee-toe-*PROE*-teen)
(AFP)

5 min.

Type of Test: Blood

Body Systems and Functions: Hematological system

BLOOD

Normal Findings: Varies with length of gestation. Screening tests are done from 16 to 18 weeks of gestation: 30–43 µg/mL.

Test Results Time Frame: Within 24 hr

Test Description: AFP is present in a human fetus and in certain pathological conditions in adults. AFP is synthesized by the fetal liver and is the major protein in fetal serum. In pregnant women, AFP is measured during 16–18 weeks gestation as a screening test for neurological defects in the fetus. When the neural tube is not closed, AFP leaks into the amniotic fluid and raises the AFP level. This in turn raises levels of AFP in maternal blood.

CLINICAL ALERT:
Couples who have delivered a child with a neural tube defect should be offered the AFP during subsequent pregnancies. In addition, the AFP must be confirmed with ultrasound.

Consent Form: Not required

List of Equipment: Red-top tube or serum separator tube; needle and syringe or vacutainer; alcohol swab

Test Procedure:
1. Label the specimen tube. *Correctly identifies the client and the test to be performed.*
2. Obtain a 5-mL blood sample.
3. Do not agitate the tube. *Agitation may cause RBC hemolysis.*
4. Send tube to the laboratory.

Clinical Implications and Indications:
1. Elevated levels are found with anencephaly, encephalocele, spina bifida, myelomeningocele, fetal renal abnormalities, fetal obstructions of the GI tract, missed abortion, impending fetal death, severe Rh immunization, esophageal and duodenal atresia, and multiple gestations.
2. Some false positives have no explanation (<1%).

Nursing Care:
Before Test: Explain the test procedure and the purpose of the test. Assess the client's knowledge of the test.
During Test: Adhere to standard precautions.
After Test: Apply pressure to venipuncture site. Explain that some bruising, discomfort, and swelling may appear at the site and that warm, moist compresses can alleviate this. Monitor for signs of infection.

Potential Complications: Bleeding and bruising at venipuncture site

Interfering Factors: Miscalculation of gestational age; mother's poor health

Nursing Considerations:
Pregnancy: This test should only be done between 15 and 20 weeks gestation (note: 16–18 weeks is preferred).
Pediatric: Infants and children will need assistance in remaining still during the venipuncture and age-appropriate comfort measures following the test.

Listing of Related Tests: Ultrasound; amniocentesis

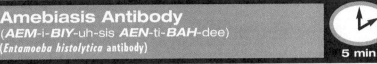

WEBLINKS

http://www.methodisthealth.com

Amebiasis Antibody
(**AEM**-i-**BIY**-uh-sis **AEN**-ti-**BAH**-dee)
(*Entamoeba histolytica* antibody)

5 min.

Type of Test: Blood

Body Systems and Functions: Gastrointestinal system

Normal Findings: Negative

Test Results Time Frame: Within 24 hr

Test Description: *Entamoeba histolytica* is a parasite of the lower intestine. This test detects serum antibodies to the presence of the parasite. The definitive test for *E. histolytica* is a stool sample, but absence of organisms in the stool does not rule out infection, since antibiotics, oil enemas, and barium interfere with identification. In addition, stool samples are insensitive and may have false-positive findings.

Consent Form: Not required

List of Equipment: Red-top tube or serum separator tube; needle and syringe or vacutainer; alcohol swab

Test Procedure:
1. Label the specimen tube. *Correctly identifies the client and the test to be performed.*
2. Obtain a 5-mL blood sample.
3. Do not agitate the tube. *Agitation may cause RBC hemolysis.*
4. Send tube to the laboratory.

Clinical Implications and Indications:
1. Titers of 128 and higher indicate recent and active infection.
2. Titers below 32 generally exclude the presence of amoebic disease.
3. Titers of 32–64 should be confirmed by other serological methods.
4. A positive test may indicate past, not current, infection.

Nursing Care:
Before Test: Explain the test procedure and the purpose of the test. Assess the client's knowledge of the test.
During Test: Adhere to standard precautions.
After Test: Apply pressure to venipuncture site. Explain that some bruising, discomfort, and swelling may appear at the site and that warm, moist compresses can alleviate this. Monitor for signs of infection.

Potential Complications: Bleeding and bruising at venipuncture site

Nursing Considerations:

Pediatric: Infants and children will need assistance in remaining still during the venipuncture and age-appropriate comfort measures following the test.

Listing of Related Tests: Stool sample; sigmoidoscopy

WEBLINKS

http://www.usyd.edu

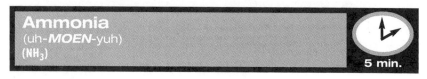

Ammonia
(uh-*MOEN*-yuh)
(NH₃)

5 min.

Type of Test: Blood

Body Systems and Functions: Metabolic system

Normal Findings: Normal laboratory findings vary among laboratory settings

Adults	11–32 µmol/L
Newborns	64–107 µmol/L

Test Results Time Frame: Within 24 hr

Test Description: Ammonia is produced in the breakdown of proteins by bacteria in the intestine. Ammonia is detoxified by the liver to urea, and circulating blood should have very low amounts. Ammonia levels are drawn to monitor liver function and metabolism.

CLINICAL ALERT:
In clients with impaired liver function, ammonia levels can be decreased in the blood by limiting protein intake and by giving antibiotics to decrease bacterial levels in the gut.

Consent Form: Not required

List of Equipment: Lavender-top, green-top, or plasma separator tube; needle and syringe or vacutainer; alcohol swab

Test Procedure:
1. Label the specimen tube. *Correctly identifies the client and the test to be performed.*
2. Obtain a 5-mL blood sample.
3. Gently invert tube several times, but do not agitate the tube. *Mixes the anticoagulant, but agitation may cause RBC hemolysis.*
4. Send tube to the laboratory.
5. Keep specimen cool. *High temperatures alter the results.*

Clinical Implications and Indications:
1. Elevated levels are found with congenital protein errors of metabolism, hemolytic disease of newborns, congestive heart failure, cor pulmonale,

Reye's syndrome, liver disease, liver failure, acute bronchitis, myelocytic and lymphocytic leukemia, exercise, and recent protein ingestion, alkalosis.
2. Decreased levels are found with kidney damage and essential hypertension.

Nursing Care:

Before Test: Explain the test procedure and the purpose of the test. Assess the client's knowledge of the test. Client must be NPO except for water for at least 8 hr and not exercise immediately before the blood is drawn.

During Test: Adhere to standard precautions.

After Test: Apply pressure to venipuncture site. Explain that some bruising, discomfort, and swelling may appear at the site and that warm, moist compresses can alleviate this. Monitor for signs of infection.

Potential Complications: Bleeding and bruising at venipuncture site

Interfering Factors: Medications that increase results are chlorothiazide, chlorthalidone, ethacrynic acid, furosemide, ammonium salts, asparaginase, barbiturates, ethanol, glucose, hydroflumethiazide, morphine, thiopental, acetazolamide, isoniazid, levoglutamide, tetracycline. and alcohol; medications that decrease results are acetohydroxamic acid, arginine, glutamic acid, diphenydramine, isocarboxazid, MAO inhibitors, *Lactobacillus acidophilus*, lactulose, kenamycin, neomycin, tetracycline, potassium salts, sodium salts, glucose, acetazolamide, secretin, and mafenide.

Nursing Considerations:

Pediatric: Infants and children will need assistance in remaining still during the venipuncture and age appropriate comfort measures following the test.

Listing of Related Tests: Bilirubin; urobilinogen; alkaline phosphatase; AST; ALT; LDH; serum protein electrophoresis; prothrombin time; cholesterol; serum immunoglobulin

WEBLINKS

http://www.methodisthealth.com

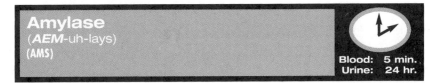

Amylase
(*AEM*-uh-lays)
(AMS)

Blood: 5 min.
Urine: 24 hr.

Type of Test: Blood; urine

Body Systems and Functions: Metabolic system

Normal Findings:

Serum	
Adults	25–125 IU/L
Newborn (2–4 days):	5–65 IU/L
Older adults (above age 70):	21–160 IU/L
Urine	0–275 U/L

BLOOD

Test Results Time Frame: Within 24 hr

Test Description: Amylase is a colloidal enzyme that breaks down starch to sugars. AMS belongs to a class of enzymes that hydrolyzes starches. Amylase is produced primarily by the pancreas but is also produced in the salivary glands, liver, fallopian tubes, and skeletal muscle. AMS is mainly used to test for pancreatic disease.

> **CLINICAL ALERT:**
> Greater than 600 IU/L values often indicate acute disorders such as pancreatitis and obstruction of bile ducts in the biliary tract.

Consent Form: Not required

List of Equipment: *Blood:* red-top tube or serum separator tube; needle and syringe or vacutainer; alcohol swab. *Urine:* sterile plastic container; ice.

Test Procedure:

Blood:
1. Label the specimen tube. *Correctly identifies the client and the test to be performed.*
2. Obtain a 5-mL blood sample.
3. Do not agitate the tube. *Agitation may cause RBC hemolysis.*
4. Send tube to the laboratory.

Urine:
1. Label a sterile urine container. *Correctly identifies the client and the test to be performed.*
2. Obtain a clean-catch specimen of urine at timed intervals (e.g., 1, 2, or 24 hr). *Ensures accurate results.*
3. Keep specimen cool. *High temperatures alter the results.*
4. Send specimen to laboratory.

Clinical Implications and Indications:
1. Elevated levels of serum amylase are found with pancreatitis, bile stones or obstruction, perforated peptic ulcer, intestinal obstruction, peritonitis, alcohol intoxication, trauma, cholecystitis, macroamylasemia, parotid gland disease, diabetic ketoacidosis, and acute respiratory insufficiency.
2. Elevated levels in urine amylase are found with acute pancreatitis, cholelithiasis, and peptic ulcer.
3. Decreased urine levels are found with hepatitis, liver cancer or cirrhosis, advanced chronic pancreatitis, and hyperglycemia.

Nursing Care:
Before Test: Explain the test procedure and the purpose of the test. Assess the client's knowledge of the test (note: obtain AMS specimen before medications or Hypaque dye is given to the patient). Instruct client not to discard any urine during designated time period.

During Test: Adhere to standard precautions. If any urine is accidentally discarded or contaminated with feces, discard entire specimen and begin test again.

After Test: Blood: Apply pressure to venipuncture site. Explain that some bruising, discomfort, and swelling may appear at the site and that warm, moist compresses can alleviate this. Monitor for signs of infection. Urine: Document urine quantity, date, and exact hours of collection on requisition.

Potential Complications: Bleeding and bruising at venipuncture site

Interfering Factors: Urine contaminated with feces; spillage or inaccurate collection of the urine specimen, including refrigeration or placing on ice; heavy bleeding during menstruation; medications that increase results are dexamethasone, furosemide, L-asparaginase, methanol, salicylates, thiazides, ethanol, bethanechol, Hypaque dye, meperidine, and chloride salts; citrate decreases result.

Nursing Considerations:
Pediatric: In neonates, the presence of amylase may indicate disease.
Blood: Infants and children will need assistance in remaining still during the venipuncture and age-appropriate comfort measures following the test.
Urine: A collection bag or insertion of a straight catheter is likely needed for infants and toddlers.

Listing of Related Tests: Serum lipase; blood glucose; calcium; potassium

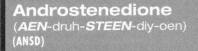

WEBLINKS

http://chorus.rad.mcw.edu

Androstenedione
(*AEN*-druh-*STEEN*-diy-oen)
(ANSD)

5 min.

Type of Test: Blood

Body Systems and Functions: Endocrine system

Normal Findings:

Age:		
0–1	F 6–78 ng/dL	M 6–78 ng/dL
1–5	F 5–51 ng/dL	M 5–51 ng/dL
6–12	F 7–68 ng/dL	M 7–68 ng/dL
13–17	F 17–51 ng/dL	M 43–221 ng/dL
Adults	F 50–250 ng/dL	M 50–250 ng/dL
Postmenopausal women	16–120 ng/dL	

Test Results Time Frame: Within 48 hr

Test Description: Androstenedione, produced by the ovary, testes, and the adrenal cortex, is a prohormone for both estrogen and testosterone. The test is used to evaluate hyperandrenergic states, including congenital adrenal hyperplasia, ovarian hyperplasia or tumor, Cushing's syndrome, and ectopic ACTH-producing tumors. Androstenedione testing is gaining favor as a test for monitoring glucocorticoid therapy as it is not subject to diurnal variation and correlates well with clinical control.

CLINICAL ALERT:
Androstenedione supplementation has become popular with male athletes because they believe they will be more powerful. Research shows no measureable effect on free or total testosterone, but HDL levels dropped and plasma estrogens rose. No measurable effect has been noted on athletic performance.

Consent Form: Not required

List of Equipment: Red-top tube or serum separator tube; needle and syringe or vacutainer; alcohol swab

Test Procedure:
1. Label the specimen tube. *Correctly identifies the client and the test to be performed.*
2. Obtain a 5-mL blood sample.
3. Do not agitate the tube. *Agitation may cause RBC hemolysis.*
4. Send tube to the laboratory.

Clinical Implications and Indications:
1. Elevated levels are found with Cushing's syndrome, some ovarian tumors, ectopic ACTH-producing tumors, ovarian hyperplasia, and congenital adrenal hyperplasia.
2. Decreased levels are found with adrenal failure and ovarian failure.

Nursing Care:
Before Test: Explain the test procedure and the purpose of the test. Assess the client's knowledge of the test.
During Test: Adhere to standard precautions.
After Test: Apply pressure to venipuncture site. Explain that some bruising, discomfort, and swelling may appear at the site and that warm, moist compresses can alleviate this. Monitor for signs of infection.

Potential Complications: Bleeding and bruising at venipuncture site

Interfering Factors: Corticosteroid therapy causes androstenedione levels to increase; nuclear scan 1 week before test.

Nursing Considerations:
Pediatric: Infants and children will need assistance in remaining still during the venipuncture and age-appropriate comfort measures following the test.

WEBLINKS

http://www.niddk.nih.gov

Angiotensin-Converting Enzyme
(*AEN*-jee-oe-*TEN*-sin k:n-*V:R*-ting) (ACE)

5 min.

Type of Test: Blood

Body Systems and Functions: Endocrine system

Normal Findings: 12–35 μ/L. Normal laboratory findings vary among laboratory settings.

Test Results Time Frame: Within 24 hr

Test Description: ACE converts angiotension I, which is inactive, to the active angiotensin II. Angiotensin II maintains blood pressure through vasoconstriction. This test measures the amount of serum angiotensin and is not commonly used except with ACE-producing disease, primarily sarcoidosis. Analysis of ACE levels may also be useful to identify people who are not taking an ACE inhibitor drug as ordered. The severity of sarcoidosis and the response to therapy can be determined by this test.

Consent Form: Not required

List of Equipment: Red-top tube or serum separator tube; needle and syringe or vacutainer; alcohol swab

Test Procedure:
1. Label the specimen tube. *Correctly identifies the client and the test to be performed.*
2. Obtain a 5-mL blood sample.
3. Do not agitate the tube. *Agitation may cause RBC hemolysis.*
4. Send tube to the laboratory.

Clinical Implications and Indications:
1. Elevated levels are found with sarcoidosis, acute and chronic bronchitis, pulmonary fibrosis, and connective tissue diseases such as lupus, leprosy, and Gaucher's disease.

Nursing Care:
Before Test: Explain the test procedure and the purpose of the test. Assess the client's knowledge of the test.
During Test: Adhere to standard precautions.
After Test: Apply pressure to venipuncture site. Explain that some bruising, discomfort, and swelling may appear at the site and that warm, moist compresses can alleviate this. Monitor for signs of infection.

Potential Complications: Bleeding and bruising at venipuncture site

Interfering Factors: Ethylenenediaminetetra-acetic acid (EDTA); hemolysis; lipemia

Nursing Considerations:
Pediatric: Infants and children will need assistance in remaining still during the venipuncture and age-appropriate comfort measures following the test. Clients below the age of 20 normally have high levels of ACE.

| WEBLINKS 🗕🗙 |

http://www.ncbi.nlm.nih.gov/entrez/query.fcgi

BLOOD

Anion Gap
(*AEN*-iy-ahn gaep)

5 min.

Type of Test: Blood

Body Systems and Functions: Metabolic system

Normal Findings: 8–18 mm/L if K^+ is used in the calculation

CRITICAL VALUES:
Values less than 8 or greater than 18 indicate problems with acid-base balance.

Test Results Time Frame: Within 24 hr

Test Description: Anion gap measures the difference between the sum of the cations Na^+ and K^+ and the sum of the anions Cl^- and HCO_3^-. These measured ions reflect the acid-base balance of the body. The "gap" in anions is the difference between measured cations and anions and reflects the unmeasured ions in body composition. The measured cations are usually more than the measured anions, so there is a gap in the amount of measured anions. The anion gap test is used to determine the cause of metabolic acidosis and may help identify a mixed rather than a simple acid-base imbalance in which changes in both anions and cations cancel one another out.

Consent Form: Not required

List of Equipment: Red-top tube or serum separator tube; needle and syringe or vacutainer; alcohol swab

Test Procedure:
1. Label the specimen tube. *Correctly identifies the client and the test to be performed.*
2. Obtain a 5-mL blood sample.
3. Do not agitate the tube. *Agitation may cause RBC hemolysis.*
4. Send tube to the laboratory.

Clinical Implications and Indications:
1. An increased anion gap diagnoses metabolic acidosis that occurs with lactic acidosis (the most common cause) when excessive metabolic acids are ingested (poisoning with methanol, salicylates, etc.) or when there is a decreased loss of metabolic acids (renal failure, diabetic ketoacidosis, etc.).
2. An anion gap in the normal range may reflect metabolic acidosis that is due to decreased serum potassium (renal tubular acidosis), increased loss of anions (severe diarrhea), or altered renal chloride reabsorption. When the anion gap is in normal range in metabolic acidosis, diabetic ketoacidosis is the most common cause.
3. Decreases in the anion gap in metabolic acidosis are most commonly due to hypoalbuminemia.

Nursing Care:
Before Test: Explain the test procedure and the purpose of the test. Assess the client's knowledge of the test.

During Test: Adhere to standard precautions.
After Test: Apply pressure to venipuncture site. Explain that some bruising, discomfort, and swelling may appear at the site and that warm, moist compresses can alleviate this. Monitor for signs of infection.

BLOOD

Potential Complications: Bleeding and bruising at venipuncture site

Interfering Factors: Iodine used in wound packing; medications that increase results are acetaminophen, ammonium chloride, antihypertensives, carbenicillin, corticosteroids, ethylene glycol, furosemide, iron, nitrates, sodium bicarbonate, sorbitol, thiazides, and toluene; medications that decrease levels are alkalis, boric acid, bromides, cortisone acetate, lithium carbonate, magnesium, phenylbutazone, and sodium chloride.

Nursing Considerations:
Pediatric: Infants and children will need assistance in remaining still during the venipuncture and age-appropriate comfort measures following the test.

WEBLINKS

http://alice.ucdavis.edu

Anthrax
(*AN*-ther-ax)

5 min.

Type of Test: Blood; x-ray; tissue

Body Systems and Functions: Hematological system; pulmonary system; integumentary system

Normal Findings: Negative for anthrax antibodies and negative for pulmonary involvement (seen in inhalation anthrax)

Test Results Time Frame: Blood: 24–48 hours; chest x-ray: 30–60 minutes; tissue: within 24 hours

Test Description: Inhalation anthrax occurs when anthrax spores are inhaled deep into the lungs, where, once embedded, they release deadly toxins into the system. Inhalation anthrax is the most serious form of the disease. Symptoms at first resemble a common cold or flu, followed by difficulty breathing, a drop in blood pressure, swelling, internal bleeding, and other symptoms. Treatment in its later stages may have no effects.
Cutaneous anthrax is much less serious but also can kill if left untreated. About 95 percent of anthrax infections take this form. Cutaneous anthrax occurs when bacteria get into a cut or break in the skin. The infection usually starts as a raised, itchy bump resembling an insect bite. Within a day or two it turns into a darkening blister or one with a dark spot in the middle. The lesion may not appear in the same spot as the break in the skin through which the spores enter, so a lesion away from a cut cannot be assumed to be harmless. An invasive procedure is performed in a surgical setting. A scraping of the infected skin area is taken to obtain body tissue and is taken under sterile technique and

examined microscopically for cell morphology and tissue anomalies.
Intestinal anthrax may occur after eating the undercooked meat of contaminated animals. Initial symptoms include nausea, loss of appetite, vomiting, and fever, followed later by abdominal pain, vomiting of blood, and severe diarrhea.
Treatment for anthrax is the use of antibiotics, such as Cipro or doxycycline, if given early. Treatment usually fails once the symptoms progress, since it does not accomplish positive results to eradicate the bacteria once they make large amounts of toxin.

CLINICAL ALERT:
Whenever anthrax exposure is questioned, the Centers for Disease Control should be immediately notified. In addition, the health care worker should practice standard precautions with vigilance. Extreme caution should be used when there is suspected inhalation anthrax exposure. Clients should be informed not to take unnecessary antibiotics if the presence of disease is not confirmed. If taking a chest x-ray, a portable x-ray machine may be brought to the nursing unit if an inpatient client cannot be moved. Clients of reproductive age should have the testes and ovaries covered with a lead shield.

Consent Form: Not required

List of Equipment: *Blood:* red-top tube or serum separator tube; needle and syringe; alcohol swab. *Pulmonary testing:* nasal swab; x-ray machine and related equipment from radiology. *Cutaneous testing:* biopsy tray.

Test Procedure:
Blood
1. Label the specimen tube. *Correctly identifies the client and the test to be performed.*
2. Obtain a 5-mL blood sample.
3. Do not agitate the tube. *Agitation may cause RBC hemolysis.*
4. Send tube to the laboratory.

Chest x-ray:
1. A routine chest x-ray is done with the patient in a standing position. If the client cannot stand, an upright position should be maintained. *X-ray films taken in the supine position will not demonstrate fluid levels.*
2. Anteroposition and left lateral views are taken.
3. The client removes street clothing to the waist and a hospital gown is worn. The hospital gown should not have buttons or snaps and all jewelry should be removed. Monitoring cables should be positioned out of view of the x-ray. *These items may obscure a clear view of the chest.*
4. The client is instructed to take a deep breath and exhale and then to take a second deep breath and hold it while the technician takes the x-ray image.

Tissue sample:
1. 1. Place client in supine position.
2. A specimen of tissue is biopsied by excision or needle biopsy. Label the specimen and place in container. *Correctly identifies the client and the test to be performed.*
3. Send specimen to laboratory.

Clinical Implications and Indications:

Blood:
Diagnoses the presence of inhalation, cutaneous, or intestinal anthrax

X-ray:
1. Abnormal chest x-rays may indicate involvement of the anthrax organisms in the lungs.
2. Inhalation anthrax is the more deadly of the types of anthrax and requires immediate treatment with the appropriately prescribed antibiotics.

Tissue:
Diagnoses the presence of cutaneous anthrax

Nursing Care:
Before Test: Explain the test procedure and the purpose of the test. Assess the client's knowledge of the test. Chest x-ray: remove jewelry and place monitoring cables off of the chest. Instruct the client that there will be no discomfort and explain the purpose and procedure of the test. Assist the x-ray technician in the proper positioning of the patient. Provide lead shields for the client and staff. *During Test:* Adhere to standard precautions. For chest x-ray, instruct the client to remain motionless and to follow breathing instructions. *After Test:* Apply pressure to venipuncture site. Explain that some bruising, discomfort, and swelling may appear at the site and that warm, moist compresses can alleviate this. Clean site of skin scraping. Provide analgesia as necessary.

Potential Complications: Unnecessary use of antibiotics when anthrax is not confirmed may cause other problems for the client (e.g., gastrointestinal complications, pseudo-colitis). Bleeding and bruising at the site of the skin scraping.

Contraindications: X-ray testing is contraindicated in pregnancy.

Interfering Factors: Obesity and lack of full inspiration may interfere with diagnosis of certain conditions.

Nursing Considerations:
Pregnancy: If an x-ray is necessary during pregnancy, the uterus should be covered with a lead shield.
Pediatric: If the anthrax disease infects infants, they are more at risk for critical complications, due to their underdeveloped immune system. Sedation is recommended for infants and children during skin scraping. Place the infant or child on a blanket for comfort. After postprocedure monitoring is completed and per health care provider's order, the pediatric client is discharged with an adult who is given instructions.
Gerontology: If the anthrax disease infects the elderly, their immune systems may be more compromised related to the aging process. This consequently makes their morbidity and mortality rates higher than persons of younger ages.
Rural: The traditional methods of contracting anthrax would be in rural farm settings. However, due to the terrorism seen in the United States, which began in September 2001, there are also increased levels of the disease in urban settings.
International: Various areas of the world have sporadic and routine anthrax contamination. There is a particularly high incidence of disease in parts of Africa and Asia.

WEBLINKS

www.cdc.gov/ncidod/dbmd/diseaseinfo; www.anthrax.osd.mil/

Anticentromere Antibody
(*AEN*-tee-*SEN*-troe-meer *AEN*-ti-*BAH*-dee)
(centromere antibody)

5 min.

Type of Test: Blood

Body Systems and Functions: Immunological system

Normal Findings: Negative

Test Results Time Frame: Within 24 hr

Test Description: Anticentromere antibody is a marker for a milder form of scleroderma called CREST sydrome (i.e., calcinosis, Raynaud's syndrome, esophageal dysfunction, sclerodactyly, and telangiectasis). Approximately 90% of people with CREST syndrome will develop anticentromere antibody. This is one of the antibodies tested to assist in the diagnosis of rheumatic diseases.

Consent Form: Not required

List of Equipment: Red-top tube or serum separator tube; needle and syringe or vacutainer; alcohol swab

Test Procedure:
1. Label the specimen tube. *Correctly identifies the client and the test to be performed.*
2. Obtain a 5-mL blood sample.
3. Do not agitate the tube. *Agitation may cause RBC hemolysis.*
4. Send tube to the laboratory.

Clinical Implications and Indications:
1. Only those with CREST syndrome or, rarely, diffuse scleroderma will have a positive test.

Nursing Care:
Before Test: Assess the client's knowledge of the test. Explain the test procedure and the purpose of the test.
During Test: Adhere to standard precautions.
After Test: Apply pressure to venipuncture site. Explain that some bruising, discomfort, and swelling may appear at the site and that warm, moist compresses can alleviate this. Monitor for signs of infection.

Potential Complications: Bleeding and bruising at venipuncture site

Nursing Considerations:
Pediatric: Infants and children will need assistance in remaining still during the venipuncture and age-appropriate comfort measures following the test.

▌ WEBLINKS ▐   🖵 ☒

http://www.methodisthealth.com

Antidiuretic Hormone
(***AEN***-tee-diy-yur-***RET***-ik)
(**ADH; vasopressin**)

5 min.

Type of Test: Blood

Body Systems and Functions: Endocrine system

Normal Findings: <1.5 pg/L (Levels vary with the osmolality of the plasma)

Test Results Time Frame: Within 24 hr

Test Description: Antidiuretic hormone (ADH) is released by the posterior pituitary in response to increased blood osmolality or decreased blood volume. When ADH is released in normal quantities, the kidneys produce small amounts of concentrated urine; when ADH is not present, the kidneys produce large quantities of dilute urine. This test helps to establish a diagnosis for people who are polyuric and/or hyponatremic.

Consent Form: Not required

List of Equipment: Red-top tube or serum separator tube; needle and syringe or vacutainer; alcohol swab

Test Procedure:
1. Label the specimen tube. *Correctly identifies the client and the test to be performed.*
2. Obtain a 5-mL blood sample in a plastic tube. *Glass causes breakdown of ADH.*
3. Do not agitate the tube. *Agitation may cause RBC hemolysis.*
4. Send tube to the laboratory.
5. Keep specimen cool. *High temperatures alter the results.*

Clinical Implications and Indications:
1. Elevated levels of ADH are found with syndrome of inappropriate antidiuretic hormone (SIADH), malignancy or pulmonary conditions, and porphyria.
2. Decreased levels are found with diabetes insipidus, nephrotic syndrome, and CNS trauma.

Nursing Care:
Before Test: Explain the test procedure and the purpose of the test. Assess the client's knowledge of the test. Teach client that it is necessary to fast and avoid strenuous exercise for 12 hr before the test. Assess pain, stress, and anxiety levels.
During Test: Adhere to standard precautions.
After Test: Apply pressure to venipuncture site. Explain that some bruising, discomfort, and swelling may appear at the site and that warm, moist compresses can alleviate this. Monitor for signs of infection.

Potential Complications: Bleeding and bruising at venipuncture site

Interfering Factors: Pain, stress, and anxiety may lead to increased ADH secretion through unknown mechanisms; exercise and eating less than 12 hr before testing; medications that alter results are antipsychotics, anticonvulsants,

BLOOD

narcotics, beta-adrenergics, acetaminophen, barbiturates, antidiuretics, ethanol, cholinergics, estrogens, nicotine, cytotoxics, antidepressants and hypoglycemics.

Nursing Considerations:
Pediatric: Infants and children will need assistance in remaining still during the venipuncture and age-appropriate comfort measures following the test.

Listing of Related Tests: Blood glucose; sodium; renin levels

WEBLINKS ⊟⊠

http://www.niddk.nih.gov

Anti-DNA Antibody
(*AEN*-tee D N A *AEN*-ti-*BAH*-dee)
(anti-DS-DNA; antibody to double-stranded DNA; double-stranded anti-DNA; antinative DNA antibody)

5 min.

Type of Test: Blood

Body Systems and Functions: Immunological system

Normal Findings: Negative at 1:10 dilution

Test Results Time Frame: Within 24 hr

Test Description: Anti-DNA antibodies measure the presence of antibodies to native DNA. In general, it is an indication of autoimmune activity. Anti-DNA antibodies are used to confirm a diagnosis of systemic lupus erythematosus (SLE) (i.e., high titers are usually found with SLE).

Consent Form: Not required

List of Equipment: Red-top tube or serum separator tube; needle and syringe or vacutainer; alcohol swab

Test Procedure:
1. Label the specimen tube. *Correctly identifies the client and the test to be performed.*
2. Obtain a 5-mL blood sample.
3. Do not agitate the tube. *Agitation may cause RBC hemolysis.*
4. Send tube to the laboratory.

Clinical Implications and Indications:
1. High titers are very specific for SLE, unlike the antinuclear antibody test, which is elevated in a number of disorders. An increased titer may occur just before a flare of SLE.
2. Lower titers are sometimes noted in other connective tissue diseases.

Nursing Care:
Before Test: Explain the test procedure and the purpose of the test. Assess the client's knowledge of the test.
During Test: Adhere to standard precautions.

BLOOD

After Test: Apply pressure to venipuncture site. Explain that some bruising, discomfort, and swelling may appear at the site and that warm, moist compresses can alleviate this. Monitor for signs of infection.

Potential Complications: Bleeding and bruising at venipuncture site

Interfering Factors: Smoking; medications that alter results are anticonvulsants, isoniazid, oral contraceptives, hydralazine, procainamide, methyldopa, oxyphenisatin, and phenothiazines.

Nursing Considerations:
Pediatric: Infants and children will need assistance in remaining still during the venipuncture and age-appropriate comfort measures following the test.

WEBLINKS

http://www.northstar.k12.ak.us

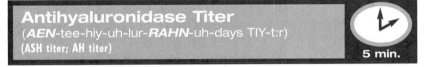

Antihyaluronidase Titer
(*AEN*-tee-hiy-uh-lur-*RAHN*-uh-days TIY-t:r)
(ASH titer; AH titer)

5 min.

Type of Test: Blood

Body Systems and Functions: Immunological system

Normal Findings: <128 Todd units/mL

Test Results Time Frame: Within 24 hr

Test Description: Antihyaluronidase (AH) titer is one of a number of streptococcal tests that check for streptococcal infection or streptococcal carrier states. The AH titer is specific for an antibody that is usually triggered by group A beta-hemolytic streptococcal infections that target hyaluronidase. The titer is often done in conjunction with a number of antistreptococcal antibody titers when the antistreptolysin O titer is low to substantiate a diagnosis of streptococcal infection. The AH titers rise in the second week of infection, and if there is successful treatment, the titers usually fall within 3–5 weeks of infection.

Consent Form: Not required

List of Equipment: Red-top tube or serum separator tube; needle and syringe or vacutainer; alcohol swab

Test Procedure:
1. Label the specimen tube. *Correctly identifies the client and the test to be performed.*
2. Obtain a 5-mL blood sample.
3. Do not agitate the tube. *Agitation may cause RBC hemolysis.*
4. Send tube to the laboratory.

Clinical Implications and Indications:
1. The test is positive when current or recent infection with streptococcal group A beta-hemolytic streptococci organisms is present.

BLOOD

2. Diagnoses: glomerulonephritis, rheumatic fever, and group A streptococcal disease.

Nursing Care:
Before Test: Explain the test procedure and the purpose of the test. Assess the client's knowledge of the test.
During Test: Adhere to standard precautions.
After Test: Apply pressure to venipuncture site. Explain that some bruising, discomfort, and swelling may appear at the site and that warm, moist compresses can alleviate this. Monitor for signs of infection.

Potential Complications: Bleeding and bruising at venipuncture site

Interfering Factors: Recent therapy with antibiotics may decrease titer levels.

Nursing Considerations:
Pediatric: Infants and children will need assistance in remaining still during the venipuncture and age-appropriate comfort measures following the test. Early antibiotic therapy is indicated where the streptococcal infections are present due to the organic damage that can ensue with this pathogen. In addition, instructing care providers to administer the entire course of the antibiotic therapy is necessary (note: to keep early discontinuing of the antibiotics from allowing the development of a more virulent infection).

Listing of Related Tests: Antistreptolysin O titer; antideoxyribonuclease B titer; antistreptokinase titer

∥WEBLINKS ▯	▤▨

http://www.mic.ki.se/Diseases/c20.html

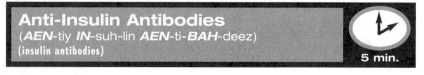

Anti-Insulin Antibodies
(*AEN*-tiy *IN*-suh-lin *AEN*-ti-*BAH*-deez)
(insulin antibodies)

5 min.

Type of Test: Blood

Body Systems and Functions: Endocrine system

Normal Findings:

Fasting:

Infant/child	<13 µU/mL
Adult	17 µU/mL

After 75 g glucose:

30 min	20–112 µU/mL
1 hr	29–88 µU/mL
2 hr	22–79 µU/mL
3 hr	4–62 µU/mL

Insulin:
glucose ratio   <0.3:1
Normal laboratory findings vary among laboratory settings.

Test Results Time Frame: Within 24 hr

Test Description: Anti-insulin antibodies are formed with clients who have diabetes and are taking exogenous insulin. When these antibodies form, clients need increasingly larger doses to maintain blood glucose levels in a normal range, which is a condition known as insulin resistance. Clients with diabetes may also develop an allergic response to insulin and therefore require larger doses. The presence of antibodies in asymptomatic persons may also predict eventual development of diabetes.

Consent Form: Not required

List of Equipment: Red-top tube or serum separator tube; needle and syringe or vacutainer; alcohol swab

Test Procedure:
1. Label the specimen tube. *Correctly identifies the client and the test to be performed.*
2. Obtain a 5-mL blood sample.
3. Do not agitate the tube. *Agitation may cause RBC hemolysis.*
4. Send tube to the laboratory.

Clinical Implications and Indications:
1. Insulin antibodies are found in the serum of people who have developed insulin resistance or insulin allergy.
2. Most commonly evidenced in the disease process of diabetes mellitus.

Nursing Care:
Before Test: Explain the test procedure and the purpose of the test. Assess the client's knowledge of the test.
During Test: Adhere to standard precautions.
After Test: Apply pressure to venipuncture site. Explain that some bruising, discomfort, and swelling may appear at the site and that warm, moist compresses can alleviate this. Monitor for signs of infection.

Potential Complications: Bleeding and bruising at venipuncture site

Interfering Factors: Radioactive scan within 1 week

Nursing Considerations:
Pediatric: Infants and children will need assistance in remaining still during the venipuncture and age-appropriate comfort measures following the test.
Home Care: Clients with diabetes who are self-treating at home need to be educated in regard to the potential allergic response that can be developed to insulin. This may lead to the need to adjust their insulin doses and can be detected in their chemistry blood glucose testing.

WEBLINKS

http://www.ncbi.nlm.nih.gov/entrez/query.fcgi

BLOOD

Anti-La(SSB)
(anti-SSB; Sjögren's antibody)

5 min.

Type of Test: Blood

Body Systems and Functions: Immunological system

Normal Findings: Negative

Test Results Time Frame: Within 24 hr

Test Description: Anti-La(SSB) is an autoantibody directed against RNA protein particles that are a cofactor in RNA polymerase III. Anti-La(SSB), in conjunction with anti-Ro, is a marker for a milder form of systemic lupus erythematosus (SLE), known as Sjögren's SLE. The test is also used in the diagnosis of different forms of connective tissue disorders.

Consent Form: Not required

List of Equipment: Red-top tube or serum separator tube; needle and syringe or vacutainer; alcohol swab

Test Procedure:
1. Label the specimen tube. *Correctly identifies the client and the test to be performed.*
2. Obtain a 5-mL blood sample.
3. Do not agitate the tube. *Agitation may cause RBC hemolysis.*
4. Send tube to the laboratory.

Clinical Implications and Indications:
1. Elevated levels are found with SLE or Sjögren's syndrome.

Nursing Care:
Before Test: Explain the test procedure and the purpose of the test. Assess the client's knowledge of the test.
During Test: Adhere to standard precautions.
After Test: Apply pressure to venipuncture site. Explain that some bruising, discomfort, and swelling may appear at the site and that warm, moist compresses can alleviate this. Monitor for signs of infection.

Potential Complications: Bleeding and bruising at venipuncture site

Nursing Considerations:
Pediatric: Infants and children will need assistance in remaining still during the venipuncture and age-appropriate comfort measures following the test.

Listing of Related Tests: Anti-Ro; anti-SSA; anti-DNA; ANA

WEBLINKS

http://www.mic.ki.se/Diseases/c20.html

Antinuclear Antibody
(*AEN*-tee-*NUE*-klee-:r *AEN*-ti-*BAH*-dee)
(ANA; fluorescent antinuclear antibody; FANA; ANF)

5 min.

Type of Test: Blood

Body Systems and Functions: Immunological system

Normal Findings: Negative at 1:20 dilution

Test Results Time Frame: Within 24 hr

Test Description: Antinuclear antibodies are produced and act against the body's own DNA and nuclear material that causes tissue damage as autoimmune disorders. This test is a fluorescent procedure that assists in differentiating among various connective tissue diseases. Antinuclear antibody testing is not diagnostic of all of the variety of diseases. However, if positive results do occur, the anti-DNA test is performed specifically to diagnose SLE.

Consent Form: Not required

List of Equipment: Red-top tube or serum separator tube; needle and syringe or vacutainer; alcohol swab

Test Procedure:
1. Label the specimen tube. *Correctly identifies the client and the test to be performed.*
2. Obtain a 2-mL blood sample.
3. Do not agitate the tube. *Agitation may cause RBC hemolysis.*
4. Send tube to the laboratory.

Clinical Implications and Indications:
1. Elevated levels are found with SLE, hepatitis, myasthenia gravis, pulmonary fibrosis, Raynaud's syndrome, and rheumatoid arthritis.

Nursing Care:
Before Test: Explain the test procedure and the purpose of the test. Assess the client's knowledge of the test. Instruct client to fast for 8 hr prior to the test.
During Test: Adhere to standard precautions.
After Test: Apply pressure to venipuncture site. Explain that some bruising, discomfort, and swelling may appear at the site and that warm, moist compresses can alleviate this. Monitor for signs of infection.

Potential Complications: Bleeding and bruising at venipuncture site

Interfering Factors: Medications that alter results are aminosalicylic acid, carbidopa, chlorpromazine, corticosteroids, gold salts, isoniazid, mephenytoin, methyldopa, oral contraceptives, phenytoin, primidone, quinidine gluconate, tetracyclines, and trimethadione.

Nursing Considerations:
Pediatric: Infants and children will need assistance in remaining still during the venipuncture and age-appropriate comfort measures following the test.

WEBLINKS

http://alice.ucdavis.edu

Antiphospholipid Antibody
(aen-tee-*FAHS*-foe-*LIP*-id *AEN*-ti-*BAH*-dee)
(APA)

5 min.

Type of Test: Blood

Body Systems and Functions: Immunological system

Normal Findings: Negative

Test Results Time Frame: Within 48 hr

Test Description: Antiphospholipid antibodies measure the antibodies of phospholipids (blood fats, which contain phosphorus). Antiphospholipid antibodies occur with coagulation problems in two separate syndromes: anticardiolipin antibodies or lupus anticoagulant. Both syndromes increase the risk of thrombosis formation, and anticardiolipin antibodies are associated with hemolytic anemia. Therefore, the production of antiphospholipid antibodies occurs most commonly with systemic lupus erythematosus. The antiphospholipid antibodies may also be associated with drugs, with other autoimmune diseases, or with aging.

Consent Form: Not required

List of Equipment: Light blue tube or serum separator tube; needle and syringe or vacutainer; alcohol swab

Test Procedure:
1. Label the specimen tube. *Correctly identifies the client and the test to be performed.*
2. Obtain a 5-mL blood sample.
3. Do not agitate the tube. *Agitation may cause RBC hemolysis.*
4. Send tube to the laboratory.

Clinical Implications and Indications:
1. Elevated levels are found with systemic lupus erythematosus, acute infection, cancer, and HIV.

Nursing Care:
Before Test: Explain the test procedure and the purpose of the test. Assess the client's knowledge of the test.
During Test: Adhere to standard precautions.
After Test: Apply pressure to venipuncture site. Explain that some bruising, discomfort, and swelling may appear at the site and that warm, moist compresses can alleviate this. Monitor for signs of infection.

Potential Complications: Bleeding and bruising at venipuncture site

Interfering Factors: Medications that alter results are phenytoin, fansidar, quinidine, quinine, hydralazine, procainamide, phenothiazines, interferon, and cocaine.

Nursing Considerations:
Pregnancy: Pregnant women with systemic lupus erythematosus who have antiphospholipid antibodies have an increased risk of miscarriage.

Pediatric: *Infants and children will need assistance in remaining still during the venipuncture and age-appropriate comfort measures following the test.*

Listing of Related Tests: PTT

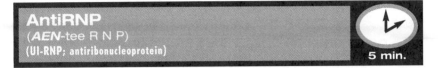

WEBLINKS

www.lupus.org

AntiRNP
(*AEN*-tee R N P)
(UI-RNP; antiribonucleoprotein)

5 min.

Type of Test: Blood

Body Systems and Functions: Immunological system

Normal Findings: Negative

Test Results Time Frame: Within 24 hr

Test Description: AntiRNP is an antinuclear antibody present in autoimmune disease detected by immunofluorescent procedures. The immunofluorescence differentiates different types of connective tissue disorders with characteristic staining patterns. AntiRNP, in conjunction with anti-Sm, is a marker for systemic lupus erythematosus (SLE), rheumatoid arthritis (RA), Sjögren's syndrome, and other connective tissue disorders.

Consent Form: Not required

List of Equipment: Red-top tube or serum separator tube; needle and syringe or vacutainer; alcohol swab

Test Procedure:
1. Label the specimen tube. *Correctly identifies the client and the test to be performed.*
2. Obtain a 5-mL blood sample.
3. Do not agitate the tube. *Agitation may cause RBC hemolysis.*
4. Send tube to the laboratory.

Clinical Implications and Indications:
1. Elevated levels are found with autoimmune disorders, such as scleroderma, discoid, and systemic lupus erythematosus.

Nursing Care:
Before Test: Explain the test procedure and the purpose of the test. Assess the client's knowledge of the test.
During Test: Adhere to standard precautions.
After Test: Apply pressure to venipuncture site. Explain that some bruising, discomfort, and swelling may appear at the site and that warm, moist compresses can alleviate this. Monitor for signs of infection.

Potential Complications: Bleeding and bruising at venipuncture site

Nursing Considerations:
Pediatric: Infants and children will need assistance in remaining still during the venipuncture and age-appropriate comfort measures following the test.

Listing of Related Tests: Anti-Ro; anti-SSA; anti-SSB; anti-DNA; ANA; anti-Sm

WEBLINKS

http://www.nlm.nih.gov

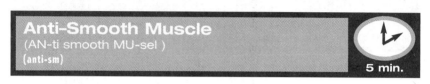

Anti–Smooth Muscle
(AN-ti smooth MU-sel)
(anti-sm)

5 min.

Type of Test: Blood

Body Systems and Functions: Immunological system

Normal Findings: Negative

Test Results Time Frame: Within 24 hr

Test Description: Anti–smooth muscle is an immunofluorescent test that detects and measures autoimmune immunoglobulins to smooth muscle. It is usually performed in conjunction with the test for antimitochondrial antibodies as an aid in differentiating various liver disorders.

Consent Form: Not required

List of Equipment: Red-top tube or serum separator tube; needle and syringe or vacutainer; alcohol swab

Test Procedure:
1. Label the specimen tube. *Correctly identifies the client and the test to be performed.*
2. Obtain a 5-mL blood sample.
3. Do not agitate the tube. *Agitation may cause RBC hemolysis.*
4. Send tube to the laboratory.

Clinical Implications and Indications:
1. Elevated levels are only found with a variety of autoimmune disorders, such as asthma, cirrhosis, hepatitis, mononucleosis, and yellow fever.
2. Differentiates between primary biliary cirrhosis and chronic active hepatitis.

Nursing Care:
Before Test: Explain the test procedure and the purpose of the test. Assess the client's knowledge of the test.
During Test: Adhere to standard precautions.
After Test: Apply pressure to venipuncture site. Explain that some bruising, discomfort, and swelling may appear at the site and that warm, moist compresses can alleviate this. Monitor for signs of infection.

Potential Complications: Bleeding and bruising at venipuncture site

Nursing Considerations:

Pediatric: *Infants and children will need assistance in remaining still during the venipuncture and age-appropriate comfort measures following the test.*

Listing of Related Tests: Anti-Ro; anti-SSA; anti-SSB; anti-DNA; ANA; anti-Sm

BLOOD

WEBLINKS

http://www.mic.ki.se/Diseases/c20.html

Anti-SS-A(Ro)
(AN-ti SS A)
(anti-SSA; anti(SSA); anti-ro(SSA); Sjögren's antibody)

5 min.

Type of Test: Blood

Body Systems and Functions: Immunological system

Normal Findings: Negative

Test Results Time Frame: Within 24 hr

Test Description: Anti-SS-A is an autoantibody that is directed against RNA protein particles that are a cofactor in RNA polymerase III. Anti-SS-A(ro), in conjunction with anti-La(SSB), is a marker for a milder form of systemic lupus erythematosus (SLE), known as Sjögren's SLE. The test is used in the diagnosis of different forms of rheumatic disease.

Consent Form: Not required

List of Equipment: Red-top tube or serum separator tube; needle and syringe or vacutainer; alcohol swab

Test Procedure:
1. Label the specimen tube. *Correctly identifies the client and the test to be performed.*
2. Obtain a 5-mL blood sample.
3. Do not agitate the tube. *Agitation may cause RBC hemolysis.*
4. Send tube to the laboratory.

Clinical Implications and Indications:
1. Elevated levels are found with systemic lupus erythematosus and forms of rheumatic disorders.

Nursing Care:

Before Test: Explain the test procedure and the purpose of the test. Assess the client's knowledge of the test.

During Test: Adhere to standard precautions.

After Test: Apply pressure to venipuncture site. Explain that some bruising, discomfort, and swelling may appear at the site and that warm, moist compresses can alleviate this. Monitor for signs of infection.

Potential Complications: Bleeding and bruising at venipuncture site

Nursing Considerations:
Pediatric: Infants and children will need assistance in remaining still during the venipuncture and age-appropriate comfort measures following the test.

Listing of Related Tests: Anti-SSB; anti-DNA; ANA

WEBLINKS 🔖

http://www.nlm.nih.gov

Antithrombin III
(**AEN**-tee-**THRAHM**-bin 3)
(At-III; heparin cofactor)

5 min.

Type of Test: Blood

Body Systems and Functions: Hematological system

Normal Findings: Plasma: 21–30 mg/dL; 85%–115% of standard; >50% of control value. Normal laboratory findings vary among the laboratory settings.

> **CRITICAL VALUES:**
> Levels 50%–70% of normal indicate risk for thrombosis and levels under 50% indicate high risk for thrombosis.

Test Results Time Frame: Within 3–5 days

Test Description: Antithrombin III inhibits the action of thrombin and four other clotting factors in the blood. Antithrombin III is an IgG immunoglobulin that is synthesized in the liver and inhibits coagulation by inactivating thrombin and other clotting factors. The action of At-III is catalyzed by heparin, which augments the activity of antithrombin III by approximately 100 times. This At-III test is done to investigate a possible deficiency of At-III in people with hypercoagulable states.

Consent Form: Not required

List of Equipment: Light-blue top tube or serum separator tube; needle and syringe or vacutainer; alcohol swab

Test Procedure:
1. Label the specimen tube. *Correctly identifies the client and the test to be performed.*
2. Obtain a 5-mL blood sample.
3. Gently invert tube several times, but do not agitate the tube. *Mixes the anticoagulant, but agitation may cause RBC hemolysis.*
4. Send tube to the laboratory.
5. Freeze sample if it cannot be sent immediately to the laboratory. *Room temperatures can alter test results.*

Clinical Implications and Indications:

1. Decreased levels are found with liver transplants and liver lobectomy, disseminated intravascular coagulation (DIC), nephrotic syndrome, hypercoagulation, deep vein thrombosis, gram-negative septicemia, protein-wasting diseases, cancer, cirrhosis, late pregnancy, and early postpartum.
2. Elevated levels are found with acute hepatitis, renal transplant, inflammation, menstruation, and vitamin K deficiency.

Nursing Care:

Before Test: Explain the test procedure and the purpose of the test. Assess the client's knowledge of the test. Instruct client to fast (except water) for 10–12 hr prior to test.
During Test: Adhere to standard precautions.
After Test: Apply pressure to venipuncture site. Explain that some bruising, discomfort, and swelling may appear at the site and that warm, moist compresses can alleviate this. Monitor for signs of infection.

Potential Complications: Bleeding and bruising at venipuncture site

Nursing Considerations:

Pregnancy: Levels decrease in late pregnancy and the early postpartum period.
Pediatric: Newborns to 6 months may have decreased levels. Infants and children will need assistance in remaining still during the venipuncture and age-appropriate comfort measures following the test.

WEBLINKS

http://www.methodisthealth.com

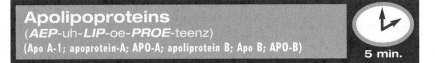

Apolipoproteins
(*AEP*-uh-*LIP*-oe-*PROE*-teenz)
(Apo A-1; apoprotein-A; APO-A; apoliprotein B; Apo B; APO-B)

5 min.

Type of Test: Blood

Body Systems and Functions: Cardiovascular system

Normal Findings:

Ratio of	A-1 to B
Women	55–100 mg/dL
Men	45–110 mg/dL

Test Results Time Frame: Within 24 hr

Test Description: Apolipoproteins are the major protein components of blood fats, of which low-density lipoprotein (LDL) and high-density lipoprotein (HDL) are examples. Apolipotroteins are an inherited alpha-1 globulin and the major protein of HDL. HDL and LDL are essential for the transport and synthesis of cholesterol for excretion/secretion in the liver and small intestine. The ratio of apolipoproteins is very useful in identifying at-risk persons for coronary artery disease (note: the HDL is significantly correlated with atherosclerotic heart disease).

BLOOD

Consent Form: Not required

List of Equipment: Red-top tube or serum separator tube; needle and syringe or vacutainer; alcohol swab

Test Procedure:
1. Label the specimen tube. *Correctly identifies the client and the test to be performed.*
2. Obtain a 5-mL blood sample.
3. Do not agitate the tube. *Agitation may cause RBC hemolysis.*
4. Send tube to the laboratory.
5. Keep specimen cool. *High temperatures alter the results.*

Clinical Implications and Indications:
1. Identifies persons at risk for atherosclerosis and coronary artery disease (CAD).
2. Elevated levels are found with acute illness, angina pectoris, CAD, and myocardial infarction.

Nursing Care:
Before Test: Explain the test procedure and the purpose of the test. Assess the client's knowledge of the test. Instruct client to fast 12 hr before test and to abstain from alcohol for 24 hr prior to test.
During Test: Adhere to standard precautions.
After Test: Apply pressure to venipuncture site. Explain that some bruising, discomfort, and swelling may appear at the site and that warm, moist compresses can alleviate this. Monitor for signs of infection.

Potential Complications: Bleeding and bruising at venipuncture site

Interfering Factors: Acute illness, which produces false positives; alcohol ingestion within 24 hr of testing; oral contraceptives, which increase levels

Nursing Considerations:
Pediatric: Infants and children will need assistance in remaining still during the venipuncture and age-appropriate comfort measures following the test.

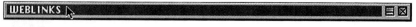

http://www.howstuffworks.com

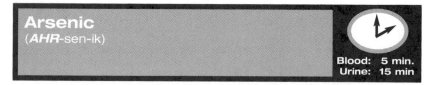

Arsenic
(*AHR*-sen-ik)

Blood: 5 min.
Urine: 15 min

Type of Test: Blood; urine; hair/nails

Body Systems and Functions: Hematological system

Normal Findings:

Blood	<0.07 µg/mL
Urine	<25 µg/specimen
Hair or nails	<1.0 µg/mL

Test Results Time Frame: Within 48 hr

Test Description: Arsenic is a heavy metal found in all tissues and is found in pesticides, environment, paints, cosmetics, and industrial chemicals. Arsenic inhibits cellular metabolism. Blood and hair/nail samples are the most reliable indicator, as urine samples can be misleading. Poisoning may be either acute or chronic.

Consent Form: Not required

List of Equipment: *Blood:* blue-top tube or serum separator tube; needle and syringe or vacutainer; alcohol swab. *Urine:* sterile acid-washed container; ice.

Test Procedure:

Blood:
1. Label the specimen tube. *Correctly identifies the client and the test to be performed.*
2. Obtain a 5-mL blood sample.
3. Gently invert tube several times, but do not agitate the tube. *Mixes the anticoagulant, but agitation may cause RBC hemolysis.*
4. Send tube to the laboratory.
5. Keep specimen cool. *High temperatures alter the results.*

Urine:
1. Label a sterile urine container. *Correctly identifies the client and the test to be performed.*
2. Obtain a clean-catch specimen of urine. *Ensures accurate results.*
3. Keep specimen cool. *High temperatures alter the results.*
4. Send specimen to laboratory.

Clinical Implications and Indications:

1. Elevated levels are found with ingested toxic food or water, pesticides with arsenic, and contaminated well water.
2. Exposure may also occur if clients work in industries that manufacture brass, bronze, ceramics, dye, or paint.

Nursing Care:

Before Test: Explain the test procedure and the purpose of the test. Assess the client's knowledge of the test. Request client not to eat shellfish or bottom-feeding seafood for 72 hr prior to the test.

During Test: Adhere to standard precautions. If any urine is accidentally discarded or contaminated with feces, discard entire specimen and begin test again the following morning.

After Test: Blood: Apply pressure to venipuncture site. Explain that some bruising, discomfort, and swelling may appear at the site and that warm, moist compresses can alleviate this. Monitor for signs of infection. Urine: Document urine quantity, date, and exact hours of collection on requisition.

Potential Complications: Bleeding and bruising at venipuncture site

BLOOD

Interfering Factors: Urine contaminated with feces; spillage or inaccurate collection of the urine specimen, including nonrefrigeration or placing on ice; heavy bleeding during menstruation

Nursing Considerations:

Pediatric: Health providers should emphasize the need to avoid contaminates that are occasionally accessible to children (e.g., paints, ceramics).

Blood: Infants and children will need assistance in remaining still during the venipuncture and age-appropriate comfort measures following the test.

Urine: A collection bag or insertion of a straight catheter is likely needed for infants and toddlers.

Rural: *Instruct clients who drink well water to have their water tested for impurities on a regular basis.*

Listing of Related Tests: CBC

WEBLINKS

http://alice.ucdavis.edu

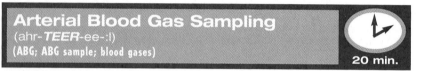

Arterial Blood Gas Sampling
(ahr-*TEER*-ee-:l)
(ABG; ABG sample; blood gases)

20 min.

Type of Test: Blood

Body Systems and Functions: Hematological system

Normal Findings:

pH:
Newborns	7.32–7.49
Adults	7.35–7.45

pO_2:
Newborns	60–70 mm Hg
Adults	75–100 mm Hg
pCO_2:	35–45 mm Hg

HCO_3:
Newborns	20–26 mEq/L
Adults	22–26 mEq/L
O_2 saturation	96%–100%
Base excess	+1 to -2

CRITICAL VALUES:
pH	<7.2 or >7.6
pO_2	
Infants	<37 mm Hg or >92 mm g
Adults	<40 mm Hg
pCO_2	<20 mm Hg or >70 mm g
HCO_3	<10 mEq/L or >40 mEq/L
O_2 saturation	<60%

BLOOD

Test Results Time Frame: Within 24 hr

Test Description: Arterial blood gas testing measures the dissolved oxygen, carbon dioxide, and pH levels in the arterial blood. The pH reflects the hydrogen ions in the circulating blood and the body has a narrow range for viability. Complex buffering systems exist in the respiratory and cardiovascular mechanisms that normally keep the different substances in balance. The lungs compensate for imbalances within 2–3 hours, while the metabolic system takes 2–3 days. When these buffering systems are not adequate, the ABGs are evaluated to assist in the assessment of cardiopulmonary dysfunctions and acid-base imbalances. The ABGs measure the effectiveness of tissue perfusion, and when imbalanced, there are serious deoxygenation and acid-base imbalance problems.

CLINICAL ALERT:
Clients with extremes in the ABG values have a high mortality rate and most likely will require critical care management.

Consent Form: Not required

List of Equipment (Arterial puncture): Blood gas collection kit; heparin if syringe is not preheparinized; lidocaine or other local anesthetic; ice in a small cup or bag; sterile dressing

Test Procedure:
1. Have the client either sit or lie supine.
2. Assess the collateral circulation to the wrist and hand prior to the radial puncture. *If the ulnar circulation is inadequate, another site must be chosen.*
3. Place the client's wrist with the dorsal side up on a small pillow, and ask the client to extend the fingers downward. *Brings the radial artery closer to the skin surface.*
4. Cleanse the site with a local antiseptic. If the client is allergic to iodine, use only alcohol. *Serious allergic reactions can result from injection of an allergen into an artery.*
5. The health care provider may choose to anesthetize the site with a local anesthetic.
6. The health care provider punctures the radial artery with a heparinized syringe. *Clots will alter results.*
7. Withdraw 2–3 mL of blood from the artery and the needle is removed.
8. Place direct pressure on the puncture site with a sterile dressing. *Arterial punctures can cause serious bleeding.*
9. Maintain digital pressure for 5 min; then apply a sterile dressing.
10. Air bubbles in the syringe are expelled, and it is placed immediately into the ice. *Waiting longer than 2 min to place the sample into ice will alter the results.*
11. Label the tube with the time the sample was collected, the client's temperature, whether the client was breathing room air, oxygen, or was ventilated. *Fever and assisted oxygen or breathing alters test interpretation.*

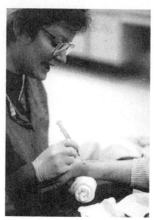

Arterial Blood Gas Procedure

Clinical Implications and Indications:

1. ABGs are drawn with critically ill clients who have altered acid-base balance and/or who have cardiopulmonary disorders such as acute respiratory disorders, hypoxia, hypocapnia, diabetic ketoacidosis, congenital heart defects, anesthesia, dysrhythmias, asthma, alkali ingestion, salicylate intoxication, emphysema, pneumonia, sepsis, and shock.
2. Evaluates and monitors the therapies offered for critical clients who often are high risk.

Nursing Care:

Before Test: Explain the test procedure and the purpose of the test. Assess the client's knowledge of the test. Explain that the radial puncture will be done after a local anesthetic or, if no anesthetic used, will cause a brief, sharp pain. Take the client's temperature.

During Test: Adhere to standard precautions.

After Test: Monitor the puncture site every 5–10 min for at least 30 min following the test for bleeding. Check for signs of nerve impairment distal to the puncture. Apply pressure for at least 5–10 min to the arterial puncture site. Explain that some bruising, discomfort, and swelling may appear at the site and that warm, moist compresses can alleviate this (note: only applied after bleeding is stopped). Monitor for signs of infection.

Potential Complications: Bleeding and bruising at arterial puncture site

Interfering Factors: Fever; suctioning; respiratory therapy treatments; exposure of the sample to room air; warming the sample; not placing the sample on ice within 2 min.

Nursing Considerations:

Pediatric: Infants and children will need assistance in remaining still during the arterial puncture and age-appropriate comfort measures following the test. Often mild sedation is recommended for infants and children.

WEBLINKS

http://www.howstuffworks.com

Aspartate Aminotransferase
(***AES***-pahr-tayt uh-mee-noe-***TRAENS***-f:r-ays)
(serum glutamic-oxaloacetic transaminase; SGOT; AST)

5 min.

BLOOD

Type of Test: Blood

Body Systems and Functions: Cardiovascular system

Normal Findings:

Newborn	15–60 U/L
6 months	20–50 U/L
1 year	16–35 U/L
5 years	19–28 U/L
Adult:	
Men	8–46 U/L
Women	7–31 U/L (note: slight increase noted with aging and exercise)

Test Results Time Frame: Within 12 hr

Test Description: Aspartate aminotransferase is an enzyme found primarily in heart muscle and liver with moderate amounts found in skeletal muscle, kidney, and pancreas. Concentration in the blood is low except with cellular damage. High levels are found following an acute MI and serum levels increase 10 times or more and remain high in liver disease. In heart ischemia AST value rises within 6–8 hr, peaks at 24–48 hr, and declines within 72–96 hr and should return to normal within 4–6 days with no further ischemia. AST is not a single indicator for MIs, as AST is associated with a multitude of drugs.

Consent Form: Not required

List of Equipment: Red-top tube or serum separator tube; needle and syringe or vacutainer; alcohol swab

Test Procedure:
1. Label the specimen tube. *Correctly identifies the client and the test to be performed.*
2. Obtain a 5-mL blood sample.
3. Do not agitate the tube. *Agitation may cause RBC hemolysis.*
4. Send tube to the laboratory.

Clinical Implications and Indications:
1. Elevated levels are found with acute myocardial infarction, severe angina, hepatitis, liver necrosis, cancer of liver, alcoholism, musculoskeletal disease, recent convulsions, heat stoke, severe burns, acute pancreatitis, strenuous exercise, toxic shock syndrome, cerebral infarction, trauma, and intramuscular injection.
2. Decreased levels are found with diabetic ketoacidosis, hemodialysis, and chronic liver disease.

BLOOD

Levels of severity for elevated AST

Elevation:
5 or more times normal
    Acute hepatocellular damage
    MI
    Shock
    Acute pancreatitis
    Infectious mononucliosis
1–5 times normal
    Biliary obsturction
    Cardiac arrythmia
    Liver tumors
    Congestive heart failure
    Muscular dystrophy
Slight elevation
    Pericarditis
    Fatty liver
    Pulmonary infarct
    CVA
    Hemolytic anemia
    Delirium tremors

Nursing Care:

Before Test: Explain the test procedure and the purpose of the test. Assess the client's knowledge of the test.
During Test: Adhere to standard precautions.
After Test: Apply pressure to venipuncture site. Explain that some bruising, discomfort, and swelling may appear at the site and that warm, moist compresses can alleviate this. Monitor for signs of infection.

Potential Complications: Bleeding and bruising at venipuncture site

Interfering Factors: Exercise increases levels; medications that increase results are antibiotics, allopurinol, anabolic steroids, barbiturates, antihypertensives, salicylates, albumin, Imuran, and flourides; pregnancy falsely decreases and increases levels.

Nursing Considerations:

Pregnancy: Levels may increase or decrease during pregnancy.
Pediatric: Infants and children will need assistance in remaining still during the venipuncture and age-appropriate comfort measures following the test.
Gerontology: Aging is a nonmodifiable cardiovascular risk factor and therefore the elderly are more at risk for problems that result in elevations of AST. In addition, there are slight increases in AST associated with increased age.

WEBLINKS

www.healthgate.com

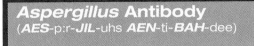

Aspergillus Antibody
(*AES*-p:r-*JIL*-uhs *AEN*-ti-*BAH*-dee)

5 min.

BLOOD

Type of Test: Blood

Body Systems and Functions: Immunological system

Normal Findings: <1:8

Test Results Time Frame: Within 24 hr

Test Description: *Aspergillus* antibody measures the *Aspergillus* fungus that lives in soil and organic materials. *Aspergillus* can be transmitted to humans by way of inhalation or a break in the skin. *Aspergillus* may cause severe respiratory infections presenting with a golden brown sputum. Persons most susceptible are those with debilitating or chronic disease or those receiving such drug therapy as steroids, prolonged antibiotics, antineoplastic agents, or oral contraceptives. Testing for *Aspergillus* antibodies assists in diagnosing an allergic bronchopulmonary condition. The test is repeated in 2–3 weeks and a positive result is best demonstrated by a fourfold or greater rise in titer between the acute exposure and convalescent specimens. In addition, the skin or infected area may be biopsied for *Aspergillus* fungal infections.

Consent Form: Not required

List of Equipment: Red-top tube or serum separator tube; needle and syringe or vacutainer; alcohol swab

Test Procedure:
1. Label the specimen tube. *Correctly identifies the client and the test to be performed.*
2. Obtain a 10-mL blood sample.
3. Do not agitate the tube. *Agitation may cause RBC hemolysis.*
4. Send tube to the laboratory.
5. Keep specimen cool. *High temperatures alter the results.*
6. Repeat 14–21 days later for convalescent sample and label the tube as convalescent sample. *Allows for separate identification of the convalescent sample, which is compared in ratio to the acute sample.*

Clinical Implications and Indications:
1. Diagnoses fungal infection by *Aspergillus*
2. Evaluates persistent pulmonary symptoms without pneumonia
3. Confirms exposure to *Aspergillus*

Nursing Care:

Before Test: Explain the test procedure and the purpose of the test. Assess the client's knowledge of the test. Determine if the client has not had a recent skin/tissue test for *Aspergillus*. If this has been done, it should be noted on the laboratory slip. Client may be required to be NPO depending on the laboratory. *During Test:* Adhere to standard precautions. Do not draw blood near skin/tissue test site.

BLOOD

After Test: Apply pressure to venipuncture site. Explain that some bruising, discomfort, and swelling may appear at the site and that warm, moist compresses can alleviate this. Monitor for signs of infection. Advise client that the test should be repeated in 2–3 weeks. If positive, the client will be treated with amphotericin B, the drug of choice.

Potential Complications: Bleeding and bruising at venipuncture site

Interfering Factors: Skin test for *Aspergillus* within the last 2 weeks; contamination of specimen

Nursing Considerations:
Pediatric: Infants and children will need assistance in remaining still during the venipuncture and age-appropriate comfort measures following the test.

Listing of Related Tests: *Aspergillus* skin test

WEBLINKS

www.medline.com; www.healthgate.com

Aspirin Tolerance
(AS-per-in tol-ur-UNS test)
(salicylate tolerance test ; ASA tolerance test)

3 hr

Type of Test: Blood

Body Systems and Functions: Hematological system

Normal Findings: Normal Ivy bleeding time of 2–7 min. After ingestion of aspirin the bleeding time may increase to 4–10 min, with a return to normal in 96 hr postingestion.

CRITICAL VALUES:
>10 min bleeding time

Test Results Time Frame: Within 4 days

Test Description: The aspirin tolerance test evaluates the changes in coagulation of the hematological system by the ingestion of aspirin. The Ivy bleeding time is done prior to and 2 hr following the ingestion of 10 g (adult) or 5 g (children under 32 kg) to assess the effects of aspirin on platelet function. In normal clients, aspirin administration has minimal influence on bleeding time.

Consent Form: Not required

List of Equipment: Skin prep; blood pressure cuff; lancet; stop watch; filter paper

Test Procedure:
1. Clean inner aspect of forearm with antiseptic solution and allow to dry. *Ensures lack of contamination.*
2. Apply blood pressure cuff and inflate to 40 mm Hg and make two small incisions 2–3 mm deep.

3. Blot blood every 15 sec until bleeding stops and note time.
4. Administer ASA according to age.
5. Wait 2 hr and repeat steps 1–3.

Clinical Implications and Indications:
1. Diagnoses collagen vascular disease, disseminated intravascular coagulation (DIC), splenomegaly, and von Willebrand's disease
2. Evaluates various anticoagulant therapies
3. Monitors thrombocytopenia caused by a suppressed immune system

Nursing Care:
Before Test: Explain the test procedure and the purpose of the test. Assess the client's knowledge of the test. Note when client last took aspirin.
During Test: Adhere to standard precautions. Provide reassurance and a calm atmosphere during the procedure.
After Test: Assess site for bleeding every 5 min for 30 min. Apply band aid to sites and advise client to watch for bleeding and signs of infection.

Potential Complications: Bleeding and bruising at puncture site

Contraindications: Platelet count <50,000; severe bleeding disorder; skin infections; ingestion of ASA within 5 days; inability to place blood pressure cuff on arm (e.g., AV fistula); restraints on extremity

Interfering Factors: ASA within 5 days; poor technique in making incisions

Nursing Considerations:
Pediatric: Infants and children will need assistance in remaining still during the venipuncture and age-appropriate comfort measures following the test.
Home Care: Health care providers must be instructed to provide safety measures for clients with increased levels of ASA tolerance times, such as wearing slippers, assessing for clinical manifestations of bleeding/bruising, and assisting client when ambulating.

| WEBLINKS |

www.healthgate.com; www.nlm.nih.gov

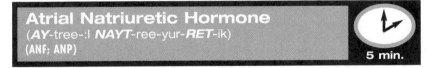

Atrial Natriuretic Hormone
(*AY*-tree-:l *NAYT*-ree-yur-*RET*-ik)
(ANF; ANP)

5 min.

Type of Test: Blood

Body Systems and Functions: Endocrine system

Normal Findings: 20–77 pg/mL

Test Results Time Frame: Within 24 hr

Test Description: Atrial natriuretic hormone (ANH) is secreted by the atria of the heart and acts as an antagonist to renin and aldosterone. The hormone is released during expansion of vessels from blood volume and produces vasodilation and increased glomerular filtration rates. It counteracts renin/angiotensin by inhibiting the action of angiotensin II and thus promoting a decrease in blood pressure. The end result is a decreased preload, afterload, and blood volume. Abnormal ANH levels can be used as a diagnostic tool to detect cardiovascular disease.

Consent Form: Not required

List of Equipment: Lavender-top tube or serum separator tube; needle and syringe or vacutainer; alcohol swab; ice

Test Procedure:
1. Label the specimen tube. *Correctly identifies the client and the test to be performed.*
2. Obtain a 5-mL blood sample.
3. Gently invert tube several times, but do not agitate the tube. *Mixes the anticoagulant, but agitation may cause RBC hemolysis.*
4. Send tube to the laboratory.
5. Keep specimen cool. *High temperatures alter the results.*

Clinical Implications and Indications: See table below.

Causes of abnormal ANH levels

Increase:
    Congestive heart failure (acute)
    Cardiovascular disease
    Dysrhythmia
    PAT
    Small cell lung carcinoma
    Subarachnoid hemorrhage
Decrease:
Chronic congestive heart failure
Drugs: Prazosin, Urapidil, Xepamide

Nursing Care:
Before Test: Explain the test procedure and the purpose of the test. Assess the client's knowledge of the test.
During Test: Adhere to Standard Precautions.
After Test: Apply pressure to venipuncture site. Explain that some bruising, discomfort, and swelling may appear at the site and that warm, moist compresses can alleviate this. Monitor for signs of infection.

Potential Complications: Bleeding and bruising at venipuncture site

Interfering Factors: Specimen not maintained on ice

Nursing Considerations:
Pediatric: Infants and children will need assistance in remaining still during the venipuncture and age-appropriate comfort measures following the test.

Rural: *If client is cared for in rural setting, the specimen may need to be sent to a regional laboratory, which could mean several additional days before results are determined.*

WEBLINKS

www.gyn.oulu.fi; http://www.oucom.ohiou.edu; www.healthgate.com

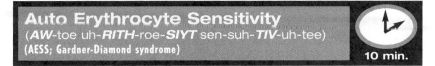

Auto Erythrocyte Sensitivity
(*AW*-toe uh-*RITH*-roe-*SIYT* sen-suh-*TIV*-uh-tee)
(AESS; Gardner-Diamond syndrome)
10 min.

Type of Test: Blood

Body Systems and Functions: Hematological system

Normal Findings: Negative

Test Results Time Frame: Within 24 hr

Test Description: Auto erythrocyte sensitization is an uncommon disorder, but well recognized in clients with severe emotional disturbances. It occurs primarily in women. Presenting factors include recurrent, purpura, and painful ecchymotic lesions of the skin, usually confined to the extremities. In most cases, hematological and immunological studies are normal. The syndrome's cause is hypothesized to be an autoimmune sensitization to erythrocyte stroma because intradermal injection of the client's own RBCs stimulates the development of ecchymosis. Blood is drawn from the client, reinjected intradermally, and observed for reaction.

Consent Form: Not required

List of Equipment: Three needles; two syringes; alcohol swabs

Test Procedure:
1 One millilter of blood is drawn from the client.
2. A new needle is placed on the syringe.
3. One milliliter of blood is injected intradermally into a purpura-free area on the thigh. Mark the area.
4. Inject 1 mL saline in a purpura-free area on the other thigh. Mark the area.
5. A positive reaction is one in which painful, edematous erythema is noted at the blood injection site.

Clinical Implications and Indications:
1. Evaluates clients with spontaneous purpura and bruising

Nursing Care:
Before Test: Explain the test procedure and the purpose of the test. Assess the client's knowledge of the test.
During Test: Adhere to standard precautions.

After Test: Apply pressure to venipuncture site. Explain that some bruising, discomfort, and swelling may appear at both the blood injection site and the control sites and that warm, moist compresses can alleviate this. Monitor for signs of infection.

Potential Complications: Bleeding and bruising at venipuncture site

Contraindications: Known coagulation disorder

Interfering Factors: Uncooperative clients

Nursing Considerations:
Pediatric: Infants and children will need assistance in remaining still during the venipuncture and age-appropriate comfort measures following the test.

Listing of Related Tests: Coagulation studies

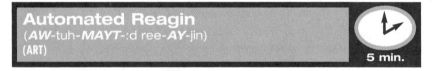

www.merck.com; www.aapa.org

Automated Reagin
(*AW*-tuh-*MAYT*-:d ree-*AY*-jin)
(ART)

5 min.

Type of Test: Blood

Body Systems and Functions: Reproductive system

Normal Findings:

Negative	Nonreactive
1:9–1:32	Primary stage of syphilis
>1:32	Secondary stage of syphilis

Test Results Time Frame: Within 24–48 hr

Test Description: Automated reagin testing measures the presence of reagin, which is produced when *Treponema pallidum* is present in the blood. This test is a nonspecific, nontreponemal test that is used to screen for syphilis and monitoring the treatment response. Syphilis is a very complex sexually transmitted disease that has a wide variety of clinical manifestations and is caused by *T. pallidum.*

Consent Form: Not required

List of Equipment: Red-top tube or serum separator tube; needle and syringe or vacutainer; alcohol swab

Test Procedure:
1. Label the specimen tube. *Correctly identifies the client and the test to be performed.*
2. Obtain a 5-mL blood sample.
3. Do not agitate the tube. *Agitation may cause RBC hemolysis.*
4. Send tube to the laboratory.

BLOOD

Clinical Implications and Indications:
1. Indicates the presence of syphilis and can be isolated 7–21 days after the first appearance of the syphilis chancre

Nursing Care:
Before Test: Explain the test procedure and the purpose of the test. Assess the client's knowledge of the test. Conduct specific sexual activity assessment prior to the ART.
During Test: Adhere to standard precautions.
After Test: Apply pressure to venipuncture site. Explain that some bruising, discomfort, and swelling may appear at the site and that warm, moist compresses can alleviate this. Monitor for signs of infection. Follow-up instructions to client who tests positive are detailed under Nursing Considerations. Instruct the client to repeat testing every 3–4 months for the next 2 years to ensure the disease is cured.

Potential Complications: Bleeding and bruising at venipuncture site

Interfering Factors: Any diseases that produce reagin; connective tissue diseases; malaria; infectious mononucleosis; hepatitis; active immunization in children; chicken pox; pneumonia; fever; measles; tuberculosis; the common cold; pregnancy; consumption of alcohol within 24 hr

Nursing Considerations:
Pregnancy: All sexual contacts within the last 90 days must be reported if there is a positive test. Use condoms for 2–4 months after treatment for a positive test. Do not become pregnant for 2 years due to the potential transmission of syphilis to the fetus.
Pediatric: Infants and children will need assistance in remaining still during the venipuncture and age-appropriate comfort measures following the test. The fetus is susceptible to congenital abnormalities in a positive test of the mother.

Listing of Related Tests: VDRL

WEBLINKS

www.healthgate.com

Bartonella Henselae Antibody
(*BAHR*-tuh-*NEL*-uh *HENZ*-lay *AEN*-ti-*BAH*-dee)
(*Rochalimaea henselae* antibody; cat-scratch antibodies)

15 min.

Type of Test: Blood

Body Systems and Functions: Integumentary system

Normal Findings: Negative

Test Results Time Frame: Within 3–7 days

Test Description: The presence of *Bartonella henselae* diagnoses cat-scratch fever, which may occur 1–3 weeks following exposure to cats, but the lymphadenopathy and other symptoms may persist for several months. The Center for Disease Control has established guidelines for cat owners to prevent cat-scratch fever. The serum immunofluorescent antibody (IFA) and the enzyme immunoassay (EIA) are currently available for *B. henselae*. The EIA is thought to be more accurate. Special cultures for the *B. henselae* bacillus can be performed to isolate it and confirm diagnosis. In addition, excisional biopsies can be histologically examined using the Warthin Starry silver stain. A skin test is also available, although the false positives and false negatives make the results less acceptable.

Consent Form: Not required

List of Equipment: Red-top tube or serum separator tube; needle and syringe or vacutainer; alcohol swab

Test Procedure:
For IFA or EIA:
1. Label the specimen tube. *Correctly identifies the client and the test to be performed.*
2. Obtain a 5-mL blood sample.
3. Do not agitate the tube. *Agitation may cause RBC hemolysis.*
4. Send tube to the laboratory.

For blood culture:
1. Label the specimen tube. *Correctly identifies the client and the test to be performed.*
2. Cleanse the venipuncture site with 70% isopropyl alcohol, followed by povidone-iodine solution.
3. Allow the site to air dry for 1–2 min. *Reduces the possibility of contamination from skin.*
4. Obtain a 10–30-mL blood sample. *The ability of the laboratory to detect bacterial growth is directly related to the amount of blood submitted for culture.*
5. Send tube to the laboratory.

Clinical Implications and Indications:
1. *Bartonella henselae* causes cat-scratch disease as a result of a cat scratch or bite or even petting a cat with cuts on one's hands. Toxoplasmosis may also be suspected.
2. Bacillary angiomatosis (BA) or bacillary epithelioid angiomatosis can result from infection. This is characterized by a proliferation of small capillaries having a close resemblance to Kaposi's sarcoma. It is more often found in persons with compromised immune systems such as HIV.
3. Peliosis hepatitis is a disseminated form of *B. henselae* occurring in HIV-compromised individuals.

Nursing Care:
Before Test: Explain the test procedure and the purpose of the test. Assess the client's knowledge of the test. Obtain an accurate history and record pertinent information on the requisition such as exposure to cat scratches or bites.
During Test: Adhere to standard precautions.
After Test: Apply pressure to venipuncture site. Explain that some bruising, discomfort, and swelling may appear at the site and that warm, moist compresses can alleviate this. Monitor for signs of infection.

BLOOD

Potential Complications: Bleeding and bruising at venipuncture site

Nursing Considerations:

Pregnancy: A differential diagnosis would include toxoplasmosis, which can cause congenital disorders.

Pediatric: Infants and children will need assistance in remaining still during the venipuncture and age-appropriate comfort measures following the test. Often young children are affected because they tend to hold and play with animals more, allowing the animal to lick them or getting scratched or bitten by kittens. One episode of cat-scratch fever usually confers lifelong immunity.

Rural: Cat-scratch fever is most often seen in the urban homeless population.

International: The Bartonella bacillus is found in arthropods such as lice, ticks, and fleas. Bartonella quintana (similar infection) causes trench fever, also known as Volhynia fever. This is a louse-borne disease occurring in Mexico and North Africa and most recently has been found with the homeless population in North America.

Listing of Related Tests: CBC; tuberculosis skin test; IFA; EIA

‖ **WEBLINKS** ⟩   ▤ ☒

www.ispub.com; www.icondata.com

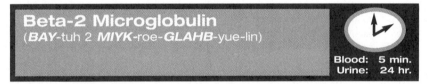

Beta-2 Microglobulin
(*BAY*-tuh 2 *MIYK*-roe-*GLAHB*-yue-lin)

Blood: 5 min.
Urine: 24 hr.

Type of Test: Blood; urine

Body Systems and Functions: Immunological system

Normal Findings: Blood: <2 µg/mL. Urine: <120 µg/24 hr.

Test Results Time Frame: Within 4 days

Test Description: Beta-2 microglobulin is a polypeptide produced and secreted by both T and B lymphocytes. Beta-2 microglobulin is metabolized by the renal tubules, so it will be elevated in renal failure. Increased levels are seen in situations were there is an inflammatory condition or when there is a rapid turnover of lymphocytes.

Consent Form: Not required

List of Equipment: *Blood:* red-top tube or serum separator tube; needle and syringe or vacutainer; alcohol swab. *Urine:* sterile plastic container; ice.

Test Procedure:

Blood:

1. Label the specimen tube. *Correctly identifies the client and the test to be performed.*
2. Obtain a 5-mL blood sample.
3. Do not agitate the tube. *Agitation may cause RBC hemolysis.*

4. Send tube to the laboratory.
5. Keep specimen cool. *High temperatures alter the results.*

Urine:
1. Label the collection container. *Correctly identifies the client and the test to be performed.*
2. Discard the first morning void. Then begin the time of the collection for the next 24 hr, including the void at the end of the 24 hr, and record the last voiding time. *An exact 24-hr count ensures accurate results.*
3. If the client has an indwelling catheter in place, keep the drainage bag on ice and empty the urine into the urine container periodically during the 24-hr period.
4. Keep urine cool during collection. *Higher temperatures alter the results.*
5. If any urine is lost, discard the entire specimen and begin collection again the next day.

Clinical Implications and Indications:
1. Evaluates and monitors HIV, lymphocytic leukemia, Crohn's disease, arthritis, hepatitis, multiple myeloma, various cancers (e.g., breast, lung), renal disease, aminoglycoside toxicity, sarcoidosis, and vasculitis
2. Detects heavy metal poisoning

Nursing Care:
Before Test: Explain the test procedure and the purpose of the test. Assess the client's knowledge of the test. For 24-hr urine, instruct client not to discard any urine. Obtain a history of recent tests using radioactive dyes.
During Test: Adhere to standard precautions.
After Test: Blood: Apply pressure to venipuncture site. Explain that some bruising, discomfort, and swelling may appear at the site and that warm, moist compresses can alleviate this. Monitor for signs of infection. Urine: Document urine quantity, date, and exact hours of collection on requisition.

Potential Complications: Bleeding and bruising at venipuncture site

Interfering Factors: Urine contaminated with feces; spillage or inaccurate collection of the 24-hr specimen, including nonrefrigeration or placing on ice; heavy bleeding during menstruation; radioactive dyes within 1 week

Nursing Considerations:
Pediatric: Blood: *Infants and children will need assistance in remaining still during the venipuncture and age-appropriate comfort measures following the test. Urine: For collection of 24-hr specimen a collection bag or indwelling catheter needs to be used for infants and toddlers.*
Rural: *If client is cared for in rural setting, the specimen may need to be sent to a regional laboratory, which could add several additional days before results are determined.*

| WEBLINKS |

http://labmed.ucsf.edu; www.nlm.nih.gov/

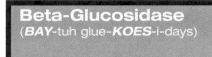

Beta-Glucosidase
(*BAY*-tuh glue-*KOES*-i-days)

5 min.

BLOOD

Type of Test: Blood

Body Systems and Functions: Metabolic system

Normal Findings: Positive for beta-glucosidase

Test Results Time Frame: Within 4 days

Test Description: Beta-glucosidase is a screening test for Gaucher's disease, a lysosomal lipid storage disorder caused by a deficiency of the enzyme beta-glucosidase. Gaucher's disease is autosomal recessive in causation. The disease has three classifications from mild to severe. In severe cases, it progresses quickly and is fatal in infants. Beta-glucosidase is an enzyme found in leukocytes that metabolizes glycolipid glucocerebroside. A decreased amount of the enzyme (at least 30% in Gaucher's disease) results in accumulation of glucocerebroside, causing splenomegaly, hepatomegaly, anemia, thrombocytopenia, erosion of long bones, and mental retardation.

Consent Form: Not required

List of Equipment: Green-top tube or plasma separator tube; needle and syringe or vacutainer; alcohol swab; ice

Test Procedure:
1. Label the specimen tube. *Correctly identifies the client and the test to be performed.*
2. Obtain a 10-mL blood sample.
3. Do not agitate the tube. *Agitation may cause RBC hemolysis.*
4. Send tube to the laboratory.
5. Keep specimen on ice. *High temperatures alter the results.*

Clinical Implications and Indications:
1. Diagnoses a family history of Gaucher's disease
2. Evaluates splenomegaly, hepatomegaly, anemia, thrombocytopenia, erosion of the long bones, and mental retardation

Nursing Care:
Before Test: Explain the test procedure and the purpose of the test. Assess the client's knowledge of the test.
During Test: Adhere to standard precautions. Provide emotional support to client and parents during the testing time.
After Test: Apply pressure to venipuncture site. Explain that some bruising, discomfort, and swelling may appear at the site and that warm, moist compresses can alleviate this. Monitor for signs of infection.

Potential Complications: Bleeding and bruising at venipuncture site

Interfering Factors: Blood not maintained on ice

BLOOD

Nursing Considerations:
Pediatric: *Infants and children will need assistance in remaining still during the venipuncture and age-appropriate comfort measures following the test.*

WEBLINKS 🔲🔲

www.acadia.net; www.medlineplus.com; www.ncbi.nlm.nih.gov

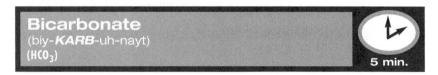

Bicarbonate
(biy-*KARB*-uh-nayt)
(HCO₃)

5 min.

Type of Test: Blood

Body Systems and Functions: Hematological system

Normal Findings:

Adult:

Venous	22–29 mEq/L or 22–29 mmol/L
Arterial	21–28 mEq/L or 21–28 mmol/L

Newborn:

Venous	16-24 mEq/L or 16–24 mmol/L

CRITICAL VALUES:
<15 or >35 mEq/L

Test Results Time Frame: Within 2 hr

Test Description: Bicarbonate testing measures the amount of bicarbonate in the venous or arterial blood. Bicarbonate is a primary substance that influences the acid-base balance of body fluids. In addition, it assists with the transport of carbon dioxide from the tissues to the lungs. Bicarbonate is considered a strong buffer when examining the arterial blood gases and is an accurate indicator of the conditions involving the regulation of the pH of the body fluids.

CLINICAL ALERT:
Extreme values of bicarbonate may be indicative of a life-threatening condition.

Consent Form: Not required

List of Equipment: Green-top tube, red-top tube, or serum separator tube; needle and syringe; alcohol swab; ice

Test Procedure:
Venous sample:
1. Label the specimen tube. *Correctly identifies the client and the test to be performed.*
2. Obtain a 10-mL blood sample.
3. Do not agitate the serum tube. *Agitation may cause RBC hemolysis.*
4. Send tube to the laboratory.

Arterial sample:
1. Label the specimen tube. *Correctly identifies the client and the test to be performed.*
2. Obtain a 10-mL blood sample from the artery (usually the radial artery).
3. Do not agitate the serum tube. *Agitation may cause RBC hemolysis.*
4. Send tube to the laboratory.

Clinical Implications and Indications:
1. Elevated levels are found with COPD, hypoventilation, Cushing's syndrome, CHF, pulmonary edema, hyperaldosteronism, compensated respiratory acidosis, gastric lavage, anoxia, metabolic alkalosis, and vomiting.
2. Decreased levels are found with diabetes mellitus, hyperventilation, burns, MI, Addison's disease, severe malnutrition, diarrhea, metabolic acidosis, compensated respiratory alkalosis, and renal failure.

Nursing Care:
Before Test: Explain the test procedure and the purpose of the test. Assess the client's knowledge of the test.
During Test: Adhere to standard precautions. For arterial blood draw provide reassurance and a calm atmosphere during the procedure.
After Test: Venous: Apply pressure to venipuncture site. Explain that some bruising, discomfort, and swelling may appear at the site and that warm, moist compresses can alleviate this. Monitor for signs of infection. Arterial: Apply pressure for 10–15 min after the specimen is obtained to ensure coagulation at the site.

Potential Complications: Bleeding and bruising at venipuncture site

Interfering Factors: Ingestion of alkaline or acidic substances; medications that increase levels are barbiturates, corticosteroids, diuretics, laxatives, opiates, and alkaline salts; medications that decrease levels are ammonium chloride, methanol, acid salts, and aspirin.

Nursing Considerations:
Pediatric: Infants and children will need assistance in remaining still during the venipuncture and age-appropriate comfort measures following the test.

| WEBLINKS | 🔲🗙 |

http://www.entnet.org

Bilirubin
(*BIL*-i-*RUE*-bin)
(direct bilirubin; indirect bilirubin; conjugated bilirubin;
unconjugated bilirubin; total bilirubin)

Blood: 5 min.
Urine: 15 min.

Type of Test: Blood; urine

Body Systems and Functions: Hepatobiliary system

BLOOD

Normal Findings:
Blood:

Full-term infant cord	<2.8 mg/dL
24 hr	2–6 mg/dL
48 hr	6–7 mg/dL
3–5 days	4–6 mg/dL
Direct bilirubin	0.0–0.3 mg/dL
Indirect bilirubin	0.1–1.0 mg/dL

Urine:

Negative	≤0.02 mg/dL

Test Results Time Frame: Within 24 hr

Test Description: Bilirubin is a substance that is produced in the liver, spleen, and bone marrow. It is also a by-product of hemoglobin metabolism. Bilirubin levels can be divided into direct (conjugated) and indirect (free or unconjugated) categories. The direct bilirubin is that part of the bilirubin that is excreted by the GI tract. The indirect bilirubin is the bilirubin that normally circulates in the bloodstream. A wide variety of disease processes cause increases in both direct and indirect bilirubin (see Clinical Implications and Indications). Bilirubin can be measured by both serum and urine samples. Note: There is no direct laboratory test for indirect bilirubin, but rather it is determined by subtracting the direct bilirubin from the total bilirubin.

Consent Form: Not required

List of Equipment: *Blood:* red-top tube or serum separator tube; needle and syringe or vacutainer; alcohol swab; lancet or capillary tube for heelstick. *Urine:* icotest tablets or chemstrips, sterile plastic container; ice.

Test Procedure:
Blood:
1. Label the specimen tube. *Correctly identifies the client and the test to be performed.*
2. Obtain a 1-mL blood sample for infants and children; 5–7 mL for adults.
3. Do not agitate the tube. *Agitation may cause RBC hemolysis.*
4. Send tube to the laboratory and protect from light. *Ensures accurate results.*

Urine:
1. Label a sterile urine container. *Correctly identifies the client and the test to be performed.*
2. Obtain 20 mL of urine.
3. Keep specimen cool. *High temperatures alter the results.*
4. Send specimen to laboratory.

Clinical Implications and Indications:
Blood:
1. Elevated total, direct, and indirect bilirubin levels are found with alcoholism, biliary obstruction or calculi, anemia, hepatitis, malaria, myocardial infarction, pancreatitis, cirrhosis, Gilbert's disease, pulmonary embolism, mononucleosis, and sickle cell anemia.
2. Decreased total, direct, and indirect bilirubin levels are not clinically significant.

Urine:
1. Elevated levels are found with cirrhosis, hepatitis, mononucleosis, and hyperthyroidism.

Nursing Care:

Before Test: Explain the test procedure and the purpose of the test. Assess the client's knowledge of the test. Instruct client to eat foods low in yellow foods (e.g., carrots, yams, yellow beans, pumpkin) for 3–4 days before test. Fast for 4 hr prior to testing.

During Test: Adhere to standard precautions. If any urine is accidentally discarded or contaminated with feces, discard entire specimen and begin test again.

After Test: Blood: Apply pressure to venipuncture site. Explain that some bruising, discomfort, and swelling may appear at the site and that warm, moist compresses can alleviate this. Monitor for signs of infection. Heelstick: Leave site open to air. Urine: Document urine quantity, date, and exact hours of collection on requisition.

Potential Complications: Bleeding and bruising at venipuncture site

Interfering Factors: Urine contaminated with feces; spillage or inaccurate collection of the urine specimen, including nonrefrigeration or placing on ice; heavy bleeding during menstruation; exposure to light; gross obesity; alcohol; medications that increase values are erythromycin, indomethacin, morphine, isoniazid, phenothiazines, salicylates, sulfonamides, and vitamin A; radioactive scan within 24 hr prior to the test

Nursing Considerations:

Pediatric: Infants and children will need assistance in remaining still during the venipuncture and age-appropriate comfort measures following the test. Neonate treatment for elevated serum bilirubin may be exchange transfusion or phototherapy. In addition, the jaundiced coloration of the newborn is often normal the first several days after birth. For infants, collect sample with heelstick blood in capillary tube. A collection bag or insertion of a straight catheter for the urine specimen is likely needed for infants and toddlers.

WEBLINKS

http://webmd.lycos.com

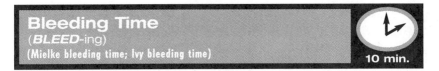

Bleeding Time
(*BLEED*-ing)
(Mielke bleeding time; Ivy bleeding time)
10 min.

Type of Test: Blood

Body Systems and Functions: Hematological system

Normal Findings:

Duke	1–3 min
Ivy	1–9 min
Template	3–6 min

CRITICAL VALUES:
>15 min

Test Results Time Frame: Immediate (note: varies depending on the method of measuring the bleeding time)

Test Description: Bleeding time is used as a screening procedure to evaluate the function of platelets and small blood vessels. Hemostasis involves a series of complex interactions among the blood vessels, platelets, and plasma proteins or coagulation factors. The blood vessels must constrict and slow the blood flow after injury. The platelets react within seconds after injury to form a plug. The coagulation factors are activated by the platelets in the injured tissue. The failure to clot may be due to the absence, deficiency, or improper function of any of the three components (vessels, platelets, plasma proteins). Bleeding time assesses the function of these components. There are three methods of measuring bleeding time: Ivy bleeding time, Duke bleeding time, and template bleeding time (each have different norms).

Consent Form: Not required

List of Equipment: Blood pressure cuff; lancet; stopwatch; alcohol swab

Test Procedure:
1. Cleanse the site chosen for puncture (often the volar aspect of the forearm).
2. Place the blood pressure cuff on the upper arm and inflate to 40 mm Hg (for Duke and template methods).
3. Make incision with lancet and simultaneously start stopwatch (note: Ivy method makes two incisions 3 mm deep; template method makes two incisions 1 mm deep and 9 mm long; Duke method makes an incision in the ear lobe).
4. Remove blood from the wound by gently blotting with filter paper, without exerting pressure on the wound.
5. When blood flow ceases, stop the stopwatch and calculate the time. If bleeding continues more than 20 min, discontinue the test.

Clinical Implications and Indications:
1. Elevated levels are found with anemia, congenital heart disease, ethyl alcohol ingestion, liver disease, DIC, Hodgkin's disease, drug sensitivity, collagen diseases, hemorrhagic disease of the newborn, hypothyroidism, uremia, idiopathic thrombocytopenic purpura, leukemia (acute), and multiple myeloma.

Nursing Care:
Before Test: Explain the test procedure and the purpose of the test. Assess the client's knowledge of the test. Instruct the client that the procedure may cause momentary discomfort when the skin is incised.
During Test: Adhere to standard precautions.
After Test: At completion of the test, a sterile dressing or band-aid is applied. If bleeding persists, ice and/or a pressure dressing may be applied. The site should be observed every 5 min for 30 min. The site should be observed twice a day for any signs of infection.

Potential Complications: If a client has a bleeding disorder, bleeding may occur up to 30 min after completion of the test.

Contraindications: Platelet counts < 50,000/mm³; clients with severe bleeding disorders

Interfering Factors: Aspirin and drugs containing aspirin taken within 5 days before the test; medications that alter results are anticoagulants, alcohol, over-the-counter cold remedies and analgesics, streptokinase, and thiazide diuretics.

WEBLINKS

www.healthgate.com

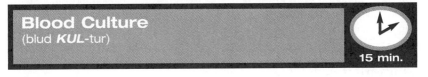

Blood Culture
(blud *KUL*-tur)

15 min.

Type of Test: Blood

Body Systems and Functions: Hematological system

Normal Findings: Negative

Test Results Time Frame: Within 48–72 hr

Test Description: Blood cultures are evaluated for the presence of bacteria in the blood. Bacteremia can be very serious, as it predisposes to the development of septic shock. The bacterial infection can be intermittent with clinical manifestations of fever, chills, and generalized weakness. The blood culture should be drawn during these symptoms to increase the chances of detection of the bacterial organisms. It is best to obtain samples from two venous sites, as they can be compared to one another. A positive bacteremia will grow organisms in both cultures.

CLINICAL ALERT:
Clients with infections can develop sepsis and therefore should assess for early symptoms (e.g., high fever, lethargy, chills) of a generalized blood infection.

Consent Form: Not required

List of Equipment: Blood culture bottles (aerobic and anaerobic); needle and syringe; alcohol swab; betadyne/iodine swab

Test Procedure:
1. Obtain blood culture bottles (aerobic and anaerobic) from the laboratory.
2. Label the blood culture bottle. *Correctly identifies the client and the test to be performed.*
3. Swab tops of bottles with alcohol and clean venipuncture site with alcohol using a circular motion beginning in the center. *Ensures accurate results.*
4. Repeat cleaning venipuncture site using betadyne/iodine swab and allow 1 min to dry. *Ensures accurate results.*
5. Obtain two 10- to 15-mL blood samples.

6. Inject the samples into prepared culture tubes, inoculate the anaerobic bottle first (if both anaerobic and aerobic cultures are required), and mix gently. *Ensures accurate results.*
7. Send bottles to the laboratory immediately.

Clinical Implications and Indications:
1. Identifies the presence of bacteria in the blood (bacteremia)

Nursing Care:
Before Test: Explain the test procedure and the purpose of the test. Assess the client's knowledge of the test.
During Test: Adhere to standard precautions.
After Test: Apply pressure to venipuncture site. Explain that some bruising, discomfort, and swelling may appear at the site and that warm, moist compresses can alleviate this. Monitor for signs of infection.

Potential Complications: Bleeding and bruising at venipuncture site

Interfering Factors: Current antibiotic therapy

Nursing Considerations:
Pregnancy: Treatment in pregnancy is difficult due to the potential harmful effects on the fetus.
Pediatric: Infants and children will need assistance in remaining still during the venipuncture and age-appropriate comfort measures following the test.
Gerontology: Elderly clients may not respond as well to antibiotic therapy, due to weakened immune systems.
Home Care: Clients who return home after bacteremia should be monitored for developing further symptomatology after the antibiotic course of therapy is completed. There is a possibility of the bacterial infection reoccurring.

║WEBLINKS║ ▧▨

www.ncbi.nlm.nih.gov

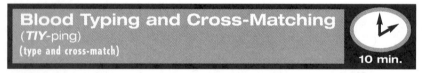

Blood Typing and Cross-Matching
(*TIY*-ping)
(type and cross-match)

10 min.

Type of Test: Blood

Body Systems and Functions: Hematological system

Normal Findings: Determination of correct blood type

Test Results Time Frame: Type and cross-match: 1 hr. Antibody screen: 2–4 hr.

Test Description: Blood typing and cross-matching involve determining the four major blood types (A, B, AB, and O). Red blood cells have A, B, AB, or no (O) surface antigens. These antigens are capable of producing antibodies. Genes determine the presence or absence of A or B antigens on chromosome 9. Red blood cells that are known as A have anti-B antibodies, while red cells B have anti-A antibodies, red cells A/B have neither antibodies and type O have both, making AB the universal recipient and O the universal donor. Most anti-A and anti-B antibodies reside in the IgM class of immunoglobulins, and some activity rests with IgG. Anti-A and anti-B antibodies are strong agglutinins causing rapid compliment-mediated destruction of incompatible cells. This clumping may plug small blood vessels and arterioles as well as accelerated red cell destruction and phagocytosis. With red cell hemolysis there is a release of free hemoglobin into the bloodstream, which can damage renal tubules and result in renal failure and death. ABO typing is an agglutination test where red cells are mixed with anti-A and anti-B serum (forward grouping). The procedure is then reversed, mixing the client's serum with A and B cell types (reverse grouping). Cross-matching detects antibodies in the serum of donors and recipients which may lead to transfusion reaction and destruction of red cells.

ABO blood type distribution

				Population distribution			
Blood group	Antigen	Antibodies	Compatible	White	Black	Native American	Asian
A	Anti-B	A, O	40	27	16	28	0
B	B	Anti-A	B, O	11	20	4	27
O	neither	Anti-A, Anti-B	O	45	49	79	40
A B	A and B	Neither A nor B	A, B, AB, O	4	4	1	5

CLINICAL ALERT:
Proper identification and labeling of the blood obtained from the client are crucial and need emphasis in clinical settings.

Consent Form: Not required

List of Equipment: Red-top tube or lavender-top tube or plasma separator tube; needle and syringe or vacutainer; alcohol swab; blood bank arm band; labeling material

Test Procedure:
1 Identify the client by name, social security number, and hospital number. *Correctly identifies the client and the test to be performed.*
2. Obtain a 25-mL blood sample and place 10 mL in red-top tube and 10 mL in lavender-top tube.
3. Label specimen with client's name, social security number, and hospital number and assign a blood bank number and place a blood bank wrist band on the client with the same information.
4. Do not agitate the tube. *Agitation may cause RBC hemolysis.*
5. Send tube to the laboratory.

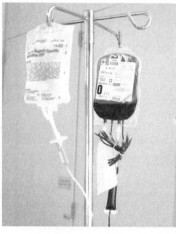

Blood Typing Equipment

Clinical Implications and Indications:

1. Identifies client's ABO type, especially prior to blood transfusion
2. Identifies donor (stored blood) ABO type
3. Determines compatibility of donor and recipient
4. Identifies maternal/infant ABO types to predict hemolytic disease in new-born
5. Determines the need for immunosuppressive therapy (RhoGAM) after pregnancy

Nursing Care:

Before Test: Explain the test procedure and the purpose of the test. Assess the client's knowledge of the test. Obtain a history of recent administration of dextran, blood or blood products, or IV contrast materials that may cause cellular aggregation resembling agglutination. Obtain history of previous blood transfusions and transfusion reactions. Obtain a history of pregnancies. Meticulously identify client by name, social security number, and hospital number and assure this information is labeled on specimen containers and client blood bank wrist band.

During Test: Adhere to standard precautions.

After Test: Apply pressure to venipuncture site. Explain that some bruising, discomfort, and swelling may appear at the site and that warm, moist compresses can alleviate this. Monitor for signs of infection. Inform client of blood type when known.

Potential Complications: Bleeding and bruising at venipuncture site

Interfering Factors: Previous administration of incompatible blood; hemolysis of specimen; type and cross-match not done in a timely fashion (must be done within 48 hr of blood draw); medications that alter results are dextran, blood or blood products, and IV contrast materials; hemodialysis; improper identification of client or blood specimen.

Nursing Considerations:
Pregnancy: *Blood typing is performed to identify mother's ABO type in the determination of Rh factor analysis.*
Pediatric: *Infants and children will need assistance in remaining still during the venipuncture and age-appropriate comfort measures following the test.*
International: *Important for travelers to know their blood type in the event of needing an emergency transfusion in the foreign country they are visiting.*

Listing of Related Tests: Rh type

║WEBLINKS 🖑   🗏🗵

www.ncbi.nlm.nih.gov; www.healthgate.com

Blood Urea Nitrogen
(yur-*REE*-uh *NIY*-troe-j:n)
(BUN)

5 min.

Type of Test: Blood

Body Systems and Functions: Renal/urological system

Normal Findings:

Newborn	4–18 mg/dL
Child	5–18 mg/dL
Adult	5–20 mg/dL
Elderly	8–21 mg/dL

CRITICAL VALUES:
>100 mg/dL

Test Results Time Frame: Within 24 hr

Test Description: The BUN test measures the nitrogen fraction of urea, the chief end product of protein metabolism. It is formed by the liver from ammonia and excreted by the kidney. BUN reflects protein intake, the liver's ability to metabolize, and the renal excretory ability. BUN exists in a normal ratio with serum creatinine and they often rise together in pathological conditions of the renal system. The BUN levels will rise first,however, which can allow interpretation of the timing of the renal disorder.

Consent Form: Not required

List of Equipment: *Adult:* red-top or serum separator tube; needle and syringe or vacutainer; alcohol swab. *Infant:* lancet; alcohol swab; glass pipette.

Test Procedure:
Adult:
1. Label the specimen tube. *Correctly identifies the client and the test to be performed.*
2. Obtain a 10-mL blood sample.

BLOOD

3. Do not agitate the tube. *Agitation may cause RBC hemolysis.*
4. Send tube to the laboratory.

Infant:
1. Use a lancet and pipette with infant sample.

Clinical Implications and indications:
See table on what causes BUN changes.

What causes BUN changes?

Increased BUN	Decreased BUN
Congestive heart failure	Hemodialysis
Shock	Inadequate protein intake
Hypovolemia (burns, starvation)	Severe liver disease
Renal disease	Water intoxication
Infection	Malabsorption syndrome
MI	Amyloidosis
Diabetes mellitus	Pregnancy
Excessive protein ingestion	Acromegaly
Neoplasms	
Addison's	
Gout	
Pancreatitis	
Tissue necrosis	
GI bleed	
Hyperalimentation	
Drugs:	Drugs:
allopurinol,	chloramphenicol,
aminoglycosides,	streptomycin,
cephalosporins,	IV dextrose
chloral hydrate,	
neoplastic drugs,	
ASA,	
thiazide diuretic,	
morphine,	
codeine,	
propranolol,	
nephrotoxic drugs.	
Long-term steroids	

Nursing Care:

Before Test: Explain the test procedure and the purpose of the test. Assess the client's knowledge of the test. Assess history of renal or liver disease. Assess dietary intake and hydration. Assess drug history and instruct client to fast for 8 hr prior to the test.

During Test: Adhere to standard precautions.

After Test: Apply pressure to venipuncture site. Explain that some bruising, discomfort, and swelling may appear at the site and that warm, moist compresses can alleviate this. Monitor for signs of infection.

Potential Complications: Bleeding and bruising at venipuncture site

Interfering Factors: Changes in protein intake; overhydration; dehydration; late-trimester pregnancy increases levels; medications that alter results are gentamycin, bactracin, and rifampin.

Nursing Considerations:
Pediatric: Infants and children will need assistance in remaining still during the venipuncture and age-appropriate comfort measures following the test.
Gerontology: Increased levels noted with aging

Listing of Related Tests: Creatinine

WEBLINKS

www.oaml.com; www.healthcentral.com; www.ncbi.nlm.nih.gov

Brucellosis Antibody
(*BRUE*-se-*LOE*-sis *AEN*-ti-*BAH*-dee)
(Bang's fever; Malta fever; undulant fever)

5 min.

Type of Test: Blood

Body Systems and Functions: Immunological system

Normal Findings: No brucellosis titers, reference values <1:80

Test Results Time Frame: Within 24–48 hr

Test Description: Brucellosis is a bacterial infection caused by gram-negative spore coccobacilli. Onset of symptomatology may occur in 5 days or as long as several weeks. Brucellosis is characterized by fever, sweating, weakness, aches, and pains and is transmitted to humans by direct contact with diseased animals or through ingestion of infected meat, milk, or cheese. Due to the long incubation period, serial titers must be drawn in order to rule out brucellosis.

CLINICAL ALERT:
Absence of agglutinins does not rule out brucellosis.

Consent Form: Not required

List of Equipment: Purple-top tube or serum separator tube; needle and syringe or vacutainer; alcohol swab

Test Procedure:
1. Label the specimen tube. *Correctly identifies the client and the test to be performed.*
2. Obtain a 10-mL blood sample.
3. Do not agitate the tube. *Agitation may cause RBC hemolysis.*
4. Send tube to the laboratory.

BLOOD

Clinical Implications and Indications:
1. Positive agglutinins are suggestive of disease.

Nursing Care:
Before Test: Explain the test procedure and the purpose of the test. Assess the client's knowledge of the test.

During Test: Adhere to standard precautions.

After Test: Apply pressure to venipuncture site. Explain that some swelling, bruising, or discomfort may occur at the site and warm, moist compresses can alleviate this. Monitor for signs of infection.

Potential Complications: Bleeding and bruising at venipuncture site

Nursing Considerations:
Pregnancy: Infants and children will need assistance in remaining still during the venipuncture and age-appropriate comfort measures following the test.

Rural: Veterinarians, farmers, and slaughterhouse workers are at higher risk for the disease.

International: Brucellosis is a widespread infectious disease that primarily affects cattle, swine, and goats. It is treated with tetracycline therapy, which may not be available in deprived countries.

WEBLINKS

www.aomc.org

Cadmium
(**KAED**-mee-:m)
(beta-2 microglobulin)

Blood: 5 min.
Urine: 24 hr.

Type of Test: Blood; urine

Body Systems and Functions: Renal/urological system

Normal Findings:
Blood:

Nonsmokers	0.4–1.2 µg/mL
Smokers	1.4–4.5 µg/mL
Urine	<1 µg/L

CRITICAL VALUES:
Urine: Irreversible renal damage may occur at levels >5 µg/g urinary creatinine.

Test Results Time Frame: Within 24–48 hr

Test Description: Cadmium is a heavy metal that is normally found in trace amounts in the human body. It is a soft bluish-white metal that is present in zinc ores. It is used industrially in electroplating and in atomic reactors. Its salts are poisonous. Cadmium anomalies may be seen with acute or chronic exposure from inhalation, dermal, ingestion, or smoking. Toxicity can lead to renal failure, pulmonary edema, interstitial pneumonia, or death. Levels can be measured from blood, urine, or hair follicles.

Consent Form: Not required

List of Equipment: *Blood:* dark-blue-top tube or plasma separator tube; needle and syringe or vacutainer; alcohol swab. *Urine:* 3-L metal-free urine collection container with toluene preservative; ice.

Test Procedure:

Blood:

1. Label the specimen tube. *Correctly identifies the client and the test to be performed.*
2. Obtain a 10-mL blood sample.
3. Gently invert tube several times, but do not agitate the tube. *Mixes the anticoagulant, but agitation may cause RBC hemolysis.*
4. Send tube to the laboratory.

Urine:

1. Label the collection container. *Correctly identifies the client and the test to be performed.*
2. Discard the first morning void. Then begin the time of the collection for the next 24 hr, including the void at the end of the 24 hr, and record the last voiding time. *An exact 24-hr count ensures accurate results.*
3. If the client has an indwelling catheter in place, keep the drainage bag on ice and empty the urine into the urine container periodically during the 24-hr period.
4. Keep urine cool during collection. *Higher temperatures alter the results.*
5. If any urine is lost, discard the entire specimen and begin collection again the next day.
6. Send a cumulative sample in a metal-free and preservative-free container. *Prevents contamination.*

Clinical Implications and Indications:

1. Elevated levels are found with industrial exposure to cadmium dust and fumes and ingestion of contaminated water or food stored in cadmium-coated containers.

Nursing Care:

Before Test: Explain the test procedure and the purpose of the test. Assess the client's knowledge of the test.

During Test: Adhere to standard precautions. If any urine is accidentally discarded or contaminated with feces, discard entire specimen and begin test again the following morning.

After Test: Blood: Apply pressure to venipuncture site. Explain that some swelling, bruising, or discomfort may occur at the site and warm, moist compresses can alleviate this. Monitor for signs of infection. Urine: Document urine quantity, date, and exact hours of collection on requisition.

Potential Complications: Bleeding and bruising at venipuncture site

Interfering Factors: Hypertension may elevate both blood and urine; prostatic and renal cancer may elevate urine levels; shellfish; urine contaminated with feces; spillage or inaccurate collection of the 24-hr specimen, including nonrefrigeration or placing on ice

Nursing Considerations:

Pediatric: *Blood: Infants and children will need assistance in remaining still during the venipuncture and age-appropriate comfort measures following the test. Urine: For collection of 24-hr specimen a collection bag or indwelling catheter needs to be used for infants and toddlers.*

WEBLINKS

www.healthgate.com

Calcitonin
(*KAEL*-suh-*TOE*-nin)
(CT; thyrocalcitonin)

5 min.

Type of Test: Blood

Body Systems and Functions: Endocrine system

Normal Findings:

Basal levels:	
Adults	<151 pg/mL
Infants (cord blood)	25–150 pg/mL
7-day-olds	77–293 pg/mL
Provocation levels:	
Males	<191 pg/mL
Females	<131 pg/mL

Test Results Time Frame: Within 24 hr

Test Description: Calcitonin is a hormone produced and secreted by C cells of the thyroid gland. Ectopic sites, such as the bladder, lungs, pituitary gland, and intestines, may also secrete calcitonin. Its action is opposite to that of parathyroid hormone, in that calcitonin increases deposition of calcium and phosphate in bone and lowers the level of calcium in the blood. A provocation test assesses for familial medullary cancer of the thyroid. Calcium chloride or pentagastrin is injected intravenously prior to the blood draw. Clients with medullary cancer will excrete elevated levels of calcitonin.

Consent Form: Not required

List of Equipment: Red-top tube or serum separator tube; needle and syringe or vacutainer; alcohol swab; calcium chloride or pentagastrin (provocation test)

Test Procedure:

1. Label the specimen tube. *Correctly identifies the client and the test to be performed.*
2. Obtain a 10-mL blood sample. If ordered, administer calcium chloride or pentagastrin per institution policy. Then obtain another 10-mL blood sample.
3. Do not agitate the tube. *Agitation may cause RBC hemolysis.*
4. Send tube to the laboratory.

Clinical Implications and Indications:

1. Elevated levels are found with alcoholic cirrhosis, thyroid cancer, chronic renal failure, pernicious anemia, cancer of the lung, breast, and pancreas, and subacute Hashimoto's thyroiditis.

Nursing Care:

Before Test: Explain the test procedure and the purpose of the test. Assess the client's knowledge of the test. Instruct client to fast for 8 hr prior to test (note: may drink water).

During Test: Adhere to standard precautions. Administer medication and monitor client.

After Test: Apply pressure to venipuncture site. Explain that some bruising, swelling, or discomfort may occur at site and that warm compresses can alleviate this. Monitor for signs of infection.

Potential Complications: Bleeding and bruising at venipuncture site

Interfering Factors: Failure to fast; term pregnancy

Nursing Considerations:

Pediatric: Infants and children will need assistance in remaining still during the venipuncture and age-appropriate comfort measures following the test.

WEBLINKS

http://www.medhlp.org

Calcium
(*KAEL*-see-:m)
(Ca^{2+}; total serum calcium)

5 min.

Type of Test: Blood

Body Systems and Functions: Endocrine system

Normal Findings: Adult: 8.5–10.5 mg/dL. Child: 8.8–10.8 mg/dL.

CRITICAL VALUES:
<7.0 or >12 mg/dL

Test Results Time Frame: Within 4 hr

Test Description: Calcium is the most abundant mineral in the body, of which over 90% is stored in the skeleton and the teeth. Calcium is essential in intra- and extracellular fluid exchange, blood clotting, maintaining a regular heartbeat, excitation of the skeletal muscles, conduction of neuromuscular impulses, and bone formation. Most of the body's calcium is stored in a usable form in the bones and teeth. The remaining calcium is found in the serum, 50% of which is ionized and available for use and the remaining 50% is bound to protein in an unusable form. Serum calcium levels include both ionized and protein-bound calcium since they cannot be measured independently. Calcium levels are largely controlled by the parathyroid gland and vitamin D.

CLINICAL ALERT:
Tourniquet use during blood draw may cause venous stasis and hemolysis, which will falsely elevate calcium levels.

Consent Form: Not required

List of Equipment: Red-top tube or serum separator tube; needle and syringe or vacutainer; alcohol swab

Test Procedure:
1. Label the specimen tube. *Correctly identifies the client and the test to be performed.*
2. Obtain a 5-mL blood sample.
3. Do not agitate the tube. *Agitation may cause RBC hemolysis.*
4. Send tube immediately to the laboratory. *Prolonged storage of specimen can falsely elevate levels.*

Clinical Implications and Indications:
1. Elevated levels (hypercalcemia) are found with hyperparathyroidism, metastatic cancer, multiple myeloma, vitamin D intoxication, overuse of calcium antacids, polycythemia vera, Paget's disease, dehydration, acidosis, and milk-alkali syndrome.
2. Decreased levels (hypocalcemia) are found with hypoparathyroidism, vitamin D deficiency, alcoholism, massive blood transfusions, acute pancreatitis, malnutrition, renal tubular disease, and alkalosis.
3. There are specific clinical manifestations to abnormal calcium levels that can be assessed (e.g., tetany, cardiac arrhythmias, carpopedal spasms).

Nursing Care:
Before Test: Explain the test procedure and the purpose of the test. Assess the client's knowledge of the test. Instruct client to fast for 8 hr prior to test (note: may drink water).
During Test: Adhere to standard precautions.
After Test: Apply pressure to venipuncture site. Explain that some swelling, bruising, or discomfort may occur at the site and warm, moist compresses can alleviate this. Monitor for signs of infection.

Potential Complications: Bleeding and bruising at venipuncture site

Interfering Factors: Calcium-containing antacids; medications which alter results: thiazides, diuretics, lithium, and anticonvulsants; increased or decreased serum protein levels; venous stasis or hemolysis

Nursing Considerations:
Pediatric: Infants and children will need assistance in remaining still during the venipuncture and age-appropriate comfort measures following the test. Calcium can be elevated during periods of bone growth.

WEBLINKS

www.sonic.net

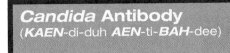

Candida Antibody
(*KAEN*-di-duh *AEN*-ti-*BAH*-dee)

5 min.

BLOOD

Type of Test: Blood

Body Systems and Functions: Immunological system

Normal Findings: Negative for *Candida*, although, this test may result in positive results in up to 25% of the normal population.

CRITICAL VALUES:
A titer >1:8 in latex agglutination is indicative of systemic infection.

Test Results Time Frame: Within 24–48 hr

Test Description: Candidiasis is usually caused by *Candida albicans*; commonly it affects the nails, mucous membranes, and skin. However, when present in the blood, this fungal infection can lead to life-threatening systemic infections. Higher risk is found with people on antibiotics, corticosteroid therapy, immunological disorders, pregnancy, diabetes, obesity, or debilitating chronic illness. When diagnosis of candidiasis cannot be made by culture or histological studies, then identification of the antibody in serum may be used.

CLINICAL ALERT:
Do not draw blood from area of skin infected with fungal infection.

Consent Form: Not required

List of Equipment: Red-top tube or serum separator tube; needle and syringe or vacutainer; alcohol swab

Test Procedure:
1. Label the specimen tube. *Correctly identifies the client and the test to be performed.*
2. Obtain a 10-mL blood sample.
3. Do not agitate the tube. *Agitation may cause RBC hemolysis.*
4. Send tube to the laboratory.

Clinical Implications and Indications:
1. Diagnoses systemic candidiasis when clinical symptoms are present

Nursing Care:
Before Test: Explain the test procedure and the purpose of the test. Assess the client's knowledge of the test.
During Test: Adhere to standard precautions.
After Test: Apply pressure to venipuncture site. Explain that some swelling, bruising, or discomfort may occur at the site and warm, moist compresses can alleviate this. Monitor for signs of infection.

Potential Complications: Bleeding and bruising at venipuncture site

Interfering Factors: Antimicrobial therapy; immunosuppression

Nursing Considerations:

Pregnancy: Vulvovaginal candidiasis, which is common in late pregnancy, can be transmitted to the infant via the birth canal.

Pediatric: Infants and children will need assistance in remaining still during the venipuncture and age-appropriate comfort measures following the test. Oral candidiasis is common and benign in children.

International: Oral candidiasis in adults may be the first sign of acquired immunodeficiency syndrome in countries where medicinal therapies are not routine.

WEBLINKS

www.thebody.com

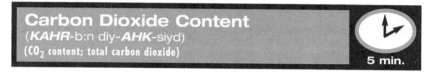

Carbon Dioxide Content
(*KAHR*-b:n diy-*AHK*-siyd)
(CO₂ content; total carbon dioxide)

5 min.

Type of Test: Blood

Body Systems and Functions: Metabolic system

Normal Findings:

Venous:

Infant–2 years old	18–29 mEq/L
2 years old–adult	22–26 mEq/L

Arterial:

2 years old–adult	23–29 mEq/L

CRITICAL VALUES:
Levels of <15 and >50 mEq/L are life threatening and mandate close monitoring.

Test Results Time Frame: Within 4 hr

Test Description: Carbon dioxide content in normal blood plasma is derived primarily (up to 95%) from bicarbonate (HCO_3), which is regulated by the kidneys. The remaining portion is from the dissolved CO_2 gas and carbonic acid (H_2CO_3), which is regulated by the respiratory system. Total CO_2 reflects the adequacy of gas exchange in the lungs and the efficiency of the acid-bicarbonate buffer system.

CLINICAL ALERT:
Blood sample may be obtained from artery or arterial line. Completely fill the tube to prevent CO_2 from diffusing out of the stopper.

Consent Form: Not required

List of Equipment: Red-top tube or serum separator tube; needle and syringe or vacutainer; alcohol swab

BLOOD

Test Procedure:
1. Label the specimen tube. *Correctly identifies the client and the test to be performed.*
2. Obtain a 10-mL blood sample.
3. Do not agitate the tube. *Agitation may cause RBC hemolysis.*
4. Send tube to the laboratory.

Clinical Implications and Indications:
1. Elevated levels are found with metabolic acidosis, respiratory acidosis, primary aldosteronism, congestive heart failure, cystic fibrosis, hypokalemia, Cushing's syndrome, and excessive vomiting.
2. Decreased levels are found with respiratory alkalosis, hyperventilation, diabetes mellitus, severe diarrhea, metabolic acidosis, dehydration, renal failure, and hypovolemia.

Nursing Care:
Before Test: Explain the test procedure and the purpose of the test. Assess the client's knowledge of the test.
During Test: Adhere to standard precautions.
After Test: Apply pressure to venipuncture site. Explain that some swelling, bruising, or discomfort may occur at the site and warm, moist compresses can alleviate this. Monitor for signs of infection. If arterial blood draw, hold direct pressure for 5 min.

Potential Complications: Bleeding and bruising at venipuncture site

Interfering Factors: Many medications increase or decrease CO_2 levels.

Nursing Considerations:
Pediatric: Infants and children will need assistance in remaining still during the venipuncture and age-appropriate comfort measures following the test.

Listing of Related Tests: Blood pH; arterial blood gases (ABGs)

WEBLINKS ⯈	

www.ocnow.com

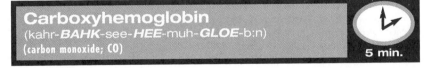

Carboxyhemoglobin
(kahr-*BAHK*-see-*HEE*-muh-*GLOE*-b:n)
(carbon monoxide; CO)

5 min.

Type of Test: Blood

Body Systems and Functions: Hematological system

Normal Findings: Nonsmoker: <2.4% of total hemoglobin. Smoker: <5.1% of total hemoglobin.

> **CRITICAL VALUES:**
> >20% total hemoglobin

BLOOD

Test Results Time Frame: Within 1–4 hr

Test Description: Carboxyhemoglobin is formed when hemoglobin and carbon monoxide are joined. Carbon monoxide affinity for hemoglobin is 218 times greater than that of oxygen. Carbon monoxide poisoning leads to anoxia since oxygen is not allowed to bind with hemoglobin. The extent of carbon monoxide poisoning is dependent upon length of exposure, age of the victim, and concentration of exposure. Symptoms may range from flulike symptoms to coma and death.

Consent Form: Not required

List of Equipment: Green-top tube or serum separator tube; needle and syringe or vacutainer; alcohol swab; ice

Test Procedure:
1. Label the specimen tube. *Correctly identifies the client and the test to be performed.*
2. Obtain a 5-mL blood sample.
3. Do not agitate the tube. *Agitation may cause RBC hemolysis.*
4. Send tube to the laboratory.
5. Keep specimen on ice. *High temperatures alter the results.*

Clinical Implications and Indications:
1. Diagnoses carbon monoxide poisoning
2. Evaluates smoke inhalation

Nursing Care:
Before Test: Explain the test procedure and the purpose of the test. Assess the client's knowledge of the test. Assess if client is a smoker.
During Test: Adhere to standard precautions.
After Test: Apply pressure to venipuncture site. Explain that some bruising, discomfort, and swelling may appear at the site and that warm, moist compresses can alleviate this. Monitor for signs of infection.

Potential Complications: Bleeding and bruising at venipuncture site

Interfering Factors: Smoking

Nursing Considerations:
Pediatric: Infants and children will need assistance in remaining still during the venipuncture and age-appropriate comfort measures following the test.
Gerontology: Carbon monoxide poisoning is potentially more life threatening in the elderly due to the higher incidence of COPD and smoking.
Rural: Exposure may occur from camp stoves or lanterns burning in tents or poorly ventilated cabins.

WEBLINKS

www.kidde.com

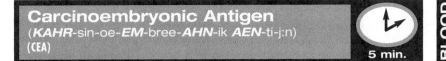

Carcinoembryonic Antigen
(*KAHR*-sin-oe-*EM*-bree-*AHN*-ik *AEN*-ti-j:n)
(CEA)

5 min.

BLOOD

Type of Test: Blood

Body Systems and Functions: Oncology system

Normal Findings: Nonsmoker: <2.5 ng/mL. Smoker: <5 ng/mL.

CRITICAL VALUES:
>6 ng/mL

Test Results Time Frame: Within 24–48 hr

Test Description: Carcinoembryonic antigen tests for the normal production of CEA that occurs in fetal development and has stopped by birth. In the presence of particular types of cancer, especially colorectal, elevated CEA levels are found. Six weeks after chemotherapy or surgical removal of the tumor, detectable CEA levels should return to the minute amount normally found in the serum. Serial blood draws are performed in order to monitor for the recurrence of the malignancy. In an individual with a previous history of colorectal cancer, serial blood draws documenting a rise in CEA have allowed detection of the recurrence before any signs or symptoms recurred. Since other factors and cancers may elevate CEA levels, it is not useful as a screening tool for colorectal cancer.

CLINICAL ALERT:
An increase in test values necessitates further diagnostic testing.

Consent Form: Not required

List of Equipment: Red-top tube or serum separator tube; needle and syringe or vacutainer; alcohol swab; ice

Test Procedure:
1. Label the specimen tube. *Correctly identifies the client and the test to be performed.*
2. Obtain a 10-mL blood sample.
3. Do not agitate the tube. *Agitation may cause RBC hemolysis.*
4. Keep specimen on ice. *High temperatures alter the results.*
5. Send tube to the laboratory.

Clinical Implications and Indications:
1. Elevated levels are found with cancer, colitis, pancreatitis, cirrhosis, peptic ulcerations, cholecystitis, and diverticulitis.
2. Monitors the effectiveness of cancer therapy.
3. Monitors for recurrence of colorectal cancer.
4. Identifies the preoperative staging of colorectal cancer.

Nursing Care:
Before Test: Explain the test procedure and the purpose of the test. Assess the client's knowledge of the test. Explain serial tests will be performed to monitor levels. Instruct the client to not smoke 24 hr prior to test.

During Test: Adhere to standard precautions.

After Test: Apply pressure to venipuncture site. Explain that some bruising, discomfort, and swelling may appear at the site and that warm, moist compresses can alleviate this. Monitor for signs of infection.

Potential Complications: Bleeding and bruising at venipuncture site

Interfering Factors: Chronic cigarette smoking; recent admission of radioisotopes; heparin; biliary obstruction

Nursing Considerations:
Pediatric: Infants and children will need assistance in remaining still during the venipuncture and age-appropriate comfort measures following the test.
Gerontology: May see elevated levels in the elderly, due to the types of causative agents and diseases of CEA.

WEBLINKS ▦ ⊠

www.thriveonline.com

Cardiac Isoenzyme
(*KAHR*-dee-aek *IY*-soe-*EN*-ziym)
(CK; LD; ALT; AST; troponin-cardiac; TNc)

5 min.

Type of Test: Blood

Body Systems and Functions: Cardiovascular system

Normal Findings:
Creatine kinase-MB (CKMB): < 7.1 U/L
Lactate dehydrogenase LDH_1 and LDH_2:
LDH_1 14%–26% of total LD level
LDH_2 29%–39% of total LD level

Test Results Time Frame: Within 45 min

Test Description: Cardiac isoenzymes are those enzymes that are specifically released from the cardiac muscle. In general, enzymes are found in all body tissues and catalyze the thousands of chemical reactions that occur in the body. Enzymes are released when tissue cells are damaged and can be detected and measured in the serum. Tissues may contain and release more than one enzyme. Some enzymes occur in more than one form, which have differing molecular details. These are called isoenzymes and are specific to a certain organ. Elevated isoenzyme levels are indicative of tissue damage to the organ to which the isoenzyme is specific. Creatine kinase has a cardiac-specific isoenzyme, CK-MB. Lactate dehydrogenase has two cardiac-specific isoenzymes LDH_1 and LDH_2. It may be necessary to obtain serial timed draws in order to monitor for changing levels of the isoenzymes.

BLOOD

CLINICAL ALERT:
CK-MB levels rise 4–8 hr after an infarction peak at 12–24 hr, and may remain elevated up to 72 hr post-infarction. LDH_1 and LDH2 peak later than CK-MB at 12–48 hr after infarction, peak in 2–5 days, and return to normal 7–10 days after infarction. CK-MB will be a greater diagnostic tool early after an infarction, whereas LDH will be a tool used later, after signs and symptoms have occurred.

Consent Form: Not required

List of Equipment: Red-top tube or serum separator tube; needle and syringe or vacutainer; alcohol swab

Test Procedure:
1. Label the specimen tube. *Correctly identifies the client and the test to be performed.*
2. Obtain a 5-mL blood sample.
3. Do not agitate the tube. *Agitation may cause RBC hemolysis.*
4. Send tube to the laboratory.

Clinical Implications and Indications:
1. CK-MB: detects, diagnoses, and monitors acute myocardial infarctions
2. LDH_1 and LDH2: supports CK-MB test results in diagnosing myocardial infarctions; aids in differential diagnosis of myocardial infarction, pulmonary infarcts, hepatic disease, and anemias

Nursing Care:
Before Test: Explain the test procedure and the purpose of the test. Assess the client's knowledge of the test. Inform client that repeat blood draws may be done.
During Test: Adhere to standard precautions.
After Test: Apply pressure to venipuncture site. Explain that some swelling, bruising, or discomfort may occur at the site and warm, moist compresses can alleviate this. Monitor for signs of infection.

Potential Complications: Bleeding and bruising at venipuncture site

Interfering Factors: Failure to draw sample at ordered time; failure to send sample to laboratory immediately

Nursing Considerations:
Pediatric: Infants and children will need assistance in remaining still during the venipuncture and age-appropriate comfort measures following the test.
Gerontology: There is a higher risk of cardiovascular disease for the elderly, due to the increasing predisposition to cardiac risk factors with aging.
Home Care: Health care providers must be aware of potential symptomatology of angina or myocardial infarctions and seek more definitive levels of health care evaluation in the event of continuing clinical manifestations.

Listing of Related Tests: Troponin

WEBLINKS

http://www.unr.edu/medlib

BLOOD

Catecholamines
(**KAET**-uh-**KOEL**-uh-meenz)
(catecholamine fractionalization; plasma)

5 min.

Type of Test: Blood

Body Systems and Functions: Renal/urological system

Normal Findings:

Norepinephrine	500 ng/L
Epinephrine	100 ng/L
Total catecholamines	1000 ng/L (excludes the diagnosis of pheochromocytoma)

Test Results Time Frame: Within 24–48 hr

Test Description: Catecholamine testing measures epinephrine, norepinephrine, and dopamine, which are neurotransmitters found in the adrenal
medulla, neurons, and the brain. Epinephrine acts during the fight-or-flight
response and increases the heart rate, dilates the bronchioles, and decreases
peripheral blood flow. Norepinephrine is secreted by the adrenal medulla and
increases blood pressure, dilates the pupils, and relaxes the GI system.
Dopamine acts to dilate renal arteries, increase the heart rate, and constrict the
peripheral vasculature. The serum catecholamine test measures norepinephrine
and epinephrine in the plasma.

Consent Form: Not required

List of Equipment: Green-top tube or serum separator tube; needle and
syringe or vacutainer; venipuncture equipment; alcohol swab; ice

Test Procedure:
1. Label the specimen tube. *Correctly identifies the client and the test to be performed.*
2. Obtain a 10-mL blood sample from IV lock. *Venipuncture procedure alone
   may cause anxiety, which may elevate catecholamines.*
3. Gently invert tube several times, but do not agitate the tube. *Mixes the anticoagulant, but agitation may cause RBC hemolysis.*
4. Send tube to the laboratory.
5. Keep specimen cool. *High temperatures alter the results.*

Clinical Implications and Indications:
1. Elevated catecholamine levels are found with pheochromocytoma. (Note: In
   borderline results, clonidine may be administered. Clonidine is an alpha-
   adrenergic agonist, which suppresses catecholamine release in normal clients
   but not in those with a secreting pheochromocytoma.)
2. Elevated plasma epinephrine levels occur exclusively in pheochromocytomas
   located in the adrenal medulla. Generally total catecholamine results >2000
   ng/L are seen only in pheochromocytoma. (Note: If the diagnosis of
   pheochromocytoma has already been made by elevated urinary catecholamines, follow-up measurement of serum catecholamines may be done
   to localize the tumor.)

Nursing Care:

Before Test: Explain the test procedure and the purpose of the test. Assess the client's knowledge of the test. Insert IV lock at least 30 min before sample of venous blood is taken. Ensure the client avoids exercise, emotional stress, smoking, and standing upright before and during the test. Ensure the client is not volume depleted. Ensure the client remains in a recumbent position and in a calm and quiet environment during the time from insertion of the IV lock to specimen collection.

During Test: Adhere to standard precautions.

After Test: Apply pressure to venipuncture site. Explain that some bruising, discomfort, and swelling may appear at the site and that warm, moist compresses can alleviate this. Monitor for signs of infection. Transport specimen to laboratory as soon as possible in a container with ice.

Potential Complications: Bleeding and bruising at venipuncture site

Interfering Factors: Emotional stress; exercise; smoking; dehydration; false-positive or false-negative results may occur if catecholamine secretion is erratic; cardiovascular system medications

Nursing Considerations:

Pediatric: In young children, plasma catecholamines are higher and more variable, thus obscuring the diagnosis between normal and pathological catecholamine secretion. Infants and children will need assistance in remaining still during the venipuncture and age-appropriate comfort measures following the test.

Listing of Related Tests: Urine catecholamine; chromogranin A plasma assay

WEBLINKS

http://www.kumc.edu

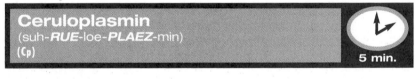

Ceruloplasmin
(suh-*RUE*-loe-*PLAEZ*-min)
(Cp)

5 min.

Type of Test: Blood

Body Systems and Functions: Hematological system

Normal Findings:

Adults	23–43 mg/dL
Newborns	2–13 mg/dL

Test Results Time Frame: Within 24 hr

Test Description: Ceruloplasmin is an alpha-2 globulin that binds and transports copper. Ceruloplasmin is decreased in Wilson's disease, thus allowing for high unbound levels of copper. This hereditary condition is characterized by degenerative changes in the liver and brain due to excessive deposition of copper. Clients with Wilson's disease have a persistently positive copper balance in spite of increased renal secretion.

Consent Form: Not required

List of Equipment: Red-top tube, yellow-top tube, or serum separator tube; needle and syringe or vacutainer; alcohol swab

Test Procedure:
1. Label the specimen tube. *Correctly identifies the client and the test to be performed.*
2. Obtain a 2-mL blood sample.
3. Do not agitate the tube. *Agitation may cause RBC hemolysis.*
4. Send tube to the laboratory.
5. Keep specimen cool. *High temperatures alter the results.*

Clinical Implications and Indications:
1. Elevated levels of ceruloplasmin are found with pregnancy, lymphomas, acute and chronic infections, rheumatoid arthritis, biliary cirrhosis, thyrotoxicosis, and copper intoxication.
2. Decreased levels of ceruloplasmin are found with Wilson's disease, nephrotic syndrome, protein malabsorption syndrome (sprue), protein malnutrition (kwashiorkor), Menkes syndrome, and hyperalimentation.

Nursing Care:
Before Test: Explain the test procedure and the purpose of the test. Assess the client's knowledge of the test.
During Test: Adhere to standard precautions.
After Test: Apply pressure to venipuncture site. Explain that some bruising , discomfort, and swelling may appear at the site and that warm, moist compresses can alleviate this. Monitor for signs of infection. Provide genetic counseling if Wilson's disease is diagnosed.

Potential Complications: Bleeding and bruising at venipuncture site

Interfering Factors: Pregnancy; oral contraceptives; medications that increase levels are estrogen, tamoxifen, methasone, and phenytoin.

Nursing Considerations:
Pregnancy: Serum ceruloplasmin levels are twice as high during parturition as those found in nonpregnant women.
Pediatric: Infants and children will need assistance in remaining still during the venipuncture and age-appropriate comfort measures following the test.

Listing of Related Tests: Copper

WEBLINKS	⊟ ☒

http://www.methodisthealth.com

Chloride
(**KLOER**-iyd)
(Cl)

5 min.

BLOOD

Type of Test: Blood

Body Systems and Functions: Renal/urological system

Normal Findings: 98–106 mmol/L

CRITICAL VALUES:
<70 or >120 mmol/L

Test Results Time Frame: Within 24 hr

Test Description: Chloride is the major extracellular anion and exists mainly in combination as sodium chloride or hydrochloric acid. Changes in serum chloride levels reflect changes in other electrolytes or acid-base balance. Chloride, in combination with sodium, maintains osmolality and water balance and is instrumental in maintaining acid-base balance. High levels of chloride in the extracellular fluid are labeled hyperchloremia. Low levels of chloride in the extracellular fluid are labeled hypochloremia.

CLINICAL ALERT:
Daily weight, fluid intake, and fluid output should be recorded in clients with abnormal electrolytes. These bodily measurements are extremely important in their reflection of the homeostatic condition of the client.

Consent Form: Not required

List of Equipment: Green-top tube or serum separator tube; needle and syringe or vacutainer; alcohol swab

Test Procedure:
1. Label the specimen tube. *Correctly identifies the client and the test to be performed.*
2. Obtain a 5-mL blood sample.
3. Gently invert tube several times, but do not agitate the tube. *Mixes the anticoagulant, but agitation may cause RBC hemolysis.*
4. Send tube to the laboratory.
5. Keep specimen cool. *High temperatures alter the results.*

Clinical Implications and Indications:
1. Decreased (hypochloremia) levels are found with loss of gastric contents due to vomiting or suction, prolonged diarrhea, excessive use of potassium-wasting diuretics, excessive sweating such as from fever or heat exhaustion, diabetic ketoacidosis, Addison's disease, acute infection, and prolonged infusion of IV dextrose solutions causing a dilutional effect.
2. The clinical manifestations of hypochloremia are hyperirritability, tetany, or muscular excitability; slowed respirations; and hypotension secondary to fluid loss.
3. Elevated levels (hyperchloremia) are found with losses of bicarbonate from the lower gastrointestinal tract in diarrhea, renal tubular acidosis,

mineralocorticoid deficiency, hyperparathyroidism, and excess administration of amino acids during hyperalimentation.

4. The clinical manifestations of hyperchloremia are weakness, lethargy, unconsciousness (a late sign), and Kussmaul respirations.

Nursing Care:

Before Test: Explain the test procedure and the purpose of the test. Assess the client's knowledge of the test.

During Test: Adhere to standard precautions.

After Test: Apply pressure to venipuncture site. Explain that some bruising, discomfort, and swelling may appear at the site and that warm, moist compresses can alleviate this. Monitor for signs of infection.

Potential Complications: Bleeding and bruising at venipuncture site

Nursing Considerations:

Pediatric: Infants usually have a higher concentration of chloride as compared to children and adults. Infants and children will need assistance in remaining still during the venipuncture and age-appropriate comfort measures following the test.

WEBLINKS

http://www.kumc.edu

Cholesterol
(koe-*LES*-t:r-ahl)
(serum lipoproteins)

5 min.

Type of Test: Blood

Body Systems and Functions: Cardiovascular system

Normal Findings:

Cholesterol:

Adult/elderly	150–200 mg/dL
Child	120–200 mg/dL
Infant	70–175 mg/dL
Newborn	53–135 mg/dl

Cholesterol lipoprotein—high-density lipoprotein (HDL):

Males	>45 mg/dL
Females	>55 mg/dL

Very low density lipoprotein (VLDL): 25%–50%

Low-density lipoprotein (LDL): 60–180 mg/dL

LDL= total cholesterol - (HDL - triglycerides/5)

Test Results Time Frame: Within 15 min

Test Description: Cholesterol is found in animal fat and is a component of cell membranes, bile acids, adrenal steroids, and hormones. Cholesterol testing is most frequently done as a screening tool for atherosclerotic coronary disease and is also a component of thyroid and liver function studies. Cholesterol lipids are combined with proteins when transported in the blood and are termed lipoproteins. HDL is mainly composed of protein. VLDL is mainly composed of triglycerides. LDL is primarily made up of cholesterol. HDL removes cholesterol and is inversely associated with coronary artery disease (CAD). High levels of HDL are associated with a decreased risk of myocardial infarction. The HDL/total cholesterol ratio should be at least 1:5. High levels of LDL have a strong association with CAD. Health care providers provide dietary and drug treatments based upon levels of LDL cholesterol levels and risk status.

Consent Form: Not required

List of Equipment: Yellow-top tube or red-top tube or serum separator tube; needle and syringe or vacutainer; alcohol swab

Test Procedure:
1. Label the specimen tube. *Correctly identifies the client and the test to be performed.*
2. Obtain a 5-mL blood sample.
3. Do not agitate the tube. *Agitation may cause RBC hemolysis.*
4. Send tube to the laboratory.

Clinical Implications and Indications:
1. Elevated levels (hypercholesterolemia) are found with type II family hypercholesterolemia, hyperlipoproteinemia, hepatocellular disease, biliary cirrhosis, cholestasis, nephrotic syndrome, glomerulonephritis, chronic renal failure, hypothyroidism, diabetes mellitus, alcoholism, obesity, and a diet high in cholesterol and fats.
2. Decreased levels (hypocholesterolemia) are found with alpha-hypoprotein deficiency, hepatocellular disease, malignant liver neoplasms, hyperthyroidism, malabsorption syndrome, malnutrition, megaloblastic anemia, severe burns, and chronic obstructive pulmonary disease.

Nursing Care:
Before Test: Explain the test procedure and the purpose of the test. Assess the client's knowledge of the test. Ensure that client is NPO for 12 hr before the test.
During Test: Adhere to standard precautions.
After Test: Apply pressure to venipuncture site. Explain that some bruising, discomfort, and swelling may appear at the site and that warm, moist compresses can alleviate this. Monitor for signs of infection. Interpret the test results and provide appropriate education regarding CAD risk factors and lifestyle changes necessary to decrease elevated levels of total cholesterol and LDL. Provide referral to dietitian as necessary. Provide educational materials from the American Heart Association and National Cholesterol Education Programs. If cholesterol testing is done in a public screening program, refer client to his health care provider for further evaluation if abnormal results are obtained. Provide education on lipid-lowering drugs if prescribed.

Potential Complications: Bleeding and bruising at venipuncture site

BLOOD

Nursing Considerations:

Pediatric: Infants and children will need assistance in remaining still during the venipuncture and age-appropriate comfort measures following the test.
Gerontology: Elderly populations are more at risk for cardiovascular complications of cholesterol abnormalities.

National Cholesterol Education Program: Adult Treatment Panel II dietary and drug treatment decisions based on LDL cholesterol levels and risk status

Risk status	Dietary treatment initiation level	Drug treatment initiation level
Without CHD; <2 risk factors	160 mg/dL	>190 mg/dL*
Without CHD; 2 risk factors	130 mg/dL	160 mg/dL
With CHD	>100 mg/dL	130 mg/dL†

*In men <35 years and premenopausal women with LDL cholesterol levels 190–219 mg/dL, drug therapy should be delayed except in high-risk patients.
†In CHD patients with LDL cholesterol levels of 100–129 mg/dL. The health care provider should exercise clinical judgment regarding drug treatment initiation.

Listing of Related Tests: Triglycerides; homocysteine

| WEBLINKS |

www.acc.org

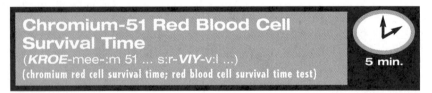

Chromium-51 Red Blood Cell Survival Time
(*KROE*-mee-:m 51 ... s:r-*VIY*-v:l ...)
(chromium red cell survival time; red blood cell survival time test)

5 min.

Type of Test: Blood

Body Systems and Functions: Hematological system

Normal Findings: Normal half survival time of chromium-51 (Cr-51) labeled red blood cells is about 25–32 days.

Test Results Time Frame: Within 3–6 weeks

Test Description: Cr-51 is a radionuclide that binds to the hemoglobin molecule. Cr-51 is injected into a sample of the client's blood and then reinjected intravenously. Cr-51 is not released until the red blood cell is removed from the circulation and the hemoglobin is degraded. Therefore the disappearance of radioactive Cr-51 corresponds to the disappearance of red blood cells. Chromated red blood cells are measured by counting blood, which is sampled at periodic intervals, and an index of the intravascular life span of red blood cells is determined. External scanning may also be done to detect sites of red blood cell destruction, such as in the spleen.

CLINICAL ALERT:
Blood transfusions should not be given during the testing time period.

Consent Form: Required

List of Equipment: Three green-top tubes or plasma separator tube; needle and syringe or vacutainer; alcohol swab

Test Procedure:
1. Label the specimen tubes. *Correctly identifies the client and the test to be performed.*
2. Obtain a 20-mL blood sample for each tube.
3. Inject Cr-51 into the blood sample and then reinject intravenously into the client.
4. Obtain blood samples from the client at 2 or 24 hr and at 1- to 3-day intervals for 10–14 days until more than 50% of the radioactivity in red cells has disappeared.
5. Gently invert tube several times, but do not agitate the tube. *Mixes the anticoagulant, but agitation may cause RBC hemolysis.*
6. Send tubes to the laboratory.

Clinical Implications and Indications:
1. Decreased times are found with chronic granulocytic leukemia, hemolytic anemia, hemoglobin C disease, hereditary spherocytosis, pernicious anemia, megaloblastic anemia of pregnancy, and sickle cell anemia.
2. Increased times are found with thalassemia minor.

Nursing Care:
Before Test: Explain the test procedure and the purpose of the test. Assess the client's knowledge of the test.
During Test: Adhere to standard precautions.
After Test: Apply pressure to venipuncture site. Explain that some bruising, discomfort, and swelling may appear at the site and that warm, moist compresses can alleviate this. Monitor for signs of infection.

Potential Complications: Bleeding and bruising at venipuncture site

Contraindications: Active bleeding

Interfering Factors: Blood loss; change in hematocrit; recent blood transfusions

Nursing Considerations:
Pediatric: Infants and children will need assistance in remaining still during the venipuncture and age-appropriate comfort measures following the test.

WEBLINKS

www.nlm.nih.gov

Chromosome Analysis
(*KROE*-muh-*SOEM* uh-*NAEL*-uh-sis)
(chromosome karyotype)

5 min.

Type of Test: Blood

Body Systems and Functions: Reproductive system

Normal Findings:

Female	44 autosomes + 2 X chromosomes	karyotype: 46, XX
Male	44 autosomes + 1 X, 1 Y chromosome	karyotype: 46, XY

A normal karyotype has 22 pairs of sex chromosomes and a pair of sex chromosomes consisting of XY for males and XX for females.

Test Results Time Frame: Preparation of cells takes a minimum of 3 days (note: some laboratories may not be equipped to perform this test, which may delay test results time frame).

Test Description: Chromosome analysis examines the leukocytes from venous blood samples because these are most easily obtained. Samples for chromosome testing may also be obtained from numerous sources: bone marrow, skin, surgical specimens, amniotic fluid, products of conception, and other tissues. Chromosome testing involves karyotyping, which is the arrangement and pairing of cell chromosomes in order of the largest to the smallest. Analysis of the chromosome structure and number is also performed. Special chromosome studies include the analysis for fragile X syndrome, one of the most common genetic causes of mental retardation. Cells undergoing evaluation for fragile X chromosome must be grown in a special medium, as the usual karyotype will not detect this abnormality.

Consent Form: Required

List of Equipment: Brown-top tube or green-top tube or plasma separator tube; needle and syringe or vacutainer; alcohol swab

Test Procedure:
1. Label the specimen tube. *Correctly identifies the client and the test to be performed.*
2. Obtain a 5-mL blood sample.
3. Gently invert tube several times, but do not agitate the tube. *Mixes the anticoagulant, but agitation may cause RBC hemolysis..*
4. Send tube to the laboratory.

Clinical Implications and Indications:
1. Diagnoses mental retardation, Down's syndrome, Turner's syndrome, Klinefelter's syndrome, cat-cry syndrome, Prader-Willi syndrome, sickle cell anemia, and chronic myelogenous leukemia
2. Evaluates translocations of chromosomes and Tay-Sachs disease

Nursing Care:
Before Test: Explain the test procedure and the purpose of the test. Assess the client's knowledge of the test. Ensure the client has received genetic counseling

from a health care professional. Provide emotional support as this test is associated with anxiety concerning test results.

During Test: Adhere to standard precautions.

After Test: Apply pressure to venipuncture site. Explain that some bruising, discomfort, and swelling may appear at the site and that warm, moist compresses can alleviate this. Monitor for signs of infection. Inform client when results will be ready. Ensure follow-up appointment with heath care provider for discussion of results and further genetic counseling.

Potential Complications: Bleeding and bruising at venipuncture site

Nursing Considerations:

Pregnancy: Special emphasis is needed for the emotional support and counseling of the pregnant client on whom this test is performed.

Pediatric: Infants and children will need assistance in remaining still during the venipuncture and age-appropriate comfort measures following the test. The majority of abnormalities involve infants and children (as delineated in Clinical Implications and Indications).

Listing of Related Tests: Chorionic villus biopsy

WEBLINKS	▤ ▣

http://www.ncbi.nlm.nih.gov/entrez/query.fcgi

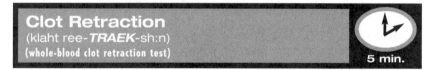

Clot Retraction
(klaht ree-*TRAEK*-sh:n)
(whole-blood clot retraction test)

5 min.

Type of Test: Blood

Body Systems and Functions: Hematological system

Normal Findings: Normal clot retraction is nearly complete in 4 hr and fully completed within 24 hr. Normal and complete clot retraction has approximately half the total volume consisting of clot and the other half consisting of serum.

Test Results Time Frame: Within 24 hr

Test Description: The clot retraction test is a measurement of the platelets' ability of contraction or retraction. Blood is allowed to clot in a tube that does not contain anticoagulant. Whole blood normally retracts from the sides of the tube and there is a subsequent separation of the contracted clot and serum. Retraction is impaired when platelets are decreased or abnormal. The fibrinogen content of plasma, ratio of plasma volume to red cell mass, and activity of a retraction-promoting principle in the serum all influence the results of the clot retraction test. An abnormal clot is soft, soggy, and easily torn. Another characteristic of an abnormal clot is that after removal from the tube it flattens out as a shapeless mass and serum continues to ooze from the clot.

Consent Form: Not required

BLOOD

List of Equipment: Red-top tube or serum separator tube; needle and syringe or vacutainer; alcohol swab

Test Procedure:
1. Label the specimen tube. *Correctly identifies the client and the test to be performed.*
2. Obtain a 5-mL blood sample.
3. Do not agitate the tube. *Agitation may cause RBC hemolysis.*
4. Send tube to the laboratory.

Clinical Implications and Indications:
1. Delayed times are found with thrombocytopenia, Glanzmann's thrombasthenia, and von Willebrand's disease.
2. Increased times are found with severe anemia and hypofibrinogenemia.

Nursing Care:
Before Test: Explain the test procedure and the purpose of the test. Assess the client's knowledge of the test.
During Test: Adhere to standard precautions.
After Test: Apply pressure to venipuncture site. Explain that some bruising, discomfort, and swelling may appear at the site and that warm, moist compresses can alleviate this. Monitor for signs of infection.

Potential Complications: Bleeding and bruising at venipuncture site

Interfering Factors: High hematocrit will cause decreased clot retraction; increased fibrinolysis will cause lysis of the clot in 10–30 min.

Nursing Considerations:
Pediatric: Infants and children will need assistance in remaining still during the venipuncture and age-appropriate comfort measures following the test.

Listing of Related Tests: Platelet count

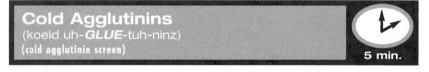

| WEBLINKS |

www.nlm.nih.gov

Cold Agglutinins
(koeld uh-*GLUE*-tuh-ninz)
(cold agglutinin screen)

5 min.

Type of Test: Blood

Body Systems and Functions: Immunological system

Normal Findings: ≤1:16 by red cell agglutination at 4°

Test Results Time Frame: Within 48 hr

Test Description: Cold agglutinins are usually IgM autoantibodies that are able to agglutinate the red blood cells at temperatures that range from 0°C–10°C. These agglutinins are normally found in small amounts and indicate infection when increased.

Consent Form: Not required

List of Equipment: Red-top tube or serum separator tube; needle and syringe or vacutainer; alcohol swab

Test Procedure:
1. Label the specimen tube. *Correctly identifies the client and the test to be performed.*
2. Obtain a 4-mL blood sample.
3. Do not agitate the tube. *Agitation may cause RBC hemolysis .*
4. Send tube to the laboratory.

Clinical Implications and Indications:
1. Elevated levels are found with viral pneumonia, influenza, infectious mononucleosis, hemolytic anemia, and Raynaud's disease.
2. Evaluates cirrhosis, chronic lymphocytic leukemia, and lymphoma.

Nursing Care:
Before Test: Explain the test procedure and the purpose of the test. Assess the client's knowledge of the test.
During Test: Adhere to standard precautions.
After Test: Apply pressure to venipuncture site. Explain that some bruising, discomfort, and swelling may appear at the site and that warm, moist compresses can alleviate this. Monitor for signs of infection.

Potential Complications: Bleeding and bruising at venipuncture site

Interfering Factors: Blood typing and cross-matching; age increases titers; antibiotic therapy

Nursing Considerations:
Pediatric: Infants and children will need assistance in remaining still during the venipuncture and age-appropriate comfort measures following the test.
Gerontology: Age causes spontaneous increases in cold agglutinins.

WEBLINKS

www.healthgate.com

Complement, Total
(*KAHM*-pluh-ment *TOE*-t:l)
(complement C3; complement C4; complement components; complement fixation; CS; complement total; CH50)

5 min.

Type of Test: Blood

Body Systems and Functions: Hematological system

Normal Findings:

Total complement	75–160 U/mL
C3	55–120 mg/dL
C4	20–50 mg/dL

Test Results Time Frame: Within 24 hr

Test Description: The total complement refers to a group of 20 proteins in the blood involved in a complex cascade system. Complement is important in the inflammatory process and is the main mediator in the antigen-antibody reactions of the cell-mediated immune response. The results associated with complement activation are cell lysis, release of mediators, vessel dilation, smooth muscle contraction, and increased vascular permeability. Complement activation consists of two major pathways: the classic and alternative pathways. The activation of the classic pathway requires antigen and complement-fixing antibody. The alternative pathway is important in the control of microbial infection and does not have an absolute requirement of an antibody. In systemic lupus erythematosus (SLE), large amounts of immune complexes are formed. These complexes activate complement and complement activation contributes to further inflammation. Complement levels decrease with SLE due to the consumption of enzymes from constant inflammation.

Consent Form: Not required

List of Equipment: Red-top tube or serum separator tube; needle and syringe or vacutainer; alcohol swab

Test Procedure:
1. Label the specimen tube. *Correctly identifies the client and the test to be performed.*
2. Obtain a 7-mL blood sample.
3. Do not agitate the tube. *Agitation may cause RBC hemolysis.*
4. Send tube to the laboratory. *The specimen must be processed within 2 hr or falsely decreased levels result.*

Clinical Implications and Indications:
1. Elevated levels are found with acute rheumatic fever, acute myocardial infarction, ulcerative colitis, and cancer.
2. Decreased levels are found with SLE, rheumatoid vasculitis, subacute bacterial endocarditis, shunt nephritis, poststreptococcal glomerulonephritis, gram-negative septicemia, anemia, malnutrition, and hepatitis.

Nursing Care:
Before Test: Explain the test procedure and the purpose of the test. Assess the client's knowledge of the test.
During Test: Adhere to standard precautions.
After Test: Apply pressure to venipuncture site. Explain that some bruising, discomfort, and swelling may appear at the site and that warm, moist compresses can alleviate this. Monitor for signs of infection.

Potential Complications: Bleeding and bruising at venipuncture site

Nursing Considerations:
Pediatric: Infants and children will need assistance in remaining still during the venipuncture and age-appropriate comfort measures following the test.

WEBLINKS

www.nlm.nih.gov

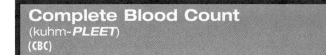

Complete Blood Count
(kuhm-*PLEET*)
(CBC)

5 min.

Type of Test: Blood

Body Systems and Functions: Hematological system

Normal Findings: Adult normal values:

Hematocrit:	
Male	41.5%–50.4%
Female	35.9%–44.6%
Hemoglobin:	
Male	14.0–17.5 g/dL
Female	12.3–15.3 g/dL
Red cell count	4.7–6.1 M/mL
White cell count	4.8–10.8 K/mL
Mean corpuscular volume (MCV)	81–99 fL
Mean corpuscular hemoglobin (MCH)	27–34 pg
Mean corpuscular hemoglobin concentration (MCHC)	32–36 g/dL
Platelet count	150–400 K/mL
Neutrophils	35%–70%
Lymphocytes	25%–45%
Monocytes	0%–12%
Eosinophils	0%–7%
Basophils	0%–2%

Test Results Time Frame: Within 24 hr

Test Description: The CBC is a combination report of a series of tests of the peripheral blood. The quantity, percentage, variety, concentrations, and quality of blood cells are identified. The tests usually included in a CBC are hematocrit, hemoglobin, red cell count, red blood cell indices, white cell count, and differential white blood cell count. Red blood cell indices consist of the following tests: MCV, MCHC, MCH, stained red cell examination, and platelet count. The differential white blood cell count consists of neutrophils, eosinophils, basophils, lymphocytes, and monocytes. The individual tests comprising a CBC are described in detail within this text.

Consent Form: Not required

List of Equipment: Purple-top tube; needle and syringe or vacutainer; alcohol swab

Test Procedure:
1. Label the specimen tube. *Correctly identifies the client and the test to be performed.*
2. Obtain a 5-mL blood sample.
3. Do not agitate the tube. *Agitation may cause RBC hemolysis.*
4. Send tube to the laboratory.

Clinical Implications and Indications:

1. The CBC is a frequently ordered outpatient and inpatient basic screening and diagnostic test that provides information about the hematological system and many other systems. It is used in routine physical examination and in the diagnosis of a wide range of conditions and diseases of children and adults (note: refer to individual tests for specific clinical implications).

Nursing Care:

Before Test: Explain the test procedure and the purpose of the test. Assess the client's knowledge of the test.

During Test: Adhere to standard precautions.

After Test: Apply pressure to venipuncture site. Explain that some bruising, discomfort, and swelling may appear at the site and that warm, moist compresses can alleviate this. Monitor for signs of infection.

Potential Complications: Bleeding and bruising at venipuncture site

Interfering Factors: Hypovolemia and fluid overload may alter results.

Nursing Considerations:

Pediatric: Infants and children will need assistance in remaining still during the venipuncture and age-appropriate comfort measures following the test.

WEBLINKS

www.healthgate.com

Coombs Antiglobulin, Direct
(kuemz *AEN*-tee-*GLAHB*-yue-l:n duh-*REKT*)
(direct antiglobulin test)

5 min.

Type of Test: Blood

Body Systems and Functions: Immunological system

Normal Findings: Negative; no agglutination

Test Results Time Frame: Within 30–40 min

Test Description: The direct Coombs test identifies autoantibodies (antigen-antibody complexes) against RBCs. The client's RBCs are mixed with Coombs serum, which contains antibodies against human serum. If the client's serum possesses autoantibodies against RBCs, agglutination will occur in the presence of Coombs serum. Agglutination indicates a positive test.

Consent Form: Not required

List of Equipment: Red-top tube or serum separator tube; needle and syringe or vacutainer; alcohol swab

Test Procedure:

1. Label the specimen tube. *Correctly identifies the client and the test to be performed.*

2. Obtain a 10-mL blood sample.
3. Do not agitate the tube. *Agitation may cause RBC hemolysis.*
4. Send tube to the laboratory.

Clinical Implications and Indications:
1. Diagnoses autoimmune hemolytic anemia
2. Evaluates transfusion reactions caused by incompatible blood
3. Diagnoses hemolytic disease of the newborn (HDN), lymphomas, lupus erythematosus, mycoplasma infection, and infectious mononucleosis

Nursing Care:
Before Test: Explain the test procedure and the purpose of the test. Assess the client's knowledge of the test.
During Test: Adhere to standard precautions.
After Test: Apply pressure to venipuncture site. Explain that some bruising, discomfort, and swelling may appear at the site and that warm, moist compresses can alleviate this. Monitor for signs of infection.

Potential Complications: Bleeding and bruising at venipuncture site

Interfering Factors: Medications that alter results are aldomet, penicillin, insulin, levodopa, cephalosporins, acetaminophen, quinidine, aspirin, and cephalothin.

Nursing Considerations:
Pregnancy: Hemolytic disease of the newborn occurs in the presence of an Rh-negative mother and Rh-positive newborn. This Rh incompatibility causes newborn jaundice.
Pediatric: Infants and children will need assistance in remaining still during the venipuncture and age-appropriate comfort measures following the test. A venous blood sample from the umbilical cord is obtained to detect antibodies in the newborn infant.

Listing of Related Tests: Indirect Coombs test

| WEBLINKS ▸ | ▤▣ |

http://www.nlm.nih.gov

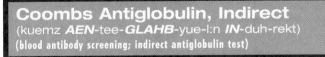

Coombs Antiglobulin, Indirect
(kuemz *AEN*-tee-*GLAHB*-yue-l:n *IN*-duh-rekt)
(blood antibody screening; indirect antiglobulin test)

5 min.

Type of Test: Blood

Body Systems and Functions: Immunological system

Normal Findings: No agglutination, indicating no antibodies against the donor's RBCs

Test Results Time Frame: Within 40 min

Test Description: The indirect Coombs test identifies serum antibodies, maternal anti-Rh antibodies during pregnancy, and incompatibilities not detected by other methods. The main purpose of this test is to determine serum antibodies to RBCs the client will receive by transfusion. This test is routinely done for blood compatibility testing or cross-matching. A small amount of the client's serum is mixed with the donor's RBCs and Coombs serum is added to the mixture. Agglutination (clumping) will occur when Coombs serum antibodies react with the client's antibodies. Agglutination will not occur if the client has no antibodies against the donor's RBCs. The absence of agglutination indicates a negative result.

Consent Form: Not required

List of Equipment: Red-top tube or serum separator tube; needle and syringe or vacutainer; alcohol swab

Test Procedure:
1. Label the specimen tube. *Correctly identifies the client and the test to be performed.*
2. Obtain a 7-mL blood sample.
3. Do not agitate the tube. *Agitation may cause RBC hemolysis.*
4. Send tube to the laboratory.

Clinical Implications and Indications:
1. Identifies the presence of recipient antibodies against a blood donor's RBCs
2. Detects the presence of antibodies from a previous transfusion or pregnancy

Nursing Care:
Before Test: Explain the test procedure and the purpose of the test. Assess the client's knowledge of the test.
During Test: Adhere to standard precautions.
After Test: Apply pressure to venipuncture site. Explain that some bruising, discomfort, and swelling may appear at the site and that warm, moist compresses can alleviate this. Monitor for signs of infection.

Potential Complications: Bleeding and bruising at venipuncture site

Nursing Considerations:
Pediatric: Infants and children will need assistance in remaining still during the venipuncture and age-appropriate comfort measures following the test.

Listing of Related Tests: Direct Coombs test; blood typing

WEBLINKS

http://www.nlm.nih.gov

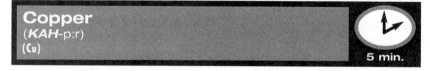

Copper
(*KAH*-p:r)
(Cu)

5 min.

Type of Test: Blood

Body Systems and Functions: Hematological system

Normal Findings:

Females	80–155 µg/dL
	13–24 µmol/L
Males	70–140 µg/dL
	11–22 µmol/L

Test Results Time Frame: Within 24 hr (note: some laboratories may not be equipped to perform this test, which may delay test results)

Test Description: Copper is an essential trace element. It is required for hemoglobin synthesis. Copper is present in the plasma in two main forms: loosely bound and firmly bound to plasma proteins. Loosely bound copper is bound predominantly to serum albumin. Firmly bound copper is incorporated into an alpha-2-globulin, which is called cerulosplasmin. The most important abnormality in copper metabolism is Wilson's disease. This hereditary condition is characterized by degenerative changes in the liver and brain, due to excessive deposition of copper. The copper is deposited in the eye, brain, liver, and kidney. An early detection of Wilson's disease makes elective therapy possible in most cases.

Consent Form: Not required

List of Equipment: Dark navy blue top metal-free tube; needle and syringe or vacutainer; alcohol swab

Test Procedure:

1. Label the specimen tube. *Correctly identifies the client and the test to be performed.*
2. Obtain a 5-mL blood sample.
3. Do not agitate the tube. *Agitation may cause RBC hemolysis.*
4. Send tube to the laboratory.

Clinical Implications and Indications:

1. Elevated levels are found with hepatic glutathione, Wilson's disease, rheumatoid arthritis, T-cell proliferation, ingestion of solutions of copper salts, contaminated water or dialysis fluids, female rheumatoid arthritis, oral contraceptives, inflammatory conditions, and Indian childhood cirrhosis.
2. Decreased serum copper levels are found with rheumatoid arthritis, Menke's steely hair disease (lack of pigmentation of skin and hair), collagen abnormalities, osteoporosis, ataxia, hypochromic anemia unresponsive to iron therapy, hypercholesteremia, impaired cardiovascular system, and an altered interleukin-2 production.

Nursing Care:

Before Test: Explain the test procedure and the purpose of the test. Assess the client's knowledge of the test.

During Test: Adhere to standard precautions.

After Test: Apply pressure to venipuncture site. Explain that some bruising, discomfort, and swelling may appear at the site and that warm, moist compresses can alleviate this. Monitor for signs of infection.

Potential Complications: Bleeding and bruising at venipuncture site

BLOOD

Interfering Factors: Medications that increase levels are oral contraceptives, methadone, and phenytoin.

Nursing Considerations:
Pregnancy: Values are increased during pregnancy.
Pediatric: Infants and children will need assistance in remaining still during the venipuncture and age-appropriate comfort measures following the test.

Listing of Related Tests: Ceruloplasmin

ⅢWEBLINKS   ▤▨

http://www.methodisthealth.com

Cordocentesis
(**KOER**-doe-sen-**TEE**-sis)
(percutaneous umbilical blood sampling)

60 min.

Type of Test: Blood

Body Systems and Functions: Reproductive system

Normal Findings: Absence of abnormal results

Test Results Time Frame: Within 24–48 hr

Test Description: Cordocentesis allows for diagnosis through fetal-blood aspiration and therapy through direct access to the fetal circulation. This test involves obtaining a sample of blood from the umbilical cord while the fetus is in utero. RBC transfusions for hemolytic disease of the newborn and platelet transfusions for severe thrombocytopenia may be done using cordocentesis. The umbilical vein is usually preferred rather than the artery because the vein is larger and straighter and has a thinner wall. The incidence of fetal bradycardia is increased when an umbilical artery is entered. Blood studies should include a Kleihauer-Betke test and a mean corpuscular RBC volume to ensure the specimen is from the fetus and not the mother.

Consent Form: Required

List of Equipment: Red-top tube or serum separator tube; needle and syringe or vacutainer; alcohol swab

Test Procedure:
1. A 20- to 25-gauge long ultrasound guided needle is used to puncture the umbilical cord at an area where it is well anchored. *Allows for minimal risk of maternal blood contamination.*
2. Label the specimen tube. *Correctly identifies the client and the test to be performed.*
3. Obtain a 5-mL blood sample.
4. Do not agitate the tube. *Agitation may cause RBC hemolysis.*
5. Send tube to the laboratory.
6. After the blood sample, the fetus is monitored by ultrasound. *Detects any significant blood leakage and fetal distress.*

Clinical Implications and Indications:

1. Diagnoses inherited and acquired blood disorders: hemoglobinopathies, coagulopathies, autoimmune and alloimmune thrombocytopenia, and inherited immunodeficiency syndromes
2. Detects infections, such as rubella, toxoplasmosis, and cytomegalovirus
3. Diagnoses inherited metabolic disorders
4. Evaluates hypoxia or acid-base imbalance found in conditions related to fetal distress

Nursing Care:

Before Test: Explain the test procedure and the purpose of the test. Assess the client's knowledge of the test. Inform the mother of the risks of the procedure. Administer antibiotics as ordered.

During Test: Adhere to standard precautions. Assist the mother with relaxation techniques.

After Test: Monitor maternal vital signs. Perform external fetal monitoring and observe for signs of fetal distress.

Potential Complications: Fetal bradycardia; blood extravasation from the puncture site; chorioamnionitis; premature labor; fetal blood loss (1%–2%)

Nursing Considerations:

Pregnancy: Cordocentesis can be performed after the 17th week of gestation.
Rural: Advisable to arrange for transportation home after recovering from procedure.

WEBLINKS

www.nlm.nih.gov

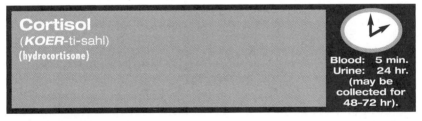

Cortisol
(**KOER**-ti-sahl)
(hydrocortisone)

Blood: 5 min.
Urine: 24 hr.
(may be
collected for
48–72 hr).

Type of Test: Blood; urine

Body Systems and Functions: Endocrine system

Normal Findings:

Blood:

Morning	7–28 µg/dL
Afternoon	2–18 µg/dL
Newborn	2–11 mcg/dL

After 1 week cortisol values equal adult levels.

Urine: 24-hr urine, 22–69 µmol (8–25 mg)

Test Results Time Frame: Blood: within 24 hr. Urine: within 24–48 hr.

Test Description: Cortisol is an adrenocortical hormone closely related to cortisone in physiological effects. Cortisone regulates metabolism, modulates the responses to many hormones and growth factors, and is involved in stress adaptation. Cortisol acts on all organ systems of the body, regulating many functional responses. Only 1% of total secretions from the adrenal gland appear as cortisol, but this small amount provides an important source of information in the diagnosis of adrenal disease. The greatest use for cortisol testing is in the diagnosis of Cushing's syndrome, a state of adrenocortical hyperfunction with excess glucocorticoids and androgens. Plasma cortisol levels are higher in the morning than in the afternoon. The cortisol stimulatory test uses an infusion of ACTH for confirmation of the diagnosis of hypofunction of the adrenal gland. The cortisol suppression test uses dexamethasone for confirmation of the diagnosis of hyperfunction of the adrenal gland.

Consent Form: Not required

List of Equipment: *Blood:* red-top tube or serum separator tube; needle and syringe or vacutainer; alcohol swab. *Urine:* sterile plastic container; ice.

Test Procedure:
Blood:
1. Label the specimen tube. *Correctly identifies the client and the test to be performed.*
2. Obtain a 3-mL blood sample.
3. Do not agitate the tube. *Agitation may cause RBC hemolysis.*
4. Send tube to the laboratory.

Urine:
1. Label the collection container. *Correctly identifies the client and the test to be performed.*
2. Discard the first morning void. Then begin the time of the collection for the next 24 hr, including the void at the end of the 24 hr, and record the last voiding time. *An exact 24-hr count ensures accurate results.*
3. If the client has an indwelling catheter in place, keep the drainage bag on ice and empty the urine into the urine container periodically during the 24-hr period.
4. Keep urine cool during collection. *Higher temperatures alter the results.*
5. If any urine is lost, discard the entire specimen and begin collection again the next day.

Clinical Implications and Indications:
1. Decreased levels are found with Addison's disease, adrenal hyperplasia, anterior pituitary hyposecretion, hypothyroidism, hepatitis, and cirrhosis.
2. Elevated levels are found with Cushing's syndrome, hyperthyroidism, stress, carcinoma, overproduction of ACTH due to tumors, adrenal adenoma, and obesity.

Nursing Care:
Before Test: Explain the test procedure and the purpose of the test. Assess the client's knowledge of the test. Instruct client not to discard any urine over the 24-hr time period. Instruct client to maintain a diet of 2–3 g salt/day for 3 days before the test. Provide written materials on sodium content of foods. Instruct client to limit physical activity for 12 hr before the test. Ensure client is free of stress and lying quietly for 30 min before the examination.

During Test: Adhere to standard precautions. Blood: Perform first venipuncture between 6 and 8 AM. For diurnal variation testing collect another sample between 4 and 6 PM. Urine: If any urine is accidentally discarded or contaminated with feces, discard entire specimen and begin test again the following morning.

After Test: Blood: Apply pressure to venipuncture site. Explain that some bruising, discomfort, and swelling may appear at the site and that warm, moist compresses can alleviate this. Monitor for signs of infection. Urine: Document urine quantity, date, and exact hours of collection on requisition.

Potential Complications: Bleeding and bruising at venipuncture site

Interfering Factors: Urine contaminated with feces; spillage or inaccurate collection of the 24-hr specimen, including nonrefrigeration or placing on ice; heavy bleeding during menstruation; renal disease; starvation; failure to refrain from certain medications; physical activity; obesity; stress; severe renal or hepatic disease; radioactive scan performed up to 1 week before test; hemolysis; medications that increase levels are amphetamines, estrogens, oral contraceptives, and cortisone; medications that decrease levels are androgens, lithium, levodopa, and dilantin.

Nursing Considerations:
Pregnancy: Cortisol levels are increased during pregnancy.
Pediatric: Blood: Infants and children will need assistance in remaining still during the venipuncture and age-appropriate comfort measures following the test. Urine: For collection of 24-hr specimen a collection bag or indwelling catheter needs to be used for infants and toddlers.

| WEBLINKS ↖ | ⊟⊠ |

www.nlm.nih.gov

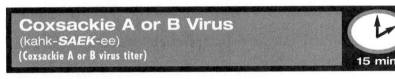

Coxsackie A or B Virus
(kahk-*SAEK*-ee)
(Coxsackie A or B virus titer)

15 min.

Type of Test: Blood; culture

Body Systems and Functions: Integumentary system

Normal Findings: Absence of Coxsackie virus

Test Results Time Frame: Within 5 days

Test Description: Coxsackie are enteroviruses that may cause vesicular skin eruptions, encephalitis, and aseptic meningitis. Enteroviruses are easily spread by the fecal-oral route. Nearly 75% of viral meningitis cases in the United States are caused by enterovirus. A routine cerebrospinal fluid (CSF) culture reveals the presence of Coxsackie virus. CSF infected with Coxsackie virus exhibits the following characteristics: usually nonpurulent, decreased mononuclear white cell count, increased lymphocytes, normal or decreased CSF glucose, and elevated CSF protein. Most viral meningitis cases typically produce nonfatal infections with a benign course. If there is brain parenchymal involvement, a more virulent course and risk of permanent sequelae are more likely. For skin eruptions caused by Coxsackie viruses, cultures are obtained from skin vesicles. In addition, blood samples can identify the presence of the disorder.

Consent Form: Required for CSF sample; not required for skin vesicle culture

List of Equipment: *Blood:* red-top tube or serum separator tube; needle and syringe or vacutainer; alcohol swab. *Culture:* skin vesicle fluid collection: collection swab; appropriate transport medium. *CSF collection:* CSF collection tray; lumbar puncture set; sterile gloves and gown; masks.

Test Procedure:
Blood:
1. Label the specimen tube. *Correctly identifies the client and the test to be performed.*
2. Obtain a 5-mL blood sample.
3. Do not agitate the tube. *Agitation may cause RBC hemolysis*
4. Send tube to the laboratory.

Culture:
1. Label collection container. *Correctly identifies the client and test to be performed.*
2. Vigorously swab squamous cells within the vesicles.

CSF specimen:
1. Follow procedure for lumbar puncture and collection of CSF specimen for culture.
2. Transport specimen immediately on ice. *Ensures accurate results.*

Clinical Implications and Indications:
1. Diagnoses hand, foot, and mouth disease
2. Diagnoses aseptic meningitis and encephalitis

Nursing Care:
Before Test: Blood and culture: Explain the test procedure and the purpose of the test. Assess the client's knowledge of the test. CSF: Explain the test procedure and the purpose of the test. Assess the client's knowledge of the test. Instruct client to have no solid foods for 12 hr prior to the lumbar puncture; fluids are usually permitted up to 3 hr prior to the test. If coagulation disorder is suspected, client will have platelet count and prothrombin/partial thromboplastin time performed. Instruct client to empty bladder and bowel prior to test. Prepare lumbar puncture set and assist client in lateral recumbent position along the edge of the bed with the knees flexed on the chest and chin touching the knees.
During Test: Adhere to standard precautions and strict aseptic technique. CSF: Assist client in maintaining lateral, recumbent position. Instruct client to remain very still and explain that movement may result in injury. Ask client to report any numbness, pain, or tingling in the legs (this may indicate nerve root damage or irritation). Apply band-aid over puncture site after lumbar needle is removed.
After Test: Blood: Apply pressure to venipuncture site. Explain that some bruising, discomfort, and swelling may appear at the site and that warm, moist compresses can alleviate this. Monitor for signs of infection. CSF: Maintain bedrest in

prone position for 1–3 hr to minimize headache after the lumbar puncture. Observe for potential complications and deterioration of mental status, sensory deficits, leg muscle weakness, and bowel or bladder incontinence or retention.

Potential Complications: Blood: bleeding and bruising at venipuncture site. CSF: traumatic lumbar puncture tap; severe headache.

Contraindications: CSF: increased intracranial pressure; cutaneous or osseous infection at site of the lumbar puncture

Nursing Considerations:
Pediatric: Coxsackie viruses cause hand-foot-mouth disease in young children and presents as vesicles on the tongue and skin of the palms and soles. Adult family members of infected children may also develop the disease. Infants and children will need assistance in remaining still during the venipuncture and the culture and will require age-appropriate comfort measures following the test.
Gerontology: The older person may find it difficult to maintain positions when required to do so for lengthy periods of time during either the culture or the CSF procedure.
Rural: Advisable to arrange for transportation home after recovering from procedure
International: Enterovirus outbreaks are most common during the summer months.

WEBLINKS

http://www.cmrinstitute.org

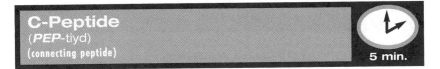

C-Peptide
(*PEP*-tiyd)
(connecting peptide)

5 min.

Type of Test: Blood

Body Systems and Functions: Endocrine system

Normal Findings: 500–2,500 pg/mL

Test Results Time Frame: Within 24 hr

Test Description: C-peptide, a biologically inactive peptide chain, is formed during the conversion of proinsulin to insulin in the pancreatic beta cells. C-peptide is secreted into the blood in almost equal concentration, as is insulin. Measurement of C-peptide gives a reliable indicator of beta and secretory function and insulin secretions. C-peptide helps to determine the variety of factors involved in the disease process of diabetes mellitus.

Consent Form: Not required

List of Equipment: Yellow-top tube or purple-top tube or serum separator tube; needle and syringe or vacutainer; alcohol swab

BLOOD

Test Procedure:

1. Label the specimen tube. *Correctly identifies the client and the test to be performed.*
2. Obtain a 10-mL blood sample.
3. Do not agitate the tube. *Agitation may cause RBC hemolysis.*
4. Send tube to the laboratory.

Clinical Implications and Indications:

1. Elevated levels are found with endogenous hyperinsulinism in diabetes and post-pancreatectomy if cancer is still present.
2. Decreased or absent levels are found with surreptitious insulin injection, no beta cell function, and remission of diabetes mellitus.

Nursing Care:

Before Test: Explain the test procedure and the purpose of the test. Assess the client's knowledge of the test. Instruct client to be NPO 8 hr prior to test (water is permitted).

During Test: Adhere to standard precautions.

After Test: Apply pressure to venipuncture site. Explain that some swelling, bruising, or discomfort may occur at the site and warm, moist compresses can alleviate this. Monitor for signs of infection.

Potential Complications: Bleeding and bruising at venipuncture site

Nursing Considerations:

Pediatric: Infants and children will need assistance in remaining still during the venipuncture and age-appropriate comfort measures following the test.

Listing of Related Tests: Insulin

WEBLINKS

www.webmd.com

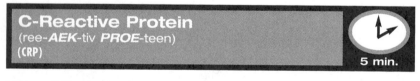

C-Reactive Protein
(ree-*AEK*-tiv *PROE*-teen)
(CRP)

5 min.

Type of Test: Blood

Body Systems and Functions: Immunological system

Normal Findings: Less than 6 mg/L

Test Results Time Frame: Within 4 hr

Test Description: C-reactive protein is a globulin that in the presence of calcium ions precipitates the C substance of pneumococcal cells. CRP is an abnormal protein that appears in the blood in the acute stages of various inflammatory disorders but is undetectable in the blood of healthy individuals. Progressive increases correlate with increases of inflammatory injury. CRP may be used to follow therapeutic response medications.

Consent Form: Not required

List of Equipment: Red-top tube or serum separator tube; needle and syringe or vacutainer; alcohol swab

Test Procedure:
1. Label the specimen tube. *Correctly identifies the client and the test to be performed.*
2. Obtain a 10mL blood sample.
3. Do not agitate the tube. *Agitation may cause RBC hemolysis.*
4. Send tube to the laboratory.

Clinical Implications and Indications:
1. Elevated levels are found with bacterial infections, active rheumatic fever, postoperative wound infections, kidney or bone marrow transplant rejection, Crohn's disease, systemic lupus erythematosus, active rheumatoid arthritis, TB, acute myocardial infarctions, and blood transfusions.

Nursing Care:
Before Test: Explain the test procedure and the purpose of the test. Assess the client's knowledge of the test. Instruct client to fast for 8 hr (note: may drink water).
During Test: Adhere to standard precautions.
After Test: Apply pressure to venipuncture site. Explain that some bruising, swelling, or discomfort may occur at site and that warm compresses can alleviate this. Monitor for signs of infection.

Potential Complications: Bleeding and bruising at venipuncture site

Interfering Factors: Nonfasting sample; oral contraceptives; some brands of intrauterine devices

Nursing Considerations:
Pregnancy: Levels are frequently elevated with pregnancy.
Gerontology: False positives may occur in clients over 60.

Listing of Related Tests: Erythrocyte sedimentation rate

WEBLINKS ▤ ☒

http://www.mc.vanderbilt.edu/histo/blood/erythrocytes.html

Creatine
(**KREE**-uh-teen)
(Cr; plasma creatinine; Pcr; serum creatinine; creatinine clearance; creatinine height index)

5 min.

Type of Test: Blood

Body Systems and Functions: Musculoskeletal system

Normal Findings:

Males	0.2–0.6 mg/dL
Females	0.6–1.0 mg/dL
Newborn	0.3–1.2 mg/dL
Infant	0.2–0.4 mg/dL
Child	0.3–0.7 mg/dL
Adolescent	0.5–1.0 mg/dL

CRITICAL VALUES:
4 mg/dL could indicate serious renal function impairment.

Test Results Time Frame: Within 24 hr

Test Description: Creatine is synthesized in a two-step process in the kidneys, small intestine, pancreas, and liver. Creatine combines readily with phosphocreatine to form creatinine. Approximately 98% of creatine is contained in muscle and about 1.7% is converted to creatinine. Serum and urine creatinine is used as an indication of renal function. The body content of creatine is proportional to muscle mass. Skeletal muscle necrosis or atrophy causes a significant increase in serum creatine. Creatine is filtered by the glomeruli and nearly or completely reabsorbed by the proximal tubules. There is a resultant very small net excretion of creatine.

Consent Form: Not required

List of Equipment: Serum separator tube; needle and syringe or vacutainer; alcohol swab

Test Procedure:
1. Label the specimen tube. *Correctly identifies the client and the test to be performed.*
2. Obtain a 1-mL blood sample.
3. Do not agitate the tube. *Agitation may cause RBC hemolysis, which increases creatine values by 100%–200%.*
4. Send tube to the laboratory.

Clinical Implications and Indications:
1. Elevated levels are found with trauma, muscular dystrophy, poliomyelitis, amyotrophic lateral sclerosis, amytonia congenita, dermatomyositis, myasthenia gravis, starvation, hyperthyroidism, and diabetic acidosis.

Nursing Care:
Before Test: Explain the test procedure and the purpose of the test. Assess the client's knowledge of the test.
During Test: Adhere to standard precautions.
After Test: Apply pressure to venipuncture site. Explain that some bruising, discomfort, and swelling may appear at the site and that warm, moist compresses can alleviate this. Monitor for signs of infection.

Potential Complications: Bleeding and bruising at venipuncture site

Nursing Considerations:
Pregnancy: Serum creatine levels are increased during the puerperium.

Pediatric: *Infants and children will need assistance in remaining still during the venipuncture and age-appropriate comfort measures following the test.*

WEBLINKS 🔍

http://www.nih.gov

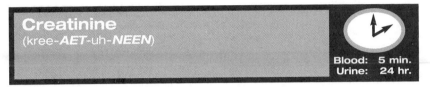

Creatinine
(kree-*AET*-uh-*NEEN*)

| Blood: | 5 min. |
| Urine: | 24 hr. |

Type of Test: Blood; urine

Body Systems and Functions: Renal/urological system

Normal Findings:

Blood: 0.4–1.5 mg/dL
Urine:
Men   <0.8–1.8 g/24 hr
Women   0.6–1.6 g /24 hr
Creatinine clearance (mL/min/1.73 m^2):

Age (years)	Males	Females
<20	88–146	81–136
20–30	88–146	81–136
30–40	82–140	75–128
40–50	75–133	69–122
50–60	68–126	64–116
60–70	61–120	58–110
70–80	55–113	52–105

Test Results Time Frame: Blood: within 24 hr. Urine: within 1–3 hr after 24-hr collection.

Test Description: Creatinine is a catabolic byproduct of muscle energy metabolism and is excreted by the kidney. Creatinine is not dramatically affected by fluid balance, nutritional status, or liver function, as is the blood urea nitrogen (BUN) test. Creatinine is dependent upon muscle mass, which does not have day-to-day major changes. Therefore the serum creatinine level remains constant and normal in the presence of normal renal function. Kidney disorders hinder creatinine excretion. Urine creatinine alone is not valuable in evaluating kidney function. Urine creatinine is done as a component of a creatinine clearance test. Creatinine clearance is equivalent to and a measurement of glomerular filtration rate (GFR), or the milliliters of filtrate produced by the kidneys per minute. Creatinine clearance may also be defined as the measurement of the rate at which the kidneys are able to clear creatinine from the blood. The creatinine clearance rate is calculated from the urine and serum creatinine levels.

Consent Form: Not required

BLOOD

List of Equipment: *Blood:* red-top tube or serum separator tube; needle and syringe or vacutainer; alcohol swab. *Urine:* sterile plastic container; ice.

Test Procedure:

Blood:

1. Label the specimen tube. *Correctly identifies the client and the test to be performed.*
2. Obtain a 5-mL blood sample.
3. Do not agitate the tube. *Agitation may cause RBC hemolysis.*
4. Send tube to the laboratory.

Urine:

1. Label the collection container and include the client's height and weight. Document the client's height and weight in the health care record. *Correctly identifies the client and the test to be performed and creatinine clearance values are based on the client's body surface area.*
2. Discard the first morning void. Then begin the time of the collection for the next 24 hr, including the void at the end of the 24 hr, and record the last voiding time. *An exact 24-hr count ensures accurate results.*
3. If the client has an indwelling catheter in place, keep the drainage bag on ice and empty the urine into the urine container periodically during the 24-hr period.
4. Keep urine cool during collection. *Higher temperatures alter the results.*
5. If any urine is lost, discard the entire specimen and begin collection again the next day.

Clinical Implications and Indications:

1. Decreased creatinine clearance is found with disorders of kidney function (e.g., acute and chronic renal failure, glomerulonephritis, pyelonephritis, amyloidosis), shock, hemorrhage, congestive heart failure, and liver failure.
2. Increased creatinine clearance is found with high cardiac output, pregnancy, burns, and carbon monoxide poisoning.
3. Increased serum creatinine is found with glomerulonephritis, pyelonephritis, acute tubular necrosis, and urinary obstruction.
4. Increased urine creatinine is found with acromegaly, gigantism, diabetes mellitus, and hyothyroidism.
5. Decreased urine creatinine is found with hyperthyroidism, anemia, muscular dystrophy, polymyositis neurogenic atrophy, inflammatory muscle disease, advanced renal disease, and leukemia.

Creatinine clearance = UV/P

where U = mg/dL of creatinine excreted in the urine over 24 hr, V = volume of urine in mL/min (total volume of urine in 24 hr is divided by 1440 min to get mL/min), and P = serum creatinine in mg/dL

Nursing Care:

Before Test: Explain the test procedure and the purpose of the test. Assess the client's knowledge of the test. Encourage fluids for optimal hydration if not contraindicated. Large urine volumes contribute to accurate test results. Instruct client to avoid consuming large amounts of meat prior to the test. Instruct client to avoid vigorous exercise during the test. Instruct client not to discard any urine over the 24-hr time period.

During Test: Adhere to standard precautions. If any urine is accidentally discarded or contaminated with feces, discard entire specimen and begin test again the following morning.

After Test: Blood: Apply pressure to venipuncture site. Explain that some bruising, discomfort, and swelling may appear at the site and that warm, moist compresses can alleviate this. Monitor for signs of infection. Urine: Document urine quantity, date, and exact hours of collection on requisition. Instruct client to resume appropriate, client-specific diet, fluid intake, and activity level.

Potential Complications: Bleeding and bruising at venipuncture site

Interfering Factors: Vigorous exercise may increase creatinine clearance; a high-meat diet may increase serum creatinine; cephalosporins decrease creatinine clearance; urine contaminated with feces; spillage or inaccurate collection of the 24-hr specimen, including nonrefrigeration or placing on ice; heavy bleeding during menstruation

Nursing Considerations:
Pregnancy: Pregnancy markedly increases creatinine clearance.
Pediatric: Blood: Infants and children will need assistance in remaining still during the venipuncture and age-appropriate comfort measures following the test. Urine: For collection of 24-hr specimen a collection bag or indwelling catheter needs to be used for infants and toddlers.

Listing of Related Tests: Blood urea nitrogen

WEBLINKS 🔲 ☒

http://www.creighton.edu

Creatinine Kinase
(kree-*AET*-uh-*NEEN KIY*-nays)
(CPK; CK)

5 min.

Type of Test: Blood

Body Systems and Functions: Cardiovascular system

Normal Findings:
Total CPK:

Adult male	12–70 µ/mL or 55–170 µ/L	
Adult female	10–55 µ/mL or 30–135 µ/L	

Isoenzymes:

CPK-MM	100%
CPK-MB	0%
CPK-BB	0%

Test Results Time Frame: Within 30 min

Test Description: CPK is an enzyme contained in the heart muscle, skeletal muscle, and brain. When heart muscle is damaged, such as in a myocardial infarction, CPK is released into the blood. This is evidenced by an increased serum level of CPK. CPK is composed of three isoenzymes: CPK-BB, CPK-MB, and CPK-MM. The CPK-MB isoenzyme is a specific marker for damaged myocardial cells. The CPK-MB level increases 3–6 hr from the onset of myocardial infarction, peaks in 12–24 hr, and returns to normal in 12–48 hr.

Consent Form: Not required

List of Equipment: Lavender-top tube or red-top tube or serum separator tube; needle and syringe or vacutainer; alcohol swab

Test Procedure:
1. Label the specimen tube. *Correctly identifies the client and the test to be performed.*
2. Obtain a 7-mL blood sample.
3. Gently invert tube several times, but do not agitate the tube. *Mixes the anticoagulant, but agitation may cause RBC hemolysis.*
4. Send tube to the laboratory.

Clinical Implications and Indications:
1. Total CPK levels are elevated with myopathy due to alcoholism, electrical cardioversion or defibrillation, cardiac catheterization, stroke, and surgery.
2. CPK-MB is elevated with myocardial infarction, cardiac surgery, myocarditis, and Reye's syndrome.
3. CPK-BB is elevated with stroke, seizure, pulmonary infarction, and intestinal ischemia.
4. CPK-MM is elevated with muscular dystrophy and skeletal muscle injury.

Nursing Care:
Before Test: Explain the test procedure and the purpose of the test. Assess the client's knowledge of the test. Inform client that slight discomfort may be experienced from needle poke. Obtain complete history of client's symptoms, including onset of chest pain, duration, severity, quality, and predisposing and alleviating factors.
During Test: Adhere to standard precautions.
After Test: Apply pressure to venipuncture site. Explain that some bruising, discomfort, and swelling may appear at the site and that warm, moist compresses can alleviate this. Monitor for signs of infection.

Potential Complications: Bleeding and bruising at venipuncture site

Interfering Factors: Intramuscular injections; strenuous exercise; recent surgery

Nursing Considerations:
Pregnancy: Levels are elevated during the first trimester of pregnancy.

Listing of Related Tests: Serum asparate aminotransferase; lactic dehydrogenase; troponin; myoglobin

WEBLINKS

http://www.howstuffworks.com

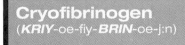

Cryofibrinogen
(*KRIY*-oe-fiy-*BRIN*-oe-j:n)

5 min.

BLOOD

Type of Test: Blood

Body Systems and Functions: Hematological system

Normal Findings: Negative

Test Results Time Frame: Within 24 hr

Test Description: Cryofibrinogen is made of fibrinogen and protein fragments that precipitate at 0°ree;–4°C and redissolve when warmed. Clients who have increased cryofibrinogen levels have an increased sensitivity to cold, urticaria, bleeding, and blood vessel damage. Positive tests require a study of cold precipitable proteins to contrast cryofibrinogen from cryoglobulins.

Consent Form: Not required

List of Equipment: Blue-top tube; needle and syringe or vacutainer; alcohol swab

Test Procedure:
1. Label the specimen tube. *Correctly identifies the client and the test to be performed.*
2. Obtain a 7-mL blood sample.
3. Do not agitate the tube. *Agitation may cause RBC hemolysis.*
4. Send tube to the laboratory.

Clinical Implications and Indications:
1. Diagnoses familial Mediterranean fever, hemophilia, hepatitis C, multiple myeloma, toxemia, and thromboembolic conditions

Nursing Care:
Before Test: Explain the test procedure and the purpose of the test. Assess the client's knowledge of the test.
During Test: Adhere to standard precautions.
After Test: Apply pressure for prolonged time (5 min) to venipuncture site. Explain that some bruising, discomfort, and swelling may appear at the site and that warm, moist compresses can alleviate this. Monitor for signs of infection.

Potential Complications: Bleeding and bruising at venipuncture site

Interfering Factors: Heparin therapy within the past 2 days

Nursing Considerations:
Pediatric: Infants and children will need assistance in remaining still during the venipuncture and age-appropriate comfort measures following the test.

WEBLINKS

http://www.entnet.org

Cryoglobulin
(KRIY-oe-*GLAHB*-yue-l:n)

5 min.

Type of Test: Blood

Body Systems and Functions: Hematological system

Normal Findings: Negative for cryoglobulins

Test Results Time Frame: Within 3–5 days

Test Description: Cryoglobulins are immunoglobulins in the blood that precipitate when cold and dissolve when rewarmed. Precipitation causes sludging within the affected vessels. Clients will exhibit symptoms of purpura, arthralgia, or Raynaud's syndrome manifested as pain, cyanosis, and coldness of the fingers. The blood sample is refrigerated for 72 hr and evaluated for precipitation. If precipitation is present, it is measured and recorded. The sample is then rewarmed and examined for dissolution of precipitation.

Consent Form: Not required

List of Equipment: Red-top tube or serum separator tube; needle and syringe or vacutainer; alcohol swab

Test Procedure:
1. Label the specimen tube. *Correctly identifies the client and the test to be performed.*
2. Obtain a 10-mL blood sample.
3. Do not agitate the tube. *Agitation may cause RBC hemolysis.*
4. Send tube to the laboratory.
5. Keep specimen cool. *High temperatures alter the results.*

Clinical Implications and Indications:
1. Diagnoses lupus erythematosus, Sjögren's syndrome, rheumatoid arthritis, multiple myeloma, leukemia, Waldenstrom's macroglobulinemia, lymphoma, acute and chronic infections, hepatitis, cirrhosis, and Raynaud's phenomenon

Nursing Care:
Before Test: Explain the test procedure and the purpose of the test. Assess the client's knowledge of the test. Instruct client to be NPO for 8 hr before the test.
During Test: Adhere to standard precautions.
After Test: Apply pressure to venipuncture site. Explain that some bruising, discomfort, and swelling may appear at the site and that warm, moist compresses can alleviate this. Monitor for signs of infection. If the test is positive, educate client to avoid cold temperatures, wear gloves, and dress warmly to prevent symptoms of Raynaud's syndrome.

Potential Complications: Bleeding and bruising at venipuncture site

Nursing Considerations:
Pediatric: Infants and children will need assistance in remaining still during the venipuncture and age-appropriate comfort measures following the test.

International: Serum cryoglobulins are present less frequently in Japanese clients than among those studied in Western countries.

WEBLINKS

www.nlm.nih.gov

Cytomegalovirus Antibody
(siy-toe-*MEG*-uh-loe-*VIY*-ruhs *AEN*-ti-*BAH*-dee)
(CMV; cytomegalovirus antibody; CMV antibody)

5 min.

Type of Test: Blood

Body Systems and Functions: Immunological system

Normal Findings: Negative:

IgM	<1:8
IgH	<1:8 for those exposed
IgG	<1:16 for those exposed

Test Results Time Frame: Within 72 hr

Test Description: The cytomegalovirus antibody test detects the presence of CMV, which is a type of herpes virus found in all body secretions. The CMV can cross the placenta and is transferred in blood. The virus is present in a large segment of the population early in life without causing apparent disease. Host factors predisposing to the presence of disease should be investigated when serum antibody test is positive. CMV may be cultured from the urine, but this method of detection has a much lower incidence of correlation with CMV disease.

> **CLINICAL ALERT:**
> A positive CMV antibody test precludes using the blood for transfusion or in organs for donation. Immunosuppressed clients are highly susceptible to CMV, particularly clients with AIDS. Acute CMV infection in the client with AIDS often leads to eye damage and blindness, and cerebral damage. Cytomegalovirus may be dangerous for pregnant women because of brain damage to the fetus (causing congenital CMV).

Consent Form: Not required

List of Equipment: Red-top tube or serum separator tube; needle and syringe or vacutainer; alcohol swab

Test Procedure:
1. Label the specimen tube. *Correctly identifies the client and the test to be performed.*
2. Obtain a 5-mL blood sample.
3. Do not agitate the tube. *Agitation may cause RBC hemolysis.*
4. Send tube to the laboratory.

BLOOD

5. Repeat 10–14 days later for convalescent sample and label the tube as convalescent sample. *Allows for separate identification of the convalescent sample that is compared in ratio to the acute sample.*

Clinical Implications and Indications:

1. Detects the presence of opportunistic disease in AIDS client.
2. CMV immune status should be performed on all organ transplant candidates before surgery.
3. CMV mononucleosis usually occurs in older adults as contrasted with Epstein-Barr mononucleosis.
4. Detects congenital CMV, which may cause a variety of neurological and developmental anomalies in the infant.

Nursing Care:

Before Test: Assess the client's knowledge of the test. Explain the test procedure and the purpose of the test. Advise the organ donor that this test is one of several that is included in the hematological assessment for their prospective organ donation.

During Test: Adhere to standard precautions.

After Test: Apply pressure to venipuncture site. Explain that some bruising, discomfort, and swelling may appear at the site and that warm, moist compresses can alleviate this. Monitor for signs of infection. Teach client that it is important to return in 10–14 days for follow-up sampling to see if infection is subsiding.

Potential Complications: Bleeding and bruising at venipuncture site

Interfering Factors: Epstein-Barr virus and rheumatoid factor, which cause false-positive results

Nursing Considerations:

Pediatric: The CMV test is not valid for infants less than 6 months of age, due to potential maternal antibodies present in the serum. Infants and children will need assistance in remaining still during the venipuncture and age-appropriate comfort measures following the test.

Listing of Related Tests: Torch test; cold agglutinin titer; bronchoscopy; Western blot assay

WEBLINKS ▮ 🗖 🗙

http://www.nlm.nih.gov

Dehydroepiandrosterone Sulfate
(dee-*HIY*-droe-*EP*-ee-aen-*DRAHS*-t:r-oen *SUHL*-fayt)
(DHEA-S)

🕐

5 min.

Type of Test: Blood

Body Systems and Functions: Endocrine system

Normal Findings: Dehydroepiandrosterone sulfate, serum:

Age	Male (µg/dL)	Female (µg/dL)
6 months–4 years	3–24	3–24
5–6 years	13–57	13–57
7–8 years	37–74	37–74
9–10 years	52–127	52–127
11–12 years	76–166	76–166
13–19 years	76–640	65–380
20–29 years	280–640	65–380
30–39 years	120–520	45–270
40–49 years	95–530	32–240
50–59 years	70–310	26–200
60–69 years	42–290	13–130
70 years & over	28–175	10–90

Test Results Time Frame: Within 24 hr

Test Description: Dehydroepiandrosterone sulfate (DHEA-S) is a weak androgen secreted primarily by the "zona reticularis" of the adrenal cortex. Secretion is controlled by ACTH and other pituitary factors. Physiologically, DHEA-S has many roles, including the development of pubic and axillary hair, the development and maintenance of immunocompetence, and as a possible tumor marker. Serum levels of DHEA-S are one thousand times greater than DHEA. DHEA levels show diurnal variation while DHEA-S does not. Levels change slowly due to slow metabolism and low renal clearance.

Consent Form: Not required

List of Equipment: Red-top tube or serum separator tube; needle and syringe or vacutainer; alcohol swab

Test Procedure:
1. Label the specimen tube. *Correctly identifies the client and the test to be performed.*
2. Obtain a 5-mL blood sample.
3. Do not agitate the tube. *Agitation may cause RBC hemolysis.*
4. Send tube to the laboratory.

Clinical Implications and Indications:
1. Diagnoses hirsutism and amenorrhea (the most common sign of increased adrenal androgen production by women)
2. Evaluates polycystic ovary syndrome where high DHEA-S levels are encountered (levels >700–800 mg/dL in women are suggestive of a hormone-secreting adrenal tumor)
3. Evaluates Cushing's syndrome, which is caused by adrenal carcinomas where DHEA-S is elevated

Nursing Care:
Before Test: Explain the test procedure and the purpose of the test. Assess the client's knowledge of the test.
During Test: Adhere to standard precautions.

After Test: Apply pressure to venipuncture site. Explain that some bruising, discomfort, and swelling may appear at the site and that warm, moist compresses can alleviate this. Monitor for signs of infection.

Potential Complications: Bleeding and bruising at venipuncture site

Nursing Considerations:
Pediatric: Infants and children will need assistance in remaining still during the venipuncture and age-appropriate comfort measures following the test. Serum concentrations of DHEA-S are high at birth (newborn range 30–250 mg/ dL) and even higher in sick and premature infants. Values decrease precipitously during the first week of life and then down to 2–24 mg/dL for children 6 months to 4 years.

⊞WEBLINKS ▮   🗏🗷

http://adam.excite.com

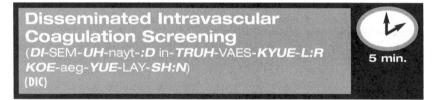

Disseminated Intravascular Coagulation Screening
(*DI*-SEM-*UH*-nayt-:*D* in-*TRUH*-VAES-*KYUE-L:R* *KOE*-aeg-*YUE*-LAY-*SH:N*)
(DIC)

5 min.

Type of Test: Blood

Body Systems and Functions: Hematological system

Normal Findings: Negative for DIC

Test Results Time Frame: Within 24–48 hr

Test Description: Disseminated intravascular screening refers to multiple coagulation related tests that are performed to rule out the process of DIC. DIC is a pathological condition whereby the coagulation mechanisms have been increased to the point of depleting the coagulation stores (e.g., platelets, clotting factors). In this process, fibrinolysis results in the formation of fibrin degradation products, which further act as anticoagulants. Intravascular sludging occurs due to fibrin clots and excessive bleeding is caused at a microvascular level due to the lack of coagulability. Overall, DIC is life threatening and has a high mortality rate even with treatment. The tests that are covered separately in this text that are part of DIC screening are bleeding time, platelet count, prothrombin time, partial thromboplastin time, coagulation factors, fibrin degradation products, red blood smear, euglobulin lysis time, and D-dimer.

> **CLINICAL ALERT:**
> DIC is a very critical condition, and when clinical manifestations are first observed, immediate action must be taken (e.g., reporting to health care provider overseeing client).

Consent Form: Not required

List of Equipment: Red-top tube or serum separator tube; needle and syringe or vacutainer; alcohol swab

Test Procedure: Overall, a wide variety of blood testing is done as part of this screening, and the following procedures are generic if taking a sample from the blood:

1. Label the specimen tube. *Correctly identifies the client and the test to be performed.*
2. Obtain a 5-mL blood sample.
3. Do not agitate the tube. *Agitation may cause RBC hemolysis.*
4. Send tube to the laboratory.

Clinical Implications and Indications:

1. Diagnoses and evaluates disseminated intravascular coagulation

Nursing Care:

Before Test: Explain the test procedure and the purpose of the test. Assess the client's knowledge of the test.

During Test: Adhere to standard precautions.

After Test: Apply pressure to venipuncture site. Explain that some bruising, discomfort, and swelling may appear at the site and that warm, moist compresses can alleviate this. Monitor for signs of infection.

Potential Complications: Bleeding and bruising at venipuncture site, which is pronounced due to the DIC process.

Nursing Considerations:

Pregnancy: DIC occurs more frequently during pregnancy.

Pediatric: Infants and children will need assistance in remaining still during the venipuncture and age-appropriate comfort measures following the test.

| WEBLINKS |

www.healthgate.com

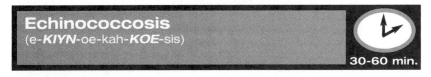

Echinococcosis
(e-*KIYN*-oe-kah-*KOE*-sis)

30-60 min.

Type of Test: Blood; tissue

Body Systems and Functions: Immunological system

Normal Findings: Negative for echinococcosis; IHA 1:2–1:64

Test Results Time Frame: Blood: within 24–48 hr. Tissue: within 72 hr.

Test Description: Echinococcosis testing is an examination of a parasitic infection of a tapeworm. Dogs are the common host for echinococcosis and humans become the intermediate host. The eggs are blood borne and form cysts in the liver and elsewhere in the body (note: the cysts may take 5–20 years to become symptomatic). Cattle and sheep also carry the parasite. The most definitive diagnosis is made by a cyst biopsy, but there is also serum testing (which is not as conclusive). The biopsy is an invasive procedure performed in a surgical setting. An excision or needle punch sample of body tissue is taken under sterile technique and examined microscopically for cell morphology and tissue anomalies. Removal of the cyst may not lower titers for years.

CLINICAL ALERT:
Leakage of infected cyst from accidental aspiration could result in an allergic reaction to the contents of the cyst. Therefore, have emergency equipment readily available in the event of an anaphylactic reaction.

Consent Form: Required

List of Equipment: *Biopsy:* biopsy equipment. *Blood:* red-top tube or serum separator tube; needle and syringe or vacutainer; alcohol swab.

Test Procedure:
Blood:
1. Label the specimen tube. *Correctly identifies the client and the test to be performed.*
2. Obtain a 7-mL blood sample.
3. Do not agitate the tube. *Agitation may cause RBC hemolysis.*
4. Send tube to the laboratory.
Biopsy:
1. Place client in supine position in surgical suite or procedure room.
2. A specimen of infected tissue is biopsied by excision or needle biopsy. Place specimen in container.
3. Send specimen to laboratory.

Clinical Implications and Indications:
1. Detects the presence of echinococcosis

Nursing Care:
Before Test: Explain the test procedure and the purpose of the test. Assess the client's knowledge of the test. Provide preprocedure sedation and analgesia as ordered. Transport client to operating or procedure room. Drape client appropriately.
During Test: Adhere to sterile technique and standard precautions. Biopsy: Provide reassurance and a calm atmosphere during the procedure.
After Test: Blood: Apply pressure to venipuncture site. Explain that some bruising, discomfort, and swelling may appear at the site and that warm, moist compresses can alleviate this. Monitor for signs of infection. Biopsy: Clean site of biopsy and apply dressing to site. Provide analgesia as necessary. Continue to offer emotional support and inform client that results of the test will take several days.

Potential Complications: Bleeding and bruising at site

Interfering Factors: False positives may result from cirrhosis, collagen diseases, SLE, and schistosomiasis.

Nursing Considerations:
Pediatric: Children are highly at risk due to the dominant host being the dog.
Rural: Those living in rural settings are at risk due to the incidence of parasite infestations in sheep and cattle.

WEBLINKS

www.healthgate.com

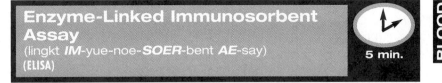

Enzyme-Linked Immunosorbent Assay
(lingkt *IM*-yue-noe-*SOER*-bent *AE*-say)
(ELISA)

5 min.

BLOOD

Type of Test: Blood

Body Systems and Functions: Immunological system

Normal Findings: Negative for HIV antibody and other autoimmune disorders

Test Results Time Frame: Within 24 hr

Test Description: ELISA detects the antibodies that result from exposure to HIV, which is the virus that causes AIDS and AIDS-related complex (ARC). The virus infects the T-helper lymphocytes and affects the ability to produce antibodies, which decreases the immune response. Antigens can be detected as early as 2 weeks after exposure to the virus, and they can remain for 2–4 months. However, the antibodies can take up to a year to be detected. A repeat testing of a positive ELISA is performed, and then follow-up tests of a Western blot (WB) and indirect fluorescent antibody (IFA) to confirm the presence of antibodies to HIV-1. The lack of confirmation of HIV with negative WB and IFA testing does not preclude infection, and therefore, repeat testing in 3–6 months is suggested.

CLINICAL ALERT:
Legal restrictions exist and vary regarding HIV testing and reporting of results. Therefore, careful consideration must be given in allowing access to the ELISA test result. However, health care workers directly involved with client care need to know whether the client tests positive to protect themselves from exposure.

Consent Form: Required

List of Equipment: Red-top tube or serum separator tube; needle and syringe or vacutainer; alcohol swab

Test Procedure:
1. Label the specimen tube. *Correctly identifies the client and the test to be performed.*
2. Obtain a 5-mL blood sample.
3. Do not agitate the tube. *Agitation may cause RBC hemolysis.*
4. Send tube to the laboratory.

Clinical Implications and Indications:
1. Diagnoses HIV infection
2. Determines infection for the use of blood transfusion

Nursing Care:
Before Test: Explain the test procedure and the purpose of the test. Assess the client's knowledge of the test.

During Test: Adhere to standard precautions.

After Test: Inform the client that other tests may be required if the ELISA is positive to confirm diagnosis. Also instruct client that a repeat test may be necessary in 3–6 months. Apply pressure to venipuncture site. Explain that some bruising, discomfort, and swelling may appear at the site and that warm, moist compresses can alleviate this. Monitor for signs of infection.

Potential Complications: Bleeding and bruising at venipuncture site

Interfering Factors: False-positive tests may result (often due to the length of time between transmission and seroconversion); negative results may occur with advanced AIDS from severe immunological disorders resulting in absence of detectable antibodies; previous exposure to HIV; the protein medium used in the test kits

Nursing Considerations:
Pediatric: Infants and children will need assistance in remaining still during the venipuncture and age-appropriate comfort measures following the test.
Home Care: Clients in home settings with ARC have many teaching needs as well as supportive emotional needs. The care provider must individualize client care and provide accurate information to family and significant others regarding transmission and exposure considerations.

Listing of Related Tests: Western blot; indirect fluorescent antibody (IFA); Genie assay; radioimmunoprecipitation

WEBLINKS

http://www.nlm.nih.gov

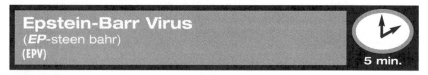

Epstein-Barr Virus
(*EP*-steen bahr)
(EPV)

5 min.

Type of Test: Blood

Body Systems and Functions: Immunological system

Normal Findings: Negative

Test Results Time Frame: Within 72 hr

Test Description: The Epstein-Barr virus is a herpes virus that is very common and is the causative agent of mononucleosis. EPV is also thought to cause Burkitt's lymphoma, nasopharyngeal cancer, and chronic fatigue syndrome. Epstein-Barr increases the formation of abnormal leukocytes in the lymph nodes and stimulates increased heterophil antibody formation. Common clinical manifestations of Epstein-Barr include fever, lethargy, pharyngitis, and lymphadenopathy. The virus is spread through direct contact and has an incubation period of 4–8 weeks.

Consent Form: Not required

List of Equipment: Red-top tube or serum separator tube; needle and syringe or vacutainer; alcohol swab

Test Procedure:
1. Label the specimen tube. *Correctly identifies the client and the test to be performed.*
2. Obtain a 3-mL blood sample.
3. Do not agitate the tube. *Agitation may cause RBC hemolysis.*
4. Send tube to the laboratory.

Clinical Implications and Indications:
1. Elevated levels are found with infectious mononucleosis, Epstein-Barr virus, head and neck tumors, infectious hepatitis, sarcoidosis, nasopharyngeal cancer, systemic lupus erythematosus, and leukemia.
2. Heterophil antibodies will remain elevated for 8–12 weeks after symptoms appear.

Nursing Care:
Before Test: Explain the test procedure and the purpose of the test. Assess the client's knowledge of the test.
During Test: Adhere to standard precautions.
After Test: Apply pressure to venipuncture site. Explain that some bruising, discomfort, and swelling may appear at the site and that warm, moist compresses can alleviate this. Monitor for signs of infection.

Potential Complications: Bleeding and bruising at venipuncture site

Interfering Factors: Posttransfusion reactions; collagen vascular diseases

Nursing Considerations:
Pediatric: Infants and children will need assistance in remaining still during the venipuncture and age-appropriate comfort measures following the test.
Gerontology: The Epstein-Barr viruses are potentially very serious to the elderly person.
Home Care: The health care provider needs to consider Epstein-Barr viruses when clients are unusually lethargic and inform clients of diagnostic testing.

Listing of Related Tests: Monospot screen

| WEBLINKS |

www.healthgate.com

Estriol
(*ES*-tree-ahl)
(estrogen fractions; E3)

Blood: 5 min.
Urine: 24 hr.

Type of Test: Blood; urine

Body Systems and Functions: Endocrine system

Normal Findings:

Blood (during pregnancy):

Week	ng/mL
34	5.3–18.3
35	5.2–26.4
36	8.2–28.1
37	8.0–30.1
38	8.6–38.0
39	7.2–34.3
40	9.6–28.9

Urine (results are determined by radioimmunoassay): Values vary considerably, but serial measurements of urine estriol levels plotted on a graph should describe a steadily rising curve.

Test Results Time Frame: Within 24–48 hr

Test Description: The estriol test measures the amount of estriol in the blood. Estriol is a specific type of estrogen hormone. The most common use of estriol measurements is in the evaluation of fetal status during pregnancy. Serial urine and blood studies for estriol excretion provide an objective means of assessing placental function and fetal normality in high-risk pregnancies. Excretion of estriol increases around the eighth week of gestation and continues to rise until shortly before delivery. Rising values indicate an adequately functioning fetus. Decreasing values suggest fetoplacental deterioration.

Consent Form: Not required

List of Equipment: *Blood:* red-top tube or serum separator tube; needle and syringe or vacutainer; alcohol swab. *Urine:* sterile plastic container; ice.

Test Procedure:

Blood:

1. Label the specimen tube. *Correctly identifies the client and the test to be performed.*
2. Obtain a 5-mL blood sample.
3. Do not agitate the tube. *Agitation may cause RBC hemolysis.*
4. Send tube to the laboratory.

Urine:

1. Label the collection container. *Correctly identifies the client and the test to be performed.*
2. Discard the first morning void. Then begin the time of the collection for the next 24 hr, including the void at the end of the 24 hr, and record the last voiding time. *An exact 24-hr count ensures accurate results.*
3. If the client has an indwelling catheter in place, keep the drainage bag on ice and empty the urine into the urine container periodically during the 24-hr period.
4. Keep urine cool during collection. *Higher temperatures alter the results.*
5. If any urine is lost, discard the entire specimen and begin collection again the next day.

◢ **mplications and Indications:**
    levels are found with adrenal tumor, multiple pregnancy, ovarian
    nd testicular tumor.
2. Decreased levels are found with adrenogenital syndrome, congenital anom-
    alies, failing pregnancy, fetal dysmaturity, fetal distress and death, hypopitu-
    itarism, menopause, placental insufficiency, preeclampsia/eclampsia, Stein-
    Leventhal syndrome, and Turner's syndrome.
3. Serum levels are used in combination with HCG and AFP serum levels to
    screen for Down's syndrome.
4. Decreased urine levels are found with congenital anomalies, such as anen-
    cephaly, fetal adrenal insufficiency, placental sulfatase deficiency, and Rh
    isoimmunization.

Nursing Care:

Before Test: Explain the test procedure and the purpose of the test. Assess the
client's knowledge of the test. For 24-hr urine, instruct client not to discard any
urine. Obtain a history of recent tests using radioactive dyes.
During Test: Adhere to standard precautions. If any urine is accidentally discarded or contaminated with feces, discard entire specimen and begin test again the
following morning.
After Test: Blood: Apply pressure to venipuncture site. Explain that some bruising, discomfort, and swelling may appear at the site and that warm, moist compresses can alleviate this. Monitor for signs of infection. Urine: Document urine
quantity, date, and exact hours of collection on requisition.

Potential Complications: Bleeding and bruising at venipuncture site

Interfering Factors: Urine contaminated with feces; spillage or inaccurate
collection of the 24-hr specimen, including nonrefrigeration or placing on ice;
heavy bleeding during menstruation; urinary tract infections; abnormal hemoglobin of mother; anemia; malnutrition; liver disease; intestinal disease; medications
that may increase levels are adrenocorticosteroids (corticosteroids), estrogen-con-
taining drugs, phenothiazines, and tetracyclines; a medication that can decrease
test measurements is clomiphene; medications that may affect urine test results
are ampicillin, cascara sagrada, corticosteroids, estrogens, hydrochlorothiazide,
meprobamate, methenamine mandelate, phenazopyridine hydrochloride, phe-
nolphthalein, phenothiazines, progesterone, senna, steroids, and tetracyclines.

Nursing Considerations:

*Pregnancy: Used in combination with other tests to determine fetal well-being and
the functioning of the fetus. Provide emotional support for client anxiety due to
concerns about the fetus.*
*Pediatric: Blood: Infants and children will need assistance in remaining still dur-
ing the venipuncture and age-appropriate comfort measures following the test.
Urine: A collection bag or indwelling catheter needs to be used for infants and toddlers.*
*Home Care: Urine test can be collected at home for 24 hr provided proper proce-
dure is followed.*

Listing of Related Tests: SalEst

WEBLINKS ▯ 🗏🗵

http://adam.excite.com

Estrodial
(es-tra-*DI*-ol)
(E2; estrogen fractions)

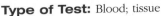

Blood: 5 min.
Biopsy: 15-30 min.

Type of Test: Blood; tissue

Body Systems and Functions: Endocrine system

Normal Findings:

		SI units
Menstruating females:		
Early cycle	20–70 pg/mL	73–626 pmol/L
Midcycle	70–500 pg/mL	258–1840 pmol/L
Late cycle	45–340 pg/mL	166–1251 pmol/L
Postmenopausal	15–18 pg/mL	18.4–66 pmol/L
Adult males	10–50 pg/mL	37–184 pmol/L
Prepubescent males	2–8 pg/mL	11–29 pmol/L

Estrodial receptor levels (in breast cancer): negative; positive levels when >10 fmol/mg cytosol protein

Test Results Time Frame: Blood: within 24 hr. Biopsy: within 2–4 days.

Test Description: Blood: Estradiol is an estrogenic hormone secreted by the ovaries. Estradiol stimulates endometrial growth in preparation for the progestational stage. Estradiol also suppresses FSH and stimulates LH. Estrodial diminishes or stops during menopause. Biopsy: Estrogen and progesterone levels are evaluated in breast cancer cells to determine whether the tissue will likely respond to hormonal therapy or to the removal of the ovaries. The biopsy is an invasive procedure that is performed with strict sterile technique. An excision or needle punch sample of body tissue is taken and examined microscopically for cell morphology and tissue anomalies.

CLINICAL ALERT:
Do not place biopsy specimen in formalin.

Consent Form: Not required

List of Equipment: *Blood:* red-top tube or serum separator tube; needle and syringe or vacutainer; alcohol swab. *Biopsy:* biopsy tray.

Test Procedure:
Blood:
1. Label the specimen tube and include the present menstrual cycle phase.
   Correctly identifies the client and the test to be performed.
2. Obtain a 3-mL blood sample.
3. Do not agitate the tube. *Agitation may cause RBC hemolysis.*
4. Send tube to the laboratory.
Biopsy:
1. Place client in supine position.

2. A 1-g specimen of breast tissue is biopsied by excision or needle biopsy. Place specimen in container.
3. Send specimen to laboratory.

Clinical Implications and Indications:
Blood:
1. Elevated levels are found with adrenal tumors, cirrhosis, hyperthyroidism, liver tumors, ovarian neoplasm, and polycystic ovary syndrome.
2. Decreased levels are found with amenorrhea, anorexia nervosa, hypopituitarism, infertility, menopause, osteoporosis, and ovarian hypofunction.

Biopsy:
1. A positive test for estrogen occurs at levels greater than 3 fmol and for progesterone binding at levels of 5 fmol and above.
2. Greater than half of positive estrogen tumors will respond to endocrine therapy.
3. Estrogen negative tumors will rarely respond to endocrine therapy.

Nursing Care:
Before Test: Explain the test procedure and the purpose of the test. Assess the client's knowledge of the test. Provide preprocedure sedation and analgesia as ordered. Transport client to operating or procedure room. Drape client appropriately.

During Test: Adhere to standard precautions. Biopsy: provide reassurance and a calm atmosphere during the procedure.

After Test: Blood: Apply pressure to venipuncture site. Explain that some bruising, discomfort, and swelling may appear at the site and that warm, moist compresses can alleviate this. Monitor for signs of infection. Biopsy: Clean site of biopsy and apply dressing to site. Provide analgesia as necessary. Continue to offer emotional support and inform client that results of the test will take several days.

Potential Complications: Bleeding and bruising at site

Interfering Factors: Antiestrogen preparations taken within previous 2 months; medications that alter results are ampicillin, cascara, cortisone, hydrochlorothiazide, meprobamates, phenazopyridine, and tetracyclines.

⌷UEBLINKS ▷

www.healthgate.com

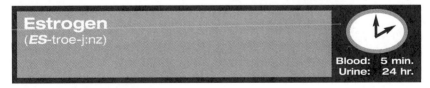

Estrogen
(***ES***-troe-j:nz)

Blood: 5 min.
Urine: 24 hr.

Type of Test: Blood; urine

Body Systems and Functions: Endocrine system

Normal Findings:

		SI units
Blood:		
Premenopausal	60–400 pg/mL	60–400 ng/L
Postmenopausal	<130 pg/mL	<130 ng/L
Males	20–80 pg/mL	10–130 ng/L
Children	<25 pg/mL	<25 ng/L
Urine:		
Females:		
Follicular phase	7–65 g/g creatinine	0.79–7.35 mg/mol creatinine
Midcycle phase	32–104 g/g creatinine	3.62–11.75 mg/mol creatinine
Luteal phase	8–135 g/g creatinine	0.90–15.26 mg/mol creatinine
Males	4–23 g/g creatinine	0.45–2.60 mg/mol creatinine

Test Results Time Frame: Within 48 hr

Test Description: Estrogen is a hormone that is made in the ovaries, testes, placenta, and adrenals. Estrogen assists in developing and maintaining the female sex organs. Estrogen levels change throughout the menstrual cycle, with the greatest amounts being produced during ovulation and the latter phase of the cycle. In addition, estrogen levels greatly decrease during pregnancy and menopause. Both serum and urine levels may be obtained individually or together for evaluation of estrogen levels.

Consent Form: Not required

List of Equipment: *Blood:* red-top tube or serum separator tube; needle and syringe or vacutainer; alcohol swab. *Urine:* sterile plastic container; ice.

Test Procedure:
Blood:
1. Label the specimen tube. Write age, sex, current menstrual cycle phase on sample. *Correctly identifies the client and the test to be performed.*
2. Obtain a 1.5-mL blood sample.
3. Do not agitate the tube. *Agitation may cause RBC hemolysis.*
4. Send tube to the laboratory.
5. Keep specimen on ice. *High temperatures alter the results.*

Urine:
1. Label the collection container. *Correctly identifies the client and the test to be performed.*
2. Discard the first morning void. Then begin the time of the collection for the next 24 hr, including the void at the end of the 24 hr, and record the last voiding time. *An exact 24-hr count ensures accurate results.*
3. If the client has an indwelling catheter in place, keep the drainage bag on ice and empty the urine into the urine container periodically during the 24-hr period.
4. Keep urine cool during collection. *Higher temperatures alter the results.*
5. If any urine is lost, discard the entire specimen and begin collection again the next day.

Clinical Implications and Indications:
1. Elevated levels are found with amenorrhea, fibrocystic disease, corpus leuteum cyst, ovarian or testicular tumors, and virilization.

BLOOD

2. Decreased levels are found with amenorrhea, anorexia nervosa, dysmenorrhea, infertility, menopause, menstruation, osteoporosis, ovarian dysfunction, and Turner's syndrome.

Nursing Care:

Before Test: Explain the test procedure and the purpose of the test. Assess the client's knowledge of the test. Instruct client not to discard any urine over the 24-hr time period.

During Test: Adhere to standard precautions. If any urine is accidentally discarded or contaminated with feces, discard entire specimen and begin test again the following morning.

After Test: Apply pressure to venipuncture site. Explain that some bruising, discomfort, and swelling may appear at the site and that warm, moist compresses can alleviate this. Monitor for signs of infection. Document urine quantity, date, and exact hours of collection on requisition.

Potential Complications: Bleeding and bruising at venipuncture site

Interfering Factors: Urine contaminated with feces; spillage or inaccurate collection of the 24-hr specimen, including nonrefrigeration or placing on ice; heavy bleeding during menstruation; radioactive scan within prior 48 hr; medications that increase results are cascara, estrogens, levodopa, oral contraceptives, phenothiazines, testosterone, tetracyclines, and vitamins; medications that decrease results are acetazolamide, cascara, glucose, hydrochlorothiazide, phenothiazines, tetracyclines, and vitamins.

Nursing Considerations:

Pregnancy: This test does not measure estriol and therefore should not be used in pregnancy or to evaluate fetal well-being.

Pediatric: Infants and children will need assistance in remaining still during the venipuncture and age-appropriate comfort measures following the test. For collection of 24-hr specimen a collection bag or indwelling catheter needs to be used for infants and toddlers.

WEBLINKS

www.ncbi.nlm.nih.gov

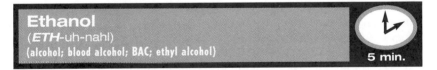

Ethanol
(*ETH*-uh-nahl)
(alcohol; blood alcohol; BAC; ethyl alcohol)

5 min.

Type of Test: Blood

Body Systems and Functions: Hematological system

Normal Findings:

		SI units
Negative		
Intoxication	>150 mg/dL	32.5 mmol/L
Coma	>300 mg/dL	>65.1 mmol/L

CRITICAL VALUES:
300 mg/dL

Test Results Time Frame: Within 24 hr

Test Description: Ethanol is absorbed very rapidly from the GI tract, with peak blood levels occurring in 40–70 min on an empty stomach. Ethanol is metabolized in the liver and when consumed in excess causes hepatocellular damage. When severe clinical manifestations of intoxication are seen in the presence of low alcohol levels, there could be a serious pathological condition. Ethanol is a central nervous system depressant, acts as an anesthetic, and is a diuretic. Ethanol may be given as an inhibitor to the labor process.

CLINICAL ALERT:
Extremely high levels may be fatal and need immediate treatment if there is an overdose (note: tolerance to alcohol occurs in chronic alcoholism).

Consent Form: Not required

List of Equipment: Red-top tube or gray-top tube or serum separator tube; needle and syringe or vacutainer; nonalcohol swab

Test Procedure:
1 Label the specimen tube. *Correctly identifies the client and the test to be performed.*
2. If specimen is being collected for legal purposes, a witness is needed for sample collection.
3. Obtain a 3-mL blood sample.
4. Do not agitate the tube. *Agitation may cause RBC hemolysis.*
5. Send tube to the laboratory.

Clinical Implications and Indications:
1. Diagnoses the severity of alcohol ingestion (note: many substances contain alcohol: shaving lotion, liniments, fluid extracts, elixirs, tinctures, and cough medicines)
2. Evaluates alcohol levels, which can also be determined with breath tests

Nursing Care:
Before Test: Explain the test procedure and the purpose of the test. Assess the client's knowledge of the test. Cleanse the site with nonalcoholic swab (e.g., povidone-iodine). Assess the overdose clinical manifestations potentially present.
During Test: Adhere to standard precautions. Continue to assess any symptomatology of further CNS deterioration.
After Test: Continue to assess for CNS depression. Apply pressure to venipuncture site. Explain that some bruising, discomfort, and swelling may appear at the site and that warm, moist compresses can alleviate this. Monitor for signs of infection.

Potential Complications: Bleeding and bruising at venipuncture site

Interfering Factors: Increased blood ketones; isopropanol; methanol

Nursing Considerations:
Pregnancy: Child-bearing-aged women should be instructed not to drink any form of alcohol due to the harm for the fetus (especially if there is suspected pregnancy).

Pediatric: Infants and children will need assistance in remaining still during the venipuncture and age-appropriate comfort measures following the test. Note: Very small amounts of alcohol consumption in children are potentially very serious.
Gerontology: The older person with alcoholism may tolerate higher alcohol levels due to tolerance to the drug.
Home Care: Health care providers need to assess the amount of alcohol consumed in their clients and evaluate their clinical manifestations for potential referral to counseling for the alcoholism.

Listing of Related Tests: Alcohol breath test

WEBLINKS

www.thriveonline.com; http://www.alcoholicsanonymous.org

Euglobulin Lysis Time
(yue-*GLAHB*-yue-*LIN LIY*-sis)
(euglobulin clot lysis; firinolysis/euglobulin lysis)

5 min.

Type of Test: Blood

Body Systems and Functions: Hematological system

Normal Findings: Lysis in 1.5–4 hr

CRITICAL VALUES:
100% lysis in 1 hr (note: lysis in less than 1 hr indicates excessive fribrinolytic activity)

Test Results Time Frame: Within 24 hr

Test Description: Euglobulin lysis time measures the clotting activities by evaluating plasminogen and plasminogen activator. These substances are proteins that prevent fibrin clot formations. Fibrinolysis is essential to normal hemostasis and clotting/dissolution is constantly occurring. When this system is dysfunctioning, a fibrin clot will dissolve immediately and result in a bleeding tendency. The effects of thrombolytic medications (e.g., streptokinase, urokinase) are assessed by euglobulin testing. In this test, the lysis time is evaluated by adding the client's plasma to a blood clot and observed for 6–24 hr (labeled the euglobulin lysis time).

CLINICAL ALERT:
If client has severely lengthened clotting times, place on bleeding precautions and monitor neurological symptoms of intracerebral bleeding.

Consent Form: Not required

List of Equipment: Three blue-top tubes; needles and syringes or vacutainers; alcohol swabs; ice

Test Procedure:
1. Label the specimen tube. *Correctly identifies the client and the test to be performed.*

BLOOD

2. Obtain a 5-mL blood sample.
3. Do not agitate the tube. *Agitation may cause RBC hemolysis.*
4. Send tube to the laboratory.
5. Keep specimen on ice. *High temperatures alter the results.*

Clinical Implications and Indications:

1. Elevated levels are found with cirrhosis, shock, DIC, incompatible blood transfusion, malignancies, and thrombolytic medications.
2. Decreased levels are found with prematurity and diabetes.

Nursing Care:

Before Test: Explain the test procedure and the purpose of the test. Assess the client's knowledge of the test. Instruct client to avoid strenuous activity for 1 hr prior to test.
During Test: Adhere to standard precautions.
After Test: Apply pressure to venipuncture site (note: may need to leave pressure on for 3–5 min if there is prolonged clotting time). Explain that some bruising, discomfort, and swelling may appear at the site and that warm, moist compresses can alleviate this. Monitor for signs of infection.

Potential Complications: Bleeding and bruising at venipuncture site

Interfering Factors: Exercising within 1 hr of test; venipuncture that is preceded by pumping the fist or massaging the vein; anticoagulants

Nursing Considerations:

Pediatric: Infants and children will need assistance in remaining still during the venipuncture and age-appropriate comfort measures following the test.

Listing of Related Tests: Diluted whole-blood clot lysis

║║WEBLINKS ☐☒

www.ncbi.nlm.nih.gov

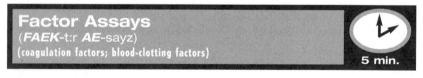

Factor Assays
(*FAEK*-t:r *AE*-sayz)
(coagulation factors; blood-clotting factors)

5 min.

Type of Test: Blood

Body Systems and Functions: Hematological system

Normal Findings:

		SI units
Factor I	200–400 mg/mL	2.0–4.0 U
Factor II	70–130 mg/100 mL	0.7–1.3 U
Factor V	70–130 mg/100 mL	0.7–1.3 U
Factor VII	70–130 mg/100 mL	0.7–1.3 U
Factor X	70–130 mg/100 mL	0.7–1.3 U
Factor VIII	50–200 mg/100 mL	0.5–2.0 U

Factor IX	70–130 mg/100 mL	0.7–1.3 U
Factor XI	70–130 mg/100 mL	0.7–1.3 U
Factor XII	30–225 mg/100 mL	0.3–2.2 U
Factor XIII	Dissolution of formed clot within 24 hr	

Normal laboratory findings vary among laboratory settings.

CRITICAL VALUES:
See individual assay test.

Test Results Time Frame: Within 24 hr

Test Description: Factor assays are tests that are definitive measurements of coagulation factors. The factor assays are used to differentiate among mild, moderate, and severe coagulation disorders and to monitor the therapies of factor inhibitors. The normal mechanisms of circulating coagulation factors are activated on the surface of the aggregated platelets, forming fibrin, which anchors the platelet plug to the site of the injury. Many factors are involved in the reaction cascade that forms fibrin. It is these individual factors that are measured in factor assays.

CLINICAL ALERT:
If client has severely lengthened clotting times, place on bleeding precautions and monitor neurological symptoms of intracerebral bleeding.

Consent Form: Not required

List of Equipment: Blood specimen tube specific to assay; needle and syringe or vacutainer; alcohol swab

Test Procedure:
1. Label the specimen tube. *Correctly identifies the client and the test to be performed.*
2. Obtain a 5-mL blood sample.
3. Gently invert tube several times, but do not agitate the tube. *Mixes the anticoagulant, but agitation may cause RBC hemolysis.*
4. Send tube to the laboratory.

Clinical Implications and Indications:
1. Definitively evaluates and monitors prolonged PT or PTT
2. Monitors the effects of disorders or drugs that are known causes of deficiencies in clotting factors

Nursing Care:
Before Test: Explain the test procedure and the purpose of the test. Assess the client's knowledge of the test. Note the time and dose of last anticoagulant, if pertinent.
During Test: Adhere to standard precautions.
After Test: Apply pressure to venipuncture site (note: may need to leave pressure on for 3–5 min if there is prolonged clotting time). Explain that some bruising, discomfort, and swelling may appear at the site and that warm, moist compresses can alleviate this. Monitor for signs of infection.

Potential Complications: Bleeding and bruising at venipuncture site

Interfering Factors: Venipuncture that is preceded by pumping the fist or massaging the vein; anticoagulants

Nursing Considerations:

Pediatric: Infants and children will need assistance in remaining still during the venipuncture and age-appropriate comfort measures following the test.

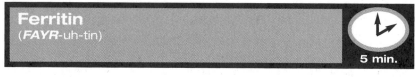

WEBLINKS

www.ncbi.nlm.nih.gov

Ferritin
(*FAYR*-uh-tin)

5 min.

Type of Test: Blood

Body Systems and Functions: Hematological system

Normal Findings:

		SI units
Adult Females:		
<40 years	11–22 ng/mL	11–22 mg/L
>40 years	12–263 ng/mL	12–263 mg/L
Adult Males:	15–200 ng/mL	15–200 mg/L
Children:		
Newborn	25–200 ng/mL	25–200 mg/L
1 month	200–600 ng/mL	20–600 mg/L
2–5 months	50–200 ng/mL	50–200 mg/L
6 months–15 years	7–140 ng/mL	7–140 mg/L

Test Results Time Frame: Within 2–4 days

Test Description: Ferritin is an iron-storing protein that is made in the liver, spleen, bone marrow, tumor cells, and inflammatory areas. This test evaluates whether iron is being adequately stored in the body, even though its production may be normal. Menstruating women are an example of persons who may have less iron storage, and the different anemias can sometimes be distinguished by the ferritin levels.

Consent Form: Not required

List of Equipment: Red-top tube or serum separator tube; needle and syringe or vacutainer; alcohol swab

Test Procedure:
1. Label the specimen tube. *Correctly identifies the client and the test to be performed.*
2. Obtain a 1-mL blood sample.
3. Do not agitate the tube. *Agitation may cause RBC hemolysis.*
4. Send tube to the laboratory.

BLOOD

Clinical Implications and Indications:

1. Increased levels are found with anemia, cancer, cirrhosis, hepatic disease, leukemia, inflammation, tissue trauma, multiple myeloma, jaundice, siderosis, thalasssemia, Hodgkin's disease, and renal disease.
2. Decreased levels are found with anemia, hemodialysis, pregnancy, and GI surgery.
3. Evaluates and differentiates among various types of anemias.

Nursing Care:

Before Test: Explain the test procedure and the purpose of the test. Assess the client's knowledge of the test.

During Test: Adhere to standard precautions.

After Test: Apply pressure to venipuncture site. Explain that some bruising, discomfort, and swelling may appear at the site and that warm, moist compresses can alleviate this. Monitor for signs of infection.

Potential Complications: Bleeding and bruising at venipuncture site

Interfering Factors: Radioactive scan within previous 48 hr

Nursing Considerations:

Pregnancy: Iron deficiencies are somewhat common and ferritin abnormalities can be anticipated in pregnancy.

Pediatric: Infants and children will need assistance in remaining still during the venipuncture and age-appropriate comfort measures following the test.

Listing of Related Tests: Serum iron; transferrin; total iron-binding capacity

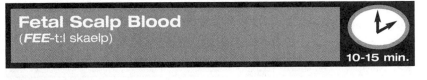

WEBLINKS

http://www.webmd.com

Fetal Scalp Blood
(*FEE*-t:l skaelp)

10-15 min.

Type of Test: Blood

Body Systems and Functions: Hematological system

Normal Findings:

pH	7.25–7.35
PO_2	18–22 mm Hg
PCO_2	40–50 mm Hg
Base excess	0–10 mEq/L
Oxygen saturation	30%–50%

Test Results Time Frame: Within 24 hr

Test Description: Fetal scalp blood testing evaluates the acid-base condition of the fetus, which is an excellent screening of fetal distress. The acid-base balance of the bloodstream is vital to fetal viability and is a physiological reflection of many systems in the fetus. Acid-base controls are particularly influenced by the combined functioning of the cardiovascular, renal, and respiratory systems. Fetal hypoxia results in an increased release of lactic acid, which decreases blood pH and causes acidosis. There is a high correlation between fetal acidosis and morbidity/mortality in the fetus. The pH is of primary consideration in evaluating the components of acid-base balance in the fetus.

Consent Form: Required

List of Equipment: Amnioscopy equipment; scalpel; capillary tubes; petroleum jelly; cotton ball

Test Procedure:
1. Place mother in lithotomy position and perform amnioscopy.
2. Apply petroleum jelly to fetal scalp. *Causes droplets of fetal blood to bead.*
3. Obtain capillary tube sample of fetal scalp blood with metal blade.
4. Apply firm pressure to bleeding area. *Stops bleeding.*
5. Send sample to laboratory.

Clinical Implications and Indications:
1. Evaluates and monitors fetal distress

Nursing Care:
Before Test: Explain the test procedure and the purpose of the test. Assess the client's knowledge of the test.
During Test: Adhere to standard precautions.
After Test: If test reveals fetal distress, provide emotional support. Client may experience menstrual-like cramping and some vaginal discomfort.

Potential Complications: Hematoma; hemorrhaging; infection; bruising

Contraindications: Premature membrane rupture; active cervical infection

Nursing Considerations:
Pediatric: Abnormalities of the fetus may be detected in time to facilitate effective interventions.

Listing of Related Tests: Fetal nonstress

WEBLINKS ▤ ☒

http://adam.excite.com

Fibrin Degradation Products
(fiy-*BRIN DEG*-ruh-*DAY*-sh:n *PRAH*-duhkts)
(FDP; fibrin breakdown products; fibrin split products)

5 min.

Type of Test: Blood

Body Systems and Functions: Hematological system

Normal Findings: <10 mg/mL or <10 mg/L (SI units)

CRITICAL VALUES:
> 40 mg/mL

Test Results Time Frame: Within 24 hr

Test Description: Fibrin degradation products is a test that directly measures the effectiveness of the clotting process. There are four products (e.g., D, E, X, Y) that are formed during the dissolving of clots. These substances are indicative of recent clotting activity. If present in increased amounts, they act as anticoagulants.

Consent Form: Not required

List of Equipment: Blue-top tube; needle and syringe or vacutainer; alcohol swab

Test Procedure:
1. Label the specimen tube. *Correctly identifies the client and the test to be performed.*
2. Obtain a 2-mL blood sample.
3. Do not agitate the tube. *Agitation may cause RBC hemolysis.*
4. Send tube to the laboratory.

Clinical Implications and Indications:
1. Elevated levels are found with blood transfusion reactions, thromboembolic states, cancer, DVT, congenital heart disease, DIC, preeclampsia, sepsis, shock, sunstroke, and extensive tissue damage.
2. Decreased levels are not significant.

Nursing Care:
Before Test: Explain the test procedure and the purpose of the test. Assess the client's knowledge of the test.
During Test: Adhere to standard precautions.
After Test: Apply pressure for prolonged time (5 min) to venipuncture site. Explain that some bruising, discomfort, and swelling may appear at the site and that warm, moist compresses can alleviate this. Monitor for signs of infection.

Potential Complications: Bleeding and bruising at venipuncture site

Interfering Factors: Traumatic venipuncture; medications that alter results are barbiturates, heparin, urokinase, and streptokinase.

Nursing Considerations:
Pediatric: Infants and children will need assistance in remaining still during the venipuncture and age-appropriate comfort measures following the test.
Home Care: Health care providers should assess for clinical manifestations of spontaneous bleeding (e.g., nosebleeds, ecchymosis).

Listing of Related Tests: Partial thromboplastin time

WEBLINKS

www.ncbi.nlm.nih.gov

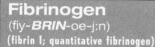

Fibrinogen
(fiy-*BRIN*-oe-j:n)
(fibrin I; quantitative fibrinogen)

5 min.

Type of Test: Blood

Body Systems and Functions: Hematological system

Normal Findings:

		SI units
Adult	200–400 mg/dL	2–4 g/L
Newborn	125-300 mg/dL	1-3 mg/L

CRITICAL VALUES:
<100 mg/dL

Test Results Time Frame: Within 24 hr

Test Description: Fibrinogen is a test that measures the effectiveness of the clotting process. Fibrinogen (factor I) is a complex polypeptide that is converted to fibrin after thrombin enzyme action and combines with platelets to clot the blood. Fibrinogen is made in the liver and is increased in disorders associated with tissue damage or inflammation. This test is determined by adding thrombin to the plasma, measuring the amount of time taken for clotting, and determining the amount of fibrin that is calculated based on the thrombin clotting time.

Consent Form: Not required

List of Equipment: Blue-top tube; needle and syringe or vacutainer; alcohol swab

Test Procedure:
1. Label the specimen tube. *Correctly identifies the client and the test to be performed.*
2. Obtain a 5-mL blood sample.
3. Do not agitate the tube. *Agitation may cause RBC hemolysis.*
4. Send tube to the laboratory.

Clinical Implications and Indications:
1. Elevated levels are found with arthritis, acute inflammation, CHD, hepatitis, menstruation, cigarette smoking, pregnancy, and trauma.
2. Decreased levels are found with abortion, liver disorders, cancer, DIC, eclampsia, malnutrition, septicemia, embolism, shock, and transfusion reaction.

Nursing Care:
Before Test: Explain the test procedure and the purpose of the test. Assess the client's knowledge of the test.
During Test: Adhere to standard precautions.
After Test: Apply pressure for prolonged time (5 min) to venipuncture site. Explain that some bruising, discomfort, and swelling may appear at the site and that warm, moist compresses can alleviate this. Monitor for signs of infection.

Potential Complications: Bleeding and bruising at venipuncture site

Interfering Factors: Blood transfusions within the month prior to this test; medications that decrease results are asparaginase, phenobarbital drug poisoning, urokinase, and streptokinase; medications that increase results are estrogen and oral contraceptives.

Nursing Considerations:
Pediatric: Infants and children will need assistance in remaining still during the venipuncture and age-appropriate comfort measures following the test.
Home Care: Health care providers should assess for clinical manifestations of spontaneous bleeding (e.g., nosebleeds, ecchymosis).

Listing of Related Tests: Partial thromboplastin time

WEBLINKS

www.ncbi.nlm.nih.gov

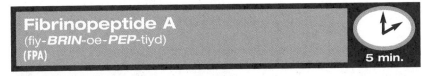

Fibrinopeptide A
(fiy-***BRIN***-oe-***PEP***-tiyd)
(FPA)   5 min.

Type of Test: Blood

Body Systems and Functions: Hematological system

Normal Findings: Negative

Test Results Time Frame: Within 24 hr

Test Description: Fibrinopeptide A reflects the amount of active intravascular blood clotting (often seen in DIC). FPA is a very sensitive assay performed to evaluate thrombin activity involved in clotting. Increases in FPA levels can occur without intravascular thrombosis, which decreases the value of a positive test.

CLINICAL ALERT:
DIC is a critical condition and the initial clinical manifestations of bleeding tendencies need immediate attention.

Consent Form: Not required

List of Equipment: Red-top tube or serum separator tube; needle and syringe or vacutainer; alcohol swab

Test Procedure:
1. Label the specimen tube. *Correctly identifies the client and the test to be performed.*
2. Obtain a 5-mL blood sample.
3. Do not agitate the tube. *Agitation may cause RBC hemolysis.*
4. Send tube to the laboratory.

BLOOD

Clinical Implications and Indications:
1. Elevated levels are found with DVT, DIC, infections, leukemia, postoperative conditions, and tumors.
2. Decreased levels are found with leukemia remissions.

Nursing Care:
Before Test: Explain the test procedure and the purpose of the test. Assess the client's knowledge of the test.
During Test: Adhere to standard precautions.
After Test: Apply pressure to venipuncture site. Explain that some bruising, discomfort, and swelling may appear at the site and that warm, moist compresses can alleviate this. Monitor for signs of infection.

Potential Complications: Bleeding and bruising at venipuncture site

Interfering Factors: Traumatic venipuncture

Nursing Considerations:
Pediatric: Infants and children will need assistance in remaining still during the venipuncture and age-appropriate comfort measures following the test.
Home Care: Health care providers should assess for clinical manifestations of spontaneous bleeding (e.g., nosebleeds, ecchymosis).

Listing of Related Tests: Partial thromboplastin time

WEBLINKS

www.ncbi.nlm.nih.gov

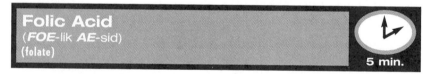

Folic Acid
(*FOE*-lik *AE*-sid)
(folate)

5 min.

Type of Test: Blood

Body Systems and Functions: Hematological system

Normal Findings:

< age 60	1.8–9 ng/mL	4.1–20.4 nmol/L
> age 60	1.2–12 ng/mL	1.2–12 nmol/L

Test Results Time Frame: Within 24 hr

Test Description: Folic acid is a vitamin/amino acid that is required for normal functioning of the red and white blood cells. Folic acid is a potent growth promoter and depends on the normal functioning of the intestinal mucosa for absorption. Folic acid is necessary for DNA production. Folic acid is hypothesized to be involved in congenital anomalies. Folic acid is formed by bacteria in the intestines, stored in the liver, and found in a variety of foods (e.g., eggs, leafy vegetables, milk, and fruits).

Consent Form: Not required

List of Equipment: Red-top tube or serum separator tube; needle and syringe or vacutainer; alcohol swab

Test Procedure:
1. Label the specimen tube. *Correctly identifies the client and the test to be performed.*
2. Obtain a 1-mL blood sample.
3. Do not agitate the tube. *Agitation may cause RBC hemolysis.*
4. Send tube to the laboratory.

Clinical Implications and Indications:
1. Elevated levels are found with vegetarian diet, pernicious anemia, and blood transfusion.
2. Decreased levels are found with alcoholism, anemia, vitamin B_{12} deficiency, blind loop syndrome, Crohn's disease, malabsorption syndrome, malnutrition, pregnancy, and renal failure.

Nursing Care:
Before Test: Explain the test procedure and the purpose of the test. Assess the client's knowledge of the test. Instruct client to fast from solid foods 8 hr prior to test.
During Test: Adhere to standard precautions.
After Test: Apply pressure to venipuncture site. Explain that some bruising, discomfort, and swelling may appear at the site and that warm, moist compresses can alleviate this. Monitor for signs of infection. Protect specimen from light.

Potential Complications: Bleeding and bruising at venipuncture site

Interfering Factors: Hemolysis; drugs that are folate antagonists (e.g., methotrexate, pentamidine); medications that decrease levels are anticoagulants, anticonvulsants, ethanol glutethimide, oral contraceptives, phenytoin, and quinine sulfate.

Nursing Considerations:
Pediatric: Infants and children will need assistance in remaining still during the venipuncture and age-appropriate comfort measures following the test.

WEBLINKS

http://www.methodisthealth.com

Follicle-Stimulating Hormone
(*FAHL*-ik-:l *STIM*-yue-*LAYT*-ing)
(FSH; follitropin)

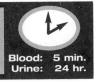

Blood: 5 min.
Urine: 24 hr.

Type of Test: Blood; urine

Body Systems and Functions: Endocrine system

Normal Findings:
Blood:

		SI units
Adult females:		
Premenopausal	4–30 mIU/mL	4–30 IU/L
Follicular phase	2–25 mIU/mL	2–25 IU/L
Midcycle phase	10–90 mIU/mL	10–90 IU/L
Luteal phase	2–25 mIU/mL	2–25 IU/L
Pregnant	low	
Menopausal	40–250 mIU/mL	40–250 IU/L
Postmenopausal	40–250 mIU/mL	40–250 IU/L
Adult males	4–25 mIU/mL	4–25 IU/L
Children	5–13 mIU/mL	5–13 IU/L

Urine:

		SI units
Adult females	3–12 mIU/mL	3–12 IU/L
Follicular phase	2–15 mIU/mL	2–15 IU/L
Midcycle phase	8–60 mIU/mL	8–60 IU/L
Luteal phase	2–10 mIU/mL	2–10 IU/L
Menopausal	35–100 mIU/mL	35–100 IU/L
Adult males	2–18 IU/24 hr	2–18 IU/day
Female children:		
Neonate–12 months	< 1.4 IU/24 hr	< 1.4 IU/L
1–8 years	< 4.0 IU/24 hr	< 4.0 IU/day
9–10 years	1–4 IU/24 hr	<1–4 IU/day
11–12 years	1–8 IU/24 hr	1–8 IU/day
13–14 years	1–10 IU/24 hr	1–10 IU/day
Male children:		
Neonate–12 months	< 1.4 IU/24 hr	< 1.4 IU/L
1–8 years	< 4.5 IU/24 hr	< 4.5 IU/day
9–10 years	1–5 IU/24 hr	< 1–5 IU/day
11–12 years	1.5–5 IU/24 hr	1.5–5 IU/day
13–14 years	2–12 IU/24 hr	2–12 IU/day

Note: Values should be compared with norms of the laboratory performing the test.

Test Results Time Frame: Within 24–48 hr

Test Description: Follicle-stimulating hormone (FSH) is released from the anterior pituitary gland. It has different functions dependent upon gender. In females, FSH promotes maturation of the ovarian follicle (produces estrogen). With the production of estrogen, luteinizing hormones are produced and together they induce ovulation. In males, FSH produces spermatogenesis and the leuteinizing hormone (produces androgens). Urine testing is very useful because the 24-hr specimen reflects both the highs and lows of the FSH secretion.

Consent Form: Not required

List of Equipment: *Blood:* red-top tube or serum separator tube; needle and syringe or vacutainer; alcohol swab. *Urine:* sterile plastic container; ice.

Test Procedure:

Blood:
1. Label the specimen tube and include last menstruation. *Correctly identifies the client and the test to be performed.*
2. Obtain a 1-mL blood sample between 6 and 7 AM.
3. Do not agitate the tube. *Agitation may cause RBC hemolysis.*
4. Send tube to the laboratory.

Urine:
1. Label the collection container. *Correctly identifies the client and the test to be performed.*
2. Discard the first morning void. Then begin the time of the collection for the next 24 hr, including the void at the end of the 24 hr, and record the last voiding time. *An exact 24-hr count ensures accurate results.*
3. If the client has an indwelling catheter in place, keep the drainage bag on ice and empty the urine into the urine container periodically during the 24-hr period.
4. Keep urine cool during collection. *Higher temperatures alter the results.*
5. If any urine is lost, discard the entire specimen and begin collection again the next day.

Clinical Implications and Indications:
1. Elevated levels are found with acromegaly, amenorrhea, gonadal failure, hypothalamic tumor, menopause, menstruation, pituitary tumors, precocious puberty, testicular disorders, and Turner's syndrome.
2. Decreased levels are found with adrenal hyperplasia, amenorrhea, anorexia nervosa, anovulatory menstrual cycle, hypophysectomy, neoplasms, and pre-pubertal child.
3. Repeat testing is necessary after positive test to confirm diagnosis.

Nursing Care:

Before Test: Explain the test procedure and the purpose of the test. Assess the client's knowledge of the test. Instruct client not to discard any urine over the 24-hr time period.

During Test: Adhere to standard precautions for both methods of collection. If any urine is accidentally discarded or contaminated with feces, discard entire specimen and begin test again the following morning.

After Test: Blood: Apply pressure to venipuncture site. Explain that some bruising, discomfort, and swelling may appear at the site and that warm, moist compresses can alleviate this. Monitor for signs of infection. Urine: Document urine quantity, date, and exact hours of collection on requisition.

Potential Complications: Bleeding and bruising at venipuncture site

Interfering Factors: Urine contaminated with feces; spillage or inaccurate collection of the 24-hr specimen, including nonrefrigeration or placing on ice; radionuclides cause decreased FSH levels.

Nursing Considerations:

Pediatric: Blood: Infants and children will need assistance in remaining still during the venipuncture and age-appropriate comfort measures following the test.

Urine: For collection of 24-hr specimen a collection bag or indwelling catheter needs to be used for infants and toddlers.

WEBLINKS ⬚⊠

http://www.niddk.nih.gov

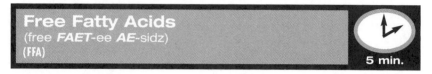

Free Fatty Acids
(free *FAET*-ee *AE*-sidz)
(FFA)

5 min.

Type of Test: Blood

Body Systems and Functions: Hematological system

Normal Findings:

	SI units
8–25 mg/dL	0.30–0.90 mmol/L

Test Results Time Frame: Within 24 hr

Test Description: Free fatty acids (FFA) are transported through the blood in a nonesterified fatty acid form and they are combined with albumin. Normally, there are 3 fatty acid molecules combined with each molecule of albumin, but that number can increase to 30 when the need for fatty acid transport is great (lack of carbohydrates for energy). The same things that increase FFA will usually increase triglycerides and change lipoprotein levels.

Consent Form: Not required

List of Equipment: Red-top tube or serum separator tube; needle and syringe or vacutainer; alcohol swab

Test Procedure:
1. Label the specimen tube. *Correctly identifies the client and the test to be performed.*
2. Obtain a 5-mL blood sample.
3. Do not agitate the tube. *Agitation may cause RBC hemolysis.*
4. Send tube to the laboratory.

Clinical Implications and Indications:
1. Elevated levels are found with diabetes, malnutrition, alcohol intoxication, hypothermia, pheochromocytoma, acute renal failure, and chronic hepatitis.

Nursing Care:
Before Test: Explain the test procedure and the purpose of the test. Assess the client's knowledge of the test. Instruct client to abstain from alcohol for 24 hr and from food for 8 hr prior to test.
During Test: Adhere to standard precautions.
After Test: Apply pressure to venipuncture site. Explain that some bruising, discomfort, and swelling may appear at the site and that warm, moist compresses can alleviate this. Monitor for signs of infection.

Potential Complications: Bleeding and bruising at venipuncture site

Interfering Factors: Ingestion of alcohol within 24 hr; failure to follow dietary restrictions; medications that decrease levels are aspirin, clofibrate, glucose, insulin, neomycin, and streptozocin.

Nursing Considerations:
Pediatric: Infants and children will need assistance in remaining still during the venipuncture and age-appropriate comfort measures following the test.

Listing of Related Tests: Triglycerides; cholesterol

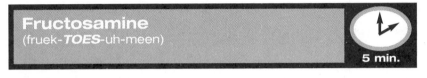

WEBLINKS

www.globind.com

Fructosamine
(fruek-*TOES*-uh-meen)

5 min.

Type of Test: Blood

Body Systems and Functions: Hematological system

Normal Findings:
Adult:

Diabetic	>2.0–5.0 mmol/L
Nondiabetic	1.5–2.7 mmol/L
Child	5% below adult levels

Test Results Time Frame: Within 24 hr

Test Description: Fructosamine reflects the concentration of glucose in the blood. It elevates in 2–3 weeks as contrasted with glycated hemoglobin (hemoglobin AIC), which takes 4–8 weeks. The fructosamine is used as a method of evaluating the longer control therapies used in diabetes rather than just glucose measurements. As a test, fructosamine provides greater breadth of diagnostics for the diabetic client.

CLINICAL ALERT:
Potential clinical manifestations of hypoglycemia should be monitored (due to the fasting prior to test).

Consent Form: Not required

List of Equipment: Red-top tube or serum separator tube; needle and syringe or vacutainer; alcohol swab

Test Procedure:
1. Label the specimen tube. *Correctly identifies the client and the test to be performed.*
2. Obtain a 5-mL blood sample.

3. Do not agitate the tube. *Agitation may cause RBC hemolysis.*
4. Send tube to the laboratory.

Clinical Implications and Indications:

1. Evaluates diabetic control measures
2. Evaluates and monitors gestational diabetes, type I diabetes in children, and diabetic clients with abnormal hemoglobin

Nursing Care:

Before Test: Explain the test procedure and the purpose of the test. Assess the client's knowledge of the test. Instruct client to fast for 12 hr prior to test.
During Test: Adhere to standard precautions.
After Test: Apply pressure to venipuncture site. Explain that some bruising, discomfort, and swelling may appear at the site and that warm, moist compresses can alleviate this. Monitor for signs of infection.

Potential Complications: Bleeding and bruising at venipuncture site

Interfering Factors: Albumin levels <3.0 g/dL; hemoglobin; ascorbic acid; ceruloplasmin

Nursing Considerations:

Pediatric: Infants and children will need assistance in remaining still during the venipuncture and age-appropriate comfort measures following the test.

Listing of Related Tests: Glucose testing; glycated hemoglobin

WEBLINKS

http://alice.ucdavis.edu

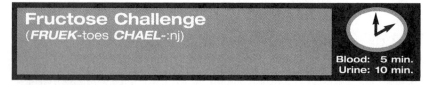

Fructose Challenge
(*FRUEK*-toes *CHAEL*-:nj)

Blood: 5 min.
Urine: 10 min.

Type of Test: Blood; urine

Body Systems and Functions: Hematological system

Normal Findings: Serum: normal levels of glucose, carbon dioxide, phosphate, potassium, uric acid, and magnesium. Urine: normal levels of phosphorus, urine urate, lactate, alanine, and magnesium.

Test Results Time Frame: Within 24 hr

Test Description: Fructose testing measures fructose, which is a carbohydrate and a product of sucrose hydrolysis and is found in fruit and honey. Fructose testing administers IV fructose and measures the change in serum and urine values of the components it is known to affect (see normal values). The urine values are obtained from the urinary output obtained from an indwelling urinary catheter.

CLINICAL ALERT:
If client experiences hypoglycemic clinical manifestations (shaky, agitated, cool or clammy skin) during preprocedure care, inform client to ingest instant glucose and report symptomatology to health care provider.

Consent Form: Required

List of Equipment: *Blood:* red-top tube or serum separator tube; needle and syringe or vacutainer; alcohol swab; IV equipment. *Urine:* sterile plastic container.

Test Procedure:
1. Initiate an IV line with solution per protocol (usually 0.9% sterile saline).
2. Insert an indwelling urinary catheter 2 hr prior to test.
3. Label a sterile urine container. *Correctly identifies the client and the test to be performed.*
4. Obtain 60 mL of urine. *Provides a baseline.*
5. Label the specimen tube. *Correctly identifies the client and the test to be performed.*
6. Obtain a 10-mL blood sample. *Provides a baseline.*
7. Administer fructose per protocol (usually 200 mg/kg of body weight).
8. Obtain 10-mL blood samples immediately after fructose and at 5, 10, 15, 20, 30, 45, 60, 90, and 120 min.
9. Obtain 60 mL of urine 2 hr postinjection of fructose.
10. Do not agitate the tubes. *Agitation may cause RBC hemolysis.*
11. Send urine and blood specimens to laboratory.

Clinical Implications and Indications:
1. Diagnoses hereditary fructose intolerance

Nursing Care:
Before Test: Explain the test procedure and the purpose of the test. Assess the client's knowledge of the test. Instruct client to not eat fructose or sucrose for 3 weeks prior to test and fast foods for 8 hr before test.
During Test: Adhere to standard precautions.
After Test: Apply pressure to venipuncture site. Explain that some bruising, discomfort, and swelling may appear at the site and that warm, moist compresses can alleviate this. Monitor for signs of infection.

Potential Complications: Bleeding and bruising at venipuncture site; profound hypoglycemia

Contraindications: Alcohol consumption; dizziness

Interfering Factors: Diet with too much fructose and sucrose for 3 weeks before test

Nursing Considerations:
Pediatric: Infants and children will need assistance in remaining still during the venipuncture and age-appropriate comfort measures following the test. Infants fed with sucrose-containing formula will have more severe symptoms than breast-fed infants.

Rural: *If client lives a distance from health care facility during fasting from fructose and sucrose, instruct client how to treat hypoglycemia and who to notify with concerns.*

WEBLINKS

www.ncbi.nlm.nih.gov

Fungal Antibody Screen
(*FUHNG*-g:l *AEN*-ti-*BAH*-dee)
(histoplasmosis; blastomycosis; coccidioidomycosis; fungal antibody tests)

5 min.

Type of Test: Blood

Body Systems and Functions: Immunological system

Normal Findings: Negative

Test Results Time Frame: Within 24 hr

Test Description: A fungal antibody screen measures fungi, which are eukaryotic organisms that exist on living and nonliving organic materials. There are limited numbers of fungi that live in humans. The antibodies are present soon after the fungi invade the person and may be detected by the fungal antibody screen. A second convalescent blood sample confirms the client as host to the identified organism.

Consent Form: Not required

List of Equipment: Red-top tube or serum separator tube; needle and syringe or vacutainer; alcohol swab

Test Procedure:
1. Label the specimen tube. *Correctly identifies the client and the test to be performed.*
2. Obtain a 5-mL blood sample.
3. Do not agitate the tube. *Agitation may cause RBC hemolysis.*
4. Send tube to the laboratory.
5. Repeat 10–14 days later for convalescent sample and label the tube as convalescent sample. *Allows for separate identification of the convalescent sample, which is compared in ratio to the acute sample.*

Clinical Implications and Indications:
1. Detects antifungal antibodies and monitors the therapy used for fungal infections
2. Evaluates fungal infections associated with malnutrition, invasive lines, parenteral nutrition, surgery, trauma, steroid therapy, and chemotherapy

Nursing Care:
Before Test: Explain the test procedure and the purpose of the test. Assess the client's knowledge of the test. Instruct client to fast for 12 hr before test.

BLOOD

During Test: Adhere to standard precautions.

After Test: Apply pressure to venipuncture site. Explain that some bruising, discomfort, and swelling may appear at the site and that warm, moist compresses can alleviate this. Monitor for signs of infection.

Potential Complications: Bleeding and bruising at venipuncture site

Interfering Factors: Recent fungal antigen skin testing; immunosuppression from blastomycosis and histoplasmosis

Nursing Considerations:
Pediatric: Infants and children will need assistance in remaining still during the venipuncture and age-appropriate comfort measures following the test.

║║WEBLINKS ▷   ▣▢

http://adam.excite.com

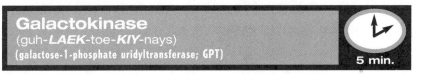

Galactokinase
(guh-*LAEK*-toe-*KIY*-nays)
(galactose-1-phosphate uridyltransferase; GPT)

5 min.

Type of Test: Blood

Body Systems and Functions: Hematological system

Normal Findings: 12.1–39.7 U/g of hemoglobin

Test Results Time Frame: Within 24 hr

Test Description: Galactokinase measures the enzyme, which functions by metabolizing galactose to glucose in the liver. When there are low levels of galactokinase, this is labeled galactosemia. This condition is a relatively rare autosomal recessive disorder, which results from an inherited error of galactose metabolism.

Consent Form: Not required

List of Equipment: Green-top tube; needle and syringe or vacutainer; alcohol swab; ice

Test Procedure:
1. Label the specimen tube. *Correctly identifies the client and the test to be performed.*
2. Obtain a 5-mL blood sample.
3. Do not agitate the tube. *Agitation may cause RBC hemolysis.*
4. Keep specimen on ice. *High temperatures alter the results.*
5. Send tube to the laboratory.

Clinical Implications and Indications:
1. Diagnoses galactosemia
2. Evaluates juvenile (infantile/childhood) cataracts, which result from the low-galactokinase condition and the resulting accumulation of galactose-1-phosphate

Nursing Care:

Before Test: Explain the test procedure and the purpose of the test. Assess the client's knowledge of the test. Refer to genetic counselor.

During Test: Adhere to standard precautions.

After Test: Apply pressure to venipuncture site. Explain that some bruising, discomfort, and swelling may appear at the site and that warm, moist compresses can alleviate this. Monitor for signs of infection.

Potential Complications: Bleeding and bruising at venipuncture site

Interfering Factors: Specimen not placed on ice

Nursing Considerations:

Pediatric: Infants and children will need assistance in remaining still during the venipuncture and age-appropriate comfort measures following the test. Instruct parents whose children have positive test results to reduce galactose-containing foods (e.g., milk). Encourage them that the liver and lens changes are reversible.

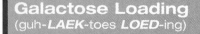 **WEBLINKS**

http://www.med.stanford.edu/

Galactose Loading
(guh-*LAEK*-toes *LOED*-ing)

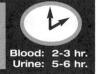

Blood: 2-3 hr.
Urine: 5-6 hr.

Type of Test: Blood; urine

Body Systems and Functions: Hematological system

Normal Findings: Galactose tolerance test (urine or oral):

Blood:

		SI units
1-hr specimen	40–60 mg/dL	2.22–3.33 mmol/L
Timed specimens	<110 mg/dL	<6.11 mmol/L

Urine:

Normal	<2 g/5 hr	<5.45 mmol/L
Borderline	2–3 g/5 hr	11.1–16.7 mmol/5 hr
Abnormal	>3 g/5 hr	>16.7 mmol/5 hr

Galactose clearance test (blood):

		SI units
45 min	<99 mg/dL	5.45 mmol/L
60 min	<43 mg/dL	<2.34 mmol/L
75 min	Minimal	Minimal
2 hr	<0 mg/dL	0 mmol/L

Test Results Time Frame: Within 24 hr

Test Description: Galactose testing measures the monosaccharide that is obtained from lactose after metabolism by the lactase enzyme. The galactose loading test involves the administration of either oral or intravenous galactose and is followed by the timed measurements of blood and urine galactose. The liver normally maintains blood glucose levels by converting carbohydrates to glucose, with one method being to convert galactose to glucose, which is then stored as glycogen. In pathologies, the conversion to galactose is delayed and thus the reason for this testing. The galactose loading test is not often used due to its lack of specificity.

Consent Form: Not required

List of Equipment: *Blood:* five green-top tubes; needles and syringes or vacutainer; alcohol swabs; galactose. *Urine:* four green-top tubes; needles and syringes or vacutainer; alcohol swabs; urine collection container; galactose.

Test Procedure:
Blood:
1. Label the specimen tube. *Correctly identifies the client and the test to be performed.*
2. Administer IV galactose per protocol and record time of administration.
3. After 45 min, obtain a 5-mL blood sample. Then repeat the blood sample collection at 60, 75, and 120 min. Record each collection time.
4. Do not agitate the tubes. *Agitation may cause RBC hemolysis.*
5. Send tubes to the laboratory.

Urine:
1. Label the specimen tube. *Correctly identifies the client and the test to be performed.*
2. Administer oral galactose per protocol and record time.
3. After 30 min, obtain a 5-mL blood sample. Then repeat the blood sample collection at 60, 75, and 120 min. Record each collection time.
4. For the 5 hr after the galactose ingestion, collect all urine and keep refrigerated. *Ensures accurate results.*
5. Send tubes and urine to the laboratory.

Clinical Implications and Indications:
1. Elevated levels are found with hepatitis, cirrhosis, hyperthyroidism, and hepatocellular jaundice.
2. Evaluates liver function during pathology.

Nursing Care:
Before Test: Explain the test procedure and the purpose of the test. Assess the client's knowledge of the test. Instruct client to fast for 8 hr prior to test. Instruct client not to discard any urine over the 5 hr.
During Test: Adhere to standard precautions. If any urine is accidentally discarded or contaminated with feces, instruct client to notify health care provider.
After Test: Apply pressure to venipuncture site. Explain that some bruising, discomfort, and swelling may appear at the site and that warm, moist compresses can alleviate this. Monitor for signs of infection. Carefully document the times of the specimen collections.

Potential Complications: Bleeding and bruising at venipuncture site

Interfering Factors: GI tract abnormalities elevates levels; renal failure delays excretion of galactose; ascorbic acid elevate levels; urine contaminated with feces; spillage or inaccurate collection of the urine specimen, including nonrefrigeration or placing on ice; heavy bleeding during menstruation

Nursing Considerations:
Pediatric: Infants and children will need assistance in remaining still during the venipuncture and age-appropriate comfort measures following the test. A collection bag or insertion of a straight catheter is likely needed for infants and toddlers.

Listing of Related Tests: Glucose tolerance test; fructose tolerance test

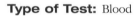

www.healthgate.com

Gamma-Glutamyl Transpeptidase
(*GAEM*-uh glue-*TAEM*-:l traens-*PEP*-tuh-days)
(GGT; GGTP; GTP)

5 min.

Type of Test: Blood

Body Systems and Functions: Hepatobiliary system

Normal Findings: GGT is present in the serum of healthy individuals. The normal range is 5–38 IU/L. Most studies have found values to be comparable in men and women. Children older than age 4 have levels similar to adults.

Test Results Time Frame: Within 60 min

Test Description: Gamma-glutamyl transpeptidase is an enzyme that aids amino acids and peptides across cellular membranes. Gamma-glutamyl transpeptidase catalyzes the transfer of the gamma-glutamyl group from gamma-glutamyl peptides to other peptides and to L-amino acids. GGT is an isoenzyme of alkaline phosphatase. It is located in the liver, kidney, pancreas, brain, heart, salivary glands, and prostate. Carcinoma is evaluated by the varying levels of GGT.

CLINICAL ALERT:
An isolated elevation in serum GGT or a GGT elevation out of proportion to that of other enzymes may be an indicator of alcohol abuse or alcoholic liver disease.

Consent Form: Not required

List of Equipment: Green-top tube or plasma separator tube; needle and syringe or vacutainer; alcohol swab

Test Procedure:
1. Label the specimen tube. *Correctly identifies the client and the test to be performed.*
2. Obtain a 5-mL blood sample.
3. Gently invert tube several times, but do not agitate the tube. *Mixes the anticoagulant, but agitation may cause RBC hemolysis.*

4. Send tube to the laboratory.
5. Keep specimen cool. *High temperatures alter the results.*

Clinical Implications and Indications:
1. The major clinical value of serum GGT is in conferring organ specificity to an elevated value for alkaline phophatase, since GGT activity is not increased in clients with bone disease.
2. Elevated levels are found with hepatobiliary tract disorders, hepatocellular carcinoma, hepatitis, congestive heart failure, acute myocardial infarction (after 4–10 days), diabetes mellitus with hypertension, seizure disorder, and hyperlipoproteinemia (type IV).
3. Diagnoses obstructive jaundice in neonates.

Nursing Care:
Before Test: Explain the test procedure and the purpose of the test. Assess the client's knowledge of the test. Assess client's intake of drugs or alcohol. Instruct client to fast for 8 hr before the test with the exception of water (varies with different laboratory procedures). Studies show there is no significant difference according to gender, age, or fasting.
During Test: Adhere to standard precautions.
After Test: Apply pressure to venipuncture site. Explain that some bruising, discomfort, and swelling may appear at the site and that warm, moist compresses can alleviate this. Monitor for signs of infection.

Potential Complications: Bleeding and bruising at venipuncture site

Interfering Factors: Medications that alter results are barbiturates, phenytoin, and alcohol.

Nursing Considerations:
Pregnancy: Serum enzyme activity does not rise during the course of normal pregnancy.
Pediatric: This test may be elevated in neonates with obstructive jaundice. Infants and children will need assistance in remaining still during the venipuncture and age-appropriate comfort measures following the test.

Listing of Related Tests: Hepatic function panel; liver profile

WEBLINKS
http://catalog.lib.ncsu.edu

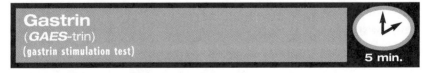

Gastrin
(***GAES***-trin)
(gastrin stimulation test)

5 min.

Type of Test: Blood

Body Systems and Functions: Gastrointestinal system

BLOOD

Normal Findings:

Adults aged 16–60	25–90 ng/L
Over age 60	<100 ng/L
Children	<10–125 ng/L

Test Results Time Frame: Within 12 hr

Test Description: Serum gastrin levels may be elevated in conditions in which gastric acid secretion is very low or absent or in conditions in which there is gastric acid hypersecretion. Gastric acid is made of hydrochloric acid, electrolytes, and mucus. The gastric acid is secreted by the stomach during the gastric stage of digestion. During disease states, the acid can increase or decrease, which causes increased pathology.

Consent Form: Not required

List of Equipment: Red-top tube or serum separator tube; needle and syringe or vacutainer; alcohol swab

Test Procedure:

1. Label the specimen tube. *Correctly identifies the client and the test to be performed.*
2. Obtain a 5-mL blood sample.
3. Do not agitate the tube. *Agitation may cause RBC hemolysis.*
4. Send tube to the laboratory.

Clinical Implications and Indications:

1. Gastrin is a hormone that is secreted by the stomach and duodenum with vagal stimulation.
2. Elevated levels are found with Zollinger-Ellison syndrome, pernicious anemia, gastric carcinoma, uremia, and chronic gastritis.
3. Decreased levels are found with stress ulcers, hypothyroidism, and gastric hyperacidity.

Nursing Care:

Before Test: Explain the test procedure and the purpose of the test. Assess the client's knowledge of the test. Instruct client to fast from food 12 hr before the study and to abstain from alcoholic beverages or caffeine 12–24 hr before the test.
During Test: Adhere to standard precautions.
After Test: Apply pressure to venipuncture site. Explain that some bruising, discomfort, and swelling may appear at the site and that warm, moist compresses can alleviate this. Monitor for signs of infection.

Potential Complications: Bleeding and bruising at venipuncture site

Interfering Factors: Ingestion of any food containing protein and calcium infusion elevates gastrin levels.

Nursing Considerations:

Pediatric: Infants and children will need assistance in remaining still during the venipuncture and age-appropriate comfort measures following the test.

WEBLINKS ▨ ⊟ ⊠

http://www.usyd.edu

Globulin
(*GLAHB*-yue-lin)

5 min.

Type of Test: Blood

Body Systems and Functions: Immunological system

Normal Findings: Total globulin 2.3–3.5 g/dL. Test results give levels of total protein (or globulin), alpha-1, alpha-2, beta, and gamma globulins that include the antibodies.

Test Results Time Frame: Within 24 hr

Test Description: Globulin measures the group of proteins (globulins) that are produced by the liver and lymphoid tissue. The word globulin refers to the nonalbumin portion of serum protein. Most globulin molecules are considerably larger than albumin and form the main transport system for substances and constitute the antibody system, the clotting proteins, complement, and certain "acute reaction" proteins. Electrophoresis divides globulins into alpha, beta, and gamma fractions.

Consent Form: Not required

List of Equipment: Red-top tube or serum separator tube; needle and syringe or vacutainer; alcohol swab

Test Procedure:
1. Label the specimen tube. *Correctly identifies the client and the test to be performed.*
2. Obtain a 5-mL blood sample.
3. Do not agitate the tube. *Agitation may cause RBC hemolysis.*
4. Send tube to the laboratory.

Clinical Implications and Indications:
1. Globulin measurement is often performed along with protein, albumin, and the albumin-globulin (A:G) ratio.
2. Elevated levels are found with acute inflammation, tissue necrosis, malignancies (alpha-1), acute infections, allergies, rheumatic fever, rheumatoid arthritis, ulcerative colitis, nephrotic syndrome (alpha-2), hypothroidism, Cushing's disease, iron deficiency anemia, sarcoidosis (beta), connective tissue diseases, leukemia, and Crohn's disease.
3. Decreased levels are found with hepatitis, malnutrition, malabsorption, lupus erythematosus, and asthma.

Nursing Care:
Before Test: Explain the test procedure and the purpose of the test. Assess the client's knowledge of the test. Instruct client to fast for 8 hr before the test.
During Test: Adhere to the standard precautions.
After Test: Apply pressure to venipuncture site. Explain that some bruising, discomfort, and swelling may appear at the site and that warm, moist compresses can alleviate this. Monitor for signs of infection.

Potential Complications: Bleeding and bruising at venipuncture site

Interfering Factors: High serum lipid levels can cause abnormal results; medications that alter results are ACTH, corticosteroids, growth hormone, acetaminophen, estrogen, and niacin.

Nursing Considerations:
Pediatric: Infants and children will need assistance in remaining still during the venipuncture and age-appropriate comfort measures following the test.

Listing of Related Tests: Total protein; A:G ratio; albumin; gamma globulins

WEBLINKS

http://www.nlm.nih.gov

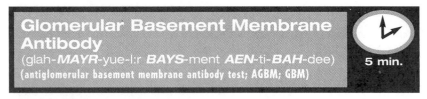

Glomerular Basement Membrane Antibody
(glah-*MAYR*-yue-l:r *BAYS*-ment *AEN*-ti-*BAH*-dee)
(antiglomerular basement membrane antibody test; AGBM; GBM)

5 min.

Type of Test: Blood

Body Systems and Functions: Renal/urological system

Normal Findings: Negative or <0.03 nmol/L

Test Results Time Frame: Within 24 hr

Test Description: Glomerular basement membrane (GBM) antibody is a test used to identify the presence of circulating GBM antibodies. GBM is often used in the differential diagnosis of glomerular nephritis and Goodpasture's syndrome. Antibodies specific for renal structural components of the kidney can bind to respective tissue-fixed antigens and produce an immune response.

Consent Form: Not required

List of Equipment: Red-top tube or serum separator tube; needle and syringe or vacutainer; alcohol swab

Test Procedure:
1. Label the specimen tube. *Correctly identifies the client and the test to be performed.*
2. Obtain a 5-mL blood sample.
3. Do not agitate the tube. *Agitation may cause RBC hemolysis.*
4. Send tube to the laboratory.

Clinical Implications and Indications:
1. Detects antibodies in anti-GBM glomerular nephritis and Goodpasture's syndrome
2. Elevated level with tubulointerstitial nephritis

Nursing Care:

Before Test: Explain the test procedure and the purpose of the test. Assess the client's knowledge of the test.
During Test: Adhere to standard precautions.
After Test: Apply pressure to venipuncture site. Explain that some bruising, discomfort, and swelling may appear at the site and that warm, moist compresses can alleviate this. Monitor for signs of infection.

Potential Complications: Bleeding and bruising at venipuncture site

Nursing Considerations:

Pediatric: Infants and children will need assistance in remaining still during the venipuncture and age-appropriate comfort measures following the test.

Listing of Related Tests: BUN; creatinine; renal ultrasound; IVP

WEBLINKS

http://www.mic.ki.se/Diseases/c20.html

Glucagon
(*GLUE*-kuh-gahn)

5 min.

Type of Test: Blood

Body Systems and Functions: Endocrine system

Normal Findings: 30–210 mg/L (SI units)

Test Results Time Frame: Within 24 hr

Test Description: Glucagon is a polypeptide hormone secreted by the alpha cells of the islets of Langerhans in the pancreas in response to hypoglycemia. It acts on the liver to promote glucose production and glucose storage. Glucagon also increases the use of fats and excess amino acids for energy production. Glucagon is obtained from pork and beef pancrease glands. Glucagon testing test measures quantitative serum glucagon levels by radioimmunoassay.

Consent Form: Not required

List of Equipment: Lavender-top tube or plasma separator tube; needle and syringe or vacutainer; alcohol swab

Test Procedure:
1. Label the specimen tube. *Correctly identifies the client and the test to be performed.*
2. Obtain a 5-mL blood sample.
3. Gently invert tube several times, but do not agitate the tube. *Mixes the anticoagulant, but agitation may cause RBC hemolysis.*
4. Send tube to the laboratory.
5. Keep specimen cool. *High temperatures alter the results.*

BLOOD

Clinical Implications and Indications:

1. Evaluates glucagonoma and renal transplant rejection.
2. Elevated levels are found with renal failure, acute pancreatitis, uncontrolled diabetes mellitus, servere stress, and pheochromocytoma.
3. Decreased levels are found with chronic pancreatitis, cancer of the pancreas, and cystic fibrosis.

Nursing Care:

Before Test: Explain the test procedure and the purpose of the test. Assess the client's knowledge of the test.
During Test: Adhere to standard precautions.
After Test: Apply pressure to venipuncture site. Explain that some bruising, discomfort, and swelling may appear at the site and that warm, moist compresses can alleviate this. Monitor for signs of infection.

Potential Complications: Bleeding and bruising at venipuncture site

Interfering Factors: Some beta-blocker medications may cause falsely decreased levels.

Nursing Considerations:

Pediatric: Infants and children will need assistance in remaining still during the venipuncture and age-appropriate comfort measures following the test.

Listing of Related Tests: Random blood sugar; serum amylase; BUN; creatinine

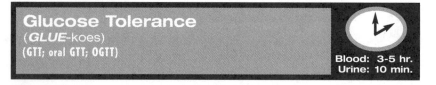

http://www.niddk.nih.gov

Glucose Tolerance
(*GLUE*-koes)
(GTT; oral GTT; OGTT)

Blood: 3-5 hr.
Urine: 10 min.

Type of Test: Blood; urine

Body Systems and Functions: Endocrine system

Normal Findings:

Fasting	70–150 mg/dL
1 hr	160 mg/dL
2 hr	115 mg/dL
3 hr	70–150 mg/dL

Test Results Time Frame: Within 24 hr

Test Description: A glucose tolerance test measures the blood glucose levels after administration of an oral carbohydrate challenge (note: urine samples may be taken as well). Glucose is the most important carbohydrate in body metabolism. It is formed during digestion from the hydrolysis of disaccharides and starch. Excess glucose is converted to glycogen in the liver (glycogenesis). Glucose is the primary source of energy within most cells and is oxidized in cell respiration into carbon dioxide and water in the form of adenosine triphosphate (ATP). The glucose tolerance test determines the body's ability to metabolize glucose and when abnormal aids in the confirmation of diabetes mellitus.

CLINICAL ALERT:
Clients with a fasting blood sugar (FBS) of greater than 150 mg/dL may not need the full GTT for confirmation of diabetes. Whatever the etiology of the abnormal FBS, the GTT will also be abnormal.

Consent Form: Not required

List of Equipment: Green-top tube or serum separator tube; needle and syringe or vacutainer; alcohol swab (note: urine collection containers if needed)

Test Procedure:
Blood:
1. Label the specimen tube. *Correctly identifies the client and the test to be performed.*
2. Obtain a 7-mL blood sample.
3. Administer 75 mg of glucose or dextrose (usually a commercial preparation) for nonpregnant persons and 100 g for pregnant women. The dose may be calculated from body weight at 1.75 g/kg. The dose should be consumed within 5 min.
4. Blood specimens are then taken at 30 min, 1hr, 2 hr, and 3 hr after glucose ingestion. If urine samples are ordered, they are taken at the same intervals. If the test is extended to 5 hr, samples are collected at 4 and 5 hr intervals.
5. Do not agitate the serum tubes. *Agitation may cause RBC hemolysis.*
6. Send tubes to the laboratory.

Urine:
1. Label a sterile urine container. *Correctly identifies the client and the test to be performed.*
2. Obtain a clean-catch specimen of urine. *Ensures accurate results.*
3. Keep specimen cool. *High temperatures alter the results.*
4. Send specimen to laboratory.

Clinical Implications and Indications:
1. Elevated levels are found with diabetes mellitus, gestational diabetes, Cushing's syndrome, pheochromocytomas, primary aldosteronism, hyperthyroidism, acromegaly, acute pancreatitis, chronic renal disease with azotemia, liver disease, burns, stress, and infections.
2. Decreased levels are found with Addison's disease, hypoparathyroidism, hypothyroidism, alcoholism, and hyperinsulinism.

Nursing Care:
Before Test: Explain the test procedure and the purpose of the test. Assess the client's knowledge of the test. Instruct client to eat adequate amounts of carbohydrates at least 3 days before the test. Inform the client to fast from food after midnight the day before the test and to refrain from smoking and strenuous exercise after midnight until the test is completed. If a double-voided urine specimen is ordered, the second void is collected 30 min after the first void. A

glass of water is advised before each urine sample is collected to ensure adequate output.

During Test: Adhere to standard precautions. Adhere to required times for blood and urine collection.

After Test: Apply pressure to venipuncture site. Explain that some bruising, discomfort, and swelling may appear at the site and that warm, moist compresses can alleviate this. Monitor for signs of infection.

Potential Complications: Bleeding and bruising at venipuncture site

Interfering Factors: Urine contaminated with feces; spillage or inaccurate collection of the specimen, including nonrefrigeration or placing on ice; heavy bleeding during menstruation; medications that alter results are glucagon, corticosteroids, oral contraceptives, estrogens, thyroid hormones, thiazide, loop diuretics, and niacin.

Nursing Considerations:
Pregnancy: The client is to receive the 100g glucose load.
Pediatric: Blood: Infants and children will need assistance in remaining still during the venipuncture and age-appropriate comfort measures following the test. Urine: A collection bag or insertion of a straight catheter is likely needed for infants and toddlers. For children suspected of juvenile diabetes, the health care provider must begin assessing the client and family members as to their ability for self-care of this complicated disease process (i.e., diabetes mellitus).
Gerontology: Carefully observe client if certain drugs need to be withheld before the test, such as diuretics.

Listing of Related Tests: Fasting blood sugar; glycosylated hemoglobin; intravenous glucose tolerance test

WEBLINKS

http://www.niddk.nih.gov

Glucose, Blood
(**GLUE**-koes)
(blood sugar; fasting glucose; FBS; random glucose; serum or plasma glucose)

Fasting: 5 min.
Capillary: 15 min.

Type of Test: Blood

Body Systems and Functions: Endocrine system

Normal Findings:

Serum, fasting	<110 mg/dL in the adult
	<60–100 mg/dL in children
	<40–80 mg/dL in newborns
Impaired fasting glucose (IFG)	110–125 mg/dL
Diagnostic value for diabetes mellitus	>125 mg/dL

CRITICAL VALUES:
In the adult a random or fasting blood glucose over 700 mg/dL is a life-threatening value; in the newborn a random or fasting blood glucose over 300 mg/dL is a life-threatening value. Emergency treatment measures are needed immediately.

Test Results Time Frame: Within 12 hr

Test Description: Glucose testing (fasting) measures the blood glucose level after a 12-hr fast. Blood glucose may be measured with venous whole blood or finger puncture blood as a fast way to diagnose hypoglycemia and hyperglycemia in ill clients or for self-adjustment of insulin dosage at home. Glucose is the most important carbohydrate in body metabolism. It is formed during digestion from the hydrolysis of disaccharides and starch. Excess glucose is converted to glycogen in the liver (glycogenesis). Glucose is the primary source of energy within most cells and is oxidized in cell respiration into carbon dioxide and water in the form of adenosine triphosphate (ATP).

Consent Form: Not required

List of Equipment: *Fasting glucose:* red-top tube or serum separator tube; needle and syringe or vacutainer; alcohol swab. *Capillary blood glucose:* reflectance monitor and kit.

Test Procedure:
Fasting blood glucose:
1. Label the specimen tube. *Correctly identifies the client and the test to be performed.*
2. Obtain a 5-mL blood sample.
3. Do not agitate the tube. *Agitation may cause RBC hemolysis.*
4. Send tube to the laboratory.
Capillary blood sugar:
1. Obtain blood drop sample by fingerstick method.
2. Interpret blood sugar level following individual reflectance monitor instructions (e.g., glucometer, Accu check).

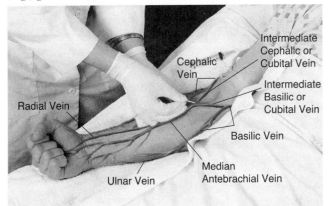

Venipuncture

Clinical Implications and Indications:
1. Elevated levels are found with diabetes mellitus, hyperthyroidism, Cushing's syndrome, pancreatitis, pregnancy (gestational diabetes), severe liver disease,

BLOOD

shock, trauma, and drugs such as glucagon, adrenal corticosteroids, oral contraceptives, and some diuretics.

2. Decreased levels are found with Addison's disease, insulinoma, hypopituitarism, insulin-producing tumors, acute alcohol ingestion, myxedema, and drugs such as insulin, salicylates, sulfonamides, and MAO inhibitors.

Nursing Care:

Before Test: Explain the test procedure and the purpose of the test. Assess the client's knowledge of the test. Instruct client to withhold food for 12 hr before a fasting test (note: 8 hr is acceptable). For those clients on injectable insulin or oral hypoglycemics, they will need to have the test performed before taking these.

During Test: Adhere to standard precautions.

After Test: Apply pressure to venipuncture site. Explain that some bruising, discomfort, and swelling may appear at the site and that warm, moist compresses can alleviate this. Monitor for signs of infection.

Potential Complications: Bleeding and bruising at venipuncture site

Interfering Factors: Uremia and elevated urea levels may lead to a false elevation of the glucose level.

Nursing Considerations:

Pediatric: Infants and children will need assistance in remaining still during the venipuncture and age-appropriate comfort measures following the test. For children suspected of juvenile diabetes, the health care provider must begin assessing the client and family members as to their ability for self-care of this complicated disease process (i.e., diabetes mellitus).

Gerontology: Those clients with impaired fasting plasma glucose are at increased risk for macrovascular disease (e.g., myocardial infarction, stroke, peripheral vascular disease).

Listing of Related Tests: Urine glucose; glycosylated hemoglobin; capillary blood sugar

WEBLINKS

http://www.ncbi.nlm.nih.gov/entrez/query.fcgi

Glucose, Postprandial
(*GLUE*-koes poest-*PRAEN*-dee-:l)
(2-hr postprandial glucose; PPBS)

2.5 hr.

Type of Test: Blood

Body Systems and Functions: Endocrine system

Normal Findings:

Children	65–120 mg/dL
Adults	65–120 mg/dL
Older adults	65–140 mg/dL

BLOOD

Test Results Time Frame: Within 12 hr

Test Description: Postprandial glucose testing measures the blood glucose 2 hr after the client ingests 100 g of carbohydrate. Most investigators believe that the 2-hr level is the most crucial. Normally, the blood sugar returns to the fasting level within 2 hr. Glucose is the most important carbohydrate in body metabolism. It is formed during digestion from the hydrolysis of disaccharides and starch. Excess glucose is converted to glycogen in the liver (glycogenesis). Glucose is the primary source of energy within most cells and is oxidized in cell respiration into carbon dioxide and water in the form of adenosine triphosphate (ATP). The postprandial method of testing adds confirmation and specific diagnostics when diabetes is suspected.

Consent Form: Not required

List of Equipment: Red-top tube or serum separator tube; needle and syringe or vacutainer; alcohol swab

Test Procedure:
1. Have the client ingest 100 g of carbohydrate 2 hr before the test.
2. Label the specimen tube. *Correctly identifies the client and the test to be performed.*
3. Obtain a 5-mL blood sample.
4. Do not agitate the tube. *Agitation may cause RBC hemolysis.*
5. Send tube to the laboratory.

Clinical Implications and Indications:
1. Screens for diabetes mellitus
2. Evaluates an abnormal fasting blood glucose
3. Diagnoses abnormal glucose metabolism
4. Monitors response to hyperglycemic agents

Nursing Care:
Before Test: Explain the test procedure and the purpose of the test. Assess the client's knowledge of the test. Instruct client to fast for 8–12 hr and then ingest a 100-g carbohydrate meal or drink.
During Test: Adhere to standard precautions.
After Test: Apply pressure to venipuncture site. Explain that some bruising, discomfort, and swelling may appear at the site and that warm, moist compresses can alleviate this. Monitor for signs of infection.

Potential Complications: Bleeding and bruising at venipuncture site

Interfering Factors: Smoking and drinking coffee during the 2-hr period can lead to falsely elevated values; strenuous exercise during the 2-hr test period can lead to falsely decreased levels.

Nursing Considerations:
Pediatric: Infants and children will need assistance in remaining still during the venipuncture and age-appropriate comfort measures following the test. For children suspected of juvenile diabetes, the health care provider must begin assessing the client and family members as to their ability for self-care of this complicated disease process (i.e., diabetes mellitus).

Listing of Related Tests: Fasting blood sugar; capillary blood sugar; urine glucose; GTT

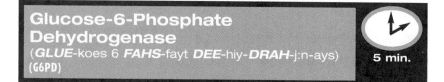

Glucose-6-Phosphate Dehydrogenase
(*GLUE*-koes 6 *FAHS*-fayt *DEE*-hiy-*DRAH*-j:n-ays) (G6PD)

5 min.

Type of Test: Blood

Body Systems and Functions: Hematological system

Normal Findings: Some laboratories report G6PD levels as units per gram of hemoglobin while others report qualitative results. Levels should be above 3 U/g Hgb.

Test Results Time Frame: Within 10 days

Test Description: Glucose-6 phosphate dehydrogenase tests for a G6PD deficiency, which is a genetic disease that predisposes to hemolytic anemia. G6PD is involved with the metabolism of reduced glutathione (GSH), which is important in protecting RBCs from damage by oxidizing agents. G6PD defect is a sex-linked genetic abnormality carried on the female (X) chromosome. The defect centers in the pentose phosphate glucose metabolic cycle of RBCs. Susceptible persons do not have anemia before exposure to oxidant drugs, including those commonly used in clients with HIV infection.

Consent Form: Not required

List of Equipment: Lavender-top tube or plasma separator tube; needle and syringe or vacutainer; alcohol swab

Test Procedure:
1. Label the specimen tube. *Correctly identifies the client and the test to be performed.*
2. Obtain a 5-mL blood sample.
3. Do not agitate the tube. *Agitation may cause RBC hemolysis.*
4. Send tube to the laboratory.

Clinical Implications and Indications:
1. G6PD screening is for those most likely to have a defect. The most frequent are found in 10% of black men and 1%–2% of black women.
2. Diagnoses the occasional case of hemolytic anemia following exposure to potential offending agents (e.g., dapsone and primaquine, occasionally sulfonamides, nitrofurantoin family, and aspirin and similar analgesics, such as phenacetin), and in populations known to have a high incidence of G6PD.
3. Detects nonspecific acute hemolysis.

BLOOD

Nursing Care:
Before Test: Explain the test procedure and the purpose of the test. Assess the client's knowledge of the test.
During Test: Adhere to standard precautions.
After Test: Apply pressure to venipuncture site. Explain that some bruising, discomfort, and swelling may appear at the site and that warm, moist compresses can alleviate this. Monitor for signs of infection.

Potential Complications: Bleeding and bruising at venipuncture site

Interfering Factors: Testing should be delayed for 30 days following discontinuation of the possible offending drug; blood transfusions may temporarily invalidate all tests for G6PD deficiency in blacks and whites.

Nursing Considerations:
Pediatric: Infants and children will need assistance in remaining still during the venipuncture and age-appropriate comfort measures following the test.
International: There is a higher incidence of G6PD in men from the Mediterranean area, India, and southeast Asia.

Listing of Related Tests: Haptoglobin; methemoglobin; reticulocyte count; serum bilirubin; LDH

║WEBLINKS ║   ▤▨

http://www.methodisthealth.com

Glycosylated Hemoglobin
(gliy-*KOES*-uh-*LAYT*-:d *HEE*-muh-*GLOE*-b:n)
(glycohemoglobin; GHB; hemoglobin A1c;Hgb A1c; HbA1c)

5 min.

Type of Test: Blood

Body Systems and Functions: Endocrine system

Normal Findings: Normal laboratory findings vary among laboratory settings; there have been problems in the standardization of HbA1c assays.

Hgb A1c	3.5%–6.0% in the nondiabetic
Hgb A1c	7.5%–11.4% in the controlled diabetic
Hgb A1c	>15% in the uncontrolled diabetic

CRITICAL VALUES:
>15% of total Hb is an out-of-control diabetic; 14.3%–20% of total Hg reflects ketoacidosis.

Test Results Time Frame: Within 72 hr

Test Description: Hemoglobin A constitutes about 97%–98% of normal adult hemoglobin. About 4%–6% of HbA consists of HbA molecules that have been somewhat modified by attachment of a glucose molecule onto its beta chain. This subgroup is called HbA1c. Glycosylated hemoglobin is the amount of glucose permanently bound to hemoglobin, and its function depends on the

BLOOD

blood sugar level. The level of glycosylated hemoglobin reflects the average blood sugar over a period of approximately 8–12 weeks. High levels reflect inadequate diabetic control. After normoglycemic levels are stabilized, HgbA1c levels return to normal in about 3 weeks.

CLINICAL ALERT:

In clients suspected of hyperglycemia, the potential for diabetic ketoacidosis (DKA) can develop. The health care provider needs to be alert to early clinical manifestations of DKA (e.g., blood glucose levels > 250 mg/dL, ketones in urine, dehydration, and alteration in level of consciousness).

Consent Form: Not required

List of Equipment: Lavender-top tube or plasma separator tube; needle and syringe or vacutainer; alcohol swab

Test Procedure:
1. Label the specimen tube. *Correctly identifies the client and the test to be performed.*
2. Obtain a 5-mL blood sample.
3. Gently invert tube several times, but do not agitate the tube. *Mixes the anticoagulant, but agitation may cause RBC hemolysis.*
4. Send tube to the laboratory.

Clinical Implications and Indications:
1. Monitors blood glucose levels and related control in clients with known diabetes
2. Evaluates client's degree of adherence to the therapeutic regimen for glucose control that is prescribed

Nursing Care:
Before Test: Explain the test procedure and the purpose of the test. Assess the client's knowledge of the test.
During Test: Adhere to standard precautions.
After Test: Apply pressure to venipuncture site. Explain that some bruising, discomfort, and swelling may appear at the site and that warm, moist compresses can alleviate this. Monitor for signs of infection. Provide the client with information concerning the test results and any needed changes in diabetic regimen and self-care.

Potential Complications: Bleeding and bruising at venipuncture site

Interfering Factors: Clients with hemolytic or megaloblastic anemia produce falsely low glycosylated hemoglobin values due to the shortened life span of the RBCs; chronic renal failure has been reported to produce falsely high results.

Nursing Considerations:
Pregnancy: Pregnancy can elevate levels.
Pediatric: Infants and children will need assistance in remaining still during the venipuncture and age-appropriate comfort measures following the test. For children suspected of a new onset of juvenile diabetes, the health care provider must begin assessing the client and family members as to their ability for self-care of this complicated disease process (i.e., diabetes mellitus).

Gerontology: Heparin therapy can elevate levels.

Listing of Related Tests: Fasting blood sugar; postprandial glucose

WEBLINKS	⊟⊠

www.med.stanford.edu

Growth Hormone
(*GROTH HOR*-mon)
(GH; hGH; STH; SH; somatotropin)

5 min.

Type of Test: Blood

Body Systems and Functions: Endocrine system

Normal Findings:

Newborns	15–40 ng/mL
Children	0–20 ng/mL
Adults	0–10 ng/mL

Test Results Time Frame: Within 72 hr

Test Description: Growth hormone is a polypeptide anterior pituitary hormone that is required for general body growth. Growth hormone secretion is pulsatile, mediated by reduction in tonic inhibition by somatostatin. Growth hormone is synthesized and controlled by the hypothalamus. Peak GH secretory activity occurs within an hour after the onset of deep sleep. Exercise, physical activity, trauma, and sepsis are associated with increased GH secretion. Ultrasensitive GH assays facilitate detailed studies of GH secretory dynamics.

> **CLINICAL ALERT:**
> Client will usually have two consecutive blood draws between the hours of 6 and 8 AM.

Consent Form: Not required

List of Equipment: Red-top tube or serum separator tube; needle and syringe or vacutainer; alcohol swab

Test Procedure:
1. Label the specimen tube. *Correctly identifies the client and the test to be performed.*
2. Obtain a 5-mL blood sample on two consecutive days between the hours of 6 and 8 AM. Another method is to observe the client until deep sleep occurs, wake the client 60–90 min later, and quickly draw a blood sample. *Ensures accurate results.*
3. Do not agitate the tube. *Agitation may cause RBC hemolysis.*
4. Send tube to the laboratory.

Clinical Implications and Indications:
1. GH deficiency is suspected or questioned as part of the differential diagnosis of retarded growth or short stature.

2. Evaluates multihormone pituitary dysfunction.
3. Monitors response to treatment of growth retardation.
4. Diagnoses gigantism in children with increased levels indicative of pituitary etiology.
5. Diagnoses acromegaly in adults.

Nursing Care:

Before Test: Explain the test procedure and the purpose of the test. Assess the client's knowledge of the test. The client should be awake but not yet out of bed. Instruct client to fast and avoid strenuous activity for 8 hr before the test (note: basal levels will be determined in the morning after an overnight fast). *During Test:* Adhere to standard precautions. *After Test:* Apply pressure to venipuncture site. Explain that some bruising, discomfort, and swelling may appear at the site and that warm, moist compresses can alleviate this. Monitor for signs of infection.

Potential Complications: Bleeding and bruising at venipuncture site

Interfering Factors: Hyperglycemia treated with medications can cause falsely decreased levels; hypoglycemia can cause falsely elevated levels; radioactive scanning performed within 48 hr of the test; medications that alter results are amphetamines, beta blockers, and histamines.

Nursing Considerations:

Pediatric: Infants and children will need assistance in remaining still during the venipuncture and age-appropriate comfort measures following the test. Early assessment of growth abnormalities could make the health care provider suspect growth hormone disturbances (e.g., gigantism).

Listing of Related Tests: Growth hormone stimulation test; growth hormone suppression test

WEBLINKS

www.thriveonline.com

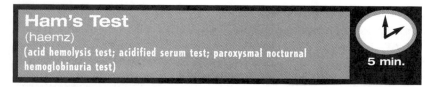

Ham's Test
(haemz)
(acid hemolysis test; acidified serum test; paroxysmal nocturnal hemoglobinuria test)

5 min.

Type of Test: Blood

Body Systems and Functions: Hematological system

Normal Findings: Negative

Test Results Time Frame: Within 48 hr

Test Description: Ham's test is performed to test the stability of the RBC membrane. The client's blood sample is mixed with its own serum and the serum of an ABO-compatible donor. This combined sample is acidified and examined for lysis, which, if present, is definitive for abnormality in RBC membrane. RBCs are sensitive to carbon dioxide, which increases plasma pH, especially during sleep.

Consent Form: Not required

List of Equipment: Lavender-top tube or plasma separator tube; needle and syringe or vacutainer; alcohol swab

Test Procedure:
1. Label the specimen tube. *Correctly identifies the client and the test to be performed.*
2. Obtain a 7-mL blood sample.
3. Gently invert tube several times, but do not agitate the tube. *Mixes the anticoagulant, but agitation may cause RBC hemolysis.*
4. Send tube to the laboratory.

Clinical Implications and Indications:
1. Diagnoses hemolytic anemia and paroxysmal nocturnal hemoglobinuria
2. Evaluates the cause of bone marrow aplasia

Nursing Care:
Before Test: Explain the test procedure and the purpose of the test. Assess the client's knowledge of the test.
During Test: Adhere to standard precautions.
After Test: Apply pressure to venipuncture site. Explain that some bruising, discomfort, and swelling may appear at the site and that warm, moist compresses can alleviate this. Monitor for signs of infection.

Potential Complications: Bleeding and bruising at venipuncture site

Interfering Factors: A false-negative result can occur if the client has received a blood transfusion of RBCs within 3 weeks of the test.

Nursing Considerations:
Pediatric: *Infants and children will need assistance in remaining still during the venipuncture and age-appropriate comfort measures following the test.*

Listing of Related Tests: Hemoglobin; hematocrit; Heinz bodies

WEBLINKS

http://alice.ucdavis.edu

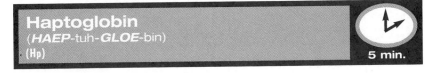

Haptoglobin
(*HAEP*-tuh-*GLOE*-bin)
(Hp)

5 min.

Type of Test: Blood

Body Systems and Functions: Metabolic system

Normal Findings:

Newborns	0–30 mg/dL
Children	0–10 mg/dL
Adults	60–270 mg/dL

Test Results Time Frame: Within 24 hr

Test Description:
Haptoglobin is an alpha-2 globulin that binds any free hemoglobin released into the blood from intravascular or extravascular RBC destruction. Under ordinary conditions a decreased serum haptoglobin level suggests that hemolysis has lowered available haptoglobin through the binding of free hemoglobin.

Consent Form: Not required

List of Equipment:
Red-top tube or serum separator tube; needle and syringe or vacutainer; alcohol swab

Test Procedure:
1. Label the specimen tube. *Correctly identifies the client and the test to be performed.*
2. Obtain a 5-mL blood sample.
3. Do not agitate the tube. *Agitation may cause RBC hemolysis.*
4. Send tube to the laboratory.

Clinical Implications and Indications:
1. Decreased levels are found with hemolysis, severe liver disease, extravascular hematomas, estrogen therapy, infectious mononucleosis, prostatic heart valves, and transfusion reactions.
2. Elevated levels are found with inflammatory diseases, such as arthritis, myocardial infarction, biliary obstruction, ulcerative colitis, burns, and cancers.

Nursing Care:
Before Test: Explain the test procedure and the purpose of the test. Assess the client's knowledge of the test.
During Test: Adhere to standard precautions.
After Test: Apply pressure to venipuncture site. Explain that some bruising, discomfort, and swelling may appear at the site and that warm, moist compresses can alleviate this. Monitor for signs of infection.

Potential Complications: Bleeding and bruising at venipuncture site

Interfering Factors: Steroid use can result in elevated levels.

Nursing Considerations:
Pediatric: Infants and children will need assistance in remaining still during the venipuncture and age-appropriate comfort measures following the test.

Listing of Related Tests: Red blood cell count; hemoglobin; alpha-2 globulin

Heinz Bodies
(hiynz)
(Heinz granules)

5 min.

BLOOD

Type of Test: Blood

Body Systems and Functions: Hematological system

Normal Findings: Negative; absent

Test Results Time Frame: Within 24 hr

Test Description: Heinz bodies are small, scattered, dotlike structures of size in the RBCs derived from denatured hemoglobin, which attach to the RBC membrane. They are visualized with stains such as methylene blue. Their presence indicates an abnormal hemoglobin structure. Hemoglobin is responsible for carrying oxygen, and therefore pathology will result in an anemic condition with associated clinical manifestations of anemia (e.g., fatigue, lethargy).

Consent Form: Not required

List of Equipment: Lavender-top tube or plasma separator tube; needle and syringe or vacutainer; alcohol swab

Test Procedure:
1. Label the specimen tube. *Correctly identifies the client and the test to be performed.*
2. Obtain a 3-mL blood sample.
3. Gently invert tube several times, but do not agitate the tube. *Mixes the anticoagulant, but agitation may cause RBC hemolysis.*
4. Send tube to the laboratory.

Clinical Implications and Indications:
1. Assists in determining the etiology of hemolytic anemia

Nursing Care:
Before Test: Explain the test procedure and the purpose of the test. Assess the client's knowledge of the test.
During Test: Adhere to standard precautions.
After Test: Apply pressure to venipuncture site. Explain that some bruising, discomfort, and swelling may appear at the site and that warm, moist compresses can alleviate this. Monitor for signs of infection.

Potential Complications: Bleeding and bruising at venipuncture site

Interfering Factors: Sulfonamides; antimalarial medications

Nursing Considerations:
Pediatric: Infants and children will need assistance in remaining still during the venipuncture and age-appropriate comfort measures following the test.

Listing of Related Tests: Hemoglobin and hematocrit; CBC differential

WEBLINKS

http://alice.ucdavis.edu

BLOOD

Hematocrit
(*HEM*-uh-toe-krit)
(Hct)

5 min.

Type of Test: Blood

Body Systems and Functions: Hematological system

Normal Findings:

Children, 1–10 years	31%–41%
Adults:	
Men	40%–54%
Women	38%–47%

CRITICAL VALUES:
<15% or >60%

Test Results Time Frame: Within 24 hr

Test Description: Hematocrit is the percentage of RBC mass to original blood volume. After centrifugation, the height of the RBC column is measured and compared with the height of the column of original whole blood. The hematocrit depends on the number of RBCs as well as the average size of the RBCs. In general, losing blood from whatever causes will cause hematocrit levels to decrease. In addition, hemoglobin and hematocrit (H&H) are often obtained together to evaluate a wide variety of hematological disorders.

CLINICAL ALERT:
Severely increased levels could indicate life-threatening crises, such as hemoconcentration (evidenced by decreased pulse pressure, tachycardia, thirst, and weakness) or a polycythemia overtransfusion (with symptoms of extremity pain or redness, facial flushing, irritability). Severely decreased levels could also indicate life-threatening crises, such as hemodilution or blood loss (could exhibit clinical manifestations of hemorrhagic shock).

Consent Form: Not required

List of Equipment: Lavender-top tube or plasma separator tube; needle and syringe or vacutainer; alcohol swab

Test Procedure:
1. Label the specimen tube. *Correctly identifies the client and the test to be performed.*
2. Obtain a 5-mL blood sample.
3. Gently invert tube several times, but do not agitate the tube. *Mixes the anticoagulant, but agitation may cause RBC hemolysis.*
4. Send tube to the laboratory.

Clinical Implications and Indications:
1. Routine screening of the complete blood count
2. Diagnoses suspected anemia and monitors treatment of anemia
3. Monitors blood loss

Nursing Care:
Before Test: Explain the test procedure and the purpose of the test. Assess the client's knowledge of the test.
During Test: Adhere to standard precautions.
After Test: Apply pressure to venipuncture site. Explain that some bruising, discomfort, and swelling may appear at the site and that warm, moist compresses can alleviate this. Monitor for signs of infection.

Potential Complications: Bleeding and bruising at venipuncture site

Interfering Factors: Abnormalities in the RBC size as well as high WBC count may alter values; elevated serum sodium levels may produce elevated levels due to swelling of the erythrocytes.

Nursing Considerations:
Pediatric: Infants and children will need assistance in remaining still during the venipuncture and age-appropriate comfort measures following the test.

Listing of Related Tests: Hemoglobin; complete blood count

WEBLINKS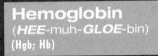

http://www.methodisthealth.com

Hemoglobin
(*HEE*-muh-*GLOE*-bin)
(Hgb; Hb)

5 min.

Type of Test: Blood

Body Systems and Functions: Hematological system

Normal Findings:

Newborns	14–27 g/dL
<1 year	10–15 g/dL
Children, 1–10 years	11–16 g/dL
Adults:	
Men	14–18 g/dL
Women	12–16 g/dL

CRITICAL VALUES:
<5 g/dL

Test Results Time Frame: Within 24 hr

Test Description: Hemoglobin, the main intracellular protein of erythrocytes, is the oxygen-carrying compound contained in RBCs. The amount of hemoglobin per 100 mL of blood can be used as an index of the oxygen-carrying capacity of the blood. Pathology of hemoglobin will result in deoxygenation symptomatology (e.g., fatigue, lethargy, pallor), and consequently continued blood samples are often drawn on clients with deficient levels. Hematocrit levels are often obtained with hemoglobin (labeled H&H) as both are commonly affected with many hematological disorders.

> **CLINICAL ALERT:**
> Severely increased levels could indicate life-threatening crises, such as hemoconcentration (evidenced by decreased pulse pressure, tachycardia, thirst, and weakness) or a polycythemia overtransfusion (with symptoms of extremity pain or redness, facial flushing, and irritability). Severely decreased levels could also indicate life-threatening crises, such as hemodilution or blood loss (could exhibit clinical manifestations of hemorrhagic shock).

Consent Form: Not required

List of Equipment: Lavender-top tube or plasma separator tube; needle and syringe or vacutainer; alcohol swab

Test Procedure:
1. Label the specimen tube. *Correctly identifies the client and the test to be performed.*
2. Obtain a 7-mL blood sample.
3. Gently invert tube several times, but do not agitate the tube. *Mixes the anticoagulant, but agitation may cause RBC hemolysis.*
4. Send tube to the laboratory.

Clinical Implications and Indications:
1. Diagnoses suspected anemia
2. Evaluates treatment for anemia
3. Monitors blood loss and replacement

Nursing Care:
Before Test: Explain the test procedure and the purpose of the test. Assess the client's knowledge of the test.
During Test: Adhere to standard precautions.
After Test: Apply pressure to venipuncture site. Explain that some bruising, discomfort, and swelling may appear at the site and that warm, moist compresses can alleviate this. Monitor for signs of infection.

Potential Complications: Bleeding and bruising at venipuncture site

Interfering Factors: Delayed testing without sample refrigeration; medications that decrease levels are antibiotics, sulfonamides, aspirin, and antineoplastics.

Nursing Considerations:
Pediatric: Neonatal hemoglobin is checked by heelstick (capillary) and is higher than venous blood values. The difference becomes less each day and disappears by the fifth day of life. Neonatal hemoglobin concentration is dependent on the amount of blood received from the umbilical cord. Infants and children will need assistance in remaining still during the venipuncture and age-appropriate comfort measures following the test.

Listing of Related Tests: Complete blood count; hematocrit

WEBLINKS

http://alice.ucdavis.edu

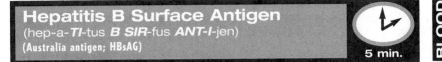

Hepatitis B Surface Antigen
(hep-a-*TI*-tus *B SIR*-fus *ANT-I*-jen)
(Australia antigen; HBsAG)

5 min.

BLOOD

Type of Test: Blood

Body Systems and Functions: Immunological system

Normal Findings: Negative

Test Results Time Frame: Within 5 days

Test Description: Hepatitis B surface antigen is the earliest indicator of hepatitis B and often precedes symptoms. The presence of hepatitis B surface antigen may indicate acute or chronic (carrier) hepatitis B. The test may be positive 2–24 weeks after exposure, with the average time being 4–8 weeks. This test is required for all blood donors, and if positive, the blood will be discarded and the donor notified of results.

Consent Form: Not required

List of Equipment: Red-top tube or serum separator tube; needle and syringe or vacutainer; alcohol swab

Test Procedure:
1. Label the specimen tube. *Correctly identifies the client and the test to be performed.*
2. Obtain a 5-mL blood sample.
3. Do not agitate the tube. *Agitation may cause RBC hemolysis.*
4. Send tube to the laboratory.

Clinical Implications and Indications:
1. Screens for the presence of hepatitis B
2. Blood donor screening
3. Identifies hepatitis B carriers
4. Evaluates and monitors the progress of hepatitis management

Nursing Care:
Before Test: Explain the test procedure and the purpose of the test. Assess the client's knowledge of the test. Ascertain history of hepatitis or exposure history. Ascertain if client has had test requiring radioactive materials in the past week.
During Test: Adhere to standard precautions.
After Test: Apply pressure to venipuncture site. Explain that some bruising, discomfort, and swelling may appear at the site and that warm, moist compresses can alleviate this. Monitor for signs of infection. If client has hepatitis, instruct client regarding the importance of a balanced diet, adequate fluid intake, and adequate rest.

Potential Complications: Bleeding and bruising at venipuncture site

Interfering Factors: Injection of radioactive materials in the past week may falsely elevate the test; HBsAG may be present in 5% of clients with Down's syndrome, hemophilia, Hodgkin's disease, and leukemia.

Nursing Considerations:

Pediatric: Infants and children will need assistance in remaining still during the venipuncture and age-appropriate comfort measures following the test.

WEBLINKS

http://cpmcnet.columbia.edu

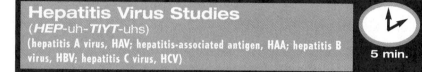

Hepatitis Virus Studies
(*HEP*-uh-*TIYT*-uhs)
(hepatitis A virus, HAV; hepatitis-associated antigen, HAA; hepatitis B virus, HBV; hepatitis C virus, HCV)

5 min.

Type of Test: Blood

Body Systems and Functions: Hepatobiliary system

Normal Findings: Nondectable findings for hepatitis A antibody (IgM) (HAVM); hepatitis B core antibody (IgM) (HBCIGM); hepatitis B surface antigen (HBSAG); hepatitis B surface antibody (AHBS); and hepatitis C antibody (HEPC)

Test Results Time Frame: Within 72 hr

Test Description: There are at least three antigenically distinct members of the group called hepatitis virus, and they are labeled hepatitis A, B, and C. Serological testing is the best method for diagnosis of hepatitis A (HAV). Two types of antibody to HAV antigen are produced, IgM and IgG. The hepatitis screen advocated is for the hepatitis B surface antigen (HbsAG) and hepatitis B core antibody (anti-HBc). Enzyme immunoassay (EIA) is used to detect anti-HVC. The best approach to confirm the diagnosis of hepatitis C is to test for HCV RNA using a sensitive polymerase chain reaction (PCR) assay. The presence of HCV RNA in serum indicates an active infection.

CLINICAL ALERT:
Emphasize adherence to standard precautions, as HBV can be transmitted with a very small amount of blood.

Consent Form: Not required

List of Equipment: Red-top tube or serum separator tube; needle and syringe or vacutainer; alcohol swab

Test Procedure:
1. Label the specimen tube. *Correctly identifies the client and the test to be performed.*
2. Obtain a 7- to 10-mL blood sample.
3. Do not agitate the tube. *Agitation may cause RBC hemolysis.*
4. Send tube to the laboratory.

Clinical Implications and Indications:
1. Diagnoses hepatitis A, B, and C
2. Evaluates and monitors the treatment of the types of hepatitis

BLOOD

Nursing Care:
Before Test: Explain the test procedure and the purpose of the test. Assess the client's knowledge of the test.
During Test: Adhere to standard precautions.
After Test: Apply pressure to venipuncture site. Explain that some bruising, discomfort, and swelling may appear at the site and that warm, moist compresses can alleviate this. Monitor for signs of infection.

Potential Complications: Bleeding and bruising at venipuncture site

Interfering Factors: Heparin therapy may yield false-positive results; injection of radionuclides within 7 days of testing with radioimmunoassay techniques; presence of competing IgG antibody

Nursing Considerations:
Pediatric: Infants and children will need assistance in remaining still during the venipuncture and age-appropriate comfort measures following the test.

Listing of Related Tests: Hepatic function panel

WEBLINKS ▶	▤☒

http://chorus.rad.mcw.edu

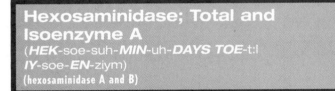

Hexosaminidase; Total and Isoenzyme A
(*HEK*-soe-suh-*MIN*-uh-*DAYS TOE*-t:l *IY*-soe-*EN*-ziym)
(hexosaminidase A and B)

5 min.

Type of Test: Blood

Body Systems and Functions: Hematological system

Normal Findings: Total hexosaminidase: 10.4–23.8 U/L; hexosaminidase A: 56%–80% of total hexosaminidase

Test Results Time Frame: Within 72 hr

Test Description: Hexosaminidase A is a lysosymal enzyme needed for the metabolism of gangliosides. These are water-soluble glycolipids found in brain tissue. A deficiency of these enzymes results in the buildup of gangliosides in the brain tissue with demylination and destruction of central nervous system cells. Hexosaminidase B is made up of two beta subunits.

Consent Form: Not required

List of Equipment: Red-top tube or serum separator tube; needle and syringe or vacutainer; alcohol swab

Test Procedure:
1. Label the specimen tube. *Correctly identifies the client and the test to be performed.*

BLOOD

2. Obtain a 5-mL blood sample (note: in neonates, the sample may be obtained from the umbilical cord).
3. Do not agitate the tube. *Agitation may cause RBC hemolysis.*
4. Send tube to the laboratory.

Clinical Implications and Indications:
1. Diagnoses Tay-Sachs disease

Nursing Care:
Before Test: Explain the test procedure and the purpose of the test. Assess the client's knowledge of the test.
During Test: Adhere to standard precautions.
After Test: Apply pressure to venipuncture site. Explain that some bruising, discomfort, and swelling may appear at the site and that warm, moist compresses can alleviate this. Monitor for signs of infection.

Potential Complications: Bleeding and bruising at venipuncture site

Interfering Factors: Enzyme levels decrease during pregnancy; oral contraceptives

Nursing Considerations:
Pregnancy: Levels decrease in pregnancy.
Pediatric: In neonates, the sample may be obtained from the umbilical cord. Infants and children will need assistance in remaining still during the venipuncture and age-appropriate comfort measures following the test.

WEBLINKS	◱◨

http://alice.ucdavis.edu

Histoplasmosis Antibody
(*HIS*-toe-plaez-*MOE*-sis *AEN*-ti-*BAH*-dee)
(fungal antibody test; *Histoplasma* antibody)

5 min.

Type of Test: Blood

Body Systems and Functions: Immunological system

Normal Findings: Complement fixation titer for *Histoplasma capsulatum:* <1:8. Immunodiffusion test: negative.

CRITICAL VALUES:
Titers of 1:8–1:16 indicate infection. Titers of 1:32 indicate active disease.

Test Results Time Frame: Within 1 week

Test Description: Histoplasmosis antibody is a fungal antibody test that assists in detecting the presence of antibodies to *Histoplasma capsulatum* (as well as other fungal etiology for infection). The test monitors the extent of infection by determining the titer. Several assay techniques are used to determine the presence of antibodies. Complement fixation titers persist for months or years if the disease remains active. The titers appear during the third to sixth week.

Latex agglutination titers become positive in 2–3 weeks and revert to negative in 5–8 months, even with persistent disease. There are few false positives. A biopsy can be made of skin and mucosal lesions, bone marrow, and the reticuloendothelial system.

Consent Form: Not required

List of Equipment: Red-top tube or serum separator tube; needle and syringe or vacutainer; alcohol swab

Test Procedure:
1. Label the specimen tube. *Correctly identifies the client and the test to be performed.*
2. Obtain a 5-mL blood sample.
3. Do not agitate the tube. *Agitation may cause RBC hemolysis.*
4. Send tube to the laboratory.

Clinical Implications and Indications:
1. Diagnoses fungal infection (note: histoplasmosis is the most common systemic fungal infection).
2. Histoplasmosis begins with a small primary focus of lung infection much like the early lesion of pulmonary tuberculosis, and chronic pulmonary histoplasmosis clinically resembles chronic pulmonary tuberculosis.

Nursing Care:
Before Test: Explain the test procedure and the purpose of the test. Assess the client's knowledge of the test.
During Test: Adhere to standard precautions.
After Test: Apply pressure to venipuncture site. Explain that some bruising, discomfort, and swelling may appear at the site and that warm, moist compresses can alleviate this. Monitor for signs of infection.

Potential Complications: Bleeding and bruising at venipuncture site

Nursing Considerations:
Pediatric: Infants and children will need assistance in remaining still during the venipuncture and age-appropriate comfort measures following the test.

Listing of Related Tests: Blood cultures; sputum culture

WEBLINKS

http://www.mic.ki.se/Diseases/c20.html

HIV Antibody
(HIV *AEN*-ti-*BAH*-dee)
(AIDS Western blot test; Western immunoblast assay; WB)

5 min.

Type of Test: Blood

Body Systems and Functions: Immunological system

Normal Findings: Absence of AIDS virus; no bands present

BLOOD

CRITICAL VALUES:
Presence of antibodies to the disease, positive for the virus

Test Results Time Frame: Within 1–2 weeks

Test Description: The Western blot assay is a test that determines the presence of antibodies for human T-cell lymphotrophic virus type III AIDS virus. AIDS is caused by human immunodeficiency virus (HIV), which is a cytoplasmic retrovirus. There are several strains of HIV and all of them attack the T lymphocytes, which are important in cell-mediated immunity. HIV is a tremendous worldwide disorder of epidemic proportions in specific populations and cultures. The HIV-enzyme immunoassay (HIV-EIA) is a fast, sensitive, and exacting method for identifying the presence of antibodies to HIV. A negative result does not prove that the client does not have the disease, nor does a positive result prove the client will develop the disease. The CDC has proven a very strong relationship between a strong immunoassay (EIA) reactivity, Western blot positive results, and a positive culture for HIV.

CLINICAL ALERT:
Due to the social stigma and fears related to AIDS, confidentiality is of high concern. The health care worker has a right to know if the client being cared for is positive for the disease. Counseling becomes an issue with this client before and after testing (if positive) due to the lasting physical, social, emotional, and financial implications of this disease. Clients have lost jobs, insurance has been canceled, and social segregation has occurred due to the knowledge of positive test results. An informed consent must be obtained prior to testing. Positive and negative results are recorded in the patient record and again confidentiality is a concern. State and local rules and requirements must be followed regarding reporting of positive results.

Consent Form: Required

List of Equipment: Red-top tube or serum separator tube; needle and syringe or vacutainer; alcohol swab

Test Procedure:
1. Label the specimen tube. *Correctly identifies the client and the test to be performed.*
2. Obtain a 5-mL blood sample.
3. Do not agitate the tube. *Agitation may cause RBC hemolysis.*
4. Send tube to the laboratory.

Clinical Implications and Indications:
1. Relative certainty of the presence of the AIDS virus.
2. HIV is spreading in epidemic proportions on a worldwide basis. The modes of transmission are body fluid related, and a tremendous amount of research is currently funded to explore continued therapeutic regimens. The financial implications of persons infected with HIV is critical, as well as the societal implications of this disease.

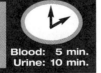

Nursing Care:

Before Test: Explain the test procedure and the purpose of the test. Assess the client's knowledge of the test. An informed and witnessed consent must be obtained prior to the test. The consent may be required to stay with the specimen. Counseling offered prior to the test should include modifications to lifestyles that may spread the disease, including unprotected sex, sharing needles, and donating blood.

During Test: Adhere to standard precautions.

After Test: Apply pressure to venipuncture site. Explain that some bruising , discomfort, and swelling may appear at the site and that warm, moist compresses can alleviate this. Monitor for signs of infection. Inform the client that if tests are positive, they must contact their health care provider immediately. Explain to the client that a positive test does not always mean there is an infection with the AIDS virus. Inform the client to observe for signs and symptoms of the disease (i.e., respiratory and skin infections, fatigue, cough, fever, and swollen lymph glands). Inform pregnant women that the disease can be passed to their unborn child.

Potential Complications: Increased bleeding may occur due to increased bleeding time.

Interfering Factors: Infection with the disease prior to the development of antibodies results in false-negative results; proteins in certain test kits

Nursing Considerations:

Pregnancy: HIV is transmitted in utero to the fetus. Therefore, at-risk populations should be instructed in this regard.

Pediatric: Maternal antibodies may be present in infants until 18 months of age. Therefore, CD4 counts, viral culture, and PCR followed by antibody detection are necessary after 18 months of age. Infants and children will need assistance in remaining still during the venipuncture and age-appropriate comfort measures following the test.

Home Care: Health care providers must use strict standard precautions when caring for HIV-positive clients to avoid contracting the disease.

Listing of Related Tests: ELISA test; Genie assay; T- and B-lymphocyte subset assay

WEBLINKS ▷		▤ ▨

http://www.med.stanford.edu/

Human Chorionic Gonadotropin
(*HYUE*-m:n *KOER*-ee-*AHN-IK GAHN*-uh-doe-*TROEP*-:n)
(HCG; pregnancy test; qualitative HCG)

Blood: 5 min.
Urine: 10 min.

Type of Test: Blood; urine

Body Systems and Functions: Reproductive system

Normal Findings: Blood: negative if not pregnant; positive in pregnant women within 8–10 days. Urine: negative if not pregnant.

Test Results Time Frame: Within 60 min

Test Description: Human chorionic gonadotropin (HCG) is a hormone secreted by the placenta and can be detected in urine or serum within 8–10 days after conception. The level peaks at 8 to 12 weeks gestation, then falls to less than 10% of the first-trimester levels by the end of the pregnancy. HCG is a very common test used to establish whether the client is pregnant.

Consent Form: Not required

List of Equipment: *Blood:* Red-top tube or serum separator tube; needle and syringe or vacutainer; alcohol swab. *Urine:* sterile plastic container; ice.

Test Procedure:
Blood:
1. Label the specimen tube. *Correctly identifies the client and the test to be performed.*
2. Obtain a 5-mL blood sample.
3. Do not agitate the tube. *Agitation may cause RBC hemolysis.*
4. Send tube to the laboratory.

Urine:
1. Label a sterile urine container. *Correctly identifies the client and the test to be performed.*
2. Obtain a clean-catch specimen of urine (note: first morning voiding preferred, at least 60 mL). *Ensures accurate results.*
3. Keep specimen cool. *High temperatures alter the results.*
4. Send specimen to laboratory.

Clinical Implications and Indications:
1. Confirms pregnancy
2. Confirms threatened or incomplete abortion
3. Assists in the diagnosis of HCG producing tumors, such as choriocarcinoma or hydatiform moles

Nursing Care:
Before Test: Explain the test procedure and the purpose of the test. Assess the client's knowledge of the test.
During Test: Adhere to standard precautions.
After Test: Blood: Apply pressure to venipuncture site. Explain that some bruising, discomfort, and swelling may appear at the site and that warm, moist compresses can alleviate this. Monitor for signs of infection. Urine: Document urine quantity, date, and exact hours of collection on requisition.

Potential Complications: Bleeding and bruising at venipuncture site

Interfering Factors: Excessive leutinizing hormone production by the pituitary gland; absence of gonadal hormones in menopausal women may cause false-positive results; radionuclide scan within 1 week may invalidate the results; urine contaminated with feces; spillage or inaccurate collection of the urine specimen, including nonrefrigeration or placing on ice; heavy bleeding during menstruation; medications that increase levels are hypnotics, tranquilizers,

BLOOD

anticonvulsants, antiparkinsonians; medications that decrease levels are diuretics and promethazines.

Nursing Considerations:
Pregnancy: The urine analysis for pregnancy can be performed 2 days after a missed menstrual period for a period of up to 3 weeks.
Pediatric: Blood: Infants and children will need assistance in remaining still during the venipuncture and age-appropriate comfort measures following the test.
Urine: A collection bag or insertion of a straight catheter is likely needed for infants and toddlers (rarely obtained from this age range).

Listing of Related Tests: 24-hr urine for HCG; qualitative HCG

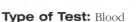

WEBLINKS

http://www.ncbi.nlm.nih.gov/entrez/query.fcgi

Human Leukocyte Antigen
(*HYUE*-m:n *LUE*-koe-siyt *AEN*-tuh-j:n)
(HLA; tissue typing; HLA-B27 antigen; white blood cell antigen; histocompatibility A antigen)

20 min.

Type of Test: Blood

Body Systems and Functions: Immunological system

Normal Findings: Human leukocyte antigens are classified into five series, designated A, B, C, D, and D related, with each series containing 10–20 distinct antigens. The HLA combinations vary according to certain races and populations. The most common B antigens in American whites are B7, B8, and B12. In American blacks, the B series are Bw17, Bw35, and a specificity characterized as IAG.

Test Results Time Frame: Within 1 week

Test Description: This test detects human leukocyte antigens (HLAs) on the surface membranes of leukocytes, platelets, and tissue cells. Each site of location is called a locus and each locus has four subloci, each containing one gene. Each sublocus (gene) has multiple alleles, or a pool of several genes. The major subloci are designated A, B, C, D, and DR, or D related. The HLA system has been closely identified with tissue transplant compatability and is used in bone marrow and renal transplantation. Also, certain HLAs have been found to occur with increased frequency in various diseases. The B27 antigen is associated with rheumatoid arthritis and variants. The incidence of HLA-B27 in ankylosing spondylitis is 90%–95% in whites. The B8 antigen is associated with myasthenia gravis and celiac disease as examples.

Consent Form: Not required

List of Equipment: *Donor specimen:* two green-top tubes or plasma separator tubes; needles and syringes or vacutainers; alcohol swabs. *Recipient specimen:* red-top tube or serum separator tube; needle and syringe or vacutainer; alcohol swab.

BLOOD

Test Procedure:

1. Label the specimen tubes. *Correctly identifies the client and the test to be performed.*
2. Obtain a 7-mL blood sample. If testing is done for tissue compatibility, obtain a 7-mL sample in a red-top tube with the recipient blood and a 7-mL sample in two green-top tubes with donor blood.
3. Do not agitate the red-top tube. *Agitation may cause RBC hemolysis.*
4. Gently invert the green-top tube several times, but do not agitate the tube. *Mixes the anticoagulant, but agitation may cause RBC hemolysis.*
5. Send tubes to the laboratory.

Clinical Implications and Indications:

1. Determines donor-recipient compatibility for transplantation
2. Determines compatibility of donor platelets in clients who will receive multiple transfusions over a long period of time
3. Assists in the diagnosis of HLA-associated diseases

Nursing Care:

Before Test: Explain the test procedure and the purpose of the test. Assess the client's knowledge of the test.
During Test: Adhere to standard precautions.
After Test: Apply pressure to venipuncture site. Explain that some bruising, discomfort, and swelling may appear at the site and that warm, moist compresses can alleviate this. Monitor for signs of infection.

Potential Complications: Bleeding and bruising at venipuncture site

Interfering Factors: Delay in sending the tubes to the laboratory can cause lymphocytes to die.

Nursing Considerations:

Pediatric: Infants and children will need assistance in remaining still during the venipuncture and age-appropriate comfort measures following the test.
International: HLA combinations vary according to certain races and populations. For example, African blacks are found to have B antigens of B7, Bw17, and IAG. Similar variations among the A antigens also have been found among various races and populations.

Listing of Related Tests: RBC antigens; CBC; blood typing and cross-matching

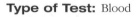

WEBLINKS

http://www.mic.ki.se/Diseases/c20.html

Human Placental Lactogen

(*HYUE*-m:n pluh-*SEN*-t:l *LAEK*-toe-j:n)
(**HPL; human chorionic somatotropin, HCS**)

5 min.

Type of Test: Blood

Body Systems and Functions: Reproductive system

Normal Findings: With pregnancy (normal laboratory findings vary among laboratory settings):

5–27 weeks	< 4.6 µg/mL
28–31 weeks	2.4–6.1 µg/mL
32–35 weeks	3.7–7.7 µg/mL
36 weeks to term	5.0–8.6 µg/mL
Diabetic at term	10–12 µg/mL

Test Results Time Frame: Within 24 hr

Test Description: Human placental lactogen is produced by the placenta and causes decreased maternal sensitivity to insulin and utilization of glucose. This increases glucose availability to the developing fetus. HPL also promotes release of maternal free fatty acids for utilization by the fetus. HPL has a role in promoting breast growth and preparation for lactation and maintenance of the pregnancy by altering the endometrium.

Consent Form: Not required

List of Equipment: Red-top tube or serum separator tube; needle and syringe or vacutainer; alcohol swab

Test Procedure:
1. Label the specimen tube. *Correctly identifies the client and the test to be performed.*
2. Obtain a 7-mL blood sample.
3. Do not agitate the tube. *Agitation may cause RBC hemolysis.*
4. Send tube to the laboratory.

Clinical Implications and Indications:
1. Detects placental insufficiency, as evidenced by low HPL levels in relation to gestational age
2. Assists in the detection of intrauterine growth retardation due to placental insufficiency, as evidenced by HPL levels less than 4.6 µg/mL
3. Supports diagnosis of hydatidiform mole and choriocarcinoma, as indicated by decreased levels of HPL
4. Monitors treatment effectiveness of cancers associated with ectopic HPL production, as indicated by decreasing levels

Nursing Care:
Before Test: Explain the test procedure and the purpose of the test. Assess the client's knowledge of the test.
During Test: Adhere to standard precautions.
After Test: Apply pressure to venipuncture site. Explain that some bruising, discomfort, and swelling may appear at the site and that warm, moist compresses can alleviate this. Monitor for signs of infection.

Potential Complications: Bleeding and bruising at venipuncture site

Interfering Factors: Incorrect interpretation of gestational age of the developing baby

Nursing Considerations:

Pregnancy: Determination of gestational age of the fetus is necessary to establish normal values.

Pediatric: Growth retardation of the fetus can be detected with low levels of HPL.

Listing of Related Tests: Blood estrogen levels; fasting blood sugar; glycosylated hemoglobin

WEBLINKS ▷	▤ ▨

http://biocrs.biomed.brown.edu

Human T-Cell Lymphotrophic (HTLV) I/II Antibody
(*HYUE*-m:n ... *LIM*-foe-*TROE*-fik ... *AEN*-ti-*BAH*-dee)
(human T-cell lymphotrophic virus I antibody)

5 min.

Type of Test: Blood

Body Systems and Functions: Immunological system

Normal Findings: Negative

Test Results Time Frame: Within 72 hr

Test Description: Human T-cell lymphotrophic (HTLV) I/II antibody is a test that detects the presence of antibody to human T-cell lymphotrophic virus 1. T lymphocytes mature in the thymus gland or the precortical areas of the lymph nodes and are responsible for cell-mediated immunity. Human T-cell lymphotrophic virus is a retrovirus associated with adult T-cell leukemia and demyelinating neurological disorders.

Consent Form: Not required

List of Equipment: Red-top tube or serum separator tube; needle and syringe or vacutainer; alcohol swab

Test Procedure:
1. Label the specimen tube. *Correctly identifies the client and the test to be performed.*
2. Obtain a 5-mL blood sample.
3. Do not agitate the tube. *Agitation may cause RBC hemolysis.*
4. Send tube to the laboratory.

Clinical Implications and Indications:
1. Diagnoses HTLV-1 infection (note: transmission of infection to recipients of HTLV-1 infected blood is well documented).
2. HTLV-1 has been detected in clients with adult T-cell leukemia (ATL), IV drug users, healthy persons, and donated blood products. The finding of these antibodies has no relationship to the presence of antibodies to HIV-1 and does not imply any risk of AIDS.

BLOOD

Nursing Care:
Before Test: Explain the test procedure and the purpose of the test. Assess the client's knowledge of the test.
During Test: Adhere to standard precautions.
After Test: Apply pressure to venipuncture site. Explain that some bruising, discomfort, and swelling may appear at the site and that warm, moist compresses can alleviate this. Monitor for signs of infection.

Potential Complications: Bleeding and bruising at venipuncture site

Nursing Considerations:
Pediatric: Infants and children will need assistance in remaining still during the venipuncture and age-appropriate comfort measures following the test.
International: HTLV-1 is endemic in the Caribbean, southeastern Japan, and some areas of Africa.

Listing of Related Tests: Western blot

WEBLINKS

http://www.vgernet.net

Hydroxybutyrate Dehydrogenase
(hiy-***DRAHK***-see-***BYUET***-:r-***AYT DEE***-hiy-***DRAH***-j:n-ays)
(HBDH; alpha-hydroxybutyric dehydrogenase)

5 min.

Type of Test: Blood

Body Systems and Functions: Metabolic system

Normal Findings: 140–350 U/mL (normal laboratory findings vary among laboratory settings)

Test Results Time Frame: Within 24 hr

Test Description: Alpha-hydroxybutyrate dehydrogenase is an enzyme found in the brain, heart muscle, kidney, and red blood cells. The enzyme is released into the bloodstream following organ damage or ischemia. This enzyme level remains elevated for 18 days following acute myocardial infarction. HBDH is also an enzyme similar to lactate dehydrogenase (LD) 1. This test is usually used because it is less costly than a complete LD isoenzyme battery and simpler to perform than LD electrophoresis.

Consent Form: Not required

List of Equipment: Red-top tube or serum separator tube; needle and syringe or vacutainer; alcohol swab

Test Procedure:
1. Label the specimen tube. *Correctly identifies the client and the test to be performed.*

BLOOD

2. Obtain a 7-mL blood sample.
3. Do not agitate the tube. *Agitation may cause RBC hemolysis.*
4. Send tube to the laboratory.

Clinical Implications and Indications:

1. Assists in the diagnosis of myocardial infarction in the client with symptoms occurring some time before seeking care or with atypical symptoms.
2. Elevated levels are found with anemia, muscular dystrophy, leukemia, lymphoma, malignant melanoma, nephrotic syndrome, orthopedic hip surgery, and acute hepatocellular damage.

Nursing Care:

Before Test: Explain the test procedure and the purpose of the test. Assess the client's knowledge of the test.

During Test: Adhere to standard precautions.

After Test: Apply pressure to venipuncture site. Explain that some bruising, discomfort, and swelling may appear at the site and that warm, moist compresses can alleviate this. Monitor for signs of infection.

Potential Complications: Bleeding and bruising at venipuncture site

Interfering Factors: Surgery; cardioversion; frozen sample; traumatic venipuncture

Nursing Considerations:

Pediatric: Bleeding and bruising at venipuncture site

Listing of Related Tests: LDH; myoglobin; troponin I; CPK

| WEBLINKS ▶ | 🗖🗙 |

http://www.entnet.org

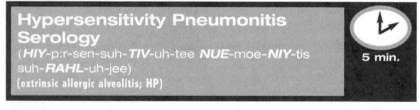

Hypersensitivity Pneumonitis Serology

(*HIY*-p:r-sen-suh-*TIV*-uh-tee *NUE*-moe-*NIY*-tis suh-*RAHL*-uh-jee)
(extrinsic allergic alveolitis; HP)

5 min.

Type of Test: Blood

Body Systems and Functions: Pulmonary system

Normal Findings: Absence of serum precipitins or negative

Test Results Time Frame: Within 48 hr

Test Description: Hypersensitivity pneumonitis serology identifies the presence of hypersensitivity pneumonitis, which is a complex syndrome. It is an inflammatory, interstitial pneumonia that results from an immunological reaction to numerous inciting agents. Known exposure to offending antigen(s) may be identified by the presence of IgG antibodies (e.g., *Aspergillus fumigatus*, *Micropolyspora faeni*, and *Thermoactino-myces vulgaris*) in serum against the

BLOOD

identified antigen. The positive precipitin test even in the presence of a clear history of exposure to the identified antigen is merely suggestive, rather than diagnostic, of a potential etiology. There is a high rate of false-negative results.

Consent Form: Not required

List of Equipment: Red-top tube or serum separator tube; needle and syringe or vacutainer; alcohol swab

Test Procedure:
1. Label the specimen tube. *Correctly identifies the client and the test to be performed.*
2. Obtain a 7-mL blood sample.
3. Do not agitate the tube. *Agitation may cause RBC hemolysis.*
4. Send tube to the laboratory.

Clinical Implications and Indications:
1. Diagnoses hypersensitivity pneumonitis
2. Assists in the diagnosis of extrinsic allergic alveolitis
3. Diagnoses asthma and farmer's lung

Nursing Care:
Before Test: Explain the test procedure and the purpose of the test. Assess the client's knowledge of the test.
During Test: Adhere to standard precautions.
After Test: Apply pressure to venipuncture site. Explain that some bruising, discomfort, and swelling may appear at the site and that warm, moist compresses can alleviate this. Monitor for signs of infection.

Potential Complications: Bleeding and bruising at venipuncture site

Interfering Factors: Commercial assays test for only a small fraction of the potential causative antigens and the test may be nonreactive in some cases even if the correct antigen is included; chylous; contaminated samples

Nursing Considerations:
Pediatric: Infants and children will need assistance in remaining still during the venipuncture and age-appropriate comfort measures following the test.

Listing of Related Tests: Inhalation challenge; bronchoalveolar lavage; lung biopsy; CBC with differential

WEBLINKS ▷   ▤ ☒

http://www.rcjournal.com

IgE Antibody, Single Allergen, IRMA Panel
([*IM*-yue-noe-*GLAHB*-yue-l:n E] *AEN*-ti-*BAH*-dee *SING*-g:l *AEL*-:r-j:n ... *PAEN*-:l)
(RAST)

⤹ 5 min.

Type of Test: Blood

BLOOD

Body Systems and Functions: Immunological system

Normal Findings: Negative

Test Results Time Frame: Within 24 hr

Test Description: IgE antibody is a panel that measures the increase and quantity of allergen-specific immunoglobulin-E antibodies. IgE antibody proteins are primarily released during allergic reactions. The IgE antibody test assists in the diagnosis of a reaction to such things as certain respiratory and food allergy stimulants. Measurable allergen-specific antibodies can be identified only by radioallergosorbent tests (RASTs).

Consent Form: Not required

List of Equipment: Red-top tube or serum separator tube; needle and syringe or vacutainer; alcohol swab

Test Procedure:
1. Label the specimen tube. *Correctly identifies the client and the test to be performed.*
2. Obtain a 5-mL blood sample.
3. Do not agitate the tube. *Agitation may cause RBC hemolysis.*
4. Send tube to the laboratory.

Clinical Implications and Indications:
1. Assists in the diagnosis of clients, especially children, with extrinsic asthma, hay fever, and atopic eczema.
2. An accurate alternative to skin testing.
3. Elevated levels are found with alcoholism, bronchitis, food and drug allergies, hay fever, parasitic infections, sinusitis, and rhinitis.
4. Decreased levels are found with advanced carcinoma, ataxia-telangiectasia, and IgE deficiency.

Nursing Care:
Before Test: Explain the test procedure and the purpose of the test. Assess the client's knowledge of the test.
During Test: Adhere to standard precautions.
After Test: Apply pressure to venipuncture site. Explain that some bruising, discomfort, and swelling may appear at the site and that warm, moist compresses can alleviate this. Monitor for signs of infection.

Potential Complications: Bleeding and bruising at venipuncture site

Interfering Factors: Gold compounds increase levels; drugs with phenytoin sodium decrease levels; radionuclide testing within the past 72 hr

Nursing Considerations:
Pediatric: Infants and children will need assistance in remaining still during the venipuncture and age-appropriate comfort measures following the test.

Listing of Related Tests: Immunoglobulins; CBC

WEBLINKS ▤▨

http://health.indiamart.com

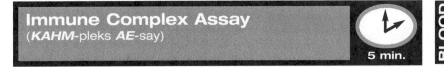

Immune Complex Assay
(*KAHM*-pleks *AE*-say)

5 min.

BLOOD

Type of Test: Blood

Body Systems and Functions: Immunological system

Normal Findings: Negative

Test Results Time Frame: Within 24 hr

Test Description: The immune complex assay is a radioimmunoassay test that helps diagnose autoimmune and infectious inflammatory disease processes. Immune complexes are antigens and antibodies capable of activating the complement cascade. This process results in the formulation of the membrane attack complex. This is an important immunological enzyme system that affects vascular permeability, chemotaxis, phagocystosis, immune adherence, and immune cell lysis.

Consent Form: Not required

List of Equipment: Red-top tube or serum separator tube; needle and syringe or vacutainer; alcohol swab

Test Procedure:
1. Label the specimen tube. *Correctly identifies the client and the test to be performed.*
2. Obtain a 7-mL blood sample.
3. Do not agitate the tube. *Agitation may cause RBC hemolysis.*
4. Send tube to the laboratory.

Clinical Implications and Indications:
1. Diagnoses immune disorders, such as Hodgkin's disease, SLE, rheumatoid arthritis, endocarditis, leukemia, and malignant melanoma
2. Detects allergic reactions to drugs as indicated by the presence of immune complexes

Nursing Care:
Before Test: Explain the test procedure and the purpose of the test. Assess the client's knowledge of the test.
During Test: Adhere to standard precautions.
After Test: Apply pressure to venipuncture site. Explain that some bruising, discomfort, and swelling may appear at the site and that warm, moist compresses can alleviate this. Monitor for signs of infection.

Potential Complications: Bleeding and bruising at venipuncture site

Interfering Factors: Heparin therapy; cold agglutinins; paraproteins; certain cryoglobulins

Nursing Considerations:
Pediatric: Infants and children will need assistance in remaining still during the venipuncture and age-appropriate comfort measures following the test.

Listing of Related Tests: Serum complement; gamma globulin; IgE antibody; Raji cell C14

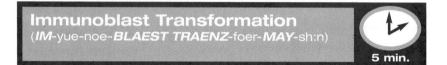

WEBLINKS

http://www.nlm.nih.gov

Immunoblast Transformation
(*IM*-yue-noe-*BLAEST TRAENZ*-foer-*MAY*-sh:n)

5 min.

Type of Test: Blood

Body Systems and Functions: Immunological system

Normal Findings: Negative

Test Results Time Frame: Within 24 hr

Test Description: Immunoblast transformation testing evaluates the capability of lymphocytes to change to proliferative cells and to respond normally to antigenic challenge. B lymphocytes are carriers of humoral immunity and are directly responsible for producing antibodies. After antigenic stimulation, activation, proliferation, and transformation of B cells occur in the germinative center. Transformed B lymphocyte leaves the germinative center as a large immunoblast. Immunoblast transformation testing detects the change that is made in these B lymphocytes. In addition, T lymphocytes change after encountering specific antigens in cell-mediated immunities, and this change is evaluated by the immunoblast transformation testing. Overall, both T and B lymphocytes can be distinguished by immunoblast transformation testing methods and not by morphology alone.

Consent Form: Not required

List of Equipment: Red-top tube or serum separator tube; needle and syringe or vacutainer; alcohol swab

Test Procedure:
1. Label the specimen tube. *Correctly identifies the client and the test to be performed.*
2. Obtain a 5-mL blood sample.
3. Do not agitate the tube. *Agitation may cause RBC hemolysis.*
4. Send tube to the laboratory.

Clinical Implications and Indications:
1. Diagnoses immunoglobulin deficiency
2. Identifies microorganisms to which the client was exposed to in an antigen-specific transformation reaction
3. Identifies compatible organ donors and recipients as indicated by nonresponsiveness on mixed lymphocyte cultures

Nursing Care:
Before Test: Explain the test procedure and the purpose of the test. Assess the client's knowledge of the test.

During Test: Adhere to standard precautions.

After Test: Apply pressure to venipuncture site. Explain that some bruising, discomfort, and swelling may appear at the site and that warm, moist compresses can alleviate this. Monitor for signs of infection (particularly due to the client potentially being immunosuppressed).

Potential Complications: Bleeding and bruising at venipuncture site

Interfering Factors: Radioisotope studies performed within 1 week of the test; pregnancy; oral contraceptives

Nursing Considerations:
Pediatric: Infants and children will need assistance in remaining still during the venipuncture and age-appropriate comfort measures following the test.

Listing of Related Tests: Immunoglobulins; T-cell count

WEBLINKS

www.chronolab.com

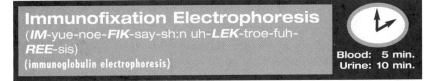

Immunofixation Electrophoresis
(*IM*-yue-noe-*FIK*-say-sh:n uh-*LEK*-troe-fuh-*REE*-sis)
(immunoglobulin electrophoresis)

Blood: 5 min.
Urine: 10 min.

Type of Test: Blood; urine

Body Systems and Functions: Immunological system

Normal Findings: Blood: Curves may be analyzed and interpreted by a pathologist if there are abnormal protein levels in the serum. Quantitative findings include age-dependent values:

IgG	700–1500 mg/dL
IgA	140–400 mg/dL
IgM	35–375 mg/dL
IgD	0–8 mg/dL
IgE	4.2–592 IU/mL

Urine: Requires individual interpretation in the presence of abnormal urinary protein levels.

Test Results Time Frame: Within 72 hr

Test Description: Immunoglobulin electrophoresis is a qualitative technique that provides a detailed separation of the individual immunoglobulins according to their electrical charges. This test can identify even slight deficiencies of monoclonal proteins and its type. Results are revealed on a printout by changes in the individual bands.

Consent Form: Not required

List of Equipment: *Blood:* red-top tube or serum separator tube; needle and syringe or vacutainer; alcohol swab. *Urine:* sterile plastic container; ice.

Test Procedure:

Blood:
1. Label the specimen tube. *Correctly identifies the client and the test to be performed.*
2. Obtain a 5-mL blood sample.
3. Do not agitate the tube. *Agitation may cause RBC hemolysis.*
4. Send tube to the laboratory.

Urine:
1. Label a sterile urine container. *Correctly identifies the client and the test to be performed.*
2. Obtain a clean-catch specimen of urine (note: this is a random urine specimen, with at least 60 mL). *Ensures accurate results.*
3. Keep specimen cool. *High temperatures alter the results.*
4. Send specimen to laboratory.

Clinical Implications and Indications:
1. Diagnoses protein abnormalities
2. Assists in the diagnosis of suspected immunodeficiency
3. Supports diagnosis of renal failure
4. Assists in the diagnosis of immune disorders, such as Hodgkin's disease, multiple myeloma, and amyloidosis

Nursing Care:

Before Test: Explain the test procedure and the purpose of the test. Assess the client's knowledge of the test.

During Test: Adhere to standard precautions.

After Test: Blood: Apply pressure to venipuncture site. Explain that some bruising, discomfort, and swelling may appear at the site and that warm, moist compresses can alleviate this. Monitor for signs of infection. Urine: Document urine quantity, date, and exact hours of collection on requisition.

Potential Complications: Bleeding and bruising at venipuncture site

Interfering Factors: Chemotherapy and radiation therapy may alter the width of the bands and make interpretation difficult; urine contaminated with feces; spillage or inaccurate collection of the urine specimen, including nonrefrigeration or placing on ice; heavy bleeding during menstruation; medications that increase levels are oral contraceptives, anticoagulants, and hydralazine.

Nursing Considerations:

Pediatric: Blood: *Infants and children will need assistance in remaining still during the venipuncture and age-appropriate comfort measures following the test.*
Urine: A collection bag or insertion of straight catheter is likely needed for infants and toddlers.

Listing of Related Tests: Serum protein; renal function tests

WEBLINKS ▮

http://www.mic.ki.se/Diseases/c20.html

Immunoglobulins
(*IM*-yue-noe-*GLAHB*-yue-linz)
(IgA; IG; IgG; IgD; IgE; IgM; gamma globulin; immune serum globulin)

5 min.

Type of Test: Blood

Body Systems and Functions: Immunological system

Normal Findings:

IgA:

Adults	90–400 mg/dL
Children:	
Newborn	0–5 mg/dL
Infant	0–11 mg/dL
3 years	50% of adult
12–16 years	85–211 mg/dL

IgA: Antibodies not present.

IgD:

Adults	0–8.0 mg/dL
Children	< 1.0 mg/dL

IgG comprises 75% of total immunoglobulins:

Adults	565–1765 mg/dL
Children:	
Cord	650–1600 mg/dL
1 year	340–1200 mg/dL
>6 years	650–1600 mg/dL

IgM normally comprises 5%–10% of total immunoglobulins:

Adults	35–375 mg/dL
Children:	
Cord	0–19 mg/dL
1–2 years	19–148 mg/dL
12–16 years	26–221 mg/dL

Test Results Time Frame: Within 24–48 hr

Test Description: The immunoglobulins referred to in these tests form specific antibodies to the specific immunoglobulin (IgA, IgD, IgE, IgG, IgM). Each of the immunoglobulins is introduced into the bloodstream when its specific antibody/antigen reactions occur. IgA reflects the immunoglobulin A when it is recognized as a foreign antigen, with the resultant action of IgG antibodies attacking it. Testing for IgA should occur in all anaphylactic transfusion reactions. IgD is a protein that acts as an autoimmune antibody in clients with collagen diseases. IgE is the antibody protein that is responsible for activation in allergic reactions. IgG makes up 75% of all immunoglobulins. It posseses antibody activity against viruses, bacteria, and toxins. IgG is also important in autoimmune diseases. IgM comprises 5%–10% of the immunoglobulins and is the first antibody to be activated when an antigen enters the body.

BLOOD

CLINICAL ALERT:
There are normal values for various age ranges in children that are best found in laboratories. Clients who are immunosuppressed need special precautions to prevent infections.

Consent Form: Not required

List of Equipment: Red-top tube or serum separator tube; needle and syringe or vacutainer; alcohol swab

Test Procedure:
1. Label the specimen tube. *Correctly identifies the client and the test to be performed.*
2. Obtain a 1- to 7-mL blood sample.
3. Do not agitate the tube. *Agitation may cause RBC hemolysis.*
4. Send tube to the laboratory.

Clinical Implications and Indications:
1. Detects serum globulin abnormalities.
2. Detects acute inflammatory response pattern, acute stress pattern, or acute-phase protein pattern.
3. IgG immunoglobulins constitute the majority of the antibodies.
4. Decreased levels are found with hypoglobulinemia, agammaglobulinemia (which may be either primary or secondary), long-term steroid treatment, nephrotic syndrome, severe infections, chronic lymphocytic leukemia, and multiple myeloma.
5. Evaluates myocardial infarction, rheumatoid collagen disease, nephrotic syndrome, and cirrhosis.
6. Chronic infections typically produce antibody responses that are prolonged and substantial enough to increase immunoglobulin values above reference limits.

Nursing Care:
Before Test: Explain the test procedure and the purpose of the test. Assess the client's knowledge of the test.
During Test: Adhere to standard precautions.
After Test: Apply pressure to venipuncture site. Explain that some bruising, discomfort, and swelling may appear at the site and that warm, moist compresses can alleviate this. Monitor for signs of infection.

Potential Complications: Bleeding and bruising at venipuncture site

Contraindications: Radionuclide testing within the past 72 hr

Interfering Factors: Not keeping specimen at the correct temperature

Nursing Considerations:
Pediatric: IgG crosses the placental barrier. Infants and children will need assistance in remaining still during the venipuncture and age-appropriate comfort measures following the test.
Gerontology: Many of the immunoglobulins are increased in the types of disease processes that are prevalent in the elderly (e.g., arthritis, cancer, chronic infections).

WEBLINKS

http://www.nlm.nih.gov

Immunoperoxidase Procedures
(*IM*-yue-noe-puh-*RAKS*-uh-days proe-*SEE*-j:rz)
(peroxidase; HRP; PAP)

5 min.

BLOOD

Type of Test: Blood

Body Systems and Functions: Immunological system

Normal Findings: Peroxidase activities have traditionally been expressed in units based upon the rate of oxidation of pyrogallol.

Test Results Time Frame: Within 48 hr

Test Description: Immunoperoxidase procedures consist of measuring a wide variety of hydrogen donors that have been utilized in peroxidase assay systems. A stain is used to localize and identify antigens in tissues. The reaction rate is determined by measuring an increase in absorbance at 510 nm, which results from the decomposition of hydrogen peroxide. One unit results in the decomposition of 1 μmol/min hydrogen peroxide at 25°C and pH 7.0 under the specified conditions.

One unit = one micromole of hydrogen peroxide/minute at 25°C and pH = 7.0

Consent Form: Not required

List of Equipment: Red-top tube or serum separator tube; needle and syringe or vacutainer; alcohol swab

Test Procedure:
1. Label the specimen tube. *Correctly identifies the client and the test to be performed.*
2. Obtain a 5-mL blood sample.
3. Do not agitate the tube. *Agitation may cause RBC hemolysis.*
4. Send tube to the laboratory.

Clinical Implications and Indications:
1. Assists in the diagnosis of immunoglobulin disorders.
2. Detects and measures antigens and antibodies.
3. Rapid diagnosis of herpes encephalitis.
4. Elevated levels are found with endocrine tumors, Hodgkin's disease, Rocky Mountain spotted fever, splenomegaly, and G-cell hyperplasia.

Nursing Care:
Before Test: Explain the test procedure and the purpose of the test. Assess the client's knowledge of the test.
During Test: Adhere to standard precautions.
After Test: Apply pressure to venipuncture site. Explain that some bruising, discomfort, and swelling may appear at the site and that warm, moist compresses can alleviate this. Monitor for signs of infection.

Potential Complications: Bleeding and bruising at venipuncture site

Nursing Considerations:
Pediatric: Infants and children will need assistance in remaining still during the venipuncture and age-appropriate comfort measures following the test.

BLOOD

Listing of Related Tests: Assay using 4-aminoantipyrine as hydrogen donor; matrix-supported horseradish peroxidase

WEBLINKS

www.worthington-biochem.com

Infertility Screen
(*IN*-f:r-*TIL*-uh-tee)
(male infertility; hypogonadism; female infertility)

5 min.

Type of Test: Blood

Body Systems and Functions: Reproductive system

Normal Findings: Normal levels of pituitary gonadotropins. Males: normal levels of FSH, LH, and serum testosterone. Females: normal levels of CBC, erythrocyte sedimentation rate, blood chemistries, thyroid function test, serum levels of prolactin, FSH, LH and total estrogens, and serum estradiol and estriol.

Test Results Time Frame: Within 72 hr

Test Description: Infertility screening tests begin with several months of recording the woman's basal body temperature (BBT) and analysis of one or two semen specimens from the male. Other tests performed include postcoital test, endometrial biopsy, hysterosalpingogram, and laparoscopy. Serum levels of testosterone and gonadotropins can differentiate between primary testicular abnormality and pituitary or hypothalamic dysfunction.

Consent Form: Not required

List of Equipment: Red-top tube or serum separator tube (lavender-top tube for CBC and ESR); needle and syringe or vacutainer; alcohol swab

Test Procedure:
1. Label the specimen tube. *Correctly identifies the client and the test to be performed.*
2. Obtain a 5-mL blood sample.
3. Do not agitate the tube. *Agitation may cause RBC hemolysis.*
4. Send tube to the laboratory.

Clinical Implications and Indications:
1. Determines presence of gonadal dysfunction.
2. Evaluates estradiol in menstrual abnormalities; all studies mentioned will help evaluate fertility problems.
3. Assists in evaluation of estrogen-producing tumors in women and testicular or adrenal tumors in men.

Nursing Care:
Before Test: Explain the test procedure and the purpose of the test. Assess the client's knowledge of the test.
During Test: Adhere to standard precautions.

After Test: Apply pressure to venipuncture site. Explain that some bruising, discomfort, and swelling may appear at the site and that warm, moist compresses can alleviate this. Monitor for signs of infection.

Potential Complications: Bleeding and bruising at venipuncture site

Interfering Factors: Radionuclide scan within 48 hr can alter some infertility tests.

Nursing Considerations:
Pregnancy: *The potential options, such as adoption and foster parenting, are viable alternatives to infertility that the health care provider should present.*

Listing of Related Tests: FSH; LH; hysterosalpingogram; diagnostic laparoscopy

▐▐WEBLINKS ▖   ▤▨

http://www.pstcc.cc.tn.us/ost/2910/pronun/c14

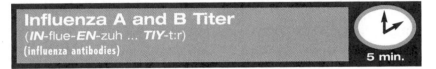

Influenza A and B Titer
(*IN*-flue-*EN*-zuh ... *TIY*-t:r)
(influenza antibodies)

5 min.

Type of Test: Blood

Body Systems and Functions: Immunological system

Normal Findings: <1:8 titer (demonstrates previous exposure); positive titer = influenza; negative titer = bacterial infection

Test Results Time Frame: Within 72 hr

Test Description: Influenza A and B titer is done primarily to screen for influenza for epidemiological reasons. It helps to assess for bacterial infection versus viral in the symptomatic client as well as risk for transmission of the virus in the positive titer client. The value of the initial sample is limited, without a convalescent sample drawn 14 days after the initial/acute sample. Influenza is a highly contagious viral respiratory disease that is characterized by coryza, fever, cough, and consitutional manifestations such as headache and malaise. Influenza A and B are responsible for periodic epidemics with yearly outbreaks affecting about 48 million Americans each winter and causing 20,000 deaths (most often due to bacterial pneumonia).

Consent Form: Not required

List of Equipment: Red-top tube or serum separator tube; needle and syringe or vacutainer; alcohol swab

Test Procedure:
1. Label the specimen tube. *Correctly identifies the client and the test to be performed.*
2. Obtain a 7-mL blood sample.
3. Do not agitate the tube. *Agitation may cause RBC hemolysis.*

4. Send tube to the laboratory.
5. Draw a convalescent sample 14 days later following the same procedure.

Clinical Implications and Indications:

1. Epidemiological screening tool for influenza viruses A and B. The B virus occurs locally, whereas the A virus spreads rapidly to all areas.
2. Differentiates influenza from bacterial infection in the symptomatic client.
3. Diagnoses the etiology of pulmonary infections and complications, such as pneumonia.

Nursing Care:

Before Test: Explain the test procedure and the purpose of the test. Assess the client's knowledge of the test.
During Test: Adhere to standard precautions.
After Test: Apply pressure to venipuncture site. Explain that some bruising, discomfort, and swelling may appear at the site and that warm, moist compresses can alleviate this. Monitor for signs of infection.

Potential Complications: Bleeding and bruising at venipuncture site

Interfering Factors: A convalescent sample is necessary for added validity of the acute sample.

Nursing Considerations:

Pediatric: Infants and children will need assistance in remaining still during the venipuncture and age-appropriate comfort measures following the test. Children under the age of 5 are particularly at risk for increased morbidity/mortality.
Gerontology: Persons 65 years of age or older are at increased risk for influenza-related complications, such as bacterial pneumonia. The elderly that have a history of chronic cardiac or pulmomary problems are at greatest risk.
Home Care: Home health care provider should be educated to the value of referral (and corresponding laboratory tests) if their clients have symptomatology that is potentially an influenza infection.
Rural: Educating clients that live distances from health care that they may not seek care for something they believe is a common cold virus when in fact it may be influenza, which potentially leads to more complications.

Listing of Related Tests: CBC with differential; sputum culture; nasopharyngeal secretions culture

| **WEBLINKS** |

http://www.nlm.nih.gov

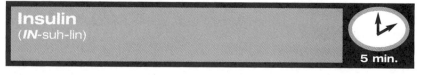

Insulin
(*IN*-suh-lin)

5 min.

Type of Test: Blood

Body Systems and Functions: Endocrine system

Normal Findings:

Fasting:

Infants/children	<13 µU/mL
Adults	17 µU/mL

After 75 g glucose:

30 min	20–112 µU/mL
1 hr	29–88 µU/mL
2 hr	22–79 µU/mL
3 hr	4–62 µU/mL
Insulin-glucose ratio	<0.3:1

Note: Normal laboratory findings vary among laboratory settings.

CRITICAL VALUES:
>30 µU/mL

Test Results Time Frame: Within 24 hr

Test Description: Insulin testing measures the rate of insulin secreted by the cells of the islets of Langerhans in the pancreas. Insulin is a hormone that is secreted normally in response to elevated blood glucose. It promotes glucose utilization, carbohydrate metabolism, and energy storage. Insulin preparations are derived from beef or pork pancreas or synthesized in the laboratory from either an alteration of pork insulin or recombinant DNA technology to form a biosynthetic human insulin. Insulin comes in rapid-acting (regular), intermediate-acting (NPH), or long-acting (Ultralente) preparations. Insulin therapy is mandatory for type I diabetics and provides life-giving medication for clients with diabetes mellitus.

CLINICAL ALERT:
When client is fasting prior to insulin testing, have a glucose source readily available in the event of severe hypoglycemia.

Consent Form: Not required

List of Equipment: Red-top tube or serum separator tube; needle and syringe or vacutainer; alcohol swab

Test Procedure:
1. Label the specimen tube. *Correctly identifies the client and the test to be performed.*
2. Obtain a 7-mL blood sample.
3. Do not agitate the tube. *Agitation may cause RBC hemolysis.*
4. Send tube to the laboratory.

Clinical Implications and Indications:
1. Diagnoses early noninsulin-dependent diabetes mellitus. There will be an excessive production of insulin in relation to blood glucose levels.
2. Confirms functional hypoglycemia.
3. Evaluates postprandial or reactive hypoglycemia of uncertain etiology.
4. Diagnoses insulinoma and assists in the diagnosis of pheochromocytoma.

Nursing Care:

Before Test: Explain the test procedure and the purpose of the test. Assess the client's knowledge of the test. Pretest fasting can lead to severe hypoglycemia and therefore have a glucose source readily available.
During Test: Adhere to standard precautions.
After Test: Apply pressure to venipuncture site. Explain that some bruising, discomfort, and swelling may appear at the site and that warm, moist compresses can alleviate this. Monitor for signs of infection.

Potential Complications: Bleeding and bruising at venipuncture site

Interfering Factors: Administration of insulin or oral hypoglycemic agents within 8 hr of the test can lead to falsely elevated levels; estrogen therapy and progesterone therapy elevate levels; quinine and insulin increase levels.

Nursing Considerations:

Pediatric: Infants and children will need assistance in remaining still during the venipuncture and age-appropriate comfort measures following the test. Careful attention needs to be given to suspected juvenile - onset diabetics. Caregivers and client must be instructed together in the educational processes of managing the disorder of the diabetic condition.

Home Care: Health care providers must be prepared to assess for clinical manifestations of hypoglycemia during pretest fasting and to have a form of glucose available.

Rural: Clients living a considerable distance from laboratory facilities should consider staying near the laboratory if pretest fasting, especially if they have a history of hypoglycemia.

Listing of Related Tests: Fasting blood glucose; postprandial blood sugar; insulin antibodies

WEBLINKS

http://www.niddk.nih.gov

Insulin Assay and Insulin Antibody
(*IN*-suh-lin ae-say *IN*-suh-lin *AEN*-ti-*BAH*-dee)
(insulin antibody)

5 min.

Type of Test: Blood

Body Systems and Functions: Endocrine system

Normal Findings: <3% binding of labeled beef and pork insulin by patient's serum 0–29 µ/mL, or 0–208 pmol/L (SI units)

Test Results Time Frame: Within 24 hr

Test Description: Insulin assay and insulin antibody measure the antibodies formed in diabetics to the insulin they are given. These insulin antibodies are immunoglobulins, called anti-insulin AB, and act as insulin-transporting proteins. The most common type is IgG but is found in all five classes of immunoglobulins in insulin-treated clients. These immunoglobulins, especially IgE, may be responsible for allergic manifestations; IgM may cause insulin resistance. This insulin-antibody level is helpful in determining the most appropriate therapeutic agent in treating diabetic clients. Insulin is secreted by the cells of the islets of Langerhans in the pancreas and is a hormone that is secreted normally in response to elevated blood glucose. It promotes glucose utilization, carbohydrate metabolism, and energy storage. Insulin preparations are derived from beef or pork pancreas or synthesized in the laboratory from either an alteration of pork insulin or recombinant DNA technology to form a biosynthetic human insulin. Insulin comes in rapid-acting (regular), intermediate-acting (NPH), or long-acting (Ultralente) preparations. Insulin therapy is mandatory for type I diabetics and provides life-giving medication for clients with diabetes mellitus.

Consent Form: Not required

List of Equipment: Red-top tube or serum separator tube; needle and syringe or vacutainer; alcohol swab

Test Procedure:
1. Label the specimen tube. *Correctly identifies the client and the test to be performed.*
2. Obtain a 5-mL blood sample.
3. Do not agitate the tube. *Agitation may cause RBC hemolysis.*
4. Send tube to the laboratory.

Clinical Implications and Indications:
1. Identifies insulin resistance
2. Identifies allergic manifestations to insulin
3. Differentiates hypoglycemia from chronic pancreatitis or insulinoma
4. Identifies insulin abuse

Nursing Care:
Before Test: Explain the test procedure and the purpose of the test. Assess the client's knowledge of the test. Fasting is not required.
During Test: Adhere to standard precautions.
After Test: Apply pressure to venipuncture site. Explain that some bruising, discomfort, and swelling may appear at the site and that warm, moist compresses can alleviate this. Monitor for signs of infection.

Potential Complications: Bleeding and bruising at venipuncture site

Interfering Factors: Radioactive scan within 7 days of test will alter test results; certain drugs (e.g., insulin, oral hypoglycemics, quinine) can increase or decrease levels.

Nursing Considerations:
Pediatric: Infants and children will need assistance in remaining still during the venipuncture and age-appropriate comfort measures following the test. Careful attention needs to be given to suspected juvenile-onset diabetics. Caregivers and client must be instructed together in the educational processes of managing the disorder of the diabetic condition.
Home Care: This testing time provides an opportunity for educating home health care providers as to the consequences of the diabetic condition and the appropriate health measures to administer.

BLOOD

Rural: *Clients living a considerable distance from laboratory facilities should consider staying near the laboratory if pretest fasting, especially if they have a history of hypoglycemia.*

Listing of Related Tests: C-peptide test (if insulin abuse suspected); random blood sugar; fasting blood glucose

WEBLINKS

http://www.entnet.org

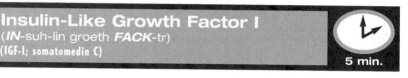

Insulin-Like Growth Factor I
(***IN***-suh-lin groeth ***FACK***-tr)
(IGF-I; somatomedin C)

5 min.

Type of Test: Blood

Body Systems and Functions: Endocrine system

Normal Findings:

Adults:		SI units
Female	24–253 ng/mL	24–253 m/L
Male	43–178 ng/mL	43–178 m/L
Children:		SI units
0–2 years		
Male	14–56 ng/mL	14–56 m/L
Female	14–60 ng/mL	14–60 m/L
3–5 years		
Male	13–83 ng/mL	13–83 m/L
Female	18–97 ng/mL	18–97 m/L
6–9 years		
Male	29–108 ng/mL	29–108 m/L
Female	34–137 ng/mL	34–137 m/L
10–12 years		
Male	44–207 ng/mL	44–207 m/L
Female	66–215 ng/mL	66–215 m/L
13–15 years		
Male	98–319 ng/mL	98–319 m/L
Female	132–305 ng/mL	132–305 m/L
16–18 years		
Male	136–293 ng/mL	136–293 m/L
Female	132–305 ng/mL	132–305 m/L

Test Results Time Frame: Within 3–4 days

Test Description: Insulin-like growth factor I measures a small polypeptide that is produced in the liver, transported in the plasma, and bound by carrier proteins. Insulin-like growth factor I is directly responsible for stimulating growth and proliferation of normal cells. It is affected by growth hormone levels and it affects growth metabolism. Levels of IGF-I are assessed when dwarfism is treated with growth hormone, and IGF-I levels are highest during the growth increases.

Consent Form: Not required

List of Equipment: Lavender-top tube; needle and syringe or vacutainer; alcohol swab

Test Procedure:
1. Label the specimen tube. *Correctly identifies the client and the test to be performed.*
2. Obtain a 2-mL blood sample.
3. Do not agitate the tube. *Agitation may cause RBC hemolysis.*
4. Send tube to the laboratory.
5. Keep specimen cool. *High temperatures alter the results.*

Clinical Implications and Indications:
1. Elevated levels are found with diabetic retinopathy, acromegaly, hyperpituitarism, obesity, pituitary gigantism, pregnancy, and precocious puberty.
2. Decreased levels are found with cirrhosis, chronic illness, diabetes mellitus, anorexia nervosa, hypopituitarism, nutritional deficiency, and pituitary tumors.

Nursing Care:
Before Test: Explain the test procedure and the purpose of the test. Assess the client's knowledge of the test.
During Test: Adhere to standard precautions.
After Test: Apply pressure to venipuncture site. Explain that some bruising, discomfort, and swelling may appear at the site and that warm, moist compresses can alleviate this. Monitor for signs of infection.

Potential Complications: Bleeding and bruising at venipuncture site

Interfering Factors: Pregnancy elevates levels.

Nursing Considerations:
Pregnancy: Levels are higher in pregnancy than in nonpregnancy.
Pediatric: Parents should be educated to look for growth abnormalities to initiate diagnostic testing. IGF-I is an important regulator of fetal growth, and its levels remain constant after the first year of life. Infants and children will need assistance in remaining still during the venipuncture and age-appropriate comfort measures following the test.

Listing of Related Tests: Growth hormone

WEBLINKS

http://www.entnet.org

BLOOD

Intravascular Coagulation Screen
(*IN*-truh-*VAES*-kyue-l:r *KOE*-aeg-yue-*LAY*-sh:n)
(disseminated intravascular coagulation profile; DIC; thrombotic
disease screen; thrombotic risk profile; coagulation profiles)

5 min.

Type of Test: Blood

Body Systems and Functions: Hematological system

Normal Findings: Normal production of fibrin thrombi

Test Results Time Frame: Within 24–48 hr

Test Description: Intravascular coagulation screening are tests that assess the potential presence of disseminated intravascular coagulation (DIC). DIC causes the disruption of hemostasis through the uncontrolled production of thrombi. Profuse bleeding occurs and coagulation factors are used more quickly than they can be produced. DIC is also complicated by fibrinolysis. The causes of internal bleeding, bruising (spontaneous and from slight contact), failure to clot, frequent nosebleeds, petechiae, and heavy menstrual flow may be assessed by screening for DIC. The test allows for the evaluation of prothrombin time, partial thromboplastin time, bleeding time, fibrinogen levels, platelet count, fibrinolysin activation, fibrin split products, thrombin time, clotting factors II, V, VIII, and X, fibrinopeptide A, D-dimer, and antithrombin III.

CLINICAL ALERT:
Clients with DIC are seriously ill and require critical care nursing. Clients must have close supervision, as spontaneous or uncontrolled bleeding may occur. If multiple blood tests are required, the DIC should be taken last. The presence of a lupus anticoagulant in the client's blood requires special precautions.

Consent Form: Not required

List of Equipment: Blue-top tube or plasma separator tube; needle and syringe or vacutainer; alcohol swab

Test Procedure:
1. Label the specimen tube. *Correctly identifies the client and the test to be performed.*
2. Obtain a 5- to 20-mL blood sample.
3. Do not agitate the tube. *Agitation may cause RBC hemolysis.*
4. Send tube to the laboratory.

Clinical Implications and Indications:
1. Detects DIC, which may result from cancer and malignant tumors, sickle cell disease, malaria, trauma or severe injury, cold hemoglobinuria, snake and brown recluse spider bites, cirrhosis, septicemia, severe obstetric complications, blood transfusions, and diseases of the connective tissue
2. Diagnoses lupus anticoagulant, which may confirm the following conditions: systemic lupus erythematosus, autoimmune diseases, thromboembolism, and spontaneous abortions

BLOOD

Nursing Care:

Before Test: Explain the test procedure and the purpose of the test. Assess the client's knowledge of the test. Counsel client to not take warfarin (Coumadin) 2 weeks before the test or heparin 2 days before the test.

During Test: Adhere to standard precautions.

After Test: Apply pressure to venipuncture site. Explain that some bruising, discomfort, and swelling may appear at the site and that warm, moist compresses can alleviate this. Monitor for signs of infection.

Potential Complications: Prolonged bleeding and bruising at venipuncture site

Interfering Factors: Improperly stored blood (must be at room temperature) or plasma (must be frozen if the turnaround time is long); hemolysis; clotted blood; a contaminated sample (such as heparin or IV solutions); tubes that contain the wrong ratio of blood to sodium citrate; lack of sodium citrate in PT, PTT, and TT; warfarin or heparin

Nursing Considerations:

Pediatric: Infants and children will need assistance in remaining still during the venipuncture and age-appropriate comfort measures following the test.

Listing of Related Tests: Bleeding time

‖ WEBLINKS ↳	▤ ⊠

www.labcorp.com

Intrinsic Factor Antibody
(in-*TRIN*-zik *FAEK*-t:r *AEN*-ti-*BAH*-dee)
(APCA; antiparietal cell antibody test)

5 min.

Type of Test: Blood

Body Systems and Functions: Gastrointestinal system

Normal Findings: No presence of intrinsic factor antibodies

Test Results Time Frame: Within 24 hr

Test Description: The intrinsic factor antibodies test measures the intrinsic factor, which is produced by the gastric cells of the stomach mucosa. The test aids in the identification of anemia, as it determines whether the anemia is autoimmune (positive to APCA) or megaloblastic in origin. For example, in pernicious anemia, antibodies to intrinsic factor are produced, which inhibit its normal function. Gastointestinal disease may also be a concern for clients with APCAs. This may require a gastric biopsy.

Consent Form: Not required

List of Equipment: Red-top tube or serum separator tube; needle and syringe or vacutainer; alcohol swab

Test Procedure:

1. Label the specimen tube. *Correctly identifies the client and the test to be performed.*
2. Obtain a 7-mL blood sample.
3. Do not agitate the tube. *Agitation may cause RBC hemolysis.*
4. Send tube to the laboratory.

Clinical Implications and Indications:

1. Detects and monitors atrophic gastritis, diabetes mellitus, gastric cancer or ulcerations, and thyroid disease
2. Assesses for anemia caused by a low B_{12} level (due to the loss of the intrinsic factor)

Nursing Care:

Before Test: Explain the test procedure and the purpose of the test. Assess the client's knowledge of the test.

During Test: Adhere to standard precautions.

After Test: Apply pressure to venipuncture site. Explain that some bruising, discomfort, and swelling may appear at the site and that warm, moist compresses can alleviate this. Monitor for signs of infection.

Potential Complications: Bleeding and bruising at venipuncture site

Interfering Factors: Increased age

Nursing Considerations:

Gerontology: False-positive results may occur over the age of 60 years.

Listing of Related Tests: Schilling test; vitamin B_{12} .

WEBLINKS

http://www.entnet.org

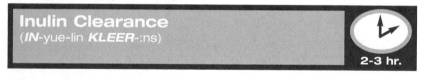

Inulin Clearance
(*IN*-yue-lin *KLEER*-:ns)

2-3 hr.

Type of Test: Blood; urine

Body Systems and Functions: Renal/urological system

Normal Findings:

Birth–10 years	82–122 mL/min
11–20 years	86–126 mL/min
21 years and older	90–130 mL/min
Over 70 years	Clearance may decrease up to 45%

Test Results Time Frame: Within 3–4 days

Test Description: Inulin clearance is a test that assesses the glomerular filtration rate (GFR) of the kidneys. The GFR is an accurate means of determining the functioning status of the kidneys. Many disorders affect the GFR, and early detection of pathology is essential. Inulin is a plant polysaccharide that after IV injection is freely and almost completely filtered by the glomeruli. This test measures both the blood and the urine to determine the rate at which inulin is being cleared through the kidney. Five separate blood and urine tests are taken at five intervals within a 2- to 3-hr period. The blood may be drawn from the arm or obtained by pricking the earlobe, heel, or finger with a lancet. The urine is collected through a catheter. The specimens are examined by radioimmunoassay.

> **CLINICAL ALERT:**
> Caution is required with those who are susceptible to congestive heart failure.

Consent Form: Not required

List of Equipment: *Blood:* five red-top tubes or plasma separator tubes; five needles and syringes or five lancets; alcohol swab. *Urine:* sterile plastic container; straight catheter kit.

Test Procedure:
Blood:
1. Label the specimen tubes. *Correctly identifies the client and the test to be performed.*
2. Obtain a 10-mL blood specimen from arm, heel, earlobe, or finger.
3. Do not agitate the blood tubes. *Agitation may cause hemolysis.*
4. Continue to collect four additional blood samples in heparinized tubes at measured intervals within a 2- to 3-hr period.
5. Inulin will be infused via IV route, as prescribed by clinician at specific times during the test.
6. Send tubes to laboratory.

Urine:
1. Have client drink 32 oz of water prior to the test and every 15 min throughout the test.
2. Label the collection container. *Correctly identifies the client and the test to be performed.*
3. Carefully insert the catheter into the client's urethra and collect 10-mL urine specimens.
4. Continue to collect four additional 10-mL urine samples at measured intervals within a 2- to 3-hr period.
5. Inulin will be infused via IV route, as prescribed by clinician at specific times during the test.
6. Send specimen containers to laboratory.

Clinical Implications and Indications:
1. Elevated levels are found with diuresis.
2. Decreased levels are found with bilateral urethral obstruction, congestive heart failure, advanced chronic bilateral pyelonephritis, acute or chronic glomerulonephritis, active tubular necrosis, low blood flow through the kidneys, dehydration, advanced kidney lesions, and nephrosclerosis.

Nursing Care:
Before Test: Explain the test procedure and the purpose of the test. Assess the client's knowledge of the test. Instruct client to fast 12 hr prior to the test (note:

1 L of water should be consumed 1 hr before the test). Advise the client not to engage in physical activity the morning of the test.

During Test: Adhere to standard precautions. Instruct client to drink 8 oz of water every 15 min during the test.

After Test: Blood: Apply pressure to venipuncture site. Explain that some bruising, discomfort, and swelling may appear at the site and that warm, moist compresses can alleviate this. Monitor for signs of infection.

Urine: Encourage client to void within 2–3 hr after the test. If urine is discolored, inform health care provider.

Potential Complications: Bleeding and bruising at venipuncture site; clinical manifestations of congestive heart failure in susceptible clients

Contraindications: Urinary tract infection; congestive heart failure

Interfering Factors: Urine contaminated with feces; heavy bleeding during menstruation; inaccurate results may occur if client does not fast or abstain from exercise the morning of the test.

Nursing Considerations:

Pediatric: Infants and children will need assistance in remaining still during the venipuncture and catheterization and age-appropriate comfort measures following the test.

Gerontology: Assessing client for specfic clinical manifestations of congestive heart failure prior to this test could prevent complications.

Listing of Related Tests: BUN; serum creatinine; creatinine clearance; urine concentration/clearance test

WEBLINKS

http://www3.healthgate.com

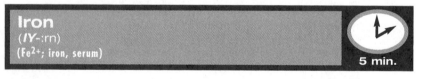

Iron
(IY-:rn)
(Fe²⁺; iron, serum)

5 min.

Type of Test: Blood

Body Systems and Functions: Hematological system

Normal Findings:

Men	75–175 μg/L
Women	65–165 μg/L
Children	50–120 μg/L
Newborns	100–250 μg/L

CRITICAL VALUES:
For poisoned child: 280–2550 μg/dL. Child may be vomiting and have convulsions, diarrhea with blood, cyanosis, and intense stomach pain. False values are >1,800 μg/dL.

Test Results Time Frame: Within 24–48 hr

Test Description: Serum iron testing assesses for iron levels in the blood. Serum iron is used for evaluating suspected iron deficiencies or to aid the diagnosis of conditions characterized by abnormally high levels of iron.

CLINICAL ALERT:
Iron serum test should be performed in the morning, as iron values are highest at this time.

Consent Form: Not required

List of Equipment: Red-top tube or serum separator tube; needle and syringe or vacutainer; alcohol swab

Test Procedure:
1. Label the specimen tube. *Correctly identifies the client and the test to be performed.*
2. Obtain a 10-mL blood sample.
3. Do not agitate the tube. *Agitation may cause RBC hemolysis.*
4. Send tube to the laboratory.

Clinical Implications and Indications:
1. Increased levels are found with acute iron poisoning, lead poisoning, acute hepatitis, acute leukemia, hemochromatosis, hemolytic anemias, thalassemia, nephrosis, iron overload syndromes, and hepatic necrosis.
2. Decreased levels are found with iron deficiency; severe, frequent, or prolonged blood loss; pregnancy (third trimester); hypothyroidism; systemic lupus erythematosus; rheumatoid arthritis; and pernicious anemia.

Nursing Care:
Before Test: Explain the test procedure and the purpose of the test. Assess the client's knowledge of the test. Instruct client to fast 8 hr prior to test. Also, inform client that rest and relaxation are less likely to disrupt iron levels.
During Test: Adhere to standard precautions.
After Test: Apply pressure to venipuncture site. Explain that some bruising, discomfort, and swelling may appear at the site and that warm, moist compresses can alleviate this. Monitor for signs of infection. Client may require follow-up for further testing. Inform laboratory if the client is on oral birth control or takes estrogen therapy.

Potential Complications: Bleeding and bruising at venipuncture site

Contraindications: Postpone test for 4 days if the client has recently had a transfusion.

Interfering Factors: Failure to fast; lack of rest before examination; intense stress; iron supplements; iron-chelating drugs

Nursing Considerations:
Pediatric: Infants and children will need assistance in remaining still during the venipuncture and age-appropriate comfort measures following the test.

Listing of Related Tests: Ferritin; total iron-binding capacity; transferrin

WEBLINKS

http://medline.cos.com

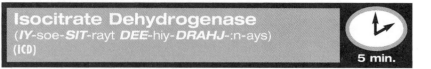

Type of Test: Blood

Body Systems and Functions: Hepatobiliary system

Normal Findings: 1.2–7 U/L at 86°F (30°C). Birth–2 weeks: Levels may be up to 4 times higher than 1.2–7 U/L.

Test Results Time Frame: Within 24–48 hr

Test Description: Isocitrate dehydrogenase is an enzyme located in the tissue. ICD is a catalyst for isocitrate acid (enabling it to convert to alpha-ketoglutaric acid). The test assesses the degree to which tissue damage has occurred in the liver, allows the identification of a viral hepatitis infection and infectious mononucleosis, and confirms liver disease when symptoms are similar to myocardial infarction (SGOT must be high).

Consent Form: Not required

List of Equipment: Red-top tube or serum separator tube; needle and syringe or vacutainer; alcohol swab

Test Procedure:
1. Label the specimen tube. *Correctly identifies the client and the test to be performed.*
2. Obtain a 5- to 7-mL blood sample.
3. Do not agitate the tube. *Agitation may cause RBC hemolysis.*
4. Send tube to the laboratory.

Clinical Implications and Indications:
1. Elevated levels are found with acute viral hepatitis, cirrhosis, malignancies in the liver, and mononucleosis.

Nursing Care:
Before Test: Explain the test procedure and the purpose of the test. Assess the client's knowledge of the test. Instruct client to be NPO 12 hr prior to the test and not to consume alcohol 24 hr prior to the test. Client may be required to stop taking any medications before the test.
During Test: Adhere to standard precautions.
After Test: Apply pressure to venipuncture site. Explain that some bruising, discomfort, and swelling may appear at the site and that warm, moist compresses can alleviate this. Monitor for signs of infection.

Potential Complications: Bleeding and bruising at venipuncture site

Interfering Factors: Failure to fast; alcohol consumption; application of tourniquet on the client's arm for more than 1 min; medications that alter results are aminosalicylic acid, isoniazid, methotrexate, and phenylbutazone.

Nursing Considerations:
Pediatric: Infants and children will need assistance in remaining still during the venipuncture and age-appropriate comfort measures following the test.

Listing of Related Tests: Hepatitis tests; lactate dehydrogenase (enzymes)

WEBLINKS

http://alice.ucdavis.edu/IMD/420A/course.htm

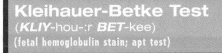

Kleihauer-Betke Test
(*KLIY*-hou-:r *BET*-kee)
(fetal hemoglobulin stain; apt test)

5 min.

Type of Test: Blood

Body Systems and Functions: Reproductive system

Normal Findings: Maternal blood does not contain fetal cells.

Test Results Time Frame: Within 24 hr

Test Description: The Kleihauer-Betke test determines the amount of feto-maternal hemorrhaging in an Rh1-negative mother and the amount of RhIG necessary to prevent antibody production. This test is performed after full-term delivery, if newborn anemia is present, or when the mother is Rh negative or slightly negative. In addition, this test is also performed after an invasive procedure, such as amniocentesis.

Consent Form: Not required

List of Equipment: Lavender-top tube or serum separator tube; needle and syringe or vacutainer; alcohol swab

Test Procedure:
1. Label the specimen tube. *Correctly identifies the client and the test to be performed.*
2. Obtain a 7-mL blood sample.
3. Do not agitate the tube. *Agitation may cause RBC hemolysis.*
4. Send tube to the laboratory.

Clinical Implications and Indications:
1. Results indicate moderate to great fetomaternal hemorrhage (50%–90% of fetal red cells contain HgF). Performed after trauma, miscarriage, and amniocentesis.
2. Optimizes detection and quanitification of fetal cells on a maternal blood smear to distinguish between various types of congenital and acquired increases in fetal hemoglobin.

Nursing Care:
Before Test: Explain the test procedure and the purpose of the test. Assess the client's knowledge of the test.
During Test: Adhere to standard precautions.
After Test: Apply pressure to venipuncture site. Explain that some bruising, discomfort, and swelling may appear at the site and that warm, moist compresses can alleviate this. Monitor for signs of infection. Ensure that client understands

BLOOD

that administration of RhIG may be required and that the client should contact her health care provider immediately for test results.

Potential Complications: Bleeding and bruising at venipuncture site

Interfering Factors: Clotting of blood sample; extended time between sample collection and laboratory analysis; improper temperature storage of sample

WEBLINKS

http://www.webmd.com

Lactate Dehydrogenase
(*LAEK*-tayt *DEE*-hiy-*DRAHJ*-:n-ays)
(LD; LDH; lactate dehydrogenase isoenzymes; lactate LDHI-5)

5 min.

Type of Test: Blood

Body Systems and Functions: Hematological system

Normal Findings:

Normal range 48–115 U/L:

LDH1	17.5%–28.3% heart
LDH2	30.4%–36.4% heart
LDH3	19.2%–24.8% lungs
LDH4	9.6%–15.6% lungs
LDH5	5.5%–12.7% liver and muscles

CRITICAL VALUES:
Peak value may reach 300–800 U/L following a myocardial infarction.

Test Results Time Frame: Within 1–24 hr

Test Description: Lactate dehydrogenase (LDH) is an intracellular enzyme found in almost all body tissues and it is released after tissue damage. The highest concentrations are found in organs such as the heart, liver, kidneys, and skeletal muscle cells. Therefore, when body tissue is damaged from trauma, ischemia, or acid-base imbalance, LDH is released into the bloodstream. A serum sample of LDH assists in diagnosing the amount of tissue damage; however, the specific location of the injury may need to be determined by other means.

CLINICAL ALERT:
Isoenzyme electrophoresis is usually necessary for definitive diagnoses of suspected disorders (since many factors may cause elevation of LDH).

Consent Form: Not required

List of Equipment: Red-top tube or serum separator tube; needle and syringe or vacutainer; alcohol swab

BLOOD

Test Procedure:
1. Label the specimen tube. *Correctly identifies the client and the test to be performed.*
2. Obtain a 7-mL blood sample.
3. Do not agitate the tube. *Agitation may cause RBC hemolysis.*
4. Send tube to the laboratory.

Clinical Implications and Indications:
1. Diagnoses suspected myocardial infarction
2. Diagnoses anemia and hepatic disorders
3. Monitors client response to some forms of chemotherapy

Nursing Care:
Before Test: Explain the test procedure and the purpose of the test. Assess the client's knowledge of the test. Instruct clients suspected of an MI that they will have the test repeated in the next 2 days to monitor progressive changes.
During Test: Adhere to standard precautions.
After Test: Apply pressure to venipuncture site. Explain that some bruising, discomfort, and swelling may appear at the site and that warm, moist compresses can alleviate this. Monitor for signs of infection.

Potential Complications: Bleeding and bruising at venipuncture site

Interfering Factors: Prolonged tourniquet application; recent pregnancy or surgery; prosthetic heart valves; medications that increase levels are alcohol, anabolic steroids, anesthetics, aspirin, bismuth salts, carbenicillin, chlorpromazine, clindamycin, clofibrate, codeine, dicumarol, floxuridine, fluorides, holothane, imipramine, levadopa, lithium, lorazepam, meperidine hydrochloride, methotrexate, methyltestorerone, metaprolol tartrate, mithramycin, morphine, niacin, nitrofurantoin, norethindrone, procainamide hydrochloride, propranolol, quinidine, sulfamethoxazole, and thryoid hormone; medications that decrease levels are ascorbic acid and oxablates.

Nursing Considerations:
Pregnancy: *Recent pregnancy may cause elevated LDH levels.*
Pediatric: *Normal values differ for pediatrics:*

Neonate	160–1500 U/L
Infant	150–360 U/L
Child	150–300 U/L

Infants and children will need assistance in remaining still during the venipuncture and age-appropriate comfort measures following the test.

Listing of Related Tests: Creatinine kinase (CK); asparate aminotransferase (AST)

WEBLINKS

http://www.healthgate.com

Lactose Tolerance
(**LAEK**-toes)
(breath hydrogen test)

1-2 hr.

Type of Test: Blood; breath

Body Systems and Functions: Gastrointestinal system

Normal Findings:
Blood:

Normal value	>30 mg/dL
Abnormal value	<20 mg/dL
Inconclusive	20–30 mg/dL
Hydrogen breath test	<25 ppm from baseline; absence of abdominal pain or cramping

CRITICAL VALUES:
Blood glucose values may rise significantly (720 mg/dL) in diabetics even though lactose is malabsorbed.

Test Results Time Frame: Several hours to 1 day (test is positive if client experiences abdominal discomfort, cramping, or diarrhea).

Test Description: A lactose tolerance test indicates the deficiency of intestinal disaccharidase in the blood. The hydrogen breath test indicates the presence of undigested lactose in the intestinal tract. The lactose ferments in the intestinal tract and thus produces higher levels of hydrogen in the patient's breath. This can be directly measured as the amount of H_2 in the breath equals the amount of undigested test dose lactose.

CLINICAL ALERT:
Abnormal values indicate the need for prompt further testing of glucose or galactose intolerance.

Consent Form: Not required

List of Equipment: Four gray-top tubes or serum separator tubes; needles and syringes or vacutainer; alcohol swab; breath-collecting mechanism

Test Procedure:
Blood:
1. Label the specimen tubes. *Correctly identifies the client and the test to be performed.*
2. Obtain a 5-mL blood sample.
3. The client drinks a mixture of 20 mL water and 50 g of lactose.
4. Blood lactose samples are taken at 30, 60, and 90 min after the ingestion of lactose mixture.
5. Do not agitate the tubes. *Agitation may cause RBC hemolysis.*
6. Send tube to the laboratory.
7. Keep specimen cool. *High temperatures alter the results.*

Hydrogen breath:
1. Samples are taken at the same intervals as blood sampling.

BLOOD

Clinical Implications and Indications:

1. Detects lactose intolerance if glucose levels do not rise (note: indicates a lack of sugar-splitting enzymes).
2. Identifies irritable bowel syndrome (IBS).
3. A glucose and galactose test should be given to verify symptoms.

Nursing Care:

Before Test: Explain the test procedure and the purpose of the test. Assess the client's knowledge of the test. Instruct client to be NPO 12 hr before test and to not smoke 8 hr before or during test.

During Test: Adhere to standard precautions.

After Test: Apply pressure to venipuncture site. Explain that some bruising, discomfort, and swelling may appear at the site and that warm, moist compresses can alleviate this. Monitor for signs of infection.

Potential Complications: Abdominal discomfort, gas, diarrhea, constipation

Interfering Factors: Intense exercise; smoking; diabetes; enterogenous steatorrhea; poor gastric emptying or small bowel transit; certain foods eaten within 24 hr of test (i.e., high fiber, dark bread, peas, sugars); medications that alter results are antibiotics taken 14 days prior to test, benzodiazepines, insulin, oral contraceptives, propranolol hydrochloride, and thiazide diuretics.

Nursing Considerations:

Pediatric: Infants and children will need assistance in remaining still during the venipuncture and age-appropriate comfort measures following the test. Lactose intolerance is often a congenital condition and may be present in newborns. The child's weight determines strength of lactose mixture for treatment.

Home Care: Clients in the home settings need to be taught that symptoms such as IBS, gas, bloating, abdominal discomfort, constipation, and diarrhea are indicative of lactose intolerance. Consequently, the clients should report these clinical manifestations to their health care provider.

International: There is a higher prevalence of lactose tolerance in Native Americans, African Americans, Asians, and Jews.

Listing of Related Tests: Glucose tolerance test; hydrogen breath test

WEBLINKS

http://chorus.rad.mcw.edu

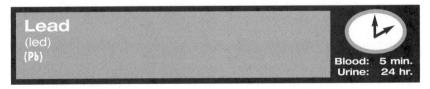

Lead
(led)
(Pb)

Blood: 5 min.
Urine: 24 hr.

Type of Test: Blood; urine

Body Systems and Functions: Hematological system

Normal Findings:

		SI units
Whole blood:		
Adults	<20 mg/dL	<1.0 μmol/L
Children	<10 mg/dL	<1.5 μmol/L
Lead encephalopathy, children	>100 mg/dL	0.39 mmol/L

Test Results Time Frame: Within 24 hr

Test Description: Lead is a heavy metal that when ingested or breathed can be highly toxic. Lead is found in paint, insecticides, pottery glaze, and the fumes of old painted wood. Lead measurements are obtained from whole-blood specimens. Both blood and 24-hr urine samples are collected simultaneously to evaluate the presence of lead.

> **CLINICAL ALERT:**
> Clients with lead poisoning are critically ill and need emergency treatment (usually lavage). Early clinical manifestations are anorexia, apathy, headache, dizziness, sleep disturbances, anemia, and weight loss.

Consent Form: Not required

List of Equipment: *Blood:* lead-free royal-blue-top EDTA tube; needle and syringe or vacutainer; alcohol swab. *Urine:* acid-washed (lead-free) container; ice.

Test Procedure:

Blood:
1. Label the specimen tube. *Correctly identifies the client and the test to be performed.*
2. Obtain a 3-mL blood sample.
3. Do not agitate the tube. *Agitation may cause RBC hemolysis.*
4. Send tube to the laboratory.

Urine:
1. Label the collection container. *Correctly identifies the client and the test to be performed.*
2. Discard the first morning void. Then begin the time of the collection for the next 24 hr, including the void at the end of the 24 hr, and record the last voiding time. *An exact 24-hr count ensures accurate results.*
3. If the client has an indwelling catheter in place, keep the drainage bag on ice and empty the urine into the urine container periodically during the 24-hr period.
4. Keep urine cool during collection. *Higher temperatures alter the results.*
5. If any urine is lost, discard the entire specimen and begin collection again the next day.

Clinical Implications and Indications:

1. Elevated levels are found with ataxia, metal poisoning (lead), microcytic anemia, and neuropathy.
2. Urine uric acid levels and blood erythropoietin levels may be elevated in lead exposure.

BLOOD

Nursing Care:

Before Test: Explain the test procedure and the purpose of the test. Assess the client's knowledge of the test. Explain the test procedure and the purpose of the test. Assess the client's knowledge of the test. Instruct client not to discard any urine over the 24-hr time period.

During Test: Adhere to standard precautions. If any urine is accidentally discarded or contaminated with feces, discard entire specimen and begin test again the following morning.

After Test: Apply pressure to venipuncture site. Explain that some bruising, discomfort, and swelling may appear at the site and that warm, moist compresses can alleviate this. Monitor for signs of infection. Document urine quantity, date, and exact hours of collection on requisition.

Potential Complications: Bleeding and bruising at venipuncture site

Interfering Factors: Urine contaminated with feces; spillage or inaccurate collection of the 24-hr specimen, including nonrefrigeration or placing on ice; heavy bleeding during menstruation; high-calcium diet; fingerstick methods of obtaining specimen

Nursing Considerations:

Pediatric: Infants and children will need assistance in remaining still during the venipuncture and age-appropriate comfort measures following the test. Toddlers often put things in their mouths and should be prevented from ingesting lead products.

WEBLINKS

www.healthgate.com

Legionella pneumophila Antibody
(*LEE*-juh-*NEL*-uh *NEU*-moe-*FIL*-uh)
(Legionnaires' disease antibodies; direct FA smear)

5 min.

Type of Test: Blood; culture; sputum

Body Systems and Functions: Respiratory system

Normal Findings: No *Legionella* antibody titer by IFA or ELISA testing

CRITICAL VALUES:
Test is species specific (there are more than 20 species of *Legionella*); antibody response requires more than fourfold increase in titer to ≥1:128. Between acute (1 week) and convalescent (3 weeks) presumptive diagnosis is ≥1:256.

Test Results Time Frame: Within 3–7 days

Test Description: *Legionella pneumophila* testing measures the antibodies of *Legionella* by various methods. The presence of IgM reflects a current infection status, and the presence of IgG is evidence of previous infection. DFA (*Legionella* antigen detection) is performed by making slides of tissue or lower respiratory secretions. They are stained by DFA and observed microscopically. *Legionella* cultures examine the specimen (tissue or respiratory secretions) and observe for growth over a time period of about 10 days. In addition, *L. pneumophila* is detected by throat swabs or sputum examination for respiratory involvement.

CLINICAL ALERT:
The blood testing needs to be reserved for use when sputum culture is not available or if culture produces negative results.

Consent Form: Not required

List of Equipment: *Blood:* red-top tube or serum separator tube; needle and syringe or vacutainer; alcohol swab. *Culture:* swab; culture medium. *Sputum:* sterile sputum container.

Test Procedure:
Blood:
1. Label the specimen tube. *Correctly identifies the client and the test to be performed.*
2. Obtain a 5-mL blood sample.
3. Do not agitate the tube. *Agitation may cause RBC hemolysis.*
4. Send tube to the laboratory.
5. Repeat 3 weeks later for convalescent sample and label the tube as convalescent sample. *Allows for separate identification of the convalescent sample, which is compared in ratio to the acute sample.*

Culture:
1. Obtain specimen and place on culture medium.

Sputum:
1. Have client expectorate deep lung specimen into sterile sputum container.

Clinical Implications and Indications:
1. Diagnoses *L. pneumophila* with a rise in titer to >1:128 in the interval between acute and convalescent phase.
2. Confirms *L. pneumophila* infection and may also indicate retrospective values.
3. Diagnoses *L. pneumophila* in clients receiving immunosuppressive therapy.
4. *Legionella pneumophila* can be transmitted through shower heads, whirlpools, and air conditioning.

Nursing Care:
Before Test: Explain the test procedure and the purpose of the test. Assess the client's knowledge of the test.
During Test: Adhere to standard precautions.
After Test: Apply pressure to venipuncture site. Explain that some bruising, discomfort, and swelling may appear at the site and that warm, moist compresses can alleviate this. Monitor for signs of infection. Inform client that a follow-up appointment (for the convalescent sample) is usually needed in approximately 3 weeks.

Nursing Considerations:
Pediatric: Infants and children will need assistance in remaining still during these testing procedures and age-appropriate comfort measures following the test.

Gerontology: Client education that positive results are most frequently seen in middle-aged to older men, smokers, and people with chronic diseases
Rural: People living or working near soil excavations are at risk.

WEBLINKS

http://www.methodisthealth.com

Leptospira
(*LEP*-toe-*SPIY*-ruh)
(*Leptospira* serodiagnosis)

Blood: 5 min.
Culture: 10 min.

Type of Test: Blood; urine

Body Systems and Functions: Immunological system

Normal Findings: No evidence of *Leptospira* in blood, cerebrospinal fluid, or urine

Test Results Time Frame: Within 2–4 weeks

Test Description: *Leptospira* culture is a test for the presence of several serotypes of *Leptospira interrogans. Leptospira* is a pathogenic spirochete that causes human infection (leptospirosis). Common hosts are cattle, rats, raccoons, and skunks. It is not usually transmitted from human to human. *Leptospira* may be in contaminates of food and water. *Leptospira* is an occupational hazard for veterinarians, butchers, fish handlers, and animal caretakers. A blood culture should be taken at the same time as the urine culture. An antibodies serum is evaluated for the presence of antibodies to *Leptospira.*

Consent Form: Not required

List of Equipment: *Blood:* two tubes of Fletcher's medium, green- or light-blue-top tube or serum separator tube; needle and syringe or vacutainer; alcohol swab. *Urine:* sterile plastic container.

Test Procedure:
Blood:
1. Label the specimen tube. *Correctly identifies the client and the test to be performed.*
2. Obtain a 5-mL blood sample.
3. Do not agitate the tube. *Agitation may cause RBC hemolysis.*
4. Send tube to the laboratory.
5. Keep specimen cool. *High temperatures alter the results.*
Blood cultures:
1. Label the culture bottle. *Correctly identifies the client and test to be performed.*
2. Obtain blood specimen.
3. Send tube to the laboratory.
Urine:
1. Label a sterile urine container. *Correctly identifies the client and the test to be performed.*

BLOOD

2. Obtain a clean-catch specimen of urine (note: first morning voiding preferred, at least 50 mL). *Ensures accurate results.*
3. Keep specimen cool. *High temperatures alter the results.*
4. Send specimen to laboratory.

Clinical Implications and Indications:
1. Diagnoses *Leptospira* disease.
2. *Leptospira* disease is usually accompanied by muscular pains, fever, jaundice, and liver and spleen enlargement (note: WBC count may be normal or < 40,000).

Nursing Care:
Before Test: Explain the test procedure and the purpose of the test. Assess the client's knowledge of the test. Before drawing blood, call the microbiology laboratory to ensure that Fletcher's medium is available. Determine onset of symptoms as blood cultures are not usually successful after the first week of illness.
During Test: Adhere to standard precautions. If any urine is accidentally discarded or contaminated with feces, discard entire specimen and begin test again.
After Test: Blood: Apply pressure to venipuncture site. Explain that some bruising, discomfort, and swelling may appear at the site and that warm, moist compresses can alleviate this. Monitor for signs of infection. Urine: Document urine quantity, date, and exact hours of collection on requisition.

Potential Complications: Bleeding and bruising at venipuncture site

Interfering Factors: Urine contaminated with feces; spillage or inaccurate collection of the urine specimen, including nonrefrigeration or placing on ice; heavy bleeding during menstruation; acidic urine; greater than 30-min time period between obtaining specimen and innoculation process with the laboratory medium

Nursing Considerations:
Pediatric: Blood: Infants and children will need assistance in remaining still during the venipuncture and age-appropriate comfort measures following the test. Urine: A collection bag needs to be used for infants and toddlers.
Rural: The common hosts are animals in "country settings," and therefore, health prevention education in rural settings is advocated. Specific areas of contamination would require assistance from local and regional public health departments.

WEBLINKS

http://adam.excite.com

Leukoagglutinin
(*LUE*-koe-uh-*GLUET*-uh-nin)

5 min.

Type of Test: Blood

Body Systems and Functions: Hematological system

Normal Findings: No leukoagglutinins present

Test Results Time Frame: Within 24–48 hr

Test Description: The leukoagglutinin test is performed in blood recipients who develop transfusion reactions or in blood donors after transfusion causes a reaction. Donor plasma contains an antibody that reacts with the recipient white cells to produce an acute clinical syndrome of fever, dyspnea, cough, and if severe, cyanosis and hypertension within 1–4 hr.

CLINICAL ALERT:
Initially, if a transfusion reaction is suspected, the transfusion is stopped, vital signs are taken frequently, and the primary physician is notified. If a transfusion recipient has a positive leukoagglutinin and further transfusions are needed, prevent further reactions with acetaminophen and/or leukocyte-reduced blood.

Consent Form: Not required

List of Equipment: Red-top tube or serum separator tube; needle and syringe or vacutainer; alcohol swab

Test Procedure:
1. Label the specimen tube. *Correctly identifies the client and the test to be performed.*
2. Obtain a 5-mL blood sample.
3. Do not agitate the tube. *Agitation may cause RBC hemolysis.*
4. Send tube to the laboratory.

Clinical Implications and Indications:
1. Elevated levels are found with a nonhemolytic transfusion reaction in the recipient or an acute noncardiogenic pulmonary edema.

Nursing Care:
Before Test: Explain the test procedure and the purpose of the test. Assess the client's knowledge of the test.
During Test: Adhere to standard precautions.
After Test: Apply pressure to venipuncture site. Explain that some bruising, discomfort, and swelling may appear at the site and that warm, moist compresses can alleviate this. Monitor for signs of infection.

Potential Complications: Bleeding and bruising at venipuncture site

Interfering Factors: Recent administration of dextran; IV contrast media; blood transfusion within past 3 months

Nursing Considerations:
Pregnancy: Febrile reactions more common in pregnant women.
Pediatric: Infants and children will need assistance in remaining still during the venipuncture and age-appropriate comfort measures following the test.

WEBLINKS

www.healthgate.com

Leukocyte Alkaline Phosphatase (LAP) Stain

(*LUE*-koe-siyt *AEL*-kuh-liyn *FAHS*-fayt)
(LAP; neutrophil alkaline phosphatase; NAP)

5 min.

Type of Test: Blood

Body Systems and Functions: Hematological system

Normal Findings: 20–100 staining score (LAP units) out of a possible of 400

> **CRITICAL VALUES:**
> Low values 0–13 LAP units; high values more than 180 LAP units

Test Results Time Frame: Within 4 hr

Test Description: Leukocyte alkaline phosphatase is an enzyme found in all tissues. Leukocyte alkaline phosphatase (LAP) is located in neutrophils and is involved in intracellular metabolism. LAP is stained to determine the presence of certain diseases. It is especially important in distinguishing between chronic granulocytic leukemia and a leukemoid (leukemia-like) reaction. A venous blood sample is stained and LAP is counted. Levels may be detected in arterial, capillary (earlobe), bone marrow, and venous blood (the specimen described below).

Consent Form: Not required

List of Equipment: Green-top tube (see individual laboratory for specific instructions on collection containers) or serum separator tube; needle and syringe or vacutainer; alcohol swab; blood smear equipment; bone marrow smear equipment

Test Procedure:
1. Label the specimen tube. *Correctly identifies the client and the test to be performed.*
2. Obtain a 2-mL blood sample, usually from the hand or inside the elbow.
3. Wrap tube in foil. *Ensures accurate results.*
4. Do not agitate the tube. *Agitation may cause RBC hemolysis.*
5. Send tube to the laboratory.

Clinical Implications and Indications:
1. Decreased levels are found with nephrotic syndrome, chronic granulocytic leukemia, infectious mononucleosis, paroxysmal nocturnal hemoglobinuria, chronic myelogenous leukemia, thrombocytopenic purpura, and sickle cell anemia.
2. Elevated levels are found with polycythemic vera, leukemoid reactions, myelofibrosis, Down's syndrome, Hodgkin's disease, aplastic leukemia, thrombocytopenia, and multiple myeloma.

Nursing Care:
Before Test: Explain the test procedure and the purpose of the test. Assess the client's knowledge of the test. Instruct client to fast for 6 hr before test.

During Test: Adhere to standard precautions.

After Test: Apply pressure to venipuncture site. Explain that some bruising, discomfort, and swelling may appear at the site and that warm, moist compresses can alleviate this. Monitor for signs of infection.

Potential Complications: Bleeding and bruising at venipuncture site

Interfering Factors: Medications that alter results are some antibiotics, steroid therapy, narcotics, methyldopa, propranolol, allopurinol, tricyclic antidepressants, oral contraceptives, anti-inflammatory medications, androgens, tranquilizers, and antidiabetic drugs; severe physical exercise; pregnancy labor

Nursing Considerations:

Pediatric: *Infants and children will need assistance in remaining still during the venipuncture and age-appropriate comfort measures following the test. May choose to use fingerstick method or earlobe for infants and children.*

Listing of Related Tests: White blood cell count

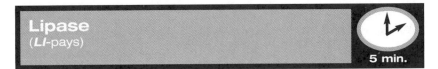

WEBLINKS

http://www.methodisthealth.com

Lipase
(*LI*-pays)

5 min.

Type of Test: Blood

Body Systems and Functions: Gastrointestinal system

Normal Findings:

Infants	9–105 IU/L
Children	20–136 IU/L
Adults	0–1.5 U/mL or 0–417 U/L (SI units)
	20–180 IU/L or 14–280 U/L (SI units)

CRITICAL VALUES:
Elevated values (>600 IU/L) may indicate acute pancreatitis or pancreatic-duct obstruction, which could require immediate interventions.

Test Results Time Frame: Within 12 hr

Test Description: Lipase is an enzyme secreted by the pancreas and participates in fat digestion by breaking down triglycerides into fatty acids and gylcerol. Lipase is secreted into the blood when there is damage to the pancreatic acinar cells. In addition, lipase is excreted in the kidneys.

Consent Form: Not required

List of Equipment: Red-top tube or serum separator tube; needle and syringe or vacutainer; alcohol swab

Test Procedure:

1. Label the specimen tube. *Correctly identifies the client and the test to be performed.*
2. Obtain a 5-mL blood sample.
3. Do not agitate the tube. *Agitation may cause RBC hemolysis.*
4. Send tube to the laboratory.

Clinical Implications and Indications:

1. Diagnoses acute pancreatitis, particularly if the client is ill for more than 3 days. Serum amylase returns to normal within 3 days, but serum lipase remains elevated for 5–7 days.
2. Diagnoses pancreatic carcinoma, especially if combined with a sustained moderate elevation of serum lipase.
3. Elevated levels are found with acute cholecystitis, early renal failure, perforated peptic, biliary obstruction, and cirrhosis.
4. Decreased levels are found with advanced chronic pancreatitis, cystic fibrosis, viral hepatitis, disorders with decreased bile salts, and advanced pancreatic carcinoma.

Nursing Care:

Before Test: Explain the test procedure and the purpose of the test. Assess the client's knowledge of the test. Instruct client to be NPO, except water, 8–12 hr prior to the test.

During Test: Adhere to standard precautions.

After Test: Apply pressure to venipuncture site. Explain that some bruising, discomfort, and swelling may appear at the site and that warm, moist compresses can alleviate this. Monitor for signs of infection.

Interfering Factors: Endoscopic retrograde cholangiopancreatography (ERCP) procedure may increase values; traumatic venipuncture may decrease values; medications that increase levels are morphine, meperidine, heparin, bethanechol, cholinergics, codeine, indomethacin, and methacholine; medications that decrease levels are protamine, calcium ions, and IV saline infusions.

Nursing Considerations:

Pediatric: Infants and children will need assistance in remaining still during the venipuncture and age-appropriate comfort measures following the test.

Listing of Related Tests: Amylase

WEBLINKS ⬚	🗖🗙

www.healthgate.com

Lipid-Associated Sialic Acid

(*LIP*-id uh-*SOE*-shee-*AYT*-:d siy-*AEL*-ik *AE*-sid)
(LASA; LASA (serial monitor); lipid-bound sialic acid)

5 min.

Type of Test: Blood

Body Systems and Functions: Oncology system

Normal Findings: 10–24 mg/dL

Test Results Time Frame: Within 24 hr

Test Description: Lipid-associated sialic acid is a tumor marker. Tumor markers are substances produced and secreted by tumor cells. In cancer, elevated concentrations of sialic acid occur because of the release and accumulation of sialyl compounds from malignant cells. Tumor markers allow evaluation of treatment and a specific method for identifying the presence of the cancer cells. The tumor markers are measured as prevention to the cancer or as follow-up for return of the proliferation of cancer cells.

Consent Form: Not required

List of Equipment: Red-top tube or serum separator tube; needle and syringe or vacutainer; alcohol swab

Test Procedure:
1. Label the specimen tube. *Correctly identifies the client and the test to be performed.*
2. Obtain a 5-mL blood sample.
3. Do not agitate the tube. *Agitation may cause RBC hemolysis.*
4. Keep specimen cool. *High temperatures alter the results and samples lose up to 25% LASA.*
5. Send tube to the laboratory.

Clinical Implications and Indications:
1. Elevated levels are found with mammary, gastroenteric, pulmonary, and ovarian neoplasms, leukemia, lymphoma, melanoma, sarcoma, and Hodgkin's disease.
2. LASA levels can also be elevated in benign diseases, including inflammatory disorders or tissue necrosis, so the test alone does not confirm cancer.
3. The test is useful in monitoring cancer after therapy.

Nursing Care:
Before Test: Explain the test procedure and the purpose of the test. Assess the client's knowledge of the test.
During Test: Adhere to standard precautions.
After Test: Apply pressure to venipuncture site. Explain that some bruising, discomfort, and swelling may appear at the site and that warm, moist compresses can alleviate this. Monitor for signs of infection. Inform client that they may be required to have test repeated to monitor the effectiveness of treatment.

Potential Complications: Bleeding and bruising at venipuncture site

Nursing Considerations:
Pediatric: Infants and children will need assistance in remaining still during the venipuncture and age-appropriate comfort measures following the test.

Listing of Related Tests: Various tumor markers (alpha-fetoprotein; CA-15-3; CA-19-9; CA-50; CA-72-4 TAG; CA-125; C-549)

WEBLINKS

BLOOD

Lipoprotein Electrophoresis
(*LIP*-oe-*PROE*-teen uh-*LEK*-troe-fuh-*REE*-sis)
(lipids; lipoproteins)

5 min.

Type of Test: Blood

Body Systems and Functions: Cardiovascular system

Normal Findings:

Chylomicrons	0%–2%
Beta of LDL	28%–53% (0.28–0.53)
Prebeta or VLDL	3%–32% (0.03–0.32)
Alpha or HDL	24%–40% (0.24–0.40)
Plasma appearance	Clear
HDL women	>45mg/dL or >0.75 mmol/L
HDL men	>55 mg/dL or >0.91 mmol/L
LDL	60–180 mg/dL or <3.37 mmol/L
VLDL	25%–50%

Test Results Time Frame: Within 24 hr

Test Description: Lipoprotein electrophoresis measures the fractions of lipoproteins. This test determines the abnormal distribution and concentration of lipoproteins in the serum, which is a good predictor of coronary artery disease. The lipoproteins are considered a major modifiable risk factor and are especially important correlates to cardiovascular disease when combined with other risk factors (e.g., hypertension, obesity, smoking). Lipids are fat substances, consisting of cholesterol, cholesterol esters, triglycerides, nonesterified fatty acids, and phospholipids. The lipoprotein fractions are chylomicrons, very low density lipoproteins (VLDLs), low-density lipoproteins (LDLs), and high-density lipoproteins (HDLs). Chylomicrons and VLDLs lower cholesterol and protein. LDLs and HDLs contain relatively high amounts of cholesterol and protein.

Consent Form: Not required

List of Equipment: Red-top tube or serum separator tube; needle and syringe or vacutainer; alcohol swab

Test Procedure:
1. Label the specimen tube. *Correctly identifies the client and the test to be performed.*
2. Obtain a 5-mL blood sample.
3. Do not agitate the tube. *Agitation may cause RBC hemolysis.*
4. Send tube to the laboratory.

Clinical Implications and Indications:
1. Elevated levels are correlated with cardiovascular disease.
2. Elevations indicate a need for dietary and lifestyle changes to reduce risk of heart disease.

Nursing Care:

Before Test: Explain the test procedure and the purpose of the test. Assess the client's knowledge of the test. Instruct client to fast for 12 hr prior to the test, to abstain from alcohol for 24 hr before the test, and to avoid strenuous exercise before the test.

During Test: Adhere to standard precautions.

After Test: Apply pressure to venipuncture site. Explain that some bruising, discomfort, and swelling may appear at the site and that warm, moist compresses can alleviate this. Monitor for signs of infection. Inform client regarding the dietary management of fat intake based on the test results and the value of exercise in lowering HDL cholesterol levels.

Potential Complications: Bleeding and bruising at venipuncture site

Interfering Factors: Levels may significantly decrease as long as 3 months after MI; HDL is elevated in hypothyroidism and diminished in hyperthyroidism; medications that increase levels are anabolic steroids, bromides, chlorpromazine, corticosteroids, epinephrine, ergocalciferol, iodides, levodopa, oral contraceptives, phenytoin, sulfonamides, thiazides, trifluoperazine, hydrochloride, trimethadione, and vitamins A, C, D, and E; medications that decrease levels are allopurinol, aminosalicylic acid, asparaginase, azathioprine, cholestryamine, chlorpropamide, chlortetracycline, clofibrate, clomiphine citrate, colchicine, colestipol hydrocholide, dextrothyroxine, erythromycin, estrogens, glucagon, haloperidol, heparin, isoniazid, kanamycin, levothyroxine sodium, MOA inhibitors, neomycin sulfate, niacin, phenformin, and tetracyclines.

Nursing Considerations:

Pediatric: Infants and children will need assistance in remaining still during the venipuncture and age-appropriate comfort measures following the test.
Gerontology: Normal results are slightly higher in the elderly.

Listing of Related Tests: Triglycerides; cholesterol

| WEBLINKS |

http://webmd.lycos.com

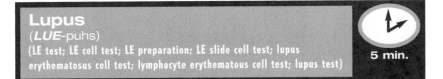

Lupus
(LUE-puhs)
(LE test; LE cell test; LE preparation; LE slide cell test; lupus
erythematosus cell test; lymphocyte erythematous cell test; lupus test)

5 min.

Type of Test: Blood

Body Systems and Functions: Immunological system

Normal Findings: No LE cells present in the blood

Test Results Time Frame: Within 72 hr

Test Description: The lupus test is a blood test that assists in the diagnosis of lupus erythematosus. Approximately 75% of clients who have lupus erythematosus will have circulating LE cells. The LE cells are a result of immunological activity directed against nucleoproteins. The LE cell test is the first test to be used to assist in the diagnosis of lupus. It is only positive in about 50% of clients, and a number of disorders cause false-positive results. The antinuclear antibody (ANA) test is the most frequently used laboratory test for assisting in the diagnosis of suspected cases of systemic lupus erythematosus.

Consent Form: Not required

List of Equipment: Red-top tube or serum separator tube; needle and syringe or vacutainer; alcohol swab

Test Procedure:
1. Label the specimen tube. *Correctly identifies the client and the test to be performed.*
2. Obtain a 5-mL blood sample.
3. Do not agitate the tube. *Agitation may cause RBC hemolysis.*
4. Send tube to the laboratory.

Clinical Implications and Indications:
1. Elevated levels are found with systemic lupus erythematosus (SLE), arthritis, hepatitis, hepatitis, and scleroderma.
2. A positive test does not necessarily mean the client has SLE because there is a risk of false-positive results and the test may be positive in only 50%–75% of clients who do have SLE.

Nursing Care:
Before Test: Explain the test procedure and the purpose of the test. Assess the client's knowledge of the test.
During Test: Adhere to standard precautions.
After Test: Apply pressure to venipuncture site. Explain that some bruising, discomfort, and swelling may appear at the site and that warm, moist compresses can alleviate this. Monitor for signs of infection.

Potential Complications: Bleeding and bruising at venipuncture site

Interfering Factors: False positives may occur in clients with rheumatoid arthritis, scleroderma, and some types of hepatitis; medications that may alter results are clofibrate, hydralazine, isoniazid, mesantoin, methyldopa, methylsergide, oral contraceptives, penicillin, phylbutazone, phenytoin, procainamide, quinidine, reserpine, streptomycin, sulfonamides, tetracycline, and tridione.

Nursing Considerations:
Pediatric: Infants and children will need assistance in remaining still during the venipuncture and age-appropriate comfort measures following the test.

Listing of Related Tests: Antinuclear antibody (ANA) test; anti-DNA antibody test; anti-Sm antibody test

WEBLINKS	

http://www.hamline.edu; http://www.mtio.com

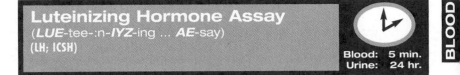

Luteinizing Hormone Assay
(LUE-tee-:n-*IYZ*-ing ... *AE*-say)
(LH; ICSH)

Blood: 5 min.
Urine: 24 hr.

BLOOD

Type of Test: Blood; urine

Body Systems and Functions: Endocrine system

Normal Findings:

Blood:	
Men	6–23 mIU/mL
Women:	
Follicular phase	5–30 mIU/mL
Midcycle	75–150 mIU/mL
Postmenopausal phase	30–200 mIU/mL
Urine:	
Men	13–60 IU/mL
Women:	
Follicular phase	2–25 IU/day
Midcycle peak	Over 3 X baseline
Postmenopausal	>24 IU/day

Test Results Time Frame: Blood: within 24 hr. Urine: within 24–48 hr.

Test Description: The luteinizing hormone assay measures luteinizing hormones (LHs), which are related to either gonadal dysfunction or failure of the pituitary gland or hypothalamus. LH may provide an indication of whether the low levels of luteinizing hormone are of a primary origin or a result of weak stimulation by pituitary hormones. These hormone levels are often used to evaluate infertility in men and women.

Consent Form: Not required

List of Equipment: *Blood:* red-top tube or serum separator tube; needle and syringe or vacutainer; alcohol swab. *Urine:* sterile plastic container.

Test Procedure:

Blood:
1. Label the specimen tube. *Correctly identifies the client and the test to be performed.*
2. Obtain a 5-mL blood sample.
3. Do not agitate the tube. *Agitation may cause RBC hemolysis.*
4. Send tube to the laboratory.

Urine:
1. Label the collection container. *Correctly identifies the client and the test to be performed.*
2. Discard the first morning void. Then begin the time of the collection for the next 24 hr, including the void at the end of the 24 hr, and record the last voiding time. An exact 24-hr count ensures accurate results.

BLOOD

3. If the client has an indwelling catheter in place, keep the drainage bag on ice and empty the urine into the urine container periodically during the 24-hr period.
4. Keep urine cool during collection. *Higher temperatures alter the results.*
5. If any urine is lost, discard the entire specimen and begin collection again the next day.

Clinical Implications and Indications:

1. Elevated levels are found with primary gonadal failure, complete testicular feminization syndrome, and precocious puberty.
2. Decreased levels are found with primary or secondary gonadal insufficiency, anovulation, amenorrhea, hypothalamic disfunction, adrenal hyperplasia, and tumors.

Nursing Care:

Before Test: Explain the test procedure and the purpose of the test. Assess the client's knowledge of the test. Instruct client not to discard any urine over the 24-hr time period.

During Test: Adhere to standard precautions. If any urine is accidentally discarded or contaminated with feces, discard entire specimen and begin test again the following morning.

After Test: Blood: Apply pressure to venipuncture site. Explain that some bruising, discomfort, and swelling may appear at the site and that warm, moist compresses can alleviate this. Monitor for signs of infection. Urine: Document urine quantity, date, and exact hours of collection on requisition.

Potential Complications: Bleeding and bruising at venipuncture site

Interfering Factors: Urine contaminated with feces; spillage or inaccurate collection of the 24-hr specimen, including nonrefrigeration or placing on ice; heavy bleeding during menstruation; hormones that affect LH levels; oral contraceptives

Nursing Considerations:

Pregnancy: Provide emotional support for clients experiencing infertility problems and consider referral to genetic counseling or other appropriate health care providers.

Pediatric: Blood:Infants and children will need assistance in remaining still during the venipuncture and age-appropriate comfort measures following the test. Urine: For collection of 24-hr specimen a collection bag or indwelling catheter needs to be used.

Listing of Related Tests: Follicle-stimulating hormone

WEBLINKS

http://webmd.lycos.com

Lyme Disease
(liym duh-*ZEEZ*)
(*Borrelia burgdorferi*)

5 min.

BLOOD

Type of Test: Blood

Body Systems and Functions: Immunological system

Normal Findings: Negative for *Borrelia burgdorferi*

Test Results Time Frame: Within 24 hr

Test Description: Lyme disease is caused by *Borrelia burgdorferi* (a spirochete), which is transmitted to a person by a deer tick bite. The disease is found mostly in the northeastern, upper midwestern, and western United States. The clinical manifestations are a characteristic rash and flulike symptoms, occurring within 1 week of the tick bite; then later (i.e., 3–24 weeks) symptoms can develop (e.g., carditis, arthritis, and CNS disturbances). False-positive and false-negative results may occur in 40%–60% of the cases because of a lack of detectable antibody response. IgM antibodies can be detected by ELISA in the early stage and by the Western blot in the later stage. Tissue biopsy, cerebrospinal fluid examination, and DNA identification may also be used for diagnosis.

Consent Form: Not required

List of Equipment: Red-top tube or serum separator tube; needle and syringe or vacutainer; alcohol swab

Test Procedure:
1. Label the specimen tube. *Correctly identifies the client and the test to be performed.*
2. Obtain a 3-mL blood sample.
3. Do not agitate the tube. *Agitation may cause RBC hemolysis.*
4. Send tube to the laboratory.

Clinical Implications and Indications:
1. Diagnoses Lyme disease
2. Determines the potential cause of carditis, peripheral neuropathy, central nervous system changes, and arthritis

Nursing Care:
Before Test: Explain the test procedure and the purpose of the test. Assess the client's knowledge of the test.
During Test: Adhere to standard precautions.
After Test: Apply pressure to venipuncture site. Explain that some bruising, discomfort, and swelling may appear at the site and that warm, moist compresses can alleviate this. Monitor for signs of infection.

Potential Complications: Bleeding and bruising at venipuncture site

Interfering Factors: False-positive results may occur with high rheumatoid factor titers and treponemal diseases; antibiotics; high lipid levels

Nursing Considerations:

Pediatric: *Infants and children will need assistance in remaining still during the venipuncture and age-appropriate comfort measures following the test.*
Rural: *Client education for persons in at-risk geographical settings. Inform persons that tick bites in their locations need to be seen by their health care providers. Emphasize prevention precautions (e.g., wearing proper clothing when in areas infested by ticks and deer).*

Listing of Related Tests: ELISA; Western blot

WEBLINKS ⏷	▣ ☒

http://www.nlm.nih.gov

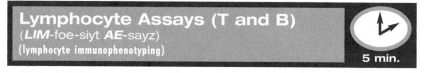

Lymphocyte Assays (T and B)
(***LIM***-foe-siyt ***AE***-sayz)
(lymphocyte immunophenotyping)

5 min.

Type of Test: Blood

Body Systems and Functions: Hematological system

Normal Findings: Total lymphocyte count ranges from 1,500 to 3,000/mm³. Normal T-cell count ranges from 1,400 to 2,700/mm³ (68%–75% of total lymphocytes). Normal B-cell count ranges from 270 to 620/mm³. Normal laboratory findings vary among laboratory settings.

> **CRITICAL VALUES:**
> Progressive depletion of CD4 T lymphocytes is associated with an increased likelihood of clinical complications from AIDS; if CD4 cell count exceeds 500 cells/mm³ in the past 6 months, there is a low probability that these symptoms result from opportunistic infections.

Test Results Time Frame: Within 24 hr

Test Description: Lymphocyte assays determine the percentage of T and B lymphocytes. Lymphocytes usually arrive at sites of infection within 24–48 hr and are responsible for cell- and humoral-mediated immunity. Lymphocytes evolve from precursor cells in the bone marrow. T lymphocytes become further differentiated in the thymus gland and are essential for the specific immune response. B lymphocytes are formed from the pluripotent stem cells in the bone marrow and migrate to the spleen, lymph nodes, and other peripheral lymphoid tissue. Mature B cells are able to identify foreign antigens and are vital to cell-mediated immunity.

> **CLINICAL ALERT:**
> Do not refrigerate or freeze the sample as this interferes with accurate results.

Consent Form: Not required

List of Equipment: Lavender-top tube or plasma separator tube; needle and syringe or vacutainer; alcohol swab

Test Procedure:

1. Label the specimen tube. *Correctly identifies the client and the test to be performed.*
2. Obtain a 5-mL blood sample.
3. Gently invert tube several times, but do not agitate the tube. *Mixes the anticoagulant, but agitation may cause RBC hemolysis.*
4. Send tube to the laboratory.

Clinical Implications and Indications:

1. Elevated levels are found with multiple myeloma, infectious mononucleosis, chronic infections, and viral infections.
2. Decreased levels are found with chronic or acute lymphocytic leukemia, HIV, immunoglobulin deficiency disease, and congenital T-cell deficiency disease.

Nursing Care:

Before Test: Explain the test procedure and the purpose of the test. Assess the client's knowledge of the test.

During Test: Adhere to standard precautions.

After Test: Apply pressure to venipuncture site. Explain that some bruising, discomfort, and swelling may appear at the site and that warm, moist compresses can alleviate this. Monitor for signs of infection.

Potential Complications: Bleeding and bruising at venipuncture site

Interfering Factors: Immunosuppressive drug therapy; steroids; chemotherapy; x-rays; presence of immunoglobulins as in autoimmune diseases; recent viral cold or use of nicotine could decrease T-cell counts.

Nursing Considerations:

Pediatric: Infants and children will need assistance in remaining still during the venipuncture and age-appropriate comfort measures following the test. Children have slightly higher T- and B-cell counts than adults.

Gerontology: The elderly with compromised immune systems, as indicated by abnormal lymphocyte assays, have much higher morbity/mortality incidence.

WEBLINKS

www.thriveonline.com

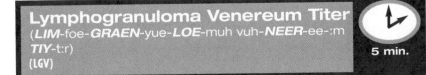

Lymphogranuloma Venereum Titer
(*LIM*-foe-*GRAEN*-yue-*LOE*-muh vuh-*NEER*-ee-:m
TIY-t:r)
(LGV)

5 min.

Type of Test: Blood

Body Systems and Functions: Immunological system

Normal Findings: No genital lesions; no presence of *Chlamydia trachomatis* serotypes L1, L2, or L3

BLOOD

CRITICAL VALUES:
Clinical symptoms (lesions; swollen lymph nodes) and a rise in antibody IgG and IgM titers of 1:16 or higher is indicative of LGV.

Test Results Time Frame: Within 24–48 hr

Test Description: Lymphogranuloma venereum titer is an indirect fluorescent and enzyme immunoassay test. This test allows for the detection of *C. trachomatis* serotypes L1, L2, and L3. Sexually transmitted disease detection requires particularly skilled communication from health care providers. In addition, data about sexually active persons reveal they are emotionally sensitive and require acquiring and maintaining a trusting relationship between the client and the health care providers.

CLINICAL ALERT:
A detailed client history is imperative. It is very common that a client presenting with one sexually transmitted disease (STD) may have other types of venereal diseases (note: many STDs are asymptomatic).

Consent Form: Not required

List of Equipment: Red-top tube or serum separator tube; needle and syringe or vacutainer; alcohol swab

Test Procedure:
1. Label the specimen tube. *Correctly identifies the client and the test to be performed.*
2. Obtain a 10-mL blood sample.
3. Do not agitate the tube. *Agitation may cause RBC hemolysis.*
4. Send tube to the laboratory.
5. Repeat 10–14 days later for convalescent sample and label the tube as convalescent sample. *Allows for separate identification of the convalescent sample that is compared in ratio to the acute sample.*

Clinical Implications and Indications:
1. Diagnoses lymphoma venereum.
2. Visible symptoms (e.g., lesions, swollen lymph nodes) are of critical importance to the diagnosis of LGV.
3. The primary lesion may only be apparent for the first 3 days of the infection and adenopathy may be visible within 1–3 weeks.

Nursing Care:
Before Test: Explain the test procedure and the purpose of the test. Assess the client's knowledge of the test. Perform a complete health and sexual history of the client.

During Test: Adhere to standard precautions.

After Test: Apply pressure to venipuncture site. Explain that some bruising, discomfort, and swelling may appear at the site and that warm, moist compresses can alleviate this. Monitor for signs of infection. Counsel the client regarding the importance of communication with sexual partner. Due to the sensitive nature of STDs, it is especially important to maintain a nonjudgmental attitude toward the client. Allow the client to describe his concerns regarding the test and the possible positive results.

Potential Complications: Bleeding and bruising at venipuncture site

Interfering Factors: Antibiotics produce false negative results.

Nursing Considerations:
Pregnancy: Infected women may transfer the pathogen to the baby during delivery.
Pediatric: Infants and children will need assistance in remaining still during the venipuncture and age-appropriate comfort measures following the test.
International: LGV is more common in tropical and subtropical regions.

Listing of Related Tests: *Chlamydia* culture

WEBLINKS

www.healthgate.com.

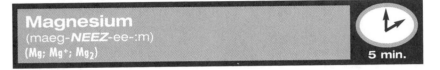

Magnesium
(maeg-*NEEZ*-ee-:m)
(Mg; Mg⁺; Mg₂)

5 min.

Type of Test: Blood

Body Systems and Functions: Metabolic system

Normal Findings:

Adult	1.6–2.6 mg/dL or 0.66–1.07 mmol/L
Child	1.7–2.1 mg/dL or 0.70–0.86 mmol/L
Newborn	1.5–2.2 mg/dL or 0.62–0.91 mmol/L

CRITICAL VALUES:
Values that reflect very serious conditions are:

Hypomagnesemia	<1.0 mg/dL
Hypermagnesemia	>5.0 mg/dL

Test Results Time Frame: Within 24–48 hr

Test Description: Magnesium tests for the level of the electrolyte magnesium. Magnesium is a white mineral element found in soft tissue, muscles, bones, and to some extent body fluids. It is a naturally occurring element, and the human body contains approximately 25 g of magnesium. Magnesium is obtained in sufficient quantities in whole grains, fruits, and vegetables. Abnormal levels of magnesium can reflect pathology in the following arenas of its normal function: metabolic activity of the body, renal function, blood coagulation, metabolism of calcium, and regulation of neuromuscular irritability.

CLINICAL ALERT:
There are significant "panic-level" categories for clients with either high or low values of magnesium. The clinical manifestations are lethargy, flushing, hypotension, and nausea/vomiting for high levels and twitching, muscle tremors, and tetany for low levels.

Consent Form: Not required

List of Equipment: Red-top tube or serum separator tube; needle and syringe or vacutainer; alcohol swab

Test Procedure:
1. Label the specimen tube. *Correctly identifies the client and the test to be performed.*
2. Obtain a 5-mL blood sample.
3. Do not agitate the tube. *Agitation may cause RBC hemolysis.*
4. Send tube to the laboratory.

Clinical Implications and Indications:
1. Magnesium levels vary in many pathological disorders. Refer to table for the wide variety of specific diseases and the corresponding hypomagnesemia or hypermagnesemia.

Pathological disorders in hypomagnesemia vs. hypermagnesemia

Hypomagnesemia seen in:	Hypermagnesemia seen in:
Hypercalcemia	Renal failure or poor renal function
Diabetic acidosis	Dehydration
Chronic renal disease	Hypothyroidism
Hyperaldosteronism	Addison's disease
Pregnancy	Adrenalectomy
Hypoparathyroidism	Severe diabetic ketoacidosis
Hemodialysis	Consumption of Mg-rich antacids
Chronic pancreatitis	IV therapy of magnesium sulfate
Severe dehydration	
Malabsorption problems	
Severe alcoholism	
Long-term hyperalimentation	
Malnutrition	
Hyperthyroidism	
Ulcerative colitis	

Nursing Care:
Before Test: Explain the test procedure and the purpose of the test. Assess the client's knowledge of the test.
During Test: Adhere to standard precautions. Place client in a prone position as blood is drawn, as the Mg level can increase by 4% in an upright position.
After Test: Apply pressure to venipuncture site. Explain that some bruising, discomfort, and swelling may appear at the site and that warm, moist compresses can alleviate this. Monitor for signs of infection.

Potential Complications: Bleeding and bruising at venipuncture site

Contraindications: Low levels of Mg may create a digitalis toxicity; tourniquet use while drawing blood; heavy wheat fiber and alcohol may lessen the absorbtion of Mg.

Interfering Factors: Medications that increase levels are aminoglycerides, cathartics, lithium, aldurox, digel, epsom salts, milk of magnesia, magnesium citrate, alcohol, Mylanta, Maalox, loop diuretics, salicylates, and thyroid medications; medications that decrease levels are mercurial and ethacrynic diuretics, calcium gluconate, amphotericin B, neomycin, insulin, aminoglycerides, amphotericin, cisplatin, corticosteroids, and cyclosporine.

Nursing Considerations:
Pediatric: Infants and children will need assistance in remaining still during the venipuncture and age-appropriate comfort measures following the test. Pediatric age ranges have different normal findings than adults.

WEBLINKS ▸

http://www.adam.com

Malaria
(muh-*LAYR*-ee-uh)
(malaria smear; *Plasmodium falciparum*; *Plasmodium malariae*; *Plasmodium ovale*; *Plasmodium vivax*)

5 min.

Type of Test: Blood; culture

Body Systems and Functions: Hematological system

Normal Findings: No morphological changes in erythrocytes and negative for blood smear for malaria parasites

Test Results Time Frame: Within 48–72 hr

Test Description: Malaria blood testing assesses for the presence of four species of blood parasites of the genus *Plasmodium* carried by *Anopheles* mosquito. These are *P. falciparum*, *P. vivax*, *P. ovale*, and *P. malariae*. The usual approach to detecting malaria antibody is the indirect fluorescent antibody (IFA) test, which detects most antibody responses. However, serological testing is useful for screening blood donors if there is a case of transfusion-induced malaria and if there is a suspected case of malaria in a client who has febrile illness and if the repeated blood smears are negative.

> **CLINICAL ALERT:**
> Travelers to countries where a malaria risk is anticipated should contact their nearest Tropical Diseases Center to discuss prophylaxis. Untreated malaria can progress to severe forms that can be fatal. The most frequent symptoms include fever and chills, headache, myalgia, arthralgia, weakness, vomiting, diarrhea, as well as splenomegaly, anemia, thrombocytopenia, hypoglycemia, pulmonary or renal dysfunction, and neurological changes. Clinical treatment will vary according the species, the level of parasitemia, and the immune status of the client.

Consent Form: Not required

BLOOD

List of Equipment: Lavender-top tube or serum separator tube; needle and syringe or vacutainer; alcohol swab

Test Procedure:
1. Label the specimen tube and include recent travel locations. *Correctly identifies the client, the test to be performed, and potential variation in treatment, depending on the geographical location.*
2. Obtain a 4-mL blood sample.
3. Gently invert tube several times, but do not agitate the tube. *Mixes the anticoagulant, but agitation may cause RBC hemolysis.*
4. Send tube to the laboratory.

Clinical Implications and Indications:
1. Detects one of four forms of *Plasmodium* species that cause malaria
2. Diagnoses trypanosomiasis

Nursing Care:
Before Test: Explain the test procedure and the purpose of the test. Assess the client's knowledge of the test. Obtain travel history from client and a history of any medication use, especially prophylactic antimalarial medications.
During Test: Adhere to standard precautions.
After Test: Apply pressure to venipuncture site. Explain that some bruising, discomfort, and swelling may appear at the site and that warm, moist compresses can alleviate this. Monitor for signs of infection.

Potential Complications: Bleeding and bruising at venipuncture site

Interfering Factors: Levels change from hour to hour, making assessment difficult.

Nursing Considerations:
Pediatric: Infants and children will need assistance in remaining still during the venipuncture and age-appropriate comfort measures following the test.
International: Malaria usually occurs in tropical or subtropical areas and at altitudes below 1,500 feet. Recent immigrants from tropical countries with febrile illness of unknown origin should be tested for malaria. Travelers to countries where a malaria risk is anticipated should contact their nearest Tropical Diseases Center to discuss prophylaxis.

WEBLINKS

http://www.dpd.cdc.gov

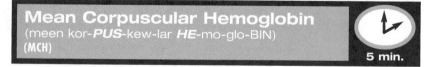

Mean Corpuscular Hemoglobin
(meen kor-*PUS*-kew-lar *HE*-mo-glo-BIN)
(MCH)

5 min.

Type of Test: Blood

Body Systems and Functions: Hematological system

Normal Findings:

Infants at 3 months	24–34 pg
Infants at 1 year	23–31 pg
Children, 10–12 years	24–30 pg
Adults	27–32 pg

CRITICAL VALUES:

Macrocytosis	>50 g
Microcytosis	15 pg (indicates iron deficiency)
Hypochromia	<27 pg

Test Results Time Frame: Within 24–48 hr

Test Description: Mean corpuscular hemoglobin (MCH) determines the mean weight of red blood cells. It is defined as picograms of hemoglobin per each red blood cell:

$$MCH = (Hgb \times 10)/(RBCs \times 10^6 \ \mu L).$$

Hemoglobin, the main intracellular protein of erythrocytes, is the oxygen-carrying compound contained in RBCs. The amount of hemoglobin per 100 mL of blood can be used as an index of the oxygen-carrying capacity of the blood. Neonatal hemoglobin is checked by heelstick (capillary) and is higher than venous blood values. The difference becomes less each day and disappears by the fifth day of life.

Consent Form: Not required

List of Equipment: Lavender-top tube or serum separator tube; needle and syringe or vacutainer; alcohol swab

Test Procedure:

1. Label the specimen tube. *Correctly identifies the client and the test to be performed.*
2. Obtain a 5-mL blood sample.
3. Gently invert tube several times, but do not agitate the tube. *Mixes the anticoagulant, but agitation may cause RBC hemolysis.*
4. Send tube to the laboratory.

Clinical Implications and Indications:

1. Evaluates and monitors macrocytic anemia, microcytic anemia, and hypochromic anemia.
2. MCH is always done as part of the complete blood count.

Nursing Care:

Before Test: Explain the test procedure and the purpose of the test. Assess the client's knowledge of the test.

During Test: Adhere to standard precautions.

After Test: Apply pressure to venipuncture site. Explain that some bruising, discomfort, and swelling may appear at the site and that warm, moist compresses can alleviate this. Monitor for signs of infection. If necessary, educate the client regarding the importance of maintaining an adequate diet or managing medications or hormone, enzyme, or congenital conditions.

Potential Complications: Bleeding and bruising at venipuncture site; clotting of blood

Interfering Factors: False elevations of RBCs may be caused by hyperlidemia, high heparin concentration, large RBC precursors, and cold agglutinins; abnormally small or large RBCs

Nursing Considerations:

Pediatric: Infants and children will need assistance in remaining still during the venipuncture and age-appropriate comfort measures following the test.

Listing of Related Tests: MCV; MCHC; CBC

WEBLINKS

http://www.vgernet.net

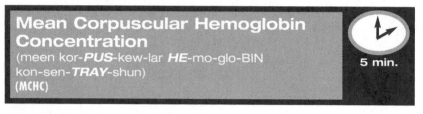

Mean Corpuscular Hemoglobin Concentration
(meen kor-*PUS*-kew-lar *HE*-mo-glo-BIN kon-sen-*TRAY*-shun)
(MCHC)

5 min.

Type of Test: Blood

Body Systems and Functions: Hematological system

Normal Findings:

Adults, the elderly, and children	32–36 g/dL
Newborns	32–33 g/dL

CRITICAL VALUES:

Increased levels	>36 g/dL
Decreased levels	<30 g/dL

Test Results Time Frame: Within 24–48 hr

Test Description: The test evaluates the hemoglobin concentration of RBCs. Hemoglobin and hematocrit are factors within MCHC and are therefore particularly useful for providing treatment for anemia. The amount of hemoglobin per unit volume of RBCs is determined by:

$$MCHC = (Hbg\ [g/dL]\ x100)/(Hct\ \%).$$

Hemoglobin, the main intracellular protein of erythrocytes, is the oxygen-carrying compound contained in RBCs. The amount of hemoglobin per 100 mL of blood can be used as an index of the oxygen-carrying capacity of the blood. Neonatal hemoglobin is checked by heelstick (capillary) and is higher than venous blood values. The difference becomes less each day and disappears by the fifth day of life.

Consent Form: Not required

List of Equipment: Lavender-top tube or serum separator tube; needle and syringe or vacutainer; alcohol swab

BLOOD

Test Procedure:
1. Label the specimen tube. *Correctly identifies the client and the test to be performed.*
2. Obtain a 5-mL blood sample.
3. Gently invert tube several times, but do not agitate the tube. *Mixes the anticoagulant, but agitation may cause RBC hemolysis.*
4. Send tube to the laboratory.

Clinical Implications and Indications:
1. Elevated levels are found with severe dehydration, xerocytosis, cold agglutin disease, hereditary spherocytosis, and intravascular hemolysis.
2. Decreased levels are found with chronic blood loss, anemia, microcytic anemia, iron anemia, severe and immediate overhydration, thalassemia, and sideroblastic anemia.
3. MCHC is always done as part of the complete blood count.

Nursing Care:
Before Test: Explain the test procedure and the purpose of the test. Assess the client's knowledge of the test.
During Test: Adhere to standard precautions.
After Test: Apply pressure to venipuncture site. Explain that some bruising, discomfort, and swelling may appear at the site and that warm, moist compresses can alleviate this. Monitor for signs of infection. If necessary, counsel the client about maintaining an adequate diet and managing medications or hormones, enzymes, or congenital conditions.

Potential Complications: Bleeding and bruising at venipuncture site

Interfering Factors: False elevated readings result from rouleaux, cold agglutins, lipemia, and high heparin concentrations (note: the reading is incorrect if it is higher than 37 g/dL, as this is the highest concentration of Hbg within RBCs)

Nursing Considerations:
Pediatric: Values are higher in newborns and infants. Infants and children will need assistance in remaining still during the venipuncture and age-appropriate comfort measures following the test.

Listing of Related Tests: MCV; MCH; CBC

| WEBLINKS | |

http://adam.excite.com

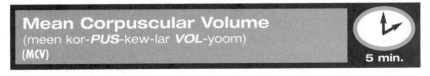

Mean Corpuscular Volume
(meen kor-*PUS*-kew-lar *VOL*-yoom)
(MCV)

5 min.

Type of Test: Blood

Body Systems and Functions: Hematological system

Normal Findings:

Children	75–85 fl µL; value increases during childhood
Adults	80–98 fl µL (x3 exponentially)

CRITICAL VALUES:

Microcytic anemia	<80 µL
Macrocytic anemia	>100 µL

Test Results Time Frame: Within 24 hr

Test Description: Mean corpuscular volume is a calculated value of the average volume of an erythrocyte. The identification of anemia relies on RBC counts. The equation for assessing the volume of a single RBC can reveal whether the RBCs are normocytic, microcytic, or macrocytic. The measurements are in cubic micrometers (femtoliters) of the mean volume. The MCV is calculated by:

$$MCV = (Hct \% \times 10)/(RBCs \times 10^{12} \text{ L}).$$

Consent Form: Not required

List of Equipment: Lavender-top tube or serum separator tube; needle and syringe or vacutainer; alcohol swab

Test Procedure:

1. Label the specimen tube. *Correctly identifies the client and the test to be performed.*
2. Obtain a 5-mL blood sample.
3. Gently invert tube several times, but do not agitate the tube. *Mixes the anticoagulant, but agitation may cause RBC hemolysis.*
4. Send tube to the laboratory.

Clinical Implications and Indications:

1. Elevated levels are found with pregnancy, oral birth control, reticulocytosis, myeloplastic anemia, aplastic anemia, pure red cell aplasia, vitamin B_{12} or folate deficiency, alcohol consumption, liver disease, Down's syndrome, and severe hypoglycemia.
2. Decreased levels are found with iron deficiency, thalassemia, anemia, hemoglobin E disease, lead poisoning, and hyperthyroidism.
3. MCV is always done as part of the complete blood count.

Nursing Care:

Before Test: Explain the test procedure and the purpose of the test. Assess the client's knowledge of the test.

During Test: Adhere to standard precautions

After Test: Apply pressure to venipuncture site. Explain that some bruising, discomfort, and swelling may appear at the site and that warm, moist compresses can alleviate this. Monitor for signs of infection. If necessary, counsel the client about maintaining a proper diet and managing medications or hormone, enzyme, or congenital conditions.

Potential Complications: Bleeding and bruising at venipuncture site; miscalculation of MCV; clotting of blood sample

Interfering Factors: High altitude; a false "normal" size may result from a mixed presence of macrocytes and microcytes; high readings result from increased reticulocytes and marked leukocytosis; medications that increase levels are cyclophosphamide, azathioprine, and vidarabine.

Nursing Considerations:
Pediatric: *Infants and children will need assistance in remaining still during the venipuncture and age-appropriate comfort measures following the test.*
International: *Hemoglobin E disease is more common in Burma, East Asia, and Veddes in Sri Lanka.*

Listing of Related Tests: MCH; MCHC; CBC

WEBLINKS

http://adam.excite.com

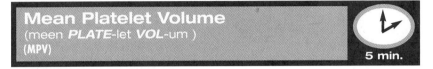

Mean Platelet Volume
(meen *PLATE*-let *VOL*-um)
(MPV)

5 min.

Type of Test: Blood

Body Systems and Functions: Hematological system

Normal Findings: MPV: 8.6–11.7 fl mL
Adults, platelet count   140–400 x 10^3/mm³
Children, platelet count   150–450 x 10^3/mm³

> **CRITICAL VALUES:**
> Decrease in platelets to <20 x 10^3/mm³ places clients at high risk of spontaneous bleeding.

Test Results Time Frame: Within 24 hr

Test Description: Mean platelet volume tests the platelet count. Platelets are the basic elements of the blood, which promote coagulation. Abnormally high or low platelets indicate serious disease states. Platelets are counted by microscopy or by an automated method. The MPV is also calculated at the same time. The MPV indicates the uniformity of the platelet distribution and is used in the differential diagnosis of thrombocytopenia. A blood smear is done to evaluate the size, shape, and clumping of the platelets. Clients who are suspected of having thrombocytopenia, uremia, liver disease, cancer, or bone marrow failure will have platelet counts to assess risk of bleeding.

> **CLINICAL ALERT:**
> Clients with increased platelet count may have a malignancy. Clients with decreased or elevated platelet values are at risk for serious bleeding.

Consent Form: Not required

List of Equipment: Lavender-top tube (EDTA) or plasma separator tube; needle and syringe or vacutainer; alcohol swab

Test Procedure:
1. Label the specimen tube. *Correctly identifies the client and the test to be performed.*
2. Obtain a 7-mL blood sample.
3. Gently invert tube several times, but do not agitate the tube. *Mixes the anticoagulant, but agitation may cause RBC hemolysis.*
4. Send tube to the laboratory.

Clinical Implications and Indications:
1. Increased levels are found with thrombocytopenia; thrombocytosis; chronic myelogenous and granulocytic leukemia; myeloproliferative diseases; polycythemia vera; primary thrombocytosis; splenectomy; iron-deficiency anemia; asphyxiation; collagen diseases such as rheumatoid arthritis, acute blood loss, or hemolytic anemia; acute infections or inflammatory disease; Hodgkin's disease; lymphomas; malignancies;chronic pancreatitis; tuberculosis; inflammatory bowel disease; renal failure; and recovery from bone marrow suppression.
2. Decreased levels are found with idiopathic thrombocytopenic purpura; neonatal purpura; pernicious, aplastic, and hemolytic anemia; massive blood transfusion; viral, bacterial, and rickettsial infections; congestive heart disease; thrombopoietin deficiency; chemotherapy; HIV infection; cancer; DIC and thrombotic thrombocytopenic purpura; toxemia of pregnancy; eclampsia; alcohol toxicity; ethanol abuse; hypersplenism; and renal insufficiency.
3. MPV is routinely done with the complete blood count.

Nursing Care:
Before Test: Assess client's knowledge of the test. Explain the test procedure and the purpose of the test.
During Test: Adhere to standard precautions.
After Test: Apply pressure to venipuncture site. Explain that some bruising, discomfort, and swelling may appear at the site and that warm, moist compresses can alleviate this. Monitor for signs of infection. Inform client to inform their health care provider immediately if site starts to bleed or bruise. Instruct client to avoid injury and using sharp objects (razor), hard tooth brush, and over-the-counter drugs with anticoagulant effects.

Potential Complications: Bleeding from venipuncture site

Interfering Factors: False positives are found with high altitudes, oral contraceptives, strenous exercise, trauma, excitement, hyperthyroidism, and diabetes; false negatives are found with menstruation and during pregnancy; epinephrine causes an increased platelet count; medications that cause a decreased platelet count are chloromycetin, streptomycin, sulfonamides, salicylates, quinidine, quinine, acetaxolamide, amidopyrine, thiazide diuretics, meprobamate, phylbutazone, tolbutamide, vaccine injections, chemotherapy, and radiation therapy.

Nursing Considerations:
Pediatric: Infants and children will need assistance in remaining still during the venipuncture and age-appropriate comfort measures following the test.

Listing of Related Tests: Prothrombin time

‖ WEBLINKS ‖

http://www.methodisthealth.com

Methemoglobin, Hemoglobin M
(met-*HEE*-muh-*GLOE*-bin *HEE*-muh-*GLOE*-bin)
(hemoglobin M)

5 min.

BLOOD

Type of Test: Blood

Body Systems and Functions: Hematological system

Normal Findings: 0.4%–1.5% of total hemoglobin

CRITICAL VALUES:
>10%

Test Results Time Frame: Within 24 hr

Test Description: Methemoglobin M is a blood test used to diagnose hereditary or acquired methemoglobinemia in clients who have symptoms of anoxia or cyanosis. Usually there is no evidence of cardiovascular or pulmonary disease. Hemoglobin M is an inherited disease that produces cyanosis.

Consent Form: Not required

List of Equipment: Lavender-top tube or plasma separator tube; needle and syringe or vacutainer; alcohol swab

Test Procedure:
1. Label the specimen tube. *Correctly identifies the client and the test to be performed.*
2. Obtain a 5-mL blood sample.
3. Gently invert tube several times, but do not agitate the tube. *Mixes the anticoagulant, but agitation may cause RBC hemolysis.*
4. Send tube to the laboratory.
5. Keep specimen cool. *High temperatures alter the results.*

Clinical Implications and Indications:
1. The most common cause of methemoglobinemia is induced by the toxic effects of drugs or chemicals, including: dapsone (most common drug causing the problem), analgesics; sulfonamide derivatives, nitrates and nitrites, nitroglycerin, antimalarials, isoniazid, quinones, potassium chloride, benzocaine, and lidocaine.

Nursing Care:
Before Test: Explain the test procedure and the purpose of the test. Assess the client's knowledge of the test.
During Test: Adhere to standard precautions.
After Test: Apply pressure to venipuncture site. Explain that some bruising, discomfort, and swelling may appear at the site and that warm, moist compresses can alleviate this. Monitor for signs of infection. If test is positive, instruct client that there will be treatment and follow-up therapy for the identified disorder.

Potential Complications: Bleeding and bruising at venipuncture site

Interfering Factors: Consumption of foods rich in nitrates prior to the test (e.g., sausage, bacon, smoked meats); absorption of silver nitrate used to treat burns; excessive use of Bromo-Seltzer; smoking; bismuth preparations for diarrhea

Nursing Considerations:

Pregnancy: Pregnant women should be advised about drinking well water containing nitrates or taking bismuth preparations for diarrhea.

Pediatric: Fetal hemoglobin is more readily converted to methemoglobin than in adults, so infants are more susceptible to methemoglobinemia. Infants and children will need assistance in remaining still during the venipuncture and age-appropriate comfort measures following the test.

Listing of Related Tests: Hemoglobin

WEBLINKS

http://www.webmd.com

Microfilaria, Peripheral
(*MIYK*-roe-fi-*LAYR*-ee-uh p:r-*RIF*-:r-:l)
(peripheral blood preparation; trypanosomiasis; helminths)

5 min.

Type of Test: Blood

Body Systems and Functions: Hematological system

Normal Findings: No indication of parasitic infestation

Test Results Time Frame: Within 24 hr

Test Description: Microfilaria is the test used to identify parasitic infestations. A blood sample is taken and immediately examined in the laboratory using both thick and thin blood smears. The parasite may be identified by the motility of the microfiliriae and the extent to which they cause movement of surrounding erythrocytes. Blood samples should be drawn at noon and at midnight to distinguish between nocturnal parasites and those that circulate during the day.

> **CLINICAL ALERT:**
> Blood samples should be drawn while the client's fever is high.

Consent Form: Not required

List of Equipment: Fingersticks; slides or lavender-top tubes; cotton ball

Test Procedure:
1. Label the specimen tube. *Correctly identifies the client and the test to be performed.*
2. Obtain a blood sample with the fingerstick and collect on a slide or in a heparinized tube.
3. Send specimen immediately to the laboratory. *Ensures accurate results.*

Clinical Implications and Indications:
1. Diagnoses trypsanosomiasis, microfilariasis, and parasitic infestation.
2. Further testing required for the confirmation of elephantitis.

3. Skin biopsy diagnoses *Onchocera volvulus* and *Diptalonema streptocera.*

Nursing Care:
Before Test: Explain the test procedure and the purpose of the test. Assess the client's knowledge of the test.
During Test: Adhere to standard precautions.
After Test: Apply pressure to blood sample site. Explain that some bruising, discomfort, and swelling may appear at the site and that warm, moist compresses can alleviate this. Monitor for signs of infection.

Potential Complications: Bleeding at blood sample site

Interfering Factors: Clotting of blood; false-negatives results; failure to identify nocturnal and daytime nature of parasite

Nursing Considerations:
Pediatric: Infants and children will need assistance in remaining still during the fingerstick or biopsy and age-appropriate comfort measures following the test.
International: A detailed history is important, particularly if the client has been traveling in areas that are high risk for parasitic infections. The possible parasite, dates, places, and nature of the traveling should be recorded.

Listing of Related Tests: Bacteremia detection; filariasis serologic test; red blood cell morphology

WEBLINKS

http://www.methodisthealth.com/pathology/hemato.htm

Migration Inhibition
(miy-*GRAY*-sh:n in-hi-*BISH*-:n)
(lymphocyte marker assay)
5 min.

Type of Test: Blood

Body Systems and Functions: Lymphatic system

Normal Findings: Values of T- and B-surface markers:

Percentage of B cells (CD19)	5%–20%
Percentage of T cells (CD3)	53%–88%
Percentage of helper T cells (CD4)	32%–61%
Percentage of suppressor/cytotoxic T cells (CD8)	18%–42%
Percentage of natural killer cells (CD16)	4%–32%
Lymphocyte counts	660–4,600 cells/μL
B-cell count (CD19)	99–426 cells/μL
T-cell count (CD3)	812–2,318 cells/μL
Helper T-cell count (CD4)	589–1,505 cells/μL
Suppressor/cytotoxic T-cell count (CD8)	325–977 cells/μL
CD4–CD8 ratio	≥1.0

Test Results Time Frame: Within 24–48 hr

Test Description: Migration inhibition is a test that examines the functioning of T and B cells. The values of these cells are defined as the absolute number of cells per microliter. The diagnoses of a variety of autoimmune disorders (e.g., acquired immunodeficiency virus, chronic infections, lymphoma) are facilitated by evaluating how these cells function within the immune system.

> **CLINICAL ALERT:**
> The results of the test may be emotionally difficult for the client to hear. Sensitivity and consideration toward the feelings and concerns of the client are very important.

Consent Form: May be required

List of Equipment: Red-top tube or serum separator tube; needle and syringe or vacutainer; alcohol swab

Test Procedure:
1. Label the specimen tube. *Correctly identifies the client and the test to be performed.*
2. Obtain a 7-mL blood sample.
3. Do not agitate the tube. *Agitation may cause RBC hemolysis.*
4. Send tube to the laboratory.

Clinical Implications and Indications:
1. Diagnoses T-cell lymphocytic leukemia, lymphoblastic lymphoma, AIDS, malignant T cells, T-cell leukemia, lymphoid malignancy, and autoimmune disorders
2. Monitors AIDS and its treatment regimen

Nursing Care:
Before Test: Explain the test procedure and the purpose of the test. Assess the client's knowledge of the test.
During Test: Adhere to standard precautions.
After Test: Apply pressure to venipuncture site. Explain that some bruising, discomfort, and swelling may appear at the site and that warm, moist compresses can alleviate this. Monitor for signs of infection. Client may need referral for support if diagnosis of serious illness is confirmed.

Potential Complications: Bleeding and bruising at venipuncture site

Interfering Factors: Inability to keep sample at room temperature (colder temperatures affect results)

Nursing Considerations:
Pediatric: Infants and children will need assistance in remaining still during the venipuncture and age-appropriate comfort measures following the test.

Listing of Related Tests: OKT 4; Leu 3

WEBLINKS 🗕🗙

http://webmd.lycos.com

Milk Precipitins
(milk pree-*SIP*-uh-tinz)
(beta-lactoglobulin antibodies screen)

5 min.

Type of Test: Blood

Body Systems and Functions: Immunological system

Normal Findings: No elevated presence of serum antibodies IgA and IgG to beta-lactoglobulin

CRITICAL VALUES:
Elevated IgA specific antibodies: present or recent reaction to beta-lactoglobulin. Elevated IgG-specific antibodies indicates that the mucosal layer of the digestive tract has experienced trauma due to the body's inability to digest beta-lactoglobulin.

Test Results Time Frame: Within 24–48 hr

Test Description: Milk precipitin test detects the presence of serum antibodies IgG and IgA to beta-lactoglobulin, a protein present in cows' milk. Certain individuals may possess a sensitivity to beta-lactoglobulin antigens. A sensitivity is indicated by elevated levels of IgG and IgA in blood serum. The serum levels are measured by ELISA. Gastrointestinal difficulties after the consumption of a milk product also aid in the diagnosis of this condition.

Consent Form: Not required

List of Equipment: Red-top tube or serum separator tube; needle and syringe or vacutainer; alcohol swab

Test Procedure:
1. Label the specimen tube. *Correctly identifies the client and the test to be performed.*
2. Obtain a 7-mL blood sample.
3. Do not agitate the tube. *Agitation may cause RBC hemolysis .*
4. Send tube to the laboratory.

Clinical Implications and Indications:
1. Evaluates adrenal fatigue
2. Diagnoses rheumatoid arthritis, canker sores, celiac disease, colitis, constipation, diarrhea, pyrosis, and irritable bowel syndrome
3. Monitors diabetes mellitus, joint and muscle pain, chronic bladder infections, and chronic persistent headaches

Nursing Care:
Before Test: Explain the test procedure and the purpose of the test. Assess the client's knowledge of the test.
During Test: Adhere to standard precautions.
After Test: Apply pressure to venipuncture site. Explain that some bruising, discomfort, and swelling may appear at the site and that warm, moist compresses can alleviate this. Monitor for signs of infection.

Potential Complications: Bleeding and bruising at venipuncture site

Nursing Considerations:

Pediatric: Children are particularly sensitive to beta-lactoglobulin. Infants and children will need assistance in remaining still during the venipuncture and age-appropriate comfort measures following the test.

Listing of Related Tests: Lactose intolerance; gliadin; IgG and IgA test

WEBLINKS

http://www.nlm.nih.gov/medlineplus/immunesystem

Mononucleosis Spot Test
(mah-noe-*NUEK*-lee-*OE*-sis)
(heterophile antibodies; heterophil agglutinins; monospot)

5 min.

Type of Test: Blood

Body Systems and Functions: Immunological system

Normal Findings: Negative; titer <1:56

Test Results Time Frame: Within 24 hr

Test Description: Mononucleosis spot testing detects antibodies that react to antigens from phylogenetically unrelated species. They agglutinate sheep red blood cells, horse red blood cells (used in the "Monospot" test), and ox and goat erythrocytes. In contrast to atypical lymphocytes, heterophile antibodies are both sensitive and specific for infectious mononucleosis; their detection is the diagnostic test of choice in most clinical situations. Heterophile antibodies appear within 1 week of the onset of clinical symptoms, peak in weeks 2–5, and may persist at low levels for up to 1 year.

CLINICAL ALERT:
Clinical manifestations are more severe in adults than children. HIV clients are especially at risk for this virus. Clients who are immunocompromised from organ transplants may contract fatal primary infections.

Consent Form: Not required

List of Equipment: Red-top tube or serum separator tube; needle and syringe or vacutainer; alcohol swab

Test Procedure:
1. Label the specimen tube. *Correctly identifies the client and the test to be performed.*
2. Obtain a 5-mL blood sample.
3. Do not agitate the tube. *Agitation may cause RBC hemolysis.*
4. Send tube to the laboratory.

Clinical Implications and Indications:
1. The detection of heterophile antibodies is the diagnostic test of choice in most clinical situations of suspected infectious mononucleosis.

2. Assists in diagnosis of EBV infection, systemic lupus erythematosus, and syphilis.

Nursing Care:
Before Test: Explain the test procedure and the purpose of the test. Assess the client's knowledge of the test.
During Test: Adhere to standard precautions.
After Test: Apply pressure to venipuncture site. Explain that some bruising, discomfort, and swelling may appear at the site and that warm, moist compresses can alleviate this. Monitor for signs of infection

Potential Complications: Bleeding and bruising at venipuncture site

Interfering Factors: False-positives tests have been reported in clients with leukemia, pancreatic cancer, and rubella (note: this is rare).

Nursing Considerations:
Pediatric: Infants and children will need assistance in remaining still during the venipuncture and age-appropriate comfort measures following the test.

Listing of Related Tests: IgM and IgG antibodies; CBC

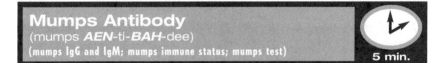

| WEBLINKS |

http://www.nlm.nih.gov

Mumps Antibody
(mumps *AEN*-ti-*BAH*-dee)
(mumps IgG and IgM; mumps immune status; mumps test)

5 min.

Type of Test: Blood

Body Systems and Functions: Immunological system

Normal Findings: Negative for IgG, <1:10 for IgM

Test Results Time Frame: Within 1–4 days

Test Description: Mumps antibodies form as a result of infection. Testing is done through enzyme-linked immunoassay (ELISA or EIA). Blood samples should be taken as early as possible after exposure to mumps and results compared to a sample taken 10–14 days later. It takes 7–14 days for the appearance of an IgM antibody response. Mumps is an acute contagious febrile disease that is known for inflammation of the parotid glands and other salivary glands. The disease is caused by a virus that has an incubation period of 12–25 days.

CLINICAL ALERT:
Infection with mumps virus can lead to meningitis or meningoencephalitis, which can lead to neurological damage, mental retardation, and mortality.

Consent Form: Not required

BLOOD

List of Equipment: Red-top tube or serum separator tube; needle and syringe or vacutainer; alcohol swab

Test Procedure:

1. Label the specimen tube. *Correctly identifies the client and the test to be performed.*
2. Obtain a 3-mL blood sample.
3. Do not agitate the tube. *Agitation may cause RBC hemolysis.*
4. Send tube to the laboratory.
5. Repeat 10–14 days later for convalescent sample and label the tube as convalescent sample. *Allows for separate identification of the convalescent sample, which is compared in ratio to the acute sample.*

Clinical Implications and Indications:

1. Diagnoses recent or current infection with the mumps virus
2. Indicates recent immunization

Nursing Care:

Before Test: Explain the test procedure and the purpose of the test. Assess the client's knowledge of the test.
During Test: Adhere to standard precautions.
After Test: Apply pressure to venipuncture site. Explain that some bruising, discomfort, and swelling may appear at the site and that warm, moist compresses can alleviate this. Monitor for signs of infection. If convalescent serum is required, explain to client the importance of returning for second sample.

Potential Complications: Bleeding and bruising at venipuncture site

Interfering Factors: On rare occassions, parainfluenza increases mumps antibody levels; recent immunization may also result in titer >1:10.

Nursing Considerations:

Pediatric: Infants and children will need assistance in remaining still during the venipuncture and age-appropriate comfort measures following the test. Children need to be immunized with the MMR vaccine at 15 months and again at 4–6 years. If mumps occur, the child should be isolated to promote recovery and prevent transmission of the disease.
Gerontology: Orchitis occurs in 20%–30% of adult males who contract the mumps virus.

WEBLINKS

http://www.nlm.nih.gov

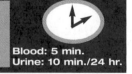

Muramidase
(myur-*RAEM*-uh-days)
(lysozyme)

Blood: 5 min.
Urine: 10 min./24 hr.

Type of Test: Blood; urine

Body Systems and Functions: Immunological system

BLOOD

Normal Findings:
Blood: females, 2.5–12.9 µg/mL; males, 3–12.8 µg/mL. Urine: 0–2.9 mg/L.

Test Results Time Frame: Within 1 week

Test Description: Muramidase tests for the presence of the enzyme that destroys bacteria by breaking down its walls. Muramidase is found in blood cells of the granulocytic and monocytic series (e.g., neutrophils, phagocytes, and macrophages). Muramidase is also present in the saliva, sweat, and tears. Muramidase was formerly named lysozyme.

Consent Form: Not required

List of Equipment: *Blood:* red-top tube or serum separator tube; needle and syringe or vacutainer; alcohol swab. *Urine:* sterile plastic container; ice.

Test Procedure:
Blood:
1. Label the specimen tube. *Correctly identifies the client and the test to be performed.*
2. Obtain a 5-mL blood sample.
3. Do not agitate the tube. *Agitation may cause RBC hemolysis.*
4. Send tube to the laboratory.

Urine (random sample):
1. Label a sterile urine container. *Correctly identifies the client and the test to be performed.*
2. Obtain a clean-catch specimen of urine (note: first morning voiding preferred, at least 15 mL). *Ensures accurate results.*
3. Keep specimen cool. *High temperatures alter the results.*
4. Send specimen to laboratory.

Urine (24 hour):
1. Label the collection container. *Correctly identifies the client and the test to be performed.*
2. Discard the first morning void. Then begin the time of the collection for the next 24 hr, including the void at the end of the 24 hr, and record the last voiding time. *An exact 24-hr count ensures accurate results.*
3. If the client has an indwelling catheter in place, keep the drainage bag on ice and empty the urine into the urine container periodically during the 24-hr period.
4. Keep urine cool during collection. *Higher temperatures alter the results.*
5. If any urine is lost, discard the entire specimen and begin collection again the next day.

Clinical Implications and Indications:
1. Assists in confimation of diagnosis and monitoring of progression of acute monocytic and myelogenous leukemias. Response to treatment may also be reflected in test results.
2. Evaluates renal tubular function.
3. Detects rejection of kidney transplant.
4. Indicates activity related to tuberculosis, sarcoidosis, Crohn's disease, and polycythemia vera.

Nursing Care:

Before Test: Explain the test procedure and the purpose of the test. Assess the client's knowledge of the test. Instruct client not to discard any urine over the 24-hr time period.

During Test: Adhere to standard precautions. If any urine is accidentally discarded or contaminated with feces, discard entire specimen and begin test again the following morning (24-hr sample).

After Test: Blood: Apply pressure to venipuncture site. Explain that some bruising, discomfort, and swelling may appear at the site and that warm, moist compresses can alleviate this. Monitor for signs of infection. Urine: Document urine quantity, date, and exact hours of collection on requisition.

Potential Complications: Bleeding and bruising at venipuncture site

Interfering Factors: Urine contaminated with feces; spillage or inaccurate collection of the 24-hr specimen, including nonrefrigeration or placing on ice; heavy bleeding during menstruation

Nursing Considerations:

Pediatric: Blood: Infants and children will need assistance in remaining still during the venipuncture and age-appropriate comfort measures following the test. Urine (random sample): A collection bag or insertion of a straight catheter is likely needed for infants and toddlers.
Urine (24 hr): A collection bag or indwelling catheter needs to be used for infants and toddlers.

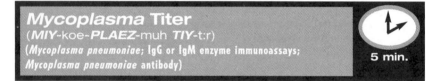

Mycoplasma Titer
(*MIY*-koe-*PLAEZ*-muh *TIY*-t:r)
(*Mycoplasma pneumoniae*; IgG or IgM enzyme immunoassays; *Mycoplasma pneumoniae* antibody)

5 min.

Type of Test: Blood

Body Systems and Functions: Pulmonary system

Normal Findings: Negative or complement fixation <1:64; seradyn color vue agglutination <1:320

Test Results Time Frame: Within 7–10 days

Test Description: *Mycoplasma* titer tests are used to diagnose *Mycoplasma pneumoniae*. *Mycoplasma* are a group of bacteria that lack cell walls and are highly pleomorphic. There are more than 70 organisms in this group, which includes at least 12 that infect humans. Due to the timing of the test itself and the subsequent time frame needed to process the sample, diagnosis is often confirmed serologically after the acute phase of the disease is over. Acute and convalescent sera may be ordered.

Consent Form: Not required

List of Equipment: Red-top tube or serum separator tube; needle and syringe or vacutainer; alcohol swab

BLOOD

Test Procedure:
1. Label the specimen tube. *Correctly identifies the client and the test to be performed.*
2. Obtain a 5-mL blood sample.
3. Do not agitate the tube. *Agitation may cause RBC hemolysis.*
4. Send tube to the laboratory.
5. Keep specimen cool. *High temperatures alter the results.*
6. Repeat 10–14 days later for convalescent sample and label the tube as convalescent sample. *Allows for separate identification of the convalescent sample, which is compared in ratio to the acute sample.*

Clinical Implications and Indications:
1. Diagnoses recent or current infection with *M. pneumoniae.*

Nursing Care:
Before Test: Explain the test procedure and the purpose of the test. Assess the client's knowledge of the test.
During Test: Adhere to standard precautions.
After Test: Apply pressure to venipuncture site. Explain that some bruising, discomfort, and swelling may appear at the site and that warm, moist compresses can alleviate this. Monitor for signs of infection. Notify client of when they are to return for follow-up testing if convalescent sample is to be collected.

Potential Complications: Bleeding and bruising at venipuncture site

Interfering Factors: Acute inflammatory diseases cause false positives.

Nursing Considerations:
Pediatric: Infants and children will need assistance in remaining still during the venipuncture and age-appropriate comfort measures following the test.
Gerontology: Elderly clients are more susceptible to complications if they contract M. pneumoniae.

Listing of Related Tests: Cold agglutinins; indirect Coombs' test

WEBLINKS

http://RespiratoryCare.medscape.com

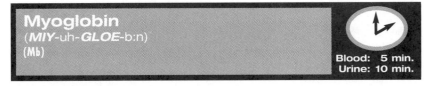

Myoglobin
(*MIY*-uh-*GLOE*-b:n)
(Mb)

Blood: 5 min.
Urine: 10 min.

Type of Test: Blood; urine

Body Systems and Functions: Musculoskeletal system

Normal Findings: Blood: <70 ng/mL. Urine: 0–2 mg/mL.

Test Results Time Frame: Within 24 hr

Test Description: Myoglobin is an oxygen-binding protein found in skeletal muscle and myocardium. It is released into circulation after damage to either the heart or skeletal muscle. It is filtered from the blood in the kidneys and high levels can occlude kidney structures. Peak levels are found in the blood 8–12 hr after muscle tissue is damaged and up to 7 days in the urine.

Consent Form: Not required

List of Equipment: *Blood:* red-top tube or serum separator tube; needle and syringe or vacutainer; alcohol swab. *Urine:* sterile plastic container; ice.

Test Procedure:
Blood:
1. Label the specimen tube. *Correctly identifies the client and the test to be performed.*
2. Obtain a 7-mL blood sample.
3. Do not agitate the tube. *Agitation may cause RBC hemolysis.*
4. Send tube to the laboratory.

Urine:
1. Label a sterile urine container. *Correctly identifies the client and the test to be performed.*
2. Obtain a clean-catch specimen of urine (note: first morning voiding preferred, at least 5 mL). *Ensures accurate results.*
3. Keep specimen cool. *High temperatures alter the results.*
4. Send specimen to laboratory.

Clinical Implications and Indications:
1. Diagnoses muscle enzyme deficiencies, injury, and dystrophy.
2. Diagnoses myocardial infarction if taken between 2 and 12 hr after myocardial infarction. Will not be elevated until after 2 hr and will begin to return to normal levels after 12 hr.
3. Elevated levels are found with renal failure, malignant hyperthermia, severe burns, systemic lupus erythematosus, surgery, trauma, delirium tremens, and seizures.

Nursing Care:
Before Test: Explain the test procedure and the purpose of the test. Assess the client's knowledge of the test.
During Test: Adhere to standard precautions. If any urine is accidentally discarded or contaminated with feces, discard entire specimen and begin test again with the next voiding sample.
After Test: Blood: Apply pressure to venipuncture site. Explain that some bruising, discomfort, and swelling may appear at the site and that warm, moist compresses can alleviate this. Monitor for signs of infection.
Urine: Document urine quantity, date, and exact hours of collection on requisition.

Potential Complications: Bleeding and bruising at venipuncture site

Interfering Factors: Urine contaminated with feces; spillage or inaccurate collection of the urine specimen, including nonrefrigeration or placing on ice; heavy bleeding during menstruation; recent nuclear scan; recent intramuscular injection

Nursing Considerations:

Pediatric: *Blood: Infants and children will need assistance in remaining still during the venipuncture and age-appropriate comfort measures following the test. Urine: A collection bag or insertion of a straight catheter is likely needed for infants and toddlers.*

Listing of Related Tests: Creatine kinase; lactic dehydrogenase; asparate aminotransferase

⬛❙WEBLINKS 🖱   🗔☒

www.adam.com

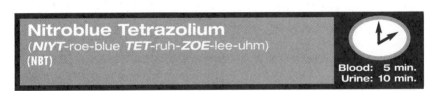

Nitroblue Tetrazolium
(***NIYT***-roe-blue ***TET***-ruh-***ZOE***-lee-uhm)
(NBT)

Blood: 5 min.
Urine: 10 min.

Type of Test: Blood; urine

Body Systems and Functions: Immunological system

Normal Findings: <10% for blood; color change to blue-violet is positive for urine

Test Results Time Frame: Within 1–3 days

Test Description: Nitroblue tetrazolium testing is usually performed as a blood test; the sample identifies poor neutrophil functioning such as that found in chronic granulomatous disease. It is also used on occasion to differentiate bacterial infections from other conditions that may present similarly. NBT may also be used as a urine sample and may be used to detect inflammatory cells and confirm the diagnosis of a urinary tract infection (UTI). Urinary tract infections can be of serious consequence when they are undetected or untreated and their pathogens progress to infecting the surrounding renal system or even the serious result of sepsis.

Consent Form: Not required

List of Equipment: *Blood:* yellow-top tube or serum separator tube; needle and syringe or vacutainer; alcohol swab. *Urine:* sterile plastic container; ice.

Test Procedure:
Blood:
1. Label the specimen tube. *Correctly identifies the client and the test to be performed.*
2. Obtain a 5-mL blood sample.
3. Do not agitate the tube. *Agitation may cause RBC hemolysis.*
4. Send tube to the laboratory.

Urine:
1. Label a sterile urine container. *Correctly identifies the client and the test to be performed.*

BLOOD

2. Obtain a clean-catch specimen of urine (note: first morning voiding preferred, at least 15–30 mL). *Ensures accurate results.*
3. Keep specimen cool. *High temperatures alter the results.*
4. Send specimen to laboratory.

Clinical Implications and Indications:

1. Diagnoses chronic granulomatous disease, systemic lupus erythematosus, sickle cell anemia, chronic myelogenous leukemia, and agammaglobulinemias based on failure of NBT reduction
2. Differentiates types of infections from other conditions: *Nocardia*, miliary TB and TB meningitis, some parasitic infections, and malaria
3. Evaluates oncology disorders, tissue transplantation, and leukocytosis unrelated to bacterial infection (e.g., rheumatoid arthritis)
4. Confirms diagnosis of UTI

Nursing Care:

Before Test: Assess the client's knowledge of the test. Explain the test procedure and the purpose of the test.
During Test: Adhere to standard precautions. If any urine is accidentally discarded or contaminated with feces, discard entire specimen and begin test again.
After Test: Blood: Apply pressure to venipuncture site. Explain that some bruising, discomfort, and swelling may appear at the site and that warm, moist compresses can alleviate this. Monitor for signs of infection. Urine: Document urine quantity, date, and exact hours of collection on requisition.

Potential Complications: Bleeding and bruising at venipuncture site

Interfering Factors: Oral contraceptives; decreased with postoperative condition; corticosteroids; normal or decreased with antibiotics; immunosuppressive drugs; localized infections

Nursing Considerations:

Pregnancy: Increases in normal states of pregnancy and is decreased or normal during postpartum period
Pediatric: Increased in infants in first 2 months of life. Blood: Infants and children will need assistance in remaining still during the venipuncture and age-appropriate comfort measures following the test. Urine: A collection bag or insertion of a straight catheter is likely needed for infants and toddlers.

Listing of Related Tests: Urine cultures

⬛ WEBLINKS ⬛   🗐🗙

www.magicbydesign.com

Ornithine Carbamoyltransferase
(*OER*-nuh-theen *KAHR*-buh-moyl-*TRAENS*-f:r-ays)
(ornithine transcarbamylase; OTC; OCT)

5 min.

Type of Test: Blood

Body Systems and Functions: Metabolic system

BLOOD

Normal Findings: Undetectable to 500 SI units/mL

Test Results Time Frame: Within 1–2 weeks

Test Description: Ornithine carbamoyltransferase (OCT) is the blood test that is useful in detecting alterations in the synthesis of urea which occurs almost completely in the liver. Deficiency of OCT is also called hyperammonemia type I and may require a liver biopsy sample to confirm. Increases in OCT serum levels are related to disease, altered function, or cancer of the liver.

Consent Form: Not required

List of Equipment: Green-top tube or plasma separator tube; needle and syringe or vacutainer; alcohol swab

Test Procedure:
1. Label the specimen tube. *Correctly identifies the client and the test to be performed.*
2. Obtain a 5-mL blood sample.
3. Gently invert tube several times, but do not agitate the tube. *Mixes the anticoagulant, but agitation may cause RBC hemolysis.*
4. Send tube to the laboratory.
5. Keep specimen cool. *High temperatures alter the results..*

Clinical Implications and Indications:
1. Elevated levels are found with liver disease or cancer, drug toxicity, alcoholism, and viral hepatitis.
2. Determines whether deficient OCT may require liver biopsy.

Nursing Care:
Before Test: Explain the test procedure and the purpose of the test. Assess the client's knowledge of the test. Instruct client to fast for 12 hr prior to test.
During Test: Adhere to standard precautions.
After Test: Apply pressure to venipuncture site. Explain that some bruising, discomfort, and swelling may appear at the site and that warm, moist compresses can alleviate this. Monitor for signs of infection. Instruct client to resume eating and taking fluids.

Potential Complications: Bleeding and bruising at venipuncture site

Interfering Factors: Failure to fast for 12 hr prior to test; medications that alter results are acetaminophen, anabolic steroids, antithyroids, carbamazepine, daunorubicin, disulfiram, doxorubicin, erythromycin, estrogens, etretinate, gold compounds, isoniazid, recent anesthetic, methotrexate, mercaptopurine, methyldopa, nitrofurantoins, estrogen, phenothiazines, phenytoin, piperacillin, rifampin, sulfonamides, IV tetracycline, and valproic acid.

Nursing Considerations:
Pediatric: *Infants and children will need assistance in remaining still during the venipuncture and age-appropriate comfort measures following the test.*

Listing of Related Tests: Blood ammonia level; enzyme assay from needle biopsy of liver; orotic acid urine level; plasma glutamine and glutamic acid; citrulline concentration

WEBLINKS

Osmolality, Blood
(ahz-moe-*LAEL*-uh-tee)
(serum osmolality; serum OS)

5 min.

Type of Test: Blood

Body Systems and Functions: Hematological system

Normal Findings:

Adults	280–295 mOsm/kg H_2O
Children	275–290 mOsm/kg H_2O

CRITICAL VALUES:
>360 mOsm/kg found in pending respiratory arrest; <265 mOsm/kg H_2O

Test Results Time Frame: Within 24 hr

Test Description: Serum osmolality tests for serum concentration, specifically the number of dissolved particles per unit of fluid. Ninety percent of the changes in serum osmolality are caused by sodium concentration variation. Generally stated, serum osmolality decreases in hydrated conditions and increases in states of dehydration.

Consent Form: Not required

List of Equipment: Red-top tube or serum separator tube; needle and syringe or vacutainer; alcohol swab

Test Procedure:
1. Label the specimen tube. *Correctly identifies the client and the test to be performed.*
2. Obtain a 7-mL blood sample.
3. Do not agitate the tube. *Agitation may cause RBC hemolysis.*
4. Send tube to the laboratory.

Clinical Implications and Indications:
1. Provides an indicator of the status of fluid and electrolyte balance.
2. Increased levels are found with nonketotic hyperglycemic coma, diabetes insipidus, uremia, renal tubular necrosis, severe pyelonephritis, azotemia, dehydration, and hypernatremia.
3. Levels may increase in response to mannitol therapy or after ingestion of ethanol, methanol, or ethylene glycol.
4. Decreased levels are found with hyponatremia, overhydration, SIADH, Addison's disease, lung cancer, and cirrhosis.

Nursing Care:
Before Test: Explain the test procedure and the purpose of the test. Assess the client's knowledge of the test.
During Test: Adhere to standard precautions.
After Test: Apply pressure to venipuncture site. Explain that some bruising, discomfort, and swelling may appear at the site and that warm, moist compresses can alleviate this. Monitor for signs of infection.

Potential Complications: Bleeding and bruising at venipuncture site

Interfering Factors: Hemolyzed blood sample; drug therapy with mineralocorticoids, osmotic diuretics; cerebrovascular accident and brain tumors may stimulate secretion of ADH; hyperglycemia

Nursing Considerations:
Pediatric: Infants and children will need assistance in remaining still during the venipuncture and age-appropriate comfort measures following the test.

Listing of Related Tests: Serum sodium; BUN; urine osmolality

WEBLINKS

http://www.methodisthealth.com

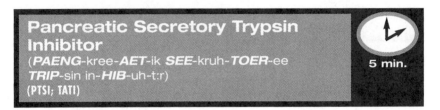

Pancreatic Secretory Trypsin Inhibitor
(*PAENG*-kree-*AET*-ik *SEE*-kruh-*TOER*-ee *TRIP*-sin in-*HIB*-uh-t:r)
(PTSI; TATI)

5 min.

Type of Test: Blood

Body Systems and Functions: Gastrointestinal system

Normal Findings: 3–20 µg/L

Test Results Time Frame: Within 24 hr

Test Description: Pancreatic trypsin inhibitor tests the naturally occurring substance of PTSI, which is produced by the pancreas. PTSI protects the mucosal cells from proteolytic breakdown and may be capable of promoting growth activity. PTSI is found in the stomach. This test acts as a marker for inflammatory diseases of the bowel and other diseases of the gut. The test is performed by radioimmunoassay. The pancreas is both an exocrine and endocrine organ that is located behind the stomach in front of the first and second lumbar vertebrae. The pancreas is responsible for secreting glucagon and insulin and the pancreatic juices that contribute to the digestion of all foods in the small intestine.

Consent Form: Not required

List of Equipment: Red-top tube or serum separator tube; needle and syringe or vacutainer; alcohol swab

Test Procedure:
1. Label the specimen tube. *Correctly identifies the client and the test to be performed.*
2. Obtain a 5-mL blood sample.
3. Do not agitate the tube. *Agitation may cause RBC hemolysis.*
4. Send tube to the laboratory.

Clinical Implications and Indications:
1. Diagnoses Crohn's disease, pancreatitis, and severe infections of the GI tract
2. Acts as a tumor marker for certain cancers (e.g., lung, ovarian) and as a marker for threatened organ rejection

Nursing Care:

Before Test: Explain the test procedure and the purpose of the test. Assess the client's knowledge of the test.
During Test: Adhere to standard precautions.
After Test: Apply pressure to venipuncture site. Explain that some bruising, discomfort, and swelling may appear at the site and that warm, moist compresses can alleviate this. Monitor for signs of infection.

Potential Complications: Bleeding and bruising at venipuncture site

Interfering Factors: Oral contraceptives; steroids

Nursing Considerations:

Pediatric: Infants and children will need assistance in remaining still during the venipuncture and age-appropriate comfort measures following the test.

WEBLINKS

http://www.niddk.nih.gov

Parathyroid Hormone
(*PAYR*-uh-*THIY*-royd)
(parathormone; PTH; PTH-C terminal; parathyrin;
parathyroid hormone radioimmunoassay)

5 min.

Type of Test: Blood

Body Systems and Functions: Endocrine system

Normal Findings:

Intact	10–60 pg/mL
N-terminal	8–24 pg/mL
C-terminal	50–330 pg/mL

Normal laboratory findings vary among laboratory settings.

Test Results Time Frame: Within 2–3 days

Test Description: Parathyroid testing is often taken in conjunction with calcium levels and is an indicator of hypocalcemia. Parathyroid hormone (PTH) normally increases calcium absorption from the GI tract, stimulates osteoclasts causing reabsorption of Ca and phosphate from bone, inhibits phosphate reabsorption by the proximal renal tubules, and enhances renal tubular calcium reabsorption. Decreased calcium stimulates PTH secretion and a rise in Ca inhibits PTH secretion. Although three forms of PTH exist (intact, multiple N-terminal fragments, and multiple C-terminal fragments), the intact form is the one most commonly evaluated.

> ### CLINICAL ALERT:
> PTH levels vary and must be interpreted in association with calcium levels.

Consent Form: Not required

List of Equipment: Red-top tube or serum separator tube; needle and syringe or vacutainer; alcohol swab; ice

Test Procedure:
1. Label the specimen tube. *Correctly identifies the client and the test to be performed.*
2. Obtain a 10-mL blood sample. The sample must be collected in the morning upon waking. *Diurnal rhythms will affect PTH levels.*
3. A serum Ca level may be requested at the same time. *Allows for comparison.*
4. Do not agitate the tube. *Agitation may cause RBC hemolysis.*
5. Send tube to the laboratory.
6. Keep specimen cool. *High temperatures alter the results.*

Clinical Implications and Indications:
1. Elevated levels are found with hyperparathyroidism, pseudohyperparathyroidism, malabsorption or vitamin D deficiency, lactation, and pregnancy.
2. Decreased levels are found with hypoparathyroidism, response to sarcoidosis, vitamin A and D intoxication, diGeorge syndrome, and post-parathyroidectomy.

Nursing Care:
Before Test: Explain the test procedure and the purpose of the test. Assess the client's knowledge of the test. Instruct client to fast 8–10 hr prior to the test. Instruct client that sample needs to be taken in the morning upon awakening.
During Test: Adhere to standard precautions.
After Test: Apply pressure to venipuncture site. Explain that some bruising, discomfort, and swelling may appear at the site and that warm, moist compresses can alleviate this. Monitor for signs of infection.

Potential Complications: Bleeding and bruising at venipuncture site

Interfering Factors: Milk ingestion; medications that alter results are thiazide diuretics, anticonvulsants, steroids, lithium, rifampin, cimetidine, and propranolol; recent radioisotope studies; failure to fast 8–10 hr; failure to collect sample in AM

Nursing Considerations:
Pregnancy: Pregnancy and lactation may alter results.
Pediatric: Infants and children will need assistance in remaining still during the venipuncture and age-appropriate comfort measures following the test.

Listing of Related Tests: Serum Ca

WEBLINKS

http://www.ncbi.nlm.nih.gov/entrez/query.fcgi

Partial Thromboplastin Time
(**PAHR**-sh:l **THRAHM**-boe-**PLAES**-tin)
(PTT; APTT; partial thromboplastin time; activated partial thromboplastin time)

5 min.

Type of Test: Blood

Body Systems and Functions: Hematological system

Normal Findings: APTT 21–35 sec; PTT 60–70 sec

CRITICAL VALUES:
PTT >100 sec; danger of spontaneous bleeding (in the case of bleed due to a high dose of heparin, protamine sulfate 1 mg/100 U heparin may reverse the process); APTT > 70 sec

Test Results Time Frame: Within 24–48 hr

Test Description: Prolongation of the partial thromboplastin time (PTT) or the activated partial thromboplastin time (APTT) is an indicator of the effectiveness of anticoagulant therapy and a screening test for bleeding tendencies and identifies deficiencies in most of the intrinsic and final common clotting pathways. Frequently, a prothrombin time (PT) is ordered in combination with an APTT because if both are prolonged, the pathology is probably in the final common clotting pathway (factors I, II, V, X) , while if only the APTT is prolonged, the abnormality is related to the extrinsic pathway (factors VIII, IX, X, XI, XII). The actual process of testing for PTT involves determining the length of time it takes for a fibrin clot to form. The APTT includes addition of an activator that speeds up the clotting time and results in a narrower range of normal. APTT is often one of the tests of choice when monitoring effectiveness of heparin therapy.

Consent Form: Not required

List of Equipment: Blue-top tube or plasma separator tube; needle and syringe or vacutainer; alcohol swab; ice

Test Procedure:
1. Label the specimen tube. *Correctly identifies the client and the test to be performed.*
2. Obtain a 7-mL blood sample.
3. Clients on intermittent heparin therapy should have the sample timed an hour in advance of administration of heparin. *To decrease effects on the result.*
4. Gently invert tube several times, but do not agitate the tube. *Mixes the anticoagulant, but agitation may cause RBC hemolysis.*
5. Send tube to the laboratory.
6. Keep specimen cool. *High temperatures alter the results.*

Clinical Implications and Indications:
1. Screens for coagulation abnormalities
2. Evaluates effectiveness of drug therapy (e.g., heparin)
3. Assesses integrity of the intrinsic and final common clotting pathways

BLOOD

Nursing Care:
Before Test: Explain the test procedure and the purpose of the test. Assess the client's knowledge of the test.
During Test: Adhere to standard precautions.
After Test: Apply gentle pressure to venipuncture site until site stops oozing blood. Explain that some bruising, discomfort, and swelling may appear at the site and that warm, moist compresses should not be used due to the potential bleeding tendencies of this client. Monitor for signs of infection. In clients with bleeding disorders or on anticoagulant therapy, this time frame will be extended from the norm. Teaching related to prolonged APTT will include observation for spontaneous bleeding of the gums or extended bleeding times from wounds, blood in the urine, low-back pain, nosebleeds, and bruising (spontaneous or with gentle contact). Advise against salicylates unless the client is being monitored by a health care provider. If client is on anticoagulant therapy, remind that repeat samples will be required on a regular basis.

Potential Complications: Extended bleeding and bruising at venipuncture site

Interfering Factors: Sample drawn from heparin lock or heparinized catheter; medications that alter results are aspirin, antibiotics, ascorbic acid, asparaginase, antihistamines, chlorpromazine, heparin, naloxone, phenytoin, tolmetin, oral contraceptives, and anticoagulants.

Nursing Considerations:
Pediatric: Infants and children will need assistance in remaining still during the venipuncture and age-appropriate comfort measures following the test.

Listing of Related Tests: PT; APTT inhibitor/deficiency screen

WEBLINKS	

www-med.stanford.edu

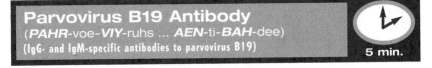

Parvovirus B19 Antibody
(*PAHR*-voe-*VIY*-ruhs ... *AEN*-ti-*BAH*-dee)
(IgG- and IgM-specific antibodies to parvovirus B19)

5 min.

Type of Test: Blood

Body Systems and Functions: Immunological system

Normal Findings: ≤0.90 IV (index value) is interpreted as negative for IgG- and IgM-specific antibodies to parvovirus B19 (by ELISA and IFA); 0.91–1.09 IV is classified equivocal and retesting is done in 10–14 days.

Test Results Time Frame: Within 1–5 days

Test Description: Parvovirus 19 IgG antibodies are present in up to 70% of adult populations. A person infected with parvovirus may be asymptomatic or have mild symptoms. Parvovirus B19 enters bone marrow erythroid precursor cells and stops erythropoiesis for up to 1 week. The result can be an aplastic crisis for those who are immunocompromised. The presence of virus in the blood disappears when the specific antibodies are detectable in serum. In non-compromised individuals, the infection is clear within several weeks and they have gained lifelong immunity to reinfection. For those who are immunocompromised, the infection becomes persistent and is accompanied by chronic anemia. Detection of specific IgG and IgM antibodies signals recent or current infection, but these will not be detected until 7–14 days after the onset of the disease.

Consent Form: Not required

List of Equipment: Red-top tube or serum separator tube; needle and syringe or vacutainer; alcohol swab

Test Procedure:
1. Label the specimen tube. *Correctly identifies the client and the test to be performed.*
2. Obtain a 5-mL blood sample.
3. Do not agitate the tube. *Agitation may cause RBC hemolysis.*
4. Send tube to the laboratory.
5. Repeat 10–14 days later for convalescent sample and label the tube as convalescent sample. *Allows for separate identification of the convalescent sample, which is compared in ratio to the acute sample.*

Clinical Implications and Indications:
1. Diagnoses chronic anemia in an immunocompromised host.
2. Detects erythema infectiosum ("fifth disease"), which is usually seen in children.
3. Detects joint arthralgia and arthropathy, which are usually most common in women.
4. Screening test for pregnant women since 7% of parvovirus B19 IgM-positive pregnant women will have a stillbirth due to related hydrops fetalis.
5. Evaluates an aplastic crisis in clients with chronic hemolytic anemias.
6. Screening test for organ transplant donor due to increased risk of aplastic anemia in organ recipient.

Nursing Care:
Before Test: Explain the test procedure and the purpose of the test. Assess the client's knowledge of the test.
During Test: Adhere to standard precautions.
After Test: Apply pressure to venipuncture site. Explain that some bruising, discomfort, and swelling may appear at the site and that warm, moist compresses can alleviate this. Monitor for signs of infection.

Potential Complications: Bleeding and bruising at venipuncture site

Nursing Considerations:
Pregnancy: Stillbirth increases for parvovirus 19 antibodies present during pregnancy.
Pediatric: Erythema infectiosum ("fifth disease") is usually seen in children. Infants and children will need assistance in remaining still during the venipuncture and age-appropriate comfort measures following the test.

Listing of Related Tests: Parvovirus B19 DNA blood test; bone marrow blot; polymerase chain reaction (PCR)

BLOOD

WEBLINKS

www.arup-lab.com

Pemphigus Antibodies
(*PEM*-fuh-guhs *AEN*-ti-*BAH*-deez)

5 min.

Type of Test: Blood

Body Systems and Functions: Immunological system

Normal Findings: <1:10 titer

Test Results Time Frame: Within 1 week

Test Description: Pemphigus antibody testing detects the presence of pemphigus, which is an autoimmune disease that is acute or chronic in nature. Three types of pemphigus have been identified: vulgaris (PV), foliaceus (PF), and paraneoplastic (PNP). A loss of keratinocyte cell-to-cell adhesion occurs and crops of bullous lesions appear suddenly on previously normal skin. In the case of PV, lesions may also occur in the mouth. When the skin lesions disappear, they leave pigmented areas. There is a direct correlation between disease activity and circulating levels of antibodies.

Consent Form: Not required

List of Equipment: Red-top tube or serum separator tube; needle and syringe or vacutainer; alcohol swab

Test Procedure:
1. Label the specimen tube. *Correctly identifies the client and the test to be performed.*
2. Obtain a 5-mL blood sample.
3. Do not agitate the tube. *Agitation may cause RBC hemolysis.*
4. Send tube to the laboratory.

Clinical Implications and Indications:
1. Diagnoses active pemphigus disease in absence of other signs or symptoms
2. Identifies lesions associated with myasthenia gravis or malignancies
3. Identifies lesions of neonates whose mothers are pemphigus vulgaris positive

Nursing Care:
Before Test: Explain the test procedure and the purpose of the test. Assess the client's knowledge of the test.
During Test: Adhere to standard precautions.
After Test: Apply pressure to venipuncture site. Explain that some bruising, discomfort, and swelling may appear at the site and that warm, moist compresses can alleviate this. Monitor for signs of infection.

BLOOD

Potential Complications: Bleeding and bruising at venipuncture site

Nursing Considerations:

Pediatric: Infants and children will need assistance in remaining still during the venipuncture and age-appropriate comfort measures following the test.

Listing of Related Tests: Oral cytology

WEBLINKS

http://www.nlm.nih.gov

Pepsinogen
(pep-*SIN*-oe-jen)
(pepsinogen 1; PG1; pepsinogen A; PGA)

5 min.

Type of Test: Blood

Body Systems and Functions: Gastrointestinal system

Normal Findings:

Infants/children	20–118 ng/mL (laboratory will specify normal values by age)
Adults	124–142 ng/mL

Test Results Time Frame: Within 7 days

Test Description: Pepsinogen tests for the presence of pepsinogens, which are classified into two groups (pepsinogens 1 and 2), which are precursors of pepsins. PG1 is produced only in the fundic portion of the stomach and responds to the same stimulators as hydrochloric acid. While the factors that influence PG1 levels are not completely understood, some association has been identified between individuals with a familial history of duodenal ulcer and elevated PG1, suggesting an inherited autosomal dominant trait. PG1 levels are determined by serum assays.

Consent Form: Not required

List of Equipment: Red-top tube or serum separator tube; needle and syringe or vacutainer; alcohol swab

Test Procedure:

1. Label the specimen tube. *Correctly identifies the client and the test to be performed.*
2. Obtain a 5-mL blood sample.
3. Do not agitate the tube. *Agitation may cause RBC hemolysis.*
4. Send tube to the laboratory.

Clinical Implications and Indications:

1. Decreased levels are found with gastric cancer, atrophic gastritis, pernicious anemia, Addison's disease, and hypopituitarism.
2. Elevated levels are found with duodenal ulcer, acute gastritis, Zollinger-Ellison syndrome, and hypergastrinemia.

Nursing Care:

Before Test: Explain the test procedure and the purpose of the test. Assess the client's knowledge of the test. Instruct client to fast 8–12 hr prior to test. If client is experiencing gastric discomfort, record details.

During Test: Adhere to standard precautions.

After Test: Apply pressure to venipuncture site. Explain that some bruising , discomfort and swelling may appear at the site and that warm moist compresses can alleviate this. Monitor for signs of infection.

Potential Complications: Bleeding and bruising at venipuncture site

Interfering Factors: Decreased renal output (causes false elevation of PG1); failure to fast the required time

Nursing Considerations:

Pediatric: Infants and children will need assistance in remaining still during the venipuncture and age-appropriate comfort measures following the test.

Listing of Related Tests: BUN; serum creatinine; serum gastrin; *Helicobacter pylori* antibody

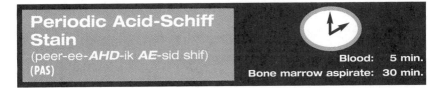

http://chorus.rad.mcw.edu

Periodic Acid-Schiff Stain

(peer-ee-*AHD*-ik *AE*-sid shif)

(PAS)

Blood:	5 min.
Bone marrow aspirate:	30 min.

Type of Test: Blood

Body Systems and Functions: Hematological system

Normal Findings: A negative result (cell being examined does not stain)

Test Results Time Frame: Within 2–3 days

Test Description: A blood or bone marrow aspirate sample, when subjected to the PAS stain, provides information used to differentiate specific cell origins. Various patterns and density of stains are indicative of malignant blasts (e.g., acute lymphocyctic leukemia reveals a fine or coarse granular pattern). PAS positivity increases with increasing myeloid differentiation but may test negative in pathological situations depending on the target cell (e.g., megaloblastic anemia).

Consent Form: Required for bone marrow aspiration

List of Equipment: Red-top tube or serum separator tube or slides; needle and syringe or vacutainer; alcohol swab; bone marrow aspiration tray

Test Procedure:

1. Label the specimen tube. *Correctly identifies the client and the test to be performed.*

2. Obtain a 1-mL blood sample.
3. Do not agitate the tube. *Agitation may cause RBC hemolysis.*
4. Send tube to the laboratory.
5. Alternately, a bone marrow aspirate sample is obtained (see bone marrow examination) and the first slides are sent for microscopic examination.

Clinical Implications and Indications:

1. Assists in diagnosing acute lymphocytic leukemia. A minority of acute myelogenous leukemia cases also test positive, but staining is diffuse versus the clumps of PAS positive material found with ALL. (This test cannot be used to differentiate between AML and ALL.)
2. Assists in diagnosing erythroleukemia, with erythroblasts testing strongly PAS positive.
3. Assists in diagnosing thalassemia and folate and B_{12} deficiencies.

Nursing Care:

Before Test: Explain the test procedure and the purpose of the test. Assess the client's knowledge of the test.

During Test: Adhere to standard precautions. If done as bone marrow aspirate, assist client in maintaining position and provide reassurance and a calm atmosphere during the procedure.

After Test: Apply pressure to venipuncture site. Explain that some bruising, discomfort, and swelling may appear at the site and that warm, moist compresses can alleviate this. Monitor for signs of infection.

Potential Complications: Bleeding and bruising at venipuncture site

Nursing Considerations:

Pediatric: Children may have difficulty cooperating in providing either blood or bone marrow samples. Use distraction techniques and, if necessary, ordered sedation for the bone marrow aspiration. (Some institutions do their bone marrow aspirations on children under short-acting anesthetic with the appropriate personnel and support systems in place). EMLA application 1 ½ hr prior to blood sampling is an option to reduce pain related to venipuncture.

Gerontology: The older person may find it difficult to maintain positions when required to do so for lengthy periods of time during the periodic acid-Schiff stain testing.

Listing of Related Tests: Other histochemical stains; Sudan black B; peroxidase; naphthol ASD acetate esterase inhibition by flouride

WEBLINKS

http://www.methodisthealth.com

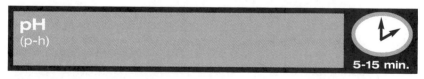

pH
(p-h)

5-15 min.

Type of Test: Blood; urine; stool

Body Systems and Functions: Hematological system, pulmonary system; gastrointestinal system; metabolic system; renal/urological system

Normal Findings:

Blood	7.35–7.45 (arterial)
	7.31–7.41 (venous)
Stool	6.5–7.5 (adult)
	5.0–7.5 (newborn)
Urine	4.6–8.0 (averages around 6.0)

Test Results Time Frame:

Blood	Within 1 hr
Stool	Within 24 hr
Urine	Immediate (dipstick)

Test Description: The measurement of the pH of a substance provides information related to body acidity or alkalinity. Increasing pH indicates increasing alkalinity. Decreasing pH equals increasing acidity.

Blood: The measurement of body alkalinity/acidity with blood sampling correlates with the client's metabolic and respiratory status. The pH is the negative logarithm of the hydrogen ion concentration. A pH greater than 7.35 occurs with acidosis, while a pH less than 7.45 equals alkalosis. The buffering system of carbonic acid to bicarbonate must be in a 20:1 ratio to be balanced. When the pH of blood is measured from an arterial blood sample, PCO_2, HCO_3, base excess/deficit, PO_2, O_2, and SO_2 are also measured so that all of the information related to acid-base balance can be analyzed. (See Arterial Blood Sampling)

Stool: The pH in stool is determined by the efficacy of digestive processes in the small bowel. As bacterial fermentation occurs, carbohydrate breakdown will increase the acidity, while protein breakdown will increase the alkalinity of the stool.

Urine: The pH is an indicator of whether normal hydrogen ion concentration is being maintained in the plasma and the extracellular fluid. The pH provides information regarding renal tubule function as well as whether a constant body pH is being maintained. If the body is retaining sodium or acid, the urine will become increasingly acidic. If the body has an excess of base or alkali, then the urine will become alkaline.

Consent Form: Not required

List of Equipment: *Blood:* blood gas heparanized needle and syringe; alcohol swab; ice water in bag. *Stool:* clean, dry container to collect stool; tongue depressor; gloves; rectal swab; clean, dry bedpan. *Urine:* reagent strip with color chart; sterile plastic container; ice.

Test Procedure:

Blood (see also Arterial Blood Gas Sampling):

1. Label the specimen tube. *Correctly identifies the client and the test to be performed* (note: the requisiton indicates if client is receiving O_2 plus flow rate, administration method, and client temperature). *Ensures accurate results.*
2. Obtain a minimum of 1 mL arterial blood sample. There should be no air in the syringe and an airtight cap/cork is placed over the tip of the syringe after the sample is collected. *Prevents hemolysis.*
3. Do not agitate the tube. *Agitation may cause RBC hemolysis.*
4. Send tube to the laboratory.

5. Keep specimen on ice. *High temperatures alter the results.*
6. Pressure is applied to the client's arterial stab site for at least 5 min. *Minimizes hematoma at arterial site.*

Stool:

1. Have client defecate into a clean bedpan, bedside commode, or toilet hat. *Decreases contamination and aids in obtaining stool specimen.*
2. Do not use the stool if it is contaminated with urine or menstrual blood. *Urine and menstrual blood affect stool culture results.*
3. Do not have the client place toilet paper on the stool after defecation. *Toilet paper affects stool culture results.*
4. Use a clean tongue depressor to place 2–3 cm of formed stool or 15 mL of liquid stool in a specimen container. *This amount is necessary for obtaining proper stool culture.*
5. Dispose of remaining stool and tongue depressor. *Decreases chance of spread of pathogen.*
6. Include visible mucus, pus, or blood in the specimen. *These may be indicative of disease or contain pathogens.*
7. Label the specimen container and send to laboratory as soon as possible. *Ensures accurate results.*

Urine:

1. Label a sterile urine container. *Correctly identifies the client and the test to be performed.*
2. Obtain a minimum of 5 mL of urine. *Ensures accurate results.*
3. A reagent strip is dipped in the urine and results compared against the color-coded table that comes with the strip.

Clinical Implications and Indications:

Blood:

1. Assesses disturbances in acid-base balance associated with respiratory or metabolic disorders (see Arterial Blood Gas Sampling)

Stool:

1. Diagnoses malabsorption syndromes and disaccharidase deficiency (decreased pH)
2. Diagnoses colitis or villous adenoma (increased pH)
3. Monitors side effects of antibiotic use and results of secretory diarrhea (increased pH)

Urine:

1. Assesses urine pH during management of infections with specific antibiotics that require alkaline urine to be effective
2. Monitors and controls pH of urine to maintain alkalinity during sulfa treatment to prevent crystal formation
3. Maintains alkaline urine pH with salicylate intoxication, during extensive blood transusion, and during antineoplastic therapy

Nursing Care:

Before Test: Explain the test procedure and the purpose of the test. Assess the client's knowledge of the test. Stool: Inform client that they should not use laxatives for a week prior to sampling. Check that no barium procedures were performed in the week prior to sampling. Explain that urine should not be mixed with the stool in the sample. Urine: Explain to client that the sample should be tested immediately to prevent change in pH that will occur if sample left standing. If the client is testing their own urine, inform them that there should be no urine splash from the protein to the pH area of the reagent strip, as this may cause the pH to read falsely acidic.

During Test: Adhere to standard precautions. If any urine is accidentally discarded or contaminated with feces, discard entire specimen and begin test again.

After Test: Blood: Apply pressure to puncture site for 5 min or until bleeding has stopped. Explain that some bruising, discomfort, and swelling may appear at the site and that warm, moist compresses can alleviate this. Monitor for signs of infection. Urine: Document urine quantity, date, and exact hours of collection on requisition.

Potential Complications: Bleeding and bruising at arterial puncture site

Interfering Factors:
Blood: improper handling of sample; medications that alter results are sodium bicarbonate, narcotics, and sedatives; antacids; suctioning; blood transfusion; O_2 therapy; diarrhea or vomiting
Stool: barium studies in week prior to test; laxative use in week prior to test; contamination of sample with urine
Urine: contamination with feces; spillage or inaccurate collection of the 24-hr specimen, including nonrefrigeration or placing on ice; heavy bleeding during menstruation; sample not tested immediately; contamination between protein and pH areas on reagent strip; medications that alter results are sodium bicarbonate, potassium citrate, acetazolamide, ammonium chloride, and mandelic acid; eating just prior to sampling

Nursing Considerations:
Pediatric: Infants and children will need assistance in remaining still during the procedure and age-appropriate comfort measures following the test; Stool: Breast-fed infants have acidic stools; bottle-fed infants have alkaline stools. Urine: A collection bag or insertion of a straight catheter is likely needed for infants and toddlers.

Listing of Related Tests: Arterial blood gas sampling

| WEBLINKS |

http://www.methodisthealth.com

Phenylalanine
(fen-:l-*AEL*-uh-neen)
(Guthrie screening test; bacterial inhibition test; PKU; phenylketonuria test; phenylalanine screening test)

10 min.

Type of Test: Blood

Body Systems and Functions: Metabolic system

Normal Findings:

Guthrie	Negative for bacterial growth on filter paper

Blood:

Newborn (2 or more days after birth)	<2 mg/dL
Adult	<6 mg/dL

Test Results Time Frame: Within 1–5 days

Test Description: Phenylketonuria (PKU) is an autosomal, recessive inborn error of metabolism that occurs due to an enzyme deficiency that prevents phenylalanine hydroxylase from being synthesized into tyrosine. Increased levels of phenylalanine can progressively result in irreversible severe mental retardation. Treatment for PKU is a phenylalanine-restricted diet and, although it was once thought that monitoring of phenylalanine levels did not require following after 6 years of age, it is currently recommended that men and women with PKU continue to maintain dietary restrictions and blood monitoring through adulthood. Elevated maternal levels of phenylalanine will result in fetal damage. Blood sample levels provide specific level information, while the Guthrie blood spot test and Phenistix urine testing for phenylalanine will only indicate a positive or negative status. The Guthrie spot test is usually the first test performed as a screening tool on the newborn and is followed by a serum level if positive.

CLINICAL ALERT:
If the test is performed prior to 2 days after birth (assuming normal feeding schedule with breast milk or formula), the result may be a false negative. Ideal timing is 4 days after birth but within the first week of life.

Consent Form: Not required

List of Equipment: Newborn screening card (Guthrie); lancet or one green-top serum tube; alcohol swab

Test Procedure:
Guthrie test:
1. For newborn screen label specimen with date of infant's birth and when first milk was taken. *Correctly identifies the client and the test to be performed.*
2. Warm infant's heel with moist warm cloth for 3–5 min. *Optimizes circulation to puncture site.*
3. Cleanse site with alcohol swab and dry with sterile swab or air dry.
4. Puncture heel with lancet and wipe away first drop of blood.
5. Touch one side of filter paper to next large blood drop until it soaks through and completely fills the circle.
6. Fill remaining circles in the same manner, applying gentle intermittent pressure to the heel if necessary.
7. Apply gentle pressure to puncture site for 5 min once sample is taken, while holding baby. *Stops bleeding at puncture site and attends to comfort needs of baby following painful procedure.*
8. Send specimen to the laboratory.
Blood sample variation for phenylalanine level:
1. Label the specimen tube. *Correctly identifies the client and the test to be performed.*
2. Obtain a 2-mL blood sample.
3. Do not agitate the tube. *Agitation may cause RBC hemolysis.*
4. Send tube to the laboratory.

BLOOD

Clinical Implications and Indications:
1. Diagnoses or monitors phenylketonuria in pregnancy.
2. Mandatory (or recommended) screening in the United States and Canada for phenylketonuria in the newborn.
3. Monitors phenylalanine levels to adjust dietary treatment for PKU. Scheduling may vary, but the usual is twice weekly until dietary control is attained, then weekly until 4 years of age, every 2 weeks until 6 years of age, and then monthly.
4. Low-birth-weight infants as well as individuals with galactosemia and hepatic encephalopathy will test positive.

Nursing Care:
Before Test: Explain the test procedure and the purpose of the test. Assess the client's knowledge of the test. Review the infant's feeding patterns with the caregiver. For a screening test, the requisition must indicate date of birth of infant and when milk was first taken.
During Test: Adhere to standard precautions.
After Test: Apply pressure to puncture site. Explain that some bruising, discomfort, and swelling may appear at the site and that warm, moist compresses can alleviate this. Monitor for signs of infection. If test is positive, caregiver must be informed to begin dietary changes immediately that will include a change in formula. Older infants, children, and adults will require a phenylalanine-restricted diet (balanced with the need for protein for normal growth). Consultation with a dietician is recommended.

Potential Complications: Bleeding and bruising at venipuncture site

Interfering Factors: Sample taken too early from newborn; sample taken from newborn who has not received milk in the first 24–48 hr of life; sample taken from an IV line delivering hyperalimentation or antibiotics; sample for Guthrie spot test applied from capillary tube rather than directly onto filter paper; Guthrie sample applied inaccurately to filter paper; medications that alter results are antibiotics, salicylates, and chlorpromazine; premature infant; ketonuria; infant feeding problems

Nursing Considerations:
Pregnancy: The adult woman with PKU should ideally be on a PKU diet at time of conception, but definitely once pregnancy is confirmed and throughout the pregnancy. If the mother's levels are high during pregnancy, the infant has a 90% chance of microcephaly and severe mental retardation.
Pediatric: Infants and children will need assistance in remaining still during the venipuncture and age-appropriate comfort measures following the test.
Home Care: Most PKU screening occurs in the home setting and should be performed according to agency/health care provider guidelines.

Listing of Related Tests: Phenistix urine test; serum tyrosine

WEBLINKS

www.pkunews.org

Phospholipids
(**FAHS**-foe-**LIP**-:dz)
(lipid)

5 min.

Type of Test: Blood

Body Systems and Functions: Hematological system

Normal Findings: 150–380 mg/dL

Test Results Time Frame: Within 1 week

Test Description: Phospholipids are divided into three types: lecithins, cephalins, and sphingomyelins. Phospholipids are not associated with coronary artery disease, but instead are examined when evaluating diseases related to the transport of fatty acids and lipids in the gastrointestinal tract to other body tissues and in pulmonary gas exchange (particularly neonatal). A primary function of phospholipids is their role in the formation of cellular and intracellular membranes. They are also an important part of lipoprotein and lipid transport, cephalin being a main constituent of thromboplastin and sphingomyelin acting as an insulator for the myelin sheath.

Consent Form: Not required

List of Equipment: Red-top tube or serum separator tube; needle and syringe or vacutainer; alcohol swab

Test Procedure:
1. Label the specimen tube. *Correctly identifies the client and the test to be performed.*
2. Obtain a 5-mL blood sample.
3. Do not agitate the tube. *Agitation may cause RBC hemolysis.*
4. Send tube to the laboratory.

Clinical Implications and Indications:
1. Evaluates fat metabolism
2. Diagnoses or monitors several conditions, including hypothyroidism, hypolipoproteinemia, pancreatitis, jaundice, nephrotic syndrome, and diabetes mellitus

Nursing Care:
Before Test: Explain the test procedure and the purpose of the test. Assess the client's knowledge of the test. Instruct client to fast for 12–14 hr and to not ingest alcohol for 24 hr prior to the test.
During Test: Adhere to standard precautions.
After Test: Apply pressure to venipuncture site. Explain that some bruising, discomfort, and swelling may appear at the site and that warm, moist compresses can alleviate this. Monitor for signs of infection.

Potential Complications: Bleeding and bruising at venipuncture site

Interfering Factors: Failure to fast for 12–14 hr; medications that alter results are estrogens, chlorpromazine, epinephrine, clofibrate, and other antilipemics.

BLOOD

Nursing Considerations:
Pregnancy: *Pregnant women will test in the high end of normal.*
Pediatric: *Infants and children will need assistance in remaining still during the venipuncture and age-appropriate comfort measures following the test.*

Listing of Related Tests: Serum cholesterol; fatty acids; phosphate; clotting times

WEBLINKS

www.healthgate.com

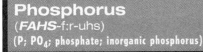

Phosphorus
(*FAHS*-f:r-uhs)
(P; PO₄; phosphate; inorganic phosphorus)

5 min.

Type of Test: Blood

Body Systems and Functions: Hematological system

Normal Findings:

Newborns	3.5–8.6 mg/dL
Infants	4.5–6.7 mg/dL
Children	4.5–6.5 mg/dL
Adults	3–4.5 mg/dL

Test Results Time Frame: Within 24 hr

Test Description: Phosphorus testing measures the amount of phosphorus found in bone and skeletal muscle and is controlled by parathyroid hormone and calcium metabolism. An inverse relation exists between phosphorus and calcium. An increase in either phosphorus or calcium will result in a decrease in the other. Most inorganic phosphorus is found in the skeletal system in combination with calcium (up to 85%), but some is also found in the blood in the form of a phosphate salt. Phosphorus participates in acid-base balance, glucose and lipid metabolism, and generation of bony tissue.

> **CLINICAL ALERT:**
> When possible, glucose transfusions should be stopped in advance of testing due to the interference of glucose with the accuracy of phosphorus results.

Consent Form: Not required

List of Equipment: Red-top tube or serum separator tube; needle and syringe or vacutainer; alcohol swab

Test Procedure:
1. Label the specimen tube. *Correctly identifies the client and the test to be performed.*
2. Obtain a 5-mL blood sample.
3. Do not agitate the tube. *Agitation may cause RBC hemolysis.*
4. Send tube to the laboratory.

Clinical Implications and Indications:

1. Elevated levels (hyperphosphatemia) are found with hypocalcemia, acute or chronic renal failure, increased tubular reabsorption (e.g., hypoparathyroidism, Addison's disease, sickle cell anemia), increased cellular release of phosphate (e.g., neoplasms, excessive tissue breakdown), bone disease (e.g., healing fractures, Paget's), increased phosphate load (e.g., hemolysis of blood, massive transfusions), magnesium deficiency, and childhood.

2. Decreased levels (hypophosphatemia) are found with renal or intestinal loss, renal tubular defects, administration of diuretics, primary hyperparathyroidism, hypokalemia, hypomagnesemia, dialysis, acute gout, primary hypophosphatemia, idiopathic hypercalciuria, decreased intestinal absorption (e.g., malabsorption, vitamin D deficiency, malnutrition, vomiting, diarrhea, antacid abuse), and intracellular shift of phosphate (e.g., alcoholism, diabetes mellitus, acidosis, total parenteral nutrition, respiratory alkalosis, salicylate poisoning, Cushing's syndome, prolonged hypothermia, administration of anabolic steroids, androgens, epinephrine, glucagon, insulin).

Nursing Care:

Before Test: Explain the test procedure and the purpose of the test. Assess the client's knowledge of the test. Instruct client to fast for 12–14 hr pretest.

During Test: Adhere to standard precautions. When possible, it is preferable to obtain sample without the use of a tourniquet.

After Test: Apply pressure to venipuncture site. Explain that some bruising, discomfort, and swelling may appear at the site and that warm, moist compresses can alleviate this. Monitor for signs of infection.

Potential Complications: Bleeding and bruising at venipuncture site

Interfering Factors: Use of tourniquet may affect result; medications that alter results are heparin, methicillin sodium, IV glucose, phenytoin, phosphate enema, anabolic steroids, androgens, antacids, diuretics, epinephrine, glucagon, insulin, mannitol, and salicylates; failure to maintain fast

Nursing Considerations:

Pediatric: Infants and children will need assistance in remaining still during the venipuncture and age-appropriate comfort measures following the test.

Gerontology: Elderly clients will have results in the low end of normal for adults or slightly lower.

International: Variations in normal levels may occur in seasonal countries (higher in summer/hot months and lower in winter/cold months).

Listing of Related Tests: Serum Ca; 25-OH vitamin D; electrolyte panel

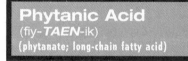

http://www.methodisthealth.com

Phytanic Acid
(fiy-*TAEN*-ik)
(phytanate; long-chain fatty acid)

5 min.

Type of Test: Blood

Body Systems and Functions: Metabolic system

Normal Findings: 0.3%–0.5%

Test Results Time Frame: Within 1–2 weeks

Test Description: Plasma phytanic acid levels are an essential tool in the diagnosis of peroxisomal disorders. Phytanic acid storage disease, also called Refsum's disease, is diagnosed by elevated levels of phytanic acid in blood plasma and tissues. Accumulation of phytanic acid affects the myelin sheath, which is the fatty covering or insulator on nerve fibers in the brain. Phytanic acid comes exclusively from the diet, so that restriction of dairy products, white bread/rice, egg yolk, stewed beef, and other items along with regular monitoring of phytanic acid levels can assist in reducing visual and hearing impairments and peripheral neuropathies. The infantile version of Refsum's is slowly progressive without dietary restriction and can result in mental retardation and failure to thrive.

Consent Form: Not required

List of Equipment: Purple-top tube or serum separator tube; needle and syringe or vacutainer; alcohol swab

Test Procedure:
1. Label the specimen tube. *Correctly identifies the client and the test to be performed.*
2. Obtain a 5-mL blood sample.
3. Do not agitate the tube. *Agitation may cause RBC hemolysis.*
4. Send tube to the laboratory.
5. Keep specimen cool. *High temperatures alter the results.*

Clinical Implications and Indications:
1. Diagnoses infantile or adult-onset Refsum's disease
2. Diagnoses peroxisomal disorders, such as Zellweger disease or adrenoleukodystrophy
3. Differentiates between possible causes of polyneuropathy

Nursing Care:
Before Test: Explain the test procedure and the purpose of the test. Assess the client's knowledge of the test. Instruct client to fast for 12–14 hr prior to the test, which should be taken in the morning.
During Test: Adhere to standard precautions.
After Test: Apply pressure to venipuncture site. Explain that some bruising, discomfort, and swelling may appear at the site and that warm, moist compresses can alleviate this. Monitor for signs of infection.

Potential Complications: Bleeding and bruising at venipuncture site

Interfering Factors: Failure to maintain fast pretest; failure to maintain phytanic acid–restricted diet; recent plasmapheresis; hemolysis of sample causes falsely elevated results; alcohol consumption in 24 hr pretest

Nursing Considerations:
Pediatric: Infants and children will need assistance in remaining still during the venipuncture and age-appropriate comfort measures following the test.

Listing of Related Tests: Fatty acid profile; serum pristanic acid; nerve conduction studies; CSF protein

www.rarediseases.org

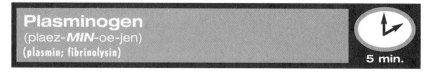

Plasminogen
(plaez-*MIN*-oe-jen)
(plasmin; fibrinolysin)

5 min.

Type of Test: Blood

Body Systems and Functions: Hematological system

Normal Findings: 20 mg/dL; 2.5–5.2 U/mL; 3.8–8.4 CTA U/mL

Test Results Time Frame: 24–96 hr (many laboratories do not do this test and it must be referred to outside agencies)

Test Description: Plasminogen is a protein found in many body tissues and fluids. It is part of the fibrinolytic system (lysis of blood clots) and is the precursor to the proteolytic enzyme plasmin. Plasmin itself cannot be directly measured. Plasmin splits fibrin and fibrinogen into fibrin degradation products (FDPs), which in turn dissolve the clot. A low level of plasminogen will cause a slowing of or ineffective clot lysis or recurrent thrombosis. An increased level is a risk factor for ineffective coagulation and bleeding. Plasminogen is also increased in malignant tumors, increasing the cancer cells' ability to invade neighboring tissues.

CLINICAL ALERT:
The results of this test are not reliable if the client is receiving IV heparin.

Consent Form: Not required

List of Equipment: Blue-top tube or serum separator tube; needle and syringe or vacutainer; alcohol swab

Test Procedure:
1. Label the specimen tube. *Correctly identifies the client and the test to be performed.*
2. Obtain a 7-mL blood sample.
3. Do not agitate the tube. *Agitation may cause RBC hemolysis.*
4. Send tube to the laboratory.
5. Keep specimen cool. *High temperatures alter the results.*

Clinical Implications and Indications:
1. Evaluates the process of fibrinolysis and the balance between coagulation and fibrinolytic systems.
2. Diagnoses hypofibrinogenemia.
3. Elevated levels are found with deep vein thrombosis, congenital defects in plasminogen inhibitors, inflammation and wound healing, surgery, stress, malignancy, and oral contraceptives.

4. Decreased levels are found with fibrinolysis, disseminated intravascular coagulation, acquired hypofibrinogenemia, liver disease, and thrombosis.

Nursing Care:
Before Test: Explain the test procedure and the purpose of the test. Assess the client's knowledge of the test.
During Test: Adhere to standard precautions.
After Test: Apply pressure to venipuncture site. Explain that some bruising, discomfort, and swelling may appear at the site and that warm, moist compresses can alleviate this. Monitor for signs of infection.

Potential Complications: After venipuncture, apply extra pressure for a longer time to site because there may be slower coagulation if plasminogen level is high.

Interfering Factors: Oral contraceptives will increase plasminogen level; medications that decrease levels are alteplase, urokinase, streptokinase, and L-asparaginase; hemolyzed specimens give altered results.

Nursing Considerations:
Pregnancy: Level is elevated during pregnancy.
Pediatric: Infants and children will need assistance in remaining still during the venipuncture and age-appropriate comfort measures following the test. Level is elevated in infants, especially in hyaline membrane disease.

Listing of Related Tests: Fibrinogen degradation products; fibrinogen testing

WEBLINKS

http://www.methodisthealth.com

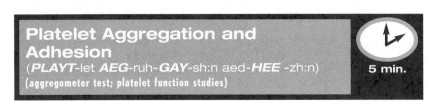

Platelet Aggregation and Adhesion
(*PLAYT*-let *AEG*-ruh-*GAY*-sh:n aed-*HEE* -zh:n)
(aggregometer test; platelet function studies)

5 min.

Type of Test: Blood

Body Systems and Functions: Hematological system

Normal Findings:

Aggregation	60%–100% aggregation within 3–5 min
Adhesion	90%–95%

Test Results Time Frame: Within 8 hr

Test Description: Platelet aggregation and adhesion tests measure the normal platelet function in coagulation. Aggregation demonstrates the ability of platelets to adhere to each other during blood clotting. The adhesion test measures the ability of platelets to adhere to foreign bodies during blood clotting.

Normal platelets adhere quickly to the damaged epithelial wall in a blood vessel. The platelets change shape and send out pseudopods, and their membranes become "stickier"; they stick to each other, forming a platelet clot. They also bind with fibrin to strengthen the clot. A platelet clot is adequate for hemostasis of a very small break; larger breaks need a blood clot (thrombus) in addition to the platelet clot. Platelet aggregation and adhesion tests expose the platelet specimen to various known agents that induce aggregation, such as thrombin, collagen, and epinephrine. The percent adhering within a set time indicates normal vs. abnormal function. Depending on the reaction to each agent, various disorders can be specifically diagnosed.

Consent Form: Not required

List of Equipment: *Aggregation test:* blue-top tube or serum separator tube; needle and syringe or vacutainer; alcohol swab. *Adhesion test:* red-top tube or serum separator tube; needle and syringe or vacutainer; alcohol swab.

Test Procedure:
1. Label the specimen tube. *Correctly identifies the client and the test to be performed.*
2. Obtain a 5-mL blood sample.
3. Do not agitate the tube. *Agitation may cause RBC hemolysis.*
4. Send tube to the laboratory.

Clinical Implications and Indications:
1. Detects abnormal aggregation associated with genetic platelet function disorders, such as Vernard-Soulier syndrome, Chediak-Higashi syndrome, von Willebrand's disease, and thrombasthenia.
2. Detects effect of medications known to decrease platelet function, such as aspirin, NSAIDs, and some antidepressants and antibiotics.
3. Detects loss of platelet function in cirrhosis and uremia.
4. Elevated levels of aggregation are found with atheromatosis, diabetes mellitus, hypercoagulability states, hyperlipidemia, and polycythemia vera.
5. Decreased aggregation levels are found with afibrinogenemia, anemia (sideroblastic), Bernard-Soulier syndrome, beta-thalassemia major, Chèdiak-Higashi syndrome, cirrhosis, idiopathic thrombocytopenia purpura (ITP), hemorrhagic thrombocytopenia, uremia, and von Willebrand's disease.

Nursing Care:
Before Test: Explain the test procedure and the purpose of the test. Assess the client's knowledge of the test. Instruct client to fast 8 hr prior to the test.
During Test: Adhere to standard precautions.
After Test: Apply pressure to venipuncture site. Explain that some bruising, discomfort, and swelling may appear at the site and that warm, moist compresses can alleviate this. Monitor for signs of infection.

Potential Complications: Bleeding and bruising at venipuncture site

Interfering Factors: Caffeine; lipemia; platelet count <100,000/mm^3; medications that decrease aggregation levels are aminophylline, antihistamines, aspirin, NSAIDs, steroids, psychotropics, phenothiazines, tricyclic antidepressants, caffeine, nitrates, nitroprusside, beta blockers, propranolol, calcium channel blockers, verapamil, diltiazem, nifedipine, penicillins, cephalosporins, pyrimidine, cocaine, marijuana, and vitamins.

BLOOD

Nursing Considerations:

Pediatric: *Infants and children will need assistance in remaining still during the venipuncture and age-appropriate comfort measures following the test.*

WEBLINKS

http://www.methodisthealth.com

Platelet Antibody Detection
(*PLAYT*-let *AEN*-ti-*BAH*-dee dee-*TEK*-sh:n)
(antiplatelet antibody detection; platelet antibody test)

5 min.

Type of Test: Blood

Body Systems and Functions: Hematological system

Normal Findings: Negative or <1,000 molecules IgG/platelet

Test Results Time Frame: Within 24 hr

Test Description: The platelet antibody detection test identifies the presence of platelet autoantibodies and isoantibodies. Autoantibodies are IgG derived and present in autoimmune disorders. Isoantibodies develop in clients who have had multiple platelet transfusions and are sensitized to the antigens on the platelets. The result is destruction of both donor platelets and the client's own platelets.

CLINICAL ALERT:
Platelet typing is important to prevent or decrease transfusion reactions (severe chilling, shaking, fever) during platelet transfusions.

Consent Form: Not required

List of Equipment: Red-top tube or serum separator tube; needle and syringe or vacutainer; alcohol swab

Test Procedure:
1. Label the specimen tube. *Correctly identifies the client and the test to be performed.*
2. Obtain a 5-mL blood sample.
3. Do not agitate the tube. *Agitation may cause RBC hemolysis.*
4. Send tube to the laboratory.

Clinical Implications and Indications:
1. Diagnoses autoimmune disorders, such as neonatal thrombocytic purpura, idiopathic thrombocytic purpura, paroxysmal hemoglobinemia, posttransfusion purpura, and drug-induced immunological thrombocytopenia (quinidine, quinine, sulfa, hydantoin, and chlordiazepoxide)
2. Determines platelet type for transfusion, especially in disorders needing frequent transfusions, such as aplastic anemia and cancer

Nursing Care:

Before Test: Explain the test procedure and the purpose of the test. Assess the client's knowledge of the test (note: specimens that cannot be processed immediately should be drawn into tubes containing acid citrate dextrose, which must be obtained from the laboratory).

During Test: Adhere to standard precautions.

After Test: Apply pressure to venipuncture site. Explain that some bruising, discomfort, and swelling may appear at the site and that warm, moist compresses can alleviate this. Monitor for signs of infection.

Potential Complications: Bleeding and bruising at venipuncture site

Interfering Factors: Anticoagulant therapy

Nursing Considerations:

Pediatric: Infants and children will need assistance in remaining still during the venipuncture and age-appropriate comfort measures following the test.

Listing of Related Tests: Quantitative antiglobin consumption test; complement fixation test

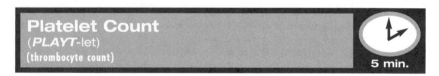

WEBLINKS

http://www.methodisthealth.com

Platelet Count
(*PLAYT*-let)
(thrombocyte count)

5 min.

Type of Test: Blood

Body Systems and Functions: Hematological system

Normal Findings:

Newborns	100,000–450,000 mm³
Neonates	150,000–390,000 mm³
Adults	150,000–450,000 mm³

CRITICAL VALUES:

A high platelet count reflects the potential for serious clinical concerns. A platelet count below 30,000 places the client at a high risk for bleeding and a level above 1,000,000 indicates a high risk for thrombosis.

Test Results Time Frame: Within 2–12 hr

Test Description: Platelet count measures the number of platelet cells. Platelets are essential for coagulation, hemostasis, and clot formation. Platelets are produced when megakaryocytes in the bone marrow mature and bud off fragments of cytoplasm. These nonnucleated fragments enter the plasma as platelets. Two-thirds of the total platelets are circulating and one-third are stored in the spleen. Platelets initiate the process of hemostasis by aggregating quickly at the site of a damaged blood vessel and adhere to the endothelium forming a platelet clot to plug the opening. Additional hemostatic processes with fibrin and clotting factors stabilize the clot.

Consent Form: Not required

List of Equipment: Red-top tube or plasma separator tube; needle and syringe or vacutainer; alcohol swab

Test Procedure:
1. Label the specimen tube. *Correctly identifies the client and the test to be performed.*
2. Obtain a 5-mL blood sample.
3. Gently invert tube several times, but do not agitate the tube. *Mixes the anticoagulant, but agitation may cause RBC hemolysis.*
4. Send tube to the laboratory.

Clinical Implications and Indications:
1. Routine blood screen, especially before surgery or other invasive procedures.
2. Confirms low or high platelet count in disease states, such as malignancy, idiopathic thrombocytopenia purpura, bone marrow failure due to cancer or medications, and liver damage.
3. Evaluates etiology of signs and symptoms of bleeding, such as epistaxis, hematuria, or bruising.
4. Elevated levels are found with living at high altitudes, exercising extensively over several months or living in chronically cold environments, anemias (posthemorrhagic, iron deficiency), carcinomatosis, chronic heart disease, cirrhosis, leukemia (chronic), pancreatitis (chronic), polycythemia vera, postsurgery, childbirth, trauma and hemorrhage, spleenectomy, and tuberculosis.
5. Decreased platelet count (thrombocytopenia) levels are found with anemias (aplastic, pernicious), antibody/HLA antigen reactions, bone marrow malignancies, burns (severe), chronic cor pulmonale, disseminated intravascular coagulation, infections (e.g., Rocky Mountain spotted fever, meningococcemia, idiopathic thrombocytopenia purpura), hemolytic disease of the newborn, leukemias (acute), lymphomas, and spleenomegaly (in liver disease).

Nursing Care:
Before Test: Explain the test procedure and the purpose of the test. Assess the client's knowledge of the test.
During Test: Adhere to standard precautions.
After Test: Apply pressure to venipuncture site. Explain that some bruising, discomfort, and swelling may appear at the site and that warm, moist compresses can alleviate this. Monitor for signs of infection. Send specimen to laboratory within 1 hr.

Potential Complications: Bleeding and bruising at venipuncture site

Interfering Factors: Dilution by increased vascular volume; traumatic venipuncture; agitated handling of specimen; variations in results depending on if hand or machine counted; hemodialysis; medications that increase levels are oral contraceptives and epinephrine; medications that decrease levels are aspirin, heparin, quinine, thiazides, alcohol, chemotherapy, anticonvulsants, chloramphenicol, isoniazid, sulfonamides, and sulfonylureas.

BLOOD

Nursing Considerations:
Pregnancy: Slight decrease in platelet count is normal. Following childbirth, platelet count may be elevated for up to 4 weeks.
Pediatric: Infants and children will need assistance in remaining still during the venipuncture and age-appropriate comfort measures following the test. There are wide variations of normal values in newborns. Capillary samples may be obtained in infants or children, although platelet count will be slightly decreased because of platelets adhering to the wound.

Listing of Related Tests: Bleeding time; prothrombin time (PT); activated partial thromboplastin time (APTT); clot retraction test

WEBLINKS

http://www.methodisthealth.com

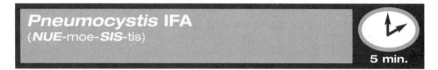

Pneumocystis IFA
(*NUE*-moe-*SIS*-tis)

5 min.

Type of Test: Blood

Body Systems and Functions: Pulmonary system

Normal Findings: <1:16 antibodies; no organisms seen

Test Results Time Frame: Within 24 hr

Test Description: *Pneumocystis* IFA measures the antibody titer for *Pneumocystis carinii*, a protozoan bacteria. *Pneumocystis carinii* is present in many mammalian species. It is spread by airborne route and usually causes an asymptomatic infection in people with intact immune systems. However, it can cause a serious pneumonia in immunosuppressed or immunodeficient persons. Premature infants may also be at risk. *Pneumocystis carinii* is the most common opportunistic infectious agent in AIDS patients, with almost 80% suffering from the infection. It is generally thought that the development of *P. carinii* pneumonia (PCP) is due to reactivation of a latent childhood or adolescent exposure to the bacteria.

CLINICAL ALERT:
Monitor respiratory status carefully as this client is likely suspected of having *P. carinii*.

Consent Form: Not required

List of Equipment: Red-top tube or serum separator tube; needle and syringe or vacutainer; alcohol swab

Test Procedure:
1. Label the specimen tube. *Correctly identifies the client and the test to be performed.*
2. Obtain a 10-mL blood sample.
3. Do not agitate the tube. *Agitation may cause RBC hemolysis.*
4. Send tube to the laboratory.

Clinical Implications and Indications:

1. A diagnostic indicator that the person may have PCP. However, presence of antibody means that a person may have been exposed and/or had an asymptomatic infection unrelated to the current problem. A definitive diagnosis for PCP depends on tissue brushings or bronchial washings from a bronchoscopy, which should be immediately scheduled if the serum test is positive.
2. Rapid diagnosis is important because the organism quickly infiltrates lung tissue, causing diffuse interstitial infiltrate with dyspnea, fever, and cough. Early treatment of PCP improves chances of survival.

Nursing Care:

Before Test: Explain the test procedure and the purpose of the test. Assess the client's knowledge of the test.
During Test: Adhere to standard precautions.
After Test: Apply pressure to venipuncture site. Explain that some bruising, discomfort, and swelling may appear at the site and that warm, moist compresses can alleviate this. Monitor for signs of infection.

Potential Complications: Bleeding and bruising at venipuncture site

Nursing Considerations:

Pediatric: Infants and children will need assistance in remaining still during the venipuncture and age-appropriate comfort measures following the test. Premature infants are at greater risk for PCP.

Listing of Related Tests: Bronchoscopy (alveolar lavage or bronchial washings); *Pneumocystitis carinii* smear; transbronchial lung biopsy (rare)

WEBLINKS

http://www.rcjournal.com

Poliomyelitis 1, 2, 3 Titer
(*POE*-lee-oe-*MIY*-uh-*LIYT*-is ... *TIYT*-:r)
(polio enterovirus)

5 min.

Type of Test: Blood; fluid analysis

Body Systems and Functions: Neurological system

Normal Findings: <8 is normal (<2 for CSF). A fourfold increase in antibody titer between the first specimen (drawn during the acute phase) and the second specimen (drawn during the convalescent phase) is diagnostic for poliomyelitis.

Test Results Time Frame: Within 24–48 hr

Test Description: Poliomyelitis titers measure the antibody titer and serotype for the poliovirus antigen. Serotypes 1, 2, and 3 can cause the symptoms of acute polio infection and also the postpolio syndrome seen in adults. Two specimens are drawn, one as soon as possible during the acute phase and the second specimen 2 weeks to 2 months later. Symptoms of acute infection begin with headache, nausea and vomiting, and back and neck pain. Symptoms may be mild and temporary or increase in severity. Paralysis, temporary or permanent, may occur if the virus attacks the brain.

> **CLINICAL ALERT:**
> Anyone suspected of having polio should be isolated from people who have not been immunized because polio is very contagious, transmitted by the fecal-oral route. In addition, anyone suspected of having polio should be carefully monitored for neurological changes, including paralysis of the respiratory nerves, which is life threatening.

Consent Form: Not required

List of Equipment: Red-top tube or serum separator tube; needle and syringe or vacutainer; alcohol swab

Test Procedure:
1. Label the specimen tube. *Correctly identifies the client and the test to be performed.*
2. Obtain an 8-mL blood sample for adults and 4 mL for children. *Different amounts for ages are required for accurate results.*
3. Do not agitate the tube. *Agitation may cause RBC hemolysis.*
4. Send tube to the laboratory.
5. Repeat 10–14 days later for convalescent sample and label the tube as convalescent sample. *Allows for separate identification of the convalescent sample, which is compared in ratio to the acute sample.*

Clinical Implications and Indications:
1. Diagnoses poliomyelitis disease

Nursing Care:
Before Test: Explain the test procedure and the purpose of the test. Assess the client's knowledge of the test.
During Test: Adhere to standard precautions.
After Test: Apply pressure to venipuncture site. Explain that some bruising, discomfort, and swelling may appear at the site and that warm, moist compresses can alleviate this. Monitor for signs of infection.

Potential Complications: Bleeding and bruising at venipuncture site

Interfering Factors: In 50% of clients with polio the first blood sample is already past the peak of the titer.

Nursing Considerations:
Pediatric: *Infants and children will need assistance in remaining still during the venipuncture and age-appropriate comfort measures following the test.*
International: *The use of oral vaccines has markedly decreased the incidence of polio since the 1950s. However, outbreaks are sporadic in countries with unimmunized groups. In the United States poliomyelitis cases have usually been associated with vaccination.*

WEBLINKS

http://www.jeffersonhealth.org

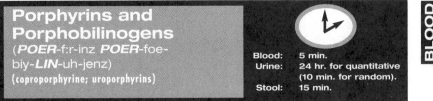

Porphyrins and Porphobilinogens
(**POER**-f:r-inz **POER**-foe-
biy-**LIN**-uh-jenz)
(coproporphyrine; uroporphyrins)

Blood:	5 min.
Urine:	24 hr. for quantitative (10 min. for random).
Stool:	15 min.

Type of Test: Blood; urine; stool

Body Systems and Functions: Hematological system

Normal Findings: Negative for porphyrins in stool and urine
Blood:

Porphyrins	<31 µg/dL
Aminolevulinic acid (ALA)	<1 mg/dL
Coproporphyrin	0.5–2.3 mg/dL
Protoporphyrin	4–52 mg/dL
Uroporphyrin	Negative to trace

Negative for porphobilinogen in urine

CRITICAL VALUES:
Clients with positive results (elevated ALA) should avoid alcohol, barbiturates, and anticonvulsants that might cause acute attack of neurological/psychotic porphyria.

Test Results Time Frame: Within 24–48 hr

Test Description: Porphyrins are intermediate products in the synthesis of hemeproteins, including hemoglobin, myoglobin, and cytochromes. Hemeproteins are found in all cells but especially in the bone marrow and liver cells. The enzyme ALA regulates the rate of heme synthesis in liver cells. Porphyrins are inherited or acquired (lead poisoning, cirrhosis, drug induced) disorders that disturb heme synthesis and cause excessive formation and excretion of porphyrin or its precursors in the blood and feces or urine. There are many types of porphyrins, but only three are clinically significant depending on the disorder: uroporphyrin in urine, coproporphyrin in feces and urine, and protoporphyrin in feces. All three porphyrins are also found in whole blood. Tests may be ordered either as a complete screen (blood, urine, and feces) or individually.

Consent Form: Not required

List of Equipment: *Blood:* green-top heparinized tube, lavender-top tube with ETDA, or black-top tube with sodium oxalate or plasma separator tube; needle and syringe or vacutainer; alcohol swab. *Urine:* 3-L dark (or foil-wrapped) bottle for quantitative porphyrins or porphobilinogen; 10- to 50-mL specimen container foil wrapped for qualitative porphyrin or porphobilinogen. *Stool:* clean, dry container to collect stool; tongue depressor; gloves; rectal swab; clean, dry bedpan.

Test Procedure:
Blood:
1. Label the specimen tube. *Correctly identifies the client and the test to be performed.*

2. Obtain a 5-mL blood sample.
3. Gently invert tube several times, but do not agitate the tube. *Mixes the anticoagulant, but agitation may cause RBC hemolysis.*
4. Send tube to the laboratory.

Urine—random sample:

1. Label a sterile urine container. *Correctly identifies the client and the test to be performed.*
2. Protect all specimens from light by wrapping container in foil if it is clear glass or plastic. *Porphyrin and prophobilinogen are unstable when exposed to light.*
3. Obtain a clean-catch specimen of urine (note: first morning voiding preferred, at least 60 mL). *Ensures accurate results.*
4. Keep specimen cool. *High temperatures alter the results.*
5. Send specimen to laboratory.
6. Refrigerate during and after collection. *Porphyrin and porpobilinogen are unstable when exposed to room temperature or heat.*

Urine—24-hr specimen (for quantitative porphyrin or prophobilinogen urine tests):

1. Label the collection container. *Correctly identifies the client and the test to be performed.*
2. Discard the first morning void. Then begin the time of the collection for the next 24 hr, including the void at the end of the 24 hr, and record the last voiding time. *An exact 24-hr count ensures accurate results.*
3. If the client has an indwelling catheter in place, keep the drainage bag on ice and empty the urine into the urine container periodically during the 24-hr period.
4. Keep urine cool during collection. *Higher temperatures alter the results.*
5. If any urine is lost, discard the entire specimen and begin collection again the next day.

Stool:

1. Have client defecate into a clean bedpan, bedside commode, or toilet hat. *Decreases contamination and aids in obtaining stool specimen.*
2. Do not use the stool if it is contaminated with urine or menstrual blood. *Urine and menstrual blood affect stool culture results.*
3. Do not have the client place toilet paper on the stool after defecation. *Toilet paper affects stool culture results.*
4. Use a clean tongue depressor to place 2–3 cm of formed stool or 15 mL of liquid stool in a specimen container. *This amount is necessary for obtaining proper stool culture.*
5. Dispose of remaining stool and tongue depressor. *Decreases chance of spread of pathogen.*
6. Include visible mucus, pus, or blood in the specimen. *These may be indicative of disease or contain pathogens.*
7. Label the specimen container and send to laboratory as soon as possible. *Ensures accurate results.*

Clinical Implications and Indications:

1. Diagnoses inherited porphyrias.
2. Diagnoses acquired porphyrias caused by drugs, heavy metal poisoning, or alcoholic cirrhosis.
3. Levels may only be elevated during acute episodes in some types of prophyria disorders. Individual enzyme assays can be done in specialized

laboratories for each of the defective enzymes, which are more definitive for diagnosing inherited porphyrias.

Nursing Care:

Before Test: Explain the test procedure and the purpose of the test. Assess the client's knowledge of the test. Instruct client to not drink alcohol for 24 hr prior to the blood draw. Instruct client not to discard any urine over the 24-hr time period.

During Test: Adhere to standard precautions. If any urine is accidentally discarded or contaminated with feces, discard entire specimen and begin test again the following morning (for 24-hr urine).

After Test: Blood: Apply pressure to venipuncture site. Explain that some bruising, discomfort, and swelling may appear at the site and that warm, moist compresses can alleviate this. Monitor for signs of infection. Urine: Document urine quantity, date, and exact hours of collection on requisition. Refrigerate urine and feces specimens and protect them from exposure to light. If results are positive, caution client to avoid alcohol, barbiturates, and anticonvulsant therapy to prevent neurological or psychotic porphyria. Instruct client to avoid sunlight.

Potential Complications: Bleeding and bruising at venipuncture site

Interfering Factors: Incorrect handling may allow feces to contaminate urine specimen as there may be high amounts of porphyrin in feces; hepatic cancer; Hodgkin's disease; infection; urine contaminated with feces; spillage or inaccurate collection of the 24-hr specimen, including nonrefrigeration or placing on ice; heavy bleeding during menstruation

Nursing Considerations:

Pregnancy: Levels may increase during menstruation or pregnancy.
Pediatric: Blood: Infants and children will need assistance in remaining still during the venipuncture and age-appropriate comfort measures following the test. Urine: For collection of 24-hr specimen a collection bag or indwelling catheter needs to be used for infants and toddlers. Random sample: A collection bag or insertion of a straight catheter is likely needed for infants and toddlers.

Listing of Related Tests: Coproporphyrin; protoporphyrin (FEP); uroporphyrin

⎹WEBLINKS⎹   ⊟⊠

http://www.methodisthealth.com/pathology/hemato.htm

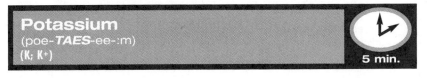

Potassium
(poe-*TAES*-ee-:m)
(K; K+)

5 min.

Type of Test: Blood

Body Systems and Functions: Hematological system

Normal Findings:

Infants	4.1–5.3 mEq/L
Children	3.4–4.7 mEq/L
Adults	3.5–5.5 mEq/L

CRITICAL VALUES:

<2.5 or >6.5 mEq/L. When potassium is outside of these parameters, cardiac electrical activity can be seriously altered with arrthymias developing, especially >7 mEq/L. At 10 mEq/L cardiac activity can cease.

Test Results Time Frame: Within 4 hr

Test Description: A potassium test measures the amount of the electrolyte potassium in the blood. The majority of potassium is found within cells where it has a major influence on the conduction of electrical impulses in cardiac and skeletal muscle. It also influences acid-base balance and numerous enzyme reactions in carbohydrate and protein metabolism. In acidosis, potassium ions move from the cells into the blood. In alkalosis, the reverse occurs. Extremes of this electrolyte potentially can be very severe and can be life threatening to the client.

Consent Form: Not required

List of Equipment: Red-top tube or serum separator tube; needle and syringe or vacutainer; alcohol swab

Test Procedure:

1. Label the specimen tube. *Correctly identifies the client and the test to be performed.*
2. Obtain a 7-mL blood sample.
3. Do not agitate the tube. *Agitation may cause RBC hemolysis.*
4. Send tube to the laboratory.

Clinical Implications and Indications:

1. Routine screening of electrolyte balance, including potassium, chloride, and sodium
2. Evaluates influence of known or suspected disorders on potassium, especially in acute or chronic renal failure, trauma, or burns
3. Evaluates influence of medications that alter potassium balance
4. Evaluates influence of acid-base imbalance on potassium
5. Evaluates response of therapy for abnormal potassium level

---

Selected factors leading to abnormal potassium levels

Increased potassium (hyperkalemia)
Acidosis
Insulin deficiency
Causes of cell destruction, i.e., trauma, necrosis, and burns
Acute or chronic renal failure
Medications:
Potassium supplements

Amphotericin B
Heparin
Isoniazid
Decreased potassium (hypokalemia)
Alkalosis
Insulin excess
GI loss through vomiting, diarrhea, fistula, or nasogastric suction
Excessive diuresis
Medications:
Furosemide
Thiazide diuretics
Cortisone
Lithium
Kayexalate
Insulin

Nursing Care:
Before Test: Explain the test procedure and the purpose of the test. Assess the client's knowledge of the test.
During Test: Adhere to standard precautions.
After Test: Apply pressure to venipuncture site. Explain that some bruising, discomfort, and swelling may appear at the site and that warm, moist compresses can alleviate this. Monitor for signs of infection.

Potential Complications: Bleeding and bruising at venipuncture site

Interfering Factors: Hemolysis; active hand pumping after tourniquet applied; medications that can increase levels are potassium supplements, amphotericin B, heparin, and isoniazid; medications that can decrease levels are furosemide, thiazide diuretics, cortisone, lithium, kayexelate, and insulin.

Nursing Considerations:
Pediatric: Infants and children will need assistance in remaining still during the venipuncture and age-appropriate comfort measures following the test.
Gerontology: Many elderly clients take diuretics, which affect potassium levels. When a client has taken a loop or thiazide diuretic, potassium levels can quickly drop unless actively replaced by eating high-potassium foods or taking potassium supplements. When potassium is outside the normal range and the client is on the medication digoxin, the heart is even more sensitive to electrical malfunction. An EKG with peaked T waves (high potassium) or depressed T or prominent U waves (low potassium) is diagnostic.

Listing of Related Tests: Serum chloride; sodium; carbon dioxide; bicarbonate

WEBLINKS

www.mayohealth.org

Prealbumin
(*PREE*-ael-*BYUE*-m:n)
(transthyretin; tryptophan-rich prealbumin)

5 min.

Type of Test: Blood

Body Systems and Functions: Hematological system

Test Results Time Frame: Within 24 hr

Test Description: The serum prealbumin concentration is used as an index of nutritional status, especially protein status. Transthyretin is an albumin precursor and has a half-life of 2–4 days, whereas albumin has a half-life of 20–22 days. Therefore, transthyretin is a more sensitive marker to detect changes in nutritional status. Transthyretin has a high tryptophan content and is an amino acid thought to be highly influential in protein synthesis.

Consent Form: Not required

List of Equipment: Red-top tube or serum separator tube; needle and syringe or vacutainer; alcohol swab

Test Procedure:
1. Label the specimen tube. *Correctly identifies the client and the test to be performed.*
2. Obtain a 1-mL blood sample.
3. Do not agitate the tube. *Agitation may cause RBC hemolysis.*
4. Send tube to the laboratory.

Clinical Implications and Indications:
1. Evaluates nutritional status. It is particularly helpful in evaluating protein balance on clients receiving albumin products to increase oncotic pressure and on clients receiving total parenteral nutrition.
2. Evaluates liver function and metabolic stress.
3. Elevated levels are found with adrenal hyperfunction and Hodgkin's disease.
4. Decreased levels are found with metabolic stress from chronic illness or metastatic malignancies, cirrhosis, and peritoneal dialysis.

Nursing Care:
Before Test: Explain the test procedure and the purpose of the test. Assess the client's knowledge of the test. Instruct client to fast for 8 hr prior to the test.
During Test: Adhere to standard precautions.
After Test: Apply pressure to venipuncture site. Explain that some bruising, discomfort, and swelling may appear at the site and that warm, moist compresses can alleviate this. Monitor for signs of infection.

Potential Complications: Bleeding and bruising at venipuncture site

Interfering Factors: Dialysis; medications that increase levels are corticosteroids and NSAIDs; medications that decrease levels are oral contraceptives, estrogens, and amiodarone.

BLOOD

Nursing Considerations:
Pediatric: Infants and children will need assistance in remaining still during the venipuncture and age-appropriate comfort measures following the test.
Gerontology: Liver function tests generally do not change in an aging client and abnormal results are usually a sign of a pathologic process.

Listing of Related Tests: Albumin; plasma protein

WEBLINKS

http://wellness.ucdavis.edu

Progesterone
(proe-*JES*-t:r-oen)
(P4)

5 min.

Type of Test: Blood

Body Systems and Functions: Endocrine system

Normal Findings: Normal laboratory findings vary among laboratory settings.

Adult males	<100 ng/dL
Menstruating females:	
Follicular phase	<150 ng/dL
Luteal phase	300–2,000 ng/dL
Pregnancy:	
7–13 weeks	1,500–5,000 ng/dL
14–72 weeks	6,500–20,000 ng/dL

Test Results Time Frame: Within 24 hr

Test Description: Progesterone testing measures the level of serum progesterone. Progesterone is produced by the ovary, placenta, and adrenals of the female and the adrenals and testes of the male. In ovulating women the progesterone follows a cyclic monthly pattern. During the follicular phase, the progesterone levels are low. The level increases slightly just before the LH peak and ovulation in midcycle, then peaks halfway through the luteal phase. If fertilization does not occur, the progesterone level falls rapidly near the end of the luteal phase before the start of menstruation. Thus, it is useful in determining when ovulation occurs. In pregnancy, progesterone is produced by the corpus luteum and the placenta in large amounts. Progesterone is necessary to prepare the endometrium for implantation of the fertilized ovum, decrease myometrial excitement, and stimulate growth of the breasts.

CLINICAL ALERT:
If the progesterone level is low during pregnancy, it indicates something is wrong in the corpus luteum function. If the level is <25 ng/dL, it indicates either an ectopic pregnancy or a nonviable pregnancy.

Consent Form: Not required

List of Equipment: Red-top tube or serum separator tube; needle and syringe or vacutainer; alcohol swab

Test Procedure:
1. Label the specimen tube. *Correctly identifies the client and the test to be performed.*
2. Obtain a 7-mL blood sample.
3. Do not agitate the tube. *Agitation may cause RBC hemolysis.*
4. Send tube to the laboratory.

Clinical Implications and Indications:
1. Determines the time of ovulation.
2. Diagnoses anovulation, oligoovulation, and luteal phase defect in low-fertile or infertile women.
3. Assesses function of corpus luteum during the first 12 weeks of pregnancy in cases of potential spontaneous abortion.
4. Diagnoses ectopic or nonviable pregnancy.
5. Progesterone is commonly a replacement hormone during menopause, and therefore progesterone levels may be drawn during this time.
6. In males, progesterone may be elevated in adrenogenital syndrome.

Nursing Care:
Before Test: Explain the test procedure and the purpose of the test. Assess the client's knowledge of the test. Document gender and the first day of the last menstrual cycle or the week of gestation on the laboratory requisition.
During Test: Adhere to standard precautions.
After Test: Apply pressure to venipuncture site. Explain that some bruising, discomfort, and swelling may appear at the site and that warm, moist compresses can alleviate this. Monitor for signs of infection. Specimen may be refrigerated for 4 days or frozen for 1 year. If serial testing is needed over several cycles, inform client of the purpose and schedule.

Potential Complications: Bleeding and bruising at venipuncture site

Interfering Factors: Recent radioactive isotope scan; medications that increase levels are estrogen, progesterone, and corticosteroid therapy.

Nursing Considerations:
Pregnancy: The client being tested for a nonviable pregnancy or threatened spontaneous abortion will need support and counseling during the process.
Pediatric: Infants and children will need assistance in remaining still during the venipuncture and age-appropriate comfort measures following the test.

Listing of Related Tests: Endometrial biopsy

WEBLINKS

http://www.niddk.nih.gov

Prolactin
(proe-*LAEK*-tin)
(HPRL; LTH; PRL; luteotropic hormone; lactogenic hormone;
lactogen; mammotropin)

5 min.

Type of Test: Blood

Body Systems and Functions: Reproductive system

Normal Findings:

Adult males	<0–10 ng/mL
Females:	
Follicular	<28 ng/mL
Luteal	5–40 ng/mL
First trimester	<80 ng/mL
Second trimester	<160 ng/mL
Third trimester	<400 ng/mL
Lactating	<40 ng/mL
Menopausal	<12 ng/mL
Newborns	> x 10 adult level
Pituitary tumor	>100 ng/mL

Test Results Time Frame: Within 24 hr

Test Description: Prolactin testing measures the level of prolactin, a peptide hormone released by the anterior pituitary. The main functions of prolactin are to promote breast tissue growth and to stimulate secretion of milk. Prolactin's production and release are controlled by a prolactin-inhibiting factor (probably dopamine) from the hypothalamus. Prolactin is also called luteotropic hormone (LTH), lactogenic hormone, and mammotropin. Prolactin is influenced by the circadian rhythm, rising in the early morning hours and peaking 2–3 hr after waking. Prolactin levels rise late in pregnancy and shortly after delivery return to a baseline value, if the woman does not breastfeed. Prolactin is mildly elevated in a breast-feeding mother.

CLINICAL ALERT:
Excessive prolactin levels disturb sexual function for both men (e.g., impotence) and women (e.g., amenorrhea, anovulation).

Consent Form: Not required

List of Equipment: Red-top tube or serum separator tube; needle and syringe or vacutainer; alcohol swab

Test Procedure:
1. Label the specimen tube. *Correctly identifies the client and the test to be performed.*
2. Obtain a 5-mL blood sample.
3. Do not agitate the tube. *Agitation may cause RBC hemolysis.*
4. Send tube to the laboratory.

Clinical Implications and Indications:

1. Evaluates oligorrhea, amenorrhea, or galactorrhea in women.
2. Evaluates impotence in men.
3. Diagnoses pituitary tumor.
4. Diagnoses prolactin-secreting ectopic tumor of the lungs or kidney.
5. Elevated levels are found with Addison's disease, anorexia nervosa, hypothalamus or pituitary tumor, hypothyroidism, chronic renal failure, liver disease, prolactin-secreting ectopic tumor, adrenal disease, acromegaly, amenorrhea, galactorrhea, pregnancy, breast feeding, sleep, and stress.
6. Decreased levels are found with pituitary infarction, hirsutism, osteoporosis, gynecomastia, and necrosis.

Nursing Care:

Before Test: Explain the test procedure and the purpose of the test. Assess the client's knowledge of the test. Schedule venous draw at 8 AM because of circadian rhythm influence on levels. Awaken client at least 2 hr before test. Instruct client to not drink alcohol for at least 24 hr before blood draw. Instruct client to fast 8–12 hr before test.
During Test: Adhere to standard precautions.
After Test: Apply pressure to venipuncture site. Explain that some bruising, discomfort, and swelling may appear at the site and that warm, moist compresses can alleviate this. Monitor for signs of infection.

Potential Complications: Bleeding and bruising at venipuncture site

Interfering Factors: Alcohol; brief increases in levels can occur due to sleep, exercise, and stress; levels are influenced by diurnal cycles and peaks in the early morning hours; hemolysis; lipemia; medications that increase levels are SRRIs, tricyclic antidepressants, oral contraceptives, meprobamate, methyldopa, isoniazid, amphetamines, haloperidol, reserpine, procainamide derivatives, estrogen, cimetidine, and metaclopramide; medications that decrease levels are dopamine, ergot alkaloids, apomorphine, and L-dopa.

Nursing Considerations:

Pregnancy: A mild elevation is expected in mothers who are breast feeding.
Pediatric: Infants and children will need assistance in remaining still during the venipuncture and age-appropriate comfort measures following the test. A newborn infant has very high levels for a short time after birth.

Listing of Related Tests: Thyrotropin assay

WEBLINKS ▤ ⊠

http://biocrs.biomed.brown.edu

Prostate-Specific Antigen
(*PRAHS*-tayt spe-*SIF*-ik *AEN*-tuh-j:n)
(PSA)

5 min.

Type of Test: Blood

Body Systems and Functions: Reproductive system

Normal Findings:

Total PSA	0–4 ng/mL
Total PSA post–radical prostectomy	0.0–0.3 ng/mL
Men over 60 years of age:	
60–69 years	0.0–5.0 ng/mL
70–79 years	0.0–6.3 ng/mL

Test Results Time Frame: Within 24 hr

Test Description: Prostate-specific antigen tests for the levels of a serum protease enzyme specific to the male prostate. It is produced by the prostate epithelium in both benign and malignant disease. Serum protease circulates in the blood in both a free form and a bound form. At this time total PSA is being used as the marker for possible cancer; research is studying whether free PSA may be a more sensitive marker once cancer is diagnosed.

Consent Form: Not required

List of Equipment: Red-top tube or serum separator tube; needle and syringe or vacutainer; alcohol swab

Test Procedure:
1. Label the specimen tube. *Correctly identifies the client and the test to be performed.*
2. Obtain a 5-mL blood sample.
3. Do not agitate the tube. *Agitation may cause RBC hemolysis.*
4. Send tube to the laboratory.

Clinical Implications and Indications:
1. PSA aids in diagnosis of prostate cancer in conjunction with the digital rectal examination (DRE) (note: the PSA specimen should be drawn before the DRE). If either the DRE or PSA is abnormal, a prostate biopsy should be done for definitive diagnosis.
2. PSA is useful in staging and monitoring treatment effects. Following a radical prostatectomy a small increase in a very low level PSA can be an early clinical marker of cancer recurrence.
3. Elevated levels are found with benign prostate hypertrophy, prostatitis, urinary retention, and osteoporosis.

Nursing Care:
Before Test: Explain the test procedure and the purpose of the test. Assess the client's knowledge of the test. Instruct client to fast for 8 hr prior to the PSA test.
During Test: Adhere to standard precautions.
After Test: Apply pressure to venipuncture site. Explain that some bruising, discomfort, and swelling may appear at the site and that warm, moist compresses can alleviate this. Monitor for signs of infection.

Potential Complications: Bleeding and bruising at venipuncture site

Interfering Factors: Vigorous exercise elevates the PSA level; ejaculation increases PSA for up to 2 days; prostate massage and prostate biopsy (note: PSA levels should not be obtained until waiting 1 week after a prostate biopsy)

Listing of Related Tests: Acid phosphatase (PAP); prostate biopsy; prostate sonography

WEBLINKS

www3.cancer.org

Protein, Blood
(**PROE**-teen)
(dip stick; uric acid; amino acids; urine hydroxyproline)

5 min.

Type of Test: Blood

Body Systems and Functions: Hematological system

Normal Findings:

Adults	6.0–8.0 g/dL
Children:	
Premature infants	4.3–7.6 g/dL
Newborns	4.6–7.4 g/dL
Infants	6.0–6.7 g/dL
Children	6.2–8.0 g/dL

Test Results Time Frame: Within 24 hr

Test Description: A serum protein test measures the total protein level in the blood. It includes measurement of albumin, globulin, and the albumin/globulin ratio. Normally, the urine contains very little protein with perhaps a trace of albumin and small amounts of alpha-1 and alpha-2 globulin. Normal people can have proteinuria with pregnancy, dehydration, and vigorous exercise. Functional proteinuria occurs in congestive heart failure, fever, and exposure to cold. Specific globulins may be increased or decreased depending on the disorder or medications. For example, trauma and burns increase alpha-2 globulin, whereas connective tissue diseases increase gamma globulin. Albumin is rarely increased except in dehydration, exercise, and the effects of some medications. However, it can be decreased in many situations when there is liver disease, malnutrition, and collagen disease.

Consent Form: Not required

List of Equipment: Red-top tube or serum separator tube; needle and syringe or vacutainer; alcohol swab

Test Procedure:
1. Label the specimen tube. *Correctly identifies the client and the test to be performed.*
2. Obtain a 5-mL blood sample.
3. Do not agitate the tube. *Agitation may cause RBC hemolysis.*
4. Send tube to the laboratory.

Clinical Implications and Indications:
1. Routine screening as part of a complete physical examination.
2. Monitors response to therapy, which alters serum protein levels.
3. Diagnoses diseases associated with altered serum protein. However, more definitive diagnosis can be done from the serum protein electrophoresis test.
4. Elevated levels are found with autoimmune collagen diseases, dehydration, macroglobulemia, multiple myeloma, and sarcoidosis,
5. Decreased levels are found with cirrhosis, ulcerative colitis, hypoalbuminemia (which is caused by acute infections, tuberculosis, trauma, burns, liver disease, congestive heart failure, diabetes, rheumatic fever, rheumatoid arthritis, and various medications: acetaminophen, azathioprin, cytoxan, estradiol), water intoxication, edema, severe burns, hemorrhage, Hodgkin's disease, hepatitis, congestive heart failure, and renal disease.

Nursing Care:
Before Test: Explain the test procedure and the purpose of the test. Assess the client's knowledge of the test. Instruct client to fast for 8 hr before the blood draw. It is also recommended the client follow a low-fat diet for several days prior to the test.
During Test: Adhere to standard precautions.
After Test: Apply pressure to venipuncture site. Explain that some bruising, discomfort, and swelling may appear at the site and that warm, moist compresses can alleviate this. Monitor for signs of infection.

Potential Complications: Bleeding and bruising at venipuncture site

Interfering Factors: High serum lipid levels; prolonged application of tourniquet; hemodialysis; medications that increase levels are ACTH, corticosteroids, growth hormone, heparin, insulin, thyroid preparations, tolbutamide, and x-ray contrast media; medications that decrease levels are ammonium ion, oral contraceptives, salicylates, dextran, and pyrazinamide.

Nursing Considerations:
Pediatric: Infants and children will need assistance in remaining still during the venipuncture and age-appropriate comfort measures following the test.

Listing of Related Tests: Serum protein electrophoresis; urine protein electrophoresis

WEBLINKS

http://webmd.lycos.com

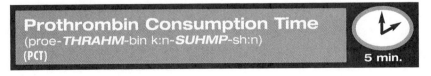

Prothrombin Consumption Time
(proe-*THRAHM*-bin k:n-*SUHMP*-sh:n)
(PCT)

5 min.

Type of Test: Blood

Body Systems and Functions: Hematological system

BLOOD

Normal Findings: 15–20 sec with more than 80% of the prothrombin consumed

CRITICAL VALUES:
Platelet count <10,000 may cause severe bleeding tendencies.

Test Results Time Frame: Within 24 hr

Test Description: Prothrombin consumption time measures the utilization of prothrombin, an alpha-2 globulin made by the liver, during clot formation. Normally the clot uses prothrombin by converting it to thrombin, which in turn causes polymerization of fibrinogen into fibrin fibers. However, clients with a deficiency in platelets, platelet factor III, or the factors used in the intrinsic coagulation pathway do not convert as much prothrombin as normal. Therefore, a higher level of prothrombin remains after the clot is formed and the prothrombin consumption time is shortened.

CLINICAL ALERT:
Severe abnormal values may indicate a potential hemorrhaging crisis.

Consent Form: Not required

List of Equipment: Red-top tube or serum separator tube; needle and syringe or vacutainer; alcohol swab

Test Procedure:
1. Label the specimen tube. *Correctly identifies the client and the test to be performed.*
2. Obtain a 7-mL blood sample.
3. Do not agitate the tube. *Agitation may cause RBC hemolysis.*
4. Send tube to the laboratory.

Clinical Implications and Indications:
1. Diagnoses deficiency of platelet factor III or factors VIII, IX, XI, and XII, which are involved in the intrinsic coagulation pathway.
2. Aids in diagnosing suspected disseminated intravascular coagulation (DIC).
3. Monitors effects of liver disease or protein deficiency on coagulation.
4. Decreased levels are found with anticoagulation therapy, cirrhosis, DIC, and hypothrombonemia.

Nursing Care:
Before Test: Explain the test procedure and the purpose of the test. Assess the client's knowledge of the test.
During Test: Adhere to standard precautions.
After Test: Apply prolonged pressure (3–5 min) to the site due to the client's high risk of bleeding if there are coagulation problems. Monitor frequently for bleeding or formation of a hematoma; if these occur, apply prolonged pressure for 10 min. Explain that some bruising, discomfort, and swelling may appear at the site and that warm, moist compresses can alleviate this. Monitor for signs of infection.

Potential Complications: Observe for excessive bleeding or hematoma at venipuncture site.

Contraindications: Generally venipuncture is not done on clients with a platelet count <10,000, a factor deficiency, or severe liver disease.

Interfering Factors: Oral anticoagulant therapy; traumatic venipuncture; excessive agitation of specimen

Nursing Considerations:
Pediatric: Infants and children will need assistance in remaining still during the venipuncture and age-appropriate comfort measures following the test.

Listing of Related Tests: Bleeding time; factor assays; partial thromboplastin time (PTT); platelet count; prothrombin consumption time (PCT); coagulation screen, which also includes clotting time; activated partial thromboplastin time (APTT)

WEBLINKS

http://webmd.lycos.com

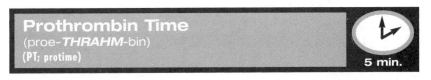

Prothrombin Time
(proe-*THRAHM*-bin)
(PT; protime)

5 min.

Type of Test: Blood

Body Systems and Functions: Hematological system

Normal Findings: Normal laboratory findings may vary among laboratory settings.

Adults	10–13.4 sec
Newborns	<17 sec
Children	11–14 sec
Anticoagulated (therapeutic level for adults):	17–24 sec or ratio of 1.5–2 times the normal value

CRITICAL VALUES:
A client with PT >30 [international normalized ratio (INR) >4.5] is at high risk for hemorrhage. A PT >40 is critical. Client must be closely monitored for signs and symptoms of bleeding in stool, hematuria, bleeding from catheter sites, and intracerebral bleeding. Intravenous vitamin K is given to correct the high protime level.

Test Results Time Frame: Within 8 hr

Test Description: Prothombin time is a coagulation test that measures the time it takes to form a firm fibrin clot after thromboplastin (factor III) and calcium are added to the serum sample. Prothrombin time evaluates the extrinsic pathway of coagulation, specifically the activation of factor X by prothrombin, factor III, and calcium. Prothrombin is a vitamin K–dependent protein produced by the liver. The findings are expressed in terms of seconds or as a percentage of normal activity. The prothrombin time is also expressed in terms of the INR using standardized thromboplastin reagents. Using both the PT and INR, the clinician can make decisions regarding the appropriate dosage of warfarin for oral anticoagulant therapy. However, the INR is not accurate in clients with liver disease.

Consent Form: Not required

List of Equipment: Light-blue-top tube or plasma separator tube; needle and syringe or vacutainer; alcohol swab

Test Procedure:
1. Label the specimen tube. *Correctly identifies the client and the test to be performed.*
2. Obtain a 4-mL blood sample. Some sources state a double-draw procedure helps prevent contamination of the sample due to the initiation of the coagulation pathway from the puncture of the vein by the needle. A double-draw procedure is only possible if vacutainer equipment is used; 2 mL of serum is drawn into a tube, which is discarded. Without withdrawing the needle a second tube is inserted for the 4-mL serum sample.
3. Gently invert tube several times, but do not agitate the tube. *Mixes the anticoagulant, but agitation may cause RBC hemolysis.*
4. Send tube to the laboratory.

Clinical Implications and Indications:
1. Prothrombin time is part of the anticoagulation screen done when client shows signs and symptoms of bleeding (e.g., at risk of bleeding during invasive procedure or surgery, oral anticoagulation therapy, and to determine dosage adequate for therapeutic level).
2. Differentiates between clients with factor V, VII, and X deficiencies, which alter the PT, and those with hemophilia A and B, which do not alter PT.
3. Elevated levels are found with liver disease, severe bone marrow depression, collagen disease, cancer, disseminated intravascular coagulation (DIC), chronic pancreatitis, and toxic shock syndrome.
4. Decreased levels are found with pulmonary embolus, thrombophlebitis, myocardial infarction, and multiple myeloma.

Nursing Care:
Before Test: Explain the test procedure and the purpose of the test. Assess the client's knowledge of the test.
During Test: Adhere to standard precautions.
After Test: When there is a possibility of a coagulation defect, apply prolonged pressure at the venipuncture site for 3–5 min if necessary. Monitor frequently in the next hour for bleeding or hematoma formation. Explain that some bruising, discomfort, and swelling may appear at the site and that warm, moist compresses can alleviate this. Monitor for signs of infection.

Potential Complications: Excessive bleeding or hematoma formation at venipuncture site

Contraindications: Generally venipuncture is not done when client has a platelet count <10,000, a factor deficiency or severe liver disease.

Interfering Factors: Concurrent therapy with heparin can lengthen the PT; medications that decrease levels are coumadin, salicylates, steroids, quinine, guanidine, alcohol, sulfonamides, phenytoin, many antibiotics, methyldopa, and indomethacin; traumatic venipuncture may activate the coagulation process;

medications that increase levels are oral contraceptives, theophylline, caffeine, barbiturates, antihistamines, vitamin K, haloperidol, meprobamate, ranitidine, rifampin, griseofulvin, and carbamazepine.

Nursing Considerations:

Pregnancy: *Therapy with the anticoagulant warfarin is teratogenetic. The medication is also in breast milk and women should not breast feed while on warfarin.*
Pediatric: *Congenital coagulation deficiencies such as hemophilia A and B will not alter the PT because this test bypasses the intrinsic pathway of coagulation. Infants and children will need assistance in remaining still during the venipuncture and age-appropriate comfort measures following the test.*

Listing of Related Tests: Bleeding time; factor assays; partial thromboplastin time (PTT); platelet count; prothrombin consumption time; coagulation screen, which also includes clotting time and activated partial thromboplastin time (APTT)

WEBLINKS ▯ ▣

http://www.webmd.lycos.com

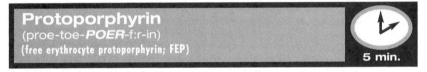

Protoporphyrin
(proe-toe-***POER***-f:r-in)
(free erythrocyte protoporphyrin; FEP)

5 min.

Type of Test: Blood

Body Systems and Functions: Hematological system

Normal Findings: 4–52 mg/dL

Test Results Time Frame: Within 24 hr

Test Description: Protoporphyrin measures the concentration of protoporphyrin in red blood cells. Protoporphyrin combines with iron to form the heme portion of hemoglobin. After hemoglobin is broken down, protoporphyrin is converted to bilirubin and circulates in the blood in the unconjugated form. In disorders affecting heme synthesis, increased amounts of protoporphyrin can be detected in the red blood cells, urine, and feces. In protoporphyria, an autosomal dominant disorder, increased amounts of protoporphyrin are secreted and excreted.

Consent Form: Not required

List of Equipment: Green-top heparinized tube, lavender-top tube with EDTA, or black-top tube containing sodium oxalate or plasma separator tube; needle and syringe or vacutainer; alcohol swab

Test Procedure:
1. Label the specimen tube. *Correctly identifies the client and the test to be performed.*
2. Obtain a 5-mL blood sample and write current hematocrit on requisition. *Test results are related to total number of red blood cells.*

BLOOD

3. Do not agitate the tube. *Agitation may cause RBC hemolysis.*
4. Protect tube from light. *Protoporphyrin is unstable in the presence of light.*
5. Send tube to the laboratory.
6. Keep specimen cool. *High temperatures alter the results.*

Clinical Implications and Indications:

1. Elevated levels are found with accelerated erythropoiesis, erythropoietic protoporphyria (>2200 mg/dL), hemolytic anemia, infection, iron deficiency, thalassemia, lead poisoning, carbon tetrachloride, and benzene toxicity.
2. Decreased levels are found with megaloblastic anemia.

Nursing Care:

Before Test: Explain the test procedure and the purpose of the test. Assess the client's knowledge of the test.
During Test: Adhere to standard precautions.
After Test: Apply pressure to venipuncture site. Explain that some bruising , discomfort, and swelling may appear at the site and that warm, moist compresses can alleviate this. Monitor for signs of infection.

Potential Complications: Bleeding and bruising at venipuncture site

Interfering Factors: Hemolysis invalidates results.

Nursing Considerations:

Pediatric: Infants and children will need assistance in remaining still during the venipuncture and age-appropriate comfort measures following the test.

Listing of Related Tests: Urine coproporphyrin (UCP); porphyrin and porphobilinogen screens

WEBLINKS ▤ ☒

www.enterprise.net

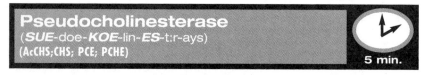

Pseudocholinesterase
(*SUE*-doe-*KOE*-lin-*ES*-t:r-ays)
(AcCHS;CHS; PCE; PCHE)

5 min.

Type of Test: Blood

Body Systems and Functions: Neurological system

Normal Findings:

RID method	0.5–1.3 pH units
Other methods:	
Male	274–532
Female	204–500
Dibucaine inhibition	81–87
Fluoride inhibition	44–54%

CRITICAL VALUES:
Low values may be due to a genetic deficiency of pseudocholinesterase (PCE) causing profound respiratory depression if succinylcholine is used to induce anesthesia, because the person is not able to inactivate the medication.

Test Results Time Frame: Within 24 hr

Test Description: Pseudocholinesterase is produced by the liver and hydrolyzes noncholine esters and inactivates acetylcholine. It is found throughout the body. It can be irreversibly inhibited by exposure to organic phosphate insecticides and reversibly inhibited by carbamate insecticides. Approximately 10% of the population carry the gene for the deficiency of PCE. Inherited deficiencies can be detected by dibucaine and fluoride inhibition tests; normal forms of PCE will not be inhibited. People with the genetic PCE deficiency cannot inactive acetylcholine and related compounds, such as the medication succinylcholine.

Consent Form: Not required

List of Equipment: Red-top tube or serum separator tube; needle and syringe or vacutainer; alcohol swab

Test Procedure:
1. Label the specimen tube. *Correctly identifies the client and the test to be performed.*
2. Obtain a 5-mL blood sample.
3. Do not agitate the tube. *Agitation may cause RBC hemolysis.*
4. Send tube to the laboratory.

Clinical Implications and Indications:
1. Diagnoses exposure to carbamate and organic phosphate insecticides.
2. The test is done prior to using succinylcholine during surgery to detect genetic deficiency of PCE.
3. Elevated levels are found with diabetes mellitus, hyperthyroidism, exposure to organic phosphate insecticides, and nephrotic syndrome
4. Decreased levels are found with cirrhosis, metastatic liver cancer, obstructive jaundice, acute infections, shock, skin diseases, uremia, and plasmaphoresis.

Nursing Care:
Before Test: Explain the test procedure and the purpose of the test. Assess the client's knowledge of the test.
During Test: Adhere to standard precautions.
After Test: Apply pressure to venipuncture site. Explain that some bruising, discomfort, and swelling may appear at the site and that warm, moist compresses can alleviate this. Monitor for signs of infection.

Potential Complications: Bleeding and bruising at venipuncture site

Interfering Factors: Medications that alter results are aminophylline, theophylline, estrogen, epinephrine, neostigmine, barbiturates, morphine, codeine, quinidine, quinine, phenothiazines, physostigmine, pyridostigmine, phospholine, folic acid, and vitamin K; anticholinergic medications alter results when testing for genetic deficiency.

Nursing Considerations:

Pregnancy: *Pregnancy decreases results by approximately 30%.*
Pediatric: *Infants and children will need assistance in remaining still during the venipuncture and age-appropriate comfort measures following the test.*

WEBLINKS 🔲🗙

http://edoc.co.za

Pyridoxal 5-Phosphate
(*PEER*-uh-*DAHK*-s:l *FAHS*-fayt)
(PLP; pyridoxine; pyridoxal; pyridoxamine)

5 min.

Type of Test: Blood

Body Systems and Functions: Metabolic system

Normal Findings: 25–80 ng/mL (Note: Normal laboratory findings vary among laboratory settings and are method dependent.)

Test Results Time Frame: Within 24 hr

Test Description: Pyridoxine, also known as vitamin B_6, is the collective name for three related compounds: pyridoxine, pyridoxal, and pyridoxamine. After absorption pyridoxine is converted into pyridoxal phosphate and pyridoxamine phosphate, the two active forms of vitamin B_6. The test measures the amount of pyridoxal phosphate in the plasma. Vitamin B_6 is readily absorbed by the intestinal tract and excreted in the urine. It is found in many foods, including meat, poultry, fish, egg yolks, wheat germ, potatoes, and vegetables. Vitamin B_6 can be partially destroyed by heat. B vitamins are important in heme synthesis and also function as coenzymes in amino acid metabolism and glycogenolysis. Pyridoxine cofactors are extremely important in their roles of converting trytophan to serotonin and play an essential role in brain function. Vitamin B_6 deficiency rarely occurs alone and is usually seen in clients with deficiencies of several B vitamins. Vitamin B_6 hypervitaminosis is rarely seen because vitamin B_6 is water soluble and readily excreted.

Consent Form: Not required

List of Equipment: Lavender-top tube or serum separator tube; needle and syringe or vacutainer; alcohol swab; foil or paper bag to cover tube

Test Procedure:

1. Label the specimen tube. *Correctly identifies the client and the test to be performed.*
2. Obtain a 7-mL blood sample.
3. Do not agitate the tube. *Agitation may cause RBC hemolysis.*
4. Immediately cover the serum tube with foil or put into a paper bag to protect the specimen from exposure to light. Write the collection time on the requisition. Specimen must be sent immediately to the laboratory where the plasma must be separated and frozen within 30 min of the blood draw. *Vitamin B is extremely unstable.*

Clinical Implications and Indications:

1. Diagnoses vitamin B_6 deficiency in alcoholism, diabetes, uremia, inadequate dietary intake, poor gastrointestinal absorption, and inflammatory bowel disease states
2. Diagnoses vitamin B_6 overdose from megavitamin supplement

Nursing Care:

Before Test: Explain the test procedure and the purpose of the test. Assess the client's knowledge of the test.
During Test: Adhere to standard precautions.
After Test: Apply pressure to venipuncture site. Explain that some bruising, discomfort, and swelling may appear at the site and that warm, moist compresses can alleviate this. Monitor for signs of infection.

Potential Complications: Bleeding and bruising at venipuncture site

Interfering Factors: Specimen is exposed to light; delay >30 min in separating and freezing plasma; medications that cause a decrease in levels are disulfiram, hydralazine, isoniazid, levodopa, oral contraceptives, penicillamine, pyrazinoic acid, some calcium channel blockers, and steroids.

Nursing Considerations:

Pediatric: Infants and children will need assistance in remaining still during the venipuncture and age-appropriate comfort measures following the test.

Listing of Related Tests: Plasma 58-phosphate; plasma pyridoxal; urinary 4-pyridoxic acid

| WEBLINKS |

http://www.methodisthealth.com

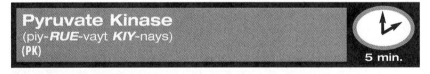

Pyruvate Kinase
(piy-*RUE*-vayt *KIY*-nays)
(PK)

5 min.

Type of Test: Blood

Body Systems and Functions: Hematological system

Normal Findings: 2.0–8.8 U/g Hgb, 0.3–0.91 mg/dL

Test Results Time Frame: Within 24 hr

Test Description: Pyruvate kinase measures the amount of pyruvic kinase (PK) present in red blood cells. Pyruvate kinase is an enzyme that functions in the formation of pyruvate and adenosine diphosphate (ADP) in glycolysis. In the presence of oxygen the process is aerobic and enters the citric acid cycle. If oxygen is absent, pyruvate is converted to lactic acid and released into the extracellular fluid. The aerobic cycle produces a much higher amount of energy. RBCs that lack PK have a low affinity for oxygen. Episodes of hemolysis in individuals lacking the enzyme are severe, chronic, and exacerbated by infections.

The inherited form is autosomal recessive. The acquired form is from either drug ingestion or metabolic liver disease.

Consent Form: Not required

List of Equipment: Lavender-top tube or serum separator tube; needle and syringe or vacutainer; alcohol swab

Test Procedure:
1. Label the specimen tube. *Correctly identifies the client and the test to be performed.*
2. Obtain a 5-mL blood sample.
3. Do not agitate the tube. *Agitation may cause RBC hemolysis.*
4. Send tube to the laboratory.

Clinical Implications and Indications:
1. Detects hemolytic anemia of unknown cause, especially in infants or young children
2. Identifies suspected G6PD or PK deficiency in individuals with positive family history or jaundice in response to oxidant drugs or foods

Nursing Care:
Before Test: Explain the test procedure and the purpose of the test. Assess the client's knowledge of the test.
During Test: Adhere to standard precautions.
After Test: Apply pressure to venipuncture site. Explain that some bruising, discomfort, and swelling may appear at the site and that warm, moist compresses can alleviate this. Monitor for signs of infection.

Potential Complications: Bleeding and bruising at venipuncture site

Interfering Factors: Hemolytic episode may cause false normal results; a transfusion gives false results.

Nursing Considerations:
Pediatric: Capillary sample may be used in infants and children. Infants and children will need assistance in remaining still during the venipuncture and age-appropriate comfort measures following the test.

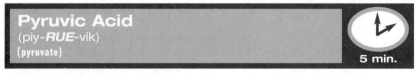

WEBLINKS

http://webmd.lycos.com

Pyruvic Acid
(piy-*RUE*-vik)
(pyruvate)

5 min.

Type of Test: Blood

Body Systems and Functions: Hematological system

Normal Findings: 0.08–0.16 mEq/L

Test Results Time Frame: Within 24 hr

Test Description: Pyruvate is a by-product of glycolysis (carbohydrate metabolism) in cells. Depending on whether the process is aerobic or anerobic, pyruvate or lactic acid, respectively, is produced. If oxygen becomes restored, the conversion of pyruvic acid to lactic acid is reversible and lactic acid is converted back to pyruvic acid or glucose. Pyruvate determination provides information for the calculation of excess lactate and general tissue oxygenation. However, pyruvic acid is unstable and difficult to measure (note: see Test Procedure).

Consent Form: Not required

List of Equipment: Grey-top tube or serum separator tube; needle and syringe or vacutainer; alcohol swab; ice; specialized equipment must be immediately available (note: see Test Procedure).

Test Procedure:
1. Label the specimen tube. *Correctly identifies the client and the test to be performed.*
2. Obtain a 5-mL blood sample.
3. Do not agitate the tube. *Agitation may cause RBC hemolysis.*
4. Ice the specimen, and send to laboratory immediately, if laboratory technician does not do procedure at bedside. *Pyruvic acid is very unstable and requires pipette procedure within 20 min.*
5. A pipetting procedure mixing 4 mL blood with percholoric acid should be done by a laboratory technician within 1 min of the draw, if performed at the bedside. The best results are obtained if the procedure is done within the first minute of obtaining the specimen. *Pyruvic acid is very unstable.*

Clinical Implications and Indications:
1. Determines cause of lactic acidosis.
2. Aids in assessment of tissue oxygenation, especially in cardiac arrest, hemorrhage, liver disease, myocardial infarction, and shock.
3. Results should be compared to blood lactate level. The normal ratio is <10:1.

Nursing Care:
Before Test: Explain the test procedure and the purpose of the test. Assess the client's knowledge of the test. Instruct client to fast overnight and to rest for 1 hr before the test. Coordinate the timing of the blood draw with the laboratory technician.
During Test: Adhere to standard precautions.
After Test: Apply pressure to venipuncture site. Explain that some bruising, discomfort, and swelling may appear at the site and that warm, moist compresses can alleviate this. Monitor for signs of infection.

Potential Complications: Bleeding and bruising at venipuncture site

Interfering Factors: Using a tourniquet or the client pumping their fist can increase levels; exercise within 1 hr; failing to ice the specimen

Nursing Considerations:
Pediatric: Infants and children will need assistance in remaining still during the venipuncture and age-appropriate comfort measures following the test.

Listing of Related Tests: Serum lactate

WEBLINKS ⬚⬚

http://webmd.lycos.com

Rabies Antibody
(*RAY*-bees *AEN*-ti-*BAH*-dee)
(fluorescent rabies antibody; FRA)

5 min.

Type of Test: Blood

Body Systems and Functions: Immunological system

Normal Findings: Negative or IFA <1:16. May require interpretation by a pathologist; animal brain is also examined for presence of rabies rhabdovirus.

Test Results Time Frame: Within 24 hr

Test Description: Rabies antibody tests examine the serum of a human exposed to the rabies rhabdovirus to identify by immunofluorescence a rise in antibody titer. The rabies rhabdovirus is introduced into the human body, usually by a bite or scratch from an infected mammal, although humans have contracted rabies from bats without skin penetration when exposed to a bat in a closed room or in a cave. The body begins the antigen-antibody response, although it is usually a week before the antibody titer is detectable. The typical incubation period is 30–50 days before symptoms begin appearing. During incubation the virus attacks the nervous system from the peripheral to the central nervous system and the brain. Once it has invaded the nervous system, the virus is relatively protected from the body's immune system. Symptoms are primarily neurological and severe with a 99% chance of death once they begin. Therefore, passive and active antibody treatment postexposure should begin immediately before any laboratory results are known. One dose of human rabies immunoglobulin HRIG is given immediately, then a series of five injections of killed rabies virus vaccine is given over a 4-week period to help stimulate the body's immune system. If this treatment is given very soon after exposure, the prognosis is excellent. Preexposure vaccination is available for those who are frequently exposed to unvaccinated mammals.

> **CLINICAL ALERT:**
> Notify clinician immediately of positive results because prophylactic treatment must be continued to prevent death (note: rabies is a reportable disease to the county health department in most areas).

Consent Form: Not required

List of Equipment: Red-top tube or serum separator tube; needle and syringe or vacutainer; alcohol swab

Test Procedure:
1. Label the specimen tube. *Correctly identifies the client and the test to be performed.*

2. Obtain a 7-mL blood sample.
3. Do not agitate the tube. *Agitation may cause RBC hemolysis.*
4. Send tube to the laboratory.

Clinical Implications and Indications:

1. Diagnoses rabies in client who has not been previously vaccinated or received passive antibody
2. Diagnoses antibody response in vaccinated person to see if titer is sufficient

Nursing Care:

Before Test: Explain the test procedure and the purpose of the test. Assess the client's knowledge of the test. Explain importance of the potentially life-saving prophylactic treatment, which must be started immediately without waiting for the test results.

During Test: Adhere to standard precautions.

After Test: Apply pressure to venipuncture site. Explain that some bruising, discomfort and swelling may appear at the site and that warm moist compresses can alleviate this. Monitor for signs of infection.

Potential Complications: Bleeding and bruising at venipuncture site

Nursing Considerations:

Pregnancy: *All rabies vaccines may be given during pregnancy.*

Pediatric: *Infants and children will need assistance in remaining still during the venipuncture and age-appropriate comfort measures following the test.*

Rural: *There may be a higher incidence in rural settings, and therefore all animal bites should be suspected as carriers of the disease.*

International: *Rabies is endemic in many areas of Africa, Asia, and Central and South America. Generally vaccination of domestic animals is not available nor is the human vaccine or immunoglobulin available for treatment of humans. Therefore it is recommended that preexposure vaccination be done for those traveling to these countries, especially if they will be in rural areas.*

❙WEBLINKS ❧   ▤▧

www.niaid.nih.gov

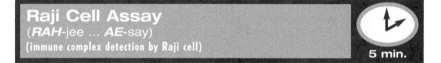

Raji Cell Assay
(*RAH*-jee ... *AE*-say)
(immune complex detection by Raji cell)

5 min.

Type of Test: Blood

Body Systems and Functions: Immunological system

Normal Findings:

Normal	<13 µg AHGeq*/mL
Borderline	13–25 µg AHGeq/mL
Abnormal	>26 µg AHGeq/mL

*AHGeq: aggregated human gamma globulin equivalents

Test Results Time Frame: Within 24 hr

Test Description: Raji cell assay detects circulating immune complexes using Raji lymphoblastoid cells that have receptors for immunoglobulin G complement and C3b. The presence of immune complexes are detected in transient antibody-antigen responses in bacterial or viral infections; prolonged elevations occur in autoimmune diseases or chronic inflammation. Results are reported in number of precipitated immune complexes. The primary usefulness of the test is in research at the present time because other tests are more standardized between laboratories and less expensive.

CLINICAL ALERT:
Immediately put specimen in ice water as warmth alters results.

Consent Form: Not required

List of Equipment: Red-top or green-top tube or serum separator tube; needle and syringe or vacutainer; alcohol swab; container with ice water

Test Procedure:
1. Label the specimen tube. *Correctly identifies the client and the test to be performed.*
2. Obtain a 5-mL blood sample.
3. Do not agitate the tube. *Agitation may cause RBC hemolysis.*
4. Send tube to the laboratory.
5. Keep specimen cool. *High temperatures alter the results.*

Clinical Implications and Indications:
1. Aids in diagnosis of autoimmune diseases, celiac disease, Crohn's disease, and chronic infections.
2. Transient elevated levels are found with drug reactions and parasitic, viral, and bacterial infections.
3. Prolonged elevated levels are found with autoimmune disorders, cirrhosis, celiac disease, Crohn's disease, cryoglobulinemia, dermatitis, herpetiforms, and sickle cell disease.

Nursing Care:
Before Test: Explain the test procedures and the purpose of the test. Assess the client's knowledge of the test.
During Test: Adhere to standard precautions.
After Test: Apply pressure to venipuncture site. Explain that some bruising, discomfort, and swelling may appear at the site and that warm, moist compresses can alleviate this. Monitor for signs of infection.

Potential Complications: Bleeding and bruising at venipuncture site

Interfering Factors: Recent scan with radioactive dye; hemolysis; failure to ice specimen

Nursing Considerations:
Pediatric: Infants and children will need assistance in remaining still during the venipuncture and age-appropriate comfort measures following the test.

Listing of Related Tests: Serum immune complex assay; serum complement components; urinary immune complex; liver function tests; viral studies

| WEBLINKS |

www.nlm.nih.gov

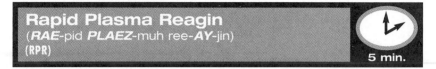

Rapid Plasma Reagin
(**RAE**-pid **PLAEZ**-muh ree-**AY**-jin)
(RPR)

5 min.

Type of Test: Blood

Body Systems and Functions: Reproductive system

Normal Findings: Negative (Note: Borderline, reactive, and weakly reactive are considered positive for syphilis antibody.)

> **CRITICAL VALUES:**
> If test is positive, state law may require filing a report with the public health department.

Test Results Time Frame: Within 24 hr

Test Description: A rapid plasma reagin is the test that measures the amount of reagin in the plasma. Reagin is the antibody relatively specific to the *Treponema pallidum* spirochete, which causes syphilis. A cardiolipin antigen to reagin is used to detect an agglutination reaction, which is positive. However, there will not be a detectable immune response for 14–21 days after exposure. This test is most useful during the secondary stage of syphilis when the presence of reagin peaks, with typical results > 1:32. It is less sensitive to primary syphilis, although there is a low level of < 1:16 in about 80% of those who come for medical intervention in the primary stage. In the late latent phase of syphilis in about one-third of clients, the RPR becomes inactive and there are no symptoms of the disease. In another third, the RPR remains reactive usually at a low level, but there are no symptoms of disease. In the remaining third, RPR is active and the symptoms of late syphilis occur. Rapid plasma reagin is an inexpensive test and used as a substitute for the VDRL for mass screening. However a definitive diagnosis of syphilis must be based on other tests, especially dark-field microscopic examinations, the FTA-ABS double stain, and MHA-TP tests. Following antibiotic treatment in the primary or secondary stage, the RPR will become negative.

Consent Form: Not required

List of Equipment: Red-top tube or serum separator tube; needle and syringe or vacutainer; alcohol swab

Test Procedure:
1. Label the serum tube. *Correctly identifies the client and the test to be performed.*
2. Obtain a 7-mL serum sample.

3. Do not agitate the serum tube. *Agitation may cause RBC hemolysis*
4. Send tube to the laboratory.

Clinical Implications and Indications:

1. Diagnoses syphilis in secondary stage in the presence of characteristic symptoms. The test has lower sensitivity for primary stage syphilis but is positive at a low level in 80% of clients with symptoms. All positives should be followed up with other diagnostic syphilis tests for confirmation.
2. Mass screening for syphilis.
3. Baseline for response to therapy.
4. The RPR will also be positive in other more rare treponeme diseases, such as yaws, bejel, and pinta.

Nursing Care:

Before Test: Explain the test procedure and the purpose of the test. Assess the client's knowledge of the test. Blood draw must be scheduled before meals because chyle alters the reaction. Instruct client to not drink alcohol for 24 hr before test.

During Test: Adhere to standard precautions.

After Test: Apply pressure to venipuncture site. Explain that some bruising, discomfort, and swelling may appear at the site and that warm, moist compresses can alleviate this. Monitor for signs of infection. Explain possibility of false positives and the importance of follow-up testing and treatment if positive. Until diagnosis is clearly negative, instruct client to abstain from sexual contact. If tests are positive, the client must be treated with antibiotic and abstain from sexual contact for 2 months until repeated testing confirms there is no active syphilis. Inform the client to use condoms for 2 more years and undergo testing every 3–4 months for 2 years.

Potential Complications: Bleeding and bruising at venipuncture site

Interfering Factors: Alcohol causes seronegative results (false negative); hemolysis of specimen; wrong time of blood draw when chyle alters results; many conditions may cause false RPR positives such as hepatitis, HIV, lyme disease, acute and chronic infections, and rheumatoid arthritis.

Nursing Considerations:

Pregnancy: Client should not become pregnant for 2 years because the spirochete can cross the placental barrier and infect the fetus.

Pediatric: Infants and children will need assistance in remaining still during the venipuncture and age-appropriate comfort measures following the test (note: heelstick may be used to collect sample).

Listing of Related Tests: Dark-field microscopy; fluorescent treponemal antibody absorbed double stain (FTA-ABS DS); microhemagglutination *Treponema pallidum* test (MHA-TP); VDRL

| WEBLINKS |

www.cdc.gov

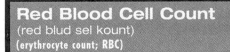
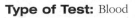

Red Blood Cell Count
(red blud sel kount)
(erythrocyte count; RBC)

5 min.

Type of Test: Blood

Body Systems and Functions: Hematological system

Normal Findings:

Newborn	4.8–7.1 million/mm³
1 month	4.1–6.1 million/mm³
6 months	3.8–5.5 million/mm³
1–10 years	4.5–4.8 million/mm³
Adults:	
Men	4.6–6.2 million/mm³
Women	4.2–5.5 million/mm³
Pregnancy	3.0–5.0 million/mm³

Test Results Time Frame: Within 24 hr

Test Description: The RBC is a component of the complete blood count (CBC) screening. The RBC is the calculation of RBCs per cubic millimeter. The RBC, known as an erythrocyte, is the major carrier of hemoglobin and thus carrier of oxygen to cells and carbon dioxide to the lungs for excretion. The average RBC has a life of 120 days and must be constantly replaced by new erythrocytes made by red bone marrow. Alterations to the normal count can be caused by blood loss, destruction of RBCs (hemolytic anemias), failure of the bone marrow to make new RBCs, and suppression of erythropoiesis by other diseases such as renal disease.

Consent Form: Not required

List of Equipment: Lavender-top tube or serum separator tube; needle and syringe or vacutainer; alcohol swab

Test Procedure:
1. Label the serum tube. *Correctly identifies the client and the test to be performed.*
2. Obtain a 7-mL serum sample.
3. Gently invert tube several times, but do not agitate the tube. *Mixes the anticoagulant, but agitation may cause RBC hemolysis.*
4. Send tube to the laboratory.

Clinical Implications and Indications:
1. Routine screening as part of the CBC.
2. Diagnoses hematological disorder involving destruction of RBCs such as hemolytic anemia.
3. Monitors effects of acute or chronic blood loss.
4. Monitors clients with elevated RBCs related to chronic hypoxia, chronic obstructive pulmonary disease (COPD), and polycythemia vera.
5. Monitors effects of disorders known for decreased erythropoiesis, such as liver disease, renal disease, and bone marrow failure.

6. Monitors response to erythropoietic therapy.
7. Elevated levels are found with burns, chronic hypoxia, COPD, dehydration, high altitude, polycythemia vera, pulmonary fibrosis, sickle cell disease, and thalassemia.
8. Decreased levels are found with bone marrow suppression, chemotherapy, chronic inflammation or infection, hemolytic anemia, hemorrhage, Hodgkin's disease, leukemia, multiple myeloma, hemodilution, systemic lupus erythematosus, and vitamin B_6, B_{12}, or folic acid deficiency.

Nursing Care:

Before Test: Explain the test procedure and the purpose of the test. Assess the client's knowledge of the test. No fasting is needed.
During Test: Adhere to standard precautions.
After Test: Apply pressure to venipuncture site. Explain that some bruising, discomfort, and swelling may appear at the site and that warm, moist compresses can alleviate this. Monitor for signs of infection.

Potential Complications: Bleeding and bruising at venipuncture site

Interfering Factors: Exercise, stress, pain, and anxiety may increase results; hemodilution by IV fluids or pregnancy will decrease results; hemolysis or traumatic venipuncture will invalidate results; medications that increase levels are methyldopa and gentamicin; medications that can cause dyscrasias are amphotericin B, aminosalicylic acid, selected sulfonamides and sulfonylureas, tetracycline and doxycycline, selected diuretics, phenyltoin, and refampin.

Nursing Considerations:

Pregnancy: *Normal pregnancy causes hemodilution of RBC with lower results.*
Pediatric: *Infants and children will need assistance in remaining still during the venipuncture and age-appropriate comfort measures following the test (note: capillary sample may be used).*

Listing of Related Tests: Hematocrit; hemoglobin, red blood cell indices; reticulocyte count and index

WEBLINKS ▸	▤ ☒

http://www.methodisthealth.com

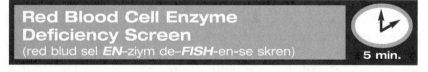

Red Blood Cell Enzyme Deficiency Screen
(red blud sel *EN*-ziym de-*FISH*-en-se skren)

5 min.

Type of Test: Blood

Body Systems and Functions: Hematological system

Normal Findings: Red blood cell enzymes are present.

Test Results Time Frame: Within 24 hr

Test Description: Red blood cell enzyme deficiency screen is a battery of tests to screen for the presence of erythrocyte enzymes that are essential for its functioning, especially in metabolic activities. There are many enzymes but three of the most important are:

1. Glucose-6-phosphate dehydrogenase (G6PD). G6PD is an enzyme in red blood cells that is important in the hexose monophosphate shunt. The majority of those with this deficiency have no symptoms until exposure to certain drugs, which may then cause hemolytic anemia. The deficiency is carried on the X chromosome.
2. Pyruvate kinase (PK). Ninety percent of the hemolytic anemias are associated with the deficiency of this enzyme. Pyruvate kinase is important in the glycolytic pathway to produce ATP energy for the red blood cell's functions. The anemia is moderate to severe, often accompanied with jaundice, splenomegaly, and aplastic crises.
3. 2,3-Diphosphoglycerate (2,3-DPG). This enzyme moderates hemoglobin-oxygen affinity and alters oxygen transport to the tissues. An increase or decrease of the enzyme causes oxyhemoglobin shifts to the right or left on the oxygen-hemoglobin dissociation curve, altering the amount of oxygen that is carried and released in the tissues. Any of the red blood cell enzymes may be congenitally deficient or become deficient due to acquired abnormalities. Some deficiencies do not exhibit any obvious clinical symptoms while others may result in hemolysis of red blood cells or in multisystem disease. G6PD deficiency affects millions worldwide while some other deficiencies affect only a few thousand people.

Consent Form: Not required

List of Equipment: Lavender-top tube or serum separator tube; needle and syringe or vacutainer; alcohol swab

Test Procedure:
1. Label the serum tube. *Correctly identifies the client and the test to be performed.*
2. Obtain a 7-mL serum sample.
3. Gently invert tube several times, but do not agitate the tube. *Mixes the anticoagulant, but agitation may cause RBC hemolysis.*
4. Send tube to the laboratory.

Clinical Implications and Indications:
1. Assists in differential diagnosis of chronic nonspherocytic hemolytic anemia

Nursing Care:
Before Test: Explain the test procedure and the purpose of the test. Assess the client's knowledge of the test.
During Test: Adhere to standard precautions.
After Test: Apply pressure to venipuncture site. Explain that some bruising, discomfort, and swelling may appear at the site and that warm, moist compresses can alleviate this. Monitor for signs of infection.

Potential Complications: Bleeding and bruising at venipuncture site

Interfering Factors: Hemolysis or clotted blood invalidates results; high altitudes increase 2,3-DPG results; banked blood decreases 2,3-DPG results;

false-normal results for G6PD may occur in blacks if sample collected during a hemolytic episode.

Nursing Considerations:
Pediatric: Capillary tube may be used. Infants and children will need assistance in remaining still during the venipuncture and age-appropriate comfort measures following the test.

Listing of Related Tests: Hematocrit; hemoglobin; red blood cell count; red blood cell morphology; red blood cell survival study; reticulocyte count and index

WEBLINKS ▣☒

http://alice.ucdavis.edu

Red Blood Cell Survival Study
(red blud sel sir-*VIY*-vl)
(chromium red cell survival; Cr-51; red blood cell survival timed study)

5 min.

Type of Test: Blood

Body Systems and Functions: Hematological system

Normal Findings:

Normal life span of RBC	120 days with average daily loss of 0.7%–0.8%
Normal half-time of RBCs	60 days
Normal half-time tagged (radioactive) RBCs	25–35 days
Scan of liver, spleen, and pericardium	None to trace radioactivity

Test Results Time Frame: 1 month

Test Description: RBC survival study is a test that tags a percentage of the client's red blood cells with radioactive Cr-51 nucleotide to determine the life span of the cells. The client's blood sample is drawn, centrifuged to remove the plasma, mixed with the nucleotide Cr-51, and reinjected into the client's bloodstream. Blood samples are taken periodically over a 4-week period and measured for radioactivity level to determine the amount of time it takes for the cells to disappear from circulation. The spleen, liver, and pericardium may also be measured for radioactivity because these organs may sequester larger than normal amounts of RBCs preventing them from returning to circulation. The spleen may also be destroying RBCs at an increased rate. A decreased RBC survival rate is seen in many hemolytic anemias, chronic lymphatic leukemia, uremia, and sickle cell disease.

Consent Form: Required

List of Equipment: Nuclear scanning equipment; red-top tube or serum separator tube; needle and syringe or vacutainer; alcohol swab

Test Procedure:

1. Label sample container with client's name. *Correctly identifies the client and the test to be performed.*
2. Intravenous access is obtained. *Allows access for radionuclide.*
3. Trained personnel administer the IV radionuclide. *Helps to minimize risk of exposure to radioactive material.*
4. Draw 30-mL blood sample, centrifuge it, and mix the RBCs with Cr-51.
5. After incubating the radioactive sample overnight, it is injected intravenously into client.
6. After 30 min, 6-mL blood sample is drawn in a tube to measure baseline radioactivity.
7. Twenty-four hours later another sample is drawn in tube.
8. Repeat blood samples will be drawn every 1–3 days for 4 weeks.
9. In addition periodic scans of the spleen, liver, and pericardium are usually done during the 4 weeks.

Clinical Implications and Indications:

1. Aids in diagnosing the cause of anemia and locating the sites of RBC sequestering/destruction in hemolytic anemias (hereditary RBC membrane defects, RBC enzyme disorders, drug-induced hemolytic anemia, sickle cell disease, secondary anemias associated with chronic lymphatic leukemia and lymphoma)
2. Aids in diagnosing disorders causing increased survival time of RBCs, such as COPD, chronic hypoxia, renal disease, and primary or secondary polycythemia

Nursing Care:

Before Test: Explain the test procedure and the purpose of the test. Assess the client's knowledge of the test.
During Test: Adhere to standard precautions.
After Test: Apply pressure to venipuncture site. Explain that some bruising, discomfort, and swelling may appear at the site and that warm, moist compresses can alleviate this. Monitor for signs of infection. No special care or precautions are needed for the radioactivity.

Potential Complications: Bleeding and bruising at venipuncture site; infection

Contraindications: Active bleeding; extended clotting time; pregnancy; breastfeeding

Interfering Factors: Recent transfusion increases results; hemorrhage decreases results; high WBC and platelet counts may invalidate results.

Nursing Considerations:

Pregnancy: Radioactivity is teratogen to fetus.
Pediatric: Infants and children will need assistance in remaining still during the venipuncture and age-appropriate comfort measures following the test.

Listing of Related Tests: Ferritin; red blood cell volume; serum iron; total iron-binding capacity (TIBC); transferrin

WEBLINKS

www.nlm.nih.gov

BLOOD

Red Cell Size, Distribution, Width
(siyz dis-truh-*BYUE*-sh:n)
(RDW)

5 min.

Type of Test: Blood

Body Systems and Functions: Hematological system

Normal Findings: 11%–15%

Test Results Time Frame: Within 24 hr

Test Description: Red cell volume distribution width (RDW) is an estimate of red blood cell size variability. It is derived from anisocytosis, the state of excessive inequality in the size of erythrocyte cells. The RDW becomes abnormal early in iron deficiency anemia. It is also abnormal in pernicious anemia. Although the RDW is an obvious symptom, it is also important to use morphological indices when determining a diagnosis. RDW is usually reported in a complete blood count.

Consent Form: Not required

List of Equipment: Lavender-top tube or serum separator tube; needle and syringe or vacutainer; alcohol swab

Test Procedure:
1. Label the specimen tube. *Correctly identifies the client and the test to be performed.*
2. Obtain a 5-mL blood sample.
3. Gently invert tube several times, but do not agitate the tube. *Mixes the anticoagulant, but agitation may cause RBC hemolysis.*
4. Send tube to the laboratory.

Clinical Implications and Indications:
1. Aids in differential diagnosis of anemias

Nursing Care:
Before Test: Explain the test procedure and the purpose of the test. Assess the client's knowledge of the test.
During Test: Adhere to standard precautions.
After Test: Apply pressure to venipuncture site. Explain that some bruising, discomfort, and swelling may appear at the site and that warm, moist compresses can alleviate this. Monitor for signs of infection.

Potential Complications: Bleeding and bruising at venipuncture site

Nursing Considerations:
Pediatric: Infants and children will need assistance in remaining still during the venipuncture and age-appropriate comfort measures following the test.
Gerontology: The elderly are more prone to anemia and therefore are a population at risk for abnormalities detected by RDW.

Listing of Related Tests: Hematocrit; hemoglobin; red blood cell count; red blood cell morphology; reticulocyte count and index

WEBLINKS

http://www.methodisthealth.com

Renin Assay
(*REN*-in *AE*-say)
(plasma renin activity; PRA; plasma renin angiotensin)

5 min.

BLOOD

Type of Test: Blood

Body Systems and Functions: Renal/urological system

Normal Findings: Values vary according to dietary sodium intake, physical activity, age, and laboratory methods.

Adult (normal sodium diet):

Supine	0.1–3.1 ng/mL/h
Standing:	
<40 years	0.1–4.3 ng/mL/h
>40 years	0.1–3.0 ng/mL/h
Adult (low-sodium diet):	
Supine	2.1–4.3 ng/mL/h
Standing:	
<40 years	2.9–24.0 ng/mL/h
>40 years	2.9–10.8 ng/mL/h
Child (normal sodium diet):	
0–3 years	16.6–15.2 ng/mL/h
3–12 years	5.9–6.7 ng/mL/h
12–18 years	<4.3 ng/mL/h

Test Results Time Frame: Within 24 hr

Test Description: Renin assay measures renin, which is an enzyme released into the renal veins by the juxtaglomerular apparatus of the kidney. Release of renin is stimulated by hypovolemia, low serum sodium, low kidney perfusion, or sympathetic stimulation, which occurs when the body is in physical stress. Renin is a catalyst in the conversion of angiotensinogen to angiotensin I, which is then converted to angiotensin II by angiotensin-converting enzyme (ACE). Angiotensin II is a powerful vasoconstrictor causing increased blood pressure and stimulating the release of aldosterone, a steroid made by the adrenal glands. Aldosterone promotes fluid and sodium retention, thereby also increasing blood pressure, and potassium excretion. Renin, angiotensin I and II, and ACE are known as the renin-angiotensin system (RAS). Under normal and many pathological situations, it is the amount of renin released by the kidney that determines the activity of the whole RAS. Renin is more easily measured since the angiotensins are unstable and difficult to measure due to short half-lives. If renal artery stenosis is suspected, the renin assay must be taken during renal vein catheterization. Blood samples from the inferior vena cava and renal vein are compared. If positive, the level is 1.4 times that of the vena cava sample.

Consent Form: Not required (Note: A consent is required for a renal vein catheterization.)

List of Equipment: Lavender-top tube or serum separator tube; needle and syringe or vacutainer; alcohol swab; ice

Test Procedure:

1. Label the specimen tube. *Correctly identifies the client and the test to be performed.*
2. Obtain a 7- to 12-mL blood sample.
3. Gently invert tube several times, but do not agitate the tube. *Mixes the anticoagulant, but agitation may cause RBC hemolysis.*
4. Send tube to the laboratory.
5. Blood may also be drawn during catheterization of the renal vein. The same procedure applies as for the blood sample described previously. Two samples are collected, one from the inferior vena cava and one from the renal vein. Clearly label each tube with collection site.

Clinical Implications and Indications:

1. Aids in evaluation of treatment of hypertension.
2. Elevated levels are found with Addison's disease, secondary aldosteronism, renovascular hypertension, chronic renal failure, cirrhosis, pheochromocytoma, and renin-producing renal tumors.
3. Decreased levels are found with Cushing's disease, essential hypertension, licorice ingestion, primary aldosteronism, and a high-sodium diet.

Nursing Care:

Before Test: Explain the test procedure and the purpose of the test. Assess the client's knowledge of the test. Instruct client to eat a 3-g/day no-added-salt sodium diet for 3–14 days prior to the test and fast for 4–8 hr before the blood draw depending on laboratory protocol. (Note: Preschedule the test with the laboratory after consulting with clinician regarding the number of days the client should be on the 3-g sodium diet and if any medications should be held.) Explain diet to client giving written materials to help with the meal planning. Caution against eating licorice. Instruct client to come to the laboratory 2 hr prior to the test and assume the sitting, lying, or standing position according to laboratory protocol. If test is to be done with renal catheterization, explain that procedure.

During Test: Adhere to standard precautions.

After Test: Apply pressure to venipuncture site. Explain that some bruising, discomfort, and swelling may appear at the site and that warm, moist compresses can alleviate this. Monitor for signs of infection. After the renal vein catheterization, vital signs, groin site, and pedal pulses need to be closely monitored per procedure protocol. Observe client for several days after test for renal thrombosis, which manifests as costovertebral tenderness, hematuria, and an elevated creatinine.

Potential Complications: Bleeding and bruising at venipuncture site

Interfering Factors: Improper position of the client; pregnancy; licorice ingestion; amount of salt intake prior to the blood draw; failure to completely fill specimen tube; failure to ice specimen or chill the tube prior to the draw if required by laboratory protocol; clients who are ambulatory have higher levels than those on bedrest; medications that decrease levels are clonidine hydrochloride, desmopressin, methyldopa, propranolol, reserpine, steroids, and vasopressin; medications that increase levels are antihypertensives, diazoxide, estrogen, furosemide, guanethidine sulfate, hydralazine hydrochloride, minoxidil, nitroprusside, spironolactone, and thiazide.

BLOOD

Nursing Considerations:

Pregnancy: *Normal pregnancy increases the level of renin.*
Pediatric: *Infants and children will need assistance in remaining still during the venipuncture and age-appropriate comfort measures following the test.*
Gerontology: *Aging decreases the level of renin.*
Rural: *Advisable to arrange for transportation home after recovering from renin assay*

Listing of Related Tests: 24-hr urinary sodium

WEBLINKS

http://www.med.nyu.edu

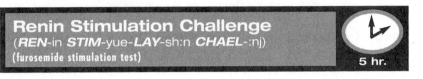

Renin Stimulation Challenge
(*REN*-in *STIM*-yue-*LAY*-sh:n *CHAEL*-:nj)
(furosemide stimulation test)

5 hr.

Type of Test: Blood

Body Systems and Functions: Endocrine system

Normal Findings: Renin increases 1–6 ng/mL/hr

Test Results Time Frame: Within 24 hr

Test Description: Renin stimulation challenge test measures the level of plasma renin activity (PRA) in response to diuresis, which decreases the extra-cellular fluid volume. It is one of several tests that should be done to clarify what is abnormal in the renin-angiotension-aldosterone system. This system is influenced by several important factors: sodium intake and extracellular fluid volume, both of which inversely influence the secretion of aldosterone and renin; physical position of the body with the upright position (sitting, standing or walking) increasing the release of aldosterone and renin; and the circadian rhythm of aldosterone secretion which is highest upon awakening and lowest in the late evening just after falling asleep.In the renin stimulation challenge test sodium intake, body position and the morning lab draws are controlled so that the effect of diuresis (extracellular fluid volume) on renin secretion can be determined. In the normal person when the furosemide dose is given, there is a two- to threefold rise in the PRA. Those with renovascular (renin-dependent) hypertension and pheochromocytoma have approximately five times the increase in PRA. Clients with primary aldosteronism have a PRA below detection by the assay. Clients with hyporeninemic hypoaldosteronism have low levels of both aldosterone and renin.

Consent Form: Not required

List of Equipment: Lavender-top tube or serum separator tube; needle and syringe or vacutainer; alcohol swab; ice

Test Procedure:
1. Label the specimen tube. *Correctly identifies the client and the test to be per-formed.*

BLOOD

2. Obtain a 7- to 12-mL blood sample.
3. Gently invert tube several times, but do not agitate the tube. *Mixes the anticoagulant, but agitation may cause RBC hemolysis.*
4. Send tube to the laboratory.
5. Keep specimen cool. *High temperatures alter the results.*
6. Administer 40–80 mg furosemide orally or intravenously.
7. Place client in the upright position (sitting, standing, or walking) for 4 hr after the dose of furosemide.
8. After 4 hr, draw a second 7- to 12-mL blood sample using the same technique and protocol as the first sample.

Clinical Implications and Indications:

1. Screening on an outpatient basis for causes of hypertension
2. Aids differential diagnosis of hypertension due to hypersecretion of aldosterone by the adrenal cortex (hyperaldosteronism) or hypersecretion of renin by the juxtaglomerular apparatus (renovascular hypertension)

Nursing Care:

Before Test: Explain the test procedure and the purpose of the test. Assess the client's knowledge of the test. Instruct client to fast for 8 hr prior to the test. Test should be done in the morning hours because of the circadian rhythm levels of aldosterone, which are highest upon awakening. Maintain a normal sodium diet in the days before the test.

During Test: Adhere to standard precautions. After receiving the dose of furosemide, instruct client to sit upright for 4 hr (lying down will increase the secretion of renin and aldosterone).

After Test: Apply pressure to venipuncture site. Explain that some bruising, discomfort, and swelling may appear at the site and that warm, moist compresses can alleviate this. Monitor for signs of infection.

Potential Complications: Bleeding and bruising at venipuncture site

Contraindications: End-stage renal disease

Interfering Factors: Sodium intake and position of the body alter the secretion of aldosterone and renin.

Nursing Considerations:

Pregnancy: Normal pregnancy increases the level of renin secretion.
Pediatric: Infants and children will need assistance in remaining still during the venipuncture and age-appropriate comfort measures following the test.

Listing of Related Tests: Renin assay; saline suppression test; 24-hr urine sodium

WEBLINKS

http://www.niddk.nih.gov

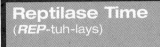

Reptilase Time
(*REP*-tuh-lays)

5 min.

BLOOD

Type of Test: Blood

Body Systems and Functions: Hematological system

Normal Findings: 18–20 sec

Test Results Time Frame: Within 24 hr

Test Description: Reptilase is an enzyme from Russell's viper venom used to test coagulation time. It detects the presence of adequate fibrinogen levels without interference from heparin. Prolonged thrombin time is confirmation that heparin is the cause of the coagulation abnormality. The test may be used in place of thrombin time in fibrinogen evaluation in client who is anticoagulated with heparin. Because it initiates coagulation by the direct activation of factor X and does not require factor VII, it can distinguish between a deficiency of either factor.

Consent Form: Not required

List of Equipment: Blue-top tube or serum separator tube; needle and two syringes or vacutainer; alcohol swab

Test Procedure:
1. A double-draw technique is recommended to prevent contamination with tissue thromboplastin from the venipuncture.
2. Label the specimen tube. *Correctly identifies the client and the test to be performed.*
3. Insert needle into vein. Draw 4 mL blood. Leave needle in place, twist off syringe, and set aside as waste sample.
4. Twist on second syringe and draw same amount of blood.
5. Gently invert tube several times, but do not agitate the tube. *Mixes the anticoagulant, but agitation may cause RBC hemolysis.*
6. Send tube to the laboratory.

Clinical Implications and Indications:
1. Diagnoses fibrinogen-related clotting defect
2. Differentially diagnoses cause of bleeding in client anticoagulated with heparin

Nursing Care:
Before Test: Explain the test procedure and the purpose of the test. Assess the client's knowledge of the test. Preschedule the test with the laboratory because blood sample may need to be sent to a regional laboratory for testing.
During Test: Adhere to standard precautions.
After Test: Apply pressure to venipuncture site. Explain that some bruising, discomfort, and swelling may appear at the site and that warm, moist compresses can alleviate this. Monitor for signs of infection.

Potential Complications: Bleeding and bruising at venipuncture site

BLOOD

Interfering Factors: Tissue thromboplastin may increase results.

Nursing Considerations:

Pediatric: Infants and children will need assistance in remaining still during the venipuncture and age-appropriate comfort measures following the test.

Listing of Related Tests: Bleeding time; coagulation screen; activated partial thromboplastin time (APTT); factor assays; partial thromboplastin time (PTT); platelet count; prothrombin time (PT)

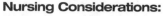

WEBLINKS

http://alice.ucdavis.edu

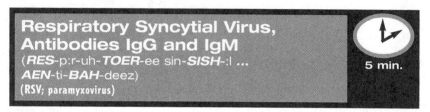

Respiratory Syncytial Virus, Antibodies IgG and IgM
(*RES*-p:r-uh-*TOER*-ee sin-*SISH*-:l ... *AEN*-ti-*BAH*-deez)
(RSV; paramyxovirus)

5 min.

Type of Test: Blood

Body Systems and Functions: Pulmonary system

Normal Findings: If client has never had RSV infection, detectable antibodies should be <1:5. For infants <6 months of age, the mother's IgG antibodies may be present, making results not reliable unless IgM antibodies are also present.

CRITICAL VALUES:
A fourfold increase in IgG antibodies or the presence of IgM antibodies

Test Results Time Frame: Within 48–72 hr

Test Description: Respiratory syncytial virus (RSV) measures the amount of the antibodies IgG and IgM by immunofluorescence. Both of these antibodies are associated with the RSV, which is the most common cause of lower respiratory tract infections. It is potentially life threatening in children under 2 years, especially in the first 6 months, and in immunosuppressed or the elderly. Most hospitalizations for RSV occur during the first 6 months of life. In older children and adults, RSV causes flu-like symptoms, bronchopneumonia, or exacerbations of chronic bronchitis. Approximately 70% of the population have antibody titers to RSV by age 5. The antibodies are not protective and reinfection can occur, although it is usually less severe and located in the upper respiratory tract. It spreads by droplets from contaminated respiratory secretions. Another method of diagnosing RSV is by obtaining nasopharyngeal washings or aspirates.

Consent Form: Not required

List of Equipment: Red-top tube or serum separator tube; needle and syringe or vacutainer; alcohol swab

Test Procedure:
1. Label the specimen tube. *Correctly identifies the client and the test to be performed.*
2. Obtain a 5-mL blood sample.
3. Do not agitate the tube. *Agitation may cause RBC hemolysis.*
4. Allow tube to rest for 1 hr at room temperature. *Allows specimen to clot.*
5. Send tube to the laboratory.

Clinical Implications and Indications:
1. Diagnoses RSV infection

Nursing Care:
Before Test: Explain the test procedures and the purpose of the test. Assess the client's knowledge of the test.
During Test: Adhere to standard precautions.
After Test: Apply pressure to venipuncture site. Explain that some bruising, discomfort, and swelling may appear at the site and that warm, moist compresses can alleviate this. Monitor for signs of infection.

Potential Complications: Bleeding and bruising at venipuncture site

Nursing Considerations:
Pediatric: In infants under 6 months, the presence of the mother's IgG antibodies is not a significant finding. However, presence of IgM antibodies is significant. Infants under 1 year need very close assessment and monitoring, as an RSV infection can quickly become life threatening due to the amount of bronchial secretions causing obstruction in small airways and severe hypoxia and respiratory fatigue with the increased effort of breathing. Infants and children will need assistance in remaining still during the venipuncture and age-appropriate comfort measures following the test.
Gerontology: Increased incidence of severe symptoms appear in the elderly. Convalescent care centers are especially susceptible to nosocomial transmission, which reinforces the need for following standard precautions.
Home Care: The virus is unstable and is readily inactivated by soap and water disinfectants. Good hand-washing techniques should be employed by those living with and caring for the client.
International: RSV is endemic on a worldwide basis and occurs in temperate climates primarily in midwinter and early spring.

Listing of Related Tests: Enzyme-linked immunosorbent assay (ELISA)

WEBLINKS

http://RespiratoryCare.medscape.com

Reticulocyte Count
(ruh-*TIK*-yue-loe-siyt)
(retic ct)

5 min.

Type of Test: Blood

BLOOD

Body Systems and Functions: Hematological system

Normal Findings:

Newborns	3.2% of total RBC
Infants	2%–5% of total RBC
Children	4%–5% of total RBC
Adults	0.5%–2% of total RBC

Note: higher in pregnant women

CRITICAL VALUES:
In polycythemia, with a reticulocyte count greater than 20%, notify health care provider immediately. The client may need a phlebotomy to decrease volume of blood and IV fluids to decrease viscosity of blood.

Test Results Time Frame: Within 24 hr

Test Description: The reticulocyte count measures the reticulocytes, which are immature red blood cells made and released by the red bone marrow in the normal erythropoietic process. The reticulocyte takes 1–2 days to mature into an erythrocyte, changing in appearance to a dense unstructured mass, with increased hemoglobin content. When there is hypoxia due to anemia or other reasons, the normal bone marrow increases the rate of erythrocyte production, resulting in an increased number of reticulocytes released. The reticulocyte count may need to be calculated as an index to account for the total decrease in mature red blood cells.

Consent Form: Not required

List of Equipment: Lavender-top tube or plasma separator tube; needle and syringe or vacutainer; alcohol swab

Test Procedure:
1. Label the specimen tube. *Correctly identifies the client and the test to be performed.*
2. Obtain a 5-mL blood sample.
3. Do not agitate the tube. *Agitation may cause RBC hemolysis.*
4. Send tube to the laboratory.

Clinical Implications and Indications:
1. Diagnoses and differentiates causes of bone marrow depression.
2. Evaluates anemia of unknown cause.
3. Evaluates response and activity of bone marrow to therapy.
4. Monitors physiological response to blood loss.
5. Elevated levels are found with erythroblastosis fetalis, hemorrhage, hemolytic anemia, leukemia, postsplenectomy, and sickle cell anemia.
6. Decreased levels are found with adrenocortical or anterior pituitary hypofunction, aplastic anemia, chronic infection, cirrhosis, folic acid deficiency, bone marrow failure, pernicious anemia, and radiation therapy.

Nursing Care:
Before Test: Explain the test procedure and the purpose of the test. Assess the client's knowledge of the test.
During Test: Adhere to standard precautions.

After Test: Apply pressure to venipuncture site. Explain that some bruising, discomfort, and swelling may appear at the site and that warm, moist compresses can alleviate this. Monitor for signs of infection.

Potential Complications: Bleeding and bruising at venipuncture site

Interfering Factors: Recent blood transfusions; pregnancy increases levels; failure to mix anticoagulant with sample; prolonged constriction of arm by tourniquet; dilution of serum sample with IV hydration solution; medications that increase levels are ATCH, antimalarials, antipyretics, levodopa, and sulfonamides; medications that decrease levels are azathioprine, chloramphenicol, dactinomycin, methotrexate, sulfonamides, and carbamazepine.

Nursing Considerations:
Pregnancy: Reticulocyte count is elevated in normal pregnancy.
Pediatric: Infants and children will need assistance in remaining still during the venipuncture and age-appropriate comfort measures following the test (note: a capillary tube may occasionally be used).

Listing of Related Tests: Hematocrit; reticulocyte production index; hemoglobin; ferritin

WEBLINKS

www.nlm.nih.gov

Reticulocyte Production Index
(ruh-*TIK*-yue-loe-*SIYT* pruh-*DUHK*-sh:n *IN*-deks) (RPI)

5 min.

Type of Test: Blood

Body Systems and Functions: Hematological system

Normal Findings: Reticulocyte index 1.0

Reticulocyte index = reticulocyte count (in %) x client's
hematocrit/normal hematocrit

Test Results Time Frame: Within 24 hr

Test Description: The reticulocyte production index is a calculated measurement relating the reticulocyte count (percentage of circulating reticulocytes) to the packed red blood cell volume (hematocrit). When anemia is present, the raw reticulocyte count can be misleading, because it does not consider that the total number of erythrocytes is decreased. In addition, the reticulocyte count does not factor in the prolonged time for reticulocytes to mature during a time of increased erythropoietic activity. Then when reticulocytes are released earlier than usual, a phenomenon occurs known as a shift. The length of maturity time increases from 1 day to 2.5 days as the hematocrit decreases. The RPI converts the reticulocyte count from a percentage to an index and corrects for the degree of anemia and for the early release (therefore a longer life span) of reticulocytes.

Consent Form: Not required

List of Equipment: The test is a calculation derived from the reticulocyte count and the hemotocrit. If these specimens have been drawn, no further specimens are needed. If not, the equipment needed is a lavender top-tube or plasma separator tube, needle and a 15- to 20-mL syringe, alcohol, and swab.

Test Procedure: (Note: Follow test procedure described below if specimens for hematocrit and reticulocyte count have not been drawn):
1. Label the specimen tube. *Correctly identifies the client and the test to be performed.*
2. Obtain a 5-mL blood sample.
3. Gently invert tube several times, but do not agitate the tube. *Mixes the anticoagulant, but agitation may cause RBC hemolysis.*
4. Send tube to the laboratory.

Clinical Implications and Indications:
1. Diagnoses and evaluates types of anemia.
2. Evaluates erythropoietic activity of bone marrow.
3. Elevated levels are found with accelerated red blood cell production.
4. Decreased levels are found with alcoholism, anemias (aplastic, iron deficiency, megaloblastic, pernicious, pure red cell), chronic infection, inability of bone marrow to increase RBC production, and radiation or chemotherapy.

Nursing Care:
Before Test: Explain the test procedure and the purpose of the test. Assess the client's knowledge of the test.
During Test: Adhere to standard precautions.
After Test: Apply pressure to venipuncture site. Explain that some bruising, discomfort, and swelling may appear at the site and that warm, moist compresses can alleviate this. Monitor for signs of infection.

Interfering Factors: Recent blood transfusions; failure to mix anticoagulant with sample; prolonged constriction of arm by tourniquet; dilution of serum sample with IV hydration solution

Nursing Considerations:
Pediatric: Infants and children will need assistance in remaining still during the venipuncture and age-appropriate comfort measures following the test.

Listing of Related Tests: Reticulocyte count; hematocrit; hemoglobin; ferritin level

WEBLINKS

www.nlm.nih.gov

Retinoblastoma Chromosome Abnormalities
(*RET*-in-oe-blaes-*TOE*-muh *KROE*-muh-*SOEM* aeb-noer-*MAEL*-uh-teez)

5 min.

Type of Test: Blood

BLOOD

Body Systems and Functions: Sensory system

Normal Findings:

Females	44 autosomes + 2 X chromosomes (46,XX)
Males	44 autosomes + 1 X and 1 Y chromosomes (46,XY)

CRITICAL VALUES:
Abnormal:

Females	46,XX,13q-
Males	46,XY,13q-

Test Results Time Frame: Within 3–5 days

Test Description: The retinoblastoma chromosome abnormalities test utilizes leukocyte screening from tissues cultured from the peripheral venous blood to determine the presence of the chromosomal defect of the retinoblastoma gene on chromosome 13, q band 14. The retinoblastoma gene is a tumor suppressor gene; when the gene is mutated, cell proliferation is unchecked. This defect is the cause of inherited autosomal dominant retinoblastoma. Retinoblastoma is a malignant tumor (glioma) of the retina of the eye. It is relatively rare accounting for 1%–3% of childhood malignancies. About 35% of retinoblastoma cases are due to the inherited chromosome defect. Two-thirds of the children with the inherited type tend to develop the disease in both eyes. Most often retinoblastoma occurs as a spontaneous uninherited mutation in the retinal cell. All cases of retinoblastoma have the potential for destroying the child's vision and metastasizing along the optic nerve to the subarachnoid space and the brain and to quickly involve the second eye unless treated early. The initial diagnostic finding is usually a white or yellow light reflex seen when examining the pupil with light.

Consent Form: Not required

List of Equipment: Green-top tube or serum separator tube; needle and syringe or vacutainer; alcohol swab

Test Procedure:
1. Label the specimen tube. *Correctly identifies the client and the test to be performed.*
2. Obtain a 10-mL blood sample.
3. Gently invert tube several times, but do not agitate the tube. *Mixes the anticoagulant, but agitation may cause RBC hemolysis.*
4. Send tube to the laboratory immediately.

Clinical Implications and Indications:
1. Screens for genetic chromosomal defect for retinoblastoma

Nursing Care:
Before Test: Explain the test procedure and the purpose of the test. Assess the client's knowledge of the test. Instruct client to fast for 3 hr before test. A morning specimen is preferred.
During Test: Adhere to standard precautions.
After Test: Apply pressure to venipuncture site. Explain that some bruising, discomfort, and swelling may appear at the site and that warm, moist compresses can alleviate this. Monitor for signs of infection.

Potential Complications: Bleeding and bruising at venipuncture site

Interfering Factors: Insufficient cells in blood sample

Nursing Considerations:
Pediatric: Infants and children will need assistance in remaining still during the venipuncture and age-appropriate comfort measures following the test. Parents of a child with chromosome abnormality will need genetic counseling.

WEBLINKS ▷   ▤ ☒

http://www.healthgate.com

Retinol Binding Protein
(*RET*-uh-nahl *BIYN*-ding *PROE*-teen)
(RBP)

5 min.

Type of Test: Blood

Body Systems and Functions: Metabolic system

Normal Findings:

Adults	3.0–6.0 mg/dL (RID method)
Newborns	1.1–3.4 mg/dL
6 months	1.8–5.0 mg/dL

Test Results Time Frame: Within 24 hr

Test Description: Retinol binding protein is a test that measures the amount of retinol binding protein (RBP) in the plasma. RBP is synthesized in the liver and is a transport protein for all-trans retinol, a form of vitamin A. While circulating in the plasma, it is bound 1:1 with transthyretin. The kidney stabilizes the retinol until it reaches the target cell where uptake of retinol is followed by dissociation and clearance of the RBP without the retinol in the kidney. Because it has a short half-life, it is a sensitive marker for current short-term changes in nutritional status. It has been correlated with nitrogen balance in severe burn patients.

Consent Form: Not required

List of Equipment: Red-top tube or serum separator tube; needle and syringe or vacutainer; alcohol swab

Test Procedure:
1. Label the specimen tube. *Correctly identifies the client and the test to be performed.*
2. Obtain a 5-mL blood sample.
3. Do not agitate the tube. *Agitation may cause RBC hemolysis.*
4. Send tube to the laboratory.

Clinical Implications and Indications:
1. Diagnoses protein malnutrition
2. Aids in diagnosis of liver dysfunction
3. RBP increases in renal disease, especially in tubular proteinuria

BLOOD

Nursing Care:
Before Test: Explain the test procedures and the purpose of the test. Assess the client's knowledge of the test.
During Test: Adhere to standard precautions.
After Test: Apply pressure to venipuncture site. Explain that some bruising, discomfort, and swelling may appear at the site and that warm, moist compresses can alleviate this. Monitor for signs of infection.

Potential Complications: Bleeding and bruising at venipuncture site

Interfering Factors: Acute or chronic renal disease increases RBP results.

Nursing Considerations:
Pediatric: Infants and children will need assistance in remaining still during the venipuncture and age-appropriate comfort measures following the test.

Listing of Related Tests: Plasma albumin

| WEBLINKS | ⊟⊠ |

www.nlm.nih.gov

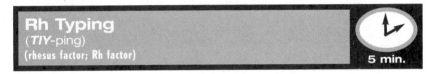

Rh Typing
(*TIY*-ping)
(rhesus factor; Rh factor)

5 min.

Type of Test: Blood

Body Systems and Functions: Hematological system

Normal Findings: Rh positive or Rh negative. The results are informational regarding blood type.

> **CRITICAL VALUES:**
> If a pregnant mother is Rh negative and the fetus she is carrying is Rh positive, the fetus is at risk of developing Rh disease (note: approximately 15% of whites and 7% of blacks are Rh negative in the American population).

Test Results Time Frame: Within 24 hr

Test Description: Rh testing measures the Rh factor, which is the system of blood typing that identifies proteins on the surface of the red blood cell. If a person's blood has an Rh antigen, the blood is Rh positive. If there are no Rh antigens, the blood is Rh negative. The Rh testing can also determine if the Rh-negative client has been sensitized to Rh-positive antigens. The most common way for the mother to be sensitized to Rh-positive antigens is during labor and delivery of her first Rh-positive child (note: it is possible for her to be sensitized after miscarriage, ectopic pregnancy, induced abortion, amniocentesis, or receiving a blood transfusion with Rh antigens). If the pregnant mother is Rh negative and is carrying an Rh-positive baby, it is possible for the mother to make antibodies that would recognize the baby's blood as foreign, which would initiate an immune response.

Consent Form: Not required

List of Equipment: Lavender-top tube or plasma separator tube; needle and syringe or vacutainer; alcohol swab

Test Procedure:

1. Label the specimen tube. *Correctly identifies the client and the test to be performed.*
2. Obtain a 5-mL blood sample.
3. Gently invert tube several times, but do not agitate the tube. *Mixes the anticoagulant, but agitation may cause RBC hemolysis.*
4. Send tube to the laboratory.
5. If obtaining other tubes of blood for testing, have a separate lavender tube solely for the Rh testing. This may mean obtaining two or more lavender-top tubes. The Rh sample is sent to the blood bank and the other tubes may be processed in a different laboratory. In addition, when drawing multiple samples, draw the lavender-top tubes last. *Prevents contamination of preservative in the other tubes.*

Clinical Implications and Indications:

1. Rh testing is routinely done on pregnant women or women who wish to become pregnant and their partners.
2. Monitors Rh antibodies, which may be done in the Rh-sensitized pregnant mother.
3. Evaluates potential for an Rh problem after a blood transfusion reaction.

Nursing Care:

Before Test: Explain the test procedure and the purpose of the test. Assess the client's knowledge of the test. Obtain accurate history regarding previous pregnancies, abortions, amniocenteses, and blood transfusions.

During Test: Adhere to standard precautions.

After Test: Apply pressure to venipuncture site. Explain that some bruising, discomfort, and swelling may appear at the site and that warm, moist compresses can alleviate this. Monitor for signs of infection. Counsel the client and her partner regarding the risks of Rh disease to the baby. Explain that RhoGAM, or RhIg, can be given by injection at 28 weeks gestation and again within 72 hr after delivery.

Potential Complications: Bleeding and bruising at venipuncture site

Nursing Considerations:

Pregnancy: It is important for the mother to know the Rh typing for herself and her partner. If the father of the baby is Rh positive, he may still have an Rh-recessive gene. Therefore, it is possible for the baby to be Rh negative, even with an Rh-positive father. An Rh-negative mother and father would have no possibility of having an Rh-positive baby. If the Rh type of the father is unable to be obtained, the Rh-negative mother would be treated as if the father is Rh positive.

Pediatric: Rh disease occurs when the Rh-negative mother's blood makes antibodies against the baby's Rh-positive blood. These antibodies destroy the baby's blood and can produce jaundice, anemia, heart failure, brain damage, and death. In severe cases of Rh disease, intrauterine blood transfusions may be performed as early as 18 weeks gestation. This would occur when the amount of antibodies in the mother's blood increases with pregnancy. Infants and children will need assistance in remaining still during the venipuncture and age-appropriate comfort measures following the test.

Listing of Related Tests: Amniocentesis; ultrasound (of the baby); cordocentesis

‖ **WEBLINKS** ⬚   ▣ ⊠

http://www.noah-health.org/

Rheumatoid Factor
(*RUE*-muh-toyd *FAEK*-t:r)
(RF; latex)

5 min.

Type of Test: Blood

Body Systems and Functions: Immunological system

Normal Findings: Rheumatoid factor negative

Test Results Time Frame: Within 24 hr

Test Description: Rheumatoid factor (RF) is an IgM antibody directed against a fragment of the IgG molecule. RF is useful as a test for autoimmune disorders and particularly in the diagnosis of rheumatoid arthritis. This is valuable in the early diagnosis of rheumatoid arthritis for potential treatment measures and inhibiting the progression of the disease.

Consent Form: Not required

List of Equipment: Red-top tube or serum separator tube; needle and syringe or vacutainer; alcohol swab

Test Procedure:
1. Label the specimen tube. *Correctly identifies the client and the test to be performed.*
2. Obtain a 5-mL blood sample.
3. Do not agitate the tube. *Agitation may cause RBC hemolysis.*
4. Send tube to the laboratory.

Clinical Implications and Indications:
1. Rheumatoid factor is present in 75% of people with rheumatoid arthritis.
2. Elevated levels are found with syphilis, sarcoidosis, tuberculosis, leprosy, infective endocarditis, parasitic infections, cancer, cirrhosis, hypertension, osteoarthritis, influenza, subacute bacterial endocarditis, tuberculosis, systemic lupus erythematosus, and advanced age.

Nursing Care:
Before Test: Explain the test procedure and the purpose of the test. Assess the client's knowledge of the test.
During Test: Adhere to standard precautions.

After Test: Apply pressure to venipuncture site. Explain that some bruising, discomfort, and swelling may appear at the site and that warm, moist compresses can alleviate this. Monitor for signs of infection.

Potential Complications: Bleeding and bruising at venipuncture site; rheumatoid vasculitis caused from venipuncture can lead to ulceration.

Nursing Considerations:
Pediatric: Infants and children will need assistance in remaining still during the venipuncture and age-appropriate comfort measures following the test. RF is often negative in juvenile rheumatoid arthritis.
Gerontology: RF may be elevated in the older adult without symptoms of rheumatoid arthritis.

Listing of Related Tests: Hematocrit; sedimentation rate; antinuclear antibody (ANA)

| WEBLINKS |

http://medlineplus.adam.com; www.nlm.nih.gov

Rocky Mountain Spotted Fever
(*RAH*-kee *MOUN*-ten *SPAHT*-:d *FEE*-v:r)
(RMSF; *Rickettsia rickettsii*)

5 min.

Type of Test: Blood

Body Systems and Functions: Immunological system

Normal Findings: Negative

Test Results Time Frame: Within 24 hr

Test Description: Specific IgG antibodies for Rocky Mountain spotted fever are detected by immunofluorescent antibody assay (IFA) and complement fixation. Serological studies may also detect virus-specific IgM . The organism can be inoculated into tissue culture and grown over 4–7 days, but this is very hazardous to personnel. The Weil-Felix test detects the production of serum antibody that is reactive against *Proteus* OX19, OX2, or OXK antigens, but it is not always reliable.

Consent Form: Not required

List of Equipment: Red-top tube or serum separator tube; needle and syringe or vacutainer; alcohol swab

Test Procedure:
1. Label the specimen tube. *Correctly identifies the client and the test to be performed.*
2. Obtain a 3-mL blood sample.
3. Do not agitate the tube. *Agitation may cause RBC hemolysis.*
4. Send tube to the laboratory.

BLOOD

5. Repeat 10–14 days later for convalescent sample and label the tube as convalescent sample. *Allows for separate identification of the convalescent sample, which is compared in ratio to the acute sample.*

Clinical Implications and Indications:

1. Diagnoses Rocky Mountain spotted fever, which is a tick-borne disease exhibiting as chills, fever, severe headache, occasional delirium, and coma. A red macular rash appears between the second and sixth days of fever.
2. Testing is often done in both the acute and convalescent stages. The convalescent sample is drawn 14–21 days after the acute event.
3. Because the initial presentation of the disease can mimic meningiococcemia, blood cultures and cerebrospinal fluid (CSF) may also be sampled. CSF pressure may be assessed at the time of the spinal tap.
4. Delay in diagnosis and treatment can occur if the client has no awareness of exposure to tick attachment. Also, reports of GI symptoms or an absence of headache may delay diagnosis. It is important to note in a history that a person has been in an endemic area, even if the client cannot recall a problem with ticks.
5. Most cases occur in spring and summer.

Nursing Care:

Before Test: Explain the test procedure and the purpose of the test. Assess the client's knowledge of the test. Inform the client that further tests may be necessary in 2–3 weeks after the onset and workup during the acute phase.
During Test: Adhere to standard precautions.
After Test: Apply pressure to venipuncture site. Explain that some bruising, discomfort, and swelling may appear at the site and that warm, moist compresses can alleviate this. Monitor for signs of infection.

Potential Complications: Bleeding and bruising at venipuncture site

Nursing Considerations:

Pediatric: Infants and children will need assistance in remaining still during the venipuncture and age-appropriate comfort measures following the test.
Gerontology: Symptoms are more severe in the elderly. There is a 70% mortality rate in the elderly if the disease is untreated.

Listing of Related Tests: CBC; platelets; sodium; CSF culture; skin biopsy; blood cultures; urinalysis

WEBLINKS

www.mayohealth.org; www.cehs.siu.edu

Rosette
(roe-*ZET*)
(fetal red cells; fetal-maternal blood test)   5 min.

Type of Test: Blood

Body Systems and Functions: Reproductive system

BLOOD

Normal Findings: Negative for fetal blood loss; no fetal red blood cells in the maternal blood

Test Results Time Frame: Within 24 hr

Test Description: The rosette test is performed to detect fetal cells in the maternal circulation. The presence of fetal red blood cells is valuable for diagnosing anemia of the newborn. There may be a risk for the mother becoming immunized against the fetal red cell groups. The rosette test is very accurate (97%) for detecting the bleeding of the fetal cells into the maternal blood. The clinical management involves the administration of RhoGAM, and the amount is determined by the rosette test.

> **CLINICAL ALERT:**
> The need for RhoGAM therapy can be evaluated by an Rh immune globulin screen (e.g., ABO, Rh typing, and microscopic Du antibody tests).

Consent Form: Not required

List of Equipment: Red-top tube or serum separator tube; needle and syringe or vacutainer; alcohol swab

Test Procedure:
1. Label the specimen tube. *Correctly identifies the client and the test to be performed.*
2. Obtain a 7-mL blood sample from the mother shortly after delivery. *Blood is examined for rosettes (mixed field agglutinins).*
3. Do not agitate the tube. *Agitation may cause RBC hemolysis.*
4. Send tube to the laboratory.

Clinical Implications and Indications:
1. Evaluates the presence and the amount of fetal blood that has been lost into the maternal circulation.
2. If there is less than 30 mL fetal blood loss, one dose of RhoGAM is given. If the fetal blood loss exceeds 35 mL, more than one vial of RhoGAM is necessary to prevent complications. In addition, if the fetal cells have not disappeared within 12–24 hr after the first RhoGAM dose, more RhoGAM is needed.

Nursing Care:
Before Test: Explain the test procedure and the purpose of the test. Assess the client's knowledge of the test. Provide emotional support due to the recent delivery of the infant.
During Test: Adhere to standard precautions. Provide reassurance and a calm atmosphere during the procedure.
After Test: Apply pressure to venipuncture site. Explain that some bruising, discomfort, and swelling may appear at the site and that warm, moist compresses can alleviate this. Monitor for signs of infection.

Potential Complications: Bleeding and bruising at venipuncture site

Nursing Considerations:
Pregnancy: Particular attention needs to be emphasized on the emotional needs of the mother during this potentially stressful event.

Pediatric: *The fetal condition may be compromised, and careful assessment of all presenting data needs consideration.*

Listing of Related Tests: Rh typing

‖WEBLINKS ⟨	⊟⊠

http://adam.excite.com

Rubella Antibody
(rue-*BEL*-uh *AEN*-ti-*BAH*-deez)
(German measles test, hemagglutination inhibition; HAI)

5 min.

Type of Test: Blood

Body Systems and Functions: Immunological system

Normal Findings:

IgM antibody	Negative
IgG antibody	<1:4; negative

Test Results Time Frame: Within 24 hr

Test Description: Rubella antibodies are a result of an RNA acute viral communicable infection, primarily seen in children and young adults. This disorder is characterized by a red or pink macular rash, lymphadenopathy, pharyngitis, and conjunctivitis. It has an incubation period of 14–21 days and is spread by droplet spray. This antibody titer stays positive for 4–5 weeks and then disappears.

CLINICAL ALERT:
It is extremely important to identify exposure to rubella in pregnant women, as congenital rubella infection during the first trimester of pregnancy is correlated with many congenital abnormalities (e.g., brain damage, heart defects, deafness), spontaneous abortion, or stillbirth.

Consent Form: Not required

List of Equipment: Red-top tube or serum separator tube; needle and syringe or vacutainer; alcohol swab

Test Procedure:
1. Label the specimen tube. *Correctly identifies the client and the test to be performed.*
2. Obtain a 5-mL blood sample.
3. Do not agitate the tube. *Agitation may cause RBC hemolysis.*
4. Send tube to the laboratory.
5. Repeat 7–10 days later for convalescent sample and label the tube as convalescent sample. *Allows for separate identification of the convalescent sample, which is compared in ratio to the acute sample.*

BLOOD

BLOOD

Clinical Implications and Indications:
1. Detects the presence of togavirus, which is the causative virus of rubella
2. Confirms congenital rubella (note: the presence of IgG antibodies in the infant is a strong indicator of the infection)

Nursing Care:
Before Test: Explain the test procedure and the purpose of the test. Assess the client's knowledge of the test.
During Test: Adhere to standard precautions.
After Test: Apply pressure to venipuncture site. Explain that some bruising, discomfort, and swelling may appear at the site and that warm, moist compresses can alleviate this. Monitor for signs of infection. Inform client that it is important to return in 7–14 days for repeat testing to see if infection is subsiding.

Potential Complications: Bleeding and bruising at venipuncture site

Interfering Factors: Rubella antibodies remain present and static for many years.

Nursing Considerations:
Pregnancy: A heelstick is acceptable, or umbilical cord blood (3-mL sample); confirmation of congenital infection requires the test be performed on the mother; women who have no antibody should be vaccinated prior to pregnancy.
Pediatric: Infants and children will need assistance in remaining still during the venipuncture and age-appropriate comfort measures following the test. Children need to be immunized with the MMR vaccine at 15 months and again at 4–6 years.

Listing of Related Tests: Torch test; ELISA; latex agglutination; LA

WEBLINKS

http://www.nlm.nih.gov

Rubeola Antibody
(rue-*BEE*-oe-luh *AEN*-ti-*BAH*-dee)
(measles; RNA myxovirus)

5 min.

Type of Test: Blood

Body Systems and Functions: Immunological system

Normal Findings: Negative viral antibodies

Test Results Time Frame: Within 24 hr

Test Description: Antibodies to the rubeola virus generally appear 1–2 weeks after exposure, when the client begins to exhibit fever, cough, headache, conjunctivitis, and an exanthematous rash on the face, trunk, and proximal extremities. Koplik's spots, mottled bright spots, appear on the buccal mucosa. These spots are pathognomonic for measles. IgM occurs first, followed a few

BLOOD

days later by IgG. The IgM antibodies generally peak in 3–6 weeks, then drop to undetectable levels. IgG titers may peak in 4–12 weeks. Atypical measles occurs in adults who received inactivated measles virus between 1963 and 1967 or who received live measles vaccine before the age of 12 months. These clients exhibit a hypersensitivity rather than an immunity to wild measles virus. Exposure is potentially fatal. Clients usually present without Koplik's spots, and the incidence of pneumonia is very high.

CLINICAL ALERT:
Women of childbearing age should not receive the measles vaccine.

Consent Form: Not required

List of Equipment: Red-top tube or serum separator tube; needle and syringe or vacutainer; alcohol swab

Test Procedure:
1. Label the specimen tube. *Correctly identifies the client and the test to be performed.*
2. Obtain a 5-mL blood sample.
3. Gently invert tube several times, but do not agitate the tube. *Mixes the anticoagulant, but agitation may cause RBC hemolysis.*
4. Send tube to the laboratory.
5. Repeat 10–14 days later for convalescent sample and label the tube as convalescent sample. *Allows for separate identification of the convalescent sample, which is compared in ratio to the acute sample.*

Clinical Implications and Indications:
1. Detects rubeola virus, which is transmitted by airborne droplets and causes measles. This is a major cause of childhood morbidity and mortality throughout the world.
2. Pneumonia and otitis media are often present with the rubeola virus.
3. Encephalitis may occur 3–7 days after the rash. In the United States, deaths are primarily due to CNS involvement.
4. Subacute sclerosing panencephalitis (SSPE) is a rare complication. This is more common in children, among males, and in rural environments. This occurs later in the disease process than the acute encephalitis.
5. Measles must be reported to the Department of Health in the United States.

Nursing Care:
Before Test: Explain the test procedure and the purpose of the test. Assess the client's knowledge of the test. Ensure that the client understands a follow-up blood test is usually done 14–21 days after the acute event.
During Test: Adhere to standard precautions.
After Test: Apply pressure to venipuncture site. Explain that some bruising, discomfort, and swelling may appear at the site and that warm, moist compresses can alleviate this. Monitor for signs of infection.

Potential Complications: Bleeding and bruising at venipuncture site

Contraindications: Clients on corticosteroid therapy should not receive measles vaccine.

Interfering Factors: PPD testing (note: PPD testing should be completed before receiving the measles vaccine or should be given 4–6 weeks after receiving the measles vaccine)

Nursing Considerations:

Pregnancy: Pregnant women should not receive the vaccine. Planned pregnancy should be avoided until 1 month following a measles vaccine.

Pediatric: Infants and children will need assistance in remaining still during the venipuncture and age-appropriate comfort measures following the test. It is recommended that children receive their first dose of measles vaccine at 12–15 months of age. A second vaccine is given at ages 4–6 years. Evidence of vaccination is required before a child begins school.

Home Care: Health care providers should be screened and vaccinated if necessary.

Rural: Subacute sclerosing panencephalitis is higher in rural boys.

International: There is a lack of vaccination in developing countries, and deaths from the disease are usually due to diarrhea and protein-losing enteropathy.

Listing of Related Tests: CBC

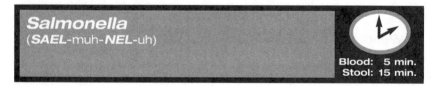

WEBLINKS

www.cdc.gov

Salmonella
(*SAEL*-muh-*NEL*-uh)

Blood: 5 min.
Stool: 15 min.

Type of Test: Blood; stool

Body Systems and Functions: Gastrointestinal system

Normal Findings: Negative

Test Results Time Frame: Within 1 week

Test Description: *Salmonella* testing of the blood or stool is the most common route of the detection of *Salmonella enteritidis*. Blood cultures show that the rate of positivity declines after the first week of symptoms, but one-fourth or more of the clients still have positive cultures in their third week of illness. This species of bacteria has three subspecies known to infect humans: *typhi, typhimurium,* and *choleraesuis.* Stool and urine cultures also test positive for *S. enteritidis.* Bone marrow may also be collected for culture. The most common form of salmonellosis is from the ingestion of contaminated food or drink. Onset of symptoms (headache, sore throat, bloody diarrhea, rose spots, leukopenia, and a fever that rises to a maximum and slowly returns to normal) can be between 8 and 48 hr. Other sources of contamination can be from handling pets or cleaning out their enclosures. Reptiles have been associated with carrying *Salmonella.*

> **CLINICAL ALERT:**
> A positive culture has transmission implications for health care providers. Maintaining strict measures of standard precautions on suspected clients with a positive *Salmonella* culture is important.

BLOOD

Consent Form: Not required

List of Equipment: *Blood:* red-top tube or serum separator tube; needle and syringe or vacutainer; alcohol swab. *Stool:* clean, dry container to collect stool; tongue depressor; gloves; rectal swab; clean, dry bedpan.

Test Procedure:

Blood:
1. Label the specimen tube. *Correctly identifies the client and the test to be performed.*
2. Obtain a 10- to 30-mL blood sample. The ability of the laboratory to detect bacteria in the specimen is directly proportional to the amount of blood sent for the culture.
3. Do not agitate the tube. *Agitation may cause RBC hemolysis.*
4. Send tube to the laboratory.

Stool:
1. Have client defecate into a clean bedpan, bedside commode, or toilet hat. *Decreases contamination and aids in obtaining stool specimen.*
2. Do not use the stool if it is contaminated with urine or menstrual blood. *Urine and menstrual blood affect stool culture results.*
3. Do not have the client place toilet paper on the stool after defecation. *Toilet paper affects stool culture results.*
4. Use a clean tongue depressor to place 2–3 cm of formed stool or 15 mL of liquid stool in a specimen container. *This amount is necessary for obtaining proper stool culture.*
5. Dispose of remaining stool and tongue depressor. *Decreases chance of spread of pathogen.*
6. Include visible mucus, pus, or blood in the specimen. *These may be indicative of disease or contain pathogens.*
7. Label the specimen container and send to laboratory as soon as possible. *Ensures accurate results.*

Clinical Implications and Indications:
1. Detects acute enterocolitis, which is caused by *S. enterica typhimurium*.
2. Enteric fever, or typhoid fever, is caused by *S. enterica typhi*. Incubation can be 5–14 days and is best diagnosed by culturing the organism from the blood. Occasionally the bone marrow is cultured.
3. *S. enterica choleraesuis* is responsible for *Salmonella* bacteremia, an infection that is characterized by recurrent fevers, bacteremia, and local infection in bones, joints, pleura, pericardium, lungs, and other sites.
4. Detects bacterial enterocolitis, *Shigella*, *Campylobacter*, protozoan enterocolitis, and parasitic enterocolitis.
5. Clients with sickle cell anemia may experience increased joint discomfort with *S. enteritidis* infections.

Nursing Care:

Before Test: Explain the test procedure and the purpose of the test. Assess the client's knowledge of the test. Prepare the client that two or three different cultures could be obtained from different sites in order to get an adequate sampling of blood. A complete history should be taken. It is important to include pertinent information on the laboratory slip regarding recent travel by the client and current antimicrobial therapy, history of bloody diarrhea, and contact with reptiles. Alfalfa sprouts can also be implicated in salmonellosis and should be included if ingested recently.

During Test: Adhere to standard precautions.

After Test: Apply pressure to venipuncture site. Explain that some bruising, discomfort, and swelling may appear at the site and that warm, moist compresses can alleviate this. Monitor for signs of infection.

Potential Complications: Bleeding and bruising at venipuncture site

Nursing Considerations:

Pediatric: *For infants and small children, 1–5 mL per culture is required. Two sets of cultures are recommended. The onset of disease symptoms may have a shorter incubation period than for adults. Infants and children will need assistance in remaining still during the venipuncture and age-appropriate comfort measures following the test.*

Gerontology: *The elderly and the immunocompromised client is at greater risk for more severe complications from salmonellosis.*

Home Care: *Good hand-washing techniques should be emphasized, especially before food preparation and after handling pets. Proper preparation and refrigeration of food are important to prevent disease.*

International: Salmonella *is often seen in countries with less means of refrigeration and decreased electricity used across the population. In addition, reptiles carry the disorder, and some countries have more chances for contamination with these animals.*

Listing of Related Tests: Complete blood test (CBC)

WEBLINKS

www.ama-assn.org; www.foodsafety.gov; www.cdc.gov

Schlichter
(*SHLIK*-t:r)
(SBT; inhibition level, antibiotic)

5 min.

Type of Test: Blood

Body Systems and Functions: Immunological system

Normal Findings: Bactericidal activity >1:8 dilution

Test Results Time Frame: Within 2–3 days

Test Description: The Schlichter test determines the amount of dilution materials necessary to be bactericidal. Recently, there have been increasing numbers of antibiotics used to treat a tremendous number of pathogens. This test provides a method of assessing whether or not the chosen antibiotic is successfully treating the organisms in selected pathological conditions.

Consent Form: Not required

List of Equipment: Red-top tube or serum separator tube; needle and syringe or vacutainer; alcohol swab; sterile aspiration tray

Test Procedure:
1. Label the specimen tube. *Correctly identifies the client and the test to be performed.*
2. Obtain a 5-mL blood sample or a 2-mL body fluid sample using sterile aspiration.
3. Do not agitate the tube. *Agitation may cause RBC hemolysis.*
4. Send tube to the laboratory.

Clinical Implications and Indications:
1. Evaluates antibiotic therapy used in the treatment of endocarditis and osteomyelitis

Nursing Care:
Before Test: Explain the test procedure and the purpose of the test. Assess the client's knowledge of the test.
During Test: Adhere to standard precautions.
After Test: Apply pressure to venipuncture site. Explain that some bruising, discomfort, and swelling may appear at the site and that warm, moist compresses can alleviate this. Monitor for signs of infection.

Potential Complications: Bleeding and bruising at venipuncture site

Nursing Considerations:
Pediatric: Infants and children will need assistance in remaining still during the venipuncture and age-appropriate comfort measures following the test.

WEBLINKS ▯   ▭▨

http://www.nlm.nih.gov

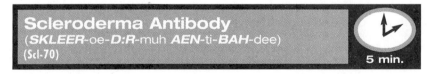

Scleroderma Antibody
(*SKLEER*-oe-*D:R*-muh *AEN*-ti-*BAH*-dee)
(Scl-70)

5 min.

Type of Test: Blood

Body Systems and Functions: Immunological system

Normal Findings: Negative

Test Results Time Frame: Within 24 hr

Test Description: The scleroderma antibody (Scl-70) is found in about 25% of clients with scleroderma. This antibody targets topoisomerase III found in clients with diffuse systemic sclerosis and 20% of those with CREST syndrome. It is highly specific but occurs late in the course of the disease and is not necessarily useful for diagnostic purposes.

Consent Form: Not required

List of Equipment: Red-top tube or serum separator tube; needle and syringe or vacutainer; alcohol swab

Test Procedure:
1. Label the specimen tube. *Correctly identifies the client and the test to be performed.*
2. Obtain a 5-mL blood sample.
3. Do not agitate the tube. *Agitation may cause RBC hemolysis.*
4. Send tube to the laboratory.

Clinical Implications and Indications:
1. Two forms of scleroderma exist and are classified as limited (80%) and diffuse (20%). The clients with limited disease often exhibit CREST syndrome, which is calcinosis cutis, Raynaud's phenomenon, esophageal involvement, sclerodactyly, and telangectasia.
2. Those with diffuse scleroderma have more internal organ involvement, and the disease course can be more rapid. The Scl-70 antibody is not present is all clients, but when it is detected, it may indicate a poorer prognosis associated with more internal organ damage (e.g., interstitial lung disease).

Nursing Care:
Before Test: Explain the test procedure and the purpose of the test. Assess the client's knowledge of the test.
During Test: Adhere to standard precautions.
After Test: Apply pressure to venipuncture site. Explain that some bruising, discomfort, and swelling may appear at the site and that warm, moist compresses can alleviate this. Monitor for signs of infection.

Potential Complications: Bleeding and bruising at venipuncture site

Nursing Considerations:
Pediatric: Infants and children will need assistance in remaining still during the venipuncture and age-appropriate comfort measures following the test.

Listing of Related Tests: Complete blood count (CBC); antinuclear antibody test (ANA); anticentromere antibodies; urinalysis

WEBLINKS

www.mayohealth.org; www.vicioso.com

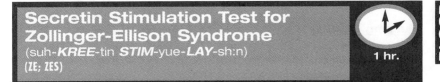

Secretin Stimulation Test for Zollinger-Ellison Syndrome
(suh-*KREE*-tin *STIM*-yue-*LAY*-sh:n)
(ZE; ZES)

1 hr.

Type of Test: Blood

Body Systems and Functions: Gastrointestinal system

Normal Findings: Serum gastrin <200 pg/mL

> **CRITICAL VALUES:**
> Greater than 2,000 pg/mL indicates Zollinger-Ellison syndrome (ZES) (note: clients with ZES often have increased fasting serum-gastrin levels of greater than 500 pg/mL).

Test Results Time Frame: Within 24 hr

Test Description: Secretin stimulation tests measure the serum gastrin. Secretin is a polypeptide secreted by the duodenal mucosa and the upper jejunum in response to gastric acids (e.g., gastrin). In this test, the serum gastrin is measured at frequent intervals following an IV injection of secretin. Peak gastrin levels usually occur 5–10 min following the administration of secretin.

> **CLINICAL ALERT:**
> EDTA tubes lower the serum gastrin values; therefore must use correct heparinized tubes.

Consent Form: Required

List of Equipment: Plasma separator tubes (6–8); IV initiation equipment; needle and syringe or vacutainer; alcohol swab; clock/timer, secretin for injection (2–3 U/kg body weight)

Test Procedure:
1. Weigh client. *Accurate calculations of secretin for injection can be calculated.*
2. Obtain a pretest blood sample. *Necessary for baseline information.*
3. Inject secretin intravenously as per formula 2-3 U/kg body weight (note exact time of injection). *All subsequent blood samples are collected from this time on.*
4. Obtain blood samples at 2.5, 5, 10, 20, and 30 min and send to laboratory with appropriate labeling. *Serial sample collection allows for assessment of the gastrin levels.*
5. Samples should be collected on ice and transported quickly to the laboratory. *Gastrin samples are unstable at room temperature.*

Clinical Implications and Indications:
1. Diagnoses Zollinger-Ellison syndrome (ZES). This syndrome is characterized by non-insulin-secreting tumors of the pancreas and duodenum, which may be either benign or malignant. Excess amounts of gastrin are produced and released, thereby stimulating the secretion of great amounts of hydrochloric acid and pepsin in the stomach.

2. Evaluates ulcers, which are resistant to standard therapy.

Nursing Care:
Before Test: Explain the test procedure and the purpose of the test. Assess the client's knowledge of the test.
During Test: Adhere to standard precautions.
After Test: Apply pressure to venipuncture site. Explain that some bruising, discomfort, and swelling may appear at the site and that warm, moist compresses can alleviate this. Monitor for signs of infection.

Potential Complications: Bleeding and bruising at venipuncture site

Nursing Considerations:
Pediatric: Infants and children will need assistance in remaining still during the venipuncture and age-appropriate comfort measures following the test.
Gerontology: Modest hypergastrinemia is often seen in older clients because of gastric mucosal atrophy and reduced gastric acid secretion.

Listing of Related Tests: Upper GI (barium study); endoscopic with biopsy of gastric mucosa; breath test for *Helicobacter pylori*

WEBLINKS

http://www.niddk.nih.gov

Sedimentation Rate, Erythrocyte
(*SED*-uh-men-*TAY*-sh:n rayt uh-*RITH*-roe-siyt)
(erythrocyte sedimentation rate; ESR)

5 min.

Type of Test: Blood

Body Systems and Functions: Hematological system

Normal Findings:

Males:	
Under 50 years old	0–15 mm/hr
Over 50 years old	0–20 mm/hr
Females:	
Under 50 years old	0–20 mm/hr
Over 50 years old	0–30 mm/hr
Children:	
Newborn	0–2 mm/hr
Up to 14 years old	0–20 mm/hr

Test Results Time Frame: Within 24 hr

Test Description: The erythrocyte sedimentation rate measures the rate of fall of red blood cells suspended in plasma. The Westergren method uses a tube that is 200 mm long with 2.5 mm diameter. The Westergren method is most sen-

BLOOD

sitive for fluctuations at higher elevations. The Wintrobe method uses a shorter tube and a different anticoagulant (note: this test is more sensitive for mild elevations and corrects for anemia). The results are reported in millimeters per hour. If individual cells stack together, the sedimentation rate is increased because the surface area of the aggregate is increased, making the travel time longer. This is called a rouleaux effect or rouleaux formation.

Consent Form: Not required

List of Equipment: Lavender-top tube or serum separator tube; needle and syringe or vacutainer; alcohol swab

Test Procedure:
1. Label the specimen tube. *Correctly identifies the client and the test to be performed.*
2. Obtain a 5-mL blood sample.
3. Gently invert tube several times, but do not agitate the tube. *Mixes the anticoagulant, but agitation may cause RBC hemolysis.*
4. Send tube to the laboratory.

Clinical Implications and Indications:
1. Elevated levels are found with conditions that have increased plasma fibrinogen, increased red blood cell size, increased plasma viscosity, or increased gamma globulins. Conditions include rheumatoid arthritis, acute MI, bacterial infection, gout, PID, lupus, burns, and some cancers.
2. Diagnoses polymyalgia rheumatica and temporal arteritis.
3. ESR can be helpful for tracking diseases ("sickness index") such as Hodgkin's disease, multiple myeloma, rheumatoid arthritis, and systemic lupus erythematosus.

Nursing Care:
Before Test: Explain the test procedure and the purpose of the test. Assess the client's knowledge of the test.
During Test: Adhere to standard precautions.
After Test: Apply pressure to venipuncture site. Explain that some bruising, discomfort, and swelling may appear at the site and that warm, moist compresses can alleviate this. Monitor for signs of infection.

Potential Complications: Bleeding and bruising at venipuncture site

Interfering Factors: ESR may be decreased by extreme leukocytosis, polycythemia, and red cell or protein abnormalities; medications that increase the ESR are theophylline, procainamide, dextran, vitamin A, and methyldopa.

Nursing Considerations:
Pregnancy: Sedimentation rate may be increased in the second and third trimesters.
Pediatric: Infants and children will need assistance in remaining still during the venipuncture and age-appropriate comfort measures following the test.
Gerontology: ESR is elevated in the elderly and in some obese clients. This may just reflect a higher degree of disease in these populations.

Listing of Related Tests: Zeta sedimentation rate (ZSR) (note: ZSR is a modification of ESR but uses capillary tubes and a centrifuge); C-reactive protein; PPD testing; chest x-ray; stool for occult blood; hematology profile (including BUN, creatinine, liver function studies); urinalysis; blood electrophoresis

---

WEBLINKS 🔍   🗕🗙

http://uwcme.org

Segmented Neutrophils
(*SEG*-ment-:d *NUET*-roe-filz)
(segmented granulocyte; polymorphonucleocytes; PMN)

5 min.

Type of Test: Blood

Body Systems and Functions: Hematological system

Normal Findings: 55%–70% (2,500–7,000 mm^3) of all leukocytes are neutrophils. Segmented neutrophils are 50%–65% (2,500–6,500 mm^3) of the total white blood cell count. Bands (immature neutrophils) account for 0%–5% (0–500 mm^3) of the total WBC.

Test Results Time Frame: Within 24 hr

Test Description: Segmented neutrophils are one of the substances in a differential white blood cell count. White blood cells are divided into granulocytes, monocytes, and lymphocytes. Then granulocytes are divided into neutrophils, eosinophils, and basophils, all of which are involved in bacterial phagocytosis. The neutrophils are divided into semented neutrophils and band neutrophils (immature neutrophils that multiply quickly in the presence of acute infection). The segmented neutrophil testing involves making a blood smear and staining it with the Wright stain and examining it under the microscope or counting it automatically using a hematology analyzer. The slide can be made manually or can be prepared using automated equipment. Neutrophils are identified by the granular or segmented appearance of the nucleus. They increase in the presence of infection and pathology.

Consent Form: Not required

List of Equipment: Lavender-top tube or serum separator tube; needle and syringe or vacutainer; alcohol swab

Test Procedure:
1. Label the specimen tube. *Correctly identifies the client and the test to be performed.*
2. Obtain a 5-mL blood sample.
3. Gently invert tube several times, but do not agitate the tube. *Mixes the anticoagulant, but agitation may cause RBC hemolysis.*
4. Send tube to the laboratory.

Clinical Implications and Indications:
1. The segmented neutrophils are part of the complete blood count or differential white blood cell count. They are responsible for pus formation, inflammation, and phagocytosis of foreign antigens.

2. The segmented neutrophils are considered in viral and bacterial infections, leukemias, anemias, inflammatory diseases, tissue damage, acute myocardial infarction, appendicitis, and other abdominal pain.

Nursing Care:
Before Test: Explain the test procedure and the purpose of the test. Assess the client's knowledge of the test.
During Test: Adhere to standard precautions.
After Test: Apply pressure to venipuncture site. Explain that some bruising, discomfort, and swelling may appear at the site and that warm, moist compresses can alleviate this. Monitor for signs of infection.

Potential Complications: Bleeding and bruising at venipuncture site

Nursing Considerations:
Pediatric: Infants and children will need assistance in remaining still during the venipuncture and age-appropriate comfort measures following the test.

Listing of Related Tests: WBC; CBC; x-ray of affected area

WEBLINKS	

http://www.mc.vanderbilt.edu; http://www-medlib.med.utah.edu

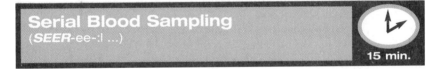

Serial Blood Sampling
(*SEER*-ee-:l ...)

15 min.

Type of Test: Blood

Body Systems and Functions: Hematological system

Normal Findings: Intact blood system

Test Results Time Frame: Within 24 hr

Test Description: Serial blood sampling is used for clients who require large amounts of blood to be obtained for laboratory studies. The advantage of this system is the reduction of client discomfort from multiple venipunctures.

CLINICAL ALERT:
Clients who are scheduled to have this procedure should be informed of its purpose. The advantages and disadvantages of a heparin lock compared to a series of venipunctures should also be discussed. To prevent coagulation, administer IV fluids slowly.

Consent Form: Not required

List of Equipment: Appropriate serum separator tubes; needles and syringes or vacutainer; alcohol swabs; stopcock

BLOOD

Test Procedure:

1. Label the appropriate specimen tubes. *Correctly identifies the client and the test to be performed.*
2. Initiate IV infusion with large-bore needle (18-gauge or larger) and attach stopcock.
3. Obtain amount of blood necessary for specified test from stopcock. *Keeps venipunctures to minimum.*
4. Do not agitate the tube. *Agitation may cause RBC hemolysis.*
5. Send tube to the laboratory.

Clinical Implications and Indications:

1. Accesses blood sample for clients with multiple and frequent laboratory blood testing
2. Decreases venipuncture numbers

Nursing Care:

Before Test: Explain the test procedure and the purpose of the test. Assess the client's knowledge of the test.

During Test: Adhere to standard precautions.

After Test: Apply pressure to venipuncture site. Explain that some bruising, discomfort, and swelling may appear at the site and that warm, moist compresses can alleviate this. Monitor for signs of infection.

Potential Complications: Bleeding and bruising at venipuncture site

Nursing Considerations:

Pediatric: Infants and children will need assistance in remaining still during the venipuncture and age-appropriate comfort measures following the test.
Gerontology: Elderly clients may benefit greatly from this type of blood sampling, due to the lack of integrity of their vessels for venipunctures.

WEBLINKS ▸

http://www.methodisthealth.com

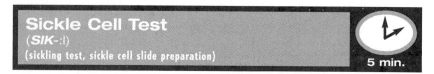

Sickle Cell Test
(*SIK*-:l)
(sickling test, sickle cell slide preparation)

5 min.

Type of Test: Blood

Body Systems and Functions: Hematological system

Normal Findings: No sickling of red blood cells

Test Results Time Frame: Within 24 hr

Test Description: The sickle cell test involves a wet preparation of red blood cells, and a reducing agent (such as metabisulfite) is examined on a slide for sickled cells. In the presence of lowered oxygen tension, the red blood cells with hemoglobin S (Hgb S) undergo a change in the globin part of the molecule and cause the transformation of shape. The number of sickled cells per 1,000 RBCs is determined and expressed as a percentage. Other tests to determine sickling include mixing red blood cells with dithionite (sickle turbidity tube test). The solution becomes opaque in the presence of Hgb S. Sickling may also be observed on a blood smear during a crisis. Electrophoresis can identify abnormal hemoglobin. A person may have sickle cell disease by inheriting a sickle cell gene from each parent (labeled SS) or by inheriting one sickle cell gene and one gene for a variety of other abnormal hemoglobins (labeled SC or S-beta-zero thalassemia). Sickle cell trait is different from sickle cell disease in that one parent contributes a sickle cell gene and one parent contributes a normal gene. Sickle cell disease is increased profoundly in African-American populations.

Consent Form: Not required

List of Equipment: Lavender-top tube or serum separator tube; needle and syringe or vacutainer; alcohol swab

Test Procedure:
1. Label the specimen tube. *Correctly identifies the client and the test to be performed.*
2. Obtain a 5-mL blood sample.
3. Gently invert tube several times, but do not agitate the tube. *Mixes the anticoagulant, but agitation may cause RBC hemolysis.*
4. Send tube to the laboratory.

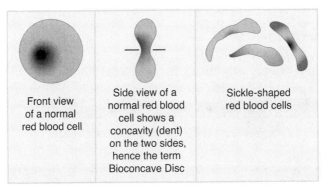

| Front view of a normal red blood cell | Side view of a normal red blood cell shows a concavity (dent) on the two sides, hence the term Bioconcave Disc | Sickle-shaped red blood cells |

Differences in shape are apparent in a normal red blood cell (bioncave disc) and sickle-shaped red blood cell (crescent shaped).

Clinical Implications and Indications:
1. Diagnoses the presence of sickle cell (hemolytic) anemia.
2. Sickle cell (hemolytic) anemia results from the destruction of the abnormal red blood cells. Sickled cells tend to obstruct the capillaries, causing tissue destruction. Thrombosis, stroke, renal damage, leg ulcers, abnormal growth patterns, and infections are some of the common problems.

Nursing Care:
Before Test: Explain the test procedure and the purpose of the test. Assess the client's knowledge of the test. Obtain accurate history regarding previous problems with anemia or a sickle cell event.

During Test: Adhere to standard precautions.

After Test: Apply pressure to venipuncture site. Explain that some bruising, discomfort, and swelling may appear at the site and that warm, moist compresses can alleviate this. Monitor for signs of infection. Refer to genetic counselor for follow-up teaching.

Potential Complications: Bleeding and bruising at venipuncture site

Nursing Considerations:

Pregnancy: *High-risk clients could be encouraged to get testing and genetic counseling before planning a pregnancy. Women with sickle cell disease may have crisis periods during the pregnancy. Early prenatal care is advised because there is a higher risk of preterm labor and low-birthweight babies. Two people with sickle cell trait could have a baby with sickle cell disease, but there is a 25% chance that the baby would not be affected at all.*

Pediatric: *Sickle cell anemia usually presents during childhood. Children with sickle cell disease have more problems with infection. Meningitis and septicemia are more severe in these children. Their survival can be enhanced by early detection. Antibiotic therapy and immunizations are encouraged. To date, 40 states include testing for newborns. Because of the tendency of the red blood cells to clump, there is a high risk of stroke in children, especially between the ages of 2 and 5 years. Blood transfusions and brain scans may be ordered on a routine basis. Some children have been treated with bone marrow transplants. Infants and children will need assistance in remaining still during the venipuncture and age-appropriate comfort measures following the test.*

International: *Sickle cell anemia is an inherited disorder predominantly found in African, African-American, and Mediterranean populations.*

Listing of Related Tests: CBC; bilirubin (often elevated from the breakdown of hemoglobin); x-rays of affected areas (especially the head of the femur); hemoglobin electrophoresis; stained blood smear; sickle turbidity test

WEBLINKS

http://www.emory.edu;http://www.noah-health.org/

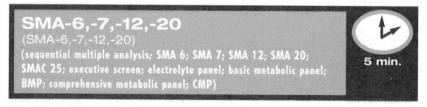

SMA-6,-7,-12,-20
(SMA-6,-7,-12,-20)
(sequential multiple analysis; SMA 6; SMA 7; SMA 12; SMA 20; SMAC 25; executive screen; electrolyte panel; basic metabolic panel; BMP; comprehensive metabolic panel; CMP)

5 min.

Type of Test: Blood

Body Systems and Functions: Hematological system

Normal Findings: See individual tests for norms.

CRITICAL VALUES:

Immediate action needs to be taken when any of the following occur:

Calcium	<6.5 or >3.5 mg/dL
Carbon dioxide	<15 or >40 mEq/L
Glucose	<40 or >500 mg/dL
Phosphorus	<1.0 mg/dL
Potassium	<3.0 or >6.0 mEq/L
Sodium	<125 or >155 mEq/L

Test Results Time Frame: Within 24 hr

Test Description: The machine called the Sequential Multiple Analyzer (SMA) is the trademark of the Technicon Corporation's automated analyzer. It is a somewhat dated panel that is often replaced with other panels of testing (e.g., basic metabolic panel, comprehensive metabolic panel). Serum can be tested for combinations of sodium, potassium, chloride, carbon dioxide, blood urea nitrogen (BUN), creatinine, glucose, calcium, phosphorus, triglycerides, direct and indirect bilirubin, uric acid, cholesterol, HDL, LDL, lactic dehydrogenase (LDH), alkaline phosphotase, serum glutamic oxaloacetic transaminase (SGOT), SGPT, iron, acid and alkaline phosphatase, and creatinine phosphokinase. The numbers following the SMA correspond to the number of tests being run. The SMA-6 includes sodium, potassium, chloride, BUN, glucose, and carbon dioxide. The other combinations vary with the laboratory used. The machine is equipped with a print-out mechanism that records the results on a graph, which includes shaded areas indicating normal ranges, thus making it possible to evaluate the results at a glance. The machine can do 60 serum specimens at one time.

Consent Form: Not required

List of Equipment: Red-top tube or serum separator tube; needle and syringe or vacutainer; alcohol swab

Test Procedure:

1. Label the specimen tube. *Correctly identifies the client and the test to be performed.*
2. Obtain a 5-mL blood sample.
3. Do not agitate the tube. *Agitation may cause RBC hemolysis*
4. Send tube to the laboratory.

Clinical Implications and Indications:

1. The SMA tests are often done for screening at the time of yearly physical examinations.
2. These test combinations are often done for hospital admission or for initial differential diagnosis.
3. SMA-6 tests are carbon dioxide, total content, blood; chloride, serum; creatinine, serum; potassium, serum; sodium, plasma or serum; and urea nitrogen, plasma or serum.
4. SMA-7 tests are carbon dioxide, total content, blood; chloride, serum; creatinine, serum; glucose, blood; potassium, serum; sodium, plasma or serum; and urea nitrogen, plasma or serum.
5. SMA-12 tests are albumin, serum; alkaline phosphatase, serum; asparte aminotransferase, serum; bilirubin, serum; calcium, serum; cholesterol, blood; glucose, blood; phosphorus, serum; protein, total, serum; urea nitrogen, plasma or serum; and uric acid, serum.

6. SMA-20 tests are alanine aminotransferase, serum; alkaline phosphatase, serum; asparte aminotransferase, serum; bilirubin, serum; calcium, serum; carbon dioxide, total content, blood; chloride, serum; cholesterol, blood; creatinine kinase, serum; creatinine, serum; gamma-glutamyl transpeptidase, blood; glucose, blood; lactate dehydrogenase, blood; phosphorus, serum; potassium, serum; protein, total, serum; sodium, plasma or serum; triglycerides, blood; urea nitrogen, plasma or serum; and uric acid, serum.

Nursing Care:

Before Test: Explain the test procedure and the purpose of the test. Assess the client's knowledge of the test. Instruct client to fast 8–12 hr prior to test.
During Test: Adhere to standard precautions.
After Test: Apply pressure to venipuncture site. Explain that some bruising, discomfort, and swelling may appear at the site and that warm, moist compresses can alleviate this. Monitor for signs of infection.

Potential Complications: Bleeding and bruising at venipuncture site

Contraindications: See individual test listing.

Interfering Factors: See individual test listing.

Nursing Considerations:

Pediatric: Infants and children will need assistance in remaining still during the venipuncture and age-appropriate comfort measures following the test.

WEBLINKS

http://websearch.about.com

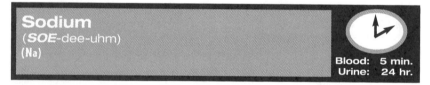

Sodium
(*SOE*-dee-uhm)
(Na)

Blood:	5 min.
Urine:	24 hr.

Type of Test: Blood: urine

Body Systems and Functions: Hematological system

Normal Findings:

Blood:

Adults	136–145 mEq/L	136–145 mmol/L
Cord	116–166 mEq/L	116–166 mmol/L
Infants	139–146 mEq/L	139–146 mmol/L
Children	138–145 mEq/L	138–145 mmol/L

Urine:

Adults	75–200 mEq/L	75–200 mmol/L
Newborns	14–40 mEq/L	14–40 mmol/L
6–10 years:		
Males	41–115 mEq/24 hr	41–115 mmol/L
Females	20–69 mEq/24 hr	20–69 mmol/L

BLOOD

10–14 years:

Males	63–177 mEq/24 hr	63–177 mmol/L
Females	48–168 mEq/24 hr	48–168 mmol/L

CRITICAL VALUES:
Blood: <110 mEq/L

Test Results Time Frame: Within 24–48 hr

Test Description: Sodium is the major cation of the extracellular fluid. Sodium functions by maintaining osmotic pressures, acid-base balances, and transmitting nerve impulses. Sodium is vital to life, and when levels are increased or decreased, there can be serious consequences. Sodium is obtained through dietary intake and is absorbed from the small intestine and excreted in the urine. Normally, sodium levels remain constant. Low levels of sodium stimulate the body to secrete aldosterone. High levels of sodium suppress aldosterone secretion. ADH and ANP are instrumental in regulating sodium and water levels in the body.

CLINICAL ALERT:
A low sodium level can be life threatening. The clinical manifestations are impaired level of consciousness and convulsions.

Consent Form: Not required

List of Equipment: *Blood:* red-top tube or serum separator tube; needle and syringe or vacutainer; alcohol swab. *Urine:* sterile plastic container; ice.

Test Procedure:
Blood:
1. Label the specimen tube. *Correctly identifies the client and the test to be performed.*
2. Obtain a 1-mL blood sample.
3. Do not agitate the tube. *Agitation may cause RBC hemolysis.*
4. Send tube to the laboratory.

Urine:
1. Label the collection container. *Correctly identifies the client and the test to be performed.*
2. Discard the first morning void. Then begin the time of the collection for the next 24 hr, including the void at the end of the 24 hr, and record the last voiding time. *An exact 24-hr count ensures accurate results.*
3. If the client has an indwelling catheter in place, keep the drainage bag on ice and empty the urine into the urine container periodically during the 24-hr period.
4. Keep urine cool during collection. *Higher temperatures alter the results.*
5. If any urine is lost, discard the entire specimen and begin collection again the next day.

Clinical Implications and Indications:
1. Elevated levels (hypernatremia) are found with Cushing's disease, congestive heart failure, dehydration, diaphoresis, diarrhea, diabetes insipidus, hypovolemia, ostomies, toxemia, vomiting, and hyperaldosteronism.
2. Decreased levels (hyponatremia) are found with adrenal insufficiency, Addison's disease, bowel obstruction, burns, hypotension, cerebral palsy, chronic renal failure, myxedema, malnutrition, and cirrhosis.

BLOOD

3. The administration of hypertonic solutions is often the cause of hypernatremia. Therefore, clinical manifestations of increased sodium levels must be
monitored carefully.

Nursing Care:

Before Test: Blood: Explain the test procedure and the purpose of the test. Assess
the client's knowledge of the test.
Urine: Instruct client not to discard any urine over the 24-hr time period.
During Test: Blood: Adhere to standard precautions.
Urine: Adhere to standard precautions. If any urine is accidentally discarded or
contaminated with feces, discard entire specimen and begin test again the following morning.
After Test: Blood: Apply pressure to venipuncture site. Explain that some bruising, discomfort, and swelling may appear at the site and that warm, moist compresses can alleviate this. Monitor for signs of infection.

Potential Complications: Bleeding and bruising at venipuncture site

Interfering Factors: Blood: intravenous solutions with sodium. Urine:
contaminated with feces; spillage or inaccurate collection of the 24-hr specimen,
including nonrefrigeration or placing on ice.

Nursing Considerations:
Pediatric: Children are more susceptible to fluctuations in electrolytes.
Blood: Infants and children will need assistance in remaining still during the
venipuncture and age-appropriate comfort measures following the test. Urine:
Document urine quantity, date, and exact hours of collection on requisition.
Gerontology: The elderly are generally more susceptible to changes in electrolytes.

Listing of Related Tests: Electrolytes; chloride; potassium; CBC; SMA

‖WEBLINKS

http://medlineplus.adam.com

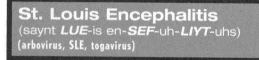

St. Louis Encephalitis
(saynt *LUE*-is en-*SEF*-uh-*LIYT*-uhs)
(arbovirus, SLE, togavirus)

5 min.

Type of Test: Blood

Body Systems and Functions: Neurological system

Normal Findings: Negative

CRITICAL VALUES:
Positive test

Test Description: Antibodies for the SLE virus are detected by the
immunofluorescent antibody assay (IFA). Serological studies may also detect
virus-specific IgM or a fourfold increase in complement-fixing or neutralizing
antibodies.

BLOOD

Consent Form: Not required

List of Equipment: Red-top tube or serum separator tube; needle and syringe or vacutainer; alcohol swab

Test Procedure:
1. Label the specimen tube. *Correctly identifies the client and the test to be performed.*
2. Obtain a 5-mL blood sample.
3. Do not agitate the tube. *Agitation may cause RBC hemolysis.*
4. Send tube to the laboratory.
5. Keep specimen cool. *High temperatures alter the results.*
6. Repeat 10–14 days later for convalescent sample and label the tube as convalescent sample. *Allows for separate identification of the convalescent sample, which is compared in ratio to the acute sample.*

Clinical Implications and Indications:
1. St. Louis encephalitis is not transmitted from person to person. Only infected mosquitoes transmit the virus. Birds and horses may serve as reservoirs of the virus.
2. Testing is often done in both the acute and convalescent stages. The convalescent sample is drawn 14–21 days after the acute event.
3. Cerebrospinal fluid (CSF) may also be sampled with serological test runs. CSF pressure may be assessed at the time of the spinal tap.

Nursing Care:
Before Test: Explain the test procedure and the purpose of the test.
During Test: Adhere to standard precautions.
After Test: Apply pressure to venipuncture site. Explain that some bruising, discomfort, and swelling may appear at the site and that warm, moist compresses can alleviate this. Monitor for signs of infection.

Potential Complications: Bleeding and bruising at venipuncture site

Nursing Considerations:
Gerontology: Symptoms are more severe in the elderly.

Listing of Related Tests: WBC; CSF pressure and protein count

WEBLINKS	⊟ ⊠

www.cdc.gov; www.mayohealth.org; www.vicioso.com

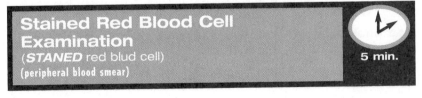

Stained Red Blood Cell Examination
(*STANED* red blud cell)
(peripheral blood smear)

5 min.

Type of Test: Blood

Body Systems and Functions: Hematological system

BLOOD

Normal Findings: No abnormalities in the RBCs

Test Results Time Frame: Within 24 hr

Test Description: Stained red blood cells are obtained by a blood smear, which is stained with the Wright stain and examined under the microscope or counted automatically using a Coulter counter. The slide can be made manually or can be prepared using automated equipment. Red blood cells are identified by their disk shape, light staining center, and lack of nucleus and organelles. Reticulocytes are not seen on normal stained blood smears and would be seen as polychromatic RBCs. Reticulocytes are immature red blood cells and may account for up to 1% of the RBCs in the peripheral smear. Cells are examined for staining ability, cytoplasmic granules, elaboration of hemoglobin, nuclear maturation, structure, cytochemistry, and changes in shape and size. Red blood cells are designed to carry oxygen to the cells of the body. Hemoglobin also contributes to the acid-base balance, acting as a buffer. Malformation of hemoglobin can cause changes in the shape of the erythrocytes (RBCs).

Consent Form: Not required

List of Equipment: Lavender-top tube; needle and syringe or vacutainer; alcohol swab

Test Procedure:
1. Label the specimen tube. *Correctly identifies the client and the test to be performed.*
2. Obtain a 5-mL blood sample.
3. Do not agitate the tube. *Agitation may cause RBC hemolysis.*
4. Send tube to the laboratory.

Clinical Implications and Indications:
1. Changes in the stained red blood cell examination could reflect problems in the development of cells (bone marrow disease/suppression or nutritional deficiencies), infection, destruction in circulation, and genetic problems (see Red Blood Cell Count).
2. Immature cells (reticulocytes) are usually stained darker blue because of a greater amount of RNA in the cytoplasm. Mature cells have a lighter stain.

Nursing Care:
Before Test: Explain the test procedure and the purpose of the test. Assess the client's knowledge of the test.
During Test: Adhere to standard precautions.
After Test: Apply pressure to venipuncture site. Explain that some bruising, discomfort, and swelling may appear at the site and that warm, moist compresses can alleviate this. Monitor for signs of infection.

Potential Complications: Bleeding and bruising at venipuncture site

Nursing Considerations:
Pediatric: Infants and children will need assistance in remaining still during the venipuncture and age-appropriate comfort measures following the test.

Listing of Related Tests: WBC; CBC; bone marrow sampling

| WEBLINKS | ▤ ▧ |

http://www.mc.vanderbilt.edu/histo/blood/erythrocytes.html

Streptococcus
(*STREP*-toe-*KAHK*-:l)
(antistreptolysin O titer (ASO); streptozyme; anti-DNAse B; ADB; streptodornase)

5 min.

Type of Test: Blood

Body Systems and Functions: Immunological system

Normal Findings: Negative for streptococcal antibodies

Test Results Time Frame: Within 24 hr

Test Description: The streptococcal test is used to diagnose streptococcal infections or illnesses by antibody testing. Rising titers over time are more indicative of infection than a single test. *Streptococcus* is a group of bacteria that are gram positive, some of which are the most common and dangerous pathogens for humans. There are several immunological groups designated by the letters A–H and K–O. More than 55 types of group A hemolytic streptocci have been identified, and they are responsible for a variety of illnesess (e.g., scarlet fever, pneumonia, acute rheumatic fever, and acute glomerulonephritis).

> **CLINICAL ALERT:**
> Clients on antibiotics may have a false negative.

Consent Form: Not required

List of Equipment: Red-top tube or serum separator tube; needle and syringe or vacutainer; alcohol swab

Test Procedure:
1. Label the specimen tube. *Correctly identifies the client and the test to be performed.*
2. Obtain a 5-mL blood sample.
3. Do not agitate the tube. *Agitation may cause RBC hemolysis.*
4. Send tube to the laboratory.

Clinical Implications and Indications:
1. ASO titer greater than 166 Todd units is considered positive (note: when run alone, the ASO and ADB tests are 80% positive for streptococcal infection; when run together, the ASO and ADB tests are 90% positive for streptococcal infection).
2. Elevated levels are found with tonsillitis, otitis media, endometritis, scarlet fever, acute rheumatic fever, glomerulonephritis, impetigo, early-onset neonatal infections, late-onset postnatal infections, urinary tract infections, bacteremia, and wound infections.

Nursing Care:
Before Test: Explain the test procedure and the purpose of the test. Assess the client's knowledge of the test.
During Test: Adhere to standard precautions.
After Test: Apply pressure to venipuncture site. Explain that some bruising, discomfort, and swelling may appear at the site and that warm, moist compresses can alleviate this. Monitor for signs of infection.

BLOOD

Potential Complications: Bleeding and bruising at venipuncture site

Interfering Factors: Antibiotic therapy; increased titers may be found in healthy carriers of *Streptococcus*.

Nursing Considerations:

Pediatric: There are a wide variety of neonatal infections related to streptococcal infections. Children also frequently have "strep throat" conditions, which need careful attention and should be cultured for the presence of the streptococcal bacteria (note: antibiotic therapy must be administered for its entire course of prescription to prevent resistance to the antibiotic and to completely eliminate the bacterial infection).

Home Care: Home health care providers should be educated to recognize streptococcal infections and consequently refer their clients for identification of the streptococcal infection.

WEBLINKS	

http://pathbox.wustl.edu

Striational Antibody
(striy-*AY*-sh:n-:l *AEN*-ti-*BAH*-dee)
(striated muscle antibody)

5 min.

Type of Test: Blood

Body Systems and Functions: Neurological system

Normal Findings: No striational antibodies

Test Results Time Frame: Within 24 hr

Test Description: The striational antibody test identifies antibodies to striational muscle, which can aid in the diagnosis of myasthenia gravis. Only 50% of persons with myasthenia gravis will have these antibodies. The acetylcholine receptor (AchR) antibody test is more accurate. Myasthenia gravis is a degenerative neurological disease that causes generalized muscle fatigue, respiratory complications usually due to a compromised diaphragm, altered speech tone, and upper extremity weakness.

Consent Form: Not required

List of Equipment: Red-top tube or serum separator tube; needle and syringe or vacutainer; alcohol swab

Test Procedure:

1. Label the specimen tube. *Correctly identifies the client and the test to be performed.*
2. Obtain a 5-mL blood sample.
3. Do not agitate the tube. *Agitation may cause RBC hemolysis.*
4. Send tube to the laboratory.

BLOOD

Clinical Implications and Indications:
1. Presence of antibodies indicates the presence of myasthenia gravis

Nursing Care:
Before Test: Explain the test procedure and the purpose of the test. Assess the client's knowledge of the test.
During Test: Adhere to standard precautions.
After Test: Apply pressure to venipuncture site. Explain that some bruising, discomfort, and swelling may appear at the site and that warm, moist compresses can alleviate this. Monitor for signs of infection.

Potential Complications: Bleeding and bruising at venipuncture site

Interfering Factors: Hemolysis of sample; plasma sample

Nursing Considerations:
Pediatric: Infants and children will need assistance in remaining still during the venipuncture and age-appropriate comfort measures following the test.

Listing of Related Tests: Acetylcholine receptor (AchR) antibodies; myasthenia gravis antibody

WEBLINKS ⬚☒

http://www.labcorp.com

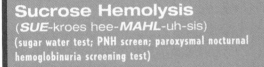

Sucrose Hemolysis
(*SUE*-kroes hee-*MAHL*-uh-sis)
(sugar water test; PNH screen; paroxysmal nocturnal hemoglobinuria screening test)

5 min.

Type of Test: Blood

Body Systems and Functions: Hematological system

Normal Findings: Negative; no hemolysis

Test Results Time Frame: Within 24 hr

Test Description: Sucrose hemolysis is the visual identification of hemolysis of a blood sample when added to a low-ionic-strength sucrose solution. Hemolysis is indicative of paroxysmal nocturnal hemoglobinuria (PNH). PNH is a form of immunodeficiency with the complement component of the immune system. Lysis of red blood cells occurs because of a lack of decay-accelerating factor, which is normally found on red blood cells.

Consent Form: Not required

List of Equipment: Blue-top tube or serum separator tube; needle and syringe or vacutainer; alcohol swab

Test Procedure:
1. Label the specimen tube. *Correctly identifies the client and the test to be performed.*

2. Obtain a 3-mL blood sample.
3. Do not agitate the tube. *Agitation may cause RBC hemolysis.*
4. Send tube to the laboratory.

Clinical Implications and Indications:
1. Hemolysis indicates the possibility of paroxysmal nocturnal hemoglobinuria.
2. The acid hemolysin (Ham test) should be performed to confirm the diagnosis.

Nursing Care:
Before Test: Explain the test procedure and the purpose of the test. Assess the client's knowledge of the test.
During Test: Adhere to standard precautions.
After Test: Apply pressure to venipuncture site. Explain that some bruising, discomfort, and swelling may appear at the site and that warm, moist compresses can alleviate this. Monitor for signs of infection.

Potential Complications: Bleeding and bruising at venipuncture site

Interfering Factors: Hemolysis of sample; clotted sample

Listing of Related Tests: Acid hemolysin (Ham test)

WEBLINKS

www.fpnotebook.com; www.health.ucsd.edu

Sulfhemoglobin
(suhlf-*HEE*-muh-*GLOE*-bin)

5 min.

Type of Test: Blood

Body Systems and Functions: Hematological system

Normal Findings: 0%–1.0% of total hemoglobin

Test Results Time Frame: Within 6 hr

Test Description: Sulfhemoglobin is an abnormal pigment on hemoglobin and is tested when cyanosis is present. The sulfhemoglobinemia is a result of hemoglobin and inorganic sulfides combining. It can lead to hypoxia and cyanosis. Hemoglobin is the iron-containing pigment consisting of the red blood cells, which carry oxygen from the lungs to the tissues. There are a variety of abnormal forms of hemoglobin that cause a number of pathologies (e.g., hemolytic anemia, sickle cell anemia).

Consent Form: Not required

List of Equipment: Red-top tube or serum separator tube; needle and syringe or vacutainer; alcohol swab

Test Procedure:
1. Label the specimen tube. *Correctly identifies the client and the test to be performed.*

2. Obtain a 5-mL blood sample.
3. Do not agitate the tube. *Agitation may cause RBC hemolysis.*
4. Send tube to the laboratory.

Clinical Implications and Indications:

1. If more than 1% of total hemoglobin is sulfhemoglobin, sulfhemoglobinemia is present.
2. Client needs to be checked for administration or ingestion of various drugs and toxins.
3. Cyanosis is usually marked.

Nursing Care:

Before Test: Explain the test procedure and the purpose of the test. Assess the client's knowledge of the test.
During Test: Adhere to standard precautions.
After Test: Apply pressure to venipuncture site. Explain that some bruising, discomfort, and swelling may appear at the site and that warm, moist compresses can alleviate this. Monitor for signs of infection. Provide management for cyanosis.

Potential Complications: Bleeding and bruising at venipuncture site

Nursing Considerations:

Pediatric: Infants and children will need assistance in remaining still during the venipuncture and age-appropriate comfort measures following the test.

Listing of Related Tests: Caroboxyhemoglobin; methemoglobin

| WEBLINKS |

www.hsc.virginia.edu; http://health.msn.com

Syphilis Detection

(*SIF*-uh-lis dee-*TEK*-sh:n)
(FTA-ABS; fluorescent treponemal antibody absorption; RPR; rapid plasma reagin; VDRL; MHA-TP; microhemagglutination assay for *Treponema pallidum* antibodies)

5 min.

Type of Test: Blood

Body Systems and Functions: Immunological system

Normal Findings: Nonreactive test means the person does not have syphilis.

Test Results Time Frame: Within 24 hr

Test Description: Syphilis testing is an antibody test that evaluates antibody production in reaction to syphilis bacteria. Syphilis is a sexually transmitted disorder that is caused by the spirochete *Treponema pallidum*. Screening for syphilis is usually performed during the first prenatal checkup for pregnant women. Syphilis is chronic and is marked by lesions that may affect any organ

BLOOD

or tissue. Typically, syphilis has cutaneous manifestations (small red papules to hard chancre) and has frequent relapses. Syphilis has three stages (i.e., primary, secondary, tertiary). Each stage has specific clinical manifestations that assist in the decisions for treatment options.

CLINICAL ALERT:
VDRL is not as accurate in clients who are immunocompromised, such as persons with HIV disease. An RPR test should be used. In addition, gonorrheal symptoms may exhibit several weeks before syphilis, and therefore the syphilis may go untreated. Therefore, management options for gonorrhea should also include treatment as though the client has contracted syphilis.

Consent Form: Not required

List of Equipment: Red-top tube or serum separator tube; needle and syringe or vacutainer; alcohol swab

Test Procedure:
1. Label the specimen tube. *Correctly identifies the client and the test to be performed.*
2. Obtain a 10-mL blood sample.
3. Do not agitate the tube. *Agitation may cause RBC hemolysis.*
4. Send tube to the laboratory.

Clinical Implications and Indications:
1. Syphilis diagnosis requires correlation of reactive or positive tests and client history.
2. Negative or nonreactive test may indicate the client does not have syphilis or has an infection that is so recent that there are not enough antibodies for reaction, the syphilis is in the latent stage, the client is immunocompromised, or the laboratory technique was poor.
3. RPR and VDRL are nonspecific tests used as screening tests. Positive results indicate the need for a confirmatory test (note: FTA-ABS and MHA-TP are confirmatory tests but do not indicate whether the disease is active, inactive, or cured).

Nursing Care:
Before Test: Explain the test procedure and the purpose of the test. Assess the client's knowledge of the test. Assess client's sexual and genitourinary history. *During Test:* Adhere to standard precautions. *After Test:* Counsel the client. Explain false positives and false negatives. If client is positive, sexual partners should be contacted and tested.

Interfering Factors: Excess chyle in the blood; alcohol consumption within 24 hr decreases reactivity of the test.

Nursing Considerations:
Pregnancy: Active syphilis during pregnancy can damage the fetus and cause anomalies.
International: Underdeveloped countries may not identify the presence of syphilis readily and also not have antibiotic treatment available.

| WEBLINKS |

www.rcpa.edu.au

T3 Uptake
(*TE*-thre *UP*-tayk)
(T3 resin uptake; resin tri-iodothyronine uptake; T3 uptake ratio; T3UR)

5 min.

BLOOD

Type of Test: Blood

Body Systems and Functions: Endocrine system

Normal Findings: 25%–35% of T3 binds to the resin (note: normal values may vary among laboratories).

Test Results Time Frame: Within 24 hr

Test Description: T3 is a hormone secreted from the thyroid gland, which affects every major body organ through its effect on metabolism and protein synthesis. T4 is the precursor to T3, which is responsible for most of the thyroid function. Nearly 99% of thyroid hormones are protein bound. This test is an indirect measurement of unsaturated thyroxine-binding globulin.

> **CLINICAL ALERT:**
> T3 uptake does not measure T3 levels but is an indirect measurement of overall binding. T4 tests should also be done to calculate free thyroxine index.

Consent Form: Not required

List of Equipment: Red-top tube or serum separator tube; needle and syringe or vacutainer; alcohol swab

Test Procedure:
1. Label the specimen tube. *Correctly identifies the client and the test to be performed.*
2. Obtain a 5-mL blood sample.
3. Do not agitate the tube. *Agitation may cause RBC hemolysis.*
4. Send tube to the laboratory.

Clinical Implications and Indications:
1. Clinical implications are limited when evaluated without T4 levels.
2. Decreased T3 uptake levels indicate a high level of unsaturated thyroxine-binding globulin.
3. Elevated T3 uptake levels indicate a high level of unsaturated thyroxine-binding globulin.

Nursing Care:
Before Test: Explain the test procedure and the purpose of the test. Assess the client's knowledge of the test. Instruct client to not take thyroid medication for 6 weeks prior to the test. Instruct client to be NPO the night before the examination.
During Test: Adhere to standard precautions.
After Test: Apply pressure to venipuncture site. Explain that some bruising, discomfort, and swelling may appear at the site and that warm, moist compresses can alleviate this. Monitor for signs of infection. Resume prescribed thyroid medications.

Potential Complications: Bleeding and bruising at venipuncture site

Interfering Factors: Pregnancy; medications that alter results are estrogrens, methadone, heparin, androgens, anabolic steroids, phenytoin, and salicylates.

Nursing Considerations:
Pregnancy: Pregnancy falsely changes T3 levels.
Pediatric: Infants and children will need assistance in remaining still during the venipuncture and age-appropriate comfort measures following the test.

Listing of Related Tests: T4; thyroxine; free thyroxine index; TSH

‖WEBLINKS‖ ▤☒

www.thriveonline.com

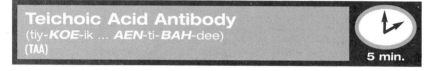

Teichoic Acid Antibody
(tiy-*KOE*-ik ... *AEN*-ti-*BAH*-dee)
(TAA)

5 min.

Type of Test: Blood

Body Systems and Functions: Immunological system

Normal Findings: No antibodies detected

Test Results Time Frame: Within 5–7 days

Test Description: Teichoic acid antibody is a standardized test to establish titers of teichoic acid, a byproduct of *Staphylococcus aureus* infections. This test is useful in diagnosing severe infections and difficult-to-treat infections. Staphylococci are gram-positive micrococci that often cause suppurative conditions by releasing endotoxins destructive to tissue cells. Some staphyloccal infections are the cause of a common food poisoning. *Staphylococcus aureus* is a species that is commonly present on the skin and mucous membranes. *Staphylococcus aureus* also causes a variety of infectious disorders and can even lead to the condition of septic shock.

Consent Form: Not required

List of Equipment: Red-top tube or serum separator tube; needle and syringe or vacutainer; alcohol swab

Test Procedure:
1. Label the specimen tube. *Correctly identifies the client and the test to be performed.*
2. Obtain a 5-mL blood sample.
3. Do not agitate the tube. *Agitation may cause RBC hemolysis.*
4. Send tube to the laboratory.

Clinical Implications and Indications:
1. Greater than 1:2 ratio is suggestive of infection.
2. High levels of antibodies indicate the possibility of endocarditis or bacteremia.

Nursing Care:

Before Test: Explain the test procedure and the purpose of the test. Assess the client's knowledge of the test.

During Test: Adhere to standard precautions.

After Test: Apply pressure to venipuncture site. Explain that some bruising, discomfort, and swelling may appear at the site and that warm, moist compresses can alleviate this. Monitor for signs of infection.

Potential Complications: Bleeding and bruising at venipuncture site

Nursing Considerations:

Pediatric: Infants and children will need assistance in remaining still during the venipuncture and age-appropriate comfort measures following the test.

Listing of Related Tests: Staphyloccal tests

WEBLINKS

www.health.ucsd.edu

Testosterone
(tes-*TAHS*-t:r-oen)
(serum testosterone)

5 min.

Type of Test: Blood

Body Systems and Functions: Reproductive system

Normal Findings:

Pediatric	6 months–8 years	<10 ng/dL
Male	8–10 years	<10–22 ng/dL
Female	8–10 years	<10–50 ng/dL
Male	11–13 years	<10–350 ng/dl
Female	11–13 years	<10 to <50 ng/dL
Male	13–15 years	15–500 ng/dL
Female	13–15 years	<10–50 ng/dL
Adult male		241–827 ng/dL
Adult female		14–76 ng/dL

Note: Normal values may vary among laboratories.

Test Results Time Frame: Within 24 hr

Test Description: Testosterone is the primary male hormone, an androgen, responsible for the development of male characteristics. Blood testing for testosterone is often done to diagnose sexual dysfunction or infertility. It may also be indicative of many hormonally influenced diseases. Recently, testosterone testing has been conducted on athletes to evaluate for the use of performance-enhancing drugs.

CLINICAL ALERT:
Testerone levels fluctuate throughout the day and are highest in the morning.

Consent Form: No

List of Equipment: Red-top tube or serum separator tube; needle and syringe or vacutainer; alcohol swab

Test Procedure:
1. Label the specimen tube. *Correctly identifies the client and the test to be performed.*
2. Obtain a 3-mL blood sample.
3. Do not agitate the tube. *Agitation may cause RBC hemolysis.*
4. Send tube to the laboratory.

Clinical Implications and Indications:

Clinical implications of testosterone

Gender	Increased levels	Decreased levels
Female	Adrenal neoplasms Hirsutism Hilar cell tumor Ovarian tumors Trophoblastic disease during pregnancy	No significance
Male	Adrenal tumors Hyperthyroidism Idiopathic CNS tumor Early puberty Syndromes of androgen resistance	Delayed puberty Down's syndrome Hepatic cirrhosis Hypogonadism Hypopituitarism Klinefelter's syndrome Orchidectomy

Nursing Care:
Before Test: Explain the test procedure and the purpose of the test. Assess the client's knowledge of the test.
During Test: Adhere to standard precautions.
After Test: Apply pressure to venipuncture site. Explain that some bruising, discomfort, and swelling may appear at the site and that warm, moist compresses can alleviate this. Monitor for signs of infection.

Potential Complications: Bleeding and bruising at venipuncture site

Interfering Factors: Alcoholism; estrogen therapy; medications that alter results are steroids and androgens.

Nursing Considerations:
Pediatric: Infants and children will need assistance in remaining still during the venipuncture and age-appropriate comfort measures following the test.
Gerontology: The elderly often have decreasing levels of testosterone.

WEBLINKS

http://pathology.uvm.edu; www.anytest.com

Thrombin Clotting Time
(*THRAHM*-bin *KLAHT*-ting)
(TCT; thrombin time; TT)

BLOOD

5 min.

Type of Test: Blood

Body Systems and Functions: Hematological system

Normal Findings: 20–30 sec (Note: Normal laboratory findings vary among laboratory settings.)

Test Results Time Frame: Within 1 hr

Test Description: Thrombin time is a measurement of stage III fibrinogen defects. The test is a measurement of the time it takes for plasma to clot when thrombin is present. Thrombin is an enzyme formed in shed blood from pro-thrombin that reacts with soluble fibrinogen when converting it to fibin. This process forms the basis of a blood clot. The longer the thrombin time, the greater the bleeding tendencies; the shorter the thrombin time, the greater the ability of the blood to coagulate.

Consent Form: Not required

List of Equipment: Light-blue-top tube or serum separator tube; needle and syringe or vacutainer; alcohol swab; ice

Test Procedure:
1. Label the specimen tube. *Correctly identifies the client and the test to be performed.*
2. Obtain a 5-mL blood sample.
3. Gently invert tube several times, but do not agitate the tube. *Mixes the anticoagulant, but agitation may cause RBC hemolysis.*
4. Send tube to the laboratory.
5. Keep specimen cool. *High temperatures alter the results.*

Clinical Implications and Indications:
1. Elevated levels are found with hypofibrinogenemia, anticoagulant therapy, disseminated intravascular coagulopathy, multiple myleoma, uremia, and severe liver disease.
2. Decreased levels are found with elevated hematocrit, hyperfibrinogenemia, and heparin therapy.

Nursing Care:
Before Test: Explain the test procedure and the purpose of the test. Assess the client's knowledge of the test. If not contraindicated, hold heparin for 48 hr prior to the test.
During Test: Adhere to standard precautions.
After Test: Apply pressure to venipuncture site. Explain that some bruising, discomfort, and swelling may appear at the site and that warm, moist compresses can alleviate this. Monitor for signs of infection.

Potential Complications: Bleeding and bruising at venipuncture site

Interfering Factors: Heparin

BLOOD

Nursing Considerations:

Pregnancy: *Changes in clotting studies need careful observation to detect the beginning clinical manifestations of disseminated intravascular coagulation (a serious complication seen during the latter stages of pregnancy).*

Pediatric: *Infants and children will need assistance in remaining still during the venipuncture and age-appropriate comfort measures following the test.*

WEBLINKS

www.mdadvice.com

Thyroglobulin
(thiy-roe-*GLAHB*-yue-lin)
(T$_g$)

5 min.

Type of Test: Blood

Body Systems and Functions: Endocrine system

Normal Findings:

Adults	3–42 ng/mL or µg/L
Newborns	36–48 ng/mL

Test Results Time Frame: Within 24 hr

Test Description: Thyroglobulin measures the iodine-containing protein, which serves as precursor to both T3 and T4. The test is used to diagnose hyperthyroidism. It is also used to measure success of treatment for thyroid cancer. Thyroglobulin levels drop with successful treatment of the cancer. The thyroid is an endocrine gland located in the anterior neck region and partially surrounds the thyroid cartilage and upper rings of the trachea. The primary action of the thyroid gland is to control the basal metabolic rate. The thyroid gland enlarges in hyperthyroidism (goiter), and it may be removed surgically. In addition, a hypothyroid state may exist (e.g., after a thyroidectomy) and the therapy is to administer a synthetic form of thyroid hormones (e.g., synthroid).

CLINICAL ALERT:
Thyroglobulin may be used instead of nuclear scans in clients with low cancer risk.

Consent Form: Not required

List of Equipment: Red-top tube or serum separator tube; needle and syringe or vacutainer; alcohol swab

Test Procedure:

1. Label the specimen tube. *Correctly identifies the client and the test to be performed.*
2. Obtain a 5-mL blood sample.
3. Do not agitate the tube. *Agitation may cause RBC hemolysis.*
4. Send tube to the laboratory.

Clinical Implications and Indications:

1. Decreased levels are found with thyrotoxicosis factitia and successful treatment of cancer.
2. Elevated levels are found with hyperthyroidism, untreated and metastatic thyroid cancer, thyroiditis, and benign adenoma.

Nursing Care:

Before Test: Explain the test procedure and the purpose of the test. Assess the client's knowledge of the test. Instruct client to not take thyroid medication for 6 weeks prior to the test.

During Test: Adhere to standard precautions.

After Test: Apply pressure to venipuncture site. Explain that some bruising, discomfort, and swelling may appear at the site and that warm, moist compresses can alleviate this. Monitor for signs of infection. Resume prescribed thyroid medications.

Potential Complications: Bleeding and bruising at venipuncture site

Interfering Factors: Autoantibodies to thyroglobulin will decrease levels.

Nursing Considerations:

Pediatric: Infants and children will need assistance in remaining still during the venipuncture and age-appropriate comfort measures following the test. Infants and children have high levels that fall to adult levels by age 2.

Listing of Related Tests: Free T4, total T4, total T3, FTI, TSH, thyroid antibodies

| WEBLINKS |

www.oncolink.upenn.edu

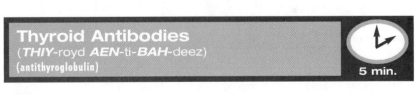

Thyroid Antibodies
(*THIY*-royd *AEN*-ti-*BAH*-deez)
(antithyroglobulin)

5 min.

Type of Test: Blood

Body Systems and Functions: Endocrine system

Normal Findings: Less than 1:100 particles by gelatin particle agglutination

Test Results Time Frame: Within 24 hr

Test Description: This test detects thyroid antibodies and is used to confirm diagnoses related to the thyroid gland. It is also used to monitor disease activity. This test is more accurate when done in conjunction with thyroid microsomal antibodies. The thyroid is an endocrine gland located in the anterior neck region and partially surrounds the thyroid cartilage and upper rings of the trachea. The primary action of the thyroid gland is to control the basal metabolic rate. The thyroid gland enlarges in hyperthyroidism (goiter) and it may be removed surgically. In addition, a hypothyroid state may exist (e.g., after a thyroidectomy) and the therapy is to administer a synthetic form of thyroid hormones (e.g., synthroid).

Consent Form: Not required

List of Equipment: Red-top tube or serum separator tube; needle and syringe or vacutainer; alcohol swab

Test Procedure:
1. Label the specimen tube. *Correctly identifies the client and the test to be performed.*
2. Obtain a 5-mL blood sample.
3. Do not agitate the tube. *Agitation may cause RBC hemolysis.*
4. Send tube to the laboratory.

Clinical Implications and Indications:
1. Elevated levels are found with autoimmune disease affecting the thyroid, hypothyroidism, Hashimoto's disease, Graves' disease, nontoxic goiter, and other autoimmune diseases.

Nursing Care:
Before Test: Explain the test procedure and the purpose of the test. Assess the client's knowledge of the test. Instruct client to not take thyroid medication for 6 weeks prior to the test.
During Test: Adhere to standard precautions.
After Test: Apply pressure to venipuncture site. Explain that some bruising, discomfort, and swelling may appear at the site and that warm, moist compresses can alleviate this. Monitor for signs of infection. Resume prescribed thyroid medications.

Potential Complications: Bleeding and bruising at venipuncture site

Interfering Factors: Up to 10% of the population may have low titers without disease.

Nursing Considerations:
Pediatric: Infants and children will need assistance in remaining still during the venipuncture and age-appropriate comfort measures following the test.

Listing of Related Tests: Thyroglobulin; thyroid microsomal antibodies

---

WEBLINKS

www.thyroid.about.com

Thyroid Antimicrosomal Antibody
(*THIY*-royd *AEN*-tiy-*MIY*-kroe-*SOEM*-:I
AEN-ti-*BAH*-dee)
(anti-TPO; thyroid peroxidase antibody)

5 min.

Type of Test: Blood

Body Systems and Functions: Endocrine system

Normal Findings: Less than 1:100 particles by gelatin particle agglutination

Test Results Time Frame: Within 24 hr

Test Description: Thyroid antimicrosomal antibody is a test to detect thyroid microsomal antibodies and is used to confirm diagnoses related to the thyroid gland. It is also used to monitor disease activity. This test is more accurate when done in conjunction with thyroid antibodies. The microsomal antibodies are a reaction to the thyroid epithelium. The thyroid is an endocrine gland located in the anterior neck region and partially surrounds the thyroid cartilage and upper rings of the trachea. The primary action of the thyroid gland is to control the basal metabolic rate. The thyroid gland enlarges in hyperthyroidism (goiter) and it may be removed surgically. In addition, a hypothyroid state may exist (e.g., after a thyroidectomy) and the therapy is to administer a synthetic form of thyroid hormones (e.g., synthroid).

Consent Form: Not required

List of Equipment: Red-top tube or serum separator tube; needle and syringe or vacutainer; alcohol swab

Test Procedure:
1. Label the specimen tube. *Correctly identifies the client and the test to be performed.*
2. Obtain a 10-mL blood sample.
3. Do not agitate the tube. *Agitation may cause RBC hemolysis.*
4. Send tube to the laboratory.

Clinical Implications and Indications:
1. Increased levels are found with autoimmune disease affecting the thyroid, hypothyroidism, Hashimoto's disease, Graves' disease, nontoxic goiter, and other autoimmune diseases.

Nursing Care:
Before Test: Explain the test procedure and the purpose of the test. Assess the client's knowledge of the test. Instruct client to not take thyroid medication for 6 weeks prior to the test.
During Test: Adhere to standard precautions.
After Test: Apply pressure to venipuncture site. Explain that some bruising, discomfort, and swelling may appear at the site and that warm, moist compresses can alleviate this. Monitor for signs of infection. Resume prescribed thyroid medications.

Potential Complications: Bleeding and bruising at venipuncture site

Interfering Factors: Up to 10% of the population may have low titers without disease; anticonvulsants and sulfonamides cause hypersensitive reactions.

Nursing Considerations:
Pediatric: Infants and children will need assistance in remaining still during the venipuncture and age-appropriate comfort measures following the test.

BLOOD

Listing of Related Tests: Thyroglobulin; thyroid antibodies; thyroid antithyroglobulin antibodies

WEBLINKS 🔲🗙

www.thyroid.about.com/health/thyroid/library/weekly/aa02169
8.htm; www.my.webmd.com

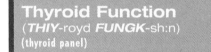

Thyroid Function
(*THIY*-royd *FUNGK*-sh:n)
(thyroid panel)

5 min.

Type of Test: Blood

Body Systems and Functions: Endocrine system

Normal Findings: See individual tests (free thyroxine index; T3; T4; TSH) for normal findings.

Test Results Time Frame: Within 24 hr

Test Description: Thyroid function tests include several different tests, which assess function of the thyroid gland. These tests are most commonly total T3, total T4, free T4, T3 uptake, and TSH (thyroid-stimulating hormone). Total T3 is a measure of triiodothyronine levels in the serum. Total T4 is a measure of the thyroxine level in the serum. Free T4 is a measure of the concentration of free thyroxine in the serum. Since most of T4 is protein bound, it is important to determine the amount of free T4. T3 uptake is a measure of the binding capacity of proteins in the serum for thyroid hormones. It is only useful if total T3 and total T4 levels are also tested. TSH measures the level of thyroid-stimulating hormone in the serum. The thyroid is an endocrine gland located in the anterior neck region and partially surrounds the thyroid cartilage and upper rings of the trachea. The primary action of the thyroid gland is to control the basal metabolic rate. The thyroid gland enlarges in hyperthyroidism (goiter), and it may be removed surgically. In addition, a hypothyroid state may exist (e.g., after a thyroidectomy), and the therapy is to administer a synthetic form of thyroid hormones (e.g., synthroid).

Consent Form: Not required

List of Equipment: Red-top tube or serum separator tube; needle and syringe or vacutainer; alcohol swab

Test Procedure:
1. Label the specimen tube. *Correctly identifies the client and the test to be performed.*
2. Obtain a 10-mL blood sample.
3. Do not agitate the tube. *Agitation may cause RBC hemolysis.*
4. Send tube to the laboratory.

Clinical Implications and Indications:
1. Total T3 is elevated in most cases of hyperthyroidism. It is more sensitive than T4.

2. T3 can be normal and T4 low, indicating hypothyroidism.
3. T3 is often low during acute illness or malnutrition.
4. Free T4 measures are not bound and so are not affected by proteins as are T4.
5. Increased free T4 levels are indicative of Graves' disease.
6. Decreased free T4 levels are indicative of hypothyroidism.
7. If T3 uptake deviates in the same direction as T4 and T3 levels, then there is a true thyroid problem. If T3 uptake deviates from T4 and T3 in the same direction, then there is a problem with binding capacity.
8. Increased levels of TSH indicate primary hypothyroidism.
9. Decreased levels of TSH may reflect hyperthyroidism, secondary or tertiary hypothyroidism, or a problem with the pituitary gland or the hypothalamus.

Nursing Care:

Before Test: Explain the test procedure and the purpose of the test. Assess the client's knowledge of the test. Instruct client to not take thyroid medication for 6 weeks prior to the test.
During Test: Adhere to standard precautions.
After Test: Apply pressure to venipuncture site. Explain that some bruising, discomfort, and swelling may appear at the site and that warm, moist compresses can alleviate this. Monitor for signs of infection. Resume prescribed thyroid medications.

Potential Complications: Bleeding or bruising at venipuncture site.

Interfering Factors: Liver disease; medications that alter results are inderal, steroids, amiodarone, and estrogen.

Nursing Considerations:

Pediatric: Infants and children will need assistance in remaining still during the venipuncture and age-appropriate comfort measures following the test.

Listing of Related Tests: T3 uptake; free T4; total T4; total T3; FTI; TSH

WEBLINKS

www.muhealth.org

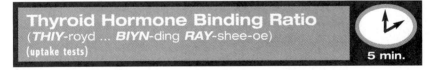

Thyroid Hormone Binding Ratio
(*THIY*-royd ... *BIYN*-ding *RAY*-shee-oe)
(uptake tests)

5 min.

Type of Test: Blood

Body Systems and Functions: Endocrine system

Normal Findings: Normal FT4 and FT3 values with a serum ratio of 1

Test Results Time Frame: Within 24 hr

Test Description: Thyroid hormone binding ratio (THBR) is also known as "uptake" tests. The T3 uptake is an indirect estimate of the thyroid binding globulin concentration and is usually presented as a percent. Recent changes recommended by the American Thyroid Association included calculating a ratio of T3 binding with normal sera having a value of 1.0. The thyroid is an endocrine gland located in the anterior neck region and partially surrounds the thyroid cartilage and upper rings of the trachea. The primary action of the thyroid gland is to control the basal metabolic rate. The thyroid gland enlarges in hyperthyroidism (goiter), and it may be removed surgically. In addition, a hypothyroid state may exist (e.g., after a thyroidectomy), and the therapy is to administer a synthetic form of thyroid hormones (e.g., synthroid).

Consent Form: Not required

List of Equipment: Red-top tube or serum separator tube; needle and syringe or vacutainer; alcohol swab

Test Procedure:
1. Label the specimen tube. *Correctly identifies the client and the test to be performed.*
2. Obtain a 10-mL blood sample.
3. Do not agitate the tube. *Agitation may cause RBC hemolysis.*
4. Send tube to the laboratory.

Clinical Implications and Indications:
1. Elevated levels are found with decreased TBG, hyperthyroidism, hypoproteinemia, liver disease, malnutrition, nephrosis, and a variety of drugs (e.g., androgens, corticotropic hormone, ACTH, penicillin).
2. Decreased levels are found with cretinism, hepatitis, hypothyroidism, pregnancy, and a variety of drugs (e.g., estrogens, heroin, lithium, methadone, and oral contraceptives).

Nursing Care:
Before Test: Explain the test procedure and the purpose of the test. Assess the client's knowledge of the test. Instruct client to not take thyroid medication for 6 weeks prior to the test.
During Test: Adhere to standard precautions.
After Test: Apply pressure to venipuncture site. Explain that some bruising, discomfort, and swelling may appear at the site and that warm, moist compresses can alleviate this. Monitor for signs of infection. Resume prescribed thyroid medications.

Potential Complications: Bleeding or bruising at venipuncture site

Nursing Considerations:
Pediatric: Infants and children will need assistance in remaining still during the venipuncture and age-appropriate comfort measures following the test.

Listing of Related Tests: T3 uptake

| WEBLINKS |

www.thyroidmanager.org

Thyroid Stimulator, Long Acting
(*THIY*-royd *STIM*-yue-*LAYT*-:r lahng *AEK*-ting)
(thyroid stimulation assay; LATS)

5 min.

BLOOD

Type of Test: Blood

Body Systems and Functions: Endocrine system

Normal Findings: No appearance of LATS in blood

Test Results Time Frame: Within 48–72 hr

Test Description: Long-acting thyroid stimulator measures the LATS-induced release of TSH. This blood test helps to diagnose Graves' disease. There is a small percentage of people who will have LATS present but do not have Graves' disease. The thyroid is an endocrine gland located in the anterior neck region and partially surrounds the thyroid cartilage and upper rings of the trachea. The primary action of the thyroid gland is to control the basal metabolic rate. The thyroid gland enlarges in hyperthyroidism (goiter), and it may be removed surgically. In addition, a hypothyroid state may exist (e.g., after a thyroidectomy), and the therapy is to administer a synthetic form of thyroid hormones (e.g., synthroid).

CLINICAL ALERT:
Only performed when simpler studies do not reveal conclusive diagnosis; laboratory values are determined by mouse bioassay.

Consent Form: Not required

List of Equipment: Red-top tube or serum separator tube; needle and syringe or vacutainer; alcohol swab

Test Procedure:
1. Label the specimen tube. *Correctly identifies the client and the test to be performed.*
2. Obtain a 5-mL blood sample.
3. Do not agitate the tube. *Agitation may cause RBC hemolysis.*
4. Send tube to the laboratory.

Clinical Implications and Indications:
1. Increased levels indicates Graves' disease.

Nursing Care:
Before Test: Explain the test procedure and the purpose of the test. Assess the client's knowledge of the test. Instruct client not to take thyroid medication for 6 weeks prior to the test.
During Test: Adhere to standard precautions.
After Test: Apply pressure to venipuncture site. Explain that some bruising, discomfort, and swelling may appear at the site and that warm, moist compresses can alleviate this. Monitor for signs of infection. Resume prescribed thyroid medications.

Potential Complications: Bleeding or bruising at venipuncture site

Nursing Considerations:

Pediatric: Infants and children will need assistance in remaining still during the venipuncture and age-appropriate comfort measures following the test.

WEBLINKS

www.thyroidmanager.org

Thyroid-Stimulating Hormone
(*THIY*-royd *STIM*-yue-*LAYT*-ing)
(TSH; thyrotropin; thyrotropin-releasing hormone stimulation test; TRH; thyroid-stimulating hormone sensation assay)

40 min.

Type of Test: Blood

Body Systems and Functions: Endocrine system

Normal Findings: After stimulation, TSH should increase about two times the baseline. Increase may be greater in women.

Test Results Time Frame: Within 24 hr

Test Description: The thyroid-stimulating hormone test helps to distinguish between primary, secondary, and tertiary hypothyroidism by testing responsiveness of the anterior lobe of the pituitary gland. TSH levels are drawn, thyrotropin is injected, and then TSH levels are redrawn. A rise in TSH levels indicates the pituitary gland is functioning. The thyroid is an endocrine gland located in the anterior neck region and partially surrounds the thyroid cartilage and upper rings of the trachea. The primary action of the thyroid gland is to control the basal metabolic rate. The thyroid gland enlarges in hyperthyroidism (goiter), and it may be removed surgically. In addition, a hypothyroid state may exist (e.g., after a thyroidectomy), and the therapy is to administer a synthetic form of thyroid hormones (e.g., synthroid).

Consent Form: Not required

List of Equipment: Two red-top tubes or two serum separator tubes; two needles and syringes or two vacutainers; alcohol swabs; IV bolus of TRH (thyrotropin-releasing hormone)

Test Procedure:
1. Label the specimen tube. *Correctly identifies the client and the test to be performed.*
2. Obtain a 5-mL blood sample.
3. Do not agitate the tube. *Agitation may cause RBC hemolysis and hemolyzed samples produce inaccurate results.*
4. Give TRH intravenously. *TRH should stimulate the pituitary to release TSH.*
5. After 30 min, draw another blood sample. *Second sample is to be evaluated for TSH level and compared to the first sample.*
6. Send tubes to the laboratory.

Clinical Implications and Indications:

1. No increase in TSH indicates hyperthyroidism and secondary hypothyroidism.
2. Two or more levels of increase are found with primary hypothyroidism.
3. A delay of TSH but then an increased level is indicative of tertiary hypothyroidism.

Nursing Care:

Before Test: Explain the test procedure and the purpose of the test. Assess the client's knowledge of the test. Client should be off thyroid medication for 6 weeks prior to the test. Instruct client to fast the night before the examination. *During Test:* Adhere to standard precautions.
After Test: Apply pressure to the venipuncture site. Explain some bruising, discomfort, and swelling may appear at the site and that warm, moist compresses can alleviate this. Monitor for signs of infection. Resume prescribed thyroid medications.

Potential Complications: Bleeding and bruising at venipuncture site

Nursing Considerations:

Pediatric: Infants and children will need assistance in remaining still during the venipuncture and age-appropriate comfort measures following the test.

Listing of Related Tests: Thyroid function tests

WEBLINKS

http://www.arup-lab.com; http://www.thriveonline.com

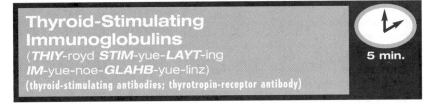

Thyroid-Stimulating Immunoglobulins
(*THIY*-royd *STIM*-yue-*LAYT*-ing *IM*-yue-noe-*GLAHB*-yue-linz)
(thyroid-stimulating antibodies; thyrotropin-receptor antibody)

5 min.

Type of Test: Blood

Body Systems and Functions: Endocrine system

Normal Findings: Less than 1:100 particles by gelatin particle agglutination

Test Results Time Frame: Within 24 hr

Test Description: Thyroid-stimulating hormone immunoglobulins are antibodies that bind to or are near the TSH receptor on thyroid cells. The thyroid-stimulating hormone immunoglobulins stimulate cyclic adenosine monophosphate production and are found in 80% of the people with Graves' disease. It is useful in monitoring progress of the disease. The thyroid is an endocrine gland located in the anterior neck region and partially surrounds the thyroid cartilage and upper rings of the trachea. The primary action of the thyroid gland is to control the basal metabolic rate. The thyroid gland enlarges in hyperthyroidism (goiter), and it may be removed surgically. In addition, a hypothyroid state may exist (e.g., after a thyroidectomy), and the therapy is to administer a synthetic form of thyroid hormones (e.g., synthroid).

Consent Form: Not required

List of Equipment: Red-top tube or serum separator tube; needle and syringe or vacutainer; alcohol swab

Test Procedure:
1. Label the specimen tube. *Correctly identifies the client and the test to be performed.*
2. Obtain a 5-mL blood sample.
3. Do not agitate the tube. *Agitation may cause RBC hemolysis.*
4. Send tube to the laboratory.

Clinical Implications and Indications:
1. Elevated levels are found with Graves' disease and hyperthyroidism.

Nursing Care:
Before Test: Explain the test procedure and the purpose of the test. Assess the client's knowledge of the test. Instruct client not to take thyroid medication for 48 hr prior to the examination.
During Test: Adhere to standard precautions.
After Test: Apply pressure to venipuncture site. Explain that some bruising, discomfort, and swelling may appear at the site and that warm, moist compresses can alleviate this. Monitor for signs of infection. Resume prescribed thyroid medications.

Potential Complications: Bleeding or bruising at venipuncture site

Nursing Considerations:
Pediatric: Infants and children will need assistance in remaining still during the venipuncture and age-appropriate comfort measures following the test.

WEBLINKS

www.arup-lab.com;
http://www.niddk.nih.gov/health/endo/endo.htm

Thyroxine
(thiy-*RAHK*-seen)
(T4; FT4; total T4)

5 min.

Type of Test: Blood

Body Systems and Functions: Endocrine system

Normal Findings:

Adults	4–11.5 µg/dL
Children	6.4–13.3 µg/dL

Note: Normal laboratory findings vary among laboratory settings.

Test Results Time Frame: Within 24 hr

Test Description: Thyroxine is also known as total T4. T4 is usually protein bound, so the T4 test is done in conjunction with the free T4, which is not protein bound. Thyroxine directly measures the level of T4 in the blood and is highly accurate when thyroxine-binding globulin is at a normal level. This test is diagnostic for hyperthyroidism or hypothyroidism and as a way to monitor thyroid replacement therapy or antithyroid drugs. The thyroid is an endocrine gland located in the anterior neck region and partially surrounds the thyroid cartilage and upper rings of the trachea. The primary action of the thyroid gland is to control the basal metabolic rate. The thyroid gland enlarges in hyperthyroidism (goiter), and it may be removed surgically. In addition, a hypothyroid state may exist (e.g., after a thyroidectomy), and the therapy is to administer a synthetic form of thyroid hormones (e.g., synthroid).

Consent Form: Not required

List of Equipment: Red-top tube or serum separator tube; needle and syringe or vacutainer; alcohol swab

Test Procedure:
1. Label the specimen tube. *Correctly identifies the client and the test to be performed.*
2. Obtain a 5-mL blood sample.
3. Do not agitate the tube. *Agitation may cause RBC hemolysis.*
4. Send tube to the laboratory.

Clinical Implications and Indications:
1. Elevated levels are found with Graves' disease, acute thyroiditis, pregnancy, and thyrotoxicosis.
2. Decreased levels are found with primary hypothyroidism, secondary hypothyroidism, protein malnutrition, renal failure, cretinism, tertiary hypothyroidism, and thyrotoxicosis.

Nursing Care:
Before Test: Explain the test procedure and the purpose of the test. Assess the client's knowledge of the test. Instruct client not to take any thyroid medications for 6 weeks prior to the test.
During Test: Adhere to standard precautions.
After Test: Apply pressure to venipuncture site. Explain that some bruising, discomfort, and swelling may appear at the site and that warm, moist compresses can alleviate this. Monitor for signs of infection. Resume prescribed thyroid medications.

Potential Complications: Bleeding and bruising at venipuncture site

Interfering Factors: Increased in infants; values are decreased in adolescents; heparin will falsely elevate values; radioisotopes interfere with the test; clients with severe or chronic illness may have fluctuation of thyroxine levels.

Nursing Considerations:
Pregnancy: Levels increase with pregnancy.
Pediatric: May perform test with as little as 0.5 mL blood. Collect specimens in newborns within 2–4 days of birth. Infants and children will need assistance in

BLOOD

remaining still during the venipuncture and age-appropriate comfort measures following the test.

Listing of Related Tests: T3 uptake, free T4, total T3, FTI, TSH, TBG

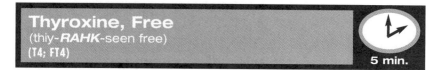

WEBLINKS

http://medline.cos.com

Thyroxine, Free
(thiy-***RAHK***-seen free)
(T4; FT4)

5 min.

Type of Test: Blood

Body Systems and Functions: Endocrine system.

Normal Findings: 280–480 pg/dL. (Note: Normal laboratory findings vary among laboratory settings.)

Test Results Time Frame: Within 24 hr

Test Description: Free thyroxine is also known as free T4. T4 is usually protein bound so the free T4 test is done in conjunction with the total T4 test. This test directly measures the level of free T4 in the blood and is used when there are suspected problems with protein binding. This test is diagnostic for hyperthyroidism or hypothyroidism and as a way to monitor thyroid replacement therapy or antithyroid drugs. The thyroid is an endocrine gland located in the anterior neck region and partially surrounds the thyroid cartilage and upper rings of the trachea. The primary action of the thyroid gland is to control the basal metabolic rate. The thyroid gland enlarges in hyperthyroidism (goiter), and it may be removed surgically. In addition, a hypothyroid state may exist (e.g., after a thyroidectomy), and the therapy is to administer a synthetic form of thyroid hormones (e.g., synthroid).

Consent Form: Not required

List of Equipment: Red-top tube or serum separator tube; needle and syringe or vacutainer; alcohol swab

Test Procedure:
1. Label the specimen tube. *Correctly identifies the client and the test to be performed.*
2. Obtain a 5-mL blood sample.
3. Do not agitate the tube. *Agitation may cause RBC hemolysis.*
4. Send tube to the laboratory.

Clinical Implications and Indications:
1. Elevated levels are found with Graves' disease and thyrotoxicosis.
2. Decreased levels are found with primary hypothyroidism, secondary hypothyroidism, tertiary hypothyroidism, and thyrotoxicosis.

BLOOD

Nursing Care:

Before Test: Explain the test procedure and the purpose of the test. Assess the client's knowledge of the test. Instruct client not to take thyroid medications for 6 weeks prior to the test.

During Test: Adhere to standard precautions.

After Test: Apply pressure to venipuncture site. Explain that some bruising, discomfort, and swelling may appear at the site and that warm, moist compresses can alleviate this. Monitor for signs of infection. Resume prescribed thyroid medications.

Potential Complications: Bleeding and bruising at venipuncture site

Interfering Factors: Increased in infants; values are decreased in adolescents; heparin will falsely elevate values; radioisotopes interfere with the test; clients with severe or chronic illness may have fluctuation of thyroxine levels.

Nursing Considerations:

Pediatric: May perform test with as little as 0.5 mL blood. Infants and children will need assistance in remaining still during the venipuncture and age-appropriate comfort measures following the test.

Listing of Related Tests: T3 uptake; free T4; total T4; total T3; FTI; TSH; thyroid antibodies

█WEBLINKS ▨   ▤▨

www.fpnotebook.com

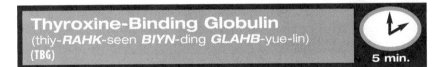

Thyroxine-Binding Globulin
(thiy-*RAHK*-seen *BIYN*-ding *GLAHB*-yue-lin)
(TBG)   5 min.

Type of Test: Blood

Body Systems and Functions: Endocrine system

Normal Findings:

Adult males	1.7–3.6 mg/dL
Adult females	1.7–3.6 mg/dL
Nonpregnant	11.5–332.2 μg/dL
First trimester of pregnancy	19.8–64.7 μg/dL
Second trimester of pregnancy	41.4–63.9 μg/dL
Third trimester of pregnancy	4.7–5.9 mg/dL
On oral contraceptives	1.5–5.5 mg/dL

Note: Normal laboratory findings vary among laboratory settings.

Test Results Time Frame: Within 24 hr

Test Description: Thyroxine-binding globulin measures the binding capacity of thyroxine to protein. It is most useful when other thyroid function tests do

BLOOD

not correlate with the metabolic status of the client, such as with pregnancy or the use of steroids. It is useful in determining causes of hyperthyroidism and hypothyroidism. The thyroid is an endocrine gland located in the anterior neck region and partially surrounds the thyroid cartilage and upper rings of the trachea. The primary action of the thyroid gland is to control the basal metabolic rate. The thyroid gland enlarges in hyperthyroidism (goiter), and it may be removed surgically. In addition, a hypothyroid state may exist (e.g., after a thyroidectomy), and the therapy is to administer a synthetic form of thyroid hormones (e.g., synthroid).

Consent Form: Not required

List of Equipment: Red-top tube or serum separator tube; needle and syringe or vacutainer; alcohol swab

Test Procedure:
1. Label the specimen tube. *Correctly identifies the client and the test to be performed.*
2. Obtain a 2-mL blood sample.
3. Do not agitate the tube. *Agitation may cause RBC hemolysis.*
4. Send tube to the laboratory.

Clinical Implications and Indications:
1. Elevated levels are found with genetic variations, hypothyroidism, infectious hepatitis or other liver disease, and estrogen-producing tumors.
2. Decreased levels are found with genetic deficiency, nephrotic syndrome, major illness or surgery, acromegaly, severe acidosis, testosterone-producing tumors, hepatic disease, and malnutrition.

Nursing Care:
Before Test: Explain the test procedure and the purpose of the test. Assess the client's knowledge of the test. Instruct client not to take thyroid medications for 6 weeks prior to the test.
During Test: Adhere to standard precautions.
After Test: Apply pressure to venipuncture site. Explain that some bruising, discomfort, and swelling may appear at the site and that warm, moist compresses can alleviate this. Monitor for signs of infection. Resume prescribed thyroid medications.

Potential Complications: Bleeding and bruising at venipuncture site

Interfering Factors: Recently administered radioisotopes; medications that increase levels are heparin, dilantin, salicylates, estrogens, and oral contraceptives; medications that decrease levels are steroids and androgens.

Nursing Considerations:
Pediatric: Neonates have higher values of thyroxine-binding globulin. Infants and children will need assistance in remaining still during the venipuncture and age-appropriate comfort measures following the test.

Listing of Related Tests: T3 uptake; free T4; total T4; total T3

| WEBLINKS |

Tolbutamide-Binding Globulin
(tahl-*BYUET*-uh-miyd *BIYN*-ding *GLAHB*-yue-lin)
(orinase)

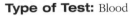

5 min.

Type of Test: Blood

Body Systems and Functions: Endocrine system

Normal Findings: Normal blood glucose levels during administration of tolbutamide

CRITICAL VALUES:
Fasting blood sugars of 50 mg/dL or less

Test Results Time Frame: Within 24 hr

Test Description: Tolbutamide is a hypoglycemic agent that produces hypoglycemia. An IV infusion of tolbutamide raises the serum insulin and causes a rapid decrease in the blood glucose level. Therefore, the test demonstrates the pancreatic beta-cell response to drug-induced stimulation. Insulin is a hormone that is secreted by the beta cells of the pancreas. Insulin is stimluated by a high blood glucose level and is essential for the use of glucose by cells to produce energy. Impaired use of glucose is characterized by hyperglycemia and may be the result of the disease pathology of diabetes mellitus. The tolbutamide testing is one of many laboratory tests performed to verify the potential presence of diabetes or a prediabetic condition.

CLINICAL ALERT:
The expected drop in blood sugars requires extreme caution on clients with fasting blood sugars of 50 mg/dL or less. If the client is allergic to sulfonylureas or sulfonamides, the test should be performed with glucagon or leucine instead of tolbutamide.

Consent Form: Not required

List of Equipment: Grey-top tube; needle and syringe or vacutainer; alcohol swab

Test Procedure:
1. Label the specimen tube. *Correctly identifies the client and the test to be performed.*
2. Take a baseline sample to determine glucose level.
3. Administer IV tolbutamide.
4. Obtain a 5-mL blood sample.
5. Do not agitate the tube. *Agitation may cause RBC hemolysis.*
6. Send tube to the laboratory.

Clinical Implications and Indications:
1. Evaluates fasting or postprandial hypoglycemia
2. Detects the presence of a suspected insulin-producing tumor of the pancreatic beta cells
3. Diagnoses a suspected prediabetic or diabetic condition that may be characterized by excessive insulin release

Nursing Care:

Before Test: Explain the test procedure and the purpose of the test. Assess the client's knowledge of the test. Instruct client to fast 8 hr before the test. *During Test:* Adhere to standard precautions.
After Test: Apply pressure to venipuncture site. Explain that some bruising, discomfort, and swelling may appear at the site and that warm, moist compresses can alleviate this. Monitor for signs of infection.

Potential Complications: Bleeding and bruising at venipuncture site

Interfering Factors: Eating within 24 hr prior to the test

Nursing Considerations:

Pediatric: Infants and children will need assistance in remaining still during the venipuncture and age-appropriate comfort measures following the test. For children suspected of juvenile diabetes, the health care provider must begin assessing the client and family members as to their ability for self-care of this complicated disease process (i.e., diabetes mellitus).

 WEBLINKS

www.medschool.com; www.labcorp.com

TORCH
(toerch)
(toxoplasmosis; rubella; cytomegalovirus; herpes simplex virus)

5 min.

Type of Test: Blood

Body Systems and Functions: Immunological system

Normal Findings: Negative for antibodies to toxoplasma, rubella, cytomegalovirus, and herpes simplex

Test Results Time Frame: Within 24 hr

Test Description: The TORCH test differentiates between acute, congenital, and intrapartum infections caused by such disorders as *Toxoplasma gondii,* rubella cytomegalovirus, and herpes virus. The presence of IgA or IgM antibodies in newborns reflects actual fetal antibody production. High levels of IgM indicates a possible intrauterine infection. TORCH is most useful in ruling out infections versus establishing etiology of infection. TORCH is an acronym derived from the first letters of toxoplasmosis, other transplacental infections, rubella, cytomegalovirus, and herpes virus.

> ### CLINICAL ALERT:
> Sample is obtained from both mother and newborn.

Consent Form: Not required

List of Equipment: Red-top tube or serum separator tube; needle and syringe or vacutainer; alcohol swab

Test Procedure:

1. Label the specimen tube. *Correctly identifies the client and the test to be performed.*
2. Obtain a 5-mL blood sample.
3. Do not agitate the tube. *Agitation may cause RBC hemolysis.*
4. Send tube to the laboratory.

Clinical Implications and Indications:

1. Diagnoses persistent rubella antibodies in infants < 6 months, which is suggestive of congenital infection. Congenital rubella is characterized by neurosensory deafness, heart anomalies, cataracts, growth retardation, and encephalitic symptoms.
2. Toxoplasmosis is diagnosed through sequential testing that reveals rising antibody titers or conversion of serological tests from negative to positive. A titer of 1:256 indicates a recent infection. Two-thirds of infants with infection will be born without symptoms. The remaining third show signs of cerebral calcifications and chorioretinitis at birth.
3. Detects the presence of cytomegalovirus and herpes virus titers that indicate infections.

Nursing Care:

Before Test: Explain the test procedure and the purpose of the test. Assess the client's knowledge of the test.
During Test: Adhere to standard precautions.
After Test: Apply pressure to venipuncture site. Explain that some bruising, discomfort, and swelling may appear at the site and that warm, moist compresses can alleviate this. Monitor infant and counsel appropriately for intrauterine or congenital infections.

Interfering Factors: History of previous infections (mother); cross-reactivity; presence of other serious illness (e.g., HIV); immunosuppression

Nursing Considerations:

Pediatric: Positive results may have serious implications related to sequela of congential infections. Infants and children will need assistance in remaining still during the venipuncture and age-appropriate comfort measures following the test.
International: Testing may not be available in underdeveloped countries.

Listing of Related Tests: Varicella zoster; HIV testing; hepatitis B; enteroviruses; parvovirus B19 (note: none of these tests are commonly included in TORCH panels)

WEBLINKS

www.bcm.tmc.edu; www.slh.wisc.edu

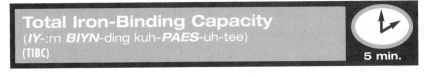

Total Iron-Binding Capacity
(IY-:rn BIYN-ding kuh-PAES-uh-tee)
(TIBC)

5 min.

Type of Test: Blood

Body Systems and Functions: Hematological system

Normal Findings:

		SI units
Children	100–350 mg/dL	18–63 mmol/L
Adults	300–360 mg/dL	54–64 mmol/L
Elderly	200–310 mg/dL	36–56 mmol/L

Test Results Time Frame: Within 24 hr

Test Description: Total iron-binding capacity measures all the proteins available for binding mobile iron. Transferrin is the largest quantity of iron-binding proteins and TIBC is an indirect measurement of transferrin. In addition, ferritin is not included in the TIBC because it binds only stored iron. TIBC only changes in small amounts with increased iron intake. TIBC is a better reflection of liver function and nutrition than iron metabolism.

CLINICAL ALERT:
Observe for clinical manifestations of anemia, such as fatigue and weakness, dizziness, tachycardia, and dyspnea.

Consent Form: Not required

List of Equipment: Red-top tube; needle and syringe or vacutainer; alcohol swab

Test Procedure:
1. Label the specimen tube. *Correctly identifies the client and the test to be performed.*
2. Obtain a 5-mL blood sample.
3. Do not agitate the tube. *Agitation may cause RBC hemolysis.*
4. Send tube to the laboratory.

Clinical Implications and Indications:
1. Elevated levels are found with oral contraceptives, pregnancy, polycythemia, and iron deficiency anemia.
2. Decreased levels are found with hypoproteinemia, cirrhosis, and anemia.

Nursing Care:
Before Test: Explain the test procedure and the purpose of the test. Assess the client's knowledge of the test. Instruct client to fast for 12 hr prior to test.
During Test: Adhere to standard precautions.
After Test: Apply pressure to venipuncture site. Explain that some bruising, discomfort, and swelling may appear at the site and that warm, moist compresses can alleviate this. Monitor for signs of infection.

Potential Complications: Bleeding and bruising at venipuncture site

Interfering Factors: Recent blood transfusion; medications that increase levels are dextran, fluorides, oral contraceptives; medications that decrease levels are ACTH and chloramphenicol.

Nursing Considerations:
Pediatric: *Infants and children will need assistance in remaining still during the venipuncture and age-appropriate comfort measures following the test.*

WEBLINKS

http://adam.excite.com

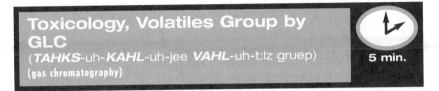

Toxicology, Volatiles Group by GLC
(*TAHKS*-uh-*KAHL*-uh-jee *VAHL*-uh-t:lz gruep)
(gas chromatography)

5 min.

Type of Test: Blood

Body Systems and Functions: Hematological system

Normal Findings: No evidence of drugs in blood

Test Results Time Frame: Variable, depending on the drug (i.e., days to weeks)

Test Description: Blood toxicology tests are performed as part of an autopsy and submitted to state laboratories for analysis. These tests are routine in death related to accidents, occupational work, or suspected criminal cases. Toxicology refers to the division of medical and biological science that is concerned with toxic substances, detecting them, studying their chemistry and pharmacological actions, and establishing antidotes and treatment toxic manifestations, prevention of poisoning, and methods for controlling exposure to harmful substances. Gas chromatography can find evidence of gaseous based toxins, just as in the cases of glue sniffing, solvent abuse, and inhalant abuse.

CLINICAL ALERT:
Usually done with an autopsy to help determine cause of death

Consent Form: Required

List of Equipment: Gray-top tube; needle and syringe or vacutainer; alcohol swab

Test Procedure:
1. Label the specimen tube. *Correctly identifies the client and the test to be performed.*
2. Obtain a 10-mL blood sample.
3. Do not agitate the tube. *Agitation may cause RBC hemolysis.*
4. Send tube to the state forensics laboratory. *State forensics laboratory has proper equipment and technicians to perform volatile toxicology analyses.*

Clinical Implications and Indications:
1. Positive results indicate the presence of inhaled gases such as acetylene, butane, fluorocarbons, toluene, benzene, trichloroethane, and trichloroethylene.

Nursing Care:

Before Test: Explain the test procedure and the purpose of the test to family members. Assess the knowledge of the test. If an autopsy is to be performed, the nurse must transport the client's body to the morgue as soon as possible to keep the body at a cool temperature.

During Test: Adhere to standard precautions.

Nursing Considerations:

Gerontology: In a suspected suicide, emotional support to the family members must be provided.

International: There may be limited access to these tests in underdeveloped countries.

Listing of Related Tests: Toxicology screens

WEBLINKS

www.undcp.org

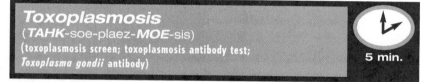

Toxoplasmosis
(*TAHK*-soe-plaez-*MOE*-sis)
(toxoplasmosis screen; toxoplasmosis antibody test; *Toxoplasma gondii* antibody)

5 min.

Type of Test: Blood

Body Systems and Functions: Immunological system

Normal Findings: Titer 1:16, no previous infection; titer 1:16–1:256, previous infection or exposure to *Toxoplasma gondii*

Test Results Time Frame: Within 24–72 hr

Test Description: Toxoplasmosis testing is a serum antibody examination, which tests for levels of antibodies against the parasite *Toxoplasma gondii.* Antibodies to *T. gondii* are prevalent in the adult population. This is because it is found in cat feces, the soil, and undercooked meats. Testing for toxoplasmosis is recommended for pregnant women and for persons with HIV disease. When the titer is greater than 1:256 or in immunocompromised clients, serial tests may be indicated for the clinician to observe for rising titers.

Consent Form: Not required

List of Equipment: Red-top tube or serum separator tube; needle and syringe or vacutainer; alcohol swab

Test Procedure:

1. Label the specimen tube. *Correctly identifies the client and the test to be performed.*
2. Obtain a 5-mL blood sample.
3. Do not agitate the tube. *Agitation may cause RBC hemolysis.*
4. Send tube to the laboratory.

Clinical Implications and Indications:

1. A positive toxoplasmosis test is associated with any value in a newborn, rising titers when serial tests are performed, a titer ratio of 1:256, which indicates recent exposure or current infection; a titer ratio of 1:1,024, which indicates active disease; and a titer ratio of 1:16 or lower, which can occur with ocular toxoplasmosis.

Nursing Care:

Before Test: Explain the test procedure and the purpose of the test. Assess the client's knowledge of the test.

During Test: Adhere to standard precautions.

After Test: Apply pressure to venipuncture site. Explain that some bruising, discomfort, and swelling may appear at the site and that warm, moist compresses can alleviate this. Monitor for signs of infection.

Potential Complications: Bleeding and bruising at venipuncture site

Interfering Factors: Immunocompromised clients

Nursing Considerations:

Pregnancy: The risk of birth defects in women with toxoplasmosis is between 3% and 5%. Toxoplasmosis crosses the placenta.

Pediatric: Congenital toxoplasmosis occurs 40% of the time in pregnant women with toxoplasmosis. Children with congenital toxoplasmosis should be treated for the infection during the first year of life and then have periodic screens thereafter. Infants and children will need assistance in remaining still during the venipuncture and age-appropriate comfort measures following the test.

| WEBLINKS |

www.aidsinfonyc.org

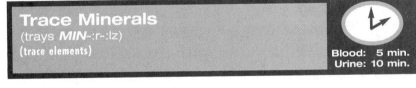

Trace Minerals
(trays *MIN*-:r-:lz)
(trace elements)

Blood: 5 min.
Urine: 10 min.

Type of Test: Blood; urine; hair or nails

Body Systems and Functions: Hematological system

Normal Findings:

Trace minerals

	Conventional units	SI units
Chromium	0.3–0.85 µg/L	5.7–16.3 nmol/L
Cobalt	1 µg/dL	1.7 nmol/L
Copper	130–230 µg/dL	20.41–36.11 µmol/L

Iodine	4–8 mg/dL	
Maganese	4–20 mg/dL	
Zinc	50–150 µg/dL	7.6–23.0 µmol/L

Test Results Time Frame: Within 24 hr

Test Description: Trace minerals are organic compounds found in minute quantities in the body. Trace minerals necessary for body function are cobalt, copper, fluorine, iodine, iron, manganese, selenium, and zinc. Some trace minerals are usually a result of exposure to toxin or poison or ingestion of medications containing a mineral, such as aluminum in aluminum-based antacids. These minerals are aluminum, antimony, arsenic, bismuth, bromine, cadmium, chromium, lead, mercury, nickel, selenium, silicon, tellurium, and thallium.

Consent Form: Not required

List of Equipment: *Blood:* dark-blue-top tube or serum separator tube; needle and syringe or vacutainer; alcohol swab. *Urine:* sterile specimen container; ice. *Hair, nails:* scissors or clippers; specimen container.

Test Procedure:
Blood:
1. Label the specimen tube. *Correctly identifies the client and the test to be performed.*
2. Obtain a 5-mL blood sample.
3. Do not agitate the tube. *Agitation may cause RBC hemolysis.*
4. Send tube to the laboratory.

Urine:
1. Label a sterile urine container. *Correctly identifies the client and the test to be performed.*
2. Obtain a clean-catch specimen of urine (note: first morning voiding preferred, at least 60 mL). *Ensures accurate results.*
3. Keep specimen cool. *High temperatures alter the results.*
4. Send specimen to laboratory.

Hair or nails:
1. Label a sterile container. *Correctly identifies the client and the test to be performed.*
2. Obtain a clean specimen of hair or nails and place in container.
3. Send specimen to laboratory.

Clinical Implications and Indications:
1. Decreased amounts typically occur in clients who are malnourished.
2. Elevated levels are most often caused by environmental contamination (e.g., water pollution, industrial pollution).
3. In more severe cases, management is the administration of parenteral nutrition.

Nursing Care:
Before Test: Explain the test procedure and the purpose of the test. Assess the client's knowledge of the test.
During Test: Adhere to standard precautions. If any urine is accidentally contaminated with feces, discard entire specimen and begin test again.

After Test: Blood: Apply pressure to venipuncture site. Explain that some bruising, discomfort, and swelling may appear at the site and that warm, moist compresses can alleviate this. Monitor for signs of infection. Urine: Document urine quantity, date, and exact hours of collection on requisition.

Potential Complications: Bleeding and bruising at venipuncture site

Interfering Factors: Urine contaminated with feces; spillage or inaccurate collection of the urine specimen; heavy bleeding during menstruation

Nursing Considerations:
*Pediatric: Blood: Infants and children will need assistance in remaining still during the venipuncture and age-appropriate comfort measures following the test.
Urine: A collection bag or insertion of a straight catheter is likely needed for infants and toddlers.*

WEBLINKS

www.arup-lab.com

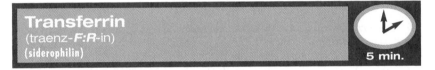

Transferrin
(traenz-*F:R*-in)
(siderophilin)

5 min.

Type of Test: Blood

Body Systems and Functions: Hematological system

Normal Findings:

Adults	200–400 mg/dL
Newborns	130–275 mg/dL
Children	203–360 mg/dL

Test Results Time Frame: Within 24 hr

Test Description: Transferrin is usually a part of iron and total iron-binding capacity blood test, which measures iron stores. Transferrin is the globulin that binds and transports iron. These tests are useful in the diagnosis of anemia and other hematological disorders.

Consent Form: Not required

List of Equipment: Red-top tube or serum separator tube; needle and syringe or vacutainer; alcohol swab

Test Procedure:
1. Label the specimen tube. *Correctly identifies the client and the test to be performed.*
2. Obtain a 5-mL blood sample.
3. Do not agitate the tube. *Agitation may cause RBC hemolysis.*
4. Send tube to the laboratory.

BLOOD

Clinical Implications and Indications:

1. Decreased levels are found with microcytic anemia, protein deficiency, severe burns, malnutrition, renal disease, and chronic infection.
2. Elevated levels are found with iron deficiency anemia, pregnancy, estrogen therapy, and oral contraceptives.

Nursing Care:

Before Test: Explain the test procedure and the purpose of the test. Assess the client's knowledge of the test. Document on laboratory slip if client is taking estrogen or oral contraceptives.

During Test: Adhere to standard precautions.

After Test: Apply pressure to venipuncture site. Explain that some bruising, discomfort, and swelling may appear at the site and that warm, moist compresses can alleviate this. Monitor for signs of infection. Observe for signs and symptoms of anemia.

Potential Complications: Bleeding and bruising at venipuncture site

Interfering Factors: Estrogen therapy; recent blood transfusions; iron-chelating drugs; hemolysis of sample

Nursing Considerations:

Pregnancy: Increased levels found in pregnant women.

Pediatric: Infants and children will need assistance in remaining still during the venipuncture and age-appropriate comfort measures following the test.

Gerontology: Elderly clients are more susceptible to complications from anemia and therefore should be assessed for clinical manifestations of anemia (e.g., fatigue, generalized weakness, and shortness of breath).

WEBLINKS ▯☒

http://pathology.uvm.edu

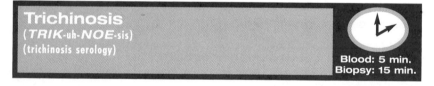

Trichinosis
(*TRIK*-uh-*NOE*-sis)
(trichinosis serology)

Blood: 5 min.
Biopsy: 15 min.

Type of Test: Blood; tissue

Body Systems and Functions: Immunological system

Normal Findings: No findings of the parasite *Trichinella spiralis* in tissue; no antibodies found in blood

Test Results Time Frame: Within 24 hr

Test Description: Trichinosis testing of the blood and tissue is diagnosing the presence of the disease caused by the helminth *Trichinella spiralis*. This helminth is often transferred to humans through the ingestion of uncooked meats, specifically pork and wild animals. The incidence of trichinosis has dropped significantly in the United States with better handling, preparation, and cooking of pork. The infection can be so severe as to cause death, but even in mild cases, symptoms may last for months.

CLINICAL ALERT:
The number of parasites reflects severity of infection.

List of Equipment: *Blood:* red-top tube or serum separator tube; needle and syringe or vacutainer; alcohol swab. *Biopsy:* biopsy tray

Test Procedure:
Blood:
1. Label the specimen tube. *Correctly identifies the client and the test to be performed.*
2. Obtain a 5-mL blood sample.
3. Do not agitate the tube. *Agitation may cause RBC hemolysis.*
4. Send tube to the laboratory.

Tissue biopsy:
1. Place client in position necessary to obtain biopsy of required tissue site.
2. A specimen of tissue is biopsied by excision or needle biopsy. Label the specimen and place in container. *Correctly identifies the client and the test to be performed.*
3. Six to seven needles are inserted into the muscle. *Each needle biopsies a different section of the muscle to increase accuracy of diagnosis.*
4. Send specimen to laboratory.

Clinical Implications and Indications:
1. Antibodies to trichinosis indicate an infection.
2. Microscopic identification of the helminth *T. spiralis* from muscle tissue indicates infection.

Nursing Care:
Before Test: Explain the test procedure and the purpose of the test. Assess the client's knowledge of the test. Provide preprocedure sedation and analgesia as ordered. Transport client to operating or procedure room. Drape client appropriately.
During Test: Adhere to sterile technique and standard precautions. Provide reassurance and a calm atmosphere during the procedure.
After Test: Blood: Apply pressure to venipuncture site. Explain that some bruising, discomfort, and swelling may appear at the site and that warm, moist compresses can alleviate this. Monitor for signs of infection. Biopsy: Clean site of biopsy. Provide analgesia as necessary.

Potential Complications: Bleeding and bruising at venipuncture site; potential bleeding and bruising from tissue biopsy site

Nursing Considerations:
Pediatric: Blood: *Infants and children will need assistance in remaining still during the venipuncture and age-appropriate comfort measures following the test. Biopsy: Sedation is recommended for infants and children. Place the infant or child on a blanket for comfort. After postprocedure monitoring is completed and per health care provider's order, the pediatric client is discharged with an adult who is given instructions.*
Gerontology: The older person may find it difficult to maintain positions when required to do so for lengthy periods of time during the biopsy.

International: Incidence is greater outside of the United States, with greater mortality rates.

║WEBLINKS ▯ ▮▮▮▮▮▮▮▮▮▮▮▮▮▮▮▮▮▮▮▮▮▮▮▮▮▮▮▮ **🗗🗵**

www.cdc.gov

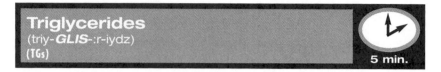

Triglycerides
(triy-**GLIS**-:r-iydz)
(TGs)

5 min.

Type of Test: Blood

Body Systems and Functions: Cardiovascular system

Normal Findings: 30–150 mg/dL

Test Results Time Frame: Within 12 hr

Test Description: Triglycerides are a combination of glycerol with different fatty acids. They are often transported in combination with proteins. The test evaluates for atherosclerosis and thus the body's ability to metabolize fats. Often triglyceride testing is used in combination with cholesterol and fatty acid testing when clients have cardiovascular disturbances. In addition, triglycerides are considered a modifiable cardiovascular risk factor that clients can incorporate into their lifestyle outcomes (i.e., lowering the triglycerides) of managing coronary artery disease.

> **CLINICAL ALERT:**
> Results are more accurate when interpreted with cholesterol levels.

Consent Form: Not required

List of Equipment: Red-top tube or serum separator tube; needle and syringe or vacutainer; alcohol swab

Test Procedure:
1. Label the specimen tube. *Correctly identifies the client and the test to be performed.*
2. Obtain a 5-mL blood sample.
3. Do not agitate the tube. *Agitation may cause RBC hemolysis.*
4. Send tube to the laboratory.

Clinical Implications and Indications:
1. Elevated levels are found with hyperlipoproteinemia, liver disease and alcoholism, nephrotic syndrome and renal disease, hypothyroidism, diabetes mellitus, pancreatitis, myocardial infarction, and gout.
2. Decreased levels are found with congenital alpha-beta-lipoproteinemia, malnutrition, and hyperthyroidism.

BLOOD

Nursing Care:
Before Test: Explain the test procedure and the purpose of the test. Assess the client's knowledge of the test. Instruct client to fast at least 12 hr prior to the test and to abstain from alcohol consumption for 24 hr before the test.
During Test: Adhere to standard precautions.
After Test: Apply pressure to venipuncture site. Explain that some bruising, discomfort, and swelling may appear at the site and that warm, moist compresses can alleviate this. Monitor for signs of infection. Interpret test results and observe for signs of cardiac disease. Instruct on dietary changes such as weight loss, low-fat diet, and exercise program.

Potential Complications: Bleeding and bruising at venipuncture site

Interfering Factors: Recent ingestion of a meal; alcohol consumption; age; oral contraceptives; pregnancy

Nursing Considerations:
Pregnancy: Values may be elevated with pregnancy.
Pediatric: Infants and children will need assistance in remaining still during the venipuncture and age-appropriate comfort measures following the test.
Gerontology: The elderly often have increased levels associated with atherosclerosis. Therefore, health care providers need to carefully assess for clinical manifestations of myocardial disease (angina, dyspnea, fatigue).
Home Care: Health care providers must carefully assess their clients for early symptomatology of heart disease and refer to more specific health care as necessary.

WEBLINKS	🗎 🗷

www.globind.com

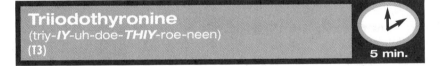

Triiodothyronine
(triy-*IY*-uh-doe-*THIY*-roe-neen)
(T3)

5 min.

Type of Test: Blood

Body Systems and Functions: Endocrine system

Normal Findings: 60–230 ng/dL

CRITICAL VALUES:
<50 ng/dL or >300 ng/dL

Test Results Time Frame: Within 48 hr

Test Description: Triiodothyronine (T3) is one of three hormones secreted by the thyroid gland. T3, in conjunction with T4, is useful in diagnosing hyperthyroidism. T3 is elevated with hyperthyroidism and thyroidtoxicosis. Thyroidtoxicosis is a form of hyperthyroidism where the T4 values are normal while the T3 levels are elevated. T3 is not usually utilized as a test for hypothyroidism.

Consent Form: Not required

List of Equipment: Red-top tube or serum separator tube; needle and syringe or vacutainer; alcohol swab

Test Procedure:

1. Label the specimen tube. *Correctly identifies the client and the test to be performed.*
2. Obtain a 5-mL blood sample.
3. Do not agitate the tube. *Agitation may cause RBC hemolysis.*
4. Send tube to the laboratory.

Clinical Implications and Indications:

1. Elevated levels are found with thyroidtoxicosis, hyperthyroidism, Graves' disease, high dosages of T4, pregnancy and use of oral contraceptives, adenoma, and goiter.
2. Decreased levels are found with hypothyroidism, starvation, recent surgery, recent injury, and kidney or liver disease.

Nursing Care:

Before Test: Explain the test procedure and the purpose of the test. Assess the client's knowledge of the test.

During Test: Adhere to standard precautions.

After Test: Apply pressure to venipuncture site. Explain that some bruising, discomfort, and swelling may appear at the site and that warm, moist compresses can alleviate this. Monitor for signs of infection.

Potential Complications: Increased bleeding may occur due to increased bleeding time.

Interfering Factors: Levels are increased in pregnancy; fasting decreases levels.

Nursing Considerations:

Pregnancy: Triiodothyronine levels are increased during pregnancy.

Pediatric: Infants and children will need assistance in remaining still during the venipuncture and age-appropriate comfort measures following the test.

Listing of Related Tests: Thyroxine (T4)

WEBLINKS

www.healthgate.com

Troponin T
(*TROE*-poe-nin)
[(cTNT); Troponin I (cTnI)]

5 min.

Type of Test: Blood

Body Systems and Functions: Cardiovascular system

Normal Findings: <0.6 ng/mL

CRITICAL VALUES:
>I ng/mL indicates current myocardial injury.

Test Results Time Frame: Within 2 hr (if requested)

Test Description: Troponin is an inhibitory protein found primarily in cardiac muscle. Calcium attaches to troponin, which permits contraction of the heart muscle. Contractility is one of the major properties of cardiac cells, and pathology occurs quickly with disturbances of troponin levels. Troponin is released with relatively small amounts of cardiac injury in as early as 1–3 hr and will remain elevated for 2 weeks postinjury.

Consent Form: Not required

List of Equipment: Red-top tube or serum separator tube; needle and syringe or vacutainer; alcohol swab

Test Procedure:
1. Label the specimen tube. *Correctly identifies the client and the test to be performed.*
2. Obtain a 5-mL blood sample within hours after onset of pain. *Ensures accurate results and efficient management.*
3. Do not agitate the tube. *Agitation may cause RBC hemolysis.*
4. Send tube to the laboratory.

Clinical Implications and Indications:
1. Elevated levels are found with myocardial infarction, chronic muscle disease, and muscle trauma.
2. Identifies severity of cardiac disorder. *Allows for correct and timely interventions.*

Nursing Care:
Before Test: Explain the test procedure and the purpose of the test. Assess the client's knowledge of the test. Explain that this test is sensitive for heart muscle damage.
During Test: Adhere to standard precautions.
After Test: Apply pressure to venipuncture site. Explain that some bruising, discomfort, and swelling may appear at the site and that warm, moist compresses can alleviate this. Monitor for signs of infection.

Potential Complications: Bleeding and bruising at venipuncture site

Interfering Factors: Increased with chronic muscle or renal disease (note: levels are not affected by orthopedic or lung surgery)

Listing of Related Tests: Cardiac isoenzymes; CPK; CK

WEBLINKS	

http://www.howstuffworks.com

BLOOD

Trypanosomiasis Serological
(tri-*PAEN*-oe-soe-*MIY*-uh-sis *SEER*-uh-*LAHJ*-ik-l)
(parasitic culture; Chagas' disease serological test)

5 min.

Type of Test: Blood

Body Systems and Functions: Hematological system

Normal Findings: Negative for parasites

CRITICAL VALUES:
Presence of parasites

Test Results Time Frame: Within 4–7 days

Test Description: Trypanosomiasis is a parasite found in blood, spinal fluid, and lymph nodes. The causative parasites are *Trypanosoma rhodesiense* and *T. gambiense*. Serum is separated from a blood sample and a smear is done to identify the presence of the parasite. Specimens should be transported to the laboratory within 1 hr of collection. It is recommended to take more than one specimen over a period of 3 days. The laboratory testing is performed by the Centers for Disease Control and Prevention or sent to a parasitology laboratory. Alternate sites are also recommended. The clinical manifestations for this disease are central nervous system (CNS) lesions, CNS changes, and meningoencephalitis in children. The course of the disease is months to years, with a high mortality rate.

CLINICAL ALERT:
Diagnosis of parasites usually requires other sites being tested. For example, trypanosomiasis parasitic infection can be tested in blood, spinal fluid, lymph node smear, and serological smear.

Consent Form: Not required

List of Equipment: Red-top serum tube; needle and syringe or vacutainer; alcohol swab

Test Procedure:
1. Label the specimen tube. *Correctly identifies the client and the test to be performed.*
2. Obtain a 5-mL blood sample.
3. Do not agitate the tube. *Agitation may cause RBC hemolysis.*
4. Place the tube on ice. *Ensures accurate results.*
5. Send tube to the laboratory.

Clinical Implications and Indications:
1. A positive smear indicates the presence of the parasite and confirmation of American trypanosomiasis.

Nursing Care:
Before Test: Explain the test procedure and the purpose of the test. Assess the client's knowledge of the test.
During Test: Adhere to standard precautions.

After Test: Ensure specimen is sent to laboratory on ice. Apply pressure to venipuncture site. Explain that some bruising, discomfort, and swelling may appear at the site and that warm, moist compresses can alleviate this. Monitor for signs of infection.

Potential Complications: Bleeding and bruising at venipuncture site

Interfering Factors: Specimen not placed on ice

Nursing Considerations:

Pediatric: Infants and children will need assistance in remaining still during the venipuncture and age-appropriate comfort measures following the test.

International: American trypanosomiasis is endemic in Latin America.

WEBLINKS

http://alice.ucdavis.edu

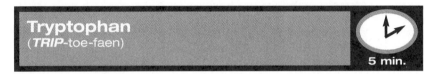

Tryptophan
(*TRIP*-toe-faen)

5 min.

Type of Test: Blood

Body Systems and Functions: Metabolic system

Normal Findings:

Adults	0.51–1.49 mg/dL
Premature infants	0.32–0.92 mg/dL
Full-term infants	0.51–1.49 mg/dL

Test Results Time Frame: Within 24 hr

Test Description: Tryptophan is an essential amino acid and it functions as a precursor for serotonin and niacin. Tryptophan is metabolized by the enzyme, tryptophan pyrrolase, which is deficient in tryptophanuria. Tryptophanuria is an inherited X-linked disorder that results in nonmetabolized trypophan. In addition, blue diaper syndrome is an autosomal recessive disorder caused by a lack of intestinal absorption of tryptophan.

Consent Form: Not required

List of Equipment: Red-top tube or serum separator tube; needle and syringe or vacutainer; alcohol swab; ice

Test Procedure:
1. Label the specimen tube. *Correctly identifies the client and the test to be performed.*
2. Obtain a 7-mL blood sample.
3. Do not agitate the tube. *Agitation may cause RBC hemolysis.*
4. Immediately place the specimen on ice. *Ensures accurate results.*
5 Send tube to the laboratory.

Clinical Implications and Indications:

1. Elevated levels are found with sepsis and tryptophanuria.
2. Decreased levels are found with blue diaper syndrome, kwashiorkor, abdominal surgery during the first 48 hr, carcinoid syndrome, hypothermia, and Hartnup disease.

Nursing Care:

Before Test: Explain the test procedure and the purpose of the test. Assess the client's knowledge of the test. Instruct the client to fast for 8 hr prior to the test.
During Test: Adhere to standard precautions.
After Test: Apply pressure to venipuncture site. Explain that some bruising, discomfort, and swelling may appear at the site and that warm, moist compresses can alleviate this. Monitor for signs of infection.

Potential Complications: Bleeding and bruising at venipuncture site

Interfering Factors: Inability to place specimen on ice immediately

Nursing Considerations:

Pediatric: Infants and children will need assistance in remaining still during the venipuncture and age-appropriate comfort measures following the test.

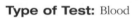

www.nlm.nih.gov

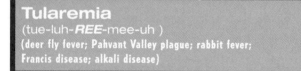

Tularemia
(tue-luh-*REE*-mee-uh)
(deer fly fever; Pahvant Valley plague; rabbit fever; Francis disease; alkali disease)

5 min.

Type of Test: Blood

Body Systems and Functions: Hematological system

Normal Findings: Negative for bacteria

CRITICAL VALUES:
Presence of *Francisella tularensis* (tularemia)

Test Results Time Frame: Within 2–4 days

Test Description: Tularemia is a bacterial infection identified by serology or enzyme immunoassay. It is named after Tulare, an area in California where the disease was first identified. It is a disease found in rodents, resembling the plague, which is transmitted by the bites of fleas, ticks, lice, and flies. It may be passed to humans through the handling of infected animals. An ulcer forms at the site of the bite, followed by inflammation of the lymph nodes, severe headache, other pains, chills, and rapid rise in temperature. Antibody levels rise after 7–21 days of exposure and peak in 60–90 days. The levels decline over several months but are still higher than normal levels. There is also a skin test for the disorder that is performed intradermally.

BLOOD

CLINICAL ALERT:
Not routinely cultured and therefore often is undetected. When the disease is present, there is a fourfold increase in titer levels.

Consent Form: Not required

List of Equipment: Red-top tube or serum separator tube; needle and syringe or vacutainer; alcohol swab

Test Procedure:
1. Label the serum tube. *Correctly identifies the client and the test to be performed.*
2. Obtain a 5-mL serum sample.
3. Do not agitate the serum tube. *Agitation may cause RBC hemolysis.*
4. Send tube to the laboratory.
5. Repeat the test in 3–5 days. *Observes for rising titer levels.*

Clinical Implications and Indications:
1. A positive smear indicates the presence of the bacteria and confirms tularemia.

Nursing Care:
Before Test: Explain the test procedure and the purpose of the test. Assess the client's knowledge of the test.
During Test: Adhere to standard precautions.
After Test: Apply pressure to venipuncture site. Explain that some bruising, discomfort, and swelling may appear at the site and that warm, moist compresses can alleviate this. Monitor for signs of infection.

Potential Complications: Bleeding and bruising at venipuncture site

Interfering Factors: *Brucella abortus; Proteus vulgaris;* drawing levels too early in the infectious process; skin testing for disease within the previous 7 days

Nursing Considerations:
Pediatric: Infants and children will need assistance in remaining still during the venipuncture and age-appropriate comfort measures following the test.
Rural: Instruct people that routinely handle animals to wear gloves as protection against this disease. Also, educate those in rural settings to cook wild animal meat thoroughly. Avoid skin contact with persons that have the disease.

WEBLINKS

http://www.methodisthealth.com

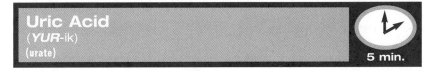

Uric Acid
(*YUR*-ik)
(urate)

5 min.

Type of Test: Blood

Body Systems and Functions: Renal/urological system

BLOOD

Normal Findings:

Adults:

Males	2.0–8.5 mg/dL
Females	2.0–8.0 mg/dL

Children:

Males	2.0–5.5 mg/dL
Females	2.0–4.0 mg/dL

CRITICAL VALUES:

Uric acid levels tend to vary from day to day and between various laboratories, and therefore uric acid levels are often repeated.

Test Results Time Frame: Within 2–3 hr

Test Description: Uric acid is the end product of protein breakdown, both dietary and body protein. The kidneys excrete uric acid as a waste product. Excess uric acid may be caused from kidney failure, which produces an increase in uric acid due to the inability of the kidneys to excrete uric acid. Some malignancies, like leukemia, cause the destruction of nucleic acid and purine products, which produces an elevation of uric acid. Gout causes increased cell breakdown, and catabolism of nucleonic acids increases the uric acid levels. Increased uric acid levels may be a warning of one of these pathological conditions.

CLINICAL ALERT:

Uric acid levels should be monitored during the treatment of leukemia, due to increased levels from the disease and from the increased uric acid from chemotherapy and radiation therapy.

Consent Form: Not required

List of Equipment: Red-top tube or serum separator tube; needle and syringe or vacutainer; alcohol swab

Test Procedure:

1. Label the specimen tube. *Correctly identifies the client and the test to be performed.*
2. Obtain a 5- to 10-mL blood sample.
3. Do not agitate the tube. *Agitation may cause RBC hemolysis.*
4. Send tube to the laboratory.

Clinical Implications and Indications:

1. Elevated levels are found with renal disease, gout, leukemia, multiple myeloma, Down's syndrome, starvation, alcoholism, lymphoma, congestive heart failure, lead poisoning, metabolic acidosis, chemotherapy, radiation therapy, and psoriasis.
2. Decreased levels are found with Fanconi's syndrome, Wilson's disease, and some malignancies.

Nursing Care:

Before Test: Explain the test procedure and the purpose of the test. Assess the client's knowledge of the test.

BLOOD

During Test: Adhere to standard precautions.

After Test: Apply pressure to venipuncture site. Explain that some bruising, discomfort, and swelling may appear at the site and that warm, moist compresses can alleviate this. Monitor for signs of infection.

Potential Complications: Bleeding and bruising at venipuncture site

Interfering Factors: Many medications can increase or decrease uric acid levels; excessive stress, exercise, and fasting cause elevations in uric acid; a diet high in purine (liver, kidney) increases uric acid levels; high doses of aspirin decrease uric acid levels.

Nursing Considerations:

Pregnancy: Levels fall about one-third, then return to normal by term.

Pediatric: Infants and children will need assistance in remaining still during the venipuncture and age-appropriate comfort measures following the test.

Listing of Related Tests: Urine uric acid

WEBLINKS

http://www.creighton.edu

Uroporphyrinogen I Synthase
(*YUR*-oe-peor-fuh-*RIN*-oe-jen ... *SIN*-thays)

5 min.

Type of Test: Blood

Body Systems and Functions: Endocrine system

Normal Findings: 8.1–16.8 nmol/L in women; 7.2–14.7 nmol/L in men

CRITICAL VALUES:
Women: <8 nmol/L; men: <7 nmol/L

Test Results Time Frame: Within 48 hr

Test Description: Uroporphyrinogen I synthase is determined by measuring the conversion of porphobilinogen to uroporphyrinogen. This test is used to identify those clients at risk for porphyria and to diagnose the disease during an episode. Porphyria is a condition where abnormal levels of porphyrins accumulate in body fluids due to a deficit in the enzymes involved in porphyrin metabolism. Clients who manifest symptoms of unexplained neurological disorders, unexplained abdominal pain, blisters on the skin, or a significant family history could be candidates for this test.

Consent Form: Not required

List of Equipment: Red-top tube or serum separator tube; needle and syringe or vacutainer; alcohol swab

BLOOD

Test Procedure:
1. Label the specimen tube. *Correctly identifies the client and the test to be performed.*
2. Obtain a 5-mL blood sample.
3. Do not agitate the tube. *Agitation may cause RBC hemolysis.*
4. Send tube to the laboratory.

Clinical Implications and Indications:
1. Decreased levels indicate porphyria (acute intermittent porphyria).
2. Test results must be combined with clinical findings to be meaningful.

Nursing Care:
Before Test: Explain the test procedure and the purpose of the test. Assess the client's knowledge of the test. Instruct client to fast at midnight prior to the test.
During Test: Adhere to standard precautions.
After Test: Apply pressure to venipuncture site. Explain that some bruising, discomfort, and swelling may appear at the site and that warm, moist compresses can alleviate this. Monitor for signs of infection.

Potential Complications: Bleeding and bruising at venipuncture site

Interfering Factors: Diet low in carbohydrates; alcohol; liver diseases; bleeding disorders; failure to fast overnight; medications that alter results are barbiturates, chlordiazepoxide, chloroquine, dichloralphenaxone, ergot, estrogens, glutethimide, gresfulvin, hydantoins, imipramine, meprobamate, methyldopa, methyprylon, phenytoin, steroid hormones, and sulfonamides

Nursing Considerations:
Pediatric: Infants and children will need assistance in remaining still during the venipuncture and age-appropriate comfort measures following the test.

Listing of Related Tests: Porphyrins; free erythrocyte protoporphyrin

WEBLINKS ▶	▤ ☒

http://www.niddk.nih.gov

Varicella-Zoster Antibody Titer
(*VAHR*-uh-*SEL*-uh *ZAHS*-t:r *AEN*-ti-*BAH*-dee *TIYT*-:r)

5 min.

Type of Test: Blood

Body Systems and Functions: Immunological system

Normal Findings: Negative findings are interpreted as the client being susceptible to the herpes zoster virus.

Test Results Time Frame: Within 3 days

Test Description: Varicella-zoster antibody titer is the test performed to determine the immunity of the herpes zoster virus, which can cause both chicken pox (varicella) and shingles (herpes zoster). These are time-limited disorders that produce skin lesions. The virus is transmitted directly from client to client, indirectly through contact with contaminated objects, or airborne spread from infected respiratory secretions. The virus multiplies in the respiratory tract and then spreads through the bloodstream to the skin and then the internal organs. To diagnose an acute infection, scrapings of the vesicles are cultured. There is a varicella vaccine.

CLINICAL ALERT:
The incubation period for chickenpox is 10–15 days. The client is infectious for 5 days after the appearance of the rash. Immunosuppressed clients should be kept away from individuals without immunity to the disease, since chickenpox can be fatal to immunosuppressed clients.

Consent Form: Not required

List of Equipment: Red-top tube or serum separator tube; needle and syringe or vacutainer; alcohol swab

Test Procedure:
1. Label the specimen tube. *Correctly identifies the client and the test to be performed.*
2. Obtain a 5-mL blood sample within hours after onset of pain.
3. Do not agitate the tube. *Agitation may cause RBC hemolysis.*
4. Send tube to the laboratory.
5. Repeat 10–14 days later for convalescent sample and label the tube as convalescent sample. *Allows for separate identification of the convalescent sample, which is compared in ratio to the acute sample.*

Clinical Implications and Indications:
1. Positive results without clinical manifestations indicate immunity to the herpes zoster virus (usually from previous infection).
2. Elevated levels are found with current infection of chickenpox and herpes zoster (shingles).

Nursing Care:
Before Test: Explain the test procedure and the purpose of the test. Assess the client's knowledge of the test.
During Test: Adhere to standard precautions.
After Test: Apply pressure to venipuncture site. Explain that some bruising, discomfort, and swelling may appear at the site and that warm, moist compresses can alleviate this. Monitor for signs of infection.

Potential Complications: Bleeding and bruising at venipuncture site; anabolic steroids increase severity of varicella-associated pneumonia.

Nursing Considerations:
Pediatric: Infants and children will need assistance in remaining still during the venipuncture and age-appropriate comfort measures following the test. Children are usually more prone to being infected with the chickenpox disease.
Gerontology: Caution needs to be emphasized with the elderly in regard to exposure to the virus, as they are more susceptible to the complications associated with the shingles disorder.

WEBLINKS

http://www.nlm.nih.gov

Vasoactive Intestinal Polypeptide
(vay-zoe-**AEK**-tiv in-**TEST**-in-:l **PAHL**-ee-**PEP**-tiyd)
(VIP)

5 min.

Type of Test: Blood

Body Systems and Functions: Endocrine system

Normal Findings: <75 pg/mL

> **CRITICAL VALUES:**
> >75 pg/mL

Test Results Time Frame: Within 5 days

Test Description: Vasoactive intestinal polypeptide performs a wide variety of functions. For example, it produces bronchial dilation of the respiratory system and vasodilatation in the cardiovascular system, stimulates GI water in the digestive tract, relaxes the intestinal smooth muscles, and stimulates the release of pancreatic islet cell hormones, including insulin and glucagon. Tumors called VIPomas are the principal cause of hypersecretion of VIP. This test is used when symptoms of hypersecretion are present.

Consent Form: Not required

List of Equipment: Lavender-top tube or plasma separator tube; needle and syringe or vacutainer; alcohol swab

Test Procedure:
1. Label the specimen tube. *Correctly identifies the client and the test to be performed.*
2. Obtain a 7-mL blood sample.
3. Gently invert tube several times, but do not agitate the tube. *Mixes the anticoagulant, but agitation may cause RBC hemolysis.*
4. Send tube to the laboratory.
5. Keep specimen cool. *High temperatures alter the results.*

Clinical Implications and Indications:
1. Diagnoses VIPomas, a group of tumors causing hypersecretion of VIP.
2. Diagnoses Verner-Morrison syndrome (a watery diarrhea condition).
3. Pancreatic cholera produces elevated VIP levels (>75 pg/mL).

Nursing Care:
Before Test: Explain the test procedure and the purpose of the test. Assess the client's knowledge of the test.
During Test: Adhere to standard precautions.
After Test: Apply pressure to venipuncture site. Explain that some bruising, discomfort, and swelling may appear at the site and that warm, moist compresses can alleviate this. Monitor for signs of infection.

Potential Complications: Bleeding and bruising at venipuncture site

Interfering Factors: Failure to ice specimen in transport

BLOOD

Nursing Considerations:
Pediatric: *Infants and children will need assistance in remaining still during the venipuncture and age-appropriate comfort measures following the test.*

Listing of Related Tests: Gastrointestinal polypeptides

WEBLINKS ▯▯

www.healthgate.com

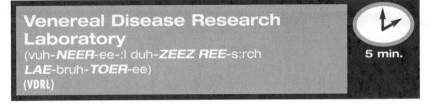

Venereal Disease Research Laboratory
(vuh-*NEER*-ee-:l duh-*ZEEZ REE*-s:rch *LAE*-bruh-*TOER*-ee)
(VDRL)

5 min.

Type of Test: Blood

Body Systems and Functions: Reproductive system

Normal Findings: Blood is nonreactive to this test.

Test Results Time Frame: Within 1–2 hr

Test Description: The VDRL detects syphilis and was named for the laboratory that developed it. Early in the course of syphilis, a globulin called reagin is produced. The VDRL test actually tests for the presence of reagin and not the spirochete, which produces the disease. Syphilis is a very complex sexually transmitted disease that has a wide variety of clinical manifestations and is caused by *Treponema pallidum*. The VDRL tests positive during the primary and secondary stages of the disease. The VDRL will test negative during treatment or during the tertiary stage of syphilis. Due to this indirect testing mechanism, there are a number of conditions that may cause a false positive due to the production of reagin. Malaria, mononucleosis, and leprosy can produce false positives.

> **CLINICAL ALERT:**
> Since excess chyle in the blood interferes with the test, blood should not be drawn immediately after a meal.

Consent Form: Not required

List of Equipment: Red-top tube or serum separator tube; needle and syringe or vacutainer; alcohol swab

Test Procedure:
1. Label the specimen tube. *Correctly identifies the client and the test to be performed.*
2. Obtain a 5-mL blood sample.
3. Do not agitate the tube. *Agitation may cause RBC hemolysis.*
4. Send tube to the laboratory.

Clinical Implications and Indications:
1. Indicates the presence of primary or secondary syphilis when combined with client history and physical findings.

2. Negative findings may indicate that the contact was too recent to have produced antibodies to the disease.

3. Positive findings need to be cross-checked with the many possible false-negative situations.

Nursing Care:

Before Test: Explain the test procedure and the purpose of the test. Assess the client's knowledge of the test. Ensure that the client has not consumed alcohol for 24 hr prior to the test. Conduct specific sexual activity assessment prior to the VDRL test.

During Test: Adhere to standard precautions.

After Test: Apply pressure to venipuncture site. Explain that some bruising, discomfort, and swelling may appear at the site and that warm, moist compresses can alleviate this. Monitor for signs of infection. Follow-up instructions to client who tests positive are detailed under Nursing Considerations.

Potential Complications: Bleeding and bruising at venipuncture site

Interfering Factors: Any diseases that produce reagin; connective tissue diseases; malaria; infectious mononucleosis; hepatitis; active immunization in children; chickenpox; pneumonia; fever; measles; tuberculosis; cold virus; pregnancy; consumption of alcohol within 24 hr

Nursing Considerations:

Pregnancy: All sexual contacts within the last 90 days must be reported if there is a positive VDRL test. Use condoms for 2–4 months after treatment for a positive VDRL. Inform client that becoming pregnant within 2 years may spread syphilis to the fetus.

Pediatric: The fetus is susceptible to congenital abnormalities in a positive VDRL test of the mother. Infants and children will need assistance in remaining still during the venipuncture and age-appropriate comfort measures following the test.

Listing of Related Tests: RPR

WEBLINKS

http://www.pstcc.cc.tn.us

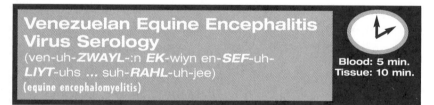

Venezuelan Equine Encephalitis Virus Serology
(ven-uh-*ZWAYL*-:n *EK*-wiyn en-*SEF*-uh-*LIYT*-uhs ... suh-*RAHL*-uh-jee)
(equine encephalomyelitis)

Blood: 5 min.
Tissue: 10 min.

Type of Test: Blood; tissue

Body Systems and Functions: Hematological system

Normal Findings: Negative for virus

CRITICAL VALUES:
Presence of virus

Test Results Time Frame: Within 3–5 days

Test Description: Venezuelan equine encephalitis virus serology tests a sample of blood or cerebrospinal fluid to identify this infection. This disease is caused by a group A arbovirus and is an intracellular parasite that must be cultured in special laboratories using animal tissue. This disease is found in horses but is communicable to humans. Symptoms include disorientation, paralysis, fever, and coma. In addition, mosquitoes transmit the virus from the host to humans.

Consent Form: Not required

List of Equipment: Red-top tube or serum separator tube; needle and syringe or vacutainer; alcohol swab; swabs; specimen cup

Test Procedure:
Blood:
1. Collect the specimen within 72 hr of infection. *Virus is in greatest numbers.*
2. Label the specimen tube. *Correctly identifies the client and the test to be performed.*
3. Obtain a 5-mL blood sample.
4. Do not agitate the tube. *Agitation may cause RBC hemolysis.*
5. Repeat 10–14 days later for convalescent sample and label the tube as convalescent sample. *Allows for separate identification of the convalescent sample, which is compared in ratio to the acute sample.*

Tissue:
1. Label specimen container. *Correctly identifies the client and the test to be performed.*
2. Obtain specimen with swab. Do not allow the specimen to dry out (if using swab). *Facilitates the virus survival.*
3. Transport the specimen to the laboratory in the appropriate solution or medium. *Keeps the virus alive.*

Clinical Implications and Indications:
1. Diagnoses Venezuelan equine encephalitis, which can lead to convulsions and coma

Nursing Care:
Before Test: Explain the test procedure and the purpose of the test. Assess the client's knowledge of the test.
During Test: Adhere to standard precautions. Avoid cross-contamination of the specimen to prevent a false positive.
After Test: Apply pressure to venipuncture site. Explain that some bruising, discomfort, and swelling may appear at the site and that warm, moist compresses can alleviate this. Monitor for signs of infection.

Potential Complications: Bleeding and bruising at venipuncture site

Interfering Factors: Not transporting the specimen in the appropriate medium (note: many viruses should be transported in a balanced salt solution)

Nursing Considerations:
Pediatric: Infants and children will need assistance in remaining still during the venipuncture and age-appropriate comfort measures following the test.
Rural: Transmission of this virus is from horses to human and therefore could be suspected more in rural settings. Wear insect-repellant spray or lotion when outdoors in areas the virus is present.
International: Occurrence of this disease is primarily in South America, Mexico, Central America, and the United States.

WEBLINKS

http://www.methodisthealth.com

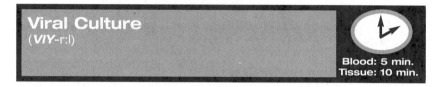

Viral Culture
(*VIY*-r:l)

Blood: 5 min.
Tissue: 10 min.

Type of Test: Blood; tissue

Body Systems and Functions: Immunological system

Normal Findings: Negative for virus

CRITICAL VALUES:
Presence of virus

Test Results Time Frame: Within 3–5 days

Test Description: A viral culture is used to identify a viral infection. Since the virus is an intracellular parasite, it must be cultured in special laboratories using animal tissue. The virus is the most common of all human infections. Viruses are made of either DNA or RNA and are surrounded by an envelope of protein. It causes some of the most deadly diseases with many viruses producing a high mortality rate. However, some viruses will only produce a mild infection.

Consent Form: Not required

List of Equipment: Equipment dependent on site of virus. *Blood:* blood tube, needle and syringe or vacutainer; alcohol swab. *Tissue:* swabs; specimen cups for urine or stool or tissue; viral transport medium for culture.

Test Procedure:
Blood:
1. Label the specimen tube. *Correctly identifies the client and the test to be performed.*
2. Obtain a 5-mL blood sample within 72 hr of infection. *Virus is in greatest numbers.*
3. Do not agitate the tube. *Agitation may cause RBC hemolysis.*
4. Send tube to the laboratory.

5. Keep specimen cool. *High temperatures alter the results.*
6. Repeat 10–14 days later for convalescent sample and label the tube as convalescent sample. *Allows for separate identification of the convalescent sample, which is compared in ratio to the acute sample.*

Tissue:
1. Label the culture tube. *Correctly identifies the client and the test to be performed.*
2. Do not allow the specimen to dry out. *Facilitates virus survival.*
3. Transport the specimen to the laboratory in the appropriate solution or medium. *Keeps the virus alive.*

Clinical Implications and Indications:
1. Virus cultures detect a wide variety of viral diseases with many etiologies.
2. Diagnoses many sexually transmitted diseases, such as AIDS, hepatitis, herpes, and human papillomavirus.
3. Detects some of the respiratory viral infections, which include influenza, rhinovirus, and adenovirus.
4. Diagnoses many disorders of the integumentary system, such as herpes simplex and varicella-zoster (these affect the skin and mucous membranes).
5. Diagnoses the presence of viral disorders of the central nervous system: rabies, polio, meningitis, and encephalitis.

Nursing Care:
Before Test: Explain the test procedure and the purpose of the test. Assess the client's knowledge of the test.
During Test: Adhere to standard precautions. Avoid cross-contamination of the specimen to prevent a false positive.
After Test: Blood: Apply pressure to venipuncture site. Explain that some bruising, discomfort, and swelling may appear at the site and that warm, moist compresses can alleviate this. Monitor for signs of infection. A convalescent blood sample is often needed 14–28 hr after the initial sample. Tissue: Dependent on the site cultured.

Potential Complications: Bleeding and bruising at venipuncture site

Interfering Factors: Not transporting the specimen in the appropriate medium (note: many viruses should be transported in a balanced salt solution)

Nursing Considerations:
Pediatric: Infants and children will need assistance in remaining still during the procedure and age-appropriate comfort measures following the test.
Gerontology: Many viral infections can be particularly affecting to the elderly population. These clients must be carefully monitored during their illness.
Home Care: Particular attention to standard precautions needs to be monitored by the health care provider in the home setting to prevent communicability.

WEBLINKS

http://adam.excite.com

Viscosity
(vis-**KAHS**-uh-tee)

5 min.

Type of Test: Blood

Body Systems and Functions: Hematological system

Normal Findings: 1.4–1.75 relative to water

Test Results Time Frame: Within 24–48 hr

Test Description: Serum viscosity is a test that determines the time it takes blood to pass through a capillary tube. Low-viscosity fluids flow freely, while high-viscosity fluids move more slowly. This measurement helps in the diagnosis of hyperviscosity diseases that produce increased protein in the blood. The test is performed by comparing the viscosity of serum to water at room temperature (note: the serum is normally more viscous than water).

Consent Form: Not required

List of Equipment: Red-top tube or serum separator tube; needle and syringe or vacutainer; alcohol swab

Test Procedure:
1. Label the specimen tube. *Correctly identifies the client and the test to be performed.*
2. Obtain a 10-mL blood sample within hours after onset of pain.
3. Do not agitate the tube. *Agitation may cause RBC hemolysis.*
4. Send tube to the laboratory.

Clinical Implications and Indications:
1. Assists in the diagnosis of multiple myeloma.
2. Hyperviscosity can lead to complications with the heart, vascular system, kidneys, and coagulation problems.
3. Elevated levels are found with arthritis, dysproteinemias, systemic lupus erythematosus, and hyperfibrinogenemia.

Nursing Care:
Before Test: Explain the test procedure and the purpose of the test. Assess the client's knowledge of the test. Explain that this test is sensitive for heart muscle damage.
During Test: Adhere to standard precautions.
After Test: Apply pressure to venipuncture site. Explain that some bruising, discomfort, and swelling may appear at the site and that warm, moist compresses can alleviate this. Monitor for signs of infection.

Potential Complications: Bleeding and bruising at venipuncture site

Nursing Considerations:
Pediatric: Infants and children will need assistance in remaining still during the venipuncture and age-appropriate comfort measures following the test.

WEBLINKS

http://www.entnet.org

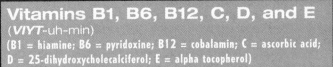

Vitamins B1, B6, B12, C, D, and E
(*VIYT*-uh-min)
(B1 = hiamine; B6 = pyridoxine; B12 = cobalamin; C = ascorbic acid;
D = 25-dihydroxycholecalciferol; E = alpha tocopherol)

5 min.

BLOOD

Type of Test: Blood

Body Systems and Functions: Gastrointestinal system

Normal Findings:

B1	10–64 ng/mL
B6	5–24 ng/mL
B12	200–1,100 pg/mL
C	28–84 µmol/L
D	60 ng/mL
E	5–17 mg/L

CRITICAL VALUES:

B1	Measured through transketolase activity, >20%
B6	<3 ng/mL
B12	<200 pg/mL, >1,100 pg/mL
C	<0.2 mg/dL, >2.0 mg/dL
D3	<10 ng/mL, >100 ng/dL
E	<3 µg/mL

Test Results Time Frame: Within 24–48 hr

Test Description: Vitamins B1, B6, B12, C, D, and E are measured with blood tests for vitamin levels to detect many abnormalities or conditions. B1, or thiamine, is essential in maintaining a healthy heart and nervous system. Thiamine deficiencies are common in third world countries, producing a disease called beriberi. Thiamine deficiencies in the United States are mostly seen in alcoholics. Deficiencies in B6 produce neurological abnormalities and iron disorders. B12 abnormalities cause such pathologies as pernicious anemia and are indicators of leukemia or liver disease. Vitamin C is sometimes thought to remedy the cold virus and when deficient vitamin C can produce such things as scurvy. Vitamin D is obtained in sunlight as well as many other sources. It is abnormal in clients with a general inadequate nutritional intake. Vitamin E alterations may indicate hemolytic anemia.

Consent Form: Not required

List of Equipment: Red-top tube, lavender-top tube, or serum separator tube; needle and syringe or vacutainer; alcohol swab

Test Procedure:

1. Label the specimen tube. *Correctly identifies the client and the test to be performed.*
2. Obtain a 5-mL blood sample for each vitamin being tested.
3. Do not agitate the tube. *Agitation may cause RBC hemolysis.*
4. Send tube to the laboratory. (The sample sent for B6 needs to be protected from light and placed on ice until transport to the laboratory.)

BLOOD

Clinical Implications and Indications:

1. B1 deficiency indicates beriberi and Wernicke-Korsakoff syndrome in alcoholics. Branched-chain ketoaciduria may also be caused from thiamine deficiency.
2. B6 is active in heme biosynthesis. Deficiencies lead to hypochromic microcytic anemia, neurological abnormalities, and iron overload. Some drugs may inhibit B6, leading to deficiency (isoniazid and penicillin).
3. B12 deficiency may indicate hyperthyroidism, pernicious anemia, and malabsorption syndromes. High levels of B12 may indicate leukemia or liver disease.
4. Lack of vitamin C will produce scurvy, leading to hemorrhage anemia, leukopenia, and sometimes thrombocytopenia. High doses of vitamin C can destroy vitamin B12, leading to B12 deficiency.
5. Deficits in vitamin D are found with children living in areas lacking in sunshine, malabsorption syndrome, pregnancy or breast feeding, chronic muscle wasting, severe burns, oral contraceptives, estrogen, liver disease, cystic fibrosis, and pancreatitis.
6. Deficiency in vitamin E may produce hemolytic anemia due to the breakdown of RBC membranes.

Nursing Care:

Before Test: Explain the test procedure and the purpose of the test. Assess the client's knowledge of the test. Instruct client to be NPO for at least 12 hr prior to the test.
During Test: Adhere to standard precautions.
After Test: Apply pressure to venipuncture site. Explain that some bruising, discomfort, and swelling may appear at the site and that warm, moist compresses can alleviate this. Monitor for signs of infection.

Potential Complications: Bleeding and bruising at venipuncture site

Interfering Factors: Pregnancy; eating or drinking 12 hr prior to test; medications that alter results are anticonvulsants, corticosteroids, colchicine, neomycin, and phenytoin.

Nursing Considerations:

Pregnancy: Vitamins are usually suggested in the prenatal time period as a means of ensuring health in the pregnant woman to both the mother and the fetus.
Pediatric: For collection of 24-hr specimen a collection bag or indwelling catheter needs to be used for infants and toddlers.
Gerontology: Vitamin deficiencies may exist among the elderly due to their inability to obtain wide varieties of food sources.
International: A variety of vitamin deficiencies may occur in countries with rampant poverty. Consequently, diseases specific to vitamin abnormalities must be assessed by health care providers.

WEBLINKS

http://chorus.rad.mcw.edu

Von Willebrand Factor Antigen
(vahn **WIL**-uh-braend **FAEK**-t:r **AEN**-tuh-jen)
(pseudohemophilia test)

5 min.

BLOOD

Type of Test: Blood

Body Systems and Functions: Hematological system

Normal Findings: Factor XIII antigen: 50–150 mg/dL

Test Results Time Frame: Within 48 hr

Test Description: Von Willebrand's is an inherited bleeding disorder, which affects a molecule of factor XIII. This disorder is a pseudohemophilia. Factor assays are done to identify a particular clotting factor abnormality. When a client history and screening indicate the possibility of an abnormality, individual factors can be evaluated. Factor XIII is screened when hemophilia or von Willebrand's disease is suspected. To be more specific for von Willebrand's disease, a cofactor called Ristocetin is performed. This determines how fast platelets aggregate. To differentiate between hemophilia and von Willebrand's, a factor XIII antigen test is performed. This will be low with von Willebrand's disease but normal in hemophilia.

CLINICAL ALERT:
If the client is taking aspirin, bleeding times are exaggerated with von Willebrand's disease. Therefore, the site of blood draw should be examined for bleeding.

Consent Form: Not required

List of Equipment: Light-blue-top tube or plasma separator tube; needle and syringe or vacutainer; alcohol swab

Test Procedure:
1. Label the specimen tube. *Correctly identifies the client and the test to be performed.*
2. Obtain a 5-mL blood sample using the two-tube method. The second tube should contain sodium citrate as an anticoagulant.
3. Gently invert tube several times, but do not agitate the tube. *Mixes the anticoagulant, but agitation may cause RBC hemolysis.*
4. Keep specimen cool. *High temperatures alter the results.*
5. Send tube to the laboratory.

Clinical Implications and Indications:
1. Factor XIII antigen will be low with von Willebrand's disease but normal with hemophilia.

Nursing Care:
Before Test: Explain the test procedure and the purpose of the test. Assess the client's knowledge of the test. Assess use of aspirin dosages and frequency of ingestion of aspirin.
During Test: Adhere to standard precautions.
After Test: Apply pressure to venipuncture site. Explain that some bruising, discomfort, and swelling may appear at the site and that warm, moist compresses

can alleviate this. Monitor for signs of infection. If bleeding persists for longer than 15 min, continue to apply pressure and report condition to primary provider.

Potential Complications: Extended bleeding and bruising at venipuncture site; taking aspirin greatly increases bleeding times.

Nursing Considerations:
Pediatric: Infants and children will need assistance in remaining still during the venipuncture and age-appropriate comfort measures following the test.

Listing of Related Tests: Bleeding time; PT; PTT; plasminogen; activated coagulation time

WEBLINKS

www.healthgate.com

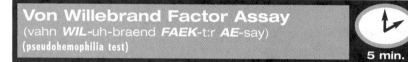

Von Willebrand Factor Assay
(vahn **WIL**-uh-braend **FAEK**-t:r **AE**-say)
(pseudohemophilia test)

5 min.

Type of Test: Blood

Body Systems and Functions: Hematological system

Normal Findings: Ristocetin 45–140 AU (or 45%–140% of normal); factor XIII 55–145 AU (or 55%–145% of normal)

Test Results Time Frame: Within 48 hr

Test Description: Von Willebrand's is an inherited bleeding disorder, which affects a molecule of factor XIII. This disorder is a pseudohemophilia. Factor assays are done to identify a particular clotting factor abnormality. When a client history and screening indicate the possibility of an abnormality, individual factors can be evaluated. Factor XIII is screened when hemophilia or von Willebrand's disease is suspected. To be more specific for von Willebrand's disease, a cofactor called Ristocetin is performed. This determines how fast platelets aggregate.

CLINICAL ALERT:
If the client is taking aspirin, bleeding times are exaggerated with von Willebrand's disease. Therefore, the site of blood draw should be examined for bleeding.

Consent Form: Not required

List of Equipment: Light-blue-top tube or plasma separator tube; needle and syringe or vacutainer; alcohol swab

Test Procedure:
1. Label the specimen tube. *Correctly identifies the client and the test to be performed.*

2. Obtain a 5-mL blood sample using the two-tube method. *The second tube should contain sodium citrate as an anticoagulant.*
3. Gently invert tube several times, but do not agitate the tube. *Mixes the anticoagulant, but agitation may cause RBC hemolysis.*
4. Send tube to the laboratory.
5. Keep specimen cool. *High temperatures alter the results.*

Clinical Implications and Indications:

1. In von Willebrand's disease both factor XIII and Ristocetin are decreased.
2. Factor XIII is decreased with hemophilia A.
3. Cofactor Ristocetin is also decreased in Bernard-Soulier disease.

Nursing Care:

Before Test: Explain the test procedure and the purpose of the test. Assess the client's knowledge of the test. Ask the client about use of aspirin dosages and frequency of ingestion of aspirin.

During Test: Adhere to standard precautions.

After Test: Apply pressure to venipuncture site. Explain that some bruising, discomfort, and swelling may appear at the site and that warm, moist compresses can alleviate this. Monitor for signs of infection. If bleeding persists for longer than 15 min, continue to apply pressure and notify primary care provider.

Potential Complications: Extended bleeding and bruising at venipuncture site; taking aspirin greatly increases bleeding times.

Nursing Considerations:

Pediatric: Infants and children will need assistance in remaining still during the venipuncture and age-appropriate comfort measures following the test.

Listing of Related Tests: Bleeding time; PT; PTT; plasminogen; activated coagulation time

| WEBLINKS |

www.healthgate.com

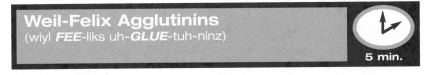

Weil-Felix Agglutinins
(wiyl *FEE*-liks uh-*GLUE*-tuh-ninz)

5 min.

Type of Test: Blood

Body Systems and Functions: Immunological system

Normal Findings: A negative titer would be <8.

> ### CRITICAL VALUES:
> 1:40 titer is considered possible for rickettsiae disease; 1:160 titer is considered presumptive evidence of infection with rickettsiae disease.

Test Results Time Frame: Within 48 hr

Test Description: Weil-Felix agglutinins involves culturing the rickettsiae in a special laboratory and is an indirect method used to test for the disease. The nonpathogenic organism *Proteus* 0X-19 is agglutinated in the presence of the serum of a person infected with rickettsiae. For example, Rocky Mountain spotted fever and typhus agglutinates *Proteus* 0X-19.

CLINICAL ALERT:
To help confirm a diagnosis of rickettsiae infection, the laboratory needs to know if the client has been exposed to lice or ticks. Since vectors spread this disease, the client is not contagious to other humans.

Consent Form: Not required

List of Equipment: Red-top tube or serum separator tube; needle and syringe or vacutainer; alcohol swab

Test Procedure:
1. Label the specimen tube. *Correctly identifies the client and the test to be performed.*
2. Obtain a 6-mL blood sample.
3. Do not agitate the tube. *Agitation may cause RBC hemolysis.*
4. Send tube to the laboratory.

Clinical Implications and Indications:
1. Identifies the presence of one of the rickettsial diseases, such as Rocky Mountain spotted fever, typhus, and *Proteus* infection.

Nursing Care:
Before Test: Explain the test procedure and the purpose of the test. Assess the client's knowledge of the test. Ascertain if the client has an infection with any *Proteus* pathogens. *Proteus* infections of the urinary tract, respiratory tract, and wounds will cause a false positive to this test. Ask the client if there has been exposure to a vector.
During Test: Adhere to standard precautions.
After Test: Apply pressure to venipuncture site. Explain that some bruising, discomfort, and swelling may appear at the site and that warm, moist compresses can alleviate this. Monitor for signs of infection.

Potential Complications: Bleeding and bruising at venipuncture site

Interfering Factors: Infections with *Proteus* pathogens give false-positive results; liver disease produces false-positive results.

Nursing Considerations:
Pediatric: Infants and children will need assistance in remaining still during the venipuncture and age-appropriate comfort measures following the test.
Rural: The rural settings and living areas are more likely areas where vectors reside and therefore should be assessed accordingly.

WEBLINKS

http://www.mic.ki.se/Diseases/c20.html*Proteus*

Western Equine Encephalitis Virus

(*WES*-t:rn *EK*-wiyn en-*SEF*-uh-*LIYT*-uhs)
(equine encephalomyelitis)

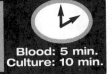

Blood: 5 min.
Culture: 10 min.

Type of Test: Blood; culture

Body Systems and Functions: Hematological system

Normal Findings: Negative for virus

CRITICAL VALUES:
Presence of virus

Test Results Time Frame: Within 3–5 days

Test Description: Western equine encephalitis virus testing involves obtaining a sample of blood, cerebrospinal fluid, or a culture that is used to identify this infection. The pathogen is caused by a group A arbovirus, specifically, togavirus, which results in meningitis, inflammation of parts of the brain and spinal cord. Since the virus is an intracellular parasite, it must be cultured in special laboratories using animal tissue. This disease is found in horses but is communicable to humans. There are three types: Western, Eastern, and Venezuelan. Clinical manifestations include lethargy, sore throat, stupor, fever, coma, and paralyis in children. Mosquitoes transmit the virus.

Consent Form: Not required

List of Equipment: Depends on site of virus. *Blood:* blood tube; needle and syringe or vacutainer; alcohol swab. *Culture:* swabs or specimen cups for urine, stool, or tissue.

Test Procedure:
Blood:
1. Collect the specimen within 72 hr of infection. *Virus is in greatest numbers.*
2. Label the specimen tube. *Correctly identifies the client and the test to be performed.*
3. Obtain a 5- to 7-mL blood sample.
4. Do not agitate the tube. *Agitation may cause RBC hemolysis.*
5. Send tube to the laboratory.
6. Repeat 10–14 days later for convalescent sample and label the tube as convalescent sample. *Allows for separate identification of the convalescent sample, which is compared in ratio to the acute sample.*

Culture:
1. Collect the specimen within 72 hr of infection. *Virus is in greatest numbers.*
2. Label the culture medium. *Correctly identifies the client and the test to be performed.*
3. Do not allow the specimen to dry out. *Facilitates the virus survival.*
4. Transport the specimen to the laboratory in the appropriate solution or medium. *Keeps the virus alive.*

BLOOD

Clinical Implications and Indications:
1. Diagnoses aseptic meningitis and meningoencephalitis.
2. Meningitis can lead to a fatal condition in 10% of its victims.

Nursing Care:
Before Test: Explain the test procedure and the purpose of the test. Assess the client's knowledge of the test.

During Test: Adhere to standard precautions. Avoid cross-contamination of the specimen to prevent a false positive.

After Test: Depends on the site cultured. Apply pressure to venipuncture site. Explain that some bruising, discomfort, and swelling may appear at the site and that warm, moist compresses can alleviate this. Monitor for signs of infection.

Potential Complications: Bleeding and bruising at venipuncture site

Interfering Factors: Not transporting the specimen in the appropriate medium (note: many viruses should be transported in a balanced salt solution)

Nursing Considerations:
Pediatric: Infants and children will need assistance in remaining still during the venipuncture and age-appropriate comfort measures following the test.

Rural: Transmission of this virus is from horses to human and therefore could be suspected more in rural settings. Wear insect-repellent spray or lotion when outdoors in areas where the virus is present.

International: Occurrence is mainly in the Western Hemisphere and in late summer through early fall.

Listing of Related Tests: Eastern equine encephalitis virus serology

WEBLINKS

http://www.methodisthealth.com

White Blood Cell Count and Differential Count
(hwit blod sel kownt and *DIF*-er-EN-shal kownt)
(WBC count; leukocyte count)

5 min.

Type of Test: Blood

Body Systems and Functions: Immunological system

Normal Findings: WBC count 4,100–10,800 cells/mm^3. Differential is reported in percentage of the total number of WBCs.

CRITICAL VALUES:
WBCs <500 cells/mm^3 or >30,000 cells/mm3 are critical values.

Test Results Time Frame: Within 24–48 hr

Test Description: White blood cell count and differential count are performed to determine the amount of WBCs in the blood. The body fights infection by using WBCs, or leukocytes. They encapsulate organisms and destroy them. The differential allows the health care providers to know the type of WBC that is involved in the client's hematological responses. Patterning of certain types of WBCs evidences some diseases. There are five types of WBCs, and the differential is the percentage of each type: neutrophils, eosinophils, basophils, lymphocytes, and monocytes.

CLINICAL ALERT:
Extremely low or high values require contacting the health care provider immediately.

Consent Form: Not required

List of Equipment: Lavender-top tube; needle and syringe or vacutainer; alcohol swab

Test Procedure:
1. Label the specimen tube. *Correctly identifies the client and the test to be performed.*
2. Obtain a 5-mL blood sample.
3. Gently invert tube several times, but do not agitate the tube. *Mixes the anticoagulant, but agitation may cause RBC hemolysis.*
4. Send tube to the laboratory.

Clinical Implications and Indications:
1. WBCs >10,000 cells/mm^3 may indicate leukemia, trauma or tissue injury, infection from most bacteria, or death of tissue (as with burns, MI, or gangrene).
2. WBCs <5,000 cells/mm^3 may indicate bone marrow depression, viral infections, bone marrow disorders (pernicious anemia, aplastic anemia), and iron deficiency anemia.

Nursing Care:
Before Test: Explain the test procedure and the purpose of the test. Assess the client's knowledge of the test.
During Test: Adhere to standard precautions.
After Test: Apply pressure to venipuncture site. Explain that some bruising, discomfort, and swelling may appear at the site and that warm, moist compresses can alleviate this. Monitor for signs of infection.

Potential Complications: Bleeding and bruising at venipuncture site

Interfering Factors: Strenuous exercise; stress; heavy meal prior to test; age (newborn and infant count is high, >10,000 cells/mm^3); medications that alter results are anticonvulsants, flucytosine, indomethacin, metronidazole, anti-inflammatories, and phenytoin.

Nursing Considerations:
Pediatric: Infants and children will need assistance in remaining still during the venipuncture and age-appropriate comfort measures following the test.
Gerontology: The elderly with elevated WBCs are more at risk for morbidity and mortality, especially in the event of respiratory infections.

BLOOD

Home Care: Health care providers need to be instructed to advise WBC assessment when clients have infections that are causing generalized inflammatory clinical manifestations (e.g., febrile response, lethargy).

WEBLINKS

http://www.nlm.nih.gov

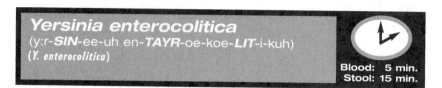

Yersinia enterocolitica
(y:r-*SIN*-ee-uh en-*TAYR*-oe-koe-*LIT*-i-kuh)
(*Y. enterocolitica*)

Blood: 5 min.
Stool: 15 min.

Type of Test: Blood; stool

Body Systems and Functions: Immunological system

Normal Findings: Blood: negative for antibody. Stool: negative for *Y. enterocolitica*.

CRITICAL VALUES:
Positive for *Y. enterocolitica*

Test Results Time Frame: Within 48 hr to several weeks

Test Description: *Yersinia enterocolitica* is the most common type of *Yersinia* pathogens. It is a fungus that is found in animals and bodies of water. *Yersinia enterocolitica* is transmitted to humans by the fecal-oral route or by consumption of the pathogen from food and water. The organism grows and develops within the hematological or gastrointestinal system and thus is identified with either a blood or stool culture. It produces headache, fever, cramps, malaise, abdominal pain, and diarrhea. In extreme cases it can produce mesenteric adenitis, reactive arthritis, or intra-abdominal abscess and septicemia.

CLINICAL ALERT:
The culture of *Y. enterocolitica* grows very slowly, especially at 37°, which is used by most laboratories. It is believed that room temperature is best for growing this organism. Due to the difficulty in culturing this organism, many laboratories may not detect it.

Consent Form: Not required

List of Equipment: *Blood:* red-top tube or serum separator tube; needle and syringe or vacutainer; alcohol swab. *Stool:* clean, dry container to collect stool; tongue depressor; gloves; rectal swab; clean, dry bedpan.

Test Procedure:
Blood:
1. Label the specimen as acute sample. *Correctly identifies the client and the test to be performed.*
2. Obtain a 5-mL blood sample.

3. Do not agitate the tube. *Agitation may cause RBC hemolysis*
4. Send tube to the laboratory.
5. Repeat 10–14 days later for convalescent sample and label the tube as convalescent sample. *Allows for separate identification of the convalescent sample, which is compared in ratio to the acute sample.*

Stool:
1. Label the specimen cup. *Correctly identifies the client and the test to be performed.*
2. Obtain three separate stool samples. *Diagnosis cannot be determined with a single sample.*
3. Send specimen to the laboratory. *Specimen must be tested within 2 hr for accuracy of levels.*

Clinical Implications and Indications:
1. Positive specimen indicates presence of the pathogen *Y. enterocolitica.*

Nursing Care:
Before Test: Explain the test procedure and the purpose of the test. Assess the client's knowledge of the test
During Test: Adhere to standard precautions.
After Test: Blood: Apply pressure to venipuncture site. Explain that some bruising, discomfort, and swelling may appear at the site and that warm, moist compresses can alleviate this. Monitor for signs of infection. Stool: Transport sample to laboratory immediately, as the test must be performed within 2 hr.

Potential Complications: Growth of this specimen may require using "cold enrichment" (incubation for several weeks).

Interfering Factors: Immunosuppresion; antifungal therapy; bleeding and bruising at venipuncture site; lengthy time for stool to be taken to laboratory

Nursing Considerations:
Pediatric: Blood: *Infants and children will need assistance in remaining still during the venipuncture and age-appropriate comfort measures following the test. Stool: Older children will need a cathartic prior to obtaining the sample.*

WEBLINKS

http://www.mic.ki.se/Diseases/c20.html

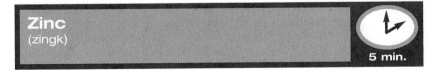

Zinc
(zingk)

5 min.

Type of Test: Blood

Body Systems and Functions: Hematological system

Normal Findings: 0.75–1.4 µg/mL

CRITICAL VALUES:
<0.70 µg/mL is considered deficiency.

Test Results Time Frame: Within 48 hr

Test Description: Zinc testing determines zinc toxicity and zinc deficiency. Zinc is a trace metal that is important to cellular growth and metabolic processes. Toxicity may occur from accidental industrial exposure or ingestion of acidic foods or beverages from galvanized containers.

CLINICAL ALERT:
Do not leave the tourniquet on the arm for more than 1 min, as this will produce an inaccurate test result.

Consent Form: Not required

List of Equipment: Red-top tube or serum separator tube; needle and syringe or vacutainer; alcohol swab

Test Procedure:
1. Label the specimen tube. *Correctly identifies the client and the test to be performed.*
2. Obtain a 5-mL blood sample.
3. Do not agitate the tube. *Agitation may cause RBC hemolysis.*
4. Send tube to the laboratory.

Clinical Implications and Indications:
1. Decreased levels are found with inadequate nutritional needs, people over 55, pregnant women, chronic wasting illness, estrogens, oral contraceptives, and diuretics.
2. Deficiencies have also been shown in alcoholics and postoperative clients who have had part of their intestinal tract removed.

Nursing Care:
Before Test: Explain the test procedure and the purpose of the test. Assess the client's knowledge of the test.
During Test: Adhere to standard precautions.
After Test: Apply pressure to venipuncture site. Explain that some bruising, discomfort, and swelling may appear at the site and that warm, moist compresses can alleviate this. Monitor for signs of infection.

Potential Complications: Bleeding and bruising at venipuncture site

Interfering Factors: A collection tube that is not metal free; zinc-chelating agents will affect test results (penicillinase and corticosteroids).

Nursing Considerations:
Pediatric: Infants and children will need assistance in remaining still during the venipuncture and age-appropriate comfort measures following the test.
Rural: Clients in rural settings may be more at risk for contaminates in well water. Instruct clients to have their water tested on an annual basis for impurities.

WEBLINKS

http://www.entnet.org

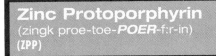

Zinc Protoporphyrin
(zingk proe-toe-*POER*-f:r-in)
(ZPP)

5 min.

BLOOD

Type of Test: Blood

Body Systems and Functions: Hematological system

Normal Findings: 0–40 μg/dL

CRITICAL VALUES:
>60 μg/dL

Test Results Time Frame: Within 24 hr

Test Description: Elevated zinc protoporphyrin (ZZP) reflects the amount of the zinc derivative of protoporphyrin released into the bloodstream. Zinc is a nutritional trace mineral that is vital to cellular growth and metabolism. Zinc levels are usually measured for heavy metal screening in clients with suspected abnormalities (e.g., lead poisoning).

CLINICAL ALERT:
Health organizations may require ZPP whole-blood testing reported in units of micrograms per deciliter.

Consent Form: Not required

List of Equipment: Lavender-top or dark-blue-top tube; needle and syringe or vacutainer; alcohol swab

Test Procedure:
1. Label the specimen tube. *Correctly identifies the client and the test to be performed.*
2. Obtain a 7-mL blood sample.
3. Do not agitate the tube. *Agitation may cause RBC hemolysis.*
4. Send tube to the laboratory and protect it from light. *Ensures accurate results.*

Clinical Implications and Indications:
1. Evaluates iron deficiency, anemia during chronic erythropoietic protoporphyria, and chronic lead poisoning

Nursing Care:
Before Test: Explain the test procedure and the purpose of the test. Assess the client's knowledge of the test.
During Test: Adhere to standard precautions.
After Test: Apply pressure to venipuncture site. Explain that some bruising, discomfort, and swelling may appear at the site and that warm, moist compresses can alleviate this. Monitor for signs of infection.

Potential Complications: Bleeding and bruising at venipuncture site

Interfering Factors: Exposure to light; not being refrigerated; elevated bilirubin or riboflavin gives false positives; false positives may occur from clotted and hemolyzed specimens.

Nursing Considerations:

Pediatric: *Infants and children will need assistance in remaining still during the venipuncture and age-appropriate comfort measures following the test. In addition, lead poisoning is an environmental hazard for children as related to consuming lead-based paints or products.*

Rural: *Older homes and buildings may expose clients to lead-based paints, which could lead to toxicity of ZPP. Therefore, health care providers should include this potential in clients living in these potentially at-risk conditions.*

WEBLINKS

http://www.methodisthealth.com

EXAMINATION BY CULTURE, TISSUE, AND MICRO-SCOPIC TESTING

Culture, tissue, and microscopic testing cover a wide variety of test types. Almost all types of body fluids or tissues are secured for one or another of these various tests. For example, cultures take specimens from the body that will be grown in the laboratory for signs of disease-producing organisms. Growing organisms from a specimen can produce a definitive diagnosis for a particular disease. In addition, tissue examinations take specimens that will be examined for cell morphology, most commonly to detect cell changes that indicate cancer. And microscopic testing involves the use of a microscope to examine body tissues and cells to diagnose malignant and premalignant conditions.

COLLECTION OF SPECIMENS

Specimen collection will differ greatly depending on the particular method of culture, tissue, or microscopic testing procedure. The methods of specimen procurement vary and the techniques for collection are very specific to the individual type of test. For example, specimens to be cultured in the laboratory will need careful collection technique, as contamination will result in inappropriate diagnosis and treatment.

Culture Specimen Collection

There are specific methods of collecting specimens for culture. The following is a procedural list of how cultures are obtained:

1. Wear appropriate personal protection against contamination; gloves are usually required, but a mask and gown might also be appropriate.
2. Collect specimens into sterile containers using sterile technique.
3. Use the appropriate collection container; for example, anaerobic organisms must be collected into containers that exclude air.
4. Attempt the collection of specimens before antibiotic or other antiorganism therapies have been initiated; label specimens accordingly if the client is taking medications that may affect results.
5. Transport specimens immediately to the laboratory; most specimens should not be either refrigerated or left at room temperature.

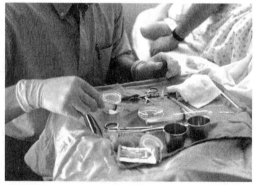

The specimen is removed from the needle

Tissue Collection Procedure

There are specific methods of collecting tissue specimens. The following is a procedural list of how tissue samples are obtained:

1. Most tissue collections are obtained for conditions that are not contagious; however, collection may require contact with blood and/or body fluids. The health care provider must observe the appropriate standard precautions.
2. The quality of the test depends on the quality of the tissue specimen. The health care provider must take special care to follow the collection procedures precisely.

Microscopic Specimen Collection

There are specific methods of using the microscopic method of examining specimens. Preparation of microscope slides requires the preparation of thin layers of cells that can be clearly visualized. Although the slides are prepared in a variety of ways, depending on the site of the specimen and the examination to be performed, careful attention to preserve cells is necessary.

CLIENT CARE IN CULTURE, TISSUE, AND MICROSCOPIC TESTING

The client care in obtaining cultures and tissue samples and using microscopic testing is varied. Overall, an explanation for the reason of the test needs to be communicated to the client. Then the actual method for implementing a specific test is explained, with an emphasis on increasing client knowledge and focusing on decreasing the stress level of the client. Some of these tests may require an informed consent. There may be certain physical body positions that the client will be placed in for the testing. In addition, some of these types of tests will allow pretesting medications to decrease the pain potential and to relax the client. Some of the tissue biopsies are somewhat painful even with the medications and relaxation techniques and emotional support needs to be maintained during the diagnostic testing. For example, a liver biopsy requires the client to be placed in a supine or left lateral position and a local anesthetic is injected into the skin prior to the biopsy. Then the biopsy needle is inserted while the client inhales for approximately 10 seconds to move the diaphragm and prevent a pneumothorax. It is important for the health care providers to realize that the validity of the testing is dependent on the manner in which the client stays in the correct position and how they breathe correctly during the procedure.

Life span implications in culture, tissue, and microscopic testing

There are different life span considerations for culture, tissue, and microscopic testing that are specifically related to the developmental age of the clients. For example, infants and children may require sedation or assistance in remaining still during the testing. In addition, the elderly might need particular assistance in positioning during the testing, depending on the individual test and the length of time the client is required to be involved.

CULTURE, TISSUE, MICROSCOPIC

Allergen Skin
(*AEL*-:r-j:n)

1 hr.

Type of Test: Tissue

Body Systems and Functions: Immunological system

Normal Findings: No raised wheal where allergen is introduced into skin

Test Results Time Frame: Within 24 hr

Test Description: Allergen skin testing is used to establish or confirm allergies when combined with a positive clinical history. Skin reactions test the IgE-mediated wheal and flare allergic response to an allergen. This response takes about 5 min after injection and peaks at 30 min. Two common methods are used: the prick-puncture, which does not involve the dermis, and the intradermal. The prick-puncture is generally the first test used because results correspond well to clinical symptoms, the test is safer (no fatal anaphylaxis has been reported, although clients sometimes report systemic reactions) and the test is highly reliable when done correctly. A positive test response varies with the method used. With the prick-puncture method, a positive response is a wheal of 1–2 mm with flare and itching within 20 min. Negative prick-puncture tests with positive clinical symptoms can be repeated with the more sensitive intradermal test.

CLINICAL ALERT:
Always have a health care provider on-site with intradermal testing as fatal anaphylactic responses have occurred with testing. Have an emergency response dose of epinephrine drawn and ready before any testing is done.

Consent Form: Not required

List of Equipment: Standardized allergen samples; standardized needles for testing (note: equipment depends on the method used)

Test Procedure:
Prick-puncture method:
1. Place a small drop of the test extract on the volar surface of the forearm.
2. Insert a 25-gauge needle into the epidural surface at a low angle. *Prevents insertion of the test material into the dermis.*
3. Gently elevate the epidermis with the needle tip so that bleeding does not occur. *Bleeding can create false-positive results.*
4. Withdraw the needle.
5. Wipe the solution away 1 min later. *Prevents mixing of extracts and contaminating test results.*
6. Place the next drop of test extract at least 2 cm away from the first test. *Avoids mixing the extracts, contaminating test results.*
7. Record the largest and smallest diameter of the wheal at 20 min.

Clinical Implications and Indications:

1. A positive test with a positive clinical history indicates an allergy to the particular allergen. Sometimes clients will have a positive skin test with no clinically significant symptoms.
2. False negatives are possible with prick-puncture testing, and the provider may choose to repeat with the more sensitive intradermal method.

Nursing Care:

Before Test: Explain the test procedure and the purpose of the test. Assess the client's knowledge of the test. Assess previous allergy history because test materials may need to be more dilute with suspected strong sensitivities. Assess medication history because a number of medications will interfere with allergic responsiveness.

During Test: Adhere to standard precautions.

After Test: Observe client for 20–30 minutes for hypersensitivity reaction.

Potential Complications: Allergic reactions ranging from localized to anaphylactic responses

Contraindications: Allergen testing should not be conducted in areas of severe psoriasis or eczema.

Interfering Factors: Medications that alter results are antihistamines, ketotifen, imipramine, phenothiazines, tranquilizers, corticosteroids, theophylline, beta-adrenergics, cromones, and dopamine (will all decrease allergic skin response); false negatives are also possible with nonstandardized test material, immunosuppression due to disease, and skin disease; false positives can be caused by skin irritation from overly forceful skin puncture and bleeding.

Nursing Considerations:

Pediatric: Infants as young as 2 months may be tested.

Gerontology: Immune response declines with age and false negatives are more likely.

CULTURE, TISSUE, MICROSCOPIC

```
WEBLINKS                                          ▣☒
```

http://www.mic.ki.se/Diseases/c20.html

Angiography
(*AEN*-jee-*AHG*-ruh-fee)
(angiogram; cardiac angiogram)

1–3 hr. (note: varies with site to be visualized)

Type of Test: Microscopic

Body Systems and Functions: Cardiovascular system

Normal Findings: Normal vessel in appearance

Test Results Time Frame: Within 24–48 hr

CULTURE, TISSUE, MICROSCOPIC

Test Description: An angiogram is a picture of a part of the cardiovascular system. The picture is taken by injecting a contrast medium into a vessel through a catheter. As the medium reaches the area of interest, a series of x-rays are taken to visualize the vessel. Common sites of angiograms are the heart, kidneys, lungs, liver, and brain.

CLINICAL ALERT:
Angiography testing involves invasive techniques that can place a client at risk. Direct injuries can occur with accidental perforation of a vessel during the test. Allergic reactions to the contrast medium can range from sneezing to cardiac collapse and death. Therefore, always have an emergency "crash cart" available during angiography procedures.

Consent Form: Required

List of Equipment: Cardiac catheterization laboratory or special studies laboratory will have specific testing equipment and personnel.

Test Procedure:
1. Administer any premedications ordered for the client. *Provides necessary anesthesia.*
2. The client is placed on an x-ray table and must lie still. *Ensures accuracy of test results.*
3. An IV line is started. Allows administration of fluids or medications if needed.
4. Local anesthetic is given at the venipuncture site.
5. A vessel is entered (can be either a vein or an artery) through puncture or cutdown. *Allows a catheter to be advanced through the vessel to reach the area to be studied.*
6. Contrast medium is injected through the catheter.
7. Angiographic films are taken as the contrast medium enters the study area.
8. The catheter is removed and pressure applied to the site for 10–15 min. *Prevents bleeding from the puncture site.*

Clinical Implications and Indications:
1. Angiograms are performed when vessels in the specific organ or vascular area (e.g., kidneys, lung, heart) need to be visualized to identify potential abnormalities or obstruction.

Nursing Care:
Before Test: Explain the test procedure and the purpose of the test. Assess the client's knowledge of the test. Inform client that angiograms are similar to minor surgery. Assess for potential allergies to contrast medium. Inform client that during injection of contrast medium, a burning sensation may be felt for a few seconds behind the eyes or in the jaw, teeth, tongue, or lips. Assess for anxiety and provide sedation as ordered. Administer preoperative medication usually 30 min before procedure. Obtain baseline vital signs and neurological assessment. Report any recent use of anticoagulants.
During Test: Adhere to standard precautions. Assess for allergic reactions to contrast medium. Continuous monitoring of vital signs and other vital physical functions is done by the laboratory staff.

After Test: Assess for allergic reactions to contrast medium. Monitor vital signs and insertion site. Teach client to report any signs of infection, fever, or pain at the insertion site.

Potential Complications: Anaphylaxis due to allergic reaction to iodinated contrast material; nausea; vomiting; cardiac collapse; hemorrhaging; respiratory arrest; death

Contraindications: Previous history of allergy to iodine, eggs, or shellfish

Interfering Factors: Inability to remain still

Nursing Considerations:
Pregnancy: Intravenous contrast should be avoided in pregnant women if possible.

WEBLINKS

http://www.howstuffworks.com

Blastomycosis Determination
(blas-to-mi-*KO*-sis de-*TER*-min-a-shun)
(Gilchrist's skin test)

Skin test: 5 min.
Biopsy: 10 min.

Type of Test: Tissue

Body Systems and Functions: Immunological system

Normal Findings: Skin test: negative. Biopsy: no growth.

Test Results Time Frame: Within 72 hr

Test Description: Blastomycosis is an uncommon chronic fungal infection. The disease is most commonly seen in males 30–60 years of age who are farmers, forestry workers, hunters, or campers in south central and midwest Canada and the United States. The fungus is thought to be inhaled, affecting the lungs and then disseminating to other body sites, especially skin and bone. A skin test is done with the specific antigen to identify an antigen-antibody response. A biopsy is performed on skin lesions and inoculated into agar for incubation and identification. The biopsy is an invasive procedure performed in a surgical setting. An excision or needle punch sample of body tissue is taken under sterile technique and examined microscopically for cell morphology and tissue anomalies.

> **CLINICAL ALERT:**
> Have emergency equipment readily available in the event of an anaphylactic reaction to the skin test.

Consent Form: Not required (note: some institutions may require a consent for biopsy)

List of Equipment: *Skin test:* tuberculin needle and syringe; alcohol swab; specific antigen; epinephrine 1:1000 in event of anaphylaxis. *Skin biopsy:* sterile container; biopsy tray; local anesthetic.

CULTURE, TISSUE, MICROSCOPIC

Test Procedure:

Skin test:
1. Cleanse skin of lower anterior forearm with alcohol and allow to dry.
2. Prepare .1 mL antigen in TB syringe and inject intradermally, causing a wheal or bleb.
3. Record site.
4. Reading: Inspect site. Measure area of any induration. A positive test is 5 mm or greater with erythema and edema.

Skin biopsy:
1. Cleanse area of skin lesion and biopsy site.
2. Place specimen in sterile container with appropriate label. *Correctly identifies the client and the test to be performed.*

Clinical Implications and Indications:

1. A method of screening clients for exposure or infection with blastomycosis

Nursing Care:

Before Test: Explain the test procedure and the purpose of the test. Assess the client's knowledge of the test. Provide preprocedure sedation and analgesia as ordered. Transport client to operating or procedure room. Drape client appropriately. Obtain history of disease exposure (e.g., occupation, recreation). Obtain history of sensitivities to other skin tests or local anesthetic if biopsy is to be done.

During Test: Adhere to sterile technique and standard precautions. Provide reassurance and a calm atmosphere during the procedure.

After Test: Skin test: Remind client to return in 48–72 hr for skin test reading. Advise client not to scratch the area. Biopsy: Clean site of biopsy. Provide analgesia as necessary.

Potential Complications: Skin test: anaphylaxis. Biopsy: infection.

Contraindications: Skin test: history of tuberculosis, previous positive skin tests or reaction to vaccinations

Interfering Factors: Improper intradermal injection; incorrect measurement at time of reading; delay of injection following drawing up of antigen; recent bacterial, viral, or fungal infection; hematological cancer; medications that alter results are immunosuppressive agents and steroids.

Nursing Considerations:

Pediatric: Infants and children will need assistance in remaining still during the venipuncture and age-appropriate comfort measures following the test.
Rural: There is an increased incidence in specific areas of the rural settings, particularly among farmers in those areas.
International: There is an increased incidence in central Canada.

WEBLINKS ▯

www.healthlink.mcw.edu; www.mc.vanderbilt.edu; http://fun-gusweb.utmb.edu

CULTURE, TISSUE, MICROSCOPIC

Bordetella pertussis
(*BOER*-duh-*TEL*-uh p:r-*TUHS*-uhs)
(whooping cough)

10 min.

Type of Test: Culture

Body Systems and Functions: Pulmonary system

Normal Findings: Absence of *Bordetella* bacteria

Test Results Time Frame:

48–72 hr	Positive diagnosis
12 days of no growth	Negative diagnosis

Test Description: *Bordetella pertussis* is an aerobic bacterium that contains very small gram-negative coccobacilli. This bacterium is metabolized in the respiratory system and produces toxins that destroy cells and cause thick mucus to collect in the airways. Droplets from the nose, mouth, or throat of an affected individual easily spread this disease. A nasopharynx culture is obtained in order to see if the *B. pertussis* bacteria grow.

CLINICAL ALERT:
Health care provider wears a mask to prevent respiratory exposure (note: requires special charcoal transport medium).

Consent Form: Not required

List of Equipment: Mask; gloves; specimen kits

Test Procedure:
1. Place client in a sitting position and obtain required specimen kit and check expiration date. *Provides correct medium for culture.*
2. Put on a mask. *Protects caregiver from exposure.*
3. Ask client to blow nose. *Helps decrease the chance of possible contamination from nares.*
4. Gently insert swab into nasal passage, being careful not to touch side of nare, and when resistance is met, gently rotate swab. *Facilitates obtaining specimen from nasopharynx.*
5. Place swab, aseptically, into provided culture tube. Cut wire off of swab so cap can be placed. *Prevents contamination from skin flora.*
6. Send specimen to laboratory.

Clinical Implications and Indications:
1. Diagnoses suspected cases of pertussis and monitors its progression and treatment

Nursing Care:
Before Test: Explain the test procedure and the purpose of the test. Assess the client's knowledge of the test. Ask client to discuss their signs and symptoms of upper respiratory infection. Obtain immunization history. Assess if client is or has recently taken any antibiotics. Instruct client not to use antiseptic mouthwash before test.

CULTURE, TISSUE, MICROSCOPIC

During Test: Adhere to standard precautions.

After Test: Label and transport specimen immediately to laboratory. Instruct client to cough or sneeze into a tissue and wash hands frequently.

Interfering Factors: Pretest antibiotic therapy, which may delay or prevent the bacteria growth; contamination of the swab from the oral cavity; inadequate amount of specimen obtained; use of antiseptic mouthwash that may decrease the amount of organisms available for culture

Nursing Considerations:

Pediatric: Place child in caregiver's lap with head and body immobilized. Provide emotional support to client and caregiver. Pertussis is most prevalent in pediatric population.

Rural: Outbreaks may occur due to incomplete immunization series or complete lack of immunization.

International: Outbreaks may occur due to incomplete immunization series or complete lack of immunization.

WEBLINKS

www.astdhpphe.org

Breast Biopsy
(brest *BIY*-ahp-see)

Needle biopsy: 30 min.
Open biopsy: 4 hr.

Type of Test: Tissue

Body Systems and Functions: Reproductive system

Normal Findings: No abnormal development of the cells or tissue elements

Test Results Time Frame: Within 24–48 hr

Test Description: A breast biopsy examines tissue or fluid that is removed from the breast lesion to diagnose or rule out malignancy. Samples may be obtained from a fine needle aspiration, core biopsy, or stereotactic guidance, all of which are performed using a local anesthetic. Open surgical biopsies are performed with the client under a general anesthetic. Needle aspiration and core biopsy do not require radiological intervention during the procedure. Open biopsies frequently have a marker wire placed into the tumor with the assistance of mammography visualization prior to surgery. Stereotactic guidance involves insertion of the needle after a three-dimensional view is obtained by mammography and computers. The abnormal tissue is located and a sample is then taken. If fluid is removed, it is placed on a slide, and if tissue is taken, it is placed into a sterile container. Frozen-section examination may also be performed.

CULTURE, TISSUE, MICROSCOPIC

CLINICAL ALERT:
Clients may experience vertigo during procedure; therefore, monitor for early signs and symptoms, such as lightheadedness, vertigo, pallor, and diaphoresis. In addition, specimen must be sent to laboratory immediately after obtaining.

Consent Form: Required

List of Equipment: Povidone-iodine; biopsy tray; local anesthetic; dry sterile dressing; needle; slides; transport container

Test Procedure:
Needle or core technique:
1. Confirm correct breast with client and chart. *Helps prevent biopsy from incorrect site.*
2. Cleanse the breast tissue with povidone-iodine and drape breast. *Promotes aseptic technique.*
3. Anesthetize site and obtain biopsy sample.
4. Specimen is placed on slides or in sterile container. *Allows evaluation of sample.*
5. Apply a dry sterile dressing over puncture site. *Helps to prevent infection.*

Stereotactic technique:
1. Client assisted into required position for mammogram machine.
2. Confirm correct breast with client and chart. *Helps prevent biopsy from incorrect site.*
3. Cleanse the breast tissue with povidone-iodine and drape breast. *Promotes aseptic technique.*
4. Anesthetize site. *Helps to decrease client's discomfort.*
5. Insertion of dye or wire marker, or obtain a core biopsy after abnormal tissue is identified. *Allows mass detection during open biopsy.*
6. Specimen is placed on slides or in sterile container. *Allows evaluation of sample.*
7. Apply a dry sterile dressing over puncture site. *Helps to prevent infection.*

Open biopsy:
1. Confirm correct breast with client and chart. *Helps prevent biopsy from incorrect site.*
2. Client is placed under general anesthetic.
3. Cleanse the breast tissue with povidone-iodine and drape breast. *Promotes aseptic technique.*
4. Obtain sample or remove complete mass.

Clinical Implications and Indications:
1. Evaluates abscesses, cysts, mastitis, calcification, and fibrocystic disease
2. Diagnoses carcinoma conditions of the breast

Nursing Care:
Before Test: Explain the test procedure and the purpose of the test. Assess the client's knowledge of the test. Provide preprocedure sedation and analgesia as ordered. Transport client to operating or procedure room. Drape client appropriately. Instruct client to remain NPO for 8 hr before test if a general anesthetic is to be used.

During Test: Adhere to sterile technique and standard precautions. Provide reassurance and a calm atmosphere during the procedure. Confirm with client and chart which breast is being biopsied. Monitor for signs of syncope.

After Test: Clean site of biopsy. Provide analgesia as necessary. Take vital signs frequently. Provide emotional support and encourage normal activity. Educate client to use warm, moist compresses for pain and to wear a supportive bra. Teach client signs and symptoms of infection.

Potential Complications: Bleeding and bruising at the site; cellulitis

Nursing Considerations:
Gerontology: The older person may find it difficult to maintain positions when required to do so for lengthy periods of time during the biopsy.
***Rural:** Advisable to arrange for transportation home after recovering from the biopsy.*

WEBLINKS 🔲🗙

www.thriveonline.com

Cathepsin-D
(kuh-*THEP*-sin)

30 min.

Type of Test: Tissue

Body Systems and Functions: Oncology system

Normal Findings: Studies define negative cases as weakly positive tumors for cathepsin-D (CD) expression, 1%–10% CD positive cells.

Test Results Time Frame: Within 48–72 hr

Test Description: Cathepsin-D is an estrogen-induced lysomal protease that is synthesized in normal tissue but may be overexpressed and secreted in certain breast cancers. Clinical studies define high levels of cathepsin-D as greater than 10% of CD immunoreaction in carcinoma cells. High-level expression of CD is determined by immunohistochemistry of breast cancer tissue and is an independent predictor of poor long-term survival in clients with negative node breast cancer. Cathepsin-D analysis is used in combination with other diagnostic tests and is recommended for investigative use.

Consent Form: Required

Test Procedure:
1. Obtain biopsy equipment.
2. Secure a specimen of solid tumor that is 0.5–1.0 g.
3. The pathologist analyzes breast cancer tissue for expression of cathepsin-D using immunohistochemical techniques.

Clinical Implications and Indications:
1. Prognostic for metastasis in breast cancer.
2. Decreased levels of cathepsin-D are not clinically significant.

CULTURE, TISSUE, MICROSCOPIC

Nursing Care:

Before Test: Explain the test procedure and the purpose of the test. Assess the client's knowledge of the test. Provide emotional support.

During Test: Adhere to standard precautions.

After Test: Ensure client has follow-up appointment to review results of cathepsin-D test. Provide referral to breast cancer support groups.

WEBLINKS	☰ ☒

www.nlm.nih.gov

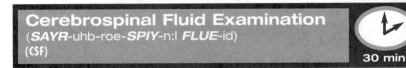

Cerebrospinal Fluid Examination
(*SAYR*-uhb-roe-*SPIY*-n:l *FLUE*-id)
(CSF)

30 min.

Type of Test: Culture

Body Systems and Functions: Neurological system

Normal Findings: The characteristics of CSF are 0–5 cells/μL lymphocytes, 14–45 mg/dL protein, 45–100 mg/dL glucose, and crystal clear color.

Test Results Time Frame: Incubation time before negative culture can be reported is 5 days.

Test Description: Cerebrospinal fluid is usually obtained by lumbar puncture but may also be collected from the ventricles of the brain if a ventriculostomy drainage bag is in place. CSF in bacterial meningitis will have increased WBCs, increased protein, and decreased glucose. CSF of enteroviral meningitis will have increased WBCs, increased protein, and normal glucose levels. CSF acts as a protective cushion type of substance to the brain and also provides nutrients to the brain and surrounding tissues.

Common bacterial agents of acute meningitis by age

Age	Organisms
Neonates–3 months	Group B streptococci: Escherichia coli; Listeria monocytogenes*; Streptococcus pneumoniae
4 months–6 years	*H. influenzae,* type B
6–45 years	*Neisseria meningitides*
>45 years	*S. pneumoniae; L. monocytogenes;* Group B streptococci

*May cause meningitis in all age groups in immunocompromised persons.

Consent Form: Required

List of Equipment: CSF collection tray; lumbar puncture set; sterile gloves and gown; masks

Test Procedure:

1. Label collection tubes. *Correctly identifies the client and test to be performed.*
2. Follow the procedure for lumbar puncture and collection of CSF specimen for culture.
3. Three samples of 2–3 mL each are placed in separate, sterile vials and labeled as number 1, chemistry and serology; number 2, microbiology studies; and number 3, hematology cell counts. *Ensures accurate results.*
4. Transport promptly to laboratory.
5. Refer to the health care institution's policy for the process of collection from the ventriculostomy if a ventriculostomy bag is in place.

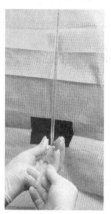

Cerebrospinal fluid examination

Clinical Implications and Indications:

1. Diagnoses meningitis and viral encephalitis
2. Evaluates the color, pressure, and specific cytological information of the CSF

Nursing Care:

Before Test: Explain the test procedure and the purpose of the test. Assess the client's knowledge of the test. Have the client empty his or her bladder; prepare lumbar puncture set; and assist client in lateral recumbent position along the edge of the bed with the knees flexed on the chest and chin touching the knees.

During Test: Adhere to strict aseptic technique and standard precautions. Assist client in maintaining appropriate position. Instruct client to lie still and provide reassurance.

After Test: Have the client lie flat in bed for 6-12 hours (note: assists in preventing headache). Monitor neurological and vital signs. Monitor injection site for CSF leak. Administer analgesics PRN for headache. Encourage fluids if not contraindicated.

Potential Complications: Traumatic lumbar puncture; severe headache; infection

Contraindications: Increased intracranial pressure; cutaneous or osseous infection at site of the lumbar puncture

Nursing Considerations:

Pediatric: *The incidence of* Hemophilus influenza, *type B meningitis, has declined due to vaccination. Enteroviruses are the most common cause of meningitis and should be considered first in a child or adolescent during the late summer or early fall. Newborns have the highest prevalence of meningitis.*

WEBLINKS 🔖   ▣ ☒

http://www.mic.ki.se/Diseases/c20.html

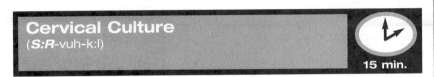

Cervical Culture
(**S:R**-vuh-k:l)

15 min.

CULTURE, TISSUE, MICROSCOPIC

Type of Test: Culture

Body Systems and Functions: Reproductive system

Normal Findings: Negative culture; no evidence of suspecting organism growth

Test Results Time Frame: Within 48 hr

Test Description: A cervical culture is performed to identify the etiological agents of cervicitis or other symptoms suggesting a sexually transmitted disease (STD) and to identify asymptomatic women with an organism that causes an STD. Endocervical cultures are obtained after the cervix is visualized with a speculum. The cervical culture test procedure is done by a health care professional with education in this procedure. The method of specimen handling varies according to the type of organism sought.

CLINICAL ALERT:
If a Papanicolaou smear is indicated, it should be collected before the cervical culture is obtained. The sample for *Neisseria gonorrhea* should be collected before the sample for *Chlamydia trachomatis* or herpes simplex virus.

Consent Form: Refer to health care facility policy.

List of Equipment: Speculum; collection swab or brush; appropriate transport medium

Test Procedure:
1. Label collection container. *Correctly identifies the client and test to be performed.*
2. Moisten the speculum with warm water. Do not use lubricants. *Lubricants may contain antibacterial agents.*
3. Remove all secretions and discharge from the cervical os.
4. Insert the swab or brush 1–2 cm into the endocervical canal and rotate firmly against the wall for 10–30 sec.
5. Withdraw the swab or brush without touching the vagina. *Avoids contamination of specimen.*

6. Place swab or brush in appropriate transport medium.
7. Deliver to laboratory as soon as possible. Do not refrigerate specimen. *Recovery of the organisms may be more difficult due to a delay in processing.*

Clinical Implications and Indications:
1. Diagnoses genital ulcers, vaginal lymphadenopathy, and pelvic inflammatory disease
2. Evaluates abnormal discharges and itching
3. Identifies the signs and symptoms of bacterial STDs, such as chlamydia, gonorrhea, and herpes simplex virus

Nursing Care:
Before Test: Explain the test procedure and the purpose of the test. Assess the client's knowledge of the test. Place client in dorsal lithotomy position. Drape client appropriately.
During Test: Adhere to standard precautions. Provide emotional support if test causes discomfort.
After Test: Provide privacy for client.

WEBLINKS

www.best4health.org

Chlamydia
(kluh-*MID*-ee-uh)
(chlamydia antibodies; chlamydia antibody IgG test; chlamydia culture; chlamydia group titer; chlamydia test)

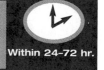

Within 24–72 hr.

Type of Test: Culture; blood; urine

Body Systems and Functions: Reproductive system

Normal Findings: *Chlamydia trachomatis:* no growth of pathological organisms in cell culture or no evidence of organism under microscopic evaluation. *Chlamydia psittaci, C. pneumoniae:* no antibodies present in serological tests.

Test Results Time Frame: Incubation of cell culture requires 48–72 hr. Polymerase chain reaction microscopic evaluation test results using endocervical swab and male urine specimens are ready in 24 hr.

Test Description: Chlamydia are intracellular parasites. Three species are pathological for humans: *C. trachomatis, C. psittaci,* and *C. pneumoniae. Chlamydia trachomatis* is the most common cause of sexually transmitted disease in the United States. *Chlamydia trachomatis* infections are divided into classic trachoma, sexually transmitted infections, and perinatal ocular and respiratory tract infections. Symptoms of classic trachoma are conjunctivitis, conjunctival scarring, and blindness. *Chlamydia trachomatis* also causes a sexually transmitted infection with lymphogranuloma venereum (LGV) strains. *Chlamydia psittaci* causes the infection psittacosis and is transmitted from infected birds to humans. Owners of pet birds make up half of the 40–60 cases reported in the

United States each year. *Chlamydia pneumoniae* is transmitted from human to human. A DNA probe from the cervix, urethra, or eye is the preferred method of diagnosis of chlamydial infections. Cell culture and polymerase chain reaction may also be used.

Consent Form: May be required

List of Equipment: *Blood:* serum separator tube; needle and syringe or vacutainer; alcohol swab (*C. psittaci, C. pneumoniae*). *Culture:* DNA probe kit (a swab for specimen collection may be used) (*C. trachomatis*). *Urine:* sterile plastic container; ice.

Test Procedure:

Blood:
1. Label the specimen tube. *Correctly identifies the client and the test to be performed.*
2. Obtain a 5-mL blood sample.
3. Do not agitate the tube. *Agitation may cause RBC hemolysis.*
4. Send tube to the laboratory.

Culture:
1. Label the swab specimen. *Correctly identifies the client and the test to be performed.*
2. Obtain specimen per health care facility protocol.
3. Provide prompt transportation of culture specimen to laboratory.

Urine:
1. Label a sterile urine container. *Correctly identifies the client and the test to be performed.*
2. Obtain a clean-catch specimen of urine (note: first morning voiding preferred, at least 15 mL). *Ensures accurate results.*
3. Keep specimen cool. *High temperatures alter the results.*
4. Send specimen to laboratory.

Specimens for detection of chlamydia trachoma Specimens for the diagnosis of infections with C. trachomatis are determined by the disease manifestation.

Disease	Specimen
Mucopurulent cervicitis	DNA probe kit or endocervical swab
Acute urethral syndrome (females)	DNA probe kit or urethral swab
Acute endometritis	Endometrial aspirate
Acute salpingitis	Fallopian tube biopsy
Nongonococcal urethritis (males)	DNA probe kit or urethral swab, urine
Inclusion conjunctivitis	DNA probe kit or conjunctival scrapings/swab
Trachoma	DNA probe kit or conjunctival scrapings/swab
Lymphogranuloma venereum	Lymph node aspirate, biopsy of ulcerated lesion, serum
Pneumonitis (infants)	Serum, tracheobronchial aspirate, nasopharyngeal swab

Clinical Implications and Indications:

1. Presence of antibody titer indicates chlamydial infection in the past. A four-fold or greater rise in antibody titers between specimens in the acute and convalescent phase in a client with symptoms supports the diagnosis of infection.
2. The presence of *C. trachomatis* organisms with DNA probe (or in culture or under microscope) confirms infection. The clinical symptoms are a small painless vesicle in the primary phase; symptoms in the secondary stage are regional lymphadenopathy, fever, chills, anorexia, headache, myalgias, arthralgias, urethritis, and cervicitis.
3. *Chlamydia psittaci* enters the body via the respiratory tract, causing chills, fever, malaise, cough with dry or blood-streaked mucus, painful myalgias, arthralgias, and a macular rash.
4. The clinical manifestations of infection with *C. pneumoniae* are mild pneumonia, pharyngitis, hoarseness, persistent cough, fever, otitis, myocarditis, bronchitis, and endocarditis.

Nursing Care:

Before Test: Explain the test procedure and the purpose of the test. Assess the client's knowledge of the test. Instruct client to not urinate at least 2 hr prior to urine specimen collection.
During Test: Adhere to standard precautions. If any urine is accidentally contaminated with feces, discard entire specimen and begin test again.
After Test: Blood: Apply pressure to venipuncture site. Explain that some bruising, discomfort, and swelling may appear at the site and that warm, moist compresses can alleviate this. Monitor for signs of infection. Urine: Document urine quantity, date, and exact hours of collection on requisition. Provide counseling as appropriate concerning sexually transmitted diseases.

Potential Complications: Bleeding and bruising at venipuncture site

Contraindications: Urine contaminated with feces; spillage or inaccurate collection of the urine specimen, including nonrefrigeration or placing on ice; heavy bleeding during menstruation; antibiotic therapy

Interfering Factors: False-positive rises in antibody titer of *C. psittaci* may occur in clients with Legionnaire's disease; too much volume of urine will dilute the specimen.

Nursing Considerations:

Pregnancy: Chlamydia trachomatis may be transmitted from an infected mother to the infant during passage through the birth canal. These infants develop conjunctivitis and interstitial pneumonitis.
Pediatric: Classic trachoma is transmitted among children via fingers, fomites, and flies. A collection bag or insertion of a straight catheter is likely needed for infants and toddlers. Infants and children will need assistance in remaining still during the venipuncture and age-appropriate comfort measures following the test.
International: Chlamydia is endemic in Asia, Africa, and South America. In the United States approximately 500 cases are reported each year. Chlamydia is most common in people of low socioeconomic status living in the southeastern states, in

homosexual men, and in people who have visited chlamydia-endemic countries. Classic trachoma is an important cause of blindness in the Middle East, North Africa, and northern India.

WEBLINKS

http://www.ncbi.nlm.nih.gov/entrez/query.fcgi

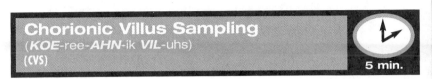

Chorionic Villus Sampling
(*KOE*-ree-*AHN*-ik *VIL*-uhs)
(CVS)

5 min.

CULTURE, TISSUE, MICROSCOPIC

Type of Test: Tissue

Body Systems and Functions: Reproductive system

Normal Findings: Absence of chromosomal abnormalities, fetal metabolic enzyme, or blood disorders

Test Results Time Frame: Within 24–48 hr

Test Description: Chorionic villus sampling (CVS) is done for prenatal diagnosis of chromosomal and genetic disorders. CVS involves obtaining a sample of tissue from the villi of the chorion, which are considered fetal cells. The sampling method includes inserting a catheter into the cervix of the mother and into the outer portion of the membranes that surround the fetus. A microscopic and chemical examination of the tissue sample is performed to detect abnormalities. The CVS should not be done before 10 weeks gestation and the chance of having a successful pregnancy outcome is less with a CVS than after amniocentesis. In addition, the accuracy of the data is less with a CVS than an amniocentesis.

CLINICAL ALERT:
CVS cannot detect neural tube defects.

Consent Form: Required

List of Equipment: Sterile speculum, antiseptic solution, biopsy tray

Test Procedure:
1. Place client in supine position. *Allows ultrasound examination of the fetus.*
2. The client is placed in a lithotomy position. *Allows for cleansing of the vagina with antiseptic solution.*
3. A sterile catheter is inserted into the vagina, through the cervical canal, and into trophoblastic tissue.
4. A small amount of tissue is extracted using a syringe.
5. Ultrasound is now employed. *Assesses fetal viability.*

Clinical Implications and Indications:
1. Appropriate test when maternal age is greater than 35 years
2. Identifies previous child with chromosomal abnormality and parent with chromosomal abnormality

3. Diagnoses fetus with risk for genetic disorders and fetal tissue abnormalities
4. Identifies chromosomal abnormalities
5. Diagnoses fetal metabolic and hematological disorders

Nursing Care:

Before Test: Explain the test procedure and the purpose of the test. Assess the client's knowledge of the test and provide genetic counseling. The client must drink 32 ounces of water 1 hr before the test and should not void until instructed. Baseline maternal vital signs and fetal heart rate are obtained. Instruct the client that she may experience cramping as the catheter passes through the cervical canal.

During Test: Adhere to standard precautions. Provide reassurance and support during the test. Assist client with relaxation techniques if cramping occurs.

After Test: Assess the client for bleeding. Monitor maternal vital signs and fetal heart rate every 15 min and PRN for 1 hr. Instruct the client to notify the health care provider if abdominal pain, bleeding, elevated temperature, or abnormal discharge occurs. Clients who are Rh-negative may receive RhoGAM.

Potential Complications: There is a slightly increased chance of spontaneous abortions with CVS as compared to amniocentesis; bleeding; intrauterine infection; limb deformities; Rh isoimmunization; fetal death

Nursing Considerations:

Pregnancy: Special emphasis is needed for the emotional support and counseling of the pregnant client with whom this test is performed. CVS can be done during the eighth–twelfth week of pregnancy, thus making possible first-trimester diagnosis.

WEBLINKS

http://biocrs.biomed.brown.edu

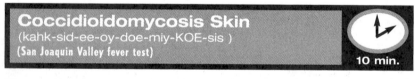

Coccidioidomycosis Skin
(kahk-sid-ee-oy-doe-miy-KOE-sis)
(San Joaquin Valley fever test)

10 min.

Type of Test: Tissue

Body Systems and Functions: Integumentary system

Normal Findings: Absence of tuberculin-type response; no induration and erythema less than 5 mm in diameter

Test Results Time Frame: Within 3–5 days

Test Description: The coccidioidomycosis test determines the presence of infection by the detection of *Coccidioides immitis*. This fungus has been isolated from the soil and from vegetation, primarily fruit. The infection is thought to occur by inhalation of dust laden with the organism. Primary pulmonary coccidioidomycosis is manifested by pulmonary symptoms and allergic skin symptoms. About 60% of infected persons are asymptomatic.

CULTURE, TISSUE, MICROSCOPIC

Consent Form: Not required

List of Equipment: Intradermal syringe and needle; coccidioidin (an antigen prepared from a culture)

Test Procedure:
1. Place client's arm in supported position with forearm exposed. *Allows for accurate injection.*
2. Inject client intradermally with coccidioidin extract.
3. Document the location, time, and date of the injection.

Clinical Implications and Indications:
1. A positive test indicates past or present infection by *C. immitis.*

Nursing Care:
Before Test: Explain the test procedure and the purpose of the test. Assess the client's knowledge of the test.
During Test: Adhere to standard precautions.
After Test: Instruct the client to return in 1–3 days for skin test evaluation.

Interfering Factors: A negative skin test does not exclude active disease; negative tests may be due to anergy, tolerance, impotent antigen, or administration before development of cell-mediated immunity; cross reactions with histoplasmin, blastomycin, and paracoccidioidin antigens may result in a false-positive reaction.

Nursing Considerations:
Pregnancy: Pregnancy may predispose to systemic disease.
Pediatric: Infants are at increased risk for severe disease.
Gerontology: The elderly are at increased risk for severe disease.
International: There is evidence that the disease is endemic in rodents, especially in the southwestern United States. A large outbreak occurred in 1994 in Ventura County, California, after the Northridge earthquake. Severe disease is several times higher in Mexicans and Native Americans and significantly higher in blacks and Filipinos. Persons with blood type B or AB and immunosuppressed clients are at increased risk for severe disease.

WEBLINKS

http://www.urmc.rochester.edu

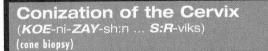

Conization of the Cervix
(*KOE*-ni-*ZAY*-sh:n ... *S:R*-viks)
(cone biopsy)

1 hr.

Type of Test: Tissue

Body Systems and Functions: Reproductive system

Normal Findings: Absence of abnormalities of the cervical tissue

Test Results Time Frame: Within 24 hr

CULTURE, TISSUE, MICROSCOPIC

Test Description: Conization of the cervix involves a diagnostic or therapeutic excision of a cone of tissue from the cervix. Often, the conization of the cervix follows abnormal PAP smears, colposcopy biopsies, and endocervical curettage. In the conization of the cervix, the tissue is examined for abnormalities by a pathologist. Sometimes lasers are used instead of the scalpel in the procedure. Cervical intraepithelial neoplasia (CIN) is the current term used to identify all epithelial abnormalities of the cervix. The epithelial cells are malignant and confined to the epithelium. CIN is divided into grade I, II, or III. In CIN I the upper two-thirds of the epithelium has undergone some cytoplasmic differentiation. In CIN II abnormal changes involve the lower two-thirds of the epithelium. CIN III lesions have full-thickness changes with undifferentiated nonstratified cells. Adenocarcinoma in situ (adenoCIS) is often associated with CIN. (Note: The biopsy in the conization of the cervix is an invasive procedure performed in a surgical setting. An excision or needle punch sample of body tissue is taken under sterile technique and examined microscopically for cell morphology and tissue anomalies.)

Consent Form: Required

List of Equipment: Biopsy tray

Test Procedure:

1. Place client in lithotomy position.
2. An incision is made into the mucous membrane of the cervix, which includes all the abnormal areas of tissue.
3. Bleeding is controlled by injecting a dilute solution of phenylephrine (Neo-Synephrine) or pitressin into the line of the incision before beginning the procedure. Bleeding is also controlled by electrocauterization.
4. A specimen of tissue is biopsied by excision or needle biopsy. Label the specimen and place in container. *Correctly identifies the client and the test to be performed.*
5. Send specimen to laboratory.

Clinical Implications and Indications:

1. Diagnoses cervical intraepithelial neoplasia and cervical glandular cell abnormalities (adenocarcinoma in situ)
2. Secondarily used as a therapeutic measure for clients who desire further fertility
3. Detects microinvasive carcinoma of the cervix by cytological testing, biopsies, or colposcopic examination
4. Evaluates postmenopausal women for the presence of abnormal cytological findings (note: lesions of postmenopausal women are usually located within the endocervical canal and cannot be evaluated with other techniques)

Nursing Care:

Before Test: Explain the test procedure and the purpose of the test. Assess the client's knowledge of the test. Provide preprocedure sedation and analgesia as ordered. Transport client to operating or procedure room. Place client in dorsal lithotomy position. Drape client appropriately.

During Test: Adhere to sterile technique and standard precautions. Provide reassurance and a calm atmosphere during the procedure.

After Test: Assess for potential complications. Instruct client about potential delayed complications and when to notify health care provider. Clean site of biopsy. Provide analgesia as necessary.

Potential Complications: Bleeding and bruising at the site; uterine perforation; continued bleeding 10–14 days after the operation; cervical stenosis; infertility; incompetent cervix; increased preterm delivery (low birth weight)

Nursing Considerations:
Pregnancy: Conization of the cervix during pregnancy may cause the major immediate complications of rupture of membranes and premature labor.
Pediatric: Sedation is recommended for infants and children. Place the infant or child on a blanket for comfort. After postprocedure monitoring is completed and per health care provider's order, the pediatric client is discharged with an adult who is given instructions. The onset of early regular sexual activity as a teenager and continued exposure to multiple sexual partners are factors associated with cervical cancer.
Gerontology: The older person may find it difficult to maintain positions when required to do so during the biopsy.
Rural: Advisable to arrange for transportation home after recovering from the conization of the cervix.
International: Women from lower socioeconomic class, blacks, and Mexican-Americans are at a higher risk for developing cervical cancer. Multiple sexual partners increase the probability of developing cervical intraepithelial neoplasia. In Europe and especially Scandinavia conization is widely used as treatment for cervical intraepitheal neoplasia.

Listing of Related Tests: Colposcopy

WEBLINKS

www.best4health.org

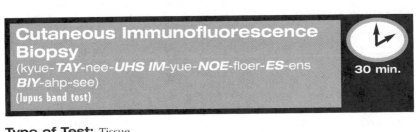

Cutaneous Immunofluorescence Biopsy
(kyue-*TAY*-nee-*UHS IM*-yue-*NOE*-floer-*ES*-ens *BIY*-ahp-see)
(lupus band test)

30 min.

Type of Test: Tissue

Body Systems and Functions: Integumentary system

Normal Findings: No abnormal patterns or antibodies

Test Results Time Frame: Within 2–5 days

Test Description: Cutaneous immunofluorescence biopsy is a laboratory technique that is applied to the evaluation of the skin of clients when an immunological source for a skin rash is suspected. In lupus erythematosus, immunoglobulins and complement components are deposited in the skin and are identified by their immunofluorescent patterns. This test confirms the histopathology of skin lesions and is also used to determine treatment result progress. In blistering diseases such as pemphigus and pemphigoid, a lesion may show the specific antibodies of these diseases. Cutaneous immunofluorescence is a biopsy that is an invasive procedure performed in a surgical setting. An excision or needle punch sample of body tissue is taken under sterile technique and examined microscopically for cell morphology and tissue anomalies.

Consent Form: Required

List of Equipment: Biopsy tray

Test Procedure:

1. Place client in supine position.
2. A specimen of tissue is biopsied by excision or needle biopsy. Label the specimen and place in container. *Correctly identifies the client and the test to be performed.*
3. Send specimen on ice to laboratory.

Clinical Implications and Indications:

1. Diagnoses systemic or discoid lupus erythematosus, pemphigus, vasculitis, bullous pemphigoid, and dermatitis herpetiforms

Nursing Care:

Before Test: Explain the test procedure and the purpose of the test. Assess the client's knowledge of the test. Provide preprocedure sedation and analgesia as ordered. Transport client to operating or procedure room. Drape client appropriately.

During Test: Adhere to sterile technique and standard precautions. Provide reassurance and a calm atmosphere during the procedure.

After Test: Clean site of biopsy. Provide analgesia as necessary.

Potential Complications: Bleeding and bruising at the site; infection

Contraindications: Anticoagulant therapy

Nursing Considerations:

Pediatric: Sedation is recommended for infants and children. Place the infant or child on a blanket for comfort. After postprocedure monitoring is completed and per health care provider's order, the pediatric client is discharged with an adult who is given instructions.

Gerontology: The older person may find it difficult to maintain positions when required to do so during the biopsy.

Rural: Advisable to arrange for transportation home after recovering from procedure.

WEBLINKS

http://www.cmrinstitute.org

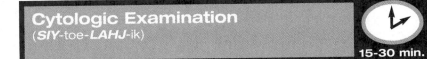

Cytologic Examination
(*SIY*-toe-*LAHJ*-ik)

15-30 min.

Type of Test: Microscopic

Body Systems and Functions: Oncology system

Normal Findings: Negative for malignant or abnormal cells or tissues

Test Results Time Frame: Within 24–48 hr (depends on specific type of cytologic examination ordered)

Test Description: Cytology of body tissues and cells involves the examination of cells in order to diagnose malignant and premalignant conditions. Specimens are evaluated for number of cells; distribution of cells; surface modification; size, shape, and appearance of cells; staining characteristics; functional adaptations; and inclusions. Sources for cytologic studies may include fine needle aspiration of superficial and palpable lesions; sputum; tissue biopsy; Papanicolaou smears; urine; cerebral spinal fluid; effusions of the pleural, pericardial, peritoneal, and abdominal cavities; and gastrointestinal fluid. Some specimens may be easy to obtain, such as a smear of the oral cavity, while others are less accessible, such as amniotic fluid. Tissue samples may be obtained in surgery.

Consent Form: May or may not be required. Refer to specific specimen source and method of collection.

List of Equipment: Sterile collection container(s) for specimen obtained. Other equipment may be necessary depending upon the specific specimen source and method of collection.

Test Procedure:
1. Refer to individual health care institution policy for collection procedure and requirements.
2. Label collection container. *Correctly identifies the client and test to be performed.*
3. Transport specimen to laboratory immediately. *Delay in processing causes a deterioration of tumor cells.*

Clinical Implications and Indications:
1. Diagnoses infectious processes, malignancies, benign atypical changes, metaplasia, viral changes and diseases, degenerative changes, fungal and parasitic diseases, hormonal cell patterns, maturation index of the major cell types, inflammatory conditions, leukemia, and meningitis

Nursing Care:
Before Test: Explain the test procedure and the purpose of the test. Assess the client's knowledge of the test.

CULTURE, TISSUE, MICROSCOPIC

During Test: Adhere to standard precautions and sterile technique as appropriate. Consult with health care institution's cytology laboratory regarding appropriate specimen collection container and procedure for collection.

After Test: Refer to nursing posttest care and monitoring according to the specific type of specimen collection procedure.

Potential Complications: Refer to specific potential complications according to the method of specimen collection for cytologic study.

Contraindications: Refer to specific contraindications associated with the type of specimen collection procedure employed.

Interfering Factors: False-negative and false-positive results may be due to a variety of reasons depending upon the specific specimen source and collection procedure; delays in processing the specimen may cause a deterioration of tumor cells, causing a false-negative result; sampling error, where diagnostic cells are not present in the specimen obtained, is another source of false-negative results.

DNA Ploidy
(*PLOY*-dee)
(stemline DNA analysis)

30-60 min.

Type of Test: Tissue

Body Systems and Functions: Oncology system

Normal Findings: Negative for malignant cells

Test Results Time Frame: Within 24–48 hr

Test Description: DNA ploidy is an invasive biopsy procedure performed in a surgical setting. An excision or needle punch sample of body tissue is taken under sterile technique and examined microscopically for cell morphology and tissue anomalies. Malignant cells have a greater proliferation than do normal cells, and the DNA ploidy test allows for detection of the cancerous cells in the breast.

Consent Form: Required

List of Equipment: Biopsy tray

Test Procedure:
1. Label specimen container. *Correctly identifies the client and the test to be performed.*
2. Place client in supine position and drape appropriately. *Allows for privacy.*
3. Obtain biopsy specimen of breast tissue.

Clinical Implications and Indications:
1. Diagnoses the presence of breast cancer

Nursing Care:
Before Test: Explain the test procedure and the purpose of the test. Assess the client's knowledge of the test. Provide preprocedure sedation and analgesia as ordered. Transport client to operating or procedure room.
During Test: Adhere to sterile technique and standard precautions. Provide reassurance and a calm atmosphere during the procedure.
After Test: Clean site of biopsy. Provide analgesia as necessary.

Potential Complications: Bleeding and bruising at the site

Interfering Factors: Inability to remain still

Nursing Considerations:
Pediatric: Sedation is recommended for infants and children. Place the infant or child on a blanket for comfort. After postprocedure monitoring is completed and per health care provider's order, the pediatric client is discharged with an adult who is given instructions.
Gerontology: The older person may find it difficult to maintain positions when required to do so for lengthy periods of times during the biopsy.
Rural: Advisable to arrange for transportation home after recovering from the biopsy

Listing of Related Tests: Physical examination of the breast; estrogen and progesterone testing

WEBLINKS
http://adam.excite.com

CULTURE, TISSUE, MICROSCOPIC

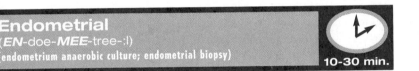

Endometrial
(EN-doe-MEE-tree-:l)
(endometrium anaerobic culture; endometrial biopsy)

10–30 min.

Type of Test: Tissue

Body Systems and Functions: Reproductive system

Normal Findings: No growth of pathogenic bacteria and normal endometrial response 3–5 days before menses

Test Results Time Frame: Within 48–72 hr

Test Description: Endometrial testing involves either obtaining a tissue culture or a biopsy specimen from the endometrium. The endometrium is the uterine layer that proliferates and sheds as it responds to the hormonal changes throughout the menstrual cycle. A biopsy is an invasive procedure performed in a surgical setting. An excision or needle punch sample of body tissue is taken under sterile technique and examined microscopically for cell morphology and tissue anomalies. The biopsy is obtained 3–5 days before menses to ensure a "secretory-like" endometrium on cellular examination. Sometimes the biopsy is performed to determine the effects of estrogen with clients who have ovarian abnormalities. A culture is obtained when there are suspected pathologies connected with the endometrium.

CLINICAL ALERT:
Procedure may cause menstrual-like cramping.

Consent Form: Required

List of Equipment: Biopsy tray

Test Procedure:
1. Place client in lithotomy position and drape. *Ensures privacy.*
2. A specimen of tissue is biopsied by excision or needle biopsy. Label the specimen and place in container. *Correctly identifies the client and the test to be performed.*
3. Send specimen to laboratory.

Clinical Implications and Indications:
1. Evaluates and monitors anovulation, endometriosis, inflammatory conditions, pelvic inflammatory disease (PID), polyps, tuberculosis, and tumors

Nursing Care:
Before Test: Explain the test procedure and the purpose of the test. Assess the client's knowledge of the test. Provide preprocedure sedation and analgesia as ordered. Transport client to operating or procedure room. Drape client appropriately.

During Test: Adhere to sterile technique and standard precautions. Provide reassurance and a calm atmosphere during the procedure.

After Test: Clean site of biopsy. Provide analgesia as necessary. Provide sanitary pad for minor spotting. Inform client to take showers (not baths) for 3–4 days. Instruct client to notify health care provider if there is excessive bleeding or purulent drainage.

Potential Complications: Uterine bleeding; infection; perforated uterus; infertility

Contraindications: Infections of cervix or vagina; abnormal positioning of the cervix

Interfering Factors: Refrigeration of specimen

Nursing Considerations:
Gerontology: The older person may find it difficult to maintain positions when required to do so for lengthy periods of time.

WEBLINKS

http://adam.excite.com

Margin tab: CULTURE, TISSUE, MICROSCOPIC

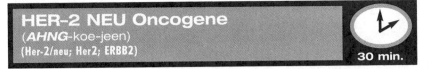

HER-2 NEU Oncogene
(**AHNG**-koe-jeen)
(Her-2/neu; Her2; ERBB2)

30 min.

CULTURE, TISSUE, MICROSCOPIC

Type of Test: Tissue

Body Systems and Functions: Oncology system

Normal Findings: Normal amplification or expression of the ERBB2 proto-oncogene

Test Results Time Frame: Within 5 days

Test Description: HER-2 NEU oncogene is an oncogene linked to breast cancer. This is a protein member of the tyrosine kinase family and is thought to be a growth factor receptor. A typical breast cell carries about 50,000 HER-2 NEU receptors on its surface. When this gene is mutated, the number jumps to between 1 and 1.5 million. The test is an immunohistochemical assay.

Consent Form: Required

Test Procedure:
1. Procedure is performed as a tissue test in pathology during biopsy of the breast tissue.
2. Tissue samples are labeled and placed in appropriate containers and sent to the pathology laboratory. *Correctly identifies the client and the test to be performed.*

Clinical Implications and Indications:
1. Diagnoses suspected breast cancer
2. Identifies prognostic information for breast, ovarian, and non–small cell lung carcinomas

Nursing Care:
Before Test: Explain the test procedure and the purpose of the test. Assess the client's knowledge of the test.
During Test: Adhere to standard precautions. Provide reassurance and a calm atmosphere during the procedure.
After Test: Clean site of biopsy. Provide analgesia as necessary.

Potential Complications: Bleeding and bruising at the site

Listing of Related Tests: Breast biopsy

Herpes Virus
(*HUR*-peez)
(HSV-1; HSV-2)

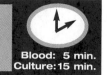

Blood: 5 min.
Culture: 15 min.

Type of Test: Culture; blood

Body Systems and Functions: Reproductive system

Normal Findings: Negative antibody of <1:10 titer; negative culture for presence of virus

Test Results Time Frame: Within 24 hr for serum; up to 4 weeks for culture

Test Description: Herpes virus testing is serological testing for the presence of antibodies for HSV-1 or HSV-2. This is often performed if cultures have been found to be positive. A blood sample may be obtained and cultures are obtained to isolate the herpes simplex virus, which includes HSV-1. HSV-1 affects the eyes, mouth, and respiratory tract, and HSV-2 affects the genital tract. Cytology confirms the presence of the virus.

Consent Form: Not required

List of Equipment: *Blood:* red-top tube or serum separator tube; needle and syringe or vacutainer; alcohol swab. *Culture:* culturette swabs; gloves; vaginal speculum (as appropriate for collection); viral transport medium.

Test Procedure:
Blood:
1. Label the specimen tube. *Correctly identifies the client and the test to be performed.*
2. Obtain a 5-mL blood sample.
3. Do not agitate the tube. *Agitation may cause RBC hemolysis.*
4. Send tube to the laboratory.
5. Keep specimen cool. *High temperatures alter the results.*

Culture specimen (lower eyelid or mouth):
1. Swab or scrape affected area with culturette swab and place onto viral medium.
2. Fix specimen to slide with appropriate spray and send to laboratory.

Culture specimen (male urethra):
1. Insert culturette swab into urethral opening and rotate swab.
2. Place into viral transport medium. Send to laboratory.

Culture specimen (female cervix):
1. Place client in lithotomy position and insert vaginal speculum.
2. Insert culturette swab into the vagina and swab the cervix.
3. Place into viral transport medium. Send to laboratory.

Clinical Implications and Indications:
1. Determines presence of HSV by culture, cytology, or serology
2. Determines the cause of lesions of eyes, mouth, and genitalia

Nursing Care:
Before Test: Explain the test procedure and the purpose of the test. Assess the client's knowledge of the test.
During Test: Adhere to standard precautions.
After Test: Apply pressure to venipuncture site. Explain that some bruising, discomfort, and swelling may appear at the site and that warm, moist compresses can alleviate this. Monitor for signs of infection.

Potential Complications: Bleeding and bruising at venipuncture site

Interfering Factors: Contamination of specimen; pretest antiviral therapy, which delays growth of pathogens

Nursing Considerations:
Pediatric: Infants and children will need assistance in remaining still during the venipuncture and age-appropriate comfort measures following the test.

Listing of Related Tests: Herpes virus antigen

WEBLINKS

http://biocrs.biomed.brown.edu

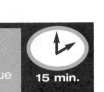

Human Papilloma Virus in Situ Hybridization
(*HYUE*-m:n *PAEP*-uh-*LOE*-muh *VIY*-ruhs in *SI*-tue
HIY-bruh-diy-*ZAY*-sh:n)   **15 min.**
(HPV; condylomata acuminata; venereal warts; genital warts)

Type of Test: Tissue

Body Systems and Functions: Reproductive system

Normal Findings: Negative for the koilocyte

Test Results Time Frame: Within 72 hr

Test Description: Human papilloma virus in situ hybridization detects the presence and types of HPVs that are the causative agents for sexually transmitted genital warts. Although vulvar lesions are most often diagnosed by appearance alone, cervical and possibly vaginal lesions are often not visible. Physical examination cannot distinguish types of HPV or precancerous or cancerous cellular changes. Therefore, the in situ hybridization technique of cytology is often recommended. The classic cytological finding in HPV is the koilocyte, or "balloon cell." This is a squamous cell, frequently enlarged, frequently binucleate or multinucleate, with dense and opaque nuclear material. Colposcopic examination of the vagina and cervix is often suggested due to high rates of cervical involvement and relatively high false-negative rates on cytology. Acetic acid application followed by magnification often reveals clinically inapparent lesions. Biopsy may be needed to confirm findings. DNA hybridization provides a more specific diagnosis of HPV infection.

CULTURE, TISSUE, MICROSCOPIC

CULTURE, TISSUE, MICROSCOPIC

Consent Form: Not required (note: required for colposcopy)

List of Equipment: Speculum; lubricant; drapes; glass slide; fixative; special containers with preservative solution for colposcopy; ViraPap test kit if available

Test Procedure:
1. Label the slides. *Correctly identify the client and the procedure to be performed.*
2. Place the client in the lithotomy position and drape. *Ensures privacy.*
3. Perform speculum examination and Pap smear of the cervix.
4. Spray fixative on slides and place in preservative.
5. With colposcopy, position the scope to focus on the cervix. Swab the cervix with 3% acetic acid. *Removes mucus.*
6. Biopsy tissues using a forceps inserted through the speculum.
7. Rinse the vagina with sterile saline or water.
8. Place samples in appropriate containers with special preservative solution and take to the laboratory.

Clinical Implications and Indications:
1. Diagnoses reported vulvar lesions, which are often asymptomatic.
2. Distinguishes the type of HPV, precancerous, or cancerous cellular changes.
3. DNA hybridizaton provides more specific diagnosis of HPV infection after histological findings in genital warts.

Nursing Care:
Before Test: Explain the test procedure and the purpose of the test. Assess the client's knowledge of the test. Provide preprocedure sedation and analgesia as ordered. Drape client appropriately.

During Test: Adhere to standard precautions. Provide for privacy during procedure. Provide reassurance and a calm atmosphere during the procedure.

After Test: Explain that some cramping and spotting may occur for a short time. Instruct client to remove vaginal tampon within 8 hr if one was inserted and to wear tampons if there is further bleeding or drainage. Provide analgesia as necessary.

Potential Complications: Persistent bleeding may warrant cautery, suturing, or application of silver nitrate.

Contraindications: Bleeding disorders; pregnancy

Interfering Factors: Scarring of the cervix

Listing of Related Tests: Gonorrhea and *Chlamydia* cultures; syphilis serology; Pap exam

WEBLINKS

http://www.pstcc.cc.tn.us/ost/2910/pronun/c14

Kidney Biopsy
(*BIY*-ahp-see)
(renal biopsy; punch biopsy of the kidney; closed kidney biopsy)

15-30 min.

Type of Test: Tissue

Body Systems and Functions: Renal/urological system

Normal Findings: No pathological conditions

Test Results Time Frame: Within 1–3 days

Test Description: A kidney biopsy is a microscopic assessment of renal tissue obtained by biopsy. The biopsy is an invasive procedure performed in a surgical setting. An excision or needle punch sample of kidney tissue is taken under sterile technique and examined microscopically for cell morphology and tissue anomalies. Tissue samples can be obtained through open renal biopsy, but the procedure is usually performed percutaneously. The procedure can be refined with ultrasonographic or fluoroscopic guidance.

CLINICAL ALERT:
There may be serious implications of a pathology result from the kidney biopsy. Consequently, there needs to be sensitivity toward the patient and acknowledgment of concerns and anxieties regarding the possible outcome of the test.

Consent Form: Required

List of Equipment: Travenol Trucut needle; Vim-Silverman needle; various needles and syringes for anesthesia; scalpel blade; lidocaine; sterile drapes; betadine gauze; gowns and masks; specimen containers

Test Procedure:
1. Place client in the prone position with a pillow placed under the abdomen. *Provides comfort and straightens the spine.*
2. The skin over the kidneys is locally anesthetized with lidocaine.
3. Client inspires and holds his or her breath during the procedure. *Prevents the kidney from moving as the biopsy needle is inserted.*
4. A specimen of tissue is biopsied by excision or needle biopsy. Label the specimen and place in container. *Correctly identifies the client and the test to be performed.*
5. Send specimen to laboratory.

Clinical Implications and Indications:
1. Evaluates and monitors acute glomerulonephritis, amyloid infiltration, chronic glomerulonephritis, disseminated lupus erythromatosus, pyelonephritis, rejection of kidney transplant, renal cell carcinoma, renal vein thrombosis, and Wilm's tumor

CULTURE, TISSUE, MICROSCOPIC

CULTURE, TISSUE, MICROSCOPIC

Nursing Care:

Before Test: Explain the test procedure and the purpose of the test. Assess the client's knowledge of the test. Provide preprocedure sedation and analgesia as ordered. Transport client to operating or procedure room. Drape client appropriately. Instruct client to be NPO 8 hr prior to test. Inform the patient that transient pain may be felt during the needle insertion into the kidney.

During Test: Adhere to sterile technique and standard precautions. Provide reassurance and a calm atmosphere during the procedure.

After Test: Clean site of biopsy. Provide analgesia as necessary. Vital signs are taken frequently and instruct client to remain supine in bed for at least 24 hr. Collect samples of client's urine for examination of hematuria (blood may be present in urine of up to 24 hr after the procedure but should be absent after this time). Also, collect blood samples for hematocrit and hemoglobin counts. Assess for symptoms of a punctured bowel or liver. Puncture site must be observed for drainage every 15 min for 4 hr, every 30 min for the following 4 hr, every hour for the following 4 hr, and then every 4 hr. Instruct client to drink fluids. Following discharge from the hospital, instruct client to not lift heavy objects, engage in intense exercise, or play contact sports for 1–2 weeks.

Potential Complications: Enlarging hematomas (indicated by a severe drop in hematocrit levels, intense pain at the biopsy site, drop in blood pressure, and gross hematuria); hemorrhage of renal tissue; accidental puncture of the bowel, aorta, or lung; infection

Contraindications: Absence of a kidney; renal artery aneurysm; polynephritis or perinephric abcess; hydronephrosis; uncontrolled hypertension; uncorrected volume depletion; coagulation disorders; operable kidney tumors; urinary tract infections; severe thrombocytopenia ($<50,000/mm^3$)

Nursing Considerations:

Pediatric: Sedation is recommended for infants and children. Place the infant or child on a blanket for comfort. After postprocedure monitoring is completed and per health care provider's order, the pediatric client is discharged with an adult who is given instructions.

Gerontology: The older person may find it difficult to maintain positions when required to do so for lengthy periods of time during the biopsy.

Home Care: Instruct client to recognize the clinical manifestations of a potential renal hemorrhage. Also, inform client to contact health care provider if there is a burning sensation in the kidney area or a generalized febrile condition.

Rural: Advisable to arrange for transportation home after recovering from the biopsy.

Listing of Related Tests: Renal ultrasonography; renal computed tomography

WEBLINKS

http://www.creighton.edu

Kidney Stone Analysis
(stoen uh-**NAEL**-uh-sis)
(stone analysis; calculi analysis)

1 hr.

CULTURE, TISSUE, MICROSCOPIC

Type of Test: Tissue

Body Systems and Functions: Renal/urological system

Normal Findings: Absence of stone formation

Test Results Time Frame: Within 1–3 days

Test Description: Kidney stone analysis is performed with infrared spectroscopy. The stones themselves are formed of cystine, oxalate, uric acid, calcium, or calcium oxalate. The type of stone determines the treatment. The kidney stone is obtained by straining the urine and examining the clean, washed stone. Clients with kidney stones typically have severe flank pain that is often treated with narcotic analgesics.

> **CLINICAL ALERT:**
> Clients with excruciating flank pain should be assessed for the possibility of renal calculi. Narcotic analgesics would typically be given as soon as possible to alleviate the discomfort.

Consent Form: Not required

List of Equipment: Sterile plastic container; meshed disposable screen

Test Procedure:
1. The client screens all voided urine with a fine meshed disposable screen. *Ensures better chances of obtaining the specimen.*
2. All sediment or calculi are saved for analysis.
3. Label the collection container. *Correctly identifies the client and the test to be performed.*
4. Send specimen to laboratory.

Clinical Implications and Indications:
1. Evaluates and monitors the presence of kidney stones

Nursing Care:
Before Test: Explain the test procedure and the purpose of the test. Assess the client's knowledge of the test. The client may require pain medication if the stone has not passed.
During Test: Adhere to standard precautions.
After Test: Counsel the client regarding fluid intake, changes in diet, and medications to prevent other stone reccurrence.

Interfering Factors: Applying adhesive tape to the stones will interfere with the infrared spectroscopy.

Nursing Considerations:
Pediatric: Children may incur renal stones from infection due to calcium phosphate and magnesium ammonium phosphate.

Home Care: *Home health care provider will need to carefully assist client in the screening of all urine samples and assess the urine for the presence of kidney stones.*

WEBLINKS

www.nlm.nih.gov

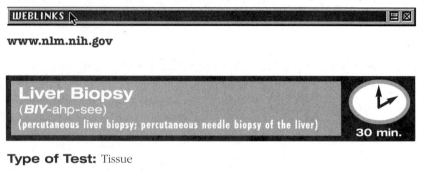

Liver Biopsy
(***BIY***-ahp-see)
(percutaneous liver biopsy; percutaneous needle biopsy of the liver)

30 min.

Type of Test: Tissue

Body Systems and Functions: Hepatobiliary system

Normal Findings: Absence of abnormal cells and tissue

Test Results Time Frame: Within 24–48 hr

Test Description: The liver biopsy is an invasive procedure performed in a surgical setting. An excision or needle punch sample of a small sample of liver tissue is taken under sterile technique and examined microscopically for cell morphology and tissue anomalies. This test is performed to diagnose or confirm the cause of chronic liver disease and liver tumors and after liver transplants to determine cause of elevated liver tests and determine if rejection is occurring. The liver biopsy may also be done using ultrasound or CT guidance.

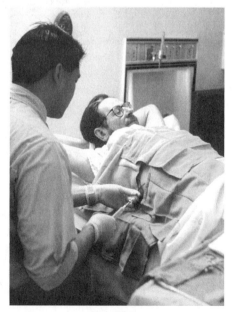

Liver Biopsy

CULTURE, TISSUE, MICROSCOPIC

CLINICAL ALERT:
Prothrombin time and hemoglobin must be checked prior to this invasive test.

Consent Form: Required

List of Equipment: Local anesthetic; biopsy needle (14–18 gauge); specimen bottle containing formalin 10%; labels

Test Procedure:
1. Place client in supine or left lateral position with right arm over head.
2. Skin is cleansed and local anesthestic is injected into skin over the biopsy site.
3. A specimen of tissue is biopsied by excision or needle biopsy. Label the specimen and place in container. *Correctly identifies the client and the test to be performed.*
4. During the insertion and biopsy, client must hold their breath for approximately 10 sec to avoid pneumothorax.
5. Send specimen to laboratory.

Clinical Implications and Indications:
1. Detects Wilson's disease, sarcoidosis, hemosiderosis, schistosomiasis, and Weil's disease
2. Evaluates and monitors benign tumors, malignant tumors, abscesses, cysts, hepatitis, diabetes, infiltrative diseases (amyloidosis, hemochromatosis), metabolic disorders, and accumulation of bile

Nursing Care:
Before Test: Explain the test procedure and the purpose of the test. Assess the client's knowledge of the test. Provide preprocedure sedation and analgesia as ordered. Transport client to operating or procedure room. Drape client appropriately. Instruct client to be NPO for 12 hr prior to the test. Inform client to hold breath for 10–15 sec. Assess the prothrombin time and hemoglobin level.
During Test: Adhere to sterile technique and standard precautions. Provide reassurance and a calm atmosphere during the procedure.
After Test: Clean site of biopsy. Provide analgesia as necessary. Apply pressure dressing and assess site for potential bleeding. Assess vital signs frequently and keep client on bedrest for observation.

Potential Complications: Bleeding and bruising at the site of the biopsy; puncture of the kidney, lung (pneumothorax), or colon; puncture of the gallbladder associated with bile leakage and peritonitis

Contraindications: Decreased prothrombin time or platelet count; inability to hold breath for 10 sec; anemia; hemangioma; infection; extrahepatic lesion; marked ascites; septic cholangitis; bleeding disorders or obstructive jaundice

Interfering Factors: Abnormal clotting time or low hemoglobin; false-negative results may occur if biopsy needle misses diseased area; degeneration or distortion of specimen may occur with faulty preparation; false-positive results may be caused by misinterpretation of markedly reactive hepatocytes.

Nursing Considerations:

Pediatric: Sedation is recommended for infants and children. Place the infant or child on a blanket for comfort. After postprocedure monitoring is completed and per health care provider's order, the pediatric client is discharged with an adult who is given instructions.

Gerontology: The older person may find it difficult to maintain positions when required to do so for lengthy periods of time during the biopsy.

Rural: Advisable to arrange for transportation home after recovering from procedure.

WEBLINKS

www.canoe.ca

Lung Biopsy
(luhng *BIY*-ahp-see)
(fine needle biopsy of the lung)

30-60 min.

Type of Test: Tissue

Body Systems and Functions: Pulmonary system

Normal Findings: No pathology evident

Test Results Time Frame: Within 3–4 days

Test Description: A lung biopsy is an invasive procedure performed in a surgical setting. An excision or a needle punch sample of lung tissue is taken under sterile technique and examined microscopically for cell morphology and tissue anomalies. The lung biopsy aids in the diagnosis of cancer, pulmonary fibrosis, sarcoidosis, and lung infections. It also helps in the identification and evaluation of lung damage caused by environmental exposure or inherited lung diseases.

Consent Form: Required

List of Equipment: Bronchoscope; IV equipment; lead markers to position for biopsy needle; sterile towels; local anesthetic; scalpel; biopsy needle; specimen bottle; dressing

Test Procedure:
1. Place client in sitting position.
2. Perform clotting time test and chest x-rays.
3. A specimen of tissue is biopsied by excision or needle biopsy. Label the specimen and place in container. *Correctly identifies the client and the test to be performed.*
4. Send specimen to laboratory.

Clinical Implications and Indications:
1. Diagnoses various diseases contracted from environmental exposure, infections of the lung (e.g., pneumonia), carcinoma of the lung (squamous cell, oat-cell, adenocarcinoma), sarcoidosis, and granuloma
2. Evaluates degenerative diseases of the lung

Nursing Care:

Before Test: Explain the test procedure and the purpose of the test. Assess the client's knowledge of the test. Provide preprocedure sedation and analgesia as ordered. Transport client to operating or procedure room. Drape client appropriately. Inform client of the importance of lying still during the biopsy to prevent injury. Instruct the client to fast for 8 hr prior to the procedure.

During Test: Adhere to sterile technique and standard precautions. Provide reassurance and a calm atmosphere during the lung biopsy.

After Test: Place client in a semi-Fowler's position. Vital signs should be closely observed, until the client is stable, the client observed for symptoms of a hemothorax or pneumothorax. Counsel the client to immediately contact health care provider if he experiences shortness of breath, bleeding, difficulty breathing, rapid pulse, or cyanosis. Place a dressing on the site of the biopsy. Provide analgesia as necessary.

Potential Complications: Bleeding and bruising at the site; hemothorax; pneumothorax; infection; empyema

Contraindications: Cysts of the lung; suspected vascular anomalies of the lung; pulmonary hypertension; respiratory insufficiency; clotting abnormalities

Interfering Factors: Obesity; anxiety; smoking; poor nutrition; recent or chronic illness; antihypertensives; muscle relaxants; sedatives; tranqulizers; insulin; beta-adrenergic blockers; cortisone; narcotics

Nursing Considerations:

Pediatric: Sedation is recommended for infants and children. Place the infant or child on a blanket for comfort. After postprocedure monitoring is completed and per health care provider's order, the pediatric client is discharged with an adult who is given instructions.

Gerontology: The older person may find it difficult to maintain positions when required to do so for lengthy periods of time during the biopsy.

Rural: Advisable to arrange for transportation home after recovering from lung biopsy.

CULTURE, TISSUE, MICROSCOPIC

WEBLINKS

http://www.rcjournal.com

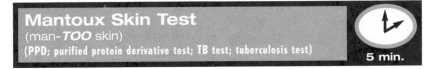

Mantoux Skin Test
(man-*TOO* skin)
(PPD; purified protein derivative test; TB test; tuberculosis test)

5 min.

Type of Test: Tissue

Body Systems and Functions: Pulmonary system

Normal Findings: Negative or minimal skin reaction (induration <5 mm in diameter)

CRITICAL VALUES:
Positive test >10 mm in diameter

Test Results Time Frame: Intradermal evaluation takes place 72 hr after injection. Two-step test: 3 days for first test results; 1–2 weeks waiting period; then 3 days for injection and evaluation of second test (total time 3 weeks).

Test Description: Mantoux skin test evaluates whether there is active or dormant tuberculosis infection. Tuberculin is a protein fraction of tubercle bacilli and is injected intradermally. The injection of tuberculin skin test solution will produce an erythema at the injection site in a positive client. Tuberculosis, as a disease, is on the rise over the past decade and is suspected more frequently when working with those at risk. The TB skin test is usually given to such persons as those whose symptoms suggest TB; those who have had a high risk of exposure, are malnourished, or are alcohol or drug abusers; the chronically ill; or health care professionals. The latter will be tested on an annual basis for preventative treatment reasons.

CLINICAL ALERT:
Have anaphylaxis equipment readily available in the event of reaction to tuberculin injection.

Consent Form: Not required

List of Equipment: Tuberculin syringe and needle; 0.1 mL (5 tuberculin units) of skin test solution; alcohol swab

Test Procedure:
1. Draw up 0.1 mL of tuberculin skin test into TB syringe according to manufacturer's directions.
2. Swab area on dorsal side of arm with alcohol swab. *Prevents contamination.*
3. When dry, pull the skin taut and inject intradermally.
4. A 6- to 10-mm pale wheal should be evident.
5. Evaluate injection site in 72 hr (or instruct client to telephone nurse with results). *Assesses for positive reaction.*

Clinical Implications and Indications:
1. Likelihood of TB infection corresponds to the intensity of the skin reaction.
2. Active and dormant cases of TB must be evaluated by sputum tests and chest x-ray.
3. Other *Mycobacterium* species or a client previously treated for TB may result in positive tests in a healthy person.
4. A negative result is good evidence against TB even in clients with symptoms of lung disease.
5. In the United States, TB rates are higher in the elderly, men, nonwhites, and immigrants.
6. Clinicians in contact with suspected or confirmed TB must wear a properly fitted, high-efficiency dust and mistproof mask.

Nursing Care:
Before Test: Explain the test procedure and the purpose of the test. Assess the client's knowledge of the test. Obtain information on past history and potential exposure to TB.
During Test: Adhere to standard precautions.

After Test: Ensure that client understands the importance of returning for reading of the skin test after 72 hr or teach client how to read the test and telephone the clinic in 72 hr. To measure, evaluate the reaction in a well-lit area. Have client flex their forearm. Look for hardening or thickening. Palpate the injection site to compare with normal skin. Circle the induration (if present) and measure the diameter (in millimeters) perpendicularly to the long axis of the arm.

Potential Complications: Allergic reaction (extremely rare)

Interfering Factors: Inexperienced reader of TB test; not read in prescribed time frame; measurement error; inaccurate antigen amount; too deep an injection of antigen; incorrect storage of antigen; active TB; low values of sensitized T lymphocytes; viruses (measles, mumps, chickenpox); Hodgkin's disease; lymphoma; chronic lymphocytic leukemia; sarcoidosis; newborns; elderly clients; corticosteroids; immunosuppresive agents

Nursing Considerations:
International: Some countries have high incidence of TB and immigrants from those countries should be retested for TB.

| WEBLINKS |

http://www.rcjournal.com

Methicillin-Resistant *Staphylococcus aureus*
(*METH*-uh-*SIL*-:n ree-*ZIST*-:nt
STAEF-uh-loe-*KAHK*-uhs *AWR*-ee-uhs)
(MRSA)

30 min.

Type of Test: Culture

Body Systems and Functions: Immunological system

Normal Findings: No *Staphylococcus aureus* grown on cultures

Test Results Time Frame: Within 48–72 hr

Test Description: *Staphylococcus aureus* is carried in the nares or skin of 20%–40% of healthy people and is rarely pathogenic. However, in acute-care hospitals and long-term care facilities, where individuals are more vulnerable to infection, a significant increase in antibiotic-resistant infections (nosocomial infections) has occurred. One of the most pathogenic is methicillin-resistant *S. aureus*, an organism especially prevalent in immunocompromised and seriously ill clients. MRSA accounts for over 12% of all nosocomial infections in the United States. MRSA testing involves cultures of the anterior nares, perineum, skin lesions, wounds, and catheter exit sites to determine if *S. aureus* is the causative organism of the infection. MRSA is no more infectious than other strains of *S. aureus*; it is just more difficult to treat (note: it is most effectively treated with IV vancomycin).

CULTURE, TISSUE, MICROSCOPIC

CLINICAL ALERT:
Any client testing positive for MRSA poses a serious health risk to other clients in the institution. Strict isolation protocol must be followed.

Consent Form: Not required

List of Equipment: Swab; culture tube

Test Procedure:
1. Obtain specimen from each potential infection site.
2. Label swab and note location (e.g., anterior nares). *Correctly identifies the client and the test performed.*
3. Send specimen to the laboratory.

Clinical Implications and Indications:
1. Diagnoses MRSA.
2. Clients at risk for MRSA infection are those who have been transferred from a nursing home or who have had a previous MRSA colonization or infection.

Nursing Care:
Before Test: Explain the test procedure and the purpose of the test. Assess the client's knowledge of the test.
During Test: Adhere to standard precautions.
After Test: If client tests positive for MRSA, isolation precautions are mandatory. Strategic planning by the institution should be implemented to detect, prevent, or control MRSA spread. If test is positive, appropriate isolation protocol must be followed, usually involving a private room, clean isolation gown, and non-sterile gloves. Scrupulous hand washing is particularly important, and visitors must be instructed on isolation procedures. Bland soap is relatively ineffective in combating MRSA. Antimicrobial soaps and waterless alcohol-based products are strongly recommended.

Potential Complications: Infection at culture site

Interfering Factors: Recent washing of the skin or wound with an antiseptic soap or cleansing solution

WEBLINKS

http://www.mic.ki.se/Diseases/c20.html; www.unc.edu

Minimum Inhibitory Concentration
(*MIN*-uh-muhm in-*HIB*-uh-*TOER*-ee *KAHN*-s:n-*TRAY*-sh:n)
(MIC; minimum bactericidal concentration; MBC; susceptibility testing)

10 min.

Type of Test: Culture

Body Systems and Functions: Immunological system

Normal Findings: Dependent on the type of bacteria isolated and each antibiotic with which it is tested

CRITICAL VALUES:
Organism grows and is resistant to antibiotics.

Test Results Time Frame: Within 2–3 days

Test Description: Minimum inhibitory concentration tests enable the appropriate treatment regimen to be implemented for bacterial infections. The pathogenic bacteria isolated from the culture is inoculated with various concentrations of different antibiotics. The degree to which the growth of the organism is or is not inhibited by a specific concentration of antimicrobial agent is defined as susceptible (S), intermediate (I), or resistant (R).

CLINICAL ALERT:
Clients with MRSA (methicillin-resistant *Staphylococcus aureus*) or VRE (vancomycin-resistant enterococcus) may need to be isolated. Gowns, gloves, and masks should be worn if these infections are suspected. Also, some bacterial infections may need to be reported to an officer of public health. Check with local public health office for specific information and guidelines.

Consent Form: Not required

List of Equipment: Depends on type of organism being cultured. For wound exudates: sterile swabs or wipes; polyester-tipped swabs; sterile container with fastenable lid; ampule of Stuart's transport medium; biohazard bag.

Test Procedure:
1. Clean the skin thoroughly with sterile wipes, starting at the location from which sample will be taken and gradually move outward. Allow the area to dry. Repeat 3–4 times with clean wipes. *Ensures accurate results.*
2. Collect the specimen with polyester swab. Specimens from the boundaries of lesions and wounds are preferable to specimens from the center of the wound. Specimens can be samples of drainage, pus, blood, sputum, feces, secretions, or blood. Attempt to retrieve a large sample if possible. Small-sample collection can be facilitated by dampening the swab with a saline solution before collection. *Ensures accurate results.*
3. Place in transport container and label appropriately (client information, source of specimen, time of collection, studies required, suspected type of bacteria, medical and immunological status and history of client, client's medications). *Correctly identifies the client and the test to be performed.*
4. Transport immediately to the laboratory.

Clinical Implications and Indications:
1. Detects the following bactericidal agents: aminoglycerides, cephalosporins, metronidazole, penicillins, quinolones, rifampin, and vancomycin
2. Detects the following bacteriostatic agents: chloramphenicol, erythromycin, sulfonamides, and tetracycline

Nursing Care:
Before Test: Explain the test procedure and the purpose of the test. Assess the client's knowledge of the test.

During Test: Adhere to standard precautions (note: caution is imperative to prevent the transmission of pathogens).

After Test: Client may need to be isolated to prevent contamination of other individuals.

Interfering Factors: Contamination of specimen during transportation; specimens obtained longer than 72 hr

Nursing Considerations:

Home Care: Health care provider needs to be instructed very specifically regarding the test procedure for collecting a specimen of a potentially contaminated area. Place great emphasis on following standard precautions.

Listing of Related Tests: Kirby Bauer test; mycobacterial infection tests

WEBLINKS

http://www.labcorp.com

Neisseria gonorrhoeae
(niy-*SEER*-ee-uh *GAHN*-uh-*REE*-uh)
(gonorrhea; genital *Neisseria gonorrhoeae*)

15 min.

Type of Test: Microscopic

Body Systems and Functions: Reproductive system

Normal Findings: Negative

Test Results Time Frame: Within 48 hr

Test Description: *Neisseria gonorrhoeae* is a pyogenic, gram-negative, oxidase-positive cocci that is a parasite of humans. It is the causative agent of the sexually transmitted infection gonorrhea. *N. gonorrhoeae* inhabits the mucous membranes of the genital tract and may also be found in the oral mucosa of clients who engage in oral sex. Specimens are obtained from the discharge (fluid) from the genital tract, external genitalia, urethra, and anorectal area to detect presence of *N. gonorrhoeae*.

CLINICAL ALERT:
Do not refrigerate specimen as *N. gonorrhoeae* is easily destroyed with cold temperatures. If the client tests positive, all sexual partners will need to be notified within 90 days.

Consent Form: Not required

List of Equipment: Culturette swab; vaginal speculum for vaginal and endocervical culture

Test Procedure:

Vaginal culture:
1. Place client in lithotomy position with appropriate draping.
2. Cleanse external genitalia and perineal area. *Prevents contamination of the specimen.*

3. Using a culturette swab, obtain sample of discharge from the urethra or vulva.
4. For vaginal and endocervical culture, lubricate and insert vaginal speculum and obtain specimen.
5. Place in culturette tube and break bottom.
6. Send to laboratory.

Urethral culture in men:
1. Retract foreskin as needed and cleanse penis.
2. Insert culturette swab into urethral orifice to obtain sample of discharge. *Ensures accurate results.*
3. Place in culturette tube; break bottom.
4. Send to laboratory.

Anorectal culture:
1. Insert culturette swab into anal canal approximately 1 in. and obtain specimen.
2. Place in culturette tube; break bottom.
3. Send to laboratory.

Clinical Implications and Indications:
1. Diagnoses the presence of gonorrhea in the client with purulent urethral and vaginal discharge.
2. Positive cultures are found with cervicitis, dysuria, endometriosis, epididymidis, pelvic inflammatory disease, salpingitis, vaginitis, and prostatitis.

Nursing Care:
Before Test: Explain procedure and purpose of the test. Assess the client's knowledge of the test. Emotional sensitivity is required, due to the potential sexual implications of a positive test.
During Test: Adhere to standard precautions.
After Test: Instruct client that if culture is positive, all sexual partners must be tested.

Interfering Factors: Pretest antibiotic therapy inhibits growth of pathogens; concomitant yeast infection; feminine hygiene sprays or douching; menses; female douching within previous 24 hr; male voiding within 1 hr of urethral culture; refrigerated specimens

Listing of Related Tests: GC screen; RPR; VDRL

WEBLINKS

http://www.pstcc.cc.tn.us/ost/2910/pronun/c14

Nerve Biopsy
(n:rv *BIY*-ahp-see)
(sural nerve biopsy; Sbx)

1 hr.

Type of Test: Tissue

Body Systems and Functions: Neurological system

CULTURE, TISSUE, MICROSCOPIC

Normal Findings: Normal nerve anatomy

Test Results Time Frame: Within 24 hr

Test Description: A nerve biopsy is a surgical procedure (usually out-patient) that involves the removal of a small portion of nerve (usually sural, but sometimes superficial radial or superficial peroneal). The sample of tissue is taken under sterile technique, and the tissue is examined microscopically for cell morphology and tissue anomalies. The nerve biopsy may identify demyelination, destruction of the axon of the nerve cell, or inflammatory nerve conditions.

Consent Form: Required

List of Equipment: Biopsy tray

Test Procedure:
1. Place client in supine position.
2. A specimen of tissue is biopsied by excision or needle biopsy. Label the specimen and place in container. *Correctly identifies the client and the test to be performed.*
3. Send specimen to laboratory.

Clinical Implications and Indications:
1. Identifies presence of inflammatory processes such as vasculitis
2. Detects disease processes that involve demyelination of nerve (e.g., multiple sclerosis)
3. Diagnoses neuropathy
4. Identifies cellular abnormalities of nerve such as those found in toxic response to chemotherapy, alcohol abuse, and vitamin E deficiency

Nursing Care:
Before Test: Explain the test procedure and the purpose of the test. Assess the client's knowledge of the test. Provide preprocedure sedation and analgesia as ordered. Transport client to operating or procedure room. Drape client appropriately.
During Test: Adhere to sterile technique and standard precautions. Provide reassurance and a calm atmosphere during the procedure.
After Test: Clean site of biopsy. Provide analgesia as necessary. Inform client that there may be alteration or loss of sensation at the operative site. A few clients may experience localized discomfort for a few days or chronically.

Potential Complications: Bleeding and bruising at the site; permanent nerve damage; infection

Contraindications: Anticoagulant use

Interfering Factors: Nerve specimen too short in length

Nursing Considerations:
Pediatric: Sedation is recommended for infants and children. Place the infant or child on a blanket for comfort. After postprocedure monitoring is completed and per health care provider's order, the pediatric client is discharged with an adult who is given instructions.
Gerontology: The older person may find it difficult to maintain positions during the biopsy when required to do so for lengthy periods of time.

Rural: *Advisable to arrange for transportation home after recovering from procedure.*

Listing of Related Tests: Muscle biopsy

WEBLINKS

www.bcm.tmc.edu

Nocardia Culture
(noe-*KAHR*-dee-uh)
(nocardia asteroides brasiliensis; transvalensis; otitidiscaviarum cultures)

10-30 min.

Type of Test: Culture

Body Systems and Functions: Immunological system

Normal Findings: Negative culture

CRITICAL VALUES:
Nocardia species found in culture of cerebrospinal fluid are potentially critical for clients.

Test Results Time Frame: Within 4 days–4 weeks

Test Description: A nocardia culture provides the opportunity to microscopically examine gram stains and modified acid-fast stains for gram-positive bacilli of the Nocardia species. Since this organism is found in soil and plant decay, infection is most frequently pulmonary. However, Nocardia can also be introduced through innoculation during trauma. Nocardiosis is usually categorized as pulmonary, systemic, CNS, extrapulmonary, cutaneous, subcutaneous, lymphocutaneous or actinomycetoma.

Consent Form: Not required

List of Equipment: (Note: Equipment is dependent on type of sample being cultured) *Blood:* red top tube or serum separator tube; needle and syringe or vacutainer; alcohol swab; culture vials. *Sputum:* sterile container or cup. *Stool:* sterile tongue blade; sterile container with lid. *Throat:* sterile swab; culture tube with medium. *Urine:* sterile plastic container; ice. *Wound:* sterile swab; culture tube with medium.

Test Procedure: (note: dependent on site of sample)
Blood:
1. Scrub skin with Betadine.
2. Cleanse top of culture bottles with iodine and leave to dry.
3. Label the specimen tube. *Correctly identifies the client and the test to be performed.*
4. Obtain a 5-mL blood sample.
5. Do not agitate the tube. *Agitation may cause RBC hemolysis.*
6. Send tube to the lab.

CULTURE, TISSUE, MICROSCOPIC

CULTURE, TISSUE, MICROSCOPIC

Sputum:
1. Obtain 5–10 mL early morning sputum sample prior to breakfast.
2. Lid should be put on sample and sample taken directly to lab.

Stool:
1. Have client defecate into a clean bedpan, bedside commode, or toilet hat. *Decreases contamination and aids in obtaining stool specimen.*
2. Do not use the stool if it is contaminated with urine or menstrual blood. *Urine and menstrual blood affects stool culture results.*
3. Do not have the client place toilet paper on the stool after defecation. *Toilet paper affects stool culture results.*
4. Use a clean tongue depressor to place 2–3 cm of formed stool or 15 cc of liquid stool in a specimen container. *This amount is necessary for obtaining proper stool culture.*
5. Dispose of remaining stool and tongue depressor. *Decreases chance of spread of pathogen.*
6. Include visible mucous, pus, or blood in the specimen. *These may be indicative of disease or contain pathogens.*
7. Label the specimen container and send to lab as soon as possible. *Ensures accurate results.*

Throat or Wound:
1. Swab area with sterile cotton swab and place in tube with culture medium.

Urine:
1. Label a sterile urine container. *Correctly identifies the client and the test to be performed.*
2. Obtain a clean catch specimen of urine (note: first morning voiding preferred, at least 60 mL). *Ensures accurate results.*
3. Keep specimen cool. *High temperatures alter the results.*
4. Send specimen to lab.

CSF:
1. Follow procedure for lumbar puncture.
2. Label a sterile container. *Correctly identifies the client and the test to be performed.*
3. Take specimen to the lab.

Clinical Implications and Indications:
1. Diagnoses infection with *Nocardia* species bacteria.

Nursing Care:
Before Test: Explain the test procedure and the purpose of the test. Assess the client's knowledge of the test.
During Test: Adhere to standard precautions. If any urine is accidentally discarded or contaminated with feces, discard entire specimen and begin test again.
After Test: Blood: apply pressure to venipuncture site. Explain that some bruising, discomfort and swelling may appear at the site and that warm moist compresses can alleviate this. Monitor for signs of infection. Urine: document urine quantity, date, and exact hours of collection on requisition.

Potential Complications: Bleeding and bruising at venipuncture site

Interfering Factors: Urine contaminated with feces; spillage or inaccurate collection of the urine specimen including nonrefrigeration or placing on ice; heavy bleeding during menstruation; sulfonamides; antibiotics; immunosuppression

Nursing Considerations:
Pediatric: Blood: infants and children will need assistance in remaining still during the venipuncture and age appropriate comfort measures following the test. Culture: sedation could be recommended for infants and children. Place the infant or child on a blanket for comfort. After post-procedure monitoring is completed and per health care provider's order, the pediatric client is discharged with an adult who is given instructions. Urine: a collection bag or insertion of a straight catheter is likely needed for infants and toddlers.

Listing of Related Tests: Nitroblue tetrazolium test

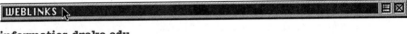

informatics.drake.edu

Ocular Cytology
(*AHK*-yue-l:r siy-*TAHL*-uh-jee)
(conjunctival; corneal or eye smear; fine needle aspiration)

5–10 min.

Type of Test: Microscopic

Body Systems and Functions: Sensory system

Normal Findings: All cells normal

Test Results Time Frame: Within 2–3 days

Test Description: Ocular cytology is the microscopic examination of cell specimen taken from the eye. The specimen may be collected by swab or fine needle aspiration. This test is likely performed when there have been such clinical manifestations as visual disturbances, eye pain, or unusual drainage from the eye region.

Consent Form: Not required for swab testing. Individual facilities may require consent for fine needle aspiration.

List of Equipment: Sterile swab; sterile ophthalmic spatula; slides and fixative

Test Procedure:
1. Swab lesion with sterile cotton-tipped applicator or scrape the lesion with sterile ophthalmic spatula. Alternately, fine needle aspiration of orbital masses may also be used for smears. *Obtains accurate sample.*
2. The sample is smeared on two glass slides and one slide is spray fixed immediately and the other left to air dry. Some laboratories use an approach in which air drying is contraindicated; therefore the individual preparing the slides must be informed in advance of procedure.

Clinical Implications and Indications:

1. Diagnoses intraocular dysplastic or malignant conjunctival lesions
2. Diagnoses trachoma-inclusion conjunctivitis
3. Diagnoses intraocular and orbital tumors

Nursing Care:

Before Test: Explain the test procedure and the purpose of the test. Assess the client's knowledge of the test. Client is unlikely to be wearing a contact lens in the affected eye, but if they are, ensure it is removed.
During Test: Adhere to standard precautions.

Interfering Factors:
Improper fixation; poor cell representation or preservation; lymphoma identification may be difficult because malignant cells may intermix with inflammatory cells.

Nursing Considerations:

Pediatric: Sedation may be recommended for infants and children. Place the infant or child on a blanket for comfort. After postprocedure monitoring is completed and per health care provider's order, the pediatric client is discharged with an adult who is given instructions.
Rural: Advisable to arrange for transportation home after recovering from procedure.

WEBLINKS

http://www.med.harvard.edu/AANLIB/hms1.html

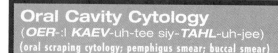

Oral Cavity Cytology
(*OER*-:l *KAEV*-uh-tee siy-*TAHL*-uh-jee)
(oral scraping cytology; pemphigus smear; buccal smear)

15 min.

Type of Test: Tissue

Body Systems and Functions: Gastrointestinal system

Normal Findings: Normal cellular structure and numbers

Test Results Time Frame: Within 1 week

Test Description: Oral cavity cytology involves taking a sample (i.e., scaping) of the oral cavity either where visible oral/buccal lesions are found or randomly. The resulting smear is evaluated for cellular abnormalities.

Consent Form: Not required

List of Equipment: Tongue-blade; culture medium; cup of water

Test Procedure:

1. Instruct client to vigorously rinse mouth with water several times before the test. *Cleanses area from excessive organisms.*
2. Scape the client's oral cavity or oral lesion with a spatula or tongue blade. If the scrape is for genetic assessment, it is taken from the lateral buccal mucosa just above the dentate line along the anterior two-thirds of the

buccal mucosa. If the scrape is for pemphigus, the lesion chould be scraped where normal and affected mucosa meet.
3. The scrape is smeared on labeled glass slides and fixed immediately with spray or liquid fixative. *Ensures accurate results.*
4. Instruct the client to rinse mouth after the scraping. *Promotes good oral hygiene.*

Clinical Implications and Indications:
1. Diagnoses dysplastic and neoplastic lesions
2. Diagnoses oral pemphigus, herpes, or *Candida*
3. Screens for trisomy 21, 13, and 18; multiple-X syndrome; Klinefelter's syndrome; and Turner's syndrome

Nursing Care:
Before Test: Explain the test procedure and the purpose of the test. Assess the client's knowledge of the test. Have client rinse mouth vigorously several times before the scrape is performed.
During Test: Adhere to standard precautions.
After Test: The requisition should indicate if the client is a smoker, has skin lesions, has been undergoing radiation or chemotherapy, or has dentures.

Contraindications: Anticoagulant therapy

Interfering Factors: Poorly fixed sample; not enough cells in sample; smoking

Nursing Considerations:
Pediatric: Infants and children will need assistance in remaining still during the oral scraping and age-appropriate comfort measures following the test.

Listing of Related Tests: Karyotyping studies

WEBLINKS

http://becker.wustl.edu/

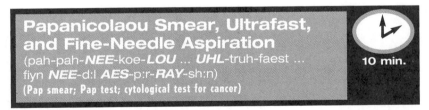

Papanicolaou Smear, Ultrafast, and Fine-Needle Aspiration
(pah-pah-*NEE*-koe-*LOU* ... *UHL*-truh-faest ... fiyn *NEE*-d:l *AES*-p:r-*RAY*-sh:n)
(Pap smear; Pap test; cytological test for cancer)

10 min.

Type of Test: Tissue

Body Systems and Functions: Reproductive system

Normal Findings: No abnormal cells

Test Results Time Frame: Within 3–5 days

Test Description: The Papanicolaou smear is a screening tool for premalignant and malignant cervical changes, rather than a diagnostic test. Cervical cells are removed from the ectocervix, transformation zone, and endocervical

CULTURE, TISSUE, MICROSCOPIC

areas. Any cellular findings that may suggest a cancerous or precancerous state are followed by biopsy. False positives and false negatives can occur, so client symptoms are also important indicators for further testing. Pap tests are currently recommended annually for all women 18 years or older (or at the onset of sexual activity, if prior to 18 years of age) until age 60–65. The time frame may be extended or decreased depending on the client's risk factors, age, and family history.

Consent Form: Not required

List of Equipment: Speculum; wooden spatula/swab/cytobrush/cytobroom; slides; fixative

Test Procedure:

1. Place client in the lithotomy position with the perineal area exposed. The examiner is seated and has an effective lighting source.
2. Select the appropriate-sized vaginal speculum, which has been warmed and lubricated in water, and insert slowly into the vagina and secure. *Lubricant jelly is not used as it will interfere with test results.*
3. Obtain the cellular sample from the cervical canal with a spatula or brush that is rotated 360°. *Rotation provides opportunity to collect cells from all areas.*
4. Immediately transfer the sample to the slide(s) and spray or otherwise fix. *Air-dried samples may alter appearance of cells.*
5. Label the slides and complete requisition with the date of last menstrual period and medication history.

Clinical Implications and Indications:

1. Screening test for cancerous and precancerous cells. Must be followed by further testing if abnormalities are found or none are found but client is symptomatic. This test is 90%–95% accurate in detection of cervical malignancies, less effective with endometrial. Current classification scale of choice is the Bethesda system (see table).
2. Presence of abnormal cells may also be representative of fungal infections, venereal disease, or an inflammatory process.
3. Monitors response to therapy for cervical cancer or infection.
4. Provides information related to hormonal cytology when assessing endocrine-associated conditions.
5. Provides a sample for cytology of gastric and prostatic secretions, sputum, and urine.

Evaluation of Papanicolaou smear

Adequacy of the specimen	Satisfactory for evaluation
	Satisfactory for evaluation but limited by (specify reason)
	Unsatisfactory for evaluation (specify reason)
General categorization (optional)	Within normal limits
	Benign cellular changes: See descriptive diagnoses
	Epithelial cell abnormality: See descriptive diagnoses

Descriptive diagnoses
Benign cellular changes

Infection
Trichomonas vaginalis
Fungal organisms morphologically consistent with *Candida* spp.
Predominance of coccobacilli consistent with shift in vaginal flora
Bacteria morphologically consistent with *Actinomyces* spp.
Cellular changes associated with herpes simplex virus
Other

Reactive changes

Reactive cellular changes associated with:
Inflammation (includes typical repair)
Atrophy with inflammation ("atrophic vaginitis")
Radiation
Intrauterine contraceptive device
Other

Epithelial cell abnormalities

Squamous cell
Atypical squamous cells of undetermined significance: Qualify further as to whether a reactive or premalignant/malignant process
Low-grade squamous intraepithelial lesion encompassing human papillomavirus or mild dysplasia/CIN (cervical intraepithelial neoplasia)
High-grade squamous intraepithelial lesion encompassing moderate and severe dysplasia, CIS (carcinoma in situ)
Squamous cell carcinoma

Glandular cell

Endometrial cells, cytologically benign, in a postmenopausal woman
Atypical glandular cells of undetermined significance: Qualify further
Endocervical adenocarcinoma
Endometrial adenocarcinoma
Extrauterine adenocarcinoma
Adenocarcinoma, not otherwise specified

Other malignant neoplasms:
Specify Hormonal evaluation
(applies to vaginal smears only)

Hormonal pattern compatible with age and history
Hormonal pattern incompatible with age and history (specify reason)
Hormonal evaluation not possible (specify reason)

CULTURE, TISSUE, MICROSCOPIC

Nursing Care:

Before Test: Explain the test procedure and the purpose of the test. Assess the client's knowledge of the test. Confirm with the client that she has not douched or had a tub bath in the 24 hr prior to the test. Confirm that the client is not menstruating and has not had sexual intercourse in the last 24 hr. Ask the client to void prior to the examination. Reassure the client that while the insertion and presence of the speculum may feel uncomfortable, there should be no sensation of pain during the procedure. Reassure the pregnant client that the Pap test is a procedure that is safe when done during pregnancy.

During Test: Adhere to standard precautions.

After Test: Instruct client that they may have a small amount of pink-to-bloody discharge after the Pap test.

Contraindications: Menstruation

Interfering Factors: Medications that alter results are digitalis and tetracycline; vaginal medications/contraceptives within 48 hr prior to test; use of lubricating jelly on the speculum; douching or tub baths in the 24 hr prior to examination; poor collection or fixation technique

Nursing Considerations:

Pregnancy: Reassure the pregnant client that the Pap test is a procedure that is safe when done during pregnancy. The cytobrush cell retrieval tool is not recommended for the pregnant client.

Listing of Related Tests: Colposcopy

WEBLINKS

www.gyncancer.com

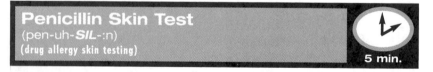

Penicillin Skin Test
(pen-uh-*SIL*-:n)
(drug allergy skin testing)

5 min.

Type of Test: Tissue

Body Systems and Functions: Immunological system

Normal Findings: No wheal or erythema

Test Results Time Frame: Within 20 min

Test Description: Penicillin skin testing of individuals with suspected IgE-mediated penicillin allergy involves a skin prick or intradermal injection with benzylpenicilloyl (BPO) compound. Immediate wheal and flare reaction is helpful in identifying those who are likely to have an anaphylactic response to drug therapy with penicillin. Because of a significantly large false-negative group, clients who test negative must be monitored during treatment with penicillin, although this group is unlikely to have a severe reaction. When testing for suspected penicillin allergy, it is advisable to test with different types of penicillins and cephalosporins.

CLINICAL ALERT:
Have emergency equipment readily available in the event of an anaphylactic reaction to the penicillin.

Consent Form: Required

List of Equipment: Penicillin extracts in saline solution; TB or 27-gauge needle and syringes; resuscitation equipment

Test Procedure:
1. Place a drop of drug/saline reagent (1:100) on the volar surface of the client's forearm.
2. The client's skin is pricked through the drop into the epidermis with a small needle.
3. Read the site at 20 min and measure in millimeters. A positive reaction is a wheal of 2 mm more than a normal saline control, with a surrounding flare (a strongly positive reaction is 5 mm or greater).
4. If the site is negative, the forearm is injected intradermally with 0.05 mL of 1:1,000–1:10,000 solution using a 27-gauge or TB needle. This is read at 20 min. A positive reaction is a wheal greater than 2 mm and flared. The wheal will be larger that the one in step 3.
5. Inject the next concentration if the site is negative again.

Clinical Implications and Indications:
1. Identifies a history of penicillin allergies, beta-lactam antibiotic allergies, and multiple antibiotic allergies

Nursing Care:
Before Test: Explain the test procedure and the purpose of the test. Assess the client's knowledge of the test. Assess for potential allergies to penicillin. Instruct client to inform health care provider if experiencing anaphylactic symptomatology (e.g., shortness of breath, itching, speech difficulties).
During Test: Adhere to standard precautions. Assess for allergic reactions to penicillin.
After Test: Tests are read 20 min after administration and recorded in millimeters. Assess for allergic reactions to penicillin. Client is advised that in rare instances symptoms may occur several hours after test, and if they do occur, the client should contact his health care provider immediately.

Potential Complications: Slight bleeding under injection site; skin irritation/itching at site; anaphylaxis due to allergic reaction to penicillin

Contraindications: History of penicillin-induced anaphylaxis; exfoliative dermatitis; history of status asthmaticus; Stevens-Johnson syndrome

Interfering Factors: False negatives from inappropriate test reagent; dialysis therapy; immunosuppression; medications that alter results are antihistamines, tricyclic antidepressants, phenothiazines, and hydroxyzine.

Nursing Considerations:
Pediatric: Younger children may have difficulty holding still during testing and may need assistance; distraction techniques during the test and comfort or distraction following the test.

CULTURE, TISSUE, MICROSCOPIC

Listing of Related Tests: Hemoagglutination assays; RAST; ELISA

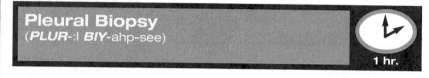

WEBLINKS

http://www.mic.ki.se/Diseases/c20.html

Pleural Biopsy
(*PLUR*-:l *BIY*-ahp-see)

1 hr.

Type of Test: Tissue

Body Systems and Functions: Pulmonary system

Normal Findings: No abnormal cells

Test Results Time Frame: 24–48 hr

Test Description: A pleural biopsy involves obtaining a small pleural tissue sample through a transthoracic needle biopsy procedure (TTNB). An excision or needle punch sample of body tissue is taken under sterile technique and examined microscopically for cell morphology and tissue anomalies. An aspiration needle with a cutting mechanism is introduced under guided fluoroscopy in the radiology department. A sample of pleural fluid for analysis is taken first before tissue is cut. The biopsy may also be done during a thoracentesis or under general anesthesia during a thoracotomy.

Consent Form: Required

List of Equipment: Biopsy tray

Test Procedure:
1. Place client in supine position.
2. A specimen of tissue is biopsied by excision or needle biopsy. Label the specimen and place in container. *Correctly identifies the client and the test to be performed.*
3. Send specimen to laboratory.
4. If the biopsy is part of a thoracentesis or an open thoracotomy surgical procedure, further explanation is needed about those procedures.

Clinical Implications and Indications:
1. Diagnoses pleural tumor for malignancy
2. Determines cause of infection involving pleura
3. Diagnoses pleural fibrosis, collagen vascular disease, and tuberculosis in the granuloma stage

Nursing Care:
Before Test: Explain the test procedure and the purpose of the test. Assess the client's knowledge of the test. Provide preprocedure sedation and analgesia as ordered. Transport client to operating or procedure room. Drape client appropriately. Client may be instructed to be NPO prior to the procedure.
During Test: Adhere to sterile technique and standard precautions. Provide reassurance and a calm atmosphere during the procedure.

After Test: Clean site of biopsy. Provide analgesia as necessary. Frequent vital signs and assessment of respiratory function, pain, and examination of the biopsy site for bleeding or infection. Postanesthesia recovery and care of thoracotomy incision are needed for surgical (open) biopsy.

Potential Complications: The biopsy is highly invasive and puts the client at risk for: pneumothorax, internal bleeding in the chest cavity, or infection.

Contraindications: Inability of the client to follow care directives during needle aspiration; bleeding disorders; ventilator therapy unless biopsy is done as an open surgical procedure

Nursing Considerations:
Pediatric: Sedation is recommended for infants and children. Place the infant or child on a blanket for comfort. After postprocedure monitoring is completed and per health care provider's order, the pediatric client is discharged with an adult who is given instructions.
Gerontology: The older person may find it difficult to maintain positions when required to do so for lengthy periods of time during the biopsy.
Rural: Advisable to arrange for transportation home after recovering from the biopsy

Listing of Related Tests: Thoracentesis; pleural fluid analysis

WEBLINKS

http://www.meddean.luc.edu

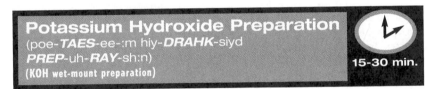

Potassium Hydroxide Preparation
(poe-*TAES*-ee-:m hiy-*DRAHK*-siyd
PREP-uh-*RAY*-sh:n)
(KOH wet-mount preparation)

15-30 min.

Type of Test: Tissue

Body Systems and Functions: Integumentary system

Normal Findings: No fungal elements present

Test Results Time Frame: Within 24 hr

Test Description: Potassium hydroxide preparation involves obtaining samples of skin, hair, nails, sputum, or wound drainage and mixing them with KOH preparation. KOH preparation washes away extraneous material so that fungal parts (mycelium, hyphae, spores, or budding yeast cells) can be more easily seen under a microscope. Fungi can grow on both living and nonliving matter. Normal integumentary defenses limit their damage on the skin, but a fungus is more likely to cause serious system infection if it is in the lungs or a wound.

Consent Form: Not required (note: some institutions may require consent for skin biopsy)

CULTURE, TISSUE, MICROSCOPIC

List of Equipment: Equipment depends on whether there will be an exci-sion of skin, a scraping of skin or nail, or a cutting of hair. Sterile gloves and sterile towels (one or two) for a sterile field are helpful for any sampling except wound or sputum. *Skin sample:* antiseptic (70% alcohol), local anesthetic if exci-sion, sterile scalpel or scissors, sterile container for excision or sterile glass slides for scraping; for slides methylene blue, 10%–20% KOH solution, and coverslips are needed. *Hair sample:* sterile scissors and sterile container; it is recommended that scalp skin scraping also be performed. *Nail sample:* antiseptic (70% alco-hol), sterile scalpel and sterile glass slide/coverslip, methylene blue, and 10%–20% KOH solution. *Wound drainage:* culture tube/sterile Q-tip. *Sputum sample:* sterile container.

Test Procedure:

1. To collect any sample, take precautions to prevent contamination by one's own fungus or by fungus in the environment. *Contamination gives false results.*

Skin excision or scraping sample:

1. Use sterile gloves and towels to set up small sterile field. *Prevents contami-nation of sample.*
2. Swab skin with antiseptic. *Prevents infection of skin.*
3. Use small amount of local anesthetic if needed. *Provides comfort.*
4. Obtain sample. Scrape outward from the peripheral erythematous margin if present. *A higher concentration of fungus is found in a reddened area.*
5. Put biopsy sample in sterile container; for scraped sample add 1 drop KOH solution and 1 drop methylene blue on slide, put sample on slide, and cover with coverslip.

Hair sample:

1. Clip several strands and place in sterile container. Several hairs should also be plucked if possible as fungus is often at base of hair shaft. It is recom-mended that skin of the scalp also be scraped.

Nail sample:

1. Swab nail with 70% alcohol. *Removes bacteria and makes visualization of fungus under microscope easier.*
2. Scrape from discolored or dystrophic parts of the nail. If subungual lesions present, debris should be collected from underneath the nail. *Characteristics of fungal growth are discoloration and changes in nail appearance.*

Sputum sample:

1. Have client perform a deep cough and expectorate into sterile container.

Wound sample:

1. Using Q-tip in culture tube, wipe wound, and insert into sterile culture tube.

All samples:

1. Label and send all containers and slides to laboratory.

Clinical Implications and Indications:

1. Diagnoses fungal infection of skin, hair, nails, sputum, or wound.
2. Detects actinomycosis, aspergillus, candidiasis, coccidiodomycosis, tinea pedis, tinea capitis (ringworm of the scalp), tinea barbae (ringworm of beard), and tinea corporis (ringworm of the body).
3. Tinea pedis can be detected with the nail scraping, but other fungi (or those that are internal) are best detected through culture.

Nursing Care:

Before Test: Explain the test procedure and the purpose of the test. Assess the client's knowledge of the test. Provide preprocedure sedation and analgesia as ordered. Transport client to operating or procedure room. Drape client appropriately. Assess skin or nail site for color and characteristic symptoms in appearance. Assess wound for color, smell, amount, and color of drainage. Caution client to remain still while sample is being obtained.

During Test: Adhere to sterile technique and standard precautions. Provide reassurance and a calm atmosphere during the procedure.

After Test: Clean site of biopsy. Provide analgesia as necessary.

Potential Complications: Bleeding and bruising at the site; infection

Interfering Factors: Results may have false positives if specimen is contaminated with cotton or cellulose fibers and cholesterol deposits.

Nursing Considerations:

Pediatric: Sedation is recommended for infants and children. Place the infant or child on a blanket for comfort. After postprocedure monitoring is completed and per health care provider's order, the pediatric client is discharged with an adult who is given instructions.

Gerontology: The older person may find it difficult to maintain positions when required to do so for lengthy periods of time during the biopsy.

Rural: Advisable to arrange for transportation home after recovering from the biopsy.

International: Many fungal infections are more common in hot, tropical climates.

Listing of Related Tests: Culture; fungal serology

WEBLINKS

http://www.cmrinstitute.org

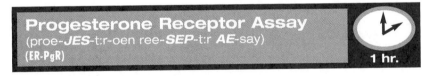

Progesterone Receptor Assay
(proe-*JES*-t:r-oen ree-*SEP*-t:r *AE*-say)
(ER-PgR)

1 hr.

Type of Test: Tissue

Body Systems and Functions: Oncology system

Normal Findings:

Negative	<3 fmol/mg cytosol protein
Borderline	3–10 fmol/mg cytosol protein
Positive	>10 fmol/mg cytosol protein

Test Results Time Frame: Within 1 week

Test Description: Progesterone receptor assay testing is performed on a breast tissue specimen from someone diagnosed with primary or metastatic breast cancer. The biopsy is an invasive procedure performed in a surgical setting. An excision or needle punch sample of body tissue is taken under sterile technique and examined microscopically for cell morphology and tissue anomalies. The purpose of the assay is to determine if the tumor would respond favorably to hormone therapy. The test is done in conjunction with an assay for estrogen receptors. An 80% response rate to hormone therapy is obtained when both estrogen and progesterone receptor levels are positive. Those clients who have a value >100 fmol/mg cytosol protein for both types of tests have the best potential for an effective hormone treatment.

Consent Form: Required

List of Equipment: Biopsy tray

Test Procedure:
1. Place client in supine position.
2. A specimen of tissue is biopsied by excision or needle biopsy. Label the specimen and place in container. *Correctly identifies the client and the test to be performed.*
3. Label specimen identifying site as right or left breast and place in container; immediately place the container in ice and take to laboratory. *Specimen must be prepared for frozen section within 15–30 min to prevent deterioration of proteins.*

Clinical Implications and Indications:
1. Identifies whether or not breast cancer tumor would be responsive to hormone therapy.
2. Clients with positive assay results during the therapy have the best prognosis.

Nursing Care:
Before Test: Explain the test procedure and the purpose of the test. Assess the client's knowledge of the test. Provide preprocedure sedation and analgesia as ordered. Transport client to operating or procedure room. Drape client appropriately.
During Test: Adhere to sterile technique and standard precautions. Provide reassurance and a calm atmosphere during the procedure.
After Test: Clean site of biopsy. Provide analgesia as necessary.

Potential Complications: Bleeding and bruising at the site of the biopsy; infection

Interfering Factors: Use of fixative on specimen; delay of transport to laboratory; medications that alter results are oral contraceptives, hormone therapy, and tamoxifen (note: alters results for as long as 2 months after stopped); massive tumor necrosis or low cellular composition will decrease levels.

Nursing Considerations:
Pediatric: Sedation is recommended for infants and children. Place the infant or child on a blanket for comfort. After postprocedure monitoring is completed and per health care provider's order, the pediatric client is discharged with an adult who is given instructions.
Gerontology: The older person may find it difficult to maintain positions when required to do so for lengthy periods of time during the biopsy.
Rural: Advisable to arrange for transportation home after recovering from the biopsy

Listing of Related Tests: Estrogen receptor assay

Prostate Biopsy
(*PRAHS*-tayt *BIY*-ahp-see)
(core biopsy of the prostate gland; fine-needle aspiration biopsy of the
prostate gland; prostate gland biopsy)

45 min.

CULTURE, TISSUE, MICROSCOPIC

Type of Test: Microscopic

Body Systems and Functions: Reproductive system

Normal Findings: No abnormal cells

Test Results Time Frame: Within 24 hr

Test Description: A prostate biopsy involves taking a small tissue sample
from the prostate. The biopsy is an invasive procedure performed in a surgical
setting. An excision or needle punch sample of body tissue is taken under sterile technique and examined microscopically for cell morphology and tissue
anomalies. One of three approaches is used: transrectal, transurethral, or perineal (note: transrectal is the most common). The tissue is microscopically examined for abnormal cells.

Consent Form: Required

List of Equipment: Biopsy tray

Test Procedure:
1. Place client in the lithotomy position for the transurethral approach on a
   urological examining table. For transrectal approach, position client on left
   side with knees pulled up toward the chest. For the perineal approach, position client in the lithotomy position. *The position depends on the method of
   the procedure so that greatest visibility and maneuverability are available.*
2. Cleanse the area with antiseptic; local anesthetic is inserted into the urethra
   for the transurethral method and injected into the perineal tissues for the
   perineal approach. *Prevents pain.*
3. Transurethral: The scope is introduced into the urethra and a biopsy of
   prostate tissue is done with a cutting loop. Transrectal: A biopsy needle
   guided by ultrasound is inserted through the side of the rectum and rotated
   to obtain a core of prostate tissue. Perineal: A small incision is made and a
   needle or punch biopsy is done. In all the methods usually four to six biopsy specimens are obtained including the suspected tumor area and the
   peripheral areas. *A greater number of specimens provides better assurance
   that cancerous cells will be detected; also the margins of the tumor are better
   defined.*
4. The tissue specimen is placed in formalin solution and the container labeled
   and sent to the laboratory. *Formalin provides tissue preservation.*

Clinical Implications and Indications:
1. Diagnoses prostate cancer
2. Diagnoses prostatic hypertrophy of unknown cause

Nursing Care:

Before Test: Explain the test procedure and the purpose of the test. Assess the client's knowledge of the test. Serum PSA or acid phosphatase (PAP) should be drawn first, as the biopsy increases PSA and PAP results. Explain to the client that premedication for relaxation may be provided. Explain which method will be used (rectal, perineal, or transurethral) and what the procedure entails. Assure client that local anesthetic is given for perineal or transurethral procedures and that transrectal needle biopsy may cause very brief periods (3–5 sec) of pain as each biopsy specimen is taken. Instruct client to remain still on the examining table, especially the needle biopsy. There are no food or drink restrictions.

During Test: Adhere to standard precautions. Provide reassurance and a calm atmosphere during the procedure.

After Test: Observe for bleeding at the site. Apply pressure to the perineal site immediately following the procedure; a dressing is usually applied for several days. Following the transurethral approach the client should monitor urine output for amount and color for 24 hr and immediately report any blood in urine.

Potential Complications: Bleeding and bruising at the site of the biopsy; infection

Contraindications: Bleeding disorder; anticoagulant therapy

Nursing Considerations:

Pediatric: Sedation is recommended for infants and children. Place the infant or child on a blanket for comfort. After postprocedure monitoring is completed and per health care provider's order, the pediatric client is discharged with an adult who is given instructions.

Gerontology: Elderly males are at risk for impotence with some prostate treatments, and therefore clients may need reassurance that the prostate biospy does not affect potency. The older person may find it difficult to maintain positions when required to do so for lengthy periods of time during the biopsy.

Rural: Advisable to arrange for transportation home after recovering from procedure.

Listing of Related Tests: Acid phosphatase (PAP); prostate-specific antigen (PSA); prostate sonogram

WEBLINKS

www.cancer.org

Rectal Biopsy
(*REK*-t:l *BIY*-ahp-see)

30 min.

Type of Test: Tissue

Body Systems and Functions: Gastrointestinal system

Normal Findings: Normal cells and tissues

Test Results Time Frame: Within 24 hr

Test Description: The rectal biopsy involves obtaining a small piece of rectal mucosa and submucosal tissue by excising a microscopic examination of cellular and tissue normality. The biopsy is an invasive procedure performed in a surgical setting. An excision or needle punch sample of body tissue is taken under sterile technique and examined microscopically for cell morphology and tissue anomalies. The tissue is excised during a protosigmoidoscopy examination using a fiber-optic endoscopic instrument. Alligator forceps is the preferred technique for anorectal lesions. Needle biopsy is used for tissue lesions, but not for large tumors (see Potential Complications). Multiple biopsies from multiple sites in the rectum and colon are preferred to better diagnose a pathological process even when an obvious lesion is apparent.

Consent Form: Required

List of Equipment: Equipment for proctological exam; rectal biopsy tray with gloves, water-soluble lubricant, fixative and specimen container

Test Procedure:
1. Label container(s) with client's name. *Correctly identifies the client and the test to be performed.*
2. Have client remove clothes from below the waist.
3. Position client on examination table in the left lateral position with knees and hips flexed. Cover client with a drape. *Provides privacy.*
4. Perform a proctological examination and administer a local anesthetic.
5. The site for the excision is located and one or more biopsies are done per endoscopic instrument, excision, or needle biopsy.
6. Put each biopsy specimen in a separate container labeled with specific location of specimen.
7. Follow laboratory instructions for fixative solution.
8. Send to laboratory immediately.

Clinical Implications and Indications:
1. Aids in diagnosis of rectal cancer of polyps and tumors
2. Aids in diagnosis and staging of Crohn's disease and ulcerative colitis
3. Aids in diagnosis of chronic infections such as amebic ulcerations and schistosomiasis mansoni
4. Aids in diagnosis of Hirschsprung's disease and aganglionosis (anal achalasia)

Nursing Care:
Before Test: Explain the test procedure and the purpose of the test. Assess the client's knowledge of the test. Explain that a local anesthetic will be given before the excision, and instruct client to remain very still while lying on side. Have client void before procedure.
During Test: Adhere to standard precautions. Provide reassurance and a calm atmosphere during the procedure. Encourage client to remain still.
After Test: Clean site of biopsy. Provide analgesia as necessary. Explain to client that a small amount of bleeding (spotting) is to be expected the first 24 hr or after the first bowel movement. Instruct client to wear a peri-pad to protect the

CULTURE, TISSUE, MICROSCOPIC

clothes. Instruct client to notify health care provider if bleeding increases or continues.

Potential Complications: Bleeding and bruising at the site; infection with needle biopsy of large tumors

Contraindications: Anticoagulant therapy; bleeding disorder such as thrombocytopenia

Interfering Factors: Unable to lie on side; inability to remain still

Nursing Considerations:
Pediatric: Infants and children will need assistance in remaining still during the biopsy and age-appropriate comfort measures following the biopsy.
Gerontology: The older person may find it difficult to maintain positions when required to do so for lengthy periods of time during the biopsy.
Rural: Advisable to arrange for transportation home after recovering from the biopsy

WEBLINKS

www.nlm.nih.gov

Rectal Culture, Swab
(*REK*-t:l ...)

5 min.

Type of Test: Culture

Body Systems and Functions: Gastrointestinal system

Normal Findings: Negative for pathogenic organisms

Test Results Time Frame: Within 24 hr

Test Description: The rectal swab culture is used as a screening for bacterial causes of diarrhea. The main advantage of the rectal swab is that testing can begin immediately for bacterial pathogens without waiting for collection of a stool specimen. However, a stool culture gives more in-depth information for diagnosis and, if negative for bacterial pathogens, can be used for detection of viruses through immunoassay and microscopy. The rectal swab culture is not diagnostic for carrier states.

Consent Form: Not required

List of Equipment: Sterile cotton-tipped swab; sterile container or culturette swab

Test Procedure:
1. Label container or culture tube with client's name, time, and date.
2. Have client disrobe from waist down.
3. Position client on side with knees flexed and place drape over client for privacy.

4. Gently insert sterile swab 2.5–3 cm into rectum. Rotate swab and move side to side; leave swab in for a few seconds. *Absorbs bacteria.*
5. Place swab into sterile container; if culturette is used, insert swab into culture tube medium compartment and crush compartment area to release solution.
6. Send to laboratory immediately. Culture specimen should be refrigerated if not immediately tested. *Ensures accurate results.*

Clinical Implications and Indications:
1. Aids in the diagnosis of abnormal pathogens causing bacterial diarrhea, such as *Campylobacter, Chlamydia, Neisseria gonorrhoeae, Salmonella, Shigella,* and *Schistosoma mansoni.*

Nursing Care:
Before Test: Explain the test procedure and the purpose of the test. Assess the client's knowledge of the test. Inform client that there is very little discomfort during the procedure and no effects after the test.
During Test: Adhere to standard precautions.

Interfering Factors: Inadequate amount to culture

Nursing Considerations:
Pediatric: Chronic diarrhea in infants or young children can dehydrate them and potentially be very serious.

Listing of Related Tests: Stool culture and sensitivity

WEBLINKS

http://www.cdc.gov

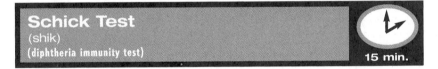

Schick Test
(shik)
(diphtheria immunity test)

15 min.

Type of Test: Tissue

Body Systems and Functions: Immunological system

Normal Findings: A negative test would exhibit little or no reaction after 3–4 days (this indicates that antibodies are present in sufficient quantities in the client's body to neutralize the diphtheria toxin).

Test Results Time Frame: Within 3–4 days

Test Description: The Schick test is a skin test that determines the degree of immunity to diphtheria. Diphtheria toxin is a potent exotoxin produced by *Cornebacterium diphtheriae.* Diphtheria affects all cells of the body, but has its greatest damage on nerves, heart, and kidneys. The Schick test involves giving an injection of 0.1 mL of dilute diphtheria toxin intradermally. The area is checked in 3–4 days, and the reaction is documented. A positive test is indicated by inflammation or induration at the point of injection. This would indicate that the client lacks antibodies to diphtheria (or has fewer than 0.03 U antitoxin/mL

CULTURE, TISSUE, MICROSCOPIC

blood) and would be susceptible to the disease. Contracting and surviving the disease do not provide immunity for life. People who have survived diphtheria still need to be vaccinated every 7–10 years.

CLINICAL ALERT:
Have emergency equipment readily available in the event of an anaphylactic reaction to the toxin.

Consent Form: Required

List of Equipment: TB syringe; alcohol swab; dilute diphtheria toxin; pen or marker

Test Procedure:
1. Swab the area on the forearm with alcohol. *Cleanses the skin before injection.*
2. Draw up 0.1 mL of diluted diphtheria toxin into a TB syringe and inject it intradermally. A small bubble should appear just under the skin. *Presence of the bubble indicates that the injection has been administered into the intradermal layer. If no bubble appears, it is possible that the injection was administered into the subcutaneous layer and would deliver inconclusive results.*
3. Draw a circle on the client's skin with a pen or marker around the injection site and document the site, amount injected, manufacturer, and lot number of the toxin. *Identifies the site of injection accurately.*
4. Have the client return in 3–4 days to have the test read by a qualified health care professional who will visually inspect the area for redness and inflammation and palpate the area for induration. Measurements should be taken and recorded. *Provides accurate information regarding the client's response to the diluted toxin.*

Clinical Implications and Indications:
1. Diagnoses diphtheria, which is an acute infectious disease that is spread by contact with a human carrier or with articles contaminated by a person with the disease.
2. Diphtheria immunization is included in the DPT (diphtheria, pertussis, and tetanus) vaccine administered to children or the DT (diphtheria toxoid) given to adults.

Nursing Care:
Before Test: Explain the test procedure and the purpose of the test. Assess the client's knowledge of the test. Obtain an accurate history regarding reaction to any previous testing or vaccines. Instruct the client as to the importance of returning on the scheduled date to have the test read and followed by the appropriate vaccination if indicated.
During Test: Adhere to standard precautions.
After Test: Read and record results. Follow up with appropriate vaccination as indicated. Assure the client that if a positive result was evident, the redness, swelling, and induration should disappear in a few days.

Potential Complications: Itching; ulceration; anaphylaxis

Nursing Considerations:
Pediatric: Vaccination in children prevents the disease and is usually in the form of DPT. If a reaction has occurred in response to this vaccine, it is possible to

receive a DT injection without the pertussis, which can decrease the possibility of the reaction occurring again. If subsequent booster vaccines are administered following a possible reaction, it is necessary for the client to stay at the medical facility for at least 20 min following the injection for observation of allergic reaction. **International:** *Proof of diphtheria immunization is not required for foreign travel. However, there have been outbreaks in areas of eastern Europe, and immunization is highly recommended.*

WEBLINKS

http://www.cdc.gov; http://www.nfid.org; http://idsc.nih.go.jp

Sexually Transmitted Disease Cultures

(*SEK*-shue-uh-*LEE* traenz-*MIT*-:d duh-zeez)
(anal culture; cervical culture; gonorrhea smear; oropharyngeal culture; urethral culture)

15 min.

CULTURE, TISSUE, MICROSCOPIC

Type of Test: Culture

Body Systems and Functions: Immunological system

Normal Findings: Negative for organism of specific sexually transmitted disease

Test Results Time Frame: Within 48 hr

Test Description: A culture for sexually transmitted diseases (STDs) is done to identify the etiologic agents of a wide number of organisms that suggest an STD and to identify asymptomatic women with an organism that causes an STD. Endocervical cultures are obtained after the cervix is visualized with a speculum. The cervical culture test procedure is done by a health care professional with education in this procedure. The method of specimen handling varies according to the type of organism sought. An anal canal culture is often performed on females after the cervical culture is negative (the same procedure is used in males). An oropharyngeal culture is obtained by inserting a swab into the mouth of a person suspected of having an STD obtained from oral sex. A urethral culture is sought when clinical manifestations of an STD are present, particularly with high-risk clients.

CLINICAL ALERT:
The sample for *Neisseria gonorrhoeae* should be collected before the sample for *Chlamydia trachomatis* or herpes simplex virus. If gonorrhea is suspected, massage the prostate to increase the number of organisms in the urethral discharge.

Consent Form: Refer to health care facility policy.

List of Equipment: Speculum; collection swab or brush; appropriate transport medium

CULTURE, TISSUE, MICROSCOPIC

Test Procedure:
1. Label collection container. *Correctly identifies the client and test to be performed.*
2. Moisten the speculum with warm water. Do not use lubricants. *Lubricants may contain antibacterial agents.*
3. Position client appropriately for location of culture (e.g., dorsal lithotomy for cervical and urethral culture). *Ensures accurate results.*
4. Remove all secretions and discharge from the suspected area of the STD with a sterile swab or brush. *Avoids contamination of specimen.*
5. Place swab or brush in appropriate transport medium.
6. Transport to laboratory as soon as possible. Do not refrigerate specimen. *Recovery of the organisms may be more difficult due to a delay in processing.*

Clinical Implications and Indications:
1. Detects a variety of sexually transmitted diseases (e.g., *C. trachomatis*, gonorrhea, genital ulcers, vaginitis)
2. Diagnoses vaginal lymphadenopathy and pelvic inflammatory disease
3. Evaluates abnormal vaginal discharges
4. Evaluates and monitors clinical manifestations of bacterial STDs specific to location of testing (e.g., cervix, oral mucosa, urethra, anus)

Nursing Care:
Before Test: Explain the test procedure and the purpose of the test. Assess the client's knowledge of the test. Place client in appropriate position for area of STD testing. Drape client appropriately.
During Test: Adhere to standard precautions. Provide emotional support if test causes discomfort.
After Test: Provide privacy for client.

Interfering Factors: Contamination of specimen from incorrect technique; false negatives for testing often require repeat testing.

Nursing Considerations:
Pregnancy: Many STD organisms are transmitted in utero to the fetus, and fetal testing is therefore necessary.
Pediatric: Infants and children are often born with congenital defects from STD pathology. Health care providers must be aware of potential anomalies and refer to pediatricians for continued evaluation.

WEBLINKS

http://www.vgernet.net

Skin Culture
(skin **KUL**-tur)
(skin fungus culture; skin mycobacteria culture)

15-30 min.

Type of Test: Culture

Body Systems and Functions: Integumentary system

Normal Findings: Negative for abnormal organisms or increases in normal skin pathogens

Test Results Time Frame: Within 2–3 days

Test Description: The skin of a healthy person has a wide variety of organisms that are normally present. As there is pathology, the numbers of these organisms increase. The following are the most common types of organisms that can be cultured: enterococci, mycobacteria, staphylococci, streptococci, yeasts and fungi, *Clostridium*, coliform, *Aspergillus*, *Penicillium*, *Proteus*, bacilli, and diphtheroids. The skin is cultured to obtain a sample of the infected area, either by scraping with a scalpel, aspirating fluid with a syringe, or swabbing with a cotton swab.

CLINICAL ALERT:
The best samples are taken from nails, hairs, and skin scrapings. Strict attention needs to be given to standard precautions. Obtain sample prior to antibiotic therapy for the most accurate organism identification.

Consent Form: Not required

List of Equipment: Sterile water; alcohol cleansing solution; sterile swab; culture medium container

Test Procedure:
1. Place client in comfortable position for obtaining culture from site.
2. Cleanse lesion with sterile water, follow with alcohol, and rinse with sterile water.
3. Scrape site with scalpel or aspirate fluid from vesicle with 25-gauge needle.
4. Place specimen in culture medium. Confirm with laboratory which culture medium is needed (e.g., anaerobic culture medium, sterile petri dish, mycobacteria culture medium).
5. Label the specimen. *Correctly identifies the client and the test to be performed.*
6. Send to laboratory.

Clinical Implications and Indications:
1. A wide variety of conditions necessitate culturing the skin to see if there is a pathogenic response. Several of the more common conditions that warrant the skin cultures are abscesses, dermatophytes (athlete's foot), carbuncles, herpes simplex, scabies, pyoderma, impetigo, erysipelas, warts, tinea cruris, furuncles, secondary invasion of burns, and other lesions.
2. Evaluates and monitors the treatments of a wide variety of skin infections.

Nursing Care:
Before Test: Explain the test procedure and the purpose of the test. Assess the client's knowledge of the test. Inform client that care will be taken to not produce discomfort and to ask for analgesics if necessary.
During Test: Adhere to standard precautions. Continue to assess the need for analgesia as skin culture is obtained.
After Test: Apply dry sterile dressing as needed.

Potential Complications: Infection from contamination during culture

Interfering Factors: Inadequate sample amount

Nursing Considerations:
Pediatric: Infants and children will need assistance in remaining still during the skin culture and age-appropriate comfort measures following the test.
Gerontology: Aging decreases the effectiveness of the immune system, and therefore careful assessment of the postprocedure wound is necessary.
Home Care: Health care provider must be instructed to continue to observe wound for clinical manifestations of infection (e.g., warmth, redness, swelling, pain).

Listing of Related Tests: Skin culture for mycobacteria; skin culture for fungus

WEBLINKS

http://www.cmrinstitute.org

Slit-Lamp Biomicroscopy
(slit laemp *BIY*-oe-miy-*KRAHS*-kuh-pee)
(slit-lamp vision test; binocular biomicroscopy)

30-60 min.

Type of Test: Microscopic

Body Systems and Functions: Sensory system

Normal Findings: Normal optic nerve and retina; normal anterior structures, including sclera, conjunctiva, lids, iris, cornea, and anterior chamber

Test Results Time Frame: Immediately

Test Description: Slit-lamp biomicroscopy is a noninvasive visualization of the anterior portion of the eye and its parts. The slit lamp is actually a binocular microscope with a light source that can be adjusted to examine the fluid, tissues, and structures of the eyes. A variety of special attachments can be added to the slit-lamp equipment, and special eye studies with detailed views can be added.

Consent Form: Required

List of Equipment: Slit-lamp apparatus; eye drops for anesthesia and dilation; ocular dye

Test Procedure:
1. Remove eye glasses and contacts.
2. Position client upright with chin resting on chin rest and forehead touching bar of slit-lamp instrument.
3. Client looks through eye of microscope as examiner proceeds with the test.
4. Eye drops may be added. *Allows pupil dilation and anesthesia for better visualization of eye structures.*

Clinical Implications and Indications:
1. Diagnoses corneal abrasions, conjunctivitis, ulcers, opacities (cataracts), and iritis
2. Detects conjunctival and corneal injuries

3. Evaluates the fit of contact lenses
4. Evaluates lacrimal apparatus dysfunction
5. Evaluates the progression of glaucoma and glaucomatous optic neuropathy

Nursing Care:
Before Test: Explain the test procedure and the purpose of the test. Assess the client's knowledge of the test. Assure client that the procedure is painless. Inform client that he will have blurred vision if ocular drops are used. Perform Snellen visual acuity test prior to slit-lamp test.
During Test: Adhere to standard precautions.
After Test: Do not allow client to drive until vision is recovered from ocular drops (2–4 hr). Wear sunglasses immediately following test.

Contraindications: Allergy to mydriatic eye drops; narrow-angle glaucoma

Interfering Factors: Inability of client to remain still; improper administration of eye drops

Nursing Considerations:
Gerontology: Chronic glaucoma increases with age.
Rural: Client should have another person accompany him/her to the test, to drive the client home.

Listing of Related Tests: Gonioscopy; intraocular pressure; Snellen acuity

WEBLINKS	

http://www.orthop.washington.edu; http://health.excite.com

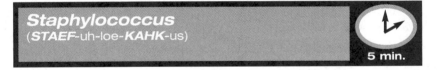

Staphylococcus
(**STAEF**-uh-loe-**KAHK**-us)

5 min.

Type of Test: Culture

Body Systems and Functions: Immunological system

Normal Findings: No pathogenic growth of *Staphylococcus* from tissue

Test Results Time Frame: Positive results reported when *Staphylococcus* grows on the culture; no growth in 48 hr indicates negative test.

Test Description: The staphylococcal test is used to diagnose staphylococcal infections or illnesses by culturing suspected sources of infection. This could include sputum, urine, wounds, and nasal cultures. Staphylococci are gram-positive micrococci that often cause suppurative conditions by releasing endotoxins destructive to tissue cells. Some staphyloccal infections are the cause of a common food poisoning. *Staphylococcus aureus* is a species that is commonly present on the skin and mucous membranes. *Staphylococcus aureus* also causes a variety of infectious disorders and can even lead to the condition of septic shock.

CULTURE, TISSUE, MICROSCOPIC

CLINICAL ALERT:
Cultures should also include a sensitivity test because of the rising incidence of methicillin-resistant *Staphylococcus aureus* (MRSA). *Staphylococcus aureus* infections are usually treated with some form of penicillin. MRSA is a nosocomial infection and usually treated with vancomycin.

Consent Form: Not required

List of Equipment: Sterile swabs; sterile specimen container

Test Procedure:
1. Label the specimen tube. *Correctly identifies the client and the test to be performed.*
2. Obtain a swabbing from the area to be tested. *Swabs are used to transfer microbes to a culture medium.*
3. Send the specimen to the laboratory as soon as possible. *Delayed transport of the specimen may alter test results.*

Clinical Implications and Indications:
1. Diagnoses the presence of infection of the staphylococcal organisms. Staphylococcal pathogens can cause such things as food poisoning and infections of the epidermis.
2. *Staphylococcus aureus* causes suppurative conditions, such as boils, carbuncles, and internal abscesses, as well as internal infectious processes (e.g., toxic shock syndrome).
3. *Staphylococcus epidermidis* is a coagulase-negative species that causes the most resistent pathologies of the skin.

Nursing Care:
Before Test: Explain the test procedure and the purpose of the test. Assess the client's knowledge of the test.
During Test: Adhere to standard precautions.
After Test: Monitor client for signs of infection.

Interfering Factors: Contamination of specimen

Nursing Considerations:
Pediatric: Children are particularly susceptible to staphyloccal infections, caused from poor hygienic practices (e.g., hand washing before eating and after voiding). Careful attention must be given to provide educational opportunities to children in this regard.
Gerontology: The elderly population are at risk for staphyloccal infections due to their risk for immunocompromised conditions. Education regarding the correct storage of foods, hand washing, and detection of early symptomatology of the presence of infection is necessary.

WEBLINKS ▯

http://infonet.med.cornell.edu

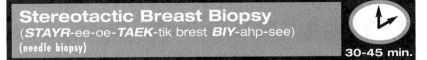

Stereotactic Breast Biopsy
(*STAYR*-ee-oe-*TAEK*-tik brest *BIY*-ahp-see)
(needle biopsy)

30-45 min.

Type of Test: Tissue

Body Systems and Functions: Reproductive system

Normal Findings: Normal breast tissue or fibrosis tissue

Test Results Time Frame: Within 48 hr

Test Description: Stereotactic breast biopsy is performance of a needle biopsy of suspicious breast lumps, which have been identified through mammography and ultrasound. Six to seven needles are inserted into the area, and each needle biopsies a piece of the tissue. This test is 99% as accurate as open surgical biopsies of breast lumps. In general, the biopsy is an invasive procedure performed in a surgical setting. An excision or needle punch sample of body tissue is taken under sterile technique and examined microscopically for cell morphology and tissue anomalies.

> **CLINICAL ALERT:**
> Client should be off anticoagulants or aspirin for 7 days prior to the procedure; performed using mammography (radiation)

Consent Form: Required

List of Equipment: Stereotactic breast biopsy table; mammography; lidocaine; betadine; biopsy needles; sterile biopsy container; gauze squares (4 x 4 to clean; 2 x 2 to cover site); ice pack

Test Procedure:
1. Client lies on a table with a hole for the breast to hang down for the test. *Prone position allows for breasts to hang for isolation of biopsy site.*
2. The area for biopsy receives local anesthetic, usually lidocaine. *Because of the depth and number of needles, local anesthetic allows for a more pain-free experience.*
3. Biopsy area is prepped using betadine or other antiseptic in the case of clients who are allergic to iodine. *Aseptic cleansing minimizes risk of infection.*
4. Immobilize the breast with plastic plates similar to mammography plates. One plate has a hole for the needles to be inserted. *Immobilizing breast assures site to be biopsied is accurately accessed.*
5. Six to seven needles are inserted into the lump, guided by radiation such as is used during a mammogram. *Each needle biopsies a different section of the lump to increase accuracy of diagnosis.*
6. Once the needles are inserted, a piece of tissue is snipped at the end of the needle and the needle is removed. *Tissue from the lump is needed for pathological evaluation.*
7. Assist the client to a sitting position. Be sure to watch for lightheadedness. Assist client to standing position. *Gradual changes in position allow the client to regain stability.*

Clinical Implications and Indications:

1. Diagnoses malignancy in breasts.
2. Eighty percent of stereotactic breast biopsy results are benign. A new form of stereotactic breast biopsy is mammotome, in which only one needle (larger bore) is used. Results are 99% as accurate as open biopsy.

Nursing Care:

Before Test: Explain the test procedure and the purpose of the test. Assess the client's knowledge of the test. Explain and discuss with client possible outcomes of the test. Check the client for allergies to iodine. Assess client for last time she had aspirin or anticoagulants. Provide preprocedure sedation and analgesia as ordered. Transport client to operating or procedure room. Drape client appropriately.

During Test: Adhere to standard precautions. Assess completeness of the local anesthetic during the test. Provide reassurance and a calm atmosphere during the procedure.

After Test: Clean biopsy site and apply 2 x 2 gauze squares or Band-Aids. Apply ice packs for 2 hr after the biopsy.

Potential Complications: Bleeding, bruising, and edema at biopsy site

Contraindications: Anticoagulants; aspirin; aspirin-containing products

Listing of Related Tests: Mammogram; breast ultrasound

WEBLINKS

http://www.idsonline.com; http://www.breastinfo.com

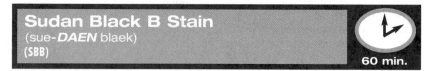

Sudan Black B Stain
(sue-*DAEN* blaek)
(SBB)

60 min.

Type of Test: Microscopic

Body Systems and Functions: Hematological system

Normal Findings: Monocytes and granulocytes stain positively; lymphocytes do not stain positively.

Test Results Time Frame: Within 24 hr

Test Description: Sudan black B stain is used on bone marrow aspirate to identify cells that indicate acute granulocytic leukemia. The leukemias are a group of chronic malignant conditions of white blood cells and white blood cell precursors. Acute granulocytic leukemia is one of the most common types of leukemia in adults and is a subtype of acute myelogenous leukemia. Common clinical manifestations are risk of infection, weakness, fatigue, bleeding, liver pain, spleen pain, headache, vomiting, and bone pain.

CULTURE, TISSUE, MICROSCOPIC

CLINICAL ALERT:
Bone marrow aspirate is used for the stain; need at least 300 µL for specimen

Consent Form: Required

List of Equipment: Sterile towels; local anesthetic; betadine solution; bone marrow aspirate kit; sterile specimen tubes

Test Procedure:
1. Place client so hip is exposed. *Position maximizes comfort and ease of obtaining biopsy.*
2. Clean bone marrow site with betadine. *Reduces likelihood of infection.*
3. Place sterile towels around the aspirate site and aspirate bone marrow. *Reduces likelihood of infection.*
4. Send aspirate to laboratory for stain and additional tests. *Ensures accurate results.*

Clinical Implications and Indications:
1. Positive stain of blast cells indicates myelogenous origin.
2. Stain is positive in acute granulocytic leukemia.
3. Stain is negative in acute lymphocytic leukemia and plasma cell leukemia.

Nursing Care:
Before Test: Explain the test procedure and the purpose of the test. Assist in positioning and prepping the client.
During Test: Adhere to standard precautions. Provide reassurance and a calm atmosphere during the procedure.
After Test: Clean site of biopsy. Provide analgesia as necessary.

Potential Complications: Bleeding and bruising at the site

Nursing Considerations:
Pediatric: Sedation is recommended for infants and children. Place the infant or child on a blanket for comfort. After postprocedure monitoring is completed and per health care provider's order, the pediatric client is discharged with an adult who is given instructions.
Gerontology: The older person may find it difficult to maintain positions when required to do so for lengthy periods of time during the aspirate. The elderly client with acute myelogenous leukemia needs particular care related to immunosuppression and generalized lethargy.
Rural: Advisable to arrange for transportation home after recovering from procedure.

Listing of Related Tests: Bone marrow aspiration; periodic acid-schiff (PAS) stain; terminal deoxynucleotidyl transferase (TDT) stain; leukocyte alkaline phosphatase (LAP) stain; tartrate-resistant acid phosphatase (TRAP) stain; buffy coat smear

WEBLINKS

www.arup-lab.com; www.hsc.virginia.edu

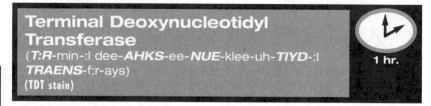

Type of Test: Microscopic

Body Systems and Functions: Hematological system

Normal Findings: Negative in blood or lymph nodes; 0%–2% in bone marrow

Test Results Time Frame: Within 24 hr

Test Description: Terminal deoxynucleotidyl transferase is a type of stain used on bone marrow aspirate to identify cells that indicate different types of leukemia and lymphoma (tumor marker). Leukemias are a neoplastic proliferation of one particular cell type (i.e., granulocytes, monocytes, lymphocytes, or megakaryocytes). The leukemias are a group of chronic malignant conditions of white blood cells and white blood cell precursors. Common clinical manifestations are risk of infection, weakness, fatigue, bleeding, liver pain, spleen pain, headache, vomiting, and bone pain. The lymphomas are neoplasms of lymphoid tissue, usually derived from B lymphocytes.

Consent Form: Required

List of Equipment: Sterile towels; local anesthetic; betadine solution; bone marrow aspirate kit; sterile specimen tubes

Test Procedure:
1. Position client so hip is exposed. *Position maximizes comfort and ease of obtaining biopsy.*
2. Bone marrow site is cleaned with betadine. *Reduces likelihood of infection.*
3. Sterile towels are placed around the aspirate site. Reduces likelihood of infection.
4. Bone marrow aspirate is performed.
5. Aspirate is sent to laboratory for stain and additional tests. *Pathologist performs stains in the laboratory.*

Clinical Implications and Indications:
1. Positive results are found with acute lymphocytic leukemia, lymphoblastic lymphoma, chronic myelogenous leukemia, blast crisis, and acute undifferentiated leukemia.

Nursing Care:
Before Test: Explain the test procedure and the purpose of the test. Assess the client's knowledge of the test. Provide preprocedure sedation and analgesia as ordered. Transport client to operating or procedure room. Drape client appropriately.
During Test: Adhere to standard precautions. Provide reassurance and a calm atmosphere during the procedure.
After Test: Clean site of biopsy. Provide analgesia as necessary.

Potential Complications: Bleeding and bruising at the site

Nursing Considerations:

Pediatric: Sedation is recommended for infants and children. Place the infant or child on a blanket for comfort. After postprocedure monitoring is completed and per health care provider's order, the pediatric client is discharged with an adult who is given instructions.

Gerontology: The older person may find it difficult to maintain positions when required to do so for lengthy periods of time during the bone marrow aspirate.

Rural: Advisable to arrange for transportation home after recovering from procedure.

Listing of Related Tests: Bone marrow aspiration; periodic acid-Schiff (PAS) stain; terminal deoxynucleotidyl transferase (TDT) stain; leukocyte alkaline phosphatase (LAP) stain; tartrate-resistant acid phosphatase (TRAP) stain; buffy coat smear

WEBLINKS

www.arup-lab.com

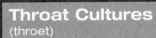

Throat Cultures
(throet)
(throat swabs; throat washings)

10 min.

Type of Test: Culture

Body Systems and Functions: Immunological system

Normal Findings: No growth of pathogenic bacteria

Test Results Time Frame: Within 24–72 hr

Test Description: Throat cultures are swabs or washings that are sent to the laboratory for determination of the presence of bacterial pathogens. For swabbing, the client is to open their mouth and a sterile swab is used to obtain secretions from the back of the throat. For washings, the client gargles with sterile saline and then expectorates into a sterile container.

> **CLINICAL ALERT:**
> The client should be told the reason for the throat culture and how the specimen will be obtained. It is important to explain to children that the procedure will be uncomfortable but that it will be done quickly (note: the nurse should wear a mask or stand to the side of the client since most clients gag or cough during this procedure).

Consent Form: Not required

List of Equipment: Swabs; specimen tubes; tongue depressor; sterile saline; specimen container

CULTURE, TISSUE, MICROSCOPIC

Test Procedure:

Swabbing:

1. Visualize client's mouth with examination light. *Assists in visualizing back of throat.*
2. Depress client's tongue with tongue depressor. *Minimizes risk of contamination of the swabs.*
3. Rotate swab firmly and gently over the back of the throat, around tonsils, and on areas of inflammation or ulceration. *Sufficient secretions are necessary for a successful culture.*
4. Do not touch swab to lips, tongue, buccal mucosa, or roof of mouth. *These areas will contaminate the specimen.*
5. Place swab in specimen tube and send to laboratory immediately. *Immediate transfer of specimen to culture medium ensures accurate results.*
6. Refrigerate culture if transport to laboratory is delayed. *Cold can delay bacterial growth in specimen.*

Washings:

1. Have client gargle with 10 mL of sterile saline and expectorate in a sterile cup. *Ten milliliters is necessary to obtain adequate volume for culture. Sterile saline is used as it is isotonic and noncontaminated.*
2. Send sterile cup to the laboratory immediately. *Immediate transfer of specimen to culture medium ensures accurate results.*
3. Refrigerate washings if transport to laboratory is delayed. *Cold can delay bacterial growth in specimen.*

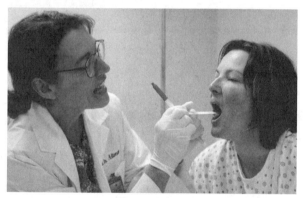

Throat Culture

Clinical Implications and Indications:

1. Positive results are found in the following infections: group A beta-hemolytic streptococci, *Neisseria gonorrhoeae*, *Neisseria meningitidis*, *Corynebacterium diptheriae*, *Bordella pertussis*, *Staphylococcus aureus*, and capnocytophaga species.

Nursing Care:

Before Test: Explain the test procedure and the purpose of the test. Assess the client's knowledge of the test.

During Test: Adhere to standard precautions (note: masks are worn as gagging and coughing are common during throat swabs).

After Test: Monitor clients for clinical manifestations of infections.

Interfering Factors: Contamination of specimen

Nursing Considerations:
Pediatric: *Infants and children will need assistance in remaining still during the procedure and age-appropriate comfort measures following the test.*

`WEBLINKS` 🔲❌

http://medline.cos.com

Thyroid Biopsy
(***THIY***-royd ***BIY***-ahp-see)
(fine-needle biopsy)

30 min.

CULTURE, TISSUE, MICROSCOPIC

Type of Test: Tissue

Body Systems and Functions: Endocrine system

Normal Findings: Normal thyroid cells

Test Results Time Frame: Within 24 hr

Test Description: A thyroid biopsy is a test that helps to determine the tissue type of thyroid cysts and tumors. Using ultrasound, the cyst or tumor is located and a sterile needle is inserted. The biopsy is an invasive procedure performed in a surgical setting. An excision or needle punch sample of body tissue is taken under sterile technique and examined microscopically for cell morphology and tissue anomalies. A thyroid biopsy is most often used to diagnose thyroid cancer (note: a thyroidectomy is curative for a high percentage of clients with thyroid cancer). The thyroid is an endocrine gland located in the anterior neck region and partially surrounds the thyroid cartilage and upper rings of the trachea. The primary action of the thyroid gland is to control the basal metabolic rate. The thyroid gland enlarges in hyperthyroidism (goiter), and it may be removed surgically. In addition, a hypothyroid state may exist (e.g., after a thyroidectomy), and the therapy is to administer a synthetic form of thyroid hormones (e.g., synthroid).

Consent Form: Required

List of Equipment: Transducer gel; ultrasound machine; local antiseptic; gauze squares; sterile biopsy needle; sterile specimen containers; tape

Test Procedure:
1. Place client in supine position with neck exposed. *Position enhances ability to obtain accurate ultrasound images.*
2. A pillow may be placed under the client's shoulder. *Allows better contact of ultrasound transducer and enhances client comfort.*
3. Warm ultrasound gel is applied over the thyroid. Warm gel is more comfortable. *Gel enhances contact between the transducer and client's skin. Allows for easier movement of the transducer.*
4. The area for biopsy receives local anesthetic, usually lidocaine. *Local anesthetic allows for client comfort and ability to be still during needle biopsy.*

5. Biopsy area is prepped using betadine or other antiseptic in the case of clients who are allergic to iodine. *Cleaning area decreases risk of infection.*
6. Needle is inserted using ultrasound to guide the practitioner. Biopsy is obtained. *Use of ultrasound to guide needle assures correct area is being biopsied.*
7. Clean site and apply pressure dressing. *Decreases likelihood of bleeding.*
8. Upon completion of the examination, clean the gel from the skin. *Promotes hygiene and client comfort.*

Clinical Implications and Indications:
1. Cancer cells indicate thyroid cancer.

Nursing Care:
Before Test: Explain the test procedure and the purpose of the test. Assess the client's knowledge of the test. Provide preprocedure sedation and analgesia as ordered. Transport client to operating or procedure room. Drape client appropriately.
During Test: Adhere to sterile technique and standard precautions. Provide reassurance and a calm atmosphere during the procedure.
After Test: Clean site of biopsy. Provide analgesia as necessary.

Potential Complications: Bleeding and bruising at the site

Nursing Considerations:
Pediatric: *Sedation is recommended for infants and children. Place the infant or child on a blanket for comfort. After postprocedure monitoring is completed and per health care provider's order, the pediatric client is discharged with an adult who is given instructions.*
Gerontology: *The older person may find it difficult to maintain positions when required to do so for lengthy periods of time during the biopsy.*
Rural: *Advisable to arrange for transportation home after recovering from the thyroid biopsy.*

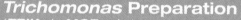

WEBLINKS

www.endocrineweb.com

Trichomonas Preparation
(***TRIK***-uh-***MOE***-nuhs)
(*Trichomonas vaginalis*; wet mount; wet preparation)

30 min.

Type of Test: Microscopic

Body Systems and Functions: Reproductive system

Normal Findings: Absence of the protozoa *Trichomonas vaginalis*

Test Results Time Frame: Within 24 hr

Test Description: *Trichomonas* preparation detects the presence of the *Trichomonas* pathogen that is responsible for this organism that causes the sexually transmitted disease. *Trichomonas* is a parasitic infection of the vaginal canal and urethra caused by the protozoa *T. vaginalis. Trichomonas* preparation is a normal part of a Pap test. Positive results occur in less than 1% of women but in 12% of the women seen at STD clinics.

CLINICAL ALERT:
The *Trichomonas* preparation test detects only the sexually transmitted disease where the sample is obtained during the Pap test and pelvic examination.

Consent Form: Not required

List of Equipment: Vaginal speculum; swabs; sterile culture tube

Test Procedure:
1. Place client in the lithotomy position. *Facilitates culture collection.*
2. Have examination light on vaginal area. *Facilitates examination and culture collection.*
3. Insert speculum into the vagina. *Allows visualization of the vaginal canal and decreases risk of contamination of swab.*
4. Use two different swabs to obtain secretions from vaginal canal. *Increases likelihood of obtaining infected specimen.*
5. Place swab in specimen tube and send to laboratory immediately. *Use of specimen tube decreases chance of contamination.*

Clinical Implications and Indications:
1. Positive identification of STD when the parasite is seen on a wet-mount preparation

Nursing Care:
Before Test: Explain the test procedure and the purpose of the test. Assess client's knowledge of the test.
During Test: Adhere to standard precautions.
After Test: Assist client with cleaning perineal area. Counsel client and monitor for vaginal discharge.

Interfering Factors: Contamination of specimen

Listing of Related Tests: Pap test

WEBLINKS

http://wdxcyber.com

Vaginal Culture
(*VAEG*-uh-n:l)

15 min.

Type of Test: Culture

Body Systems and Functions: Reproductive system

Normal Findings: Negative for pathogens

(side tab) CULTURE, TISSUE, MICROSCOPIC

CRITICAL VALUES:
Presence of pathogens

Test Results Time Frame: Within 48 hr

Test Description: A vaginal culture is used to identify organisms present in the vaginal canal. The vagina normally contains some bacteria (*Lactobacillus, Staphylococcus, Escherichia coli*) as well as some yeast. When a vaginal infection is present, a culture of the vaginal secretions may indicate the cause. If gonorrhea is suspected, an endocervical culture is indicated.

CLINICAL ALERT:
A culture may be required to confirm the identity of certain pathogens. *Candida* (fungus) and *Trichomonas* (protozoan) infections, for example, may need to be cultured for diagnosis. Gonorrhea is a communicable disease, which must be reported to the health department. Clients may not wish to name their sexual partners. Provide empathy in considering the client's concerns and assist the client in understanding the importance of notifying those infected.

Consent Form: Not required

List of Equipment: Sterile swab; culture medium

Test Procedure:
1. Label the collection container. *Correctly identifies the client and the test to be performed.*
2. Spread the vaginal opening with one hand while inserting a moistened sterile swab into the canal. *Prevents the swab from being contaminated with bacteria outside the vaginal canal.*
3. Insert the swab well inside the vagina and leave it there for 30 sec. *Allows organisms to be absorbed by the swab.*
4. Remove the swab and brush it across the medium or glass slide. *Allows the organisms to be transferred adequately.*
5. Seal the medium or spray fixative on the slide and transport the labeled container to the laboratory. *A slide is used when a smear is ordered; medium is used for a culture.*

Clinical Implications and Indications:
1. Diagnoses gonorrhea, chlamydia, herpes simplex, trichomonas, moniliasis (or other yeast infections), and bacterial vaginosis
2. Evaluates and monitors therapy for vaginal infections

Nursing Care:
Before Test: Explain the test procedure and the purpose of the test. Assess the client's knowledge of the test.
During Test: Adhere to standard precautions.

Interfering Factors: Douching prior to test; failure to send specimen to laboratory immediately; contamination of swab due to improper technique; antibiotic therapy; metronidazole

Listing of Related Tests: Vaginal culture; cervical smear

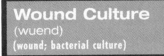

http://biocrs.biomed.brown.edu

Wound Culture
(wuend)
(wound; bacterial culture)

15 min.

CULTURE, TISSUE, MICROSCOPIC

Type of Test: Tissue

Body Systems and Functions: Integumentary system

Normal Findings: No growth of pathological organisms

Test Results Time Frame: Within 72 hr

Test Description: The wound culture is used to diagnose the presence of infection and identify the causative agent. A wide variety of wounds may exist, from which a wound culture is taken. The soft tissue infections may include any of the skin layers and may be enclosed as in an abscess. The wound may also be in an open or ulcerated state that is exposed to the environment. Organisms that grow may be either aerobic or anaerobic and may be common to the person. As the organisms increase in number, they may become pathogenic in nature. In addition, there are many organisms that are not normally found in tissue, unless in the presence of infection.

CLINICAL ALERT:
Many infected wounds have organisms that are extremely virulent and contagious (e.g., *Staphylococcus aureus*, *Pseudomonas*, *Klebsiella*). The health care provider should use extreme caution when culturing the wound and adhere to strict standard precaution techniques.

Consent Form: Not required

List of Equipment: Swab; culture tube; gloves (potentially mask, gown, eye protection device); cleansing agent (e.g., surgical soap, 70% alcohol); sterile water; sterile gauze pads; sterile petri dish

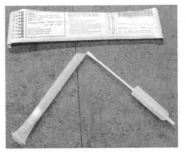

Sterile Culture Tube and Swab

Test Procedure:

1. Observe standard precautions. *Decreases chances of cross-contamination.*
2. Set up necessary equipment. *Increases efficiency of obtaining the wound culture.*
3. Assess the wound for size, color, and odor. *Provides accurate assessment of wound prior to cleaning.*
4. Irrigate the wound with sterile saline if there is drainage or pus present. *Decreases the chance of extraneous organisms in the culture.*
5. Dry culture site with sterile gauze pads. *Exposes wound to enable a good culture.*
6. Wearing sterile gloves, hold wound to enable sterile swab to be rotated over the wound area to obtain a sample. Avoid touching wound edges and surfaces with swab. *Allows for an accurate collection of the pathogens from the wound.*
7. Immediately place the swab in the sterile culture tube and label. *Decreases chance of contamination of the culture.*

Clinical Implications and Indications:

1. Detects organisms that have multiplied to excess (e.g., *Clostridium* species, enterococci, staphylococci, mycobacteria, streptococci, diptheroids, *Proteus* species, *Pseudomonas, Nocardia, Bacteriodes, Klebsiella, Escherichia coli*).
2. Evaluates samples from infections that border the mucous membranes.
3. Evaluates and monitors exudates from abscesses or deep wounds (especially if associated with foul odors or discolorations of a green or brown color).
4. Evaluates and monitors fluid draining from any wound (e.g., skin, eye, ears, nose).

Nursing Care:

Before Test: Explain the test procedure and the purpose of the test. Assess the client's knowledge of the test. Ensure client that every means will be taken to reduce client discomfort. Obtain wound culture prior to antibiotic therapy.
During Test: Adhere to standard precautions. Provide reassurance and a calm atmosphere during the procedure.
After Test: Ensure the label is correct for client name, location of client, culture site, date, clinical diagnosis, and current antibiotic therapy. Prompt transportation of culture specimen to laboratory.

Contraindications: Intense pain may prohibit the normal culturing of a deep wound without analgesia; overall trauma to the client may make wound culturing difficult (e.g., systemic burn with high percentage of body surface involvement).

Interfering Factors: Antibiotic therapy; contamination from body fluids; eschar tissue from burns does not culture easily.

Nursing Considerations:

Pediatric: Explain to the child in age-appropriate terms why the culture procedure is required. Allow older children to assist in positioning. Children may require special emotional support from family members during wound culture. Reassure child that the procedure will not hurt any more than the normal dressing change.
Gerontology: The older person may find it difficult to maintain positions when required to do so for lengthy periods of time during the wound culture.
Home Care: Health care provider may need special transportation carriers after

culture is obtained in home setting. Allow for necessary time to take specimen to laboratory.

Listing of Related Tests: Skin culture; throat culture; nasal culture; ear culture; eye culture; stool culture; sputum culture

WEBLINKS

http://www.cmrinstitute.org

CULTURE, TISSUE, MICROSCOPIC

8

Electrodiagnostic Studies

EXAMINATION BY ELECTRODIAGNOSTIC TESTS

Electrodiagnostics are noninvasive tests that involve either magnetic fields or bio-electric waves produced in the body. The electromagnetic tests measure and record bioelectrical impulses in the body. The brain, heart, nerves, and muscles all produce electrical impulses that can be diagnostic for many different conditions. Some tests will use electrical current to test body responses. Electrical sensors (electrodes) are placed at certain anatomic points to measure the tone, velocity, and direction of the impulses. The impulses are then transmitted to an oscilloscope or printed on graphic paper.

EXAMPLES OF ELECTRODIAGNOSTIC TESTING

There are a tremendous variety of electrodiagnostic tests. These tests are used to detect the presence of physiological abnormalities in many of the body systems. Some examples of these tests are electrocardiography (see figure), magnetic resonance imaging (MRI), electromyography, fetal monitoring, and sleep studies. As an example, MRIs provide cross-sectional images, which are shown on a screen and saved for analysis. No radiation exposure is involved and no known harm has been demonstrated from the use of the magnetic fields in magnetic resonance imaging. The test is primarily noninvasive and yet does have educational implications for clients receiving this type of diagnostic test.

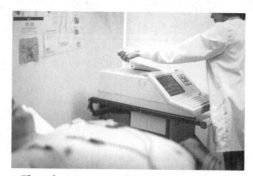

The administration of an electrocardiogram

CLIENT CARE IN ELECTRODIAGNOSTIC TESTING

Client Preparation for Electrodiagnostic Testing

The electrodiagnostic tests all tend to be noninvasive and therefore painless, with few side effects. However, there are exceptions and aspects of these types of tests that affect clients differently. For example, the MRI testing takes place in an enclosed mechanical device. This can evoke claustrophobia in susceptible people and requires a person to lie very still. The clients must be told ahead of time that they will be required to remain motionless during the MRI. Another example is electrocardiography, which can be performed on clients who are susceptible to life-threatening dysrhythmias. Clients having the need for electrocardiography may need to be prepared for the potential complications they could experience during the testing. Last, there are electrodiagnostic tests that require the insertion of needle electrodes. These tests necessitate clients learning about the needle electrodes and knowing what to expect. Because of these variations and differences among the electrodiagnostic testing, nurses need to know the specifics of how each electrodiagnostic test is performed, and then be able to care for their clients with the individual implications of each test.

Life span implications in electrodiagnostic testing

There are different life span considerations for electrodiagnostic testing that are specifically related to the developmental age of the clients. For example, infants and children may be required to be sedated or provided assistance to remain still during electrodiagnostic tests. In addition, pregnant women are usually not routinely screened with an MRI test because the effect of an MRI has not been demonstrated to be safe for a fetus, although no known harm exists. Also, the elderly might need particular assistance in positioning during electrodiagnostic testing, depending on the individual test and the length of time the client is required to be involved in the test.

Nursing Diagnoses for Electrodiagnostic Testing

Two relatively common nursing diagnoses related to electrodiagnostic tests are (1) knowledge deficit related to the test procedure and (2) anxiety related to the potential outcome of the test. First, the knowledge deficit diagnosis requires nurses to be aware of the specific implications of how electrodiagnostic tests are performed. This allows the nurse to teach clients what to expect prior to having the test, and what clinical manifestations they might have as a result of the test. The nurse must allow time for the client to ask questions and needs to be prepared to explain the test in language that is easily understood by the client. Second, it is common for clients to be anxious from their worries about the outcomes of their electrodiagnostic testing. The nurse must not give false reassurance for the potential outcomes, and should communicate genuine caring and empathy for the anxiety of the client. In addition, relaxation techniques, deep breathing exercises, and therapeutic communication need to be employed by the nurse to allay anxiety of the client.

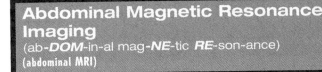

Abdominal Magnetic Resonance Imaging
(ab-*DOM*-in-al mag-*NE*-tic *RE*-son-ance)
(abdominal MRI)

30-90 min.

ELECTRODIAGNOSTIC

Type of Test: Electrodiagnostic

Body Systems and Functions: Musculoskeletal system

Normal Findings: Normal abdomen and surrounding structures

Test Results Time Frame: Within 24 hr

Test Description: An abdominal MRI test is performed to assist in the diagnosis of abdominal tissues or to measure blood flow in the area. The abdominal MRI is considered a superior test to a CT scan for detecting liver metastasis or lesions or finding ischemia in the pancreas or liver. An MRI is able to provide more detail than a CT scan, as in brain tumors of the posterior fossa. The MRI pictures take images representing magnetic characteristics of body tissues. This produces a cross-sectional image of the body and spares the client from x-ray exposure. Images can be taken at any angle, including sagittal and coronal planes. If a contrast medium is used, the material is injected through an IV before the procedure begins.

Consent Form: Required

List of Equipment: Magnetic resonance imaging equipment

Test Procedure:
1. If an IV contrast medium is used, initiate an IV site and inject the contrast before the procedure.
2. Place client in supine position and instruct client to remain completely still. *Ensures accurate results.*

3. The table with the client slides into the cylindrical scanner for the test procedure.

Clinical Implications and Indications:

1. Detects metastatic disease and lesions in liver and pancreas.
2. The MRI is used primarily for nervous and musculoskeletal problems, and therefore abdominal use is somewhat limited.

Nursing Care:

Before Test: Explain the test procedure and the purpose of the test. Assess the client's knowledge of the test. Instruct the client that during the procedure it may be uncomfortable to sit on the hard table or achieve some of the necessary positions; it is important to remain as still as possible during the test; there are no dietary restrictions prior to the test; and it is necessary to remove dental prosthesis, jewelry, eyeglasses, or other metal objects like hair clips before the procedure. Explain that some clients suffer a feeling of claustrophobia because the MRI machine has a small-diameter bore for the client's body. Inform the client that they will hear loud knocking noises emitted from the magnetic coils changing pulse direction. Mild sedation may be required to assist the client to relax as well as playing music and remaining in verbal contact with the client during the test.

During Test: Adhere to standard precautions. Instruct client to continue to remain motionless. Advise client to keep eyes closed to promote relaxation and to prevent claustraphobia. Instruct client to take deep, slow breaths in the event of nausea.

After Test: Remind the client that the test results usually take 24 hr.

Contraindications: Metal implants, such as bone screws, pacemakers, and metal surgical sutures

Interfering Factors: Inability to remain still

Nursing Considerations:

Pregnancy: MRI is not routinely done during pregnancy; fetal risk is unknown.
Pediatric: Sedation is recommended for infants and children. Place the infant or child on a blanket for comfort. After postprocedure monitoring is completed and per health care provider's order, the pediatric client is discharged with an adult who is given instructions.
Gerontology: A confused older adult may be sedated to assist in holding still.

Listing of Related Tests: CT scan of abdomen

WEBLINKS

http://chorus.rad.mcw.edu

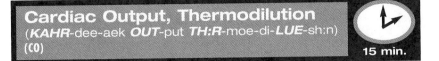

Cardiac Output, Thermodilution
(*KAHR*-dee-aek *OUT*-put *TH:R*-moe-di-*LUE*-sh:n)
(CO)

15 min.

Type of Test: Electrodiagnostic

Body Systems and Functions: Cardiovascular system

Normal Findings:

Cardiac output:

Adults	4–6 L/min
Newborns	0.8–1.0 L/min
6 months	1.0–1.3 L/min
1 year	1.3–1.5 L/min
2 years	1.5–2.0 L/min
4 years	2.3–2.75 L/min
5 years	2.5–3.0 L/min
8 years	3.4–3.6 L/min
10 years	3.8–4.0 L/min

A normal cardiac output (CO) curve starts at baseline and has a smooth rapid upstroke and a gradual downstroke.

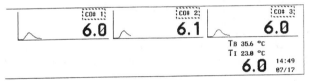

Actual normal CO curves of postoperative cardiac surgery client.
Note computer notation of temperature of blood, temperature of injectate,
and calculated mean CO.

Test Results Time Frame: Within 15 min

Test Description: Cardiac output thermography measures the CO, which is defined as the volume of blood ejected from the heart over 1 min. CO is determined by heart rate in beats per minute and the stroke volume in milliliters per beat. CO is expressed in liters per minute and is affected by preload, after-load, contractility, and heart rate. CO is measured by the critical care nurse who has demonstrated a baseline competency in this advanced skill. The conventional thermodilution bedside measurement of CO uses intermittent boluses of room temperature or iced sterile solution into the proximal port of the pulmonary artery (PA) catheter located in the right atrium. The injectate mixes with atrial blood and flows through the tricuspid valve and into the right ventricle. A thermister within the PA catheter senses the change in blood temperature as the blood flows by the catheter tip located in the pulmonary artery. The change in temperature over time is calculated by the computer and converted into a cardiac output measurement. A new modification in the measurement of CO is the continuous CO method, which uses a thermal filament located in the catheter wall. No boluses of solution are necessary in continuous CO measurement.

$$CO = \text{heart rate} \times \text{stroke volume cardiac index}$$
$$\text{Cardiac Index} = CO/\text{body surface area}$$

Consent Form: A consent is required to insert a PA catheter necessary for CO measurement. A consent is not required to perform the CO test.

List of Equipment: Specialized CO injectate syringe and tubing with stopcock; injectate solution; CO computer

Test Procedure: (Note: The measurement of CO consists of a more detailed series of important steps than outlined in this text. Refer to hospital procedure manual for an inclusive description of the CO measurement procedure.)

1. Assemble and prepare CO equipment according to manufacturer's recommendations.
2. Ensure the computation constant is correct and entered into the computer. *The computation constant programs the computer with the correct injectate volume and temperature.*
3. To obtain cardiac index, enter the client's height and weight into the computer. *Cardiac index is a more precise measurement than CO because it includes the client's body surface area.*
4. Check the pulmonary artery catheter waveform and chest x-ray for correct postioning.
5. Position the client supine with the head of bed flat or elevated no more than 20°. *Studies have shown no differences in CO measurements obtained with the head of bed flat or elevated 20°.*
6. Ensure that no other IV fluids are rapidly administered through the introducer arm of the PA catheter. *CO measurements may be affected by IV fluid administration into the introducer arm of the PA catheter.*
7. Administer the injectate within 4 sec or less. *This rate yields the most accurate results.*
8. In adults use 10 mL of injectate unless fluid restriction is necessary. *Use of fluid less than 10 mL results in more variability in measurements.*
9. Assess the CO curve.
10. Determine the mean CO by calculating the average of CO measurements that are within 10% of the medium (middle).

Clinical Implications and Indications:

1. Evaluates acute myocardial infarction that is complicated by heart failure or structural abnormalities
2. Evaluates and monitors cardiogenic, hypovolemic, or septic shock
3. Monitors cardiovascular surgery in high-risk clients and advanced stage heart failure
4. Diagnoses hemodynamic instability with multiple-organ system dysfunction
5. Assesses acute respiratory distress syndrome, acute respiratory failure, pulmonary embolism, and pulmonary infarction

Nursing Care:

Before Test: Explain the test procedure and the purpose of the test. Assess the client's knowledge of the test. Assist physician with insertion of PA catheter if not already in place. Position client supine and up to 20°.

During Test: Adhere to sterile technique and standard precautions (note: refer to hospital policy and procedures and the operational manual for CO measurement procedure).

After Test: Return client to previous head-of-bed position. Assess CO results in relation to other hemodynamic parameters, oxygenation indicators, client's clinical presentation, and other indices. Provide appropriate interventions based on all data. Consult with health care team as necessary regarding abnormal results and treatment plan.

Potential Complications: Infection at insertion site

Contraindications: Intracardiac shunts; tricuspid regurgitation; cardiac dysrhythmias

Interfering Factors: Skill level of the critical care nurse obtaining the measurement; appropriate positioning of the PA catheter; entering the correct computation constant into the computer; temperature of injectate; volume of injectate; client's body position; rapid infusions of IV fluids through the introducer side of the PA catheter

Nursing Considerations:

Pregnancy: During pregnancy CO peaks at twentieth week gestation at 30%–45% above resting nonpregnant levels. CO during labor increases up to 45% over nonpregnant values.

Pediatric: A smaller volume of injectate of 1–5 mL is used in infants and children.

Listing of Related Tests: Cardiac index

WEBLINKS

www.aacn.org

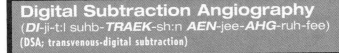

Digital Subtraction Angiography
(*DI*-ji-t:l suhb-*TRAEK*-sh:n *AEN*-jee-*AHG*-ruh-fee)
(DSA; transvenous-digital subtraction)

45–60 min.

Type of Test: Electrodiagnostic

Body Systems and Functions: Cardiovascular system

Normal Findings: Normal cardiovascular circulating system (e.g., carotid arteries, abdominal aorta, renal arteries, and peripheral vessels)

Test Results Time Frame: Within 24 hr

ELECTRODIAGNOSTIC

Test Description: Digital subtraction angiography is a computerized test that examines the arteries of the body following the IV injection of a contrast medium. A fluoroscopic image is converted from analog to digital form and the images of desired regions are seen (note: soft tissue and bone are removed from the image by the computer). This test has much less risk than an arteriogram but is not as definitive in its observations.

CLINICAL ALERT:
Have emergency equipment readily available in the event of an anaphylactic reaction to the dye.

Consent Form: Required

List of Equipment: Special monitoring equipment for electrodiagnostic testing; contrast medium; local anesthetic; IV equipment

Test Procedure:
1. Client is taken to special studies area and IV access is secured.
2. An iodine contrast medium is injected and radiographic images of the arteries are taken.

Clinical Implications and Indications:
1. Evaluates and monitors aneurysms, arterial occlusion, carotid stenosis, hepatocellular cancer, jugular tumors, pheochromocytoma, pulmonary emboli, and thoracic outlet syndrome

Nursing Care:
Before Test: Explain the test procedure and the purpose of the test. Assess the client's knowledge of the test. Assess for potential allergies to contrast medium. Inform client that during injection of contrast medium, a burning sensation may be felt for a few seconds behind the eyes or in the jaw, teeth, tongue, or lips. Assess for anxiety and provide sedation as ordered. Administer preoperative medication usually 30 minutes before procedure. Obtain baseline vital signs and neurological assessment.
During Test: Adhere to standard precautions. Assess for allergic reactions to contrast medium. Monitor vital signs every 15 min.
After Test: Assess for allergic reactions to contrast medium. Instruct client to drink fluids after test to flush contrast medium from kidneys. Monitor renal function for 48 hr following test.

Potential Complications: Anaphylaxis due to allergic reaction to iodinated contrast material; infection; hemorrhaging; hematoma; and bleeding and bruising at venipuncture site

Contraindications: Previous history of allergy to iodine, eggs, or shellfish; recent myocardial infarction; renal disorders

Interfering Factors: Inability to remain still

Nursing Considerations:

Pregnancy: *Intravenous contrast should be avoided in pregnant women if possible.*
Pediatric: *Infants and children will need assistance in remaining still during the venipuncture and age-appropriate comfort measures following the test.*
Gerontology: *The older person may find it difficult to maintain positions when required to do so for lengthy periods of time during the digital subtraction angiography.*
Rural: *Advisable to arrange for transportation home after recovering from procedure.*

Listing of Related Tests: Cardiac catheterization

⏛ WEBLINKS ⏛   ▤ ⊠

http://adam.excite.com

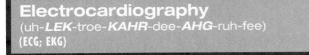

Electrocardiography
(uh-*LEK*-troe-*KAHR*-dee-*AHG*-ruh-fee)
(ECG; EKG)
15 min.

ELECTRODIAGNOSTIC

Type of Test: Electrodiagnostic

Body Systems and Functions: Cardiovascular system

Normal Findings: Normal sinus rhythm without dysrhythmias

Test Results Time Frame: Within 24 hr

Test Description: Electrocardiography is a noninvasive testing of the electrical output of the heart. This test uses all 12 electrode leads and is able to evaluate 360° of vectors that reflect the electrical functioning of the heart. The electrical activity of the heart is recorded with three primary characteristics: the P wave (atrial depolarization), QRS complex (ventricular depolarization), and T wave (ventricular repolarization). Baseline ECG readings are often performed as part of a general physical examination and used to diagnose a wide variety of cardiac problems.

> **CLINICAL ALERT:**
> A variety of dysrhythmias are life threatening and require immediate management. In general, the ventricular abnormalities are most at risk.

Consent Form: Not required

List of Equipment: Special monitoring equipment for electrodiagnostic testing

Test Procedure:

1. Place the client in a supine position.
2. Attach leads to the arms, legs, and chest using transducer gel. *Allows for conduction of all areas of the heart.*
3. ECG machine records the electrical activity of the heart in its varying vectors of analysis.

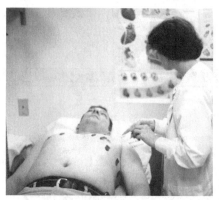

Electrocardiography Procedure

Clinical Implications and Indications:

1. Evaluates and monitors anesthesia, angina pectoris, anxiety, dysrhythmias, bradycardia, carbon monoxide poisoning, chest pain, CHF, emergency monitoring of the heart, endocarditis, MI, panic disorder, pulmonic stenosis, pacemaker function, pericarditis, respiratory distress, ventricular hypertrophy, and a wide variety of cardiac disorders.
2. Results are best interpreted when compared with other previous ECG tests.

Nursing Care:

Before Test: Explain the test procedure and the purpose of the test. Assess the client's knowledge of the test.
During Test: Adhere to standard precautions.
After Test: Clean site of transducer gel.

Interfering Factors: Inability to remain still; poor skin cleansing; improper electrode placement

Nursing Considerations:

Pediatric: Infants and children will need assistance in remaining still during the procedure and age-appropriate comfort measures following the test.

Listing of Related Tests: Holter monitoring; signal averaging electrocardiography

WEBLINKS

www.med.stanford.edu

ELECTRODIAGNOSTIC

Electrodiagnostic Study
(e-*LEK*-tro-di-ag-*NOS*-tik *STUD*-e)
(EPS; electrophysiological study; cardiac mapping)

1–8 hr.

Type of Test: Electrodiagnostic

Body Systems and Functions: Cardiovascular system

Normal Findings: Normal conduction intervals, refractive periods, and recovery times

Test Results Time Frame: Immediately

Test Description: An electrodiagnostic study is an invasive test in which fluoroscopy procedures are used to evaluate multiple-electrode catheters that are placed into the cardiac system. The electrode catheters are used to pace the heart and potentially induce arrhythmias. This allows abnormalities to be identified and evaluated as they occur. In addition, the EPS can also be used for management by inducing lesser arrhythmias, which can stop more affecting arrhythmias. The tilt-table test is a similar test that is covered individually in this text.

> **CLINICAL ALERT:**
> Have emergency equipment readily available in the event of a cardiac emergency.

Consent Form: Required

List of Equipment: Electrodiagnostic equipment

Test Procedure:
1. Attach ECG electrodes and drape client. *Ensures privacy.*
2. Catheter is placed into atrium and ventricle under fluoroscopic evaluation.
3. Record baseline ECG.
4. Stimulate cardiac electrical system. *Induces defects in electrical activity.*
5. Map the electroconduction system as defects are induced.
6. Cardiac drugs may be given. *Evaluates the medication's therapeutic effects.*

Clinical Implications and Indications:
1. Abnormal test results can indicate cardiac arrhythmias, sinoatrial node defects, vasomotor syncope syndrome, and ectopic foci.
2. Evaluates effectiveness of pacemaker.
3. Determines need for implantable cardiodefibrillator.
4. Diagnostically maps the cardiac conduction system.

Nursing Care:
Before Test: Explain the test procedure and the purpose of the test. Assess the client's knowledge of the test. Obtain baseline vital signs. Instruct client to fast from food for 6–8 hr prior to test and liquid 3 hr before test. Assess client for recent fluid volume loss.
During Test: Adhere to standard precautions. Monitor cardiovascular system responses (e.g., vital signs, arrhythmias).

ELECTRODIAGNOSTIC

After Test: Instruct client to remain on bed rest for 6–8 hr. Continue to monitor vital signs for 2–4 hr and assess for arrhythmias. Apply sterile dressing if catheter is to be left in place for future studies.

Potential Complications: Cardiac arrhythmias; perforation of the myocardium; peripheral vascular problems; hemorrhaging; infection; venous thrombosis; pericardial effusion; pulmonary embolus

Contraindications: Uncooperative clients; acute MI

Interfering Factors: Dehydration; hypovolemia; medications that alter results are antidysrhythmics, antihypertensives, analgesics, sedatives, tranquilizers, and diuretics.

Nursing Considerations:
Gerontology: The elderly may not be good candidates for this study due to their increased tendencies to cardiac abnormalities.

Listing of Related Tests: Bundle of His electrophysiology

WEBLINKS

www.healthgate.com

Electroencephalography
(uh-*LEK*-troe-en-*SEF*-:l-*AHG*-ruh-fee)
(EEG; electroencephalogram)

1–2 hr.

Type of Test: Electrodiagnostic

Body Systems and Functions: Neurological system

Normal Findings: Normal brain structure and function

Test Results Time Frame: Within 24 hr

Test Description: Electroencephalography is an electrophysiological, non-invasive study performed to evaluate the electrical activity of the brain cells. An EEG is performed to assist in diagnosing the course of structural abnormalities involving the brain. Electrodes (8–16) are placed in pairs on the scalp and recordings of waveforms are produced on paper representing patterns of specific disorders.

CLINICAL ALERT:
Study may be performed at client's bedside.

Consent Form: Not required

List of Equipment: Electrodiagnostic equipment

Test Procedure:
1. Place client in supine or sitting and upright position.
2. Attach electrodes to scalp with paste.

3. Recordings are made with client at rest.
4. Stop procedure every 5 min. *Allows client to rest.*
5. Certain activities will be asked of the client (e.g., hyperventilating, stroboscopic light stimulation, sleep induction). *Produces specific brain activity.*

Clinical Implications and Indications:

1. Diagnoses and evaluates seizure activity (e.g., grand mal, petite mal, and temporal lobe)
2. Evaluates sleep disorders and effects of drug toxicity on the brain
3. Confirms intracranial lesions, increased intracranial pressure, metabolic disorders, and inflammatory processes
4. Determines brain death and cerebral ischemia during such procedures as an endarterectomy

Nursing Care:

Before Test: Explain the test procedure and the purpose of the test. Assess the client's knowledge of the test. Instruct client to eat a meal prior to the test, but avoid caffeine for 8 hr before the test. Shampoo hair the night before the test. Limit sleep time the night before the test to 5 hr for an adult and 7 hr for a child. Inform client that there is no discomfort during this test. Instruct client to remain still during test.
During Test: Adhere to standard precautions. Carefully observe for seizure activity.
After Test: Remove electrodes and clean paste from scalp. Provide shampoo to clean head. Perform neurological assessments and provide seizure precautions as appropriate to the client situation.

Interfering Factors: Inability of client to remain still; caffeine; hypoglycemia; unclean scalp or hair; medications that alter results are sedatives, anticonvulsants, alcohol, cocaine, crack, heroin, marijuana, and tranquilizers.

Nursing Considerations:

Pediatric: Infants and children will need assistance in remaining still during the venipuncture and age-appropriate comfort measures following the test.
Gerontology: The older person may find it difficult to maintain positions when required to do so for lengthy periods of time.

Listing of Related Tests: Brain mapping; computed tomography of the brain

---

WEBLINKS

http://adam.excite.com

Electromyography
(uh-*LEK*-troe-miy-*AHG*-ruh-fee)
(EMG; electromyelogram)

1–3 hr.

Type of Test: Electrodiagnostic

Body Systems and Functions: Musculoskeletal system

ELECTRODIAGNOSTIC

Normal Findings: Normal muscle electrical activity during rest and contraction

Test Results Time Frame: Within 24–48 hr

Test Description: Electromyography is an electrophysiological study performed to determine the electrical activity of specific muscles. A comparison of the amplitude, duration, number, and configuration of muscle activity provides diagnostic data about a variety of nerve and muscle disorders. A determination of whether the pathology exists in myogenic or neurogenic causation is evaluated.

Consent Form: Required

List of Equipment: EMG equipment

Test Procedure:
1. Place client in a supine or sitting position on the examination table.
2. Attach needle electrodes to client. *Allows conduction of nerve responses.*
3. Client is asked to either remain relaxed or to tense specific muscle groups. *Allows measurement of nerve to muscle innervation.*

Clinical Implications and Indications:
1. Diagnoses muscle diseases that affect striated muscle fibers (e.g., muscular dystrophy, myasthenia gravis), poliomyelitis, thyroid toxicity, tetanus, and sarcoidosis
2. Diagnoses neuromuscular and muscular disorders, such as peripheral neuropathy from alcoholism, or diabetes, Guillain-Barrè syndrome, herniated disk, spinal stenosis, and ALS
3. Differentiates between primary and secondary muscle disorders or neuropathy
4. Evaluates neuropathies and myopathies

Nursing Care:
Before Test: Explain the test procedure and the purpose of the test. Assess the client's knowledge of the test. Inform client that the needle insertions will cause some discomfort.
During Test: Adhere to standard precautions.
After Test: Remove electrodes and cleanse skin; assess sites for hemorrhaging or infection. Administer analgesics as necessary. Allow client time to rest.

Potential Complications: Bleeding; inflammation

Contraindications: Anticoagulant therapy; infection near sites of electrode placement

Interfering Factors: Inability of client to remain still; hemorrhaging; edema; increased age; medications that alter results are muscle relaxants, cholinergics, and anticholinergics.

Nursing Considerations:
Pediatric: Infants and children will need assistance in remaining still during the procedure and age-appropriate comfort measures following the test (relatively rare to perform on this age group).

ELECTRODIAGNOSTIC

Gerontology: Responses decrease with age. The older person may find it difficult to maintain positions when required to do so for lengthy periods of time during the electromyography.

Listing of Related Tests: Electroneurography

WEBLINKS ▯

www.healthgate.com

Electroneurography
(uh-**LEK**-troe-nur-**RAHG**-ruh-fee)
(nerve conduction study)

1–3 hr.

ELECTRODIAGNOSTIC

Type of Test: Electrodiagnostic

Body Systems and Functions: Musculoskeletal system

Normal Findings: Normal nerve conduction velocity rates; no peripheral or axial nerve damage

Test Results Time Frame: Within 24–48 hr

Test Description: Electroneurography is an electrophysiological study performed to determine the nerve conduction velocity seen in peripheral nerve disease or injury. This test provides diagnostic information about the location and causation of peripheral nerve abnormalities. Electrodes are placed on the skin and electrical stimuli are recorded to peripheral nerve and muscle contraction responses. Nerve conduction velocities are slowed in diseases that affect the peripheral nerves.

Consent Form: Required

List of Equipment: Electrodiagnostic equipment

Test Procedure:
1. Place client in a supine or sitting position on the examination table.
2. Attach surface stimulating electrodes to client. *Allows conduction of electrical stimulus.*
3. Time is measured between the time the shock is delivered and the response of the muscle activity. *Allows measurement of nerve to muscle innervation time.*

Clinical Implications and Indications:
1. Diagnoses and evaluates peripheral nerve degenerative disorders and peripheral neuropathies (e.g., diabetes)
2. Differentiates muscle disease and peripheral nerve disorders
3. Evaluates nerve damage in disorders like carpel tunnel
4. Evaluates damage to nerves by toxicity of substances, such as antimicrobials, heavy metals, and solvents

Nursing Care:
Before Test: Explain the test procedure and the purpose of the test. Assess the client's knowledge of the test. Inform client that the needle insertions will cause some discomfort.
During Test: Adhere to standard precautions.
After Test: Remove electrodes and cleanse skin; assess sites for hemorrhaging or infection. Administer analgesics as necessary. Allow client time to rest.

Interfering Factors: Inability of client to remain still; increased age

Nursing Considerations:
Pediatric: Infants and children will need assistance in remaining still during the procedure and age-appropriate comfort measures following the test (relatively rare to perform on this age group).
Gerontology: Responses decrease with age. The older person may find it difficult to maintain positions when required to do so for lengthy periods of time.

Listing of Related Tests: Electromyography

WEBLINKS

www.healthgate.com

Electronystagmography
(ee-*LEK*-troe-*NIS*-tuhg-*MAHG*-ruh-fee)
(ENG; eye movement)

45–60 min.

Type of Test: Electrodiagnostic

Body Systems and Functions: Sensory system

Normal Findings: Normal nystagmic response; no hearing loss or lesions of the ocular or vestibular systems

Test Results Time Frame: Immediately

Test Description: Electronystagmography (ENG) is an electrophysiological study that measures the direction and degree of nystagmus. Nystagmus is the involuntary movement of the eye in a back-and-forth direction, which results from the initiation of the vestibular-ocular reflex. The ENG is performed by measuring the electric responses of the eye at rest and in response to various stimuli that are applied to the eye to elicit the nystagmus response. The speed and the duration of the eye movements are recorded and compared with normal values. The nystagmus response is controlled by either the CNS (the fast phase) or the vestibular system (the slow phase).

Consent Form: Not required

List of Equipment: Electrodiagnostic equipment

Test Procedure:
1. Place the client in a supine or seated position in a dark room.
2. Attach five electrodes at the outer canthus of each eye, above and below the eye center, and at the center of the forehead.
3. Instruct the client to respond to different procedures that measure the following: gaze nystagmus, pendulum tracking, positional changes, and water caloric.
4. Record the results of each test and compare them with established values.

Clinical Implications and Indications:
1. Evaluates demyelinating disorders, cerebellum lesions, brainstem lesions, dizziness, vertigo, suspected lesions of the CNS and peripheral system, and location of an abnormality.
2. Differentiates nystagmus caused by the CNS vs. the peripheral nervous system.
3. Diagnoses the etiology of hearing loss.
4. Evaluates unilateral hearing loss and vertigo due to middle ear problems or nerve injury. When the client experiences nystagmus with stimulation, the auditory nerve is working and hearing loss can be attributed to the middle ear.

Nursing Care:
Before Test: Explain the test procedure and the purpose of the test. Assess the client's knowledge of the test. Instruct client to remove makeup, eat a light meal before the study, avoid smoking, and avoid caffeine.
During Test: Adhere to standard precautions.
After Test: Remove electrodes, cleanse skin, and assess for continuing clinical manifestations of dizziness, nausea, and lethargy. If these symptoms exist, allow client to rest.

Contraindications: Pacemakers; perforated ear drum

Interfering Factors: Medications that alter results are stimulants, depressants, and antivertiginous substances; poor eyesight; blinking the eyes; loose electrodes; inability to follow commands for tests that require considerable cooperation

Nursing Considerations:
Pediatric: Infants and children will need assistance in remaining still during the procedure and age-appropriate comfort measures following the test.
Gerontology: The older person may find it difficult to maintain positions when required to do so for lengthy periods of time.

ELECTRODIAGNOSTIC

WEBLINKS

http://adam.excite.com

ELECTRODIAGNOSTIC

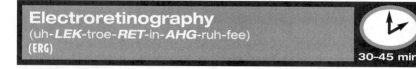

Electroretinography
(uh-*LEK*-troe-*RET*-in-*AHG*-ruh-fee)
(ERG)

30–45 min.

Type of Test: Electrodiagnostic

Body Systems and Functions: Sensory system

Normal Findings: Normal electrical responses to light; normal retina

Test Results Time Frame: Immediate

Test Description: Electroretinography (ERG) is an electrophysiological study that measures the electrical activity of the retina as it responds to a flash of light. Electrodes are positioned on a corneal contact and on the forehead, and electrical activity changes are noted. The retina is the inner part of the posterior eyeball. Its function is to convert light into activity potentials and to transmit them to the brain by way of the optic nerve. The ERG diagnoses a variety of retinal disorders.

> **CLINICAL ALERT:**
> If client begins to rub eyes or complain of pain, suspect a corneal abrasion and instruct client not to rub eye.

Consent Form: Not required

List of Equipment: Electrodiagnostic eye equipment

Test Procedure:
1. Place client in supine or sitting position in a dark room.
2. Anesthetize the eyes and then keep open with a retractor. *Ensures accurate results.*
3. Attach electrodes to receive light stimuli.
4. Bright white light is flashed in eyes. *Allows detailed eye reactions and determines the electrical response during this light stimulus.*

Clinical Implications and Indications:
1. Diagnoses retinal detachment, retinal damage caused by drugs, and retinitis
2. Evaluates color blindness and night blindness
3. Evaluates retinal condition prior to surgery
4. Detects congenital abnormalities that affect the corneal lens

Nursing Care:
Before Test: Explain the test procedure and the purpose of the test. Assess the client's knowledge of the test. Administer ocular drops per protocol. Inform client that there is little or no discomfort with this test.
During Test: Adhere to standard precautions.
After Test: Assess eyes for irritation and note any visual impairment or eye pain. Instruct client not to rub eyes and tell him that the anesthetic wears off within 1 hr.

Potential Complications: Corneal abrasion

Interfering Factors: Inability of client to remain still; improper placement of electrodes

Nursing Considerations:
Pediatric: Young children may require sedation and age-appropriate comfort measures following the test.
Rural: Advisable to arrange for transportation home after recovering from procedure.

WEBLINKS

http://www.entnet.org

Fetal Contraction
(*FEE*-t:l kuhn-*TRAEK*-sh:n)
(CST; contraction stress test)

15 min.

Type of Test: Electrodiagnostic

Body Systems and Functions: Reproductive system

Normal Findings: Negative result has no late decelerations and a normal baseline fetal heart rate associated with at least three contractions within a 10-min period.

Test Results Time Frame: Within 15 min

Test Description: A fetal contraction test is performed to assess fetal heart rate (FHR) in response to uterine contractions. It is a test to predict fetal outcome and risk for intrauterine asphyxia. FHR is assessed by using electronic fetal monitoring. FHR is monitored by using an external transducer, and a tocodynamometer is used to determine uterine activity. Negative or normal results are associated with a low risk of intrauterine death due to hypoxia and predicts fetal survival in more than 99% of cases. A negative fetal contraction test indicates that placental support is adequate and the fetus will probably survive the stress of labor if it begins in 1 week. An abnormal or positive result has persistent late decelerations with adequate challenge or persistent late decelerations with less than three uterine contractions per 10 min. A suspicious result has intermittent late decelerations with an adequate challenge; variable decelerations; and abnormal baseline fetal heart rate (<110 or >160 bpm). An unsatisfactory result has a poor quality recording and inability to achieve three contractions in 10 min.

Consent Form: Required

List of Equipment: Tocodynamometer; ultrasound transducer

Test Procedure:
1. Place the client in a semi-Fowler's position or left lateral tilt. *Minimizes supine hypotension.*
2. Record blood pressure at intervals.
3. Baseline FHR and contraction patterns are determined for 10 min prior to any stimulation of contractions.

Clinical Implications and Indications:

1. A poor fetal outcome is seen in approximately 50% of cases.
2. Confirms perinatal death.
3. Identifies a low 5-min Apgar score.
4. Detects late decelerations in labor.
5. A suspicious result may occur in a growth-retarded fetus with oligohydramnios and may be the result of the cord being compressed during contractions due to lack of protection by amniotic fluid.

Nursing Care:

Before Test: Explain the test procedure and the purpose of the test. Assess the client's knowledge of the test.

During Test: Adhere to standard precautions. Analyze tracings for good quality and minimize potential interfering factors when possible.

After Test: Interpret test outcomes. Provide counseling about meaning of fetal heart activity and movement. Report abnormal results to primary heath care provider.

Potential Complications: FHR decelerations that could cause fetal hypoxia

Contraindications: Previous classic cesarean section; placenta previa; premature rupture of membranes; multiple gestation; incompetent cervix; third-trimester unexplained bleeding

Interfering Factors: Poor quality tracings may be associated with the tocodynamometer belt placed on too loosely; the ultrasound transducer not directed at the fetal heart; maternal obesity; excessive fetal movement; small, mild, irregular contractions; high-frequency, low-amplitude contractions may be mistaken for adequate contractions; lack of uterine contractions; inadequate frequency of contractions (note: contractions may be provoked by breast stimulation or oxytocin infusion)

Listing of Related Tests: Oxytocin challenge test; nipple stimulation test; breast stimulation test

| WEBLINKS |

www.nlm.nih.gov

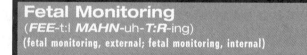

Fetal Monitoring
(*FEE*-t:l *MAHN*-uh-*T:R*-ing)
(fetal monitoring, external; fetal monitoring, internal)

10–15 min.

Type of Test: Electrodiagnostic

Body Systems and Functions: Reproductive system

Normal Findings:

Normal fetal heart rate (FHR)	120–160 bpm
Normal fetal heart rate variability	5–25 bpm
Internal monitoring only	
Prelabor	<3 contractions over 10 min
	25–40 mm Hg contraction pressure
First stage	<6 contractions over 10 min
	8–12 mm Hg baseline pressures
	30–40 mm Hg contraction pressure
Second stage	1 contraction every 2 min
	10–20 mm Hg baseline pressure
	50–80 mm Hg contraction pressure

Test Results Time Frame: Immediate

Test Description: Fetal monitoring provides immediate evaluation of the fetal heart rate (FHR), which is a valuable parameter of fetal distress. Fetal monitoring can be performed either internally or externally. The internal method is invasive and involves placement of a fetal scalp electrode through the cervical canal to measure FHR during labor (after 2–3 cm dilation). Internal monitoring is the better method of evaluating the condition of the fetus. External monitoring is a noninvasive assessment performed by placing an electronic transducer on the mother's abdomen to amplify the FRH. Both devices record fluctuations and variability of the FHR and are able to detect accelerations and decelerations as they occur with uterine contractions.

> **CLINICAL ALERT:**
> Fetal distress may be evidenced by findings and careful continual assessment is therefore required throughout testing.

Consent Form: Required for external monitor; not required for internal monitor

List of Equipment: Fetal monitoring equipment (e.g., electrodes, gel)

Test Procedure:

External monitoring:
1. Place client in semi-Fowler's or left lateral position.
2. Attach external electrodes with gel to the abdomen.
3. Set alarm limits and monitor for 10 min during active labor. *Provides baseline recording.*
4. Leave electrodes in place and monitor continuously. *Assesses fetal heart rate and variability.*

Internal monitoring:
1. Place client in lithotomy position, cleanse perineal area, and perform vaginal examination.
2. Place electrode onto fetal scalp. *Correct placement evidenced by fetal heart rate readings.*
3. Leave electrode in place and monitor continuously. *Assesses fetal heart rate and variability.*

Clinical Implications and Indications:
1. Detects fetal distress
2. Evaluates FHR during stress and nonstress
3. Evaluates fetal condition during oxytocin challenge test
4. Monitors uterine contractions

Nursing Care:
Before Test: Explain the test procedure and the purpose of the test. Assess the client's knowledge of the test.
During Test: Adhere to standard precautions. If monitoring reveals fetal distress, provide emotional support. Assess mother for clinical manifestations of fever, chills, and excessive bleeding

Potential Complications: Fetus: hematoma; hemorrhaging; infection; bruising. Mother: uterine perforation; uterine infection; bleeding.

Contraindications: Active genital herpes; lack of fetus presentation by the head

Interfering Factors: Maternal position (left-side lying promotes most efficient delivery of oxygen to fetus); medications that alter results are sympathetic and parasympathetic stimulants.

Nursing Considerations:
Pregnancy: Inform mother in third trimester that either internal or external fetal monitoring is a relatively normal method of assessing the condition of the fetus. In addition, explain how to relax by watching the condition of the contractions on the monitoring screen.
Pediatric: Abnormalities of the fetus may be detected in time to facilitate effective interventions.

Listing of Related Tests: Fetal nonstress test

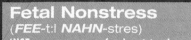

http://adam.excite.com

Fetal Nonstress
(*FEE*-t:l *NAHN*-stres)
(NST; nonstress test; fetal activity determination)

40 min.

Type of Test: Electrodiagnostic

Body Systems and Functions: Reproductive system

Normal Findings: Reactive fetal heart rate (FHR) (heart rate acceleration seen with fetal movements)

Test Results Time Frame: Immediate

Test Description: Fetal nonstress testing (NTS) is a noninvasive test that measures the fetal heart rate as it responds to fetal movement. The response is categorized as either reactive or nonreactive. A reactive response is when there

are two or more FHR accelerations with fetal movement, each of which must be at least 15 bpm for 15 sec. A nonreactive response is when there is no FHR acceleration with fetal movement during a 40-min time period. The NST is valuable in screening high-risk pregnancies and in evaluating which clients need a fetal contraction test.

CLINICAL ALERT:
Be prepared to provide intensive emotional support if test reveals fetal distress.

Consent Form: Not required

List of Equipment: External fetal monitor; transducer gel

Test Procedure:
1. Place client in Sim's position, and place an external fetal monitor on client's abdomen.
2. Observe fetal heart rate for accelerations and signs of reactivity or nonreactivity for 40 min.
3. If fetus is nonreactive for 20 min, simulate fetal activity by externally rubbing mother's abdomen or making noises near the abdomen.

Clinical Implications and Indications:
1. Detects fetal stress
2. Confirms fetal death

Nursing Care:
Before Test: Explain the test procedure and the purpose of the test. Assess the client's knowledge of the test. Instruct client to void prior to examination.
During Test: Adhere to standard precautions.
After Test: If test reveals fetal distress, provide emotional support.

Nursing Considerations:
Pregnancy: Encourage pregnant clients to report abnormalities of fetal movement, as one means of knowing when to perform the NST. If results of NST reveal a nonreactive fetus, inform client she will likely have a fetal contraction test.
Pediatric: Abnormalities of the fetus may be detected in time to facilitate effective interventions.

Listing of Related Tests: Fetal contraction

WEBLINKS ⬚⬚

http://adam.excite.com

Holter Monitoring
(*HOEL*-t:r *MAH*-nuh-*T:R*-ing)
(ambulatory monitoring)

24–48 hr.

Type of Test: Electrodiagnostic

Body Systems and Functions: Cardiovascular system

ELECTRODIAGNOSTIC

Normal Findings: Normal sinus rhythm

CRITICAL VALUES:
Extended episodes of ventricular tachycardia or profound bradycardia are arrhythmias that are potentially critical to the client.

Test Results Time Frame: Within 5 days

Test Description: The Holter monitor involves the use of a small portable ECG monitor, which the client wears. This monitor enables the continuous recording of the client's cardiac electrical activity on tape. When the client pushes a button on the recorder, due to the onset of symptoms (such as presyncopy, chest discomfort, and palpitations), an event marker is placed on the tape. A comparison is then made between symptoms noted in the journal by the client and corresponding cardiac electrical activity and the heart rhythm.

CLINICAL ALERT:
Clients will need to be oriented and have the ability to use their hands to operate a push button.

Consent Form: Not required

List of Equipment: Alcohol swabs; ECG electrodes; tape; portable Holter monitor with two lead wires; magnetic tape; journal/diary booklet

Test Procedure:
1. Cleanse the client's skin sites with an alcohol prep pad over the sites for electrode placement. These will be the fourth intercostal space to the right of the sternum (V1 position) and the fifth intercostal space at the midclavicular line (V5 position). *Ensures accurate results.*
2. Gently abrade the skin with a 4 x 4 gauze pad. *Increases skin adherence and conduction.*
3. Apply ECG electrodes over the prepared sites.
4. Attach wires with the negative electrode at the V1 position and the positive electrode at the V5 position. Attach lead wires to the monitor.
5. Insert tape into the monitor and activate.
6. Tape wires to the chest and place monitor in cover with shoulder strap or belt.

Clinical Implications and Indications:
1. Evaluates cardiac electrical activity in the client who is experiencing symptoms suggestive of a possible cardiac rhythm disturbance
2. Monitors for proarrhythmia during initiation of certain antiarrhythmic medications
3. Monitors for effectiveness of antiarrhythmic therapy

Nursing Care:
Before Test: Explain the test procedure and the purpose of the test. Assess the client's knowledge of the test. Inform the client that the monitor will be worn for 24–48 hr. Explain the use of the diary for recording daily activity and any symptoms that may occur. Instruct the client that the marker button on the machine is to be pushed when symptoms are felt. Advise the client to avoid showering or tub bathing while wearing the Holter monitor.
During Test: Adhere to standard precautions.

ELECTRODIAGNOSTIC

After Test: Instruct the client in electrode removal and returning the Holter monitor for processing.

Interfering Factors: Inadequate or improper placement of the electrodes; dislodging of the electrodes by the client; failure of the client to activate the marker button when symptoms occur; failure of the client to maintain the diary

Nursing Considerations:

Pediatric: Rarely used with younger ages due to the difficulty in adherence to wearing the Holter monitor.

Gerontology: May need the assistance of a friend or companion in maintaining the diary.

Home Care: Care providers will need instructions regarding bathing and any other activities of daily living that might cause interference with the use of the monitor. Directions concerning the use of the monitor need to be given to the care providers.

Listing of Related Tests: King of hearts event recorder; ECG rhythm strip

WEBLINKS

http://www.howstuffworks.com

ELECTRODIAGNOSTIC

Nerve Conduction Studies
(n:rv k:n-*DUHK*-sh:n)
(electromyography; electroneurography: EMG, ENG; NCS)

1 hr.

Type of Test: Electrodiagnostic

Body Systems and Functions: Neurological system

Normal Findings: Normal recorded electrode response and time relationships between nerve stimulus and response identified

Test Results Time Frame: Within 24 hr

Test Description: Nerve conduction studies measure and record electrical activity in skeletal muscles at rest and during voluntary muscle contraction. Results may aid in determining whether abnormalities are due to lower motor neuron disease or those of muscle fiber. These nerve conduction studies differentiate between diseases that cause segmental demyelination lesions and axonal losses.

CLINICAL ALERT:
Ensure that the client does not have serum enzyme tests (e.g., SGOT, LDH) ordered until 7–10 days after the nerve conduction studies (note: these enzymes are altered by the nerve conduction studies).

Consent Form: Required

List of Equipment: Specialized nerve conduction studies equipment

Test Procedure:

1. Client will be asked to sit or lie down. *Position determined by which muscles will be tested.*
2. Surface electrodes are applied with paste to the specified area being tested. Electrical current is passed through the electrode and the client experiences small shocks (note: dependent on the client's pathophysiology, if present, he will experience mild to moderate discomfort with each shock).
3. Results are recorded on tape and can be read on an oscilloscope.
4. The area is cleansed with alcohol and a small-gauge needle is then inserted and advanced slowly into the muscle. Several needles will be necessary and may be manipulated by the tester. *To identify electrical activity.*
5. Again, results will be recorded on the oscilloscope in wave forms, and sounds may be heard when the client is asked to contract their muscle. *Ensures accurate results.*
6. The needle is removed and the site is observed for obvious bleeding.

Clinical Implications and Indications:

1. Diagnoses compression and entrapment neuropathies
2. Evaluates lesions to spinal nerve root and plexus lexions
3. Evaluates site of injury where muscles has been traumatized
4. Diagnoses myopathies

Nursing Care:

Before Test: Explain the test procedure and the purpose of the test. Assess the client's knowledge of the test. Instruct clients to wear clothing that is easily removed or adjusted to provide access to area being tested.

After Test: Explain to the client that he may experience some discomfort at the site that was tested; however, over-the-counter pain relievers should be sufficient to alleviate the pain. Many working clients return to normal activity after the examination.

Contraindications: Anticoagulant therapy; pathological coagulopathies

Interfering Factors: Pain; medications that alter results are antimyasthenics, cholinergics, anticholinergics, and muscle relaxants.

Nursing Considerations:

Pediatric: Very individualized care will need to be implemented to enable this test to be performed on infants and children.

Gerontology: Elderly clients may have slower response times related to electrical activity. In addition, the older person may find it difficult to maintain positions when required to do so for lengthy periods of time during the nerve conduction studies.

Rural: Advisable to arrange for transportation home after recovering from procedure.

Listing of Related Tests: Rectal EMG

WEBLINKS

www.teleemg.com

ELECTRODIAGNOSTIC

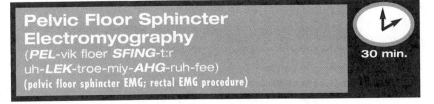

Pelvic Floor Sphincter Electromyography

(*PEL*-vik floer *SFING*-t:r uh-*LEK*-troe-miy-*AHG*-ruh-fee)

(pelvic floor sphincter EMG; rectal EMG procedure)

30 min.

Type of Test: Electrodiagnostic

Body Systems and Functions: Renal/urological system

Normal Findings: Increased EMG activity while bladder fills; electrical silence prior to and at onset of voiding; increased EMG activity with cough, crede, Valsalva, bulbocavernosus reflex, and voluntary cessation of voiding

Test Results Time Frame: Within 2 days

Test Description: Pelvic floor sphincter electromyography is a urodynamic study that measures activity in the striated muscles of the pelvic floor. It is done in conjunction with a cystometrogram (CMG). The striated sphincter should gradually increase activity during filling of the bladder and quit activity before and during bladder contraction. Surface electrode recordings can be measured from the urethral lumen in the region of the voluntary sphincter or from the anal sphincter. Needle electrodes can record from the anal sphincter, the pelvic floor musculature, or (not as successfully) the external sphincter. The most accurate information is taken from direct needle electromyography of the urethral sphincter.

Consent Form: Required

Test Procedure:

1. Surface or needle electrodes are positioned on the perianal skin or an anal plug electrode can be used. *Exact placement locations will be determined by the electromyographer or urologist.*
2. Position electrodes on the thigh. *Acts as grounding lead.*
3. Record readings with the bladder empty.
4. Reflex response to stimuli is tested in response to Crede, Valsalva maneuver, cough, or bulbocavernosus reflex.
5. Measure voluntary activity during the client contracting and relaxing the sphincter muscle. *Ensures accurate results.*
6. Fill the bladder with sterile water via catheter (CMG) and record electrical activity as the bladder fills.
7. Instruct the client to take a voiding position and the catheter is removed. Ask the client to void and record electrical activity.

Clinical Implications and Indications:

1. Differentiates between muscular and neurological causes of urinary or fecal incontinence
2. Rules out presence of detrusor striated sphincter dyssynergia
3. Assesses sacral evoked response, which provides information regarding the integrity of the pelvic and spinal cord neural pathways

Nursing Care:

Before Test: Explain the test procedure and the purpose of the test. Assess the client's knowledge of the test. Instruct client that their cooperation in response to directions will be essential. Inform client that the bulbocavernous reflex may cause some embarassment because in the male the reflex will be stimulated by squeezing the glans penis, and for a female client it is elicited by tapping the clitoris.
During Test: Adhere to standard precautions.
After Test: If needle electrodes are used, check insertion sites for bleeding or inflammation.

Contraindications: Coagulopathy

Interfering Factors: Inaccurate electrode placement; uncooperative client

Nursing Considerations:

Pediatric: Cooperation will be a challenge with the pediatric client. Infants and children will need assistance in remaining still during the procedure and age-appropriate comfort measures following the test. Patch electrodes are applied as opposed to needle electrodes. During CMG, electrical activity is recorded of the external sphincter and pelvic floor muscles in response to the bladder filling and contraction inhibition. If the child voids, this will demonstrate that the sphincter is able to relax normally.

Listing of Related Tests: Cystometrogram (CMG); detrusor pressure or flow rate

WEBLINKS ▢▢

www.springnet.com

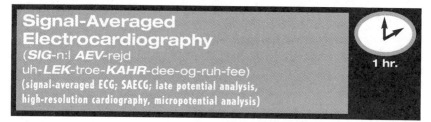

Signal-Averaged Electrocardiography
(*SIG*-n:l *AEV*-rejd uh-*LEK*-troe-*KAHR*-dee-og-ruh-fee)
(signal-averaged ECG; SAECG; late potential analysis, high-resolution cardiography, micropotential analysis)

1 hr.

Type of Test: Electrodiagnostic

Body Systems and Functions: Cardiovascular system

Normal Findings: Absence of late potentials; normal QRS complex; normal ST segment; no ventricular arrhythmias

Test Results Time Frame: Within 24 hr

Test Description: A signal-averaged electrocardiogram (SAE) is an electrodiagnostic test that is used to determine the risk for late ventricular potentials (and for arrhythmias in clients who have had an MI). The SAE is a noninvasive test that is similar to an ECG, except that the electrodes are placed in different positions and a computer is utilized to analyze the electrical output of the heart.

ELECTRODIAGNOSTIC

The SAE readings detect sensitive electrical potentials that the ECG is unable to sense. The procedure averages the cardiac cycles that are read and its results are very specific to the levels of electrical potential in the client. The SAE may be followed with the more definitive and more invasive cardiac catheterization in clients needing further testing of their cardiac condition.

Consent Form: Not required

List of Equipment: Signal-averaged ECG machine or Holter monitor; alcohol swabs, razor; electrodes

Test Procedure:
1. Place client in supine position and attach electrodes with conductive gel to the abdomen and anterior and posterior chest. *Provides good conduction of the electrodes.*
2. A transducer converts the electrical output of the heart to the SAECG machine, which in the digitalized format creates a representation of the client's cardiac cycle and compares the results to an averaged electrical set of signals. *Allows for signal averaging of the electrocardiogram.*
3. Remove the electrodes and wipe gel from client skin surfaces.

Clinical Implications and Indications:
1. Diagnoses coronary artery disease
2. Diagnoses delayed conduction in the myocardium with disorders such as myocardial infarction, cardiomyopathy, ventricular aneurysm, and congenital ventricular defects
3. Evaluates clients who have survived sudden cardiac death syndrome
4. Assists in continuing assessment of clients with pacemakers, CABG recovery, and cardiac drug therapy

Nursing Care:
Before Test: Explain the test procedure and the purpose of the test. Assess the client's knowledge of the test. Provide a quiet and calm atmosphere for the testing. Reassure client that this is a noninvasive test that causes no discomfort.
During Test: Adhere to standard precautions. Assist client to remain calm and modify breathing to reduce the interference of skeletal muscle activity.
After Test: Note and report any cardiac rhythm abnormalities evidenced on the SAE.

Interfering Factors: Improper placement of electrodes; inability to remain still; electrical equipment in area; ventricular tachycardia; lack of adequate time to detect arrhythmias

Nursing Considerations:
Pediatric: Infants and children will need assistance in remaining still during the procedure and age-appropriate comfort measures following the test. May be done following tetralogy of Fallot repair.
Gerontology: The older person may find it difficult to maintain positions when required to do so for lengthy periods of time during the SAE.

Listing of Related Tests: Programmed ventricular stimulation

WEBLINKS

http://www.howstuffworks.com/heart-diagnosis.htm

Sleep Studies
(sleep *STU*-dez)
(PSG; polysomnography; sleep apnea study)

8 hr.

Type of Test: Electrodiagnostic

Body Systems and Functions: Pulmonary system

Normal Findings: Less than five apnea episodes per hour lasting less than 10 sec each. Pulse oximetry >95%. Normal EEG and ECG.

CRITICAL VALUES:
Pulse oximetry of <88% is significant. Apnea of greater than five episodes per hour or longer than 10 sec per episode is significant.

Test Results Time Frame: Within 24 hr

Test Description: Sleep studies are tests that are used to evaluate sleep-related disorders. Typically, the client will have 5–10 episodes of apnea during the study time. During each apnea period, the client experiences bradycardia and has decreased oxygen saturation. The most common sleep disorder is sleep apnea syndrome, which is defined as a cessation of air flow during sleep. There are three types of sleep apnea (obstructive, central, and mixed). Obstructive sleep apnea is caused by pharyngeal occlusion; central sleep apnea is a cessation of air flow and respiratory movements; and mixed sleep apnea is a combination of the two. Sleep apnea clients have a history of excessive snoring, narcolepsy, insomnia, cardiac rhythm disturbances, and restless leg spasm. The diagnosis of sleep disorders is based on the clinical history and diagnostic sleep studies.

CLINICAL ALERT:
Split-night studies may be indicated, which allow the client to sleep during the first half of the night, and for the second half of the night, continuous positive airway pressure (CPAP) measures are implemented. Studies are done on-site at the sleep study laboratory. Some home monitoring devices may be available, but the reliability is compromised and visual assessment by the examiners is not done.

Consent Form: Not required

List of Equipment: Pulse oximeter; electrical encephalogram; electro-oculogram; electromyogram; electrocardiogram; CO_2 analyzer; pneumotachograph; other specific equipment to assess respiratory function, penile function, or muscle movement may be used.

Test Procedure:
1. Schedule client to participate in sleep study from 10 PM to 6 AM.
2. Attach specially designed sleep study equipment to client for PSG.
3. Darken room, make client comfortable, and monitor sleep events. *Ensures accurate results.*

ELECTRODIAGNOSTIC

Clinical Implications and Indications:

1. Diagnoses obstructive sleep apnea syndrome.
2. Sleep apnea is characterized by progressive snoring, followed by a period of silence, ending with gasping. This is due to partial or complete obstruction of the airway as the muscles of the upper airway relax. Alcohol and sedatives should be avoided because these make the sleep apnea worse.
3. Restless leg syndrome and periodic limb movement disorder are associated with sleep disorders. Once diagnosis is confirmed, treatment can include carbidopa-levodopa and clonazepam or baclofen to decrease the severity and amount of episodes.
4. Up to 25% of people with hypertension have obstructive sleep apnea. Heart and respiratory rates can change over time, often resulting in hypoxemia.
5. Metabolic disturbances such as imbalances with neurotransmitters and hormones can affect the sleep patterns.
6. Central sleep apnea occurs with cessation of chest wall movement and respiratory system airflow.

Nursing Care:

Before Test: Explain the test procedure and the purpose of the test. Assess the client's knowledge of the test. Instruct client to prepare for sleep at the normal time. Assist client in activities that promote rest and lead to sleep (e.g., comfortable position, darkened room, bath or shower, soothing music).
During Test: Adhere to standard precautions. Monitor client's sleep patterns.
After Test: Resume usual activities and routines.

Interfering Factors: Electrophysiological artifacts; defective equipment; diaphoresis; environmental noises; inability of client to sleep

Nursing Considerations:

Gerontology: Sleep complaints generally increase with age. Insomnia, an increase in wakeful periods during the night, is a common complaint. Some medications can affect the time spent in REM and non-REM sleep, thus altering the feeling of being rested.

WEBLINKS

http://www.webmd.com

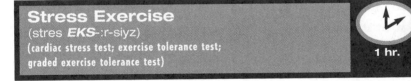

Stress Exercise
(stres *EKS*-:r-siyz)
(cardiac stress test; exercise tolerance test;
graded exercise tolerance test)

1 hr.

Type of Test: Electrodiagnostic

Body Systems and Functions: Cardiovascular system

Normal Findings: No dysrhythmias or EKG changes at 85% maximum heart rate calculated from age and gender

ELECTRODIAGNOSTIC

CRITICAL VALUES:
Life-threatening dysrhythmias that occur during the stress test (e.g., ventricular fibrillation)

Test Results Time Frame: Within 24 hr

Test Description: The stress exercise test measures cardiac efficiency while the heart is being stressed through exercise. This test is used to investigate cardiac symptoms of chest pain, valve competency, and dysrhythmias or to evaluate capacity for beginning or increasing level of exercise, especially in clients who have previously been sedentary.

CLINICAL ALERT:
Have emergency equipment readily available in the event of a life-threatening cardiac arrhythmia induced by the stress test.

Consent Form: Required

List of Equipment: Treadmill with ability to increase incline and speed; EKG pads, leads, and machine; blood pressure cuff; stethoscope

Test Procedure:
1. Prepare skin and place EKG patches in position of a 12-lead EKG (see description of EKG). Attach electrodes to EKG monitor. *Preparation prior to test.*
2. Apply blood pressure cuff. *Preparation prior to test.*
3. A resting EKG and blood pressure is taken. *Establishes baseline to compare test results*
4. The client begins walking on the treadmill at zero incline and slow pace while the computerized EKG records and monitors heart electroactivity. *Continous monitoring necessary to prevent complications.*
5. The client progressively walks at greater speeds and greater inclines to increase workload on the heart. *Increasing speed and greater inclines place stress on the heart.*
6. EKG, heart rate, and blood pressure are continually monitored for signs of abnormality. *Continuous monitoring necessary to prevent complications.*
7. Instruct client to report any chest pain, cramping, or intolerable dyspnea. *These symptoms indicate complications and the test needs to be stopped.*
8. Upon completion of the test, posttest vital signs and EKG are recorded at 3- and 10-min intervals. *Evaluates the ability of the heart to recover from exercise.*
9. The test may be stopped prior to reaching a predetermined endpoint for intolerable dyspnea, EKG abnormalities, weakness, or abnormal blood pressure changes. *Prevents potentially serious complications.*

Clinical Implications and Indications:
1. Abnormal blood pressure changes would include no rise of systolic pressure, progressive fall in systolic pressure, or elevation of diastolic pressure.
2. Abnormal changes in heart rate include either bradycardia or abnormal tachycardia.
3. EKG abnormalities include elevation or depression of ST segments from ischemia during stress and dysrhythmias, ventricular tachycardia, multifocal premature ventricular contractions, atrial tachycardia, and second- or third-degree atrioventricular block.

4. Signs and symptoms that indicate a negative test include angina, ataxia, cold sweat, cyanosis, pallor, faintness, dizziness, leg pain, lightheadedness, mottling of skin, and severe dyspnea.

Nursing Care:

Before Test: Explain the test procedure and the purpose of the test. Assess the client's knowledge of the test. Instruct client to refrain from food, coffee, or nicotine prior to the test. A light breakfast may be eaten. Instruct client to wear comfortable walking or athletic shoes and loose clothing.

During Test: Adhere to standard precautions. Monitor EKG continuously and blood pressure at designated points. Instruct client to report any chest pain, leg pain, lightheadedness, or extreme shortness of breath.

After Test: Instruct client to assume a sitting position. Record 3- and 10-min vital signs posttest. Remove EKG electrodes. Have client stay on premises until vital signs and EKG patterns have returned to baseline.

Potential Complications: Angina; cardiac dysrhythmias

Contraindications: Frequent angina; recent onset of chest pain; elevated blood pressure

Interfering Factors: Anemia; anxiety attacks; digitalis toxicity; elevated ST segment at rest; gender (higher false positives in women); hypertension; hypoxia; left-ventricular hypertrophy; Lown-Gangong-Levine syndrome; valvular heart disease; vasoregulatory asthenia

Nursing Considerations:

Gerontology: Careful observation of the elderly client is necessary due to the higher risk of cardiac complications that can occur due to aging.

Rural: Advisable to arrange for transportation home after recovering from procedure.

Listing of Related Tests: EKG

WEBLINKS

http://www.nih.gov/niams; http://www.heartsite.com; http://www.aafp.org

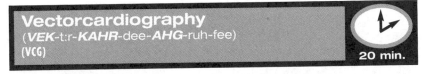

Vectorcardiography
(*VEK*-t:r-*KAHR*-dee-*AHG*-ruh-fee)
(VCG)

20 min.

Type of Test: Electrodiagnostic

Body Systems and Functions: Cardiovascular system

Normal Findings: No abnormalities noted

Test Results Time Frame: Within 24 hr

ELECTRODIAGNOSTIC

Test Description: Vectorcardiography measures the electrical activity of the heart. Unlike the electrocardiogram, which measures the electrical activity of the heart in a single plane, the vectorcardiogram measures this activity in three planes. "Vector" means that the value has magnitude as well as direction, so this test examines the direction of flow of electricity from three directions. This makes the VCG more sensitive than ECG for diagnosing a myocardial infarction. This test is often used to clarify uncertain or unclear EKGs.

CLINICAL ALERT:
If chest pain is present during the test, this should be noted and reported. If the test is to be repeated (on an inpatient in the ICU for example), then the electrode sites should be marked with ink. This will reduce the chances of nonclinical changes in readings.

Consent Form: Not required

List of Equipment: Electrodes; vectorgraph; monitor

Test Procedure:
1. Instruct the client to not move or talk during the procedure. *Affects the accuracy of the test.*
2. Place client in supine position. Attach electrodes to the chest, left leg, back, neck, and forehead (note: exact placement varies with equipment).
3. Apply conductive jelly to the lead placement sites. *Ensures a more accurate reading.*
4. Recordings are made of the electrical activity of the heart.

Clinical Implications and Indications:
1. This test will not determine the mechanical function of the heart or valves. It determines the electrical activity of the heart.
2. The measurements recorded by the VCG are rate, rhythm, position, and size of the heart. It also indicates death and ischemia of heart tissue.
3. Detects bundle branch block, myocardial infarction, and ventricular hypertrophy.

Nursing Care:
Before Test: Explain the test procedure and the purpose of the test. Assess the client's knowledge of the test.
During Test: Adhere to standard precautions. Instruct client to remain still and quiet.
After Test: No activity restrictions required.

Interfering Factors: Inability to remain still; cardiac medications such as antiarrhythmics and digitalis

Nursing Considerations:
Pediatric: Infants and children will need assistance in remaining still during the vectorcardiography and age-appropriate comfort measures following the test.

Listing of Related Tests: Electrocardiograph

WEBLINKS

http://www.howstuffworks.com

Endoscopic Studies

EXAMINATION BY ENDOSCOPY

Endoscopy involves the direct visualization of internal structures of the body through the use of special fiber-optic instruments that contain lights, and specialized tools such as suction, lavage, biopsy forceps, electrocautery, and even lasers. A camera within the endoscope records and projects images onto a monitor. Scopes are usually made from a flexible nylon that allows them to be introduced into a body cavity or organ. Procedures are performed using sterile technique, except for endoscopy of the colon. Endoscopic procedures usually take approximately 30–60 minutes and do not usually require a general anesthetic.

History of Endoscopic Procedures

The beginning of endoscopic procedures was in the early 1960s and these initial scopes were rigid in makeup. They were developed into flexible tubes, to allow their passage into body cavities. Today's fiber-optic scopes are made of strands of glass fibers. The proliferation of endoscopics began to occur in the 1980s. As their use has continued, endoscopic procedures have transformed diagnostics for a tremendous variety of conditions. For example, the sigmoidoscope is a very important instrument in screening for colon cancer in at-risk clients. It is suggested for use on a regular basis in all clients over the age of 40. And cystoscopy testing is common as a diagnostic test of the lower urinary tract.

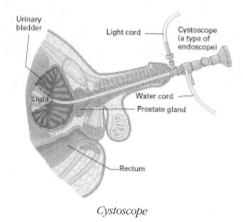

Cystoscope

COMPLICATIONS OF ENDOSCOPIC PROCEDURES

The use of endoscopic procedures does have a few complications, but their primary difficulty is an alteration in comfort. Conscious sedation and local anesthetics are most often used for the purposes of alleviating the discomfort. In addition, endoscopic procedures take the place of procedures that require more extensive diagnostic surgeries. The potential complications of endoscopy are hemorrhaging or perforation of a cavity or organ during a biopsy; potential infections from contamination during the procedure; an anaphylactic reaction (a form of distributive shock) when using a contrast medium; and arrhythmias due to the direct electrical stimulus when performed in areas that are predisposed to vagal stimulations.

Contraindications and Interfering Factors for Endoscopic Procedures

There are a variety of potential contraindications and interfering factors that accompany endoscopic procedures. For example, some contraindications are fistulas, ileus, third-trimester pregnancy, bleeding disorders, acute peritonitis, and diverticulitis. Examples of potential interfering factors are retained barium, when used as a contrast medium, and fixation of the bowel from a previous radiation therapy or surgery.

CLIENT CARE IN ENDOSCOPIC TESTING

Clients may not have much knowledge regarding endoscopic procedures and consequently need education in the preoperative phase. The following are the more typical nursing considerations for clients having endoscopic procedures: (1) often clients need to be positioned in a specific manner (e.g., Sims' position), (2) the client should be informed that there are minor pain and discomfort frequently associated with endoscopy, (3) the client should be told what to expect and the analgesia discussed, (4) informed consent is usually required and should be obtained while the client is not under the effects of preoperative sedation, (5) complications are rare, but include perforation, infection, bleeding, and allergic reactions to topical anesthetics, analgesics, or contrast media, (6) some endoscopy procedures require NPO status to prevent aspiration, (7) client education regarding premedication for the procedure, and (8) advising the client of clinical manifestations of infection (e.g., redness, warmth, swelling, pain) and to notify the health care provider with any signs/symptoms of infection.

Arthroscopy
(ahr-*THRAHS*-kuh-pee)

1 hr.

Type of Test: Endoscopic

Body Systems and Functions: Musculoskeletal system

Normal Findings: Normal structures of the joint examined; absence of tears, degeneration, cysts, deposits, or inflammation

Test Results Time Frame: Immediate

Test Description: An arthroscopy is a surgical procedure providing direct visualization of the internal structures of a joint using a fiber-optic arthroscope. The knee is the most common examination, but other joints may include shoulder, elbow, hip, waist, and ankle. This procedure is a common method used for diagnosis of injury/disorders of the knee that cannot be identified by x-ray.

Consent Form: Required

List of Equipment: Prep tray; sterile arthroscopy tray; antiseptic solution; local anesthetic; sterile stockinette; ace wrap; thigh cuff; compression dressing

Test Procedure:
1. Position client and place pneumatic cuff around the thigh (knee examination).
2. Leg is prepared with antiseptic solution and draped.
3. Elevate extremity and apply an ace wrap. *Facilitates drainage of blood from extremity.*
4. Inflate cuff to 300 mm Hg and then remove ace wrap and position extremity.
5. Small incision is made and trocar inserted.
6. Scope is manipulated within the joint and extremity manipulated as needed for maximum visualization. Cultures, biopsy, surgical repair, and removal of loose bodies and osteophytes are performed as needed.
7. Joint may be lavaged and medication instilled before removal of the scope.
8. Compression dressing is applied.

Clinical Implications and Indications:
1. Diagnoses and evaluates suspected ligament tear, damaged meniscus cartilage, bone fragments, lesions, or other problems detected by x-ray of the joint
2. Differentiates joint pain from injury or otherwise
3. Monitors progress of disease or effect of treatment

Nursing Care:

Before Test: Explain the test procedure and the purpose of the test. Assess the client's knowledge of the test. Instruct client to be NPO for a minimum of 12 hr prior to the procedure. Instruct client that they may feel discomfort with the injection of local anesthetic, but only pressure during the procedure. Teach crutch walking if appropriate.

During Test: Adhere to standard precautions.

After Test: Administer analgesics and apply ice as ordered. Provide information regarding assistive devices, activity, and exercise per physician protocol. Inform client to report fever, joint swelling, or change in color or sensation. Encourage follow-up for appropriate therapies (e.g., suture removal).

Potential Complications: Hemorrhage; infection; thrombophlebitis; reaction to anesthetic; neurovascular damage; synovial rupture; slight risk for perforated tissue, tear of muscle or ligament, or excessive bleeding

Contraindications: Infective process; fibrous ankylosis

Nursing Considerations:

Pregnancy: Performed only if benefits outweigh the risks to the fetus.

Home Care: Limited mobility may necessitate assistance with transportation and home care.

Rural: Procedure performed by a specialist, may require travel of some distance.

Listing of Related Tests: Arthrograph

WEBLINKS

www.medicinenet.com;
http://www.ncbi.nlm.nih.gov/entrez/query.fcgi

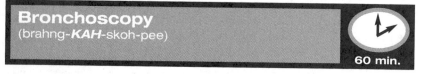

Bronchoscopy
(brahng-*KAH*-skoh-pee)

60 min.

Type of Test: Endoscopic

Body Systems and Functions: Pulmonary system

Normal Findings: Normal trachea, larynx, and bronchi

Test Results Time Frame: Dependent upon tests performed, immediate if visualization only

Test Description: Bronchoscopy allows direct visualization of the tracheobronchial tree; the client may be under either a general anesthetic or conscious sedation. Rigid bronchoscopy is usually performed in the operating room under a general anesthetic. Frequently, flexible or fiber-optic bronchoscopy is performed in different hospital units (emergency department, ICU, special studies). Rigid bronchoscopes have a larger diameter and are helpful for suctioning out large amounts of blood, retrieving foreign bodies, and dilating endobronchial strictures and for clients who require ventilation during the procedure. Flexible scopes have a smaller diameter and an additional lumen and are flexible, which allows better visualization of the smaller airways. The additional lumen can be used for tissue biopsies, bronchial washings, bronchial brushings, and medication instillation. Bronchial washings involve instillation of 100 mL of sterile water and the removal of the secretions for organism identification, especially acid-fast bacilli or fungi. Bronchial lavage entails instilling 30 mL of sterile water and removal of microorganism for identification or for thinning of thick secretions. Bronchial brushings obtain cells, for cytology, by inserting a brush and moving it around until cells adhere.

CLINICAL ALERT:
Have emergency equipment readily available in the event of the need for respiratory resuscitation. Clients may not tolerate bronchoscopy and may require general anesthesia.

Consent Form: Required

List of Equipment: Bronchoscope (flexible, rigid, or fiber optic); local anesthetic (spray, jelly, or liquid); sterile gloves; correct container for samples being taken; biopsy forceps; bronchial brush; emesis basin; suction; bag-valve mask with face mask; oral and endotracheal airways; nasal cannula; oxygen; normal saline and suction specimen canister (bronchoalveolar lavage)

Test Procedure:
Fiber optic:
1. Confirm correct client and remove dentures.
2. Confirm resuscitation equipment is present. *Medication may cause respiratory compromise.*
3. Place the client in a semi-Fowler's position. *Helps facilitate passage of the scope.*
4. Place client on oxygen if ordered. *Prevents hypoxia during the procedure.*
5. Administer local anesthetic onto the pharynx and tongue and into nose. *Helps facilitate passage of the scope.*
6. Bronchoscope is passed through the nose or mouth and lidocaine is sprayed onto the vocal cords. *Lidocaine helps abolish the gag reflex.*
7. Place samples in appropriately labeled containers and send to laboratory. *Ensures correct identification.*

Clinical Implications and Indications:
1. Determines etiology of hoarseness, abnormal chest x-rays, hemoptysis, or persistent cough
2. Evaluates respiratory distress in infants
3. Detects and stages bronchial cancer
4. Treats lung cancer through instillation of chemotherapy agents
5. Removes foreign body
6. Diagnoses lung infection, inflammation, and interstitial diseases
7. Intubates clients with cervical spine injuries
8. Evaluates possible obstruction in clients with sleep apnea

Nursing Care:
Before Test: Explain the test procedure and the purpose of the test. Assess the client's knowledge of the test. Assess for history of asthma, hypoxia, anticoagulant, or aspirin use. Check results of PT or PTT if ordered. Instruct client not to

ENDOSCOPIC

eat or drink for 8 hr. Administer atropine as ordered (decreases oral secretions). Administer premedication as ordered. Advise client that anesthetic may taste bitter.

During Test: Adhere to standard precautions. Monitor client's airway, vital signs, and oxygen saturation. Provide emotional support. Apply soft restraints if needed.

After Test: Monitor vital signs and client's airway status. Instruct client to spit out saliva into an emesis basin or suction out airway. Monitor for excessive bleeding. Advise client not to cough or clear throat (keeps clot at biopsy site). Monitor for and report immediately any subcutaneous air, stridor, or dyspnea. Educate client that sore throat, hoarseness, and blood-streaked sputum are common. Advise client to gargle or use throat lozengers for mild discomfort. Keep NPO 2 hr or until gag reflex returns.

Potential Complications: Bleeding; pneumothorax; perforation of trachea; laryngospasm; aspiration hemorrhage (after biopsy) bronchospasm; hypoxia; dysrhythmia

Contraindications: Bleeding disorders; pulmonary hypertension

Interfering Factors: Inability to extend neck; failure to obtain adequate sample

WEBLINKS

www.adam.com

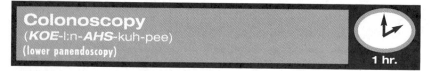

Colonoscopy
(*KOE*-l:n-*AHS*-kuh-pee)
(lower panendoscopy)

1 hr.

Type of Test: Endoscopic

Body Systems and Functions: Gastrointestinal system

Normal Findings: Normal colon

Test Results Time Frame: Within 24–48 hr

Test Description: Colonoscopy involves the examination of the large intestine from the anus to cecum with a flexible fiber-optic or video colonoscope. Air is introduced into the colon, distending the bowel walls. Photographs of the intestinal lumen may be taken. Colonoscopy is the most direct way to visualize the intestinal mucosa and can be done in clients who are actively, but not massively, bleeding. Sites of active bleeding may be treated. Foreign objects, polyps, and biopsy specimens can be removed through the colonoscope.

Consent Form: Required

List of Equipment: Endoscopic equipment; anesthetic; IV equipment

Test Procedure:
1. Place client in lateral decubitus position.
2. Colonoscope is inserted into the rectum and advanced to the cecum, and air is insufflated into the bowel, where the entire bowel is examined. *Air distends the bowel walls and improves visualization.*
3. If necessary, endoscopic surgery is performed to remove polyps or tissue is biopsied.

Clinical Implications and Indications:
1. Diagnoses polyps and tumors, ulceration and inflammation, colitis, diverticula, the origin of bleeding, diverticulosis, hemorrhoids, AV malformations, and strictures.
2. Colonoscopy is recommended for clients with high risk for colon cancer, such as a personal or family history of colon cancer, polyps, or ulcerative colitis; obvious or occult blood in stool; abdominal pain; lower gastrointestinal bleeding; and a change in bowel habits.

Nursing Care:
Before Test: Explain the test procedure and purpose of the test. Assess the client's knowledge of the test. Discontinue iron preparations 3–4 days before the examination. Discontinue aspirin and aspirin products 1 week before the test. Instruct the client regarding the appropriate bowel preparation. The 2-day bowel preparation consists of clear liquid intake for 2 days; strong cathartic such as magnesium citrate and Dulcolax; and an enema on the day of the test. The 1-day preparation consists of a glycol (CGOLyte) bowel preparation. A gallon of CGOLyte is taken orally over 4 hr. This laxative acts within 30–60 min. Instruct the client to remain NPO except for medications after midnight the day before the test. Take baseline vital signs and oxygen saturation of arterial blood. Premedicate client with analgesics and sedatives as ordered.
During Test: Adhere to standard precautions. Provide client with reassurance. Monitor vital signs and saturation of arterial oxygen.
After Test: Monitor vital signs and saturation of arterial oxygen per health care institution's protocol or for a minimum of 2 hr after the procedure and as needed. Assess client for abdominal distention and tenderness, gross blood in stools, hypotension, increased pulse, and other signs of complications of colonoscopy. Instruct client that gas pains may be experienced. Keep client NPO for 2 hr after the test and then encourage fluids to prevent dehydration associated with the bowel preparation.

Potential Complications: Bowel perforation; bleeding from biopsy sites or mucosal tears (rare); tearing of the spleen; vulvulus of the colon (rare); oversedation; respiratory depression

Contraindications: Unstable medical condition; massive intestinal bleeding; suspected perforation of the colon; toxic megacolon; recent colon anastomosis

Interfering Factors: Presence of stool and massive bleeding may obstruct the lens

ENDOSCOPIC

Nursing Considerations:
Pediatric: *Sedation is recommended for infants and children. Place the infant or child on a blanket for comfort. After postprocedure monitoring is completed and per health care provider's order, the pediatric client is discharged with an adult who is given instructions.*

Listing of Related Tests: Sigmoidoscopy

WEBLINKS

www.nlm.nih.gov

Colposcopy
(koel-*PAHS*-kuh-pee)

30 min.

Type of Test: Endoscopic

Body Systems and Functions: Reproductive system

Normal Findings: Absence of abnormalities of the cervix and vagina

Test Results Time Frame: Immediate (note: test results are dependent upon visualization and immediate identification of cervical tissue by the physician)

Test Description: Colposcopy is a macroscopic examination of the vagina and cervix with a colposcope, which is a stereoscopic binocular microscope with low magnification. Colposcopy is based on the study of the transformation zone. The transformation zone is that area of the cervix and vagina that has undergone replacement of columnar epithelium with squamous epithelium; this process is termed metaplasia. Abnormal PAP smears are further evaluated with colposcopy biopsies and endocervical curettage. Depending on the preliminary results of these tests, conization of the cervix may be indicated for further evaluation. Colposcopy is useful in identifying a suspicious lesion, but definitive diagnosis requires biopsy and examination of the tissue by a pathologist. Cervical intraepithelial neoplasia (CIN) is the current term used to identify all epithelial abnormalities of the cervix. The epithelial cells are malignant and confined to the epithelium and are divided into grade I, II, or III.

Consent Form: Required

List of Equipment: Endoscopic equipment; anesthetic; IV equipment

Test Procedure:
1. Place client in lithotomy position where a vaginal speculum is inserted to expose the vagina and cervix.
2. The cervix is sampled for cytological screening.
3. The cervix is cleansed with 3% acetic acid solution. *This removes excess mucous and cellular debris. The acetic acid solution also accentuates the difference between normal and abnormal patterns.*

4. The cervix is inspected in a clockwise manner.
5. Atypical areas are selected for biopsy.
6. Endocervical curettage is performed in nonpregnant women.

Clinical Implications and Indications:
1. Evaluates abnormal vaginal epithelial patterns
2. Diagnoses cervical lesions
3. Evaluates suspicious PAP smear results, atypical transformation zone, and dyplasia
4. Evaluates frank invasive carcinoma

Nursing Care:
Before Test: Explain the test procedure and the purpose of the test. Assess the client's knowledge of the test. Provide preprocedure sedation and analgesia as ordered. Transport client to the procedure room. Place client in lithotomy position. Drape client appropriately.
During Test: Adhere to sterile technique and standard precautions.
After Test: Assess for pain and provide pain medication as needed. Assess for potential complications. Instruct client to abstain from intercourse and not to insert tampon until healing of biopsy is confirmed.

Potential Complications: Heavy bleeding; infection

Contraindications: Heavy menstrual flow

Interfering Factors: Improper cleansing of the cervix may hinder visualization.

Nursing Considerations:
Pediatric: The onset of early regular sexual activity as a teenager and continued exposure to multiple sexual partners are factors associated with cervical cancer.
International: Women from lower socioeconomic class, blacks, and Mexican-Americans are at a higher risk for developing cervical cancer. Multiple sexual partners increase the probability of developing cervical intraepithelial neoplasia. In Europe and especially Scandinavia conization is widely used as treatment for cervical intraepitheal neoplasia.

Listing of Related Tests: Conization of the cervix

| WEBLINKS |

www.best4health.org

Culdoscopy
(kuhl-***DAHS***-kuh-pee)
(pelviscopy)

1 hr.

Type of Test: Endoscopic

Body Systems and Functions: Reproductive system

Normal Findings: Normal-appearing reproductive organs

ENDOSCOPIC

Test Results Time Frame: Within 24–48 hr

Test Description: A culdoscopy is the examination of the pelvic cavity viscera with a pelviscope that is inserted through the posterior fornix of the vagina. Culdoscopy allows the direct visualization of the uterus, fallopian tubes, broad ligaments, uterosacral ligaments, rectal wall, and sigmoid colon. This procedure is done with light sedation or an injection of local anesthetic in the vaginal cul-de-sac. Culdoscopy has been largely replaced by laparoscopy.

Consent Form: Required

Test Procedure:
1. The client is placed in the knee-chest position with the head of the table tilted downward. *Provides the best view of the pelvis and displaces the bowel from the pelvis.*
2. A small incision is made in the posterior vaginal vault and the culdoscope is passed into the cul-de-sac.
3. An examination is made of the pelvic organs.
4. Remove the scope.

Clinical Implications and Indications:
1. Evaluates and detects fallopian tube abnormalities, ectopic pregnancy, pelvic pain or masses, ovarian cysts, adhesions or scar tissue, uterine fibroids, malignancies, pelvic inflammatory disease, infection, and endometriosis

Nursing Care:
Before Test: Explain the test procedure and the purpose of the test. Assess the client's knowledge of the test. Instruct the client to be NPO after midnight. Instruct client to void before transporting to the operating room. Insert indwelling catheter and IV line with infusing solution as ordered. Provide preprocedure sedation and analgesia as ordered.
During Test: Adhere to sterile technique and standard precautions. Provide reassurance and a calm atmosphere during the procedure. Assist client with remaining in the knee-chest position.
After Test: Assess for pain and provide pain medication as needed. Assess vital signs and observe closely for potential complications. Provide education to abstain from douching and intercourse for 1–2 weeks.

Potential Complications: Infection; hemorrhage; penetration of rectum, bladder, or small intestines

Contraindications: Client's inability to assume knee-chest position; acute vaginal infection or peritonitis; masses in the cul-de-sac; adhesions of the bowel to the cul-de-sac

Listing of Related Tests: Laparoscopy

WEBLINKS

http://biocrs.biomed.brown.edu

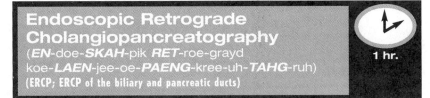

Endoscopic Retrograde Cholangiopancreatography

(**EN**-doe-**SKAH**-pik **RET**-roe-grayd
koe-**LAEN**-jee-oe-**PAENG**-kree-uh-**TAHG**-ruh)

(**ERCP; ERCP of the biliary and pancreatic ducts**)

1 hr.

ENDOSCOPIC

Type of Test: Endoscopic

Body Systems and Functions: Hepatobiliary system

Normal Findings: Normal biliary and pancreatic ducts

Test Results Time Frame: Within 24 hr

Test Description: Endoscopic retrograde cholangiopancreatography
(ERCP) is the visual and radiographic examination of the liver, gallbladder, and
pancreas using a fiber-optic duodenoscope. ERCP allows for direct imaging of
the bile ducts and periampullary region. The endoscope is inserted orally and
passes through the esophagus, stomach, and finally into the duodenum.
Intravenous glucagon is administered to paralyze the duodenum to more easily
locate the ampulla of Vater. A small catheter is advanced into the common bile
or pancreatic duct where radiographic dye is injected. X-ray films are taken to
examine the biliary tract. Tissue and pancreatic juice may be obtained for further
analysis. ERCP allows for simultaneous therapeutic intervention. ERCP is the
"gold standard" for the diagnosis of stones in the common bile duct with a high
sensitivity and specificity. The incidence of acute pancreatitis due to ERCP has
been reported to be a minimum of 5%.

Consent Form: Required

List of Equipment: Fiber-optic endoscope; anesthetic; IV equipment; x-ray
machine and related equipment from radiology

Test Procedure:
1. A flat plate of the abdomen is taken. *Ensures accurate results.*
2. Place client in supine position and drape appropriately. *Ensures privacy.*
3. Initiate IV line. *Provides access for anesthetics and medications.*
4. Insert endoscope into anesthetized oropharyngeal area and pass into duodenum.
5. Inject contrast dye and take radiographs.

Clinical Implications and Indications:
1. Diagnoses strictures, gallstones of the common bile duct, and pancreatic
   duct variations
2. Evaluates and monitors tumors, cholangitis, chronic pancreatitis, and cancer
   of the duodenum

Nursing Care:
Before Test: Explain the test procedure and the purpose of the test. Assess the
client's knowledge of the test. Assess for potential allergies to contrast medium.
Inform client that during injection of contrast medium, a burning sensation may
be felt for a few seconds behind the eyes or in the jaw, teeth, tongue, or lips.

Assess for anxiety and provide sedation as ordered. Administer preoperative medication usually 30 min before procedure. Obtain baseline vital signs and neurological assessment. Instruct client to fast for 12 hr prior to test. Instruct client to follow abdominal film guidelines. Educate client that breathing will not be impaired by the endoscope. Transport client to the surgery or special studies area.

During Test: Explain the test procedure and the purpose of the test. Assess the client's knowledge of the test. Assess for allergic reactions to contrast medium. Monitor vital signs and saturation of arterial oxygen.

After Test: Assess for allergic reactions to contrast medium. Instruct client to be NPO until gag reflex returns. Observe client for development of abdominal pain, nausea, and vomiting (symptomatology of pancreatitis). Assess for clinical manifestations of septicemia. Inform client that he/she will likely be hoarse with a sore throat for several days.

Potential Complications: Anaphylaxis due to allergic reaction to iodinated contrast material; perforation of esophagus, stomach, or duodenum; pancreatitis; aspiration of gastric contents; respiratory arrest (from oversedation); gram-negative sepsis; dysrhythmias

Contraindications: Previous history of allergy to iodine, eggs, or shellfish; perforated viscus; active pancreatitis (relative contraindication); altered anatomy, which does not allow for endoscopic access to ampulla; previous surgery such as Billroth II gastrojejunostomy or Roux-en-Y choledochojejunostomy; uncorrected coagulopathy; x-rays are usually avoided during pregnancy unless the benefit to the fetus outweighs the potential risk.

Interfering Factors: Retained barium

Nursing Considerations:

Pregnancy: *X-rays are usually avoided during pregnancy unless the benefit to the fetus outweighs the potential risk.*

Pediatric: *ERCP has been performed successfully in cholestatic neonates. A high level of technical expertise is required of the physician performing this test on infants. Most neonates require general anesthesia during the examination. Specially designed pediatric duodenoscopes are available, which allows for use of ERCP in infants with obstructive jaundice. Sedation is recommended for infants and children undergoing an x-ray (abdomenal). Place the infant or child on a blanket for comfort. After postprocedure monitoring is completed and per health care provider's order, the pediatric client is discharged with an adult who is given instructions.*

Gerontology: *The older person may find it difficult to maintain positions when required to do so for lengthy periods of time during the ERCP.*

Rural: *Advisable to arrange for transportation home after recovering from the ERCP.*

Listing of Related Tests: Cholangiography; percutaneous transhepatic cholangiography

WEBLINKS

http://adam.excite.com

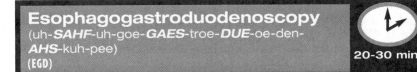

Esophagogastroduodenoscopy
(uh-***SAHF***-uh-goe-***GAES***-troe-***DUE***-oe-den-***AHS***-kuh-pee)
(EGD)

20-30 min.

Type of Test: Endoscopic

Body Systems and Functions: Gastrointestinal system

Normal Findings: Normal esophagus, stomach, and duodenum

Test Results Time Frame: Within 24 hr

Test Description: An esophagogastroduodenoscopy (EGD) is an endoscopic procedure that allows direct visualization of the upper gastrointestinal tract with a long, flexible fiber-optic lighted scope. The esophagus, stomach, and duodenum are visualized for abnormalities. The endoscope also has the capability of aspirating fluid, insufflating with air, obtaining a biopsy, using a laser to perform surgery, coagulating bleeding vessels, and injecting sclerosing agents. In addition, an enteroscopy can be performed by introducing a longer endoscope to reach into the upper small intestine. This allows for the visualization and biopsy of this area. The EGD is very sensitive in diagnosing diseases of the upper GI system and managing a variety of disorders. The biopsy is an invasive procedure performed in a surgical setting. The biopsy obtains a sample of body tissue under sterile technique, which is examined microscopically for cell morphology and tissue anomalies.

Consent Form: Required

List of Equipment: Fiber-optic endoscope; anesthetic; IV equipment

Test Procedure:
1. Place client on endoscopy table in left lateral lying position.
2. Anesthetize throat with anesthetic. *Decreases gag reflex to allow passage of endoscope.*
3. Sedate client and gently pass endoscope through the mouth into the upper GI tract.
4. Perform whatever procedure (e.g., biopsy, fluid aspiration) is necessary by what is visualized with the endoscope.
5. Aspirate excess fluids/air and remove the endoscope.

Clinical Implications and Indications:
1. Diagnoses tumors/cysts, hiatal hernia, esophagitis, gastritis, duodenitis, gastroesophageal varices, peptic ulcer, and esophageal diverticula
2. Manages upper GI bleeding and tumor or polyp removal
3. Evaluates the presence of cancer cells in the upper GI tract by biopsy

Nursing Care:
Before Test: Explain the test procedure and the purpose of the test. Assess the client's knowledge of the test. Provide preprocedure sedation and analgesia as ordered. Transport client to operating or procedure room. Drape client appropriately. Instruct client not to bite down on endoscope and remind client he will

ENDOSCOPIC

be unable to speak during the procedure. Remove dentures and eye wear. Instruct to remain NPO from midnight prior to examination.

During Test: Adhere to sterile technique and standard precautions. Provide reassurance and a calm atmosphere during the procedure.

After Test: Provide analgesia as necessary. Inform client he will likely have sore throat. Withhold fluids until completely alert with intact swallowing capabilities (usually 2–4 hr). Monitor vital signs per protocol and monitor for clinical manifestations of bleeding, abdominal pain, fever, or dysphagia.

Potential Complications: Perforation of esophagus, stomach, and duodenum; oversedation from anesthetic; hemorrhaging; pulmonary aspiration

Contraindications: Uncooperation; severe upper GI bleeding; suspected perforation; esophageal diverticula; recent GI surgery

Interfering Factors: Excessive GI bleeding; food in stomach

Nursing Considerations:

Pediatric: After postprocedure monitoring is completed and per health care provider's order, the pediatric client is discharged with an adult who is given instructions.

Gerontology: The older person may find it difficult to maintain positions when required to do so for lengthy periods of time during the EGD.

Home Care: Home health care provider will need to have warm mouthwash available for sore throat. Assess for clinical manifestations related to complications. Inform client that there is some abdominal distention, accompanied with belching and flatulence.

Rural: Advisable to arrange for transportation home after recovering from the procedure.

Listing of Related Tests: Endoscopy; upper gastrointestinal series; gastroscopy

WEBLINKS

www.ncbi.nlm.nih.gov

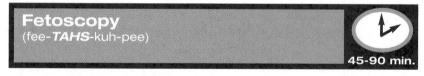

Fetoscopy
(fee-*TAHS*-kuh-pee)

45-90 min.

Type of Test: Endoscopic

Body Systems and Functions: Reproductive system

Normal Findings: No fetal stress

Test Results Time Frame: Immediate

Test Description: Fetoscopy is an endoscopic examination that directly visualizes the fetus via a small telescope-like scope. The endoscope is inserted through the abdominal wall into the uterine cavity. Besides visualization, the scope allows collection of cord blood and fetal tissue biopsies. A fetal ultrasound is ideally performed the day before the fetoscopy.

Consent Form: Required

List of Equipment: Endoscopic equipment

Test Procedure:
1. Assess fetal heart rate. *Determines a baseline.*
2. Administer meperidine (Demerol). *Prevents excessive fetal movement.*
3. Place client in supine position and perform ultrasound.
4. Insert endoscope and obtain samples per protocol.
5. Send specimens to laboratory.

Clinical Implications and Indications:
1. Detects fetal developmental defects (e.g., neural tube disorders)
2. Diagnoses blood dyscrasias of fetus (e.g, hemophilia, sickle cell anemia)

Nursing Care:
Before Test: Explain the test procedure and the purpose of the test. Assess the client's knowledge of the test. Determine fetal heart rate and administer maternal medications per protocol.
During Test: Adhere to standard precautions. Inform client that the only discomfort is the local anesthetic at the endoscopic insertion site.
After Test: Assess vital signs of mother and fetus (e.g., FHR, blood pressure, pulse). Administer RhoGAM to mother who is determined as Rh negative, unless fetus is Rh negative. Instruct mother to avoid strenuous activity for 1–2 weeks following procedure.

Potential Complications: Fetus: intrauterine fetal death; premature fetal delivery. Mother: spontaneous abortion; amnionitis; amniotic fluid leak.

Contraindications: Anteriorly placed placenta; bleeding disorders; hypertensive crisis; incompetent cervix; history of spontaneous abortion or premature labor

Interfering Factors: Excessive movement of mother

Nursing Considerations:
Pregnancy: Inform mother to report pain, bleeding, amniotic fluid loss, or febrile response.
Pediatric: Abnormalities of the fetus may be detected in time to facilitate effective interventions.

Listing of Related Tests: Fetal ultrasound

ENDOSCOPIC

| WEBLINKS |

http://adam.excite.com

Gastroscopy
(gaes-*TRAHS*-kuh-pee)

(upper gastrointestinal endoscopy; upper endoscopy; esophagogastroduo-denoscopy; EGD)

60 min.

Type of Test: Endoscopic

Body Systems and Functions: Gastrointestinal system

Normal Findings: Negative; absence of lesions; normal mucosa

Test Results Time Frame: Within 48 hr

Test Description: A gastroscopy is utilized for routine upper gastrointestinal endoscopy. The entire esophagus, stomach, and proximal duodenum are examined. A topical anesthetic is applied to the pharynx to numb the gag reflex. Intravenous sedation is administered. Fiber-optic bundles pass through the shaft of the endoscope to transmit light to the tip and the image to the endoscopist. In the handle of the endoscope are controls for maneuvering the tip as well as buttons to regulate irrigation water, air insufflation, and suction for removing air, secretions, and blood. An instrument channel allows the passage of biopsy forceps, small brushes for obtaining cytological samples, snares for removing polyps and foreign bodies, or devices to control bleeding.

Consent Form: Required

List of Equipment: Fiber-optic endoscope; topical anesthetic; patent IV line

Test Procedure:
1. Explain procedure to the client.
2. Have the client fast 6 or more hours to ensure an empty stomach. *Ensures accurate results.*
3. Assist with application of the topical anesthetic and IV sedative as needed.

Clinical Implications and Indications:
1. Evaluates dysphagia, dyspepsia, chronic abdominal pain, a change in bowel habits, acute or chronic gastrointestinal bleeding, and suspected polyps
2. Diagnoses inflammatory bowel disease and gastric cancer

Nursing Care:
Before Test: Explain the test procedure and purpose of the test. Assess the client's knowledge of the test.
During Test: Adhere to standard precautions.
After Test: Observe client for respiratory depression from the sedation for 1 hr after the procedure.

Potential Complications: Perforation of viscus; bleeding; cardiac arrhythmias; vasovagal reactions; pulmonary aspiration

Contraindications: Suspected perforated viscus; shock

Interfering Factors: Inability to remain still; uncooperative client

Nursing Considerations:

Pregnancy: *Performed if benefits outweigh the risks of the sedation.*
Pediatric: *Infants and children will need assistance in remaining still during the procedure and age-appropriate comfort measures following the test.*
Gerontology: *Low doses of sedation may cause lowered level of consciousness or respiratory depression.*
Rural: *Advisable to arrange for transportation home after recovering from EGD.*

Listing of Related Tests: Upper gastrointestinal test

WEBLINKS

http://www.usyd.edu

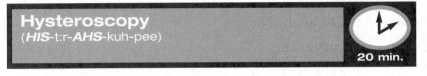

Hysteroscopy
(*HIS*-t:r-*AHS*-kuh-pee)

20 min.

ENDOSCOPIC

Type of Test: Endoscopic

Body Systems and Functions: Reproductive system

Normal Findings: Normal uterine cavity

Test Results Time Frame: Within 72 hr

Test Description: A hysteroscopy involves inserting a 4-mm hysteroscope into the vagina to the uterus to visualize the uterine cavity for abnormalities. Tissue samples are generally taken. This test is often done to ensure detection of pathology that a hysterosalpingography or curettage may miss.

Consent Form: Required

List of Equipment: Hysteroscope; speculum; carbon dioxide source or Hyskon (to distend uterine cavity); appropriate containers for tissue specimens

Test Procedure:

1. Place the client in the lithotomy position and drape. *Ensures privacy.*
2. The provider will insert the speculum and then the hysteroscope through the vagina into the uterus.
3. Carbon dioxide or Hyskon is instilled. *Distends the uterine cavity to promote easy visualization.*
4. Tissue samples are generally taken and placed in appropriate containers.
5. Label sample and send to the laboratory. *Correctly identifies the client and the test to be performed.*

Clinical Implications and Indications:

1. Evaluates pathology and biopsies endocervical tissue for analysis
2. Diagnoses and removes fibroids or adhesions

Nursing Care:

Before Test: Explain the test procedure and the purpose of the test. Assess the client's knowledge of the test.

During Test: Adhere to standard precautions and provide privacy. Provide reassurance and a calm atmosphere during the procedure.

After Test: Explain that there may be some cramping and spotting. A peripad is appropriate to use. Inform the client that they may experience shoulder pain or nausea from the carbon dioxide instillation. Provide analgesia as necessary.

Potential Complications: Bleeding; infection

Contraindications: Pregnancy; active pelvic inflammatory disease; bleeding disorders; purulent vaginal discharge

Interfering Factors: Ovulation or current menstrual period can interfere with test results and visualization.

Nursing Considerations:

Pregnancy: Clients of child-bearing ages should be assessed for the possibility of pregnancy.

Listing of Related Tests: Hysterosalpingography; curettage

WEBLINKS

http://www.pstcc.cc.tn.us

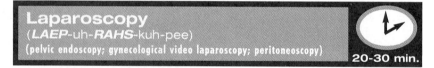

Laparoscopy
(*LAEP*-uh-*RAHS*-kuh-pee)
(pelvic endoscopy; gynecological video laparoscopy; peritoneoscopy)

20-30 min.

Type of Test: Endoscopic

Body Systems and Functions: Gastrointestinal system

Normal Findings: Abdominal/pelvic organs appear normal.

Test Results Time Frame: Within 2–3 days

Test Description: A laparoscopy uses direct visualization of the anterior intra-abdominal structures with a rigid laparoscope. It is performed with endoscopy under local anesthesia or in the operating room under general anesthesia. The laparoscopy is invaluable in both diagnostics and treatment because it has less complications than surgery that involves either general anesthesia or the excision through muscle and tissue layers of the body.

Consent Form: Required

List of Equipment: Laparoscope and biopsy instruments; sedative; CO_2 or nitrous oxide; Veres needle; specimen containers

ENDOSCOPIC

Test Procedure:

1. Place client in a supine position in the surgical setting and insert a Veres needle into the peritoneal cavity while client has general or local anesthetic.
2. A trocar and sheath are inserted into the cavity; the trocar is then removed for the insertion of the laparoscope.
3. CO_2 or nitrous oxide insufflates the peritoneum, creating a pneumoperitoneum.
4. The laparoscope is advanced into the peritoneal cavity through a small preumbilical incision and the following is visualized: omenum, surface of the liver peritoneum, gallbladder, portions of the spleen, diaphragm, a serosal surface of the small bowel and colon, and in females the ovaries, fallopian tube, and uterus.
5. Areas of pathology are noted and biopsies may be obtained.

Clinical Implications and Indications:

1. Detects ascites, portal hypertension, and liver disease of unknown etiology
2. Evaluates suspected peritoneal carcinoma or staging of cancer
3. Evaluates chronic abdominal pain (e.g., PID, adhesions, endometriosis)
4. Diagnoses suspected ectopic pregnancy, primary or secondary amenorrhea, infertility, salpingitis, hydosalpinx, and uterine fibroids
5. Suspected appendicitis or emergency evaluation of abdominal trauma
6. Detects and monitors abscess formation or infection
7. Evaluates tubal ligation, biopsy, lysis of adhesions, removal of foreign body, treatment of endometriosis, and laparoscopic surgery

ENDOSCOPIC

Nursing Care:

Before Test: Explain the test procedure and the purpose of the test. Assess the client's knowledge of the test. Instruct client to be NPO for 12 hr prior to procedure.
During Test: Adhere to standard precautions.
After Test: If client has had general anesthetic, follow standard protocol for care of the postoperative patient. Observe carefully for any other listed complications. Restrict activity for 2–7 days. Inform client that residual carbon dioxide effects may produce shoulder and abdominal pain for 1–2 days.

Potential Complications: Injury or perforation of the bowel, liver, spleen, ovary, or gallbladder; spilling of contents into peritoneum; subcutaneous emphysema; pneumomediastinum; bleeding at biopsy site; vasovagal reaction or myocardial infarction; fever; infection; peritonitis; pain, especially referred shoulder pain from diaphragmatic irritation; aortic rupture; hemorrhage; thermal burns

Contraindications: Acute peritonitis; unstable cardiac or pulmonary status; acute bowel obstruction; uncorrectable coagulopathy; history of multiple surgical procedures; formation of adhesions between viscera and abdominal wall; suspected intra-abdominal hemorrhage (blood obscures view); obstructions and hernias; chronic tuberculosis

Interfering Factors: Client movement during procedure; obesity; adhesions

WEBLINKS

www.healthgate.com

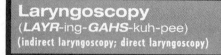

Laryngoscopy
(*LAYR*-ing-*GAHS*-kuh-pee)
(indirect laryngoscopy; direct laryngoscopy)

30 min.

Type of Test: Endoscopic

Body Systems and Functions: Pulmonary system

Normal Findings: Normal larynx with no clinical manifestations of inflammation, abnormal growths, or foreign objects

Test Results Time Frame: Immediately to several days

Test Description: A laryngoscopy is a procedure that allows for the visualization of the larynx by using either a rigid laryngoscope or a flexible fiber optic endoscope. The technique can be either indirect or direct, depending on the nature of the pathology. The laryngoscopy detects abnormalities of the larynx (vocal cords), a musculocartilaginous organ that is innervated by the laryngeal nerve and is responsible for vocalization.

CLINICAL ALERT:
Use of relaxation techniques may help the client relax and breathe more normally during the procedure.

Consent Form: Required

List of Equipment: Fiber-optic endoscope or laryngoscope; IV sedative; atropine; local or general anesthetic; sterile specimen container with formaldehyde; sterile gloves; emesis basin; resuscitation equipment

Test Procedure:
1. Administration of sedative and atropine. *Reduces secretions.*
2. Local spray anesthetic is commonly used and in some cases a general anesthetic is required.
3. Place the client in a head-tilted-back, supine position. *Enables the laryngoscope to be correctly passed through the mouth and into the larynx.*
4. Tissue is examined and biopsy of polyp, nodule, or cytology specimens taken (if necessary).
5. Send specimen to laboratory.

Clinical Implications and Indications:
1. The laryngoscopy can visualize abscesses, carcinoma, foreign body, hemorrhage, inflammation, strictures, and tuberculosis.

Nursing Care:
Before Test: Explain the test procedure and the purpose of the test. Assess the client's knowledge of the test. Provide preprocedure sedation and analgesia as ordered. Transport client to operating or procedure room. Advise the client that voice loss, hoarseness, and sore throat may occur but will be temporary. Advise client that eating or drinking is not permitted until the gag reflex returns (usually within 2 hr).
During Test: Adhere to standard precautions.
After Test: If general anesthetic is used, follow standard procedure for care of the unconscious client. If local anesthetic is used, check vital signs as required. An

ENDOSCOPIC

ice collar may minimize laryngeal edema. Instruct client to not swallow saliva or cough or clear throat, as this may dislodge blood clots and cause bleeding. Advise client that smoking should be avoided. After gag reflex has returned, normal diet may be resumed, starting with sips of water and ice chips.

Potential Complications: Bleeding; aspiration; laryngospasm

Contraindications: Severe respiratory failure; inability to tolerate interruption of high-flow oxygen

Nursing Considerations:
Pediatric: Children can become hypoxic and desaturate oxygen very quickly due to small airway lumen.

Listing of Related Tests: Bronchoscopy

| WEBLINKS |

www.healthgate.com

Mediastinoscopy
(MEE-dee-AS-ti-*NOS*-ko-pee)

45 min.

ENDOSCOPIC

Type of Test: Endoscopic

Body Systems and Functions: Oncology system

Normal Findings: Normal mediastinal structure and lymph nodes

Test Results Time Frame: Within 24–48 hr

Test Description: A mediastinoscopy is an endoscopic procedure (requiring a general anesthetic) that allows visualization and biopsy of the lymph nodes through a small suprasternal incision. It is usually performed when sputum cytology, lung scans, and x-rays have not confirmed a diagnosis. The mediastinoscopy aids in diagnosing cancer, tuberculosis, and histoplasmosis and determining whether lung cancer has spread to lymph nodes in the mediastinum.

Consent Form: Required

List of Equipment: Sterile mediastinoscopy tray; mediastinoscope; labeled specimen bottles with preservative

Test Procedure:
1. Take client to the operating room and administer a general anesthetic.
2. After the skin is prepped and draped, a small incision (1 in.; 2.4 cm) is made just above the suprasternal notch, and the mediastinoscope is then inserted and advanced into the mediastinum. *Allows visualization and biopsy of the lymph nodes.*
3. The mediastinoscope is withdrawn and the incision sutured and a bandaid or dressing applied. *Prevents bleeding.*

ENDOSCOPIC

Clinical Implications and Indications:
1. Assesses progress of lung or esophageal cancer
2. Diagnoses lymphomas (Hodgkin's disease) and other cancers
3. Obtains biopsy of mediastinal lymph nodes or intrathoracic lesions

Nursing Care:
Before Test: Explain the test procedure and the purpose of the test. Assess the client's knowledge of the test. Instruct the client to be NPO 12 hr prior to the test. Instruct the client to not drive home after the procedure. Client may be very nervous about the potential diagnosis and require emotional support from the health care provider.

During Test: Adhere to standard precautions.

After Test: Follow standard procedures for recovery from a general anesthetic. Client will usually stay in the hospital recovery area for 4 or more hours. Inform client that chest pain, tenderness at the incision site, or a sore throat may be expected but will be temporary. Inform client that they must contact their health care provider or go immediately to a hospital if side effects occur (e.g., fever, crepitus, dyspnea, cyanosis, difficulty breathing, rapid heart beat, and hemoptysis).

Potential Complications: Pneumothorax; hemoptysis; subcutaneous crepitus of the neck or face; laryngeal nerve damage (hoarseness, difficulty swallowing, changes in vocal pattern)

Contraindications: Failure to fast prior to the procedure; poor surgical risk; previous mediastinoscopy

Interfering Factors: Phenytoin hypersensitivity

WEBLINKS

http://www.healthgate.com

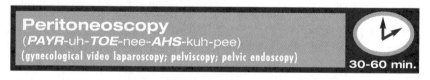

Peritoneoscopy
(*PAYR*-uh-*TOE*-nee-*AHS*-kuh-pee)
(gynecological video laparoscopy; pelviscopy; pelvic endoscopy)

30-60 min.

Type of Test: Endoscopic

Body Systems and Functions: Gastrointestinal system

Normal Findings: Normal size, shape, and appearance of uterus, fallopian tubes, ovaries, liver, gallbladder, and spleen

Test Results Time Frame: Within 2–3 days

Test Description: Peritoneoscopy is a procedure performed under general or local anesthetic to gain direct visualization of abdominal and pelvic organs. It occurs in an endoscopy suite or operating room. A scope is inserted through the abdominal wall into the peritoneum and a camera is used to generate views on a monitor. Clients have usually presented with acute or chronic abdominal or pelvic pain, an unidentified mass, or there is suspicion of advancement of cancer. Pathology can be identified and biopsies obtained if necessary. The procedure is an alternative to a laparotomy, which may still be necessary depending on pathology identified and intervention required.

Consent Form: Required

Test Procedure:

1. Place the client in supine position when first brought into the operating/examining room and induce with either general or local anesthesia. *Supine position will be maintained for most laparoscopy procedures; however, other positions may be necessary during the procedure to provide clear visualization of target organs.*
2. Insert a catheter and nasogastric tube. *Prevents distension of stomach or bladder and the danger of accidental penetration.*
3. Insert a blunt-tipped needle into the peritoneal cavity through a small periumbilical incision or a larger incision may be used to allow for direct visualization. *Choice of approach depends on purpose of procedure (e.g., adhesion lysis might be done under direct approach).*
4. Fill the abdomen with CO_2 or nitrous oxide. *Insufflation separates the abdominal wall from the intra-abdominal viscera, which provides better visualization of organs.*
5. Insert the laparoscope through a trocar and examine the organs. Biopsy is performed, if required.
6. Remove the laparoscope and allow the CO_2 or nitrous oxide to escape from the abdomen.
7. Suture the incision and apply a small bandage.

Clinical Implications and Indications:

1. Evaluates ascites or liver disease of unknown etiology
2. Investigates suspected peritoneal carcinoma and determines staging of cancer
3. Evaluates chronic or acute abdominal pain (e.g., PID, adhesions, endometriosis)
4. Confirms suspected ectopic pregnancy
5. Investigates primary or secondary amenorrhea, infertility, salpingitis, hydrosalpinx, and uterine fibroids
6. Investigates suspected appendicitis or emergency evaluation of abdominal trauma
7. Identifies cause of portal hypertension
8. Confirms abscess or infection
9. Provides access for tubal ligation, biopsy, lysis of adhesions, removal of foreign body, treatment of endometriosis, and laparoscopic surgery

Nursing Care:

Before Test: Explain the test procedure and the purpose of the test. Assess the client's knowledge of the test. Preoperative laboratory work should be available on the client's chart and will include CBC, platelets, electrolytes, prothrombin time, partial thromboplastin time, ECG, and chest x-ray. If enema or other bowel preparation is ordered preoperatively, ensure that this has been completed. Instruct client to maintain NPO status for 12 hr prior to the procedure. Complete any advance skin preparation that has been ordered (e.g., abdominal shave).

ENDOSCOPIC

Provide opportunity for client to void prior to procedure. Establish IV if requested and take baseline vital signs. Administer premedication, if ordered.
During Test: Adhere to standard precautions.
After Test: Follow standard protocol for care of the immediate postoperative patient (e.g., vital signs). Client may resume normal diet in progressive fashion. Instruct client to limit activity for 2–7 days. Teach client regarding residual effects of carbon dioxide (shoulder and subcostal pain) that may occur for 1–2 days and may be treated with over-the-counter analgesics.

Potential Complications: Injury or perforation of the bowel, liver, spleen, ovary, gallbladder; subcutaneous emphysema; pneumomediastinum; bleeding at biopsy site; vasovagal reaction or myocardial infarction; fever; infection; peritonitis; aortic rupture; hemorrhage; thermal burns; referred shoulder pain from diaphragmatic irritation

Contraindications: Acute peritonitis; unstable cardiac or pulmonary status; acute bowel obstruction; uncorrected coagulopathy; chronic tuberculosis; advanced abdominal cancer; history of multiple surgical procedures; significant abdominal hernia or mass; suspected intra-abdominal hemorrhage; pregnancy; known ruptured diaphragm; closed-head injury

Interfering Factors: Adhesions; obesity; inability to remain still

Nursing Considerations:
Pregnancy: Avoided during pregnancy unless the benefit to the fetus outweighs the potential risk.
Pediatric: Sedation is recommended for infants and children. Place the infant or child on a blanket for comfort. After postprocedure monitoring is completed and per health care provider's order, the pediatric client is discharged with an adult who is given instructions.
Rural: Advisable to arrange for transportation home after recovering from the peritoneoscopy.

| WEBLINKS ⓘ | ▤ ☒ |

www.sages.org

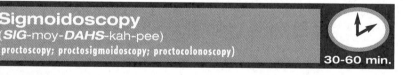

Sigmoidoscopy
(*SIG*-moy-*DAHS*-kah-pee)
(proctoscopy; proctosigmoidoscopy; proctocolonoscopy)

30-60 min.

Type of Test: Endoscopic

Body Systems and Functions: Gastrointestinal system

Normal Findings: Negative for structural or other abnormalities

Test Results Time Frame: Visual results: within 24 hr. Biopsy: within 48–72 hr.

Test Description: A sigmoidoscopy involves the insertion of an instrument into the anus and up into the colon allowing the examiner to directly view the

ENDOSCOPIC

walls of the colon. With some equipment, biopsies may be taken at the time of the examination. Polyps, fissures, hemorrhoids, and other disturbances of the lining of the colon can be viewed and samples taken for biopsy. The sigmoidoscopy is a screening test for cancer of the colon and is encouraged on a regularly scheduled basis for persons over the age of 40. There are other similar tests that examine selected portions of the lower gastrointestinal system (e.g., proctoscopy, proctosigmoidoscopy).

CLINICAL ALERT:
Test may be performed in clinic setting or hospital.

Consent Form: Required

List of Equipment: Lower gastrointestinal scope and related equipment

Test Procedure:
1. Place client in side-lying (Sims) position, usually on the left side for the flexible sigmoid examination. The rigid sigmoidoscopy may require the client to be in the knee-chest position. *Allows for easier access to the colon.*
2. The examiner performs a rectal examination, then introduces the sigmoidoscope into the colon. *The flexible sigmoidoscope may advance for about 25 in.*
3. Air may be introduced into the bowel. *Assists in viewing parts of the colon that can be difficult to assess.*
4. Biopsies can be sent to the laboratory after being put in the preservative and properly labeled.

Clinical Implications and Indications:
1. The sigmoidoscopy is an important tool in screening for colon cancer in clients who are at risk. At-risk clients are those with a family history of colon cancer, certain diets (low-residue/high-fat diets with highly refined foods), ulcerative colitis, granulomas, and familial polyposis. Colon cancer increases in people over age 40.
2. Evaluates irritable bowel syndrome or diverticular disease.
3. Locates areas of bleeding, ulceration, and irritation.

Nursing Care:
Before Test: Explain the test procedure and the purpose of the test. Assess the client's knowledge of the test. Instruct client to adhere to the dietary restrictions per protocol of facility. For example, the client may be placed on a clear liquid diet 24 hr before the test. On the evening before the test, instruct client to take oral cathartics such as Fleet Phospho-Soda, Dulcolax, or Colyte. An enema is often administered in the morning before the test. If the client is extremely anxious about the test, mild sedatives may be given. Monitor vital signs before the procedure.
During Test: Adhere to standard precautions. Provide support to the client. If the client has a history of cardiac problems, an ECG may be ordered to monitor the cardiac status during the procedure.
After Test: Instruct client to report unusual discomfort. Inform client that he may experience some flatulence and mild discomfort, relieved with change of position. Instruct client to report a rise in temperature, abdominal pain, or sustained bleeding. Take vital signs before the client is released. Clients with preexisting cardiac conditions may be given antibiotics after the test.

ENDOSCOPIC

Potential Complications: Bowel perforation; hemorrhaging; peritonitis; cardiac arrhythmias

Contraindications: Diverticulitis; fistulas; ileus; third-trimester pregnancy; sedatives; bleeding disorders; acute peritonitis; toxic megacolon

Interfering Factors: Retained barium; fixation of bowel from previous radiation therapy or surgery

Nursing Considerations:
Gerontology: The preparation for the examination may be difficult for some older clients. The elderly may not tolerate the bowel evacuation well or the cathartics may cause nausea and weakness. The older person may find it difficult to maintain positions when required to do so for lengthy periods of time during the sigmoidoscopy.
Rural: Advisable to arrange for transportation home after recovering from the sigmoidoscopy.

Listing of Related Tests: Colonoscopy; barium enema; CBC; stool examination

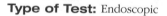

WEBLINKS

www.merck.com; www.overlakehospital.com

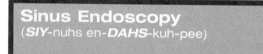

Sinus Endoscopy
(*SIY*-nuhs en-*DAHS*-kuh-pee)

30-45 min.

Type of Test: Endoscopic

Body Systems and Functions: Musculoskeletal system

Normal Findings: Normal sinuses

Test Results Time Frame: Immediate

Test Description: A sinus endoscopy uses an instrument to visualize the sinus areas. The sinuses may retain secretions that create chronic sinus infections and, even with antibiotic and allergy therapy, may not be resolved. Therefore, other treatments, such as endoscopy, are required. The sinus endoscopy's primary goal is to relieve infections and to provide diagnostics to the pathology of the sinus disorder.

CLINICAL ALERT:
If sinus problems seem to be related to dental problems, refer to dentist before performing sinus endoscopy. Severe nasal-septum defects need correction before sinus endoscopy.

Consent Form: Required

List of Equipment: Endoscopic equipment

Test Procedure:

1. Place client in upright, sitting position.
2. Anesthetize nares (often with cocaine) and insert endoscope. *Visualizes nasal sinuses.*
3. Remove endoscope.

Clinical Implications and Indications:

1. Evaluates and monitors chronic sinusitis, cysts, mucocele, sinus erosion, pathological sinus discharge, and deformities of the nasal septum area

Nursing Care:

Before Test: Explain the test procedure and the purpose of the test. Assess the client's knowledge of the test. Provide preprocedure sedation and analgesia as ordered. Transport client to operating or procedure room. Instruct client to be NPO for 8–12 hr prior to test.

During Test: Adhere to sterile technique and standard precautions. Provide reassurance and a calm atmosphere during the procedure.

After Test: Explain that some bleeding, discomfort, and swelling may accompany the postprocedure time phase of recovery. Monitor for signs of infection. Instruct client to report unusual clinical manifestations. Encourage oral fluids, particularly if client is nauseated.

Potential Complications: Excessive bleeding; nausea and vomiting; visual problems

Contraindications: Prolonged coagulation times

Interfering Factors: Deviated septum

Nursing Considerations:

Pediatric: Sedation is recommended for infants and children. Place the infant or child on a blanket for comfort. After postprocedure monitoring is completed and per health care provider's order, the pediatric client is discharged with an adult who is given instructions.

Gerontology: The older person may find it difficult to maintain positions during the sinus endoscopy due to the potential lengthy periods of time.

Home Care: Home health care providers should not let client drive after procedure. In addition, clinical manifestations of excessive bleeding, unusual pain, and infectious symptomatology should be reported at once to physician.

Rural: Advisable to arrange for transportation home after recovering from the sinus endoscopy.

Listing of Related Tests: Sinus x-ray

WEBLINKS

http://www.sinuses.com

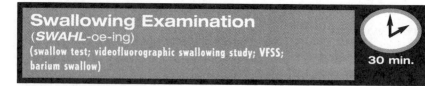

Swallowing Examination
(*SWAHL*-oe-ing)
(swallow test; videofluorographic swallowing study; VFSS; barium swallow)

30 min.

Type of Test: Endoscopic

Body Systems and Functions: Gastrointestinal system

Normal Findings: Ability to swallow all fluids without aspiration or evidence of strictures in the esophagus

Test Results Time Frame: Within 24 hr

Test Description: The swallowing examination is performed to evaluate the swallowing pattern of a client. The client is placed in a seated position and asked to drink barium while under fluoroscopy so the radiologist can observe their swallowing technique. Swallowing is essential for oral ingestion, and nutritional imbalances can exist quickly in the presence of swallowing pathology.

Consent Form: Required

List of Equipment: Fluoroscopy machine; barium in the form of liquid milkshake

Test Procedure:
1. Place client in a seated position in a fluoroscopy room. *Upright position allows for fullest view of swallowing.*
2. While the client swallows liquid barium, the fluoroscopy is utilized. *Barium is a radiopaque material, which allows for clear visualization of swallowing.*
3. After the test, give the client liberal fluids and possibly a laxative. *Enhances removal of barium from GI tract to prevent constipation or bowel obstruction.*

Clinical Implications and Indications:
1. Difficulty swallowing may be indicative of nerve damage or mechanical obstruction.
2. Difficulty in the esophageal area may be indicative of esophageal cancer, esophageal stricture, hiatal hernia, or ulcers.

Nursing Care:
Before Test: Explain the test procedure and the purpose of the test. Assess the client's knowledge of the test. Instruct client to be NPO for at least 8 hr prior to the test.
During Test: Adhere to standard precautions. Provide emotional support and reassurance. Observe for signs of aspiration.
After Test: Give client liberal amounts of fluids. Monitor bowel pattern and give a laxative if indicated. Instruct client that feces may be whitish gray for up to 72 hr after the test.

Potential Complications: Constipation; bowel obstruction; aspiration

Interfering Factors: Food in GI tract

Nursing Considerations:
Pediatric: Children will need assistance in remaining still during this procedure and age-appropriate comfort measures following the test. In addition, simple instructions for the swallowing procedures that are followed by the child are needed (note: this test is not often performed in children).

WEBLINKS ▸	🗖🗙

http://medline.cos.com; www.uwcme.org

Thoracoscopy Scan
(thoer-uh-***KAHS***-kuh-pee)
(endoscopic thoracotomy)

2-4 hr.

ENDOSCOPIC

Type of Test: Endoscopic

Body Systems and Functions: Pulmonary system

Normal Findings: Tissue in thoracic cavity is free of disease.

Test Results Time Frame: Immediate (note: written report within 24–48 hr)

Test Description: A thoracoscopy scan is an operative procedure where a surgical incision is made to allow for the insertion of a thorascope. The thorascope is used to visualize the pleura, pleural spaces, thoracic walls, mediastinum, and pericardium. It can also be used for biopsies and laser procedures.

Consent Form: Required

List of Equipment: Local anesthetic; betadine; sterile towels; thorascope; suction; sutures; chest tubes with drainage system; pressure dressing

Test Procedure:
1. Prepare client for general surgery.
2. Insert thorascope and visually examine thoracic cavity. *Less risky and almost as accurate as a thoracotomy.*
3. Chest tubes may be inserted upon completion of the procedure. *Chest tubes assist with lung reexpansion postprocedure.*
4. Follow up with postoperative procedures.

Clinical Implications and Indications:
1. Diagnoses such things as carcinoma, empyema, pleural effusion, inflammatory processes, bleeding, and infectious processes (e.g., tuberculosis, histoplasmosis)

Nursing Care:
Before Test: Explain the test procedure and the purpose of the test. Assess the client's knowledge of the test. Instruct client to fast 8 hr prior to the procedure.
During Test: Adhere to standard precautions (note: nursing care per perioperative nurses).

After Test: Postoperative chest x-ray; monitor vital signs, chest fluid drainage, respiratory status, oxygen saturation, and blood gas values; administer pain medication as necessary; encourage frequent coughing and deep breathing; splinting incision site for comfort.

Potential Complications: Heavy bleeding; tension pneumothorax; perforation of diaphragm; air emboli; respiratory distress; hypoxia; infection; empyema

Nursing Considerations:

Pediatric: Infants and children will need special assistance during the postoperative recovery time and should be referred to their normal caregivers for age-appropriate comfort measures.

Gerontology: The elderly are more at risk for developing postoperative complications after general surgery (e.g., pneumonia, arrythmias).

Listing of Related Tests: Thoracotomy

WEBLINKS

www.endosurgery.org

10

Fluid Analysis & Sputum Studies

EXAMINATION OF SPUTUM AND OTHER BODY FLUIDS

Sputum Testing

Common tests performed with sputum are gram stains, culture and sensitivity, examination for acid-fast bacilli (most commonly done to check for tuberculosis), and cytologic studies. Gram stains detect the presence of gram positive and negative bacteria and differentiate sputum from saliva. Culture and sensitivity detect the presence of many different organisms and their susceptibility to antibiotics. Tuberculosis is an acid-fast bacilli, and cytology studies are done to find cell changes due to malignancy or inflammation.

Other Body Fluid Testing

Many other fluids that may be collected for analysis are sperm, gastric acids, sweat, and bile. The procedures for collecting these different fluids vary widely and careful attention to technique and specimen handling is necessary. Sweat, bile, and gastric acids are tested for their chemical composition as an aid to diagnosis for disease states that influence their production. Some of the methods for collecting other body fluids, such as bone marrow, may be very invasive and require different forms of medications or even anesthesia.

PHYSIOLOGY OF SPUTUM FORMATION

Sputum is produced by the respiratory tract and transported to the pharynx by movement of the cilia lining the respiratory tree. The average adult produces about 100 ml per day of sputum, which is transported to the oropharynx and swallowed. Excess mucus is expectorated as sputum. A number of conditions produce excess mucus, usually from inflammation or infection in the respiratory tract. The character and consistency of sputum can provide information about the cause of the excess production. Pink, frothy sputum can result from pneumonia or acute pulmonary edema; sputum with a foul odor may be due to a lung abscess or carcinoma. Sputum may be thick, mixed with blood, sticky, and different colors, all reflecting the underlying pathophysiology. Always note these characteristics when collecting sputum (see Table).

Color	Possible Condition
pink or rust	congestive heart failure; bacterial pneumonia
blood streaks	Klebsiella pneumonia
gray or gray/black	dust or smoke inhalation
dark blood	tuberculosis, tumors
bright blood	tuberculosis, pulmonary thrombosis, brocholithiasis
green or green/yellow	pulmonary infection

HANDLING OF SPUTUM AND OTHER BODY FLUID SPECIMENS

Examine sputum specimens to determine if sputum, rather than just saliva or postnasal secretions, is present. Refrigeration is not necessary, but the sample should be taken to the laboratory as soon as possible. If the sample is sperm, it must be transported immediately to the laboratory as motility is an important aspect of the analysis. There may be specific considerations for other body fluids that will need to applied. The best method of assuring correct handling of specific body fluids is to confirm specific procedures from the associated laboratory that the specimen will be sent to for analysis.

CLIENT CONSIDERATIONS IN OBTAINING SPUTUM SPECIMENS

Obtain sputum specimens upon awakening in the morning, after secretions have pooled overnight in the lungs. Rinsing the mouth or brushing the teeth, if possible, is helpful to reduce the number of bacteria present in the mouth that may contaminate the specimen. Ask the client to sit upright, take several deep breaths, and cough deeply into a sterile specimen cup (see Figure). Warn the client not to touch the inside of the cup with the hands or mouth. The client needs to produce 1 to 3 mL of sputum. Additional methods for obtaining a sputum specimen may be attempted, as outlined:

1. Have the client drink one or two glasses of water and do postural drainage 30 minutes later. Attempt expectoration after the drainage.
2. Place a vaporizer at the bedside and do postural drainage after an hour. Attempt expectoration.
3. Request an order for an expectorant, and give it to the client with one or two glasses of water. Proceed as above.
4. If expectoration does not produce a sputum sample, it may be necessary to have a respiratory therapist obtain the sample through suctioning.

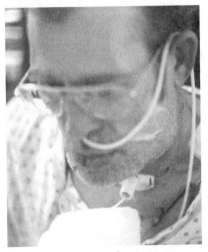

Encouraging a client to cough up a sputum specimen

CLIENT CONSIDERATIONS IN OBTAINING OTHER FLUID SPECIMENS

Specific fluid specimen collection procedures need to be carefully determined by the health care provider. There are some specimens that require precollection medications and there are some types of fluid collection that are more invasive (e.g., bone marrow, gastric aspiration, spinal fluid) and may require minor surgical procedures. The care provider implications are varied and require very specific knowledge and care procedures. The advice of this text is to consult the specific procedure manual that describes the specimen collection or to further read about the specific test in this chapter for the specific care procedures. For example, the client considerations for a thoracentesis are very specific, and individualized client education and equipment are necessary for this test.

FLUID ANALYSIS & SPUTUM

Life Span Implications for Sputum Analysis and Other Fluid Testing

Expectorated specimens may be difficult to obtain with young children, who have difficulty understanding the difference between saliva and sputum. A respiratory therapist may need to obtain the sample through suctioning. Other body fluid testing may require putting the client into specific positions (e.g., thoracentesis, paracentesis) which might be more difficult for the elderly. In addition, some of the fluids that are collected may require mild sedation for children and infants that are not necessary in other age groupings.

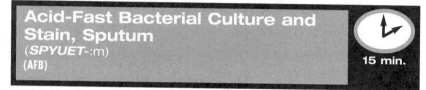

Acid-Fast Bacterial Culture and Stain, Sputum
(*SPYUET*-:m)
(AFB)

15 min.

Type of Test: Sputum

Body Systems and Functions: Pulmonary system

Normal Findings: No pathogens

CRITICAL VALUES:
Positive test results indicate clinical pathology of a contaminated culture. Health care personnel must immediately be cautious during client contact.

Test Results Time Frame: Within 1 day for stain; 6 weeks for culture

Test Description: Acid-fast bacteria are those species of bacteria that retain staining after an acid-alcohol wash. The test is primarily used to identify *Mycobacterium tuberculosis* to confirm the diagnosis of TB. Other bacteria that are acid fast include *Nocardia* species and *Actinomyces* species. The AFB stain is done to quickly identify possible *Mycobacterium*. Positive diagnosis is only possible after culture, which takes approximately 6 weeks. Tuberculosis has been more prevalent in its infection rates during recent years. Health care workers continue to be at risk for TB and are normally skin tested for its presence annually.

Consent Form: Not required

List of Equipment: Sterile sputum screw-capped container; double-walled container for transport

Test Procedure:
1. Collect specimen in the early morning. *Early-morning specimens provide the deepest sputum.*
2. Instruct client not to touch the inside or lip of the sputum cup. *Prevents introduction of nonrespiratory organisms into the sample.*
3. Have client rinse mouth. *Removes organisms from the mouth.*
4. Have client sit, breathe deeply, and cough into the sputum container.

5. Transport specimen immediately to laboratory. *Sitting at room temperature will allow overgrowth of contaminating organisms and make identification of* Mycobacterium *more difficult.*

Clinical Implications and Indications:

1. Test will be positive if *Mycobacterium* is present, indicating active respiratory tuberculosis.
2. Identifies *Nocardia* species and *Actinomyces* bacteria.

Nursing Care:

Before Test: Explain the test procedure and the purpose of the test. Assess the client's knowledge of the test.

During Test: Adhere to standard precautions. If client cannot raise sputum, the following may be helpful: increase hydration by having client drink 1–2 glasses of water; increase hydration by using a nebulizer; induce coughing by deep breathing; perform postural drainage after hydration has increased; and request physician's order for expectorant.

After Test: Send specimen cup immediately to the laboratory or refrigerate.

Interfering Factors: Obtaining saliva instead of sputum

Nursing Considerations:

International: Tuberculosis is more prevalent in underdeveloped countries.

WEBLINKS

http://RespiratoryCare.medscape.com

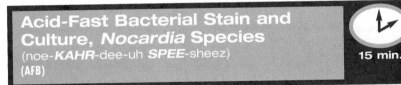

Acid-Fast Bacterial Stain and Culture, *Nocardia* Species
(noe-*KAHR*-dee-uh *SPEE*-sheez)
(AFB)

15 min.

Type of Test: Sputum

Body Systems and Functions: Respiratory system

Normal Findings: No pathogens

Test Results Time Frame: Within 1 day for stain; 6 weeks for culture

Test Description: Acid-fast bacteria are those species of bacteria that retain staining after an acid-alcohol wash. *Nocardia* species are acid-fast, although less positively than *Mycobacterium*. Sputum, transtrachael aspirates, or bronchial washes may be used to obtain a specimen. The AFB stain is done to quickly identify possible *Nocardia*. Positive diagnosis is only possible after culture, which takes approximately 6 weeks. Nocardiosis is usually found only in immunocompromised clients, including transplant recipients, people taking long-term systemic corticosteriods, and people with AIDS.

FLUID ANALYSIS & SPUTUM

CLINICAL ALERT:

If health care providers suspect active respiratory disease and the presence of *Nocardia*, then careful adherence to standard precautions is needed. This is particularly emphasized due to the fact that a positive culture is not determined for 6 weeks after the specimen is sent to the laboratory.

Consent Form: Not required

List of Equipment: Sterile sputum screw-capped container; double-walled container for transport

Test Procedure:
1. Collect specimen in the early morning. *Early-morning specimens provide the deepest sputum.*
2. Instruct client not to touch the inside or lip of the sputum cup. *Prevents introduction of nonrespiratory organisms into the sample.*
3. Have client rinse mouth. *Removes organisms from the mouth.*
4. Have client sit, breathe deeply, and cough into the sputum container.
5. If client cannot raise sputum, the following may be helpful: increase hydration by having client drink 1–2 glasses of water; increase hydration by using a nebulizer; induce coughing by deep breathing; perform postural drainage after hydration has increased; and administer expectorant.
6. Send specimen cup immediately to the laboratory or refrigerate. *Sitting at room temperature will allow overgrowth of contaminating organisms and make identification of Nocardia more difficult.*

Clinical Implications and Indications:
1. Test will be positive if *Nocardia* is present, indicating active respiratory disease.
2. Evaluates treatment of disease.

Nursing Care:
Before Test: Explain the test procedure and the purpose of the test. Assess the client's knowledge of the test.
During Test: Adhere to standard precautions.
After Test: Send specimen cup immediately to the laboratory or refrigerate the sample.

Interfering Factors: Obtaining saliva instead of sputum

Nursing Considerations:
Home Care: For clients needing a specimen from their home health care provider, specific instructions of how to collect the sample must be provided.

WEBLINKS

http://www.rcjournal.com

FLUID ANALYSIS & SPUTUM

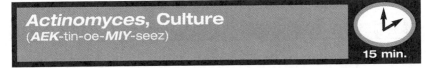

Actinomyces, Culture
(*AEK*-tin-oe-*MIY*-seez)

15 min.

Type of Test: Fluid analysis

Body Systems and Functions: Immunological system

Normal Findings: Negative

> **CRITICAL VALUES:**
> Any positive value should be reported immediately due to the potential severity in the event of an infection.

Test Results Time Frame: Within 2 weeks (note: can be longer, depending on growth of organisms)

Test Description: *Actinomyces* species are bacteria that are found as normal flora in the mouth. When they colonize traumatized tissue, they become pathogens. The most common sites of infection are the mouth and face, usually following dental procedures or trauma to the jaw. Other possible sites are the skin and the lungs and GI tract when they have been aspirated or ingested. *Actinomyces* infections are characterized by the presence of firm granules that are white or yellow.

Consent Form: Not required

List of Equipment: Sterile culture swab

Test Procedure:
1. Using sterile technique, take a sample of exudate from a granule in the infected area with a sterile swab. *Sterile technique prevents the contamination of the sample (note: granules are areas of branching bacteria in the exudate).*
2. Label the swab container that *Actinomyces* is suspected. Actinomyces *is an anaerobic organism that must be cultured in an anaerobic environment.*
3. Send sample to the laboratory.

Clinical Implications and Indications:
1. Diagnoses actinomycosis, which is a chronic suppurative disease with draining sinus tracts.
2. Confirms the presence of *Actinomyces israelii* in the infected fluid.
3. Elevated levels are found with pelvic inflammatory disease and infected abscess formation.

Nursing Care:
Before Test: Explain the test procedure and the purpose of the test. Assess the client's knowledge of the test.
During Test: Adhere to standard precautions and maintain sterility when obtaining the sample.

FLUID ANALYSIS & SPUTUM

Interfering Factors: Absence of sterile technique during collection

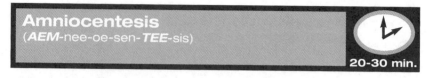

WEBLINKS

http://www.mic.ki.se/Diseases

Amniocentesis
(*AEM*-nee-oe-sen-*TEE*-sis)

20-30 min.

Type of Test: Fluid analysis

Body Systems and Functions: Reproductive system

Normal Findings: Color: clear to pale yellow late in pregnancy; chromosome analysis: normal

Bilirubin	<0.075 in first trimester
	<0.025 at term
L:S ratio	<1.6:1 before 35 weeks
	>2.0:1 at term
Alpha-fetoprotein	13–41 µg/mL at 13–14 weeks
	0.2–3.0 µg/mL at term

Test Results Time Frame: Chromosomal studies: within 2–4 weeks; other studies: within 24 hr

Test Description: Amniocentesis is the removal of fluid from the amniotic sac by needle aspiration. The following are evaluated from the amniotic fluid: fetal cells, alpha-fetoprotein, bilirubin, and lecithin:spingomyelin ratios. Overall, this testing detects fetal jeopardy or genetic disease and determination of fetal maturity.

CLINICAL ALERT:
This test may cause premature labor or fetal demise. Report any abdominal pain, cramping, vaginal bleeding, fever, contractions, or change in fetal activity immediately.

Consent Form: Required

List of Equipment: Amniocentesis tray; local anesthetic; needles; sterile dressing; antiseptic solution; swabs for antiseptic application

Test Procedure:
1. Ask woman to void. *Reduces the size of the bladder and decreases the chance of accidental puncture.*
2. Place woman in a supine position with her abdominal skin exposed.
3. Place a folded towel under her right buttock. *Moves the uterus off of the vena cava and prevents maternal supine hypotension.*

4. Attach fetal heart rate and uterine contraction monitors. *Amniocentesis can precipitate premature labor and may stress the fetus.*
5. Take maternal blood pressure and fetal heart rate baseline levels. *Provides a baseline for comparison during the procedure.*
6. Wash abdomen with an antiseptic solution
7. A sonogram guides the insertion of a needle into the amniotic sac to withdraw the fluid (note: an anesthetic is given during this time).

Clinical Implications and Indications:

1. Fetal cells are examined for chromosomal abnormalities, analysis of ABO and Rh incompatibility, and neural tube defects and to investigate fetal maturity.
2. Alpha-fetoprotein levels are measured as a confirmation of high maternal serum levels.
3. High levels of bilirubin reflect red cell destruction and may indicate hemolytic disease.
4. Low levels of bilirubin at the end of pregnancy reflect fetal maturity as the fetal liver matures and is able to conjugate bilirubin.
5. Lethicin: sphingomyelin ratios (L:S ratios) reflect fetal lung maturity, along with other surfactant phospholipids.

Nursing Care:

Before Test: Explain the test procedure and the purpose of the test. Assess the client's knowledge of the test. Explain that a sonogram will be done before the amniocentesis to assess the position of the fetus, maternal organs, and pockets of amniotic fluid. Teach client that the procedure may cause a slight feeling of pressure when the needle is inserted and a slight cramping sensation afterward. Instruct client to remain still during the test.

During Test: Adhere to standard precautions. Monitor maternal and fetal signs for indications of stress or premature labor.

After Test: Monitor maternal and fetal signs for indications of stress or premature labor for 30 min following the procedure. Instruct mother to report fever, contractions, cramping, vaginal bleeding, leaking amniotic fluid, or changes in fetal activity immediately to her health care provider.

Potential Complications: Premature labor; fetal demise

Nursing Considerations:

Pregnancy: If a maternal-fetal blood incompatibility exists, RhoGAM is given immediately following the test. The RhoGAM prevents the formation of maternal antibodies against any placental red blood cells that may have been accidentally released during the procedure.

Listing of Related Tests: AFP serum testing

WEBLINKS

http://biocrs.biomed.brown.edu

FLUID ANALYSIS & SPUTUM

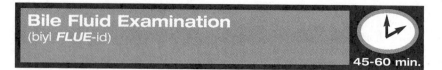

Bile Fluid Examination
(biyl *FLUE*-id)

45-60 min.

Type of Test: Fluid analysis

Body Systems and Functions: Hepatobiliary system

Normal Findings: Absent or rare cholesterol and calcium bilirubinate crystals

Test Results Time Frame: Within 24 hr

Test Description: Bile fluid is examined for substances that indicate pathology in the forms of calcium bilirubinate, calcium carbonate, and cholesterol monohydrate. Bile is continuously formed by the hepatocytes and is collected in the canaliculi and bile ducts. It is composed mainly of water, electrolytes, fatty acids, cholesterol, bilirubin, and bile salts. Bile is collected and stored in the gallbladder and is emptied into the intestine when needed for digestion.

Consent Form: Required

List of Equipment: Suction tubing; gastroduodenal tube; specimen traps, cholecystokinin

Test Procedure:
1. Establish a patent IV site.
2. Insert a gastroduodenal tube into the duodenum and confirm position with fluoroscopy.
3. Administer 100 U of cholecystokinin IV over 1 min. *Causes contraction of the gallbladder.*
4. Aspirate bile over 10–30 min.

Clinical Implications and Indications:
1. Elevated levels are found with cholecystitis, pancreatitis, and parasitism.
2. Evaluates pancreatic carcinoma.

Nursing Care:
Before Test: Explain the test procedure and the purpose of the test. Assess the client's knowledge of the test. Instruct client to fast for 8–12 hr prior to test
During Test: Adhere to standard precautions. Provide reassurance and a calm atmosphere during the procedure.
After Test: Assess client for intestinal discomfort. Administer analgesics per protocol.

Interfering Factors: Specimen pH <4.5

Nursing Considerations:
Pediatric: Infants and children will need assistance in remaining still during the procedure and may need sedation. They will require age-appropriate comfort measures following the test.

WEBLINKS

http://adam.excite.com

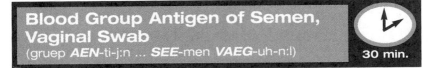

Blood Group Antigen of Semen, Vaginal Swab
(gruep *AEN*-ti-j:n ... *SEE*-men *VAEG*-uh-n:l)

30 min.

Type of Test: Fluid analysis

Body Systems and Functions: Hematological system

Normal Findings: Absence of semen

Test Results Time Frame: Within 5 days

Test Description: Blood group antigen of semen (vaginal swab) is the test used in rape trauma investigations. A high percentage of the population have secretor genes that cause the secretion of ABO antigens in body fluids, including semen. The blood type of the perpetrator may be identified by obtaining semen from the vagina of a rape victim This test is for blood type antigens only, so a suspect can only be eliminated. To identify a perpetrator, more extensive DNA testing must be performed.

CLINICAL ALERT:
Client and family involved in rape cases need tremendous emotional support from the obvious trauma.

Consent Form: Required (note: if to be used as legal evidence)

List of Equipment: Vaginal speculum; long cotton swabs; glass slides; Coplin jar of 95% ethanol; rape kit

Test Procedure:
1. Place the victim in lithotomy position and drape. *Ensures privacy.*
2. Insert speculum.
3. With long cotton swab, scrape vagina wall. *Obtains specimen.*
4. Roll swab onto two glass slides and place in 95% ethanol solution.
5. Label specimen with name, time of collection, and source of specimen and transport to laboratory. *Correctly identifies the client and the test to be performed.*

Clinical Implications and Indications:
1. Evaluates blood type in rape trauma investigations

Nursing Care:
Before Test: Explain the test procedure and the purpose of the test. Assess the client's knowledge of the test. Ascertain when the assault took place. Assure a female client that a female will be with her at all times.
During Test: Adhere to standard precautions. Remain with the client providing support and a calm atmosphere. Maintain privacy for the victim.
After Test: Offer counseling. Refer the client for sexually transmitted disease testing. The phone number for the National Coalition against Sexual Assault is (202) 483-7165.

FLUID ANALYSIS & SPUTUM

Interfering Factors: Assault over 72 hr prior to test; perpetrator has same blood type as victim; victim has bathed, douched, or defecated after the assault; perpetrator was sexually dysfunctional or has had a vasectomy; no ejaculation of perpetrator

Nursing Considerations:

Pregnancy: Follow-up for unlikely positive pregnancy test (due to the rape).
Pediatric: Special counseling and continued therapy are recommended for children and their families. Legal counsel and reporting are required with children.

Listing of Related Tests: Acid phosphates; blood typing; precipitin test against human sperm and blood

WEBLINKS

www.ncjrs.org; www.nlm.nih.gov

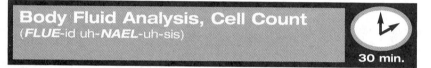

Body Fluid Analysis, Cell Count
(*FLUE*-id uh-*NAEL*-uh-sis)

30 min.

Type of Test: Fluid analysis

Body Systems and Functions: Hematological system

Normal Findings:

Table 1 Normal findings for body fluid analysis, cell count

	RBCs	WBCs	Neutrophils
Pericardial fluid	0	1000/mm^3	
Peritoneal fluid	0	<300/mm^3	<25%
Pleural fluid	0	0–1000/mm^3	
Synovial fluid	0	0–150/mm^3	<25%

Test Results Time Frame: Within 72 hr

Test Description: Aspiration of fluid is performed on a variety of areas (e.g., thoracentesis, pericentesis, pericardiocentesis, athrocentesis) to determine cell counts and cultures. The tests are done to relieve fluid accumulation and identify infections, degenerative processes, and the presence of malignant processes.

Consent Form: Required for aspiration

List of Equipment: Tray specific for area of aspiration (thoracentesis, pericentesis, pericardiocentesis, athrocentesis); skin prep; local anesthetic; 50-mL syringe; needles of various sizes or vacutainers; sterile drapes; sterile container for culture; red-top, green-top, lavender-top tubes; dressing supplies appropriate to area of aspiration

Test Procedure:

1. Label the specimen. *Correctly identifies the client and the test to be performed.*
2. Position client according to area to be aspirated.
3. Cleanse area of aspiration with appropriate skin preparation. *Ensures accurate results.*
4. Local anesthetic administered as per protocol.
5. Fluid aspiration performed.
6. Label fluid and transport to laboratory.

Clinical Implications and Indications:

Table 2 Clinical implications and indications

	Elevated RBCs	Elevated WBCs
Pericardial fluid	Hemorrhagic pericarditis	Neutrophils, bacterial pericarditis
	Dressler's syndrome	Fungal pericarditis
	Tuberculosis (TB) or fungal infection	Lymphocytes, TB or fungal infection
	Viral pericarditis	Suspect lupus
	Suspect lupus	
	Rule out carcinoma	
Peritoneal Fluid	Abdominal trauma	Ascites
	Neoplasm	Neutrophils >50% peritonitis
	TB	Tubercular peritonitis
		Cirrhosis
		Lymphoma
Pleural fluid	Trauma	Pulmonary infarction
	Pulmonary infarct	TB
	TB	Carcinoma
	Carcinoma	Pancreatitis
	Pancreatitis	Pneumonia
	Pneumonia	
Synovial fluid	Trauma	Osteoarthritis
		Rheumatoid arthritis
		Systemic lupus
		Bacterial arthritis
		TB
		Gout

Nursing Care:

Before Test: Explain the test procedure and the purpose of the test. Assess the client's knowledge of the test. Explain there may be some discomfort during the procedure. Instruct client to fast if indicated.

During Test: Adhere to standard precautions. Provide support and reassurance to the client during the procedure. Assist client in remaining still.

FLUID ANALYSIS & SPUTUM

After Test: Assess for signs of infection (e.g., redness, swelling, drainage, fever >101 degrees). Assess for bleeding and/or drainage from aspiration site. Apply appropriate dressing to the area of aspiration. Inform client to resume diet and medications as per protocol.

Potential Complications: See specific tests.

Contraindications: See specific tests.

Interfering Factors: See specific tests.

Nursing Considerations:
Pediatric: Infants and children will need assistance in remaining still during the procedure and age-appropriate comfort measures following the test.
Gerontology: The older person may find it difficult to maintain positions when required to do so for lengthy periods of time during the body fluid analysis.
Rural: Advisable to arrange for transportation home after recovering from procedure.

Listing of Related Tests: Pericentesis; pericardiocentesis; thoracentesis; arthrocentesis

WEBLINKS

www.medicinenet.com; www.ncbi.nlm.nih.gov

Bone Marrow Examination
(boen *MAYR*-oe)
(bone marrow aspiration; bone marrow biopsy; iliac crest tap; sternal tap)

30 min.

Type of Test: Fluid analysis

Body Systems and Functions: Hematological system

Normal Findings: Normal bone marrow

Test Results Time Frame: Will vary if specimen has to be sent to a hematologist for evaluation and if a bone marrow culture is ordered

Test Description: Bone marrow is located in the cancellous bone and long-bone cavities. Bone marrow is responsible for hematopoiesis (blood cell formation). Bone marrow cells can be removed for a complete microscopic hematological examination, which provides information regarding the cell's morphology. Inspection also provides information about the cause, type, and extent of abnormality present. Bone marrow cells are examined for a variety of characteristics. Cellularity indicates the number of hematopoietic cells versus fat cells. Distribution gives an estimate of the number of each different type of cell found in the specimen. The specimen is analyzed for cell maturation and the presence of any abnormal cells, such as mast cells osteoblasts, osteoclasts, and metastatic cells. The bone marrow may also be placed in a culture medium to see if any bacteria are present. The marrow sample may be taken from the aspiration technique or from the biopsy technique. Depending on the client's age, bone marrow will be taken from one of the following sites: sternum, iliac crest, proximal tibia, or vertebral bodies T10–L4.

CLINICAL ALERT:
Aspirate will be placed on slides and in tubes for aspiration technique. Marrow plug will be placed in container, with appropriate preservative, for a biopsy.

Consent Form: Required

List of Equipment: Premedication; gown; sterile drape; local anesthetic; biopsy needle; bone marrow aspiration tray; slides; thioglycolate tube (culture); preservative solution (biopsy)

Test Procedure:
1. Place client on back or side depending on site selected. *Provides correct access for procedure.*
2. Shave and cleanse the selected site with an antiseptic solution. *Helps prevent contamination.*
3. Drape the site with sterile drape. *Helps prevent contamination.*
4. Obtain sample, assist with smearing slides, and place sample in appropriate containers.
5. Label specimens according to policy and take immediately to laboratory. *Ensures correct identification.*
6. Apply direct pressure to biopsy site for 5 min; 10 min if the client has thrombocytopenia. *Helps to control bleeding.*
7. Cleanse site and apply sterile bandage. *Helps prevent contamination.*

Clinical Implications and Indications:
1. Diagnoses aplastic anemias, leukemia lymphomas, megaloblastic anemias, multiple myeloma, idiopathic thrombocytopenia purpura, and iron deficiency anemia
2. Identifies stage of carcinoma and lymphoma
3. Determines bone marrow differential
4. Monitors exposure to bone marrow depressants
5. Monitors chemotherapy treatment

Nursing Care:
Before Test: Explain the test procedure and the purpose of the test. Assess the client's knowledge of the test. Inform client 10–30 min of bed rest is required postprocedure. Administer premedication as ordered. Assist client into position (iliac crest, lateral recumbent or prone; sternal or tibial, supine; vertebral, seated position).
During Test: Adhere to standard precautions. Provide reassurance and a calm atmosphere during the procedure.
After Test: Hold direct pressure over site 5–10 min. Arrange for immediate transport of slides and specimens to the laboratory. Apply sterile bandage and monitor site. Instruct client to monitor for signs and symptoms of a bone infection (fever, headache, redness or increased pain at biopsy site, body aches). Provide analgesia as necessary.

FLUID ANALYSIS & SPUTUM

Potential Complications: Bleeding and bruising at the site; bone fracture; osteomyelitis; injury to heart and great vessels (rare)

Contraindications: Severe bleeding disorders

Interfering Factors: Recent blood transfusions; iron; liver; cytotoxic agents; failure to send specimens immediately to laboratory

Nursing Considerations:
Pediatric: Educate child about procedure and what will be felt; demonstrate procedure on a doll. Allow caregiver to be in room if they want. Provide comfort and emotional support to child and caregivers. The proximal tibia is preferred in young children and the vertebral bodies are preferred in older children. The sternum is usually not used because it is shallow and damage to the heart or great vessels may occur. Sedation is recommended for infants and children. Place the infant or child on a blanket for comfort. After postprocedure monitoring is completed and per health care provider's order, the pediatric client is discharged with an adult who is given instructions.
Gerontology: The older person may find it difficult to maintain positions when required to do so for lengthy periods of time during the biopsy.
Home Care: Monitor for signs and symptoms of infection.
Rural: Advisable to arrange for transportation home after recovering from the biopsy.

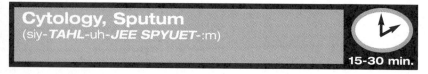

www.healthguard.com

Cytology, Sputum
(siy-*TAHL*-uh-*JEE SPYUET*-:m)

15-30 min.

Type of Test: Sputum

Body Systems and Functions: Pulmonary system

Normal Findings: Negative for abnormal findings

Test Results Time Frame: Within 24–48 hr (refer to specific health care institution laboratory guidelines)

Test Description: Cytology of sputum involves the determination of the type and number of cells present in order to diagnose pathological pulmonary conditions. Sputum is obtained from the bronchi and lungs by having the client cough up sputum or by bronchoscopy. Sputum should not be confused with saliva, which is produced by the salivary glands of the mouth. Early-morning sputum specimens are collected for usually 3 consecutive days. The client is instructed to take a deep breath and then exhale the air with a strong, deep cough. A diagnostic bronchoscopy involves the collection of bronchial secretions with the aid of a bronchoscope.

Consent Form: Not required

List of Equipment: Wide-mouthed sterile sputum collection container

Test Procedure:

1. Label collection container. *Correctly identifies the client and test to be performed.*
2. Client coughs sputum directly into container or sputum sample is obtained by physician during a bronchoscopy.
3. Transport specimen to laboratory immediately. *Delay in processing causes a deterioration of tumor cells.*

Clinical Implications and Indications:

1. Detects benign, atypical changes associated with inflammatory diseases, asthma, asbestosis, and emphysema
2. Evaluates metaplastic changes associated with chronic smoking, pneumonitis, bronchiectasis, and tuberculosis
3. Diagnoses viral pneumonia, herpes simplex infection, fungal and parasitic disease, and benign and malignant tumors

Nursing Care:

Before Test: Explain the test procedure and the purpose of the test. Assess the client's knowledge of the test. Instruct client to brush teeth and rinse well before obtaining sputum sample.

During Test: Adhere to standard precautions. Consult with health care institution's cytology laboratory if medium is required in collection container.

Interfering Factors: False-negative results may be due to delays in specimen processing.

WEBLINKS ⊟⊠

http://RespiratoryCare.medscape.com

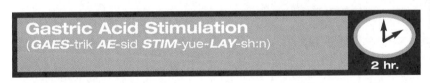

Gastric Acid Stimulation
(*GAES*-trik *AE*-sid *STIM*-yue-*LAY*-sh:n)

2 hr.

FLUID ANALYSIS & SPUTUM

Type of Test: Fluid analysis

Body Systems and Functions: Gastrointestinal system

Normal Findings:

Volume	20–100 mL
Basal acid output (BAO)	2–6 mEq/hr (note: values vary with body weight, gender, and age)
Maximal acid output (MAO)	16–26 mEq/hr
BAO/MAO ratio	0.3–0.6

Test Results Time Frame: Within 72 hr

Test Description: The gastric acid stimulation test is used as supportive data to other tests to help determine the response to substances that are administered that induce an increase in gastric acid production. Samples obtained are examined for volume, pH, and the amount of acid secretion compared with the basal gastric acidity. Gastric acid is made of hydrochloric acid, electrolytes, and mucus. The gastric acid is secreted by the stomach during the gastric stage of digestion. During disease states, the acid can increase or decrease, which causes increased pathology.

Consent Form: Not required

List of Equipment: Nasogastric (NG) tube; 50-mL syringe with male adaptor for the tube; gastric stimulant

Test Procedure:
1. Place client in sitting position.
2. An NG tube is lubricated and passed into the stomach.
3. Connect a 50-mL syringe to the NG tube and aspirate. *Confirms correct placement.*
4. Administer gastric stimulant subcutaneously.
5. If pentagastrin or histamine is used, gastric samples are obtained from the NG tube at 15-min intervals for 1 hr after injection. For histology, samples are obtained at 15-min intervals for 2 hr after injection.
6. Aspirated samples are labeled and timed and sent to the laboratory.

Clinical Implications and Indications:
1. Gastric secretory studies have enhanced the understanding of the pathophysiology of ulcer disease but are of limited clinical usefulness. The presence of hypersecretion does not predict the development of ulcer disease in an individual client.
2. Main indications are for evaluation of clients with suspected Zollinger-Ellison syndrome and in postgastrectomy clients with recurrent ulcer disease.
3. Detects duodenal ulcers as indicated by elevated BAO and MAO.
4. Assists in the detection of pernicious anemia as indicated by decreased or absent gastric acid output.
5. Diagnoses achlorhydria.

Nursing Care:
Before Test: Explain the test procedure and the purpose of the test. Assess the client's knowledge of the test. Instruct client to fast overnight and not to ingest fluids 1 hr before the test. Also, instruct client to have no nicotine after midnight the night before the test.
During Test: Adhere to standard precautions. Assist client to relax during NG tube insertion. Monitor for side effects to administered gastric stimulant, which include nausea, flushing, and dizziness.

Contraindications: Use of histamine diphosphate is contraindicated in clients with a history of suboptimally treated hypertension and asthma.

Interfering Factors: Medications that alter results are alcohol, histamine, nicotine, steroids, anticholinergic drugs, insulin, and parasympathetic drugs.

Nursing Considerations:

Pediatric: *Infants and children will need assistance in remaining still during the procedure and age-appropriate comfort measures following the test.*

Listing of Related Tests: Basal gastric acidity tests

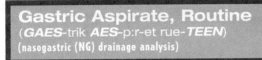 WEBLINKS

http://chorus.rad.mcw.edu

Gastric Aspirate, Routine
(*GAES*-trik *AES*-p:r-et rue-*TEEN*)
(nasogastric (NG) drainage analysis)

15-30 min.

Type of Test: Fluid analysis

Body Systems and Functions: Gastrointestinal system

Normal Findings: Negative for occult blood (i.e., blood that cannot be readily seen) and a pH of 1–7

Test Results Time Frame: Within 5 min

Test Description: Gastric aspirate screens for the presence of occult blood and determines the pH using the gastroccult slide test (note: an NG tube will likely have to be in place for this test). The slide includes both a specially buffered guaiac test for occult blood and a pH test based on the principle that certain dyes change color with changes in hydrogen ion concentration. When a gastric specimen containing blood is applied to gastroccult test paper, the hemoglobin from lysed blood cells in the sample comes in contact with the guaiac. Application of the developer (a buffered, stabilized hydrogen peroxide solution) creates a guaiac/peroxidase-like reaction that turns the test paper blue if blood is present. The pH test is based on changes in the color of dyes due to the change in hydrogen ion concentration.

Consent Form: Not required

List of Equipment: Gloves; gastroccult slides; gastroccult developer; NG tube; 50-mL syringe with male adaptor for the tube

Test Procedure:

1. Gastric aspirate is obtained by nasogastric intubation.
2. Open slide. Apply 1 drop of gastric sample to pH test circle and 1 drop to occult blood test area.
3. Determine pH of sample by visual comparison of test area to pH color comparator. This must be done within 30 sec after sample application. *Ensures accurate results.*
4. Apply 2 drops of gastroccult developer directly over the sample in the occult blood test area.
5. Read occult blood results within 60 sec and record results. *The development of any trace of blue color in the occult blood test area is regarded as a positive result.*

FLUID ANALYSIS & SPUTUM

6. Add 1 drop of gastroccult developer between the positive and negative performance monitor areas.
7. Interpret the performance monitor results. Record results. A blue color will appear in the performance monitor area within 10 sec if positive. The color will remain stable for at least 60 sec. No blue should appear in the negative performance monitor area when developer is added.

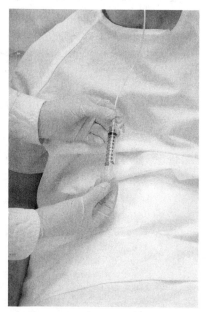

Aspirating Gastric Contents with Luer-Lok Syringe with Stylet in Place

Clinical Implications and Indications:

1. Diagnoses and manages various gastric conditions, such as Zollinger-Ellison syndrome.
2. Identifies occult blood useful in the early detection of gastric trauma or deteriorating gastric condition.
3. The pH may be of use in evaluating antacid therapy.

Nursing Care:

Before Test: Explain the test procedure and the purpose of the test. Assess the client's knowledge of the test. Instruct client to relax during insertion of nasogastric tube. Educate client not to ingest red meats, blood-containing foods, foods containing ascorbic acid, or vegetables with peroxidase activity (beets, turnips, cauliflower, broccoli) for 3 days before the test.

During Test: Adhere to standard precautions. Avoid contact of the developer with skin.

After Test: Reconnect NG tube to the suction tubing after specimen collection and ensure that suction is at the proper level (or remove NG tube if not required).

Interfering Factors: Many foods have peroxidase activity, which can produce positive gastroccult results; medications that increase levels are corticosteroids and reserpine; medications that decrease levels are Tagamet and Zantac.

Nursing Considerations:
Pediatric: Infants and children will need assistance in remaining still during the procedure and age-appropriate comfort measures following the test.

Listing of Related Tests: Hemoccult; hematest

WEBLINKS	▤ ☒

http://www.usyd.edu

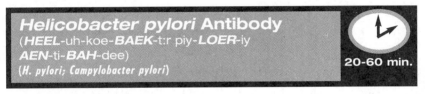

Helicobacter pylori Antibody
(*HEEL*-uh-koe-*BAEK*-t:r piy-*LOER*-iy *AEN*-ti-*BAH*-dee)
(*H. pylori; Campylobacter pylori*)

20-60 min.

Type of Test: Fluid analysis; blood; breath

Body Systems and Functions: Gastrointestinal system

Normal Findings: Negative or absent *Helicobacter pylori* growth during the culture period

Test Results Time Frame: Within 72 hr

Test Description: This is a test for *H. pylori*, a gram-negative bacilli that has been shown to play an active role as the major cause of active chronic gastritis. Endoscopy is used to obtain any microbes present in duodenal and gastric contents for culturing. Using noninvasive testing (i.e., serological or breath test) is recommended for clients less than 45 years of age without alarm symptoms (note: the method of testing discussed is for gastric content analysis).

Consent Form: Required

List of Equipment: Gloves; nasogastric tube; sterile water; sterile containers; lubricant; 50-mL syringe

Test Procedure:
1. Don gloves.
2. Lubricate and insert nasogastric tube.
3. Obtain gastric washings using sterile distilled water. *Ensures accurate results.*
4. Label and place specimens in sterile containers. *Correctly identifies the client and the test to be performed.*
5. Clamp tube and remove it.
6. Send sample to the laboratory (microbiology).

Clinical Implications and Indications:
1. Evaluates upper gastrointestinal symptoms, such as dyspepsia, early satiety, and unexplained anemia.

FLUID ANALYSIS & SPUTUM

2. Elevated levels are found with gastritis, duodenal and gastric ulcers, and gastric carcinoma.
3. Diagnoses suspected peptic ulcer.
4. Identifies bacteria in neonatal septicemia.

Nursing Care:

Before Test: Explain the test procedure and purpose of the test. Assess the client's knowledge of the test. Instruct the client to be NPO after midnight.

During Test: Adhere to standard precautions.

After Test: Advise the client that the nose may be sensitive for a few hours following the nasogastric tube placement.

Interfering Factors: Past infections without current active disease

Nursing Considerations:

Pregnancy: First-trimester pregnancy often causes nausea, which may make this client more susceptible to vomiting when having the nasogastric insertion procedure.

Pediatric: Infants and children will need assistance in remaining still during the procedure and age-appropriate comfort measures following the test.

Listing of Related Tests: Gastroscopy; upper endoscopy

WEBLINKS

www.uptodate.com

India Ink Preparation
(*IN*-dee-yuh ingk *PREP*-uh-*RAY*-sh:n)
(nigrosin preparation)

1 hr.

Type of Test: Fluid analysis

Body Systems and Functions: Hematological system

Normal Findings: Normal substances found in the cerebrospinal fluid and an absence of cryptococcus

Test Results Time Frame: Within 24 hr

Test Description: India ink particles are used in this older procedure for detection of *Cryptococcus* in cerebrospinal fluid (CSF). A lumbar puncture uses x-ray guidance to assist in the removal of a sample of CSF for analysis. Ten to 12 mL of CSF is withdrawn and tested. This test uses a wet mount and india ink particles or nigrosin. *Cryptococccus neoformans* has a thick gelatinous capsule that gives the appearance of a clear zone or halo around the organism against the dark background of india ink particles. Only about 40%-50% of cases can be detected by india ink preparations, and some of these may require repeat examinations.

> **CLINICAL ALERT:**
> Health care providers must assess whether clients have muscle movement restrictions that might make it difficult to be placed in the side-lying position for the lumbar puncture.

Consent Form: Required

List of Equipment: Cerebrospinal (LP) tray; stopcock and manometer if not in LP tray; slide and india ink particles in laboratory setting

Test Procedure:
1. Performed as a bedside procedure and may be done in the radiology department under local anesthesia.
2. Place client in the lateral recumbant position with knees drawn in toward the chest and with the head flexed with the chin toward the chest. *Enables easier access to the correct position of the spine.*
3. LP needle is passed into the L4–L5 interspace, pressure reading is taken, 10–12 mL of CSF is withdrawn, pressure readings are taken again, and the needle is withdrawn.
4. Place dressing on LP site and lie client in a side-lying position. *Prevents bleeding from the site.*

Clinical Implications and Indications:
1. Detects organisms in the spinal fluid, such as in cryptococcosis (torulosis), a fungal disease with marked predilection for lung and brain
2. Detects meningitis or brain abscess due to *Cryptococcus*

Nursing Care:
Before Test: Explain the test procedure and the purpose of the test. Assess the client's knowledge of the test. Instruct client to have no solid foods for 12 hr prior to the LP; fluids are usually permitted up to 3 hr prior to the test. If coagulation disorder is suspected, client will have platelet count and prothrombin/partial thromboplastin time performed. Instruct client to empty bladder and bowel prior to test.
During Test: Adhere to standard precautions. Assist client in maintaining lateral, recumbent position. Instruct client to remain very still and explain that movement may result in injury. Ask client to report any numbness, pain, or tingling in the legs (this may indicate nerve root damage or irritation).
After Test: Maintain bedrest in prone position for 1–3 hr to minimize post-LP headache. Observe for potential complications and deterioration of mental status, sensory deficits, leg muscle weakness, or bowel or bladder incontinence or retention.

Potential Complications: Spinal headache; local bleeding and bruising (hematoma) at LP site; immediate painful paresthesia (which usually resolves itself after the LP needle is repositioned); persistent pain or leg paresthesia

Contraindications: Increased intracranial pressure; severe degenerative vertebral joint disease; infection near the LP site

Interfering Factors: Refrigeration of LP samples; traumatic spinal tap; IV fluids containing chloride; hyperglycemia

FLUID ANALYSIS & SPUTUM

Nursing Considerations:

Pediatric: *Infants and children will need assistance in remaining still during the LP procedure and may require sedation. Health care provider must give age-appropriate comfort measures following the test.*

Gerontology: *The elderly client may have difficulty maintaining the lateral, recumbent position for the length of time for this test (note: increased sedation may be necessary).*

Rural: *Advisable to arrange for transportation home after recovering from procedure.*

Listing of Related Tests: Latex agglutination test; serological tests

WEBLINKS

http://www.methodisthealth.com

Lecithin/Sphingomyelin Ratio
(*LES*-uh-thin *SFING*-goe-*MIY*-uh-lin)
(L/S ratio)

20-30 min.

Type of Test: Fluid analysis

Body Systems and Functions: Reproductive system

Normal Findings: Ratio of 2:1 indicates pulmonary maturity; 1:2 dilution on shake test indicates lung maturity; ≥3.5:1 for fetus of women with insulin-dependent diabetes

CRITICAL VALUES:
Decreased levels indicate pulmonary immaturity and respiratory distress syndrome (RDS); L/S ratio of 1.5–1.9:1 indicates mild or moderate RDS; L/S ratio of 1–1:49 indicates moderate to severe RDS; L/S ratio <1 indicates severe RDS.

Test Results Time Frame: Within 24 hr

Test Description: The L/S ratio measures the ratio of lecithin (phospholipid) to sphingomyelin (surface-active ingredient). It is obtained by examining amniotic fluid and is used as an indicator of fetal lung maturity. In addition, decisions regarding early delivery are contemplated by the resulting values. Withdrawing amniotic fluid is usually performed no earlier than 14 weeks gestation. The fluid is examined by persons trained in chemistry, cytogenetics, and cell cultures. There are a wide variety of health care implications for issues related to the findings from amniotic fluid analysis.

CLINICAL ALERT:
If L/S ratio is <1.2:1, delivery should be delayed if possible.

Consent Form: Required

List of Equipment: Amniocentesis tray

Test Procedure:

1. Place client on back where amniocentesis is performed after skin overlying site is anesthetized locally.
2. Insert needle with stylet through the midabdominal wall and direct at an angle toward the middle of the uterine cavity (note: amniotic fluid may also be collected vaginally if the membranes have ruptured).
3. Remove stylet and attach a sterile plastic syringe and remove 5–10 mL of amniotic fluid and withdraw needle.
4. Specimen is placed in a light-resistant container that is labeled with client name, time, and date. *Prevents the breakdown of bilirubin and correctly identifies the client and the test to be performed.*
5. Apply dressing to site of insertion. *Prevents contamination and controls hemorrhaging.*
6. Take sample to laboratory.

Clinical Implications and Indications:

1. A decreased ratio after 35 weeks indicates RDS or hyaline membrane disease.

Nursing Care:

Before Test: Explain the test procedure and the purpose of the test. Assess the client's knowledge of the test. Allow client to verbalize her concerns. Advise client to follow instructions regarding emptying of bladder (before 20 weeks, keep bladder full; after 20 weeks, empty bladder).
During Test: Adhere to standard precautions.
After Test: Inspect puncture site for bleeding or amniotic fluid leak. After discharge from health care facility, instruct client to call health care provider immediately or go to emergency room if she has any fluid loss, bleeding, temperature increase, abdominal cramping, or unusual fetal movement.

Potential Complications: Puncture of bladder or bowel; miscarriage; fetal injury; leak of amniotic fluid; infection; preterm labor; maternal hemorrhage with possible maternal Rh isoimmunization; amniotic fluid embolism; abruptio placenta

Contraindications: Abruptio placenta; placenta previa; history of premature labor (before 34 weeks gestation), with an incompetent cervix

Interfering Factors: Rh disease; diabetes; severe birth asphyxia; contaminated specimens; maternal vaginal secretions or a bloody tap into the amniotic fluid may cause a false increased reading for lethicin; erythroblastosis fetalis; intrauterine growth retardation; hydrops fetalis

Nursing Considerations:

Pregnancy: The health care provider needs to use various stress management strategies and interventions due to the high propensity to anxiety related to the potential fetal complications.
Rural: Advisable to arrange for transportation home after recovering from procedure.

Listing of Related Tests: Amniocentesis

FLUID ANALYSIS & SPUTUM

WEBLINKS

http://www.pstcc.cc.tn.us/ost

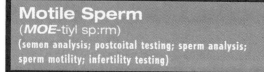

Motile Sperm
(*MOE*-tiyl sp:rm)
(semen analysis; postcoital testing; sperm analysis; sperm motility; infertility testing)

10 min.

Type of Test: Fluid analysis

Body Systems and Functions: Reproductive system

Normal Findings: 80% or more motile sperm in a total sperm count of $50–200 \times 10^6$ µL^{-1} in a volume of 2–5 mL

Test Results Time Frame: Immediately to 72 hr

Test Description: Sperm motility assessment is part of the analysis of sperm, which determines the viability of the sperm. This test is often performed to determine if clients are having difficulty conceiving. Sperm death can occur in the vagina before entering the cervix. Swabbing seminal fluid soon after intercourse (30 min or less) can provide an indication of vaginal secretion "hostility" to the sperm.

Consent Form: Not required

List of Equipment: Specimen container; microscope; aspiration syringe; glass slides

Test Procedure:
1. Clients must produce a sperm sample either by masturbation into a specimen container or by having unprotected intercourse prior to the test.
2. The sperm sample must be taken immediately to the laboratory setting for analysis or the female partner must go to the laboratory for a vaginal swab.

Clinical Implications and Indications:
1. Evaluates for possible causes of infertility.
2. Sperm count and semen volume levels increase up to 7 days during abstinence.

Nursing Care:
Before Test: Explain the test procedure and the purpose of the test. Assess the client's knowledge of the test. Clients require support and sensitivity about the nature of the test (note: many clients will find the test invasive and embarrassing). Advise female client not to wash her perineal area before or after intercourse as perfumed soaps or deodorants can be spermicidal. Instruct clients to abstain from intercourse for 72 hr before the test .
During Test: Adhere to standard precautions.
After Test: Inform client that more than one sperm test may become necessary. Sperm maturity takes 30–90 days.

Interfering Factors: Intercourse less than 72 hr pretest can reduce the number of sperm for analysis.

WEBLINKS

www.ivf.com

Mucin Clot Test

(*MYUE*-sin)

(synovial fluid mucin clot test; synovial fluid Ropes test; synovial fluid viscosity)

5 min.

Type of Test: Fluid analysis

Body Systems and Functions: Musculoskeletal system

Normal Findings: Firm clot formation with surrounding fluid having a clear appearance

Test Results Time Frame: Within 24–48 hr

Test Description: The mucin clot test measures the polymerization of synovial fluid hyaluronate and correlates it with viscosity. The synovial fluid is withdrawn from a joint and then mixed with acetic acid. The mixture of the two solutions causes a "clot" to form and the clot is graded as good, fair, or poor. Inflammation, such as with rheumatoid arthritis, degrades the quality of the mucin clot. A positive test would produce a firm clot.

Consent Form: Not required

List of Equipment: Sterile aspiration tray; lavender-top tubes; 20 mL of 5% acetic acid

Test Procedure:
1. Label the specimen tube. *Correctly identifies the client and the test to be performed.*
2. Obtain a sample of the synovial fluid.
3. Add 5 mL of synovial fluid into 20 mL of 5% acetic acid.
4. Send tube to the laboratory.
5. Sample should be refrigerated if there is a delay in analysis. *High temperatures alter the results.*

Clinical Implications and Indications:
1. Aids in the diagnosis of inflammatory joint disease (note: the mucin clot test lacks specificity (49%) and has a low positive predictive value (52%) and so should not be the only test to obtain a diagnosis).

Nursing Care:
Before Test: Explain the test procedure and the purpose of the test. Assess the client's knowledge of the test.
During Test: Adhere to standard precautions. Provide reassurance and a calm atmosphere during the procedure.
After Test: Clean site of aspiration. Provide analgesia as necessary.

Potential Complications: Bleeding and bruising at the site of fluid aspiration; infection

Interfering Factors: Lack of synovial fluid aspirate

FLUID ANALYSIS & SPUTUM

Nursing Considerations:

Pediatric: Infants and children will need assistance in remaining still during the fluid aspiration and age-appropriate comfort measures following the test.

WEBLINKS

http://www.methodisthealth.com/

Oligoclonal Banding
(*AHL*-i-goe-*KLOEN*-:l *BAEN*-ding)
(O-banding, CSF protein; immunofixation electrophoresis)

30 min.

Type of Test: Fluid analysis

Body Systems and Functions: Immunological system

Normal Findings: Negative; two or more bands (compared against negative blood serum)

Test Results Time Frame: Within 1–2 days

Test Description: O-banding involves the use of a lumbar puncture to collect cerebrospinal fluid that is then examined through electrophoresis. A blood sample is collected at the same time or within 2 hr of the lumbar puncture. Protein electrophoresis may reveal abnormal immunoglobulin bands consistent with specific nervous system disorders such as multiple sclerosis and HIV.

Consent Form: Required

List of Equipment: Lumbar puncture tray with sterile collection tubes; red-top tube or serum separator tube; needle and syringe or vacutainer; alcohol swab

Test Procedure:

1. Place client in side-lying position with knees-to-chin position and a lumbar puncture is performed. *Positioning allows access to space between lower lumbar vertebrae.*
2. A minimum of 3 mL of CSF is collected, and it is the first tube that is identified for this particular test.
3. Apply a small sterile dressing.
4. A venipuncture should be performed within 2 hr prior to or after lumbar puncture. *Serum sample is compared against CSF sample for O-banding.*
5. Place the client flat for 6 hr post–lumbar puncture. *Minimizes the occurrence of headache.*

Clinical Implications and Indications:

1. Diagnoses various nervous system disorders: multiple sclerosis, Guillain-Barrè syndrome, and cerebral infarction.
2. Detects human immunodeficiency virus, viral encephalitis, bacterial and cryptococcal meningitis, neurosyphilis, and panencephalitis.
3. Elevated levels are found with Burkitt's lymphoma and Hodgkin's disease.

Nursing Care:

Before Test: Explain the test procedure and the purpose of the test. Assess the client's knowledge of the test. Instruct client to have no solid foods for 12 hr prior to the lumbar puncture; fluids are usually permitted up to 3 hr prior to the test. If coagulation disorder is suspected, client will have platelet count and pro-thrombin/partial thromboplastin time performed. Instruct client to empty bladder and bowel prior to test. Prepare lumbar puncture set and assist client in lateral recumbent position along the edge of the bed with the knees flexed on the chest and chin touching the knees.

During Test: Adhere to standard precautions and strict aseptic technique. Assist client in maintaining lateral, recumbent position. Instruct client to lie very still and explain that movement may result in injury. Ask client to report any numbness, pain, or tingling in the legs (this may indicate nerve root damage or irritation). Apply band-aid over puncture site after lumbar needle is removed.

After Test: Maintain bedrest in prone position for 6 hr and to drink fluids to minimize post–lumbar puncture headache. Observe for potential complications and deterioration of mental status, sensory deficits, leg muscle weakness, and bowel or bladder incontinence or retention. Apply sterile dressing to puncture site and wash gently around perimeter of dressing to remove preparatory iodine or fluid. Administer analgesics if required for headache. If the serum sample has not already been collected, monitor to make sure it is collected within 2 hr of the lumbar puncture.

Potential Complications: Bleeding and bruising at puncture site

Contraindications: Increased intracranial pressure

Interfering Factors: Recent myelogram; traumatic spinal tap

Nursing Considerations:

Pediatric: Sedation is recommended for infants and children. Place the infant or child on a blanket for comfort. After postprocedure monitoring is completed and per health care provider's order, the pediatric client is discharged with an adult who is given instructions. Assistance will be required to obtain both the venipuncture sample and the lumbar puncture sample from the infant/child. To maintain the position for the lumbar puncture, the infant and young child is physically held in the knee-to-chin position, and varying degrees of assistance will be required by the older child and teenager. Parents should be monitored and supported during the procedure as they may find it particularly stressful to observe.

Gerontology: Positioning for lumbar puncture may be difficult and uncomfortable for some older clients.

Rural: Clients who have the lumbar puncture portion of this test done as an outpatient should be prepared to remain in the health care facility for a minimum of 6 hr after the test. If they leave before the 6 hr is up, they should be prepared to remain lying flat for the identified time frame. Advisable to arrange for transportation home after recovering from procedure.

Listing of Related Tests: CSF IgM and IgA

WEBLINKS

http://health.yahoo.com/

FLUID ANALYSIS & SPUTUM

Paracentesis
(**PAYR**-uh-sen-**TEE**-sis)
(peritoneal fluid analysis; abdominal paracentesis;
ascitic fluid cytology; peritoneal tap)

45 min.

Type of Test: Fluid analysis

Body Systems and Functions: Gastrointestinal system

Normal Findings: Little or no fluid in peritoneal cavity; no RBCs, bacteria, or fungi present; ammonia <50 µg/dL; amylase 138–404 U/L; glucose level equals serum level; protein 0.3–4.1 g/dL; WBC <300/µL; negative for carcinoembryonic antigen (CEA); clear to pale yellow in color

Test Results Time Frame: Within 3 days

Test Description: The purpose of the paracentesis is to remove accumulated exudative or transudative fluid from the abdominal cavity for diagnostic or therapeutic purposes. Examples of causes of exudative fluid accumulation would include inflammatory processes, such as an abscess, TB, or pancreatitis, but could also include malignancy. Transudative fluid accumulations may occur due to nephrotic syndrome, congestive heart failure, pericarditis, or inferior vena caval obstruction. Many of the transudative forms of ascites are a result of cirrhosis physiology.

CLINICAL ALERT:
Do not remove more than 750–1,000 mL at a time to prevent hypovolemia.

Consent Form: Required

List of Equipment: Purple-top and red-top tubes; aerobic and anaerobic culture media vials; sterile heparinized vacuum bottles; paracentesis tray

Test Procedure:
1. A flat or upright abdominal x-ray may be taken before the procedure. *Identifies ileus or obstruction.*
2. Instruct client to void or a Foley catheter may be inserted. *Decompresses the bladder to reduce risk of injury during procedure.*
3. Select puncture site (midline infraumbilical or lower quadrant lateral to the anterior rectus muscle). *Preferred since there are no vascular structures in the anterior abdominal wall.*
4. Place client in supine position on the examining table. Alternately, the client may be asked to maintain a sitting position with the back well supported or lie in high Fowler's. *Position will be determined by the client's ability to tolerate the position and the clinical presentation.*
5. Shave area, then cleanse, drape, and administer local anesthetic.
6. A large-gauge needle is used to enter the peritoneal cavity and fluid is withdrawn into the syringe and collection bag or directly into a vacuum bottle using a threaded catheter and IV tubing. Sometimes a small incision is made at the site and a trocar and cannula are inserted as an alternative method. If removing large amounts of fluid, it is drained slowly. *Avoids hypovolemia.*

7. Apply a bandage over the needle insertion site and maintain pressure on the site. *Prevents hemorrhaging.*

Clinical Implications and Indications:

1. Diagnoses infectious peritonitis or ascites of uncertain origin
2. Relieves respiratory distress associated with ascites
3. Identifies bleeding into the peritoneal cavity

Nursing Care:

Before Test: Explain the test procedure and the purpose of the test. Assess the client's knowledge of the test. Instruct client to void or a Foley catheter will need to be inserted. Take client's baseline vital signs, weight, and abdominal girth. Inform client that there will be a stinging sensation when the local anesthetic is given and a feeling of pressure/pain when the aspirating needle is inserted into the peritoneum. Sedation may be ordered for your client and should be timed in advance to provide the most effect possible. If infection is suspected, advise client that removal of the fluid may be accompanied by an unpleasant smell.

During Test: Adhere to standard precautions. Provide reassurance and a calm atmosphere during the procedure. Vital signs may be requested during the procedure if large amounts of fluid are being removed slowly.

After Test: Apply adhesive bandage to the site after maintaining pressure for several minutes or until obvious leakage has stopped. Take client's vital signs every 15 min for 1 hr and then as ordered. Monitor temperature 24–48 hr. Assess urinary output and presence of blood in urine. Assess the client for pain and manage as necessary. Place client on the unaffected side for 1–2 hr and then can move to whatever position is most comfortable. Documentation should include color and character of the fluid removed, the location of the site and any ongoing leakage, vital signs, and client's description of pain, feelings of dizziness, or changes in mental status. Measure abdominal girth and weight after the procedure for comparison with baselines.

Potential Complications: Intraperitoneal hemorrhage; needle perforation of abdominal viscus or solid organ; hypotension and shock from rapid removal of fluid; hepatic coma; peritonitis

Contraindications: Coagulopathy; large- or small-bowel obstruction; pregnancy

Interfering Factors: Vigorous movement of sample fluids, which damages cells; abdominal injury resulting in contamination of peritoneal fluid with blood, urine, bile, or feces

Nursing Considerations:

Pregnancy: Although paracentesis becomes more difficult and riskier to perform safely in later stages of pregnancy, it may still be necessary to reduce respiratory compromise from ascites.

Pediatric: Sedation is recommended for infants and children. Place the infant or child on a blanket for comfort. After postprocedure monitoring is completed and per health care provider's order, the pediatric client is discharged with an adult who is given instructions.

FLUID ANALYSIS & SPUTUM

Gerontology: The older person may find it difficult to maintain positions when required to do so for lengthy periods of time during the paracentesis.

Listing of Related Tests: Serum protein; glucose; amylase; LDH for comparison with sample levels; BUN; serum creatinine

WEBLINKS

www.healthgate.com

Pericardiocentesis
(payr-uh-***KAHR***-dee-oe-sen-***TEE***-sis)
(pericardial fluid analysis; pericardial effusion tap)

20 min.

Type of Test: Fluid analysis

Body Systems and Functions: Cardiovascular system

Normal Findings: Fluid will be clear or straw colored; no bacteria, RBCs, WBCs, abnormal cells present; glucose = serum level

Test Results Time Frame: Within 1–5 days (note: cultures will take longest time)

Test Description: Pericardiocentesis is the removal of fluid from the pericardial sac. It is done as a therapeutic emergency procedure in the case of cardiac tamponade, to diagnose why fluid is accumulating, or to administer medications. It is usually done in an emergency or operating room or cardiac catheterization laboratory where hemodynamic monitoring is possible. Controversy exists regarding how frequently pericardiocentesis should be chosen in nonemergency situations; however, many specialists support its use in diagnosis of selected cases of pericardial effusion. The procedure is performed only by a qualified physician (e.g., cardiologist, internist, thoracic surgeon), and the client usually receives 12–24 hr of ICU or step-down unit observation following the procedure.

CLINICAL ALERT:
Resuscitation equipment and access to oxygen/suction must be present in room in which procedure is performed. Hemodynamic monitoring capability is preferred for the procedure room.

Consent Form: Required (note: in emergency situation such as cardiac tamponade it will often not be possible to get signed consent prior to performing procedure)

List of Equipment: Pericardiocentesis tray; sterile tubes; heparinized sterile tubes; lavender- and red-top tubes; culture vials

Test Procedure:
1. When possible, pretest chest films and echocardiography should be performed. *Identifies location of fluid and organs.*
2. Place client in supine position and shave, prepare, and drape the anterior

chest and upper abdomen.

3. Apply ECG leads.
4. The site of the puncture is identified by palpating the tip of the xiphoid and moving left to the lower costal margin.
5. Administer local anesthetic.
6. Using an alligator clip the V_1 lead of the ECG is attached to an 18-gauge spinal needle on a 50-mL syringe. The needle is then advanced into the pericardium. *When advancing the needle, an ST-segment elevation on the ECG indicates epicardial contact and the needle should then be withdrawn.* The examiner may need to make several attempts from different angles to achieve success.
7. Withdraw the fluid and remove the needle.
8. Pressure is put on the puncture site until bleeding has stopped (approximately 5 min). *Prevents hemorrhaging.*
9. Apply a small dressing and take a chest x-ray. *Confirms fluid aspiration and chest status.*

Clinical Implications and Indications:
1. Removes fluid from the pericardial sac to relieve cardiac tamponade
2. Removes fluid from the pericardial sac for diagnostic purposes
3. Administers drug therapy directly to site (e.g., antineoplastics, antibiotics)

Nursing Care:
Before Test: Explain the test procedure and the purpose of the test. Assess the client's knowledge of the test. Inform client that the procedure is not painful, with the exception of the stinging sensation that may be experienced when the local anesthetic is administered. Instruct client to remain still during test, including coughing. Obtain client's baseline vital signs and attach pulse oximeter. Instruct client to limit clear fluids in the 8–12 hr prior to the procedure. Ensure chest films and echo results are available in the procedure room. Establish IV line (normal saline is usually the IV fluid of choice). Ensure emergency equipment is in room and that oxygen and suction are functioning.

During Test: Adhere to standard precautions. Monitor vital signs and observe ECG readings for changes. Provide client with reassurance.

After Test: Apply a sterile dressing to the puncture site. If continuous drainage is to be maintained, attach a closed straight drainage system. Monitor the client's vital signs, including observation of temperature in the 24 hr following the test. Hypotension or pulsus paradoxus may indicate bleeding into the pericardium. Muffled heart sounds and extended neck veins may also indicate bleeding over the heart. Assess dressing frequently for drainage.

Potential Complications: Perforation or laceration of segment of lung, heart, or liver; pneumothorax as a result of lung puncture; cardiac tamponade as a result of myocardial laceration; malignant ventricular arrhythmias; air embolism; infection; cardiac arrest

Contraindications: Coagulopathy; pericardial effusion; reaccumulation rate of blood will likely exceed rate of needle aspiration (trauma); uncooperativeness

Interfering Factors: Drug therapy with antibiotics will decrease bacteria count; contamination of specimen

FLUID ANALYSIS & SPUTUM

Nursing Considerations:

Pediatric: *Sedation is recommended for infants and children. Place the infant or child on a blanket for comfort. After postprocedure monitoring is completed and per health care provider's order, the pediatric client is discharged with an adult who is given instructions.*

Gerontology: *The older person may find it difficult to maintain positions when required to do so for lengthy periods of time during the pericardiocentesis.*

Listing of Related Tests: PT; PTT; platelet count; serum potassium; chest x-ray; echocardiogram

WEBLINKS

http://www.howstuffworks.com

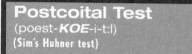

Postcoital Test
(poest-***KOE***-i-t:l)
(Sim's Huhner test)

30-60 min.

Type of Test: Fluid analysis

Body Systems and Functions: Reproductive system

Normal Findings: Mucous tenacity: stretches >10 cm; number of motile sperm >6–20/HPF

Test Results Time Frame: Within 24–48 hr

Test Description: Postcoital test is part of an examination for infertility. An examination of the postcoital endocervical mucus detects its quality and the ability of the sperm to penetrate the mucus. The postcoital test is usually accompanied by other tests when prior semen analyses have not revealed the problem. This test can also be used for medicolegal reasons in rape legal cases, but the specimen collection must be witnessed in these instances.

CLINICAL ALERT:
If this test is used for medicolegal reasons (e.g., rape), place the specimen in a sealed plastic bag and label it as legal evidence.

Consent Form: Not required

List of Equipment: Speculum; slide; coverslip; forceps or tuberculin syringe; Douglas pouch or other collection container

Test Procedure:
1. The client should be sexually abstinent for 3 days before the testing. *Allows for accurate representation of normal ejaculate.*
2. Intercourse should be performed without using a lubricant, and the woman should lie recumbent for 15–30 min after intercourse. Then the woman must come to the area for testing within the next 5 hr. *It is critical for the cervix to be examined soon after intercourse. Cervix quality is the most affected by this time limitation, but the other values are also affected.*

FLUID ANALYSIS & SPUTUM

3. In the health care facility, the client is placed in a dorsal lithotomy position and draped. *Ensures privacy.*
4. The external cervical os is wiped clear of mucus, and an endocervical specimen is obtained by aspiration in a glass cannula, which is attached by a rubber tube to a syringe.

Clinical Implications and Indications:
1. Evaluates infertility
2. Evaluates rape cases for the presence of semen (note: a female health care provider should be with the client during this testing)
3. Evaluates intrauterine insemination (IUI)

Nursing Care:
Before Test: Explain the test procedure and the purpose of the test. Assess the client's knowledge of the test. A thorough explanation of the procedures is necessary. Ensure that the client understands the time frame that is necessary for coming to the health care setting after intercourse.
During Test: Adhere to standard precautions. Assist client into the lithotomy position.
After Test: Provide emotional support, particularly in the event of a rape.

Interfering Factors: Inability to maintain appropriate time frame

Nursing Considerations:
Rural: Clients who live great distances from the health care facility need to be encouraged to take necessary measures to ensure timely transport after intercourse.

Listing of Related Tests: Antisperm antibodies; acrosomal states; biochemical analyte measurements; cervical cultures; semen analysis

WEBLINKS

http://www.ihr.com; http://www.nlm.nih.gov

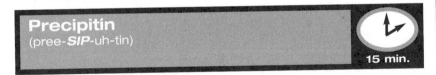

Precipitin
(pree-*SIP*-uh-tin)

15 min.

Type of Test: Fluid analysis

Body Systems and Functions: Reproductive system

Normal Findings: Negative findings

Test Results Time Frame: Within 8 hr

Test Description: Precipitin testing is performed after alleged or suspected rape to identify the presence of human semen or blood in the vagina. It is performed as soon as possible after the incident. A sample of the fluid in the vagina is mixed with antisera solution, causing an antigen/antibody reaction in the form of an insoluble precipitate if it is from a human source. An acid phosphatase test is performed due to the possibility of the attacker being infertile or sterile. Acid phosphatase is not normally present in vaginal secretions.

FLUID ANALYSIS & SPUTUM

Consent Form: Not required

List of Equipment: Rape examination tray (per institutional protocol, it may be a vaginal examination tray with speculum and normal saline)

Test Procedure:
1. State laws mandate strict procedure protocols that must be followed exactly. *The procedure constitutes legal evidence.*
2. Place client in the lithotomy position taking care to be sensitive and caring with client's emotional trauma and psychological state. *Client may still be very emotionally upset and vulnerable.*
3. After speculum is rinsed with normal saline and inserted, swab vaginal walls with nonabsorbent cotton swab.
4. Place specimen in sterile container and label. *Correctly identifies client and test. Usually signatures of witness are also required.*
5. State law may require specimen be given to the police, who forward it to a specialized laboratory. No delay should occur in getting the specimen to the laboratory or it should be frozen. *The presence of sperm is more easily identified in a fresh specimen.*

Clinical Implications and Indications:
1. Diagnoses presence of human blood or semen in vaginal canal
2. Diagnoses evidence of sexual intercourse

Nursing Care:
Before Test: Explain the test procedure and the purpose of the test. Assess the client's knowledge of the test. Instruct client to not douche before specimen is taken. Allow client to emotionally and psychologically adjust before beginning the physical examination. Provide crisis counseling immediately. Clothes must be saved for analysis of presence of semen.

During Test: Adhere to standard precautions. Provide caring support of client.

After Test: Refer client for continued counseling, continued gynecological follow-up for additional bruising, and education regarding outcomes of sexually transmitted diseases and pregnancy testing. HIV testing should be recommended over the following 6 months. If client is not on a contraceptive method, post-coital contraception should be offered and must be started within 24–72 hr of the incident. Other tests for evidence are collected, such as oral swabbing if fellatio occurred, combing of pubic hair for hair samples of the attacker, swabbing of thighs for semen of blood of the attacker, and fingernail scrapings for skin cells or blood.

Interfering Factors: Improper procedure in collecting specimen; inability of client to tolerate physical examination; douching before examination

Listing of Related Tests: Tests for sexually transmitted diseases (e.g., gonococcus and *Chlamydia* smears, serum VDRL, hepatitis B and C screen); pregnancy test; Pap smear; acid phosphatase

WEBLINKS

http://www.geocities.com

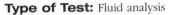

Semen Analysis

(**SEE**-m:n uh-**NAEL**-uh-sis)

(semen specimen; seminal fluid analysis; SFA)

15-30 min.

Type of Test: Fluid analysis

Body Systems and Functions: Reproductive system

Normal Findings:

Volume	≥2.0 mL; pH 7.2–7.7
Liquification	Within 30 min
Total sperm count	60–200 million
Motility	60%–80% actively motile
Morphology	70%–90% normal morphology
Viability	≥50% live
WBC	<1 million
Zinc	≥2.4 µmol per ejaculate
Citric acid	≥52 µmol per ejaculate
Fructose	≥13 µmol per ejaculate
MAR test	<10% spermatozoa with adherent particles
Immunobead test	<10% spermatozoa with adherent beads

Test Description: Semen analysis is usually part of an infertility work-up. Semen is the fluid that consists of sperm suspended in seminal plasma. It is composed of four main fractions that are contributed by the testis and epidymis, the seminal vesicle, the prostate gland, and the bulbourethral and urethral glands. In a semen analysis, the ejaculate is examined for quantity (concentration), morphology, motility, and fructose. Coagulation and liquefying properties are assessed. Viscosity, volume, pH, white blood cells, zinc, citric acid, and immunobeads are also examined.

Consent Form: Not required

List of Equipment: Sterile, leak-proof container (glass or nontoxic plastic)

Test Procedure:

1. Instruct client to be sexually abstinent for 2–5 days before the sample is collected. *Allows for accurate representation of normal ejaculate.*
2. Specimens may be collected at the laboratory or may be brought in by the client after collection outside the laboratory. If the client is not on site, he should notify the laboratory regarding the expected time for the sample to arrive. The sample must arrive within 1 hr of collection for adequate analysis. *It is critical for the specimen to be examined while it is fresh. Sperm motility is the most affected by this time limitation, but the other values are also affected.*
3. Semen specimens should be in a clean glass or nontoxic plastic container. The entire specimen is needed for analysis. *The analysis of ejaculate changes*

FLUID ANALYSIS & SPUTUM

from the initial secretions and the later secretions. Accuracy cannot be ensured if the entire sample is not collected.

4. Masturbation is the preferred method of collection. However, this method may not be acceptable to some clients. Specifically manufactured condoms, which are free of spermacides may be available. Coitus interruptus is least acceptable because some of the initial ejaculate may be lost and the sample may be contaminated by vaginal secretions.

5. If the sample is collected off-site, it must be transported at body temperature. *Ensures accurate results* (note: keeping the collected sample inside a shirt and close to the body will help to maintain the temperature).

Clinical Implications and Indications:

1. Sperm quality and quantity can be compromised by testicular trauma, inflammation (secondary to STDs, mumps, or other infection), and malignancies (e.g., leukemia, lymphoma).

2. Cryptorchidism (the failure of the testes to descend into the scrotal sac) results in elevating the temperature of the testes and compromising the sperm quality.

3. A number of congenital factors (such as Klinefelter's syndrome) can produce testicular dysfunction and subsequent changes in semen analysis.

4. It is important to get multiple samples 64–80 days apart to analyze sperm from different spermatogenic cycles.

Nursing Care:

Before Test: Explain the test procedure and the purpose of the test. Assess the client's knowledge of the test. Impress upon the client the importance of bringing the sample to the laboratory within 1 hr. If the client is unable to produce the sample on-site in the laboratory, it is necessary for him to be within a half hour of the laboratory in order to assure an adequate time to deliver the sample. An accurate history of prescription and recreational drugs, habits (such the regular use of hot tubs), injuries, and infections is important. For the evaluation of a vasectomy, instruct the client to ejaculate once or twice before the examination day.

During Test: Adhere to standard precautions. Provide adequate privacy for the collection of the specimen.

After Test: Instruct client to avoid excessive heat or cold when transporting specimen.

Interfering Factors: Recreational drugs (e.g., alcohol, opiates, marijuana); elevated scrotal temperature (this can be elevated from hot tubs, tight-fitting underwear, increased environmental temperature); inability to transport specimen in necessary time period; specimen not being kept at warm temperature;cimetidine decreases levels.

Nursing Considerations:

Home Care: The client must be within a half hour from the laboratory to ensure a fresh sample.

Rural: The client should arrange to stay close to the laboratory if he is unable to collect the specimen at the laboratory.

Listing of Related Tests: Antisperm antibodies; acrosomal states; Zonafree hamster ova penetration tests; biochemical analyte measurements; cervical mucous testing with the client's partner

WEBLINKS

http://www.ihr.com

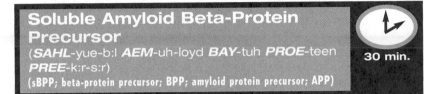

Soluble Amyloid Beta-Protein Precursor
(*SAHL*-yue-b:l *AEM*-uh-loyd *BAY*-tuh *PROE*-teen *PREE*-k:r-s:r)
(sBPP; beta-protein precursor; BPP; amyloid protein precursor; APP)

30 min.

Type of Test: Fluid analysis

Body Systems and Functions: Neurological system.

Normal Findings: Greater than 450 U/L based on ELISA

Test Results Time Frame: Within 24–48 hr

Test Description: Soluble amyloid beta-protein precursor is normally found in the cerebrospinal fluid of healthy individuals. Recently, Alzheimer's disease has been shown to have marked accumulations of soluble amyloid beta-protein precursor within the senile plaques of the brain. The sBBP has been shown to have both negative and positive effects as related to the neurological system. Therefore, this test is continuing to evolve as a diagnostic measurement of the cerebrospinal fluid.

Consent Form: Required

List of Equipment: CSF collection tray; lumbar puncture (LP) set; sterile gloves and gown; masks

Test Procedure:
1. Label collection tubes. *Correctly identifies the client and test to be performed.*
2. Follow the procedure for lumbar puncture and collection of CSF specimen for culture.
3. Transport promptly to laboratory.

Clinical Implications and Indications:
1. Decreased levels are associated with Alzheimer's disease as confirmed with autopsy-related Alzheimer's disease and with clinically diagnosed Alzheimer's disease.
2. The Alzheimer gene is located on chromosome 21, and defects of this gene are hereditary.
3. New therapeutics are on the horizon in treating Alzheimer's disease based on new findings on the relationship between soluble amyloid beta-protein precursor and plaque formation in the brain.

FLUID ANALYSIS & SPUTUM

Nursing Care:

Before Test: Explain the test procedure and the purpose of the test. Assess the client's knowledge of the test. Instruct client to have no solid foods for 12 hr prior to the LP; fluids are usually permitted up to 3 hr prior to the test. If coagulation disorder is suspected, client will have platelet count and prothrombin/partial thromboplastin time performed. Instruct client to empty bladder and bowel prior to test. Prepare LP set and assist client in lateral recumbent position along the edge of the bed with the knees flexed on the chest and chin touching the knees.

During Test: Adhere to standard precautions and strict aseptic technique. Assist client in maintaining lateral, recumbent position. Instruct client to lie very still and explain that movement may result in injury. Ask client to report any numbness, pain, or tingling in the legs (this may indicate nerve root damage or irritation). Apply band-aid over puncture site after lumbar needle is removed.

After Test: Maintain bedrest in prone position for 1–3 hr to minimize post-LP headache. Observe for potential complications and deterioration of mental status, sensory deficits, leg muscle weakness, or bowel or bladder incontinence or retention.

Potential Complications: Traumatic lumbar puncture tap; severe headache; infection

Contraindications: Increased intracranial pressure; cutaneous or osseous infection at site of the lumbar puncture

Interfering Factors: Inability to remain still

Nursing Considerations:

Pediatric: Infants and children will need assistance in remaining still during the procedure and age-appropriate comfort measures following the test.
Gerontology: The older person may find it difficult to maintain positions when required to do so for lengthy periods of time during the lumbar puncture.

Listing of Related Tests: Lumbar puncture

WEBLINKS

http://www.alzheimers.org

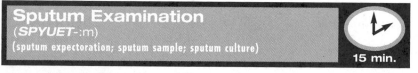

Sputum Examination
(*SPYUET*-:m)
(sputum expectoration; sputum sample; sputum culture)

15 min.

Type of Test: Sputum

Body Systems and Functions: Pulmonary system

Normal Findings: Negative pathogens in sputum

Test Results Time Frame: Within 24–48 hr

FLUID ANALYSIS & SPUTUM

Test Description: Expectorated sputum allows for examination of the lower respiratory tract secretions. There are a variety of substances that are pathogenic and develop within sputum secretions. Two such examples are fungi and *Mycobacterium*. Fungi are slow-growing eukaryotic organisms that can grow on living or nonliving organisms and are subdivided into molds and yeasts. Only a few of them grow in humans, and when they infect the respiratory system, they can cause serious infections. Mycobacteria are aerobic bacteria that resist decolorizing chemical after staining (acid fast). Mycobacteria are capable of producing a variety of diseases, such as *Mycobacterium tuberculosis*. Overall, sputum specimens are observed for mucopurulent strands, leukocytes, and blood and culture results.

CLINICAL ALERT:
Sputum may be induced if the client is unable to produce an expectorated sample. However, if saline nebulization is used, it is imperative to use saline that contains no bacteriostatic agents that would contaminate the sample.

Consent Form: Not required

List of Equipment: Sterile, leak-proof container

Test Procedure:
1. It is most desirable to obtain an early-morning expectorated specimen. *First morning specimen is most concentrated and is less likely to be contaminated with saliva and nasopharyngeal secretions.*
2. Before beginning collection, ask the client to rinse the mouth with plain water. *Removes secretions and oral plaque, which may contaminate the sample.*
3. Instruct the client to breathe deeply to stimulate coughing and expectoration. *Loosens the secretions enough to expectorate.*
4. Collect the expectorated sputum in a leak-proof sterile container. Refrigerate the container until processing takes place. *Sterility is important for culture results. Refrigeration slows other bacterial growth.*
5. Do not pool multiple samples in a 24-hr period. The client should be instructed to avoid adding saliva or nasopharyngeal secretions to the sputum sample. *Avoids contamination of the sample.*

Clinical Implications and Indications:
1. Most often, sputum is collected from clients with suspected pneumonia. Bronchoscopy, suction, and direct lung aspiration or biopsy can also be used to obtain samples.
2. It is necessary to collect the first sample before any antibiotic or antimicrobial therapy is initiated.
3. Results of smears and cultures can sometimes be difficult to interpret, because even with the most desirable specimens, some contamination from the oral flora occurs.
4. Gram stain is one of the most helpful tools in examining the sputum.
5. Induced specimens are usually inferior to the expectorated ones because they can be more dilute.

Nursing Care:
Before Test: Explain the test procedure and the purpose of the test. Assess the client's knowledge of the test. Instruct the client to try to produce the first

FLUID ANALYSIS & SPUTUM

specimen in the morning. If antimicrobial therapy is imminent, then the nurse should try to obtain a specimen as soon as possible. Obtain a recent history and a record of previous vaccinations.

During Test: Adhere to standard precautions.

Interfering Factors: Lack of nebulizing solution; unable to obtain secretions in the morning; insufficient secretions for testing

Nursing Considerations:

Gerontology: Many older people get more severely compromised with lower respiratory tract infections. Early diagnosis and treatment are essential. Vaccination for pneumonia is possible.

International: There are a greater variety of organisms that grow internationally and therefore increase the possibility of types of pathogens and the need to know which ones are specific to an area.

Listing of Related Tests: Bronchoscopy; lung biopsy

WEBLINKS

http://www.lungusa.org; http://www.multiplan.com

Sweat Test
(swet)
(pilocarpine Iontophoresis)

1 hr 15 min.

Type of Test: Fluid analysis

Body Systems and Functions: Integumentary system

Normal Findings:

Sweat sodium   16–46 mmol/L or mEq/L

Sweat chloride 8–43 mmol/L or mEq/L

Test Results Time Frame: Within 24 hr

Test Description: The sweat test is used to diagnose cystic fibrosis by looking for high levels of sodium and chloride in a child's sweat. Sweat is induced and analyzed chemically for sodium and chloride content. Sweat is a colorless, slightly turbid, salty, aqueous fluid that contains urea, fatty substances, and sodium chloride. Sweat is controlled by the sympathetic nervous system through the secretory fibers that supply the sweat glands.

CLINICAL ALERT:
Sweat potassium is not valuable diagnostically; test is used to exclude diagnosis of cystic fibrosis in siblings of persons with cystic fibrosis.

Consent Form: Not required

List of Equipment: Gauze pads or filter paper saturated with pilocarpine; electrodes to deliver a current of 4–5 mA; distilled water; sweat-collecting cups; flask; suction capillary tubes

Test Procedure:

1. Forearm (thigh back or leg in small babies) is prepared for the test. *Most surface area available in these areas.*
2. Room is to be warm or warm coverings should be placed over the collecting site. *Cool room decreases sweating and interferes with test.*
3. Pilocarpine-saturated filter paper or gauze pads are applied over the area. *Stimulates sweating.*
4. Electrodes are situated to deliver 4–5 mA at set intervals for 5 min. An area of red about 2.5 cm in diameter should be present. *Electrical impulses increase absorption of pilocarpine into the skin.*
5. Electrodes and pads are removed and the area cleaned with distilled water and dried. *Prepares area for collection of sweat specimen.*
6. Preweighed filter paper or sweat-collecting cups are secured over the red spot. Be careful not to touch the insides of the collecting device. Filter paper absorbs sweat most readily. *Contamination will interfere with the test.*
7. If paper used, it is removed after 1 hr and placed in a preweighed flask. If cups were used, they are also removed after 1 hr and suction capillary tubes are used to remove the sweat from the cups. *It takes approximately 1 hr to collect enough sweat for analysis.*
8. The filter paper or suction capillary tubes are sent to the laboratory for analysis. *Sweat is analyzed in the laboratory by medical technologists.*

Clinical Implications and Indications:

1. Sodium and chloride values greater than 60 mEq/L (mmol/L) indicate the presence of cystic fibrosis in children.
2. Sodium and chloride values between normal and 60 mEq/L are considered boderline and should be retested.
3. Chloride levels over 80 mEq/L indicate cystic fibrosis in adolescents and adults.

Nursing Care:

Before Test: Explain the test procedure and the purpose of the test. Assess the client's knowledge of the test. Inform client that they may experience a slight stinging sensation at the test site.

During Test: Adhere to standard precautions. Keep area warm and paper or cups protected.

After Test: Wash and dry the area thoroughly. Normal skin care and activity can be resumed. If results are indicative of cystic fibrosis, prepare the family for genetic counseling.

Potential Complications: Irritation and itching at test site

Interfering Factors: Dehydration; edema; a gap between sodium and chloride levels of more than 30 mmol/L indicates analysis error or contamination; false positives are caused by Addison's disease, congenital adrenal hyperplasia, diabetes insipidus, glucose-6-phosphatase deficiency, and glycogen storage disease.

Nursing Considerations:

Pediatric: Care providers must provide counseling referrals and continued follow-up for clients that test positive for cystic fibrosis.

FLUID ANALYSIS & SPUTUM

WEBLINKS

www.cff.org; www2.medsch.wisc.edu

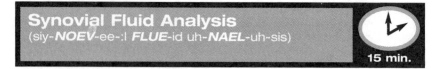

Type of Test: Fluid analysis

Body Systems and Functions: Musculoskeletal system

Normal Findings: Transparent fluid with <200 WBC and <25% neutrophils

Test Results Time Frame: Within 24 hr

Test Description: Synovial fluid analysis is a microscopic test of synovial fluid for clarity, white blood cell count, and percent of neutrophils. It is used primarily in the diagnosis of rheumatic disease and infections. Synovial fluid is a clear viscid lubricating fluid of the joint, bursa, and tendon sheaths. The synovial fluid is secreted by the synovial membrane of a joint and contains albumin, electrolytes, fat, and mucin.

Consent Form: Required

List of Equipment: Sterile towels; sterile needle with syringe; betadine; local anesthetic; gauze squares; sterile specimen container

Test Procedure:
1. Position joint with pillows. *Enhances visualization of aspiration site and for client comfort.*
2. Clean joint with betadine solution. *Reduces chance of infection.*
3. Local anesthetic is injected and needle is inserted. *Decreases level of discomfort during synovial fluid aspiration and obtains synovial fluid for examination.*
4. Remove needle and apply pressure to the knee. *Decreases bleeding or leaking.*
5. Place the synovial fluid in sterile specimen container and send to the laboratory.

Clinical Implications and Indications:
1. Noninflammatory disease is present when the fluid is transparent, WBC count is <2,000, and neutrophils are <25% of the WBCs.
2. Inflammatory disease is present when the fluid is transparent, WBC count is <75,000, and neutrophils are >50% of WBCs.
3. Sepsis is diagnosed when the fluid is opaque, WBC count is >75,000, and neutrophils are >75% of WBCs.

Nursing Care:
Before Test: Explain the test procedure and the purpose of the test. Assess the client's knowledge of the test.
During Test: Adhere to standard precautions. Provide reassurance and a calm atmosphere during the procedure.

After Test: Secure dressing over aspiration site. Evaluate client's level of comfort and offer analgesia as necessary.

Potential Complications: Bleeding, bruising, and swelling of the joint; infection

Nursing Considerations:
Pediatric: Infants and children will need assistance in remaining still during the procedure and age-appropriate comfort measures following the test.
Gerontology: The older person may find it difficult to maintain positions when required to do so for lengthy periods of time during the synovial fluid testing. In addition, elderly persons are at risk for joint pathology and therefore may have specific need of synovial fluid analysis testing.
Rural: Advisable to arrange for transportation home after recovering from the synovial fluid analysis.

WEBLINKS

http://medlineplus.adam.com; http://uwcme.org

Thoracentesis
(*THOER*-uh-sen-*TEE*-sis)
(pleural fluid aspiration; pleural fluid tap)

30 min.

Type of Test: Fluid analysis

Body Systems and Functions: Pulmonary system

Normal Findings: Normal visualization of pleural cavity and no abnormal fluid or air in pleural cavity

Test Results Time Frame: Within 24 hr

Test Description: A thoracentesis is the insertion of a needle into the thoracic cavity for the purposes of withdrawing fluid from the pleural space. The fluid could be for drainage purposes or the fluid could be sent to the laboratory for microscopic examination. A thoracentesis is also performed to insert medication into the pleural space.

> **CLINICAL ALERT:**
> If large amount of fluid is drained, client may experience shortness of breath.

Consent Form: Required

List of Equipment: Thoracentesis kit (betadine, thoracentesis needle, syringe, gauze square, sterile towels); local anesthetic; sterile specimen container(s); pressure dressing

FLUID ANALYSIS & SPUTUM

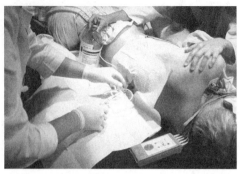

Thoracentesis

Test Procedure:

1. Place client in upright position. *Allows for maximum chest expansion.*
2. Assist with client position during thoracentesis. *Helps client to avoid moving and causing complications.*
3. Clean area with betadine and administer local anesthetic in area of thoracentesis needle insertion. *Helps with pain management and to minimize discomfort.*
4. Insertion of needle into pleural space and aspiration of pleural fluid. *Large-bore needle is used to obtain adequate amount of specimen.*
5. After needle is withdrawn, apply pressure to the area. *Pressure decreases risk of bleeding and pleural fluid leakage.*
6. Chest x-ray is obtained. *Check for pneumothorax.*

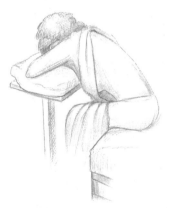

Patient Positioning

Clinical Implications and Indications:

1. High numbers of mesothelial cells indicate a chronic condition.
2. Abnormalities in serous fluid include degenerating red blood cells and red blood cell fragments, which indicate injury to a vessel.
3. Mucin is suggestive of adenocarcinoma.
4. A large number of leukocytes indicates an acute inflammatory process such as pleuritis.
5. Any abnormal cells may be indicative of inflammatory conditions or cancer.

Nursing Care:

Before Test: Explain the test procedure and the purpose of the test. Assess the client's knowledge of the test. May give sedative 20–30 min prior to the test. Obtain vital signs prior to the test. Prepare local anesthetic as ordered. Instruct client not to cough or talk during the procedure.

During Test: Adhere to standard precautions. Provide emotional reassurance throughout the procedure. Observe client's respiratory pattern and oxygenation status.

After Test: Obtain chest x-ray to assess for pneumothorax. Instruct client to remain still during the x-ray; there are no dietary restrictions prior to the test; and it is necessary to remove dental prosthesis, jewelry, eyeglasses, or other metal objects like hair clips before the procedure. Assess thoracentesis site dressing for excessive bleeding or drainage. Monitor client's comfort level and respiratory effort.

Potential Complications: Bleeding at puncture site; pain at puncture site; pneumothorax; shortness of breath

Contraindications: X-rays are usually avoided during pregnancy unless the benefit to the fetus outweighs the potential risk.

Interfering Factors: Vigorous shaking of specimen

Nursing Considerations:

Pediatric: Sedation is recommended for infants and children. Place the infant or child on a blanket for comfort. After postprocedure monitoring is completed and per health care provider's order, the pediatric client is discharged with an adult who is given instructions.

Listing of Related Tests: Chest x-ray

WEBLINKS

http://medline.cos.com

FLUID ANALYSIS & SPUTUM

11

Physical Examination, Manometric, Sensation, and Breath Studies

PHYSICAL EXAMINATION, MANOMETRIC, SENSATION, AND BREATH TESTS

This chapter covers a wide variety of tests, including such tests as visual acuity, pulmonary capacity, and cold stimulation. Most of the tests in this chapter are studies of specific organs or systems. These tests are performed to either test physiological function or to provide a diagnosis for an alteration within the body system.

Physical Examination Testing

Physical examination testing involves checking physical structures and responses to stimuli of the client. The health care provider learns to assess the normal

687

structure and function of the human body. Then the examiner applies that knowledge in working with clients and looking for the presence of abnormality. Examples of physical examination tests are otoscopy, refraction, tourniquet test, and visual acuity. Every system of the body has its identifying "tests" that can be explored by the health care provider. For example, the tourniquet test applies pressure to the arm to check for capillary fragility. The examiner follows the procedures of the physical examination and learns what changes in capillary fragility mean in regard to diagnosis of dysfunction.

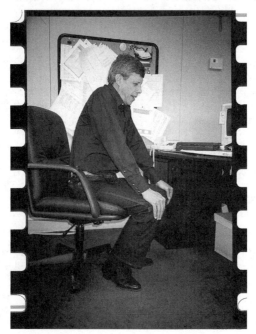

Client correctly positioned whil experiencing slight shortness of breath.

Manometric Testing

Manometric tests check the amount of pressure within a vessel or an organ. Many of these tests involve the use of specialized equipment and are not "typical" tests that are used routinely when examining clients. That is, the manometric tests are often performed after clinical manifestations are evidenced and further assessment and diagnostic information are needed by the health care provider towards the need to perform one of the manometric tests. Examples of manometric tests are cystometry, tonometry, and plethysmography. These tests confirm the function of a specific body system and provide diagnostic information that potentially leads to possible therapies for alterations.

Sensation Testing

Sensation testing involves assessing the physiological response to the application of different temperatures. These sensation tests can use cold stimulation and thermography. Examples of sensation tests are Raynaud's cold stimulation and spinal nerve root thermography. Special equipment is necessary to measure the response of skin and body temperatures to stimuli. The client responses assist in confirming the presence of specific pathophysiology. These tests are employed for the exploration and assessment of specific clinical disorders and would not be performed as a routine physical examination.

Breath Testing

Breath tests are relatively noninvasive tests, which involve collecting breath or measuring breath functions. The breath that is collected can be analyzed for various substances, such as lactose tolerance, methacholine challenge, and urea. Breath functions can measure specific pulmonary functions of the respiratory system. Breath testing is performed for specific diagnostic capabilities when suspected alterations are present in a client. Many of these breath tests require specialized equipment and may be performed in special studies laboratories or clinics. The health care provider would likely have specific education and training to allow their use of the diagnostic equipment.

CLIENT PREPARATION FOR PHYSICAL EXAMINATION, MANOMETRIC, SENSATION, AND BREATH TESTS

Physical Examination Testing

Physical examination testing tends to be painless and quickly accomplished. Prepare clients by letting them know what the test will involve and provide any needed reassurance. If the specific physical examination requires a certain positioning of the client, use good body mechanics and appropriate personnel to safely and efficiently accomplish the correct client position (see Figure). Sometimes, the condition of the client makes movement uncomfortable and special care during the physical examination is necessary.

Manometric Testing

Measuring pressures within the body may entail the insertion of a device to measure the pressure, for example into the bladder or vessel. Other tests, such as tonometry or plethysmography, are noninvasive. Tension or anxiety can increase pressure, so client reassurance and comfort are essential.

Sensation Testing

Sensation tests are noninvasive and do not invoke pain. Clients need to be reassured that the test will involve, at most, minor discomfort. Since the tests measure blood flow to an area, make certain that clients have refrained from smoking for several hours prior to the sensation test.

Breath Testing

Breath tests are relatively noninvasive and usually do not elicit a painful response. Since many different substances may be excreted in the breath, verify whether it is necessary for the client to fast for a specific time period. Then check the client's intake for the past 4 to 12 hours prior to the breath test. The pulmonary function tests may cause some shortness of breath during the testing and appropriate reassurance and positioning are necessary for the client. In addition, some pulmonary function tests may be performed with the use of bronchoinhalant medications. The specific effects of these medications need attention from the health care provider.

Life Span Implications for Physical Examination, Manometric, Sensation and Breath Testing

Most of these tests can be done on people of any age. Collecting breath requires cooperation and may not be possible on a very young child. Some manometric tests require a patient to remain very still and may only be possible with light sedation for a young child.

Nursing Diagnoses for Physical Examination, Manometric, Sensation and Breath Testing

Two common nursing diagnoses for these tests are (1) knowledge deficit related to the test procedure and (2) anxiety related to the test or to a potential outcome. Most of these tests, however, are not for life-threatening illnesses, and simple reassurance will probably be very effective prior to and during the testing. Teaching clients why a test will be done, what the test will involve, and what results to expect will help the client to manage their own health and health care decisions.

Bile Salt Absorption
(biyl sahlt uhb-*ZOERP*-sh:n)
(bile salt breath test; C-14 cholate breath test)

72 hr.

Type of Test: Breath; stool

Body Systems and Functions: Hepatobiliary system

Normal Findings: Negative breath test and negative stool specimen

Test Results Time Frame: Within 24 hr after the stool specimen collection

Test Description: Bile salt absorption is a test for diseases of bile acid malabsorption. Normally, bile salts are reabsorbed in the intestinal tract before reaching the colon. In a diseased state, some unabsorbed bile salts reach the colon and are oxidized by bacteria. Abnormal fecal fat excretion indicates a malabsorption of fats due the impaired synthesis of the bile salts. This test measures both the fecal fat excretion and the exhaled radioactive carbon dioxide released after C-14 triolein ingestion.

Consent Form: Not required

List of Equipment: Stool collection container; breath-testing equipment

PHYSICAL EXAMINATION, MANOMETRIC, SENSATION, BREATH

Test Procedure:
1. Collect and label 24-hr stool specimen. *Correctly identifies the client and the test to be performed.*
2. Gather baseline breath sample.
3. Ingest C-14 triolein test meal which contains 60 g of fat.
4. Take hourly breath samples.
5. Collect 72-hr stool sample.

Clinical Implications and Indications:
1. Assesses the bacterial overgrowth in the digestive tract, as well as diseases of the ileum, and the malabsorption of bile salts

Nursing Care:
Before Test: Explain the test procedure and the purpose of the test. Assess the client's knowledge of the test. Fast for 8 hr prior to test. Instruct client to discontinue antibiotics for 4 weeks prior to test. Obtain a history of the ingestion of H_2 receptor antagonists.

During Test: Adhere to standard precautions.

Interfering Factors: Diabetes mellitus; thyroid diseases; obesity; chronic lung disorders; hyperlipidemia; liver disease; H_2 receptor antagonists within previous 24 hr; antibiotic therapy

WEBLINKS ⊟⊠

http://adam.excite.com

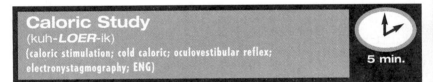

Caloric Study
(kuh-*LOER*-ik)
(caloric stimulation; cold caloric; oculovestibular reflex; electronystagmography; ENG)

5 min.

Type of Test: Physical examination

Body Systems and Functions: Neurological system

Normal Findings: A caloric study involves stimulation of the ear with cold water, which will cause rotary nystagmus away from the injected ear and back to the midline. When warm water is injected, there is rotary nystagmus toward the side of the irrigated ear canal and back to the midline, with an intact central nervous system (cerebral cortex). This response is seen for 1–3 min. If the client has a nonfunctioning cerebral cortex, the eyes will move toward the side of water injection and stay there for 1–3 min.

Test Results Time Frame: Immediate

Test Description: The caloric study involves irrigation of the ears with warm or cold water, which produces an irritation with a convection current in the inner ear (horizontal canal). This current stimulates the sensory mechanisms of the inner ear, which causes vertigo and nystagmus in an awake individual.

PHYSICAL EXAMINATION, MANOMETRIC, SENSATION, BREATH

In a comatose person, nystagmus will be produced if they have a functioning central nervous system (cerebral cortex). If the brain stem is the only working component of the brain, then the eyes will deviate toward the side of water injection and stay fixed towards that side of the head.

> **CLINICAL ALERT:**
> In comatose clients, someone will have to hold open the eyes in order to monitor for nystagmus. Cold water is usually used due to availability.

Consent Form: Not required

List of Equipment: Ice-cold water (0°C); 20-mL Luer-Lok syringe; 14- or 16-gauge angiocath (needle removed) cut to 3 cm; towels

Test Procedure:
1. Place client supine with head tilted 30° forward. *Brings horizontal canal into vertical plane.*
2. Place towels under client and on bed. *Helps to keep the client dry.*
3. Infuse 10 mL of ice-cold water into each ear and monitor for nystagmus.
4. Document procedure.

Clinical Implications and Indications:
1. Determines brain function in comatose individuals
2. Identifies brain stem inflammation, infarction, or tumor growth
3. Evaluates the vestibular and auditory systems in conscious clients

Nursing Care:
Before Test: Explain the test procedure and the purpose of the test. Assess the client's knowledge of the test. Clean ears of excessive cerumen. Instruct client to avoid tranquilizers, antivertigo medications, or alcohol 24 hr before the examination. Advise client to eat a light meal before procedure due to nausea. Have the client avoid caffeine and smoking on day of the test. Provide emotional support. *During Test:* Adhere to standard precautions. Monitor for bradycardia and vomiting.
After Test: Assess vital signs and provide emotional support to client's family.

Potential Complications: Vomiting; bradycardia

Contraindications: Tympanic membrane perforation; acute decrease of labyrinth function (i.e., Meniere's syndrome)

Interfering Factors: Cerumen

Nursing Considerations:
Pediatric: Infants and children will need assistance in remaining still during the caloric study and age-appropriate comfort measures following the test.

WEBLINKS

www.healthgate.com

Cystometry
(sis-*TAHM*-uh-tree)
(CMG; cystometrogram; urethral pressure measurments)

45 min.

Type of Test: Manometric

Body Systems and Functions: Renal/urological system

Normal Findings: Normal micturation, no residual urine, positive vesical sensation, normal volume of first urge to void (adult 150–200 mL), normal bladder capacity (adult male 350–750 mL, adult female 250–550 mL), absent bladder contractions, low intravesical pressure, positive bulbocavernosus reflex, positive saddle sensation, absent bethanechol test, positive ice water test, positive anal reflex, positive heat sensation and pain

Test Results Time Frame: Within 24–48 hr

Test Description: Cystometry is considered the cornerstone of urodynamic evaluation and involves the measurement of intravesical bladder pressure during bladder filling. Information concerning the bladder's capacity, compliance, sensation, and occurrence of involuntary contractions is obtained. The purpose of cystometry is to evaluate the detrusor muscle function and tonicity and to determine the cause of bladder dysfunction. A number of variables are measured during cystometry. Bladder access is obtained by urethral catheterization or rarely by placement of percutaneous suprapubic cystotomy tube. The filling medium may be carbon dioxide or fluid, such as saline or radiographic contrast material. If contrast material is used, a video-urodynamic study may be obtained. The temperature of fluid should be near or at body temperature. Cystometry may be performed with the client in the supine, seated, or standing position. A cystometer (a tube used to measure bladder pressure) is attached to the catheter and pressures and volumes are plotted on a graph. Supplemental cystometric tests include ice water test, bulbocavernosus reflex test, saddle sensation test, bethanechol sensitivity test, and stress incontinence test. The ice water test evaluates the integrity of vesicle reflex arc and differentiates upper from lower motor neuron lesions. The bulbocavernosus test determines the integity of the sacral portion of the spine. The saddle reflex test evaluates the reflex activity on conus medullaris. The bethanechol sensitivity test is performed to identify a neurogenic origin in the client with an acontractile bladder. The stress incontinence test evaluates loss of voluntary control of vesicourethral sphincters.

Consent Form: Required

List of Equipment: Cystometric equipment; irrigation solution

Test Procedure:
1. Ask the client to void and record the following data: time required to initiate voiding; size, force, and continuity of urinary stream; amount of urine; time of voiding; and presence of hesitancy or urine dribbling.
2. Place the client in a lithotomy or supine position. *Ensures accurate results.*
3. Insert retention catheter through the urethra and measure, record residual urine volume, and perform thermal sensation test.

PHYSICAL EXAMINATION, MANOMETRIC, SENSATION, BREATH

4. Connect cystometer to urethral catheter and instill fluid or gas into the bladder at a controlled rate with the client ideally in a standing position.
5. Ask the client to indicate the first urge to void and when the feeling that they must void is present, then ask client to void and measure and record maximal intravesical pressure.
6. Drain bladder for any residual urine and remove catheter if no additional studies are to be performed.
7. Measure urethral pressures while the catheter is withdrawn.

Clinical Implications and Indications:
1. Evaluates and monitors neurogenic bladder, urinary obstructions, and bladder hypertonicity
2. Determines decreased bladder capacity
3. Diagnoses prostatic obstruction and urinary incontinence

Nursing Care:
Before Test: Explain the test procedure and purpose of the test. Assess the client's knowledge of the test. Assess client for signs and symptoms of urinary tract infection. Clients who are catheter dependent should be placed on intermittent catheterization for a designated period of time before the test.
During Test: Adhere to standard precautions and sterile technique. Provide clear instructions. Drape client to avoid unnecessary exposure. Instruct client not to strain while voiding. Ask client to report any pain, flushing, sweating, nausea, sensation of bladder filling, and urgency to void.
After Test: Provide a warm sitz bath for comfort. Measure intake and output for 24 hr. Assess for hematuria and signs of sepsis.

Potential Complications: Sepsis

Contraindications: Urinary tract infection

Interfering Factors: Inability to follow instructions; antihistamines

Nursing Considerations:
Pediatric: Sedation is recommended for infants and children. Place the infant or child on a blanket for comfort. After postprocedure monitoring is completed and per health care provider's order, the pediatric client is discharged with an adult who is given instructions. Children require slow fill rates during cystometry. Up to 10 mL/min is considered physiological and is termed slow-fill cystometry.
Gerontology: The older person may find it difficult to maintain positions when required to do so during the cystometry.
Rural: Advisable to arrange for transportation home after recovering from the cystometry.

Listing of Related Tests: Cystourethrography; voiding cystourethrography

WEBLINKS

http://www.kumc.edu

Esophageal Acidity Test
(uh-*SAHF*-uh-*JEE*-:l ae-*SID*-uh-tee)
(Tuttle test)

30 min.

Type of Test: Manometric

Body Systems and Functions: Gastrointestinal system

Normal Findings: Esophageal pH >5.0; esophageal reflux pH <5.0

Test Results Time Frame: Immediate

Test Description: An esophageal acidity test assesses the esophageal sphincter's capability. A pH electrode measures the pH of gastric acid and the esophageal contents. The esophageal sphincter (cardiac sphincter) is a ring of smooth muscle that is the inlet to the stomach. It normally closes off the stomach from the esophagus and prevents reflux of contents.

CLINICAL ALERT:
Be prepared with emergency resuscitation equipment if client has vasovagal response.

Consent Form: Required

List of Equipment: Gastric catheter; pH electrode; 0.1% hydrochloride acid; IV initiation kit

Test Procedure:
1. Place client in sitting position
2. Insert gastric catheter with pH electrode through the mouth and have client swallow, perform the Valsalva maneuver, or lift the legs to stimulate reflux. *Allows measurement of pH.*
3. If pH is normal, pass catheter into stomach, instill 300 mL of 0.1% HCl for a 3-min period, and repeat pH testing.
4. Remove catheter.

Clinical Implications and Indications:
1. Evaluates and monitors gastroesophageal reflux

Nursing Care:
Before Test: Explain the test procedure and the purpose of the test. Assess the client's knowledge of the test. Instruct client to fast from midnight prior to test and to avoid smoking or drinking alcohol for 24 hr prior to test.
During Test: Adhere to standard precautions. Monitor for cardiac instability.
After Test: Assess vital signs frequently. Continue to evaluate for problems with vasovagal reaction.

Potential Complications: Aspiration; chemical bronchitis; vasovagal response

Contraindications: Cardiac instability

PHYSICAL EXAMINATION, MANOMETRIC, SENSATION, BREATH

Interfering Factors: Medications that decrease pH are antacids, anticholinergics, and cimetidine; medications that increase pH are adrenergic blockers, cholinergics, corticosteroids, ethanol, and reserpine.

Nursing Considerations:
Gerontology: Assess the client's cardiac status to see if he is at risk during this procedure. Evaluate for common clinical manifestations of congestive heart failure (peripheral edema, nocturnal dyspnea), or continuing symptomatology from previous myocardial infarction.

WEBLINKS

www.thriveonline.com

Exophthalmometry
(ek-*SAHF*-thael-*MAHM*-uh-tree)

30 min.

Type of Test: Physical examination

Body Systems and Functions: Sensory system

Normal Findings: 12–20 mm and eyes differ by <3 mm

Test Results Time Frame: Immediate

Test Description: Exophthalmometry is a test that measures the degree of forward protrusion of the eyeball. The exophthalmometer is a horizontal, calibrated bar that has movable 45° mirrors on both sides. Exophthalmos is a condition that accompanies hyperthyroidism and is characteristic of Graves' disease. The exophthalmic condition can dry the eyeball and potentially be damaging to the eye surface.

Consent Form: Not required

List of Equipment: Exophthalmometer

Test Procedure:
1. Place client in sitting position.
2. Measure each eye independently with the exophthalmometer and record results.
3. Repeat procedure with client's left eye fixated on the examiner's right eye.

Clinical Implications and Indications:
1. Evaluates and monitors cellulitis of the eye, hyperthyroidism, tumors of the eyes, endophthalmos, exophthalmos, periostitis, and retinoblastoma.
2. Steroid therapy causes exophthalmic condition.

Nursing Care:
Before Test: Explain the test procedure and the purpose of the test. Assess the client's knowledge of the test. Inform client that procedure is painless.
During Test: Adhere to standard precautions.

PHYSICAL EXAMINATION, MANOMETRIC, SENSATION, BREATH

Interfering Factors: Failure to set calibrated bar at baseline

Nursing Considerations:
Pediatric: Distraction techniques might be necessary for testing children.

WEBLINKS

http://health.excite.com

Methacholine Challenge
(*METH*-uh-*KOE*-leen *CHAEL*-:nj)
(bronchial provocation test; histamine challenge test; mecholyl challenge; mecholyl provocation test; methacholine provocation test; provocholine challenge)

1 hr.

Type of Test: Breath

Body Systems and Functions: Pulmonary system

Normal Findings: Minimal to no change in airway dynamics (FEV1 and/or FEF 25–75)

CRITICAL VALUES:
Positive response to inhaled antigen is >20% decrease in FEVI and/or >30% decrease in FEF 25–75.

Test Results Time Frame: Within 24–48 hr

Test Description: The methacholine challenge test identifies and characterizes the severity of nonspecific bronchial hypersensitivity or bronchospasm. This test is especially helpful in diagnosing cough-variant asthma or asthma in remission and the evaluation of the effectiveness of pharmacological agents used in the prevention of provoked bronchospasm.

CLINICAL ALERT:
Bronchospasm may occur during testing procedure.

Consent Form: Required

List of Equipment: Spirometer; mouthpiece; nose clip; gas nebulizers; 20-psi compressed gas source; dosimeter

Test Procedure:
1. Place client in sitting position. *Increases comfort level and orthopneic position.*
2. Client performs vital capacity test and FEV1 and FEF25–75 are recorded.
3. Client inhales methacholine chloride (usually 1.25 mg) via nebulizer, waits 5 min, and then repeats the FVC. If no response, the test may be repeated with increased doses of methacholine chloride.
4. Administer bronchodilator.

PHYSICAL EXAMINATION, MANOMETRIC, SENSATION, BREATH

Clinical Implications and Indications:

1. A positive response to methacholine or histamine supports the diagnosis of asthma.
2. A positive test may also occur with other diseases associated with bronchial activity, including COPD, bronchiolitis, viral upper respiratory infections, hay fever, cystic fibrosis, sarcoidosis, chemical irritant exposure, and recovery from adult respiratory distress syndrome.

Nursing Care:

Before Test: Explain the test procedure and the purpose of the test. Assess the client's knowledge of the test.
During Test: Adhere to standard precautions.
After Test: Administration of an aerosol bronchodilator and measurement of response to bronchodilator is performed on the client. Advise client that methacholine-induced bronchospasm will decline within 90 min.

Potential Complications: Severe bronchospasm

Contraindications: Severe restrictive or obstructive lung disease

Interfering Factors: Smoking; coffee; tea; cola; chocolate; significant exercise; exposure to cold air 2–48 hr prior to test; medications that alter results are sympathomimetic drugs, metaproterenol, terbutaline or salbutamol, methylxanthines, sustained-release methylxanthines, cromolyn sodium, and corticosteroids.

Nursing Considerations:

Pediatric: There is a high incidence of asthma in children, and therefore this test may be a performed with some frequency in this age population.

Listing of Related Tests: Allergy testing; bedside spirometry; flow volume loop; ingestion challenge test; spirometry

WEBLINKS

http://www.rcjournal.com

Oculoplethysmograph, Oculopneumoplethysmograph
(*AHK*-yue-loe-ple-*THIZ*-muh-graef *AHK*-yue-loe-*NUE*-moe-ple-*THIZ*-muh-graef)
(OPG; OPG-Gee; OPPG; ocular pressures)

30 min.

Type of Test: Manometric

Body Systems and Functions: Cardiovascular system

Normal Findings: *OPG:* Pulses occur in both eyes and ears simultaneously. *OPG-Gee:* Pressures in the eyes should not differ by more than 5 mm Hg, and eye pressure divided by arm pressure should not exceed 0.67.

Test Results Time Frame: Within 1–3 days

Test Description: Oculoplethysmography (OPG) provides an indirect measure of blood flow through the internal carotid artery by measuring blood flow through the opthalmic artery (the first major branch of the internal carotid). The earlobes receive their blood supply from the external carotid artery. Pulse arrival times are compared between the eyes and ears and should be the same. If stenosis of the internal carotid is occurring, then blood flow to the eye will be slower than to the ear. With oculopneumoplethysmography (OPG-Gee), eye and brachial pressures are compared following application of negative pressure to the sclera.

Consent Form: Required

List of Equipment: Specialized ocular pressure measurement equipment; blood pressure equipment; ECG equipment

Test Procedure:

Oculoplethysmography:

1. Have client remove contact lenses if applicable.
2. Place the client in supine postion on the bed or examination table.
3. Take blood pressures on both arms and apply ECG leads to client's extremities. *Establishes baseline data at time of test.*
4. Anesthetic eyedrops are applied to both eyes. *Minimizes discomfort of application of eyecups and suction.*
5. Apply photoelectric cells to earlobes. *Measures blood flow from external carotid artery.*
6. Apply eyecups to the cornea. Some laboratories differentiate between vacuum being applied (OPG-Gee) and not applied (OPG).
7. Recordings are made of pulsations in eyes and ears and comparisons are made between readings.

Variation for oculopneumoplethysmography:

1. Apply air-filled suction cups to anesthetized sclera and exert a negative pressure of 300–500 mm Hg. *Raises intraocular pressure, which, when it exceeds the ophthalmic systolic pressure, will stop blood flow.*
2. Release the vacuum slowly and record the point when pulsation returns. *This is the ophthalmic systolic arterial pressure.*
3. Compare the systolic pressures measured from the eye to the client's highest brachial systolic pressure, which is taken at the same time. *Significant pressures pointing to stenosis are a difference of 5 mm or more in the ophthalmic pressures or the difference between the ophthalmic and brachial systolics, which is calculated by dividing eye pressure by arm pressure.*

Clinical Implications and Indications:

1. Diagnoses carotid athersclerotic stenosis in clients with associated symptoms of dizziness, ataxia, syncope, and carotid bruits
2. Provides optional follow-up monitoring of clients who have had carotid endarterectomy

Nursing Care:

Before Test: Explain the test procedure and the purpose of the test. Assess the client's knowledge of the test. Instruct client that test may be performed by technician, nurse, or doctor and can be done in specified laboratories, the physician's office, or a hospital. Ascertain that client with glaucoma has taken their usual eye drops.

PHYSICAL EXAMINATION, MANOMETRIC, SENSATION, BREATH

During Test: Adhere to standard precautions.

After Test: Reassure client that slight burning of the eyes is common. Instruct client that after the eyecups are removed, the eyes may appear bloodshot for several hours, and there may be some blurring of vision for the first ½ hr. Remind client not to insert contact lenses or rub eyes for as long as the eyes are burning (minimum 2 hr posttest). Client may use artificial tears to reduce discomfort and should wear sunglasses if experiencing any photophobia. Instruct client to report severe burning or pain.

Potential Complications: Temporary photophobia; corneal abrasion; conjunctival hemorrhage

Contraindications: Eye surgery within last 6 months; uncontrolled glaucoma; client with one eye; cataracts; conjunctivitis; retinal detachment; lens implant; allergy to local anesthetic

Interfering Factors: Client is uncooperative, disoriented, or suffers from uncontrolled movement disorder; anticoagulants; hypertension

Nursing Considerations:
Pediatric: Infants and children will need assistance in remaining still during the procedure and age-appropriate comfort measures following the test.
Rural: *Advisable to arrange for transportation home after recovering from procedure.*

Listing of Related Tests: Doppler studies; B-scan ultrasound, arteriography

WEBLINKS

HTTP://webmd.lycos.com

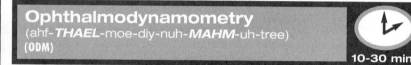

Ophthalmodynamometry
(ahf-*THAEL*-moe-diy-nuh-*MAHM*-uh-tree)
(ODM)

10-30 min.

Type of Test: Manometric

Body Systems and Functions: Cardiovascular system

Normal Findings: Normal retinal circulation or minimal retinal artery pulsation; difference of 20% or less between measurement of left and right sides

Test Results Time Frame: Immediate

Test Description: Ophthalmodynamometry involves the application of gentle pressure on the lateral aspect of the eye along with a concurrent examination with the ophthalmoscope. The overall goal is to determine whether there is impeded retinal circulation or pulsation of the central retinal artery. This is consistent with carotid artery stenosis but will only be detected if the artery is stenosed 50% or more. As a result of this test's limited sensitivity, the examiner is likely to choose other methods of carotid artery assessment. Another test may be done digitally or by exerting pressure with a spring-loaded plunger (requires two examiners).

Consent Form: Not required

List of Equipment: Ophthalmoscope

Test Procedure:
1. Dilate the client's pupils and instill a topical anesthetic.
2. Exert pressure on the sclera with the spring-loaded plunger.
3. An additional examiner observes the optic disc with indirect ophthalmoscope.
4. Note pulsation of the central retinal artery and then read diastolic pressure at the beginning of the pulsations, and read the systolic pressure at the time the pulsations cease.
5. Perform this technique on both sides and compare results (note: the digital method is less sophisticated in that the examiner watches for blocks in retinal circulation changes or the artery pulsating but does not take specific measurements).

Clinical Implications and Indications:
1. Diagnoses carotid artery stenosis.
2. Current research is determining whether this test can accurately assess space motion sickness related to increased intracranial pressures.

Nursing Care:
Before Test: Explain the test procedure and the purpose of the test. Assess the client's knowledge of the test. Reassure client that only gentle pressure will be applied to the eyeball and that the procedure will be over quickly. Instruct client to remove contact lenses.
During Test: Adhere to standard precautions.
After Test: Inform client that if dilating drops have been used, they may experience several hours of photophobia and blurred reading vision.

Contraindications: Eye surgery within last 6 months; client with one eye; cataracts; retinal detachment; lens implant

Interfering Factors: Improper placement of spring device reducing chance of reproducible results; movement of the eyeball during testing; inexperienced examiner not identifying pressure endpoints correctly

Nursing Considerations:
Pediatric: Infants and children will need assistance in remaining still during the procedure and age-appropriate comfort measures following the test (note: this test is not performed often on this age).
Rural: Advisable to arrange for transportation home after recovering from procedure (due to the dilating medications).

Listing of Related Tests: Oculopneumoplethysmography; carotid duplex scan; arteriography

WEBLINKS

http://www.med.harvard.edu/AANLIB/hms1.html

PHYSICAL EXAMINATION, MANOMETRIC, SENSATION, BREATH

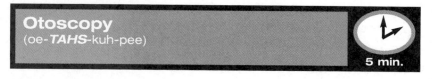

Otoscopy
(oe-*TAHS*-kuh-pee)

5 min.

Type of Test: Physical examination

Body Systems and Functions: Sensory system

Normal Findings: *External canal*: pink, minimal cerumen, hair in outer third of canal, no lesions, discharge, swelling. *Tympanic membrane*: intact, translucent, pearly grey (red if prolonged crying), slightly concave, flutters with insufflation, cone-shaped light reflex prominent at 5 o'clock in the right ear and 7 o'clock in the left, can visualize malleus.

Test Results Time Frame: Immediate

Test Description: Otoscopy is a physical examination technique that allows the visualization of the external canal of the ear and the middle ear. The otoscope is used and allows a lighted examination of the ear. The examiner develops expertise with use and a variety of disorders are able to be detected. The most common incidence of pathology are inflammatory conditions that are readily diagnosed.

Consent Form: Not required

List of Equipment: Otoscope; speculum

Test Procedure:

1. Choose the largest size of speculum that will fit comfortably in the client's ear canal.
2. Hold the otoscope upside down and along the fingers so that the outer side of the hand will be braced along the client's cheek during the examination. *Prevents damage to the client's ear canal if they move their head suddenly and also steadies the examiner's hand.*
3. Tilt the client's head slightly away from the examiner and pull the pinna up and back using the thumb and index finger. Maintain traction throughout the examination. *Positions the eardrum and straightens the canal for better visualization.*
4. Insert the otoscope slowly and examine the external canal. Reposition the client's head if only the canal wall is seen. Sometimes more traction is required. Avoid putting pressure on the inner two-thirds of the bony walls of the auditory canal. *Causes pain.*
5. Examine the tympanic membrane and there may be a need to rotate the otoscope slightly. *Allows access to full view of the eardrum.*
6. To perform insufflation, ask the client to swallow with nose pinched or to forcibly exhale with nose pinched and mouth closed (Valsalva manuever). Alternately, a pneumatic attachment to the otoscope can be used by providing gentle positive and negative pressure through puffing/sucking on the tube or squeezing the attached bulb. Watch for slight flutter of tympanic membrane. *Assesses eardrum mobility.*
7. Inspect for normal/abnormal parameters of drum and external canal.

Clinical Implications and Indications:

1. Assesses status of client as part of a general physical examination
2. Identifies infection sites, foreign bodies, or lesions in the external ear canal
3. Identifies variations from the norm of the tympanic membrane and malleus, such as amber or red color of eardrum or bubbles behind it caused by chronic or acute otitis media; bluish drum caused by blood behind eardrum consistent with head injury; dense white patch on drum caused by scarring from repeated ear infections; light reflex absent or landmarks difficult to find caused by a thickened drum due to otitis media or otitis externa; and malleus prominent caused by retraction of the drum consistent with obstructed eustachian tube

Nursing Care:

Before Test: Explain the test procedure and the purpose of the test. Assess the client's knowledge of the test. Instruct client to sit at a comfortable height for the examiner. Ask the client to hold head still throughout the examination.
During Test: Adhere to standard precautions. It is possible to explain findings to the client as the test is performed.
After Test: Ask client if he has any questions or concerns.

Contraindications: The insufflation portion of the examination is avoided for persons with upper respiratory infection since it may result in movement of infectious material into the middle ear.

Interfering Factors: Poor technique of otoscope insertion or insufflation; auditory canal obscured by excess cerumen

Nursing Considerations:

Pediatric: The pinna is pulled down and out and the speculum directed upward in children younger than 3 years of age. Restraint may be required to prevent injury and enhance visualization. Since this will likely cause the child to be combative, it should be left to the end if it is part of a full physical examination. Otoscopy is not usually performed on the newborn (for the first few days of birth) because the canal is usually filled with amniotic fluid and/or vernix caseosa. When the newborn is examined, it can be anticipated that the eardrum will be harder to visualize since the eardrum will be more horizontal (up to 1 month of age).
Home Care: Inexpensive otoscopes may be purchased and are sometimes used in the home setting. Instructions should be given to family members and nonskilled health care providers as to the safe use of these devices.

WEBLINKS

http://www.mic.ki.se/Diseases/c10.html

Oximetry
(ahk-*SIM*-uh-tree)
(pulse oximetry; ear oximetry; oxygen saturation; SaO_2)

5 min.

Type of Test: Physical examination (photodiagnostic)

Body Systems and Functions: Pulmonary system

Normal Findings: 96%–100%

Test Results Time Frame: Immediate

Test Description: Oximetry is used to monitor oxygen saturation of arterial blood noninvasively. The sensor that is attached to the finger, earlobe, or toe emits beams of red and infrared light that passes through the pulsing capillary bed, and the amount of light absorbed by the oxygenated hemoglobin is recorded. The monitor then displays the absorption rate in percentages of oxygen saturation (SaO_2). Pulse oximetry is never used in isolation as a determinant of poor oxygenation but should be viewed as an adjunct to direct observation and assessment.

CLINICAL ALERT:
Pulse oximetry will register false high readings if carboxyhemoglobin has occurred. Blood gas analysis will be necessary to assess client.

Consent Form: Not required

List of Equipment: Oxygen saturation monitor; sensor

Test Procedure:
1. Choose the site (e.g., earlobe, index finger) based on best perfusion (do not use thumb or digits that are edematous).
2. Once a location is chosen, and if circulation still appears poor, massage or apply a warm towel to site. *Increases blood flow to the site.*
3. The sensor is attached to the site and the oxygen saturation monitor is operationalized.
4. The reading is taken and is displayed on the monitor.

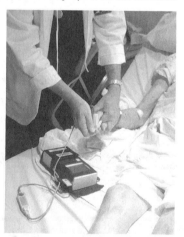

Oximetry Testing

Clinical Implications and Indications:
1. Monitors for levels on perioperative and postoperative clients
2. Evaluates individuals with respiratory compromise due to disease process or response to medication randomly, intermittently, or continuously

PHYSICAL EXAMINATION, MANOMETRIC, SENSATION, BREATH

3. Evaluates oxygen therapy involved in mechanical ventilation
4. Assesses various diagnostic testing, such as sleep studies and stress tests

Nursing Care:

Before Test: Explain the test procedure and the purpose of the test. Assess the client's knowledge of the test. Instruct client to remove any fingernail polish if applying sensor to finger. Assess client's fingernails, and if extremely long or if the client is wearing artificial nails, which are difficult to remove, use the wrap-around style of sensor versus the clip sensor. With artificial nails, the best site is the nail bed. Ensure that you have access to the right type of sensor for the right body part (e.g., ear, finger, forehead tapes). Remind client that there is no discomfort with this test. Warm sensor site prior to applying if peripheral circulation appears compromised (e.g., massage or warm towel).

During Test: Adhere to standard precautions. Ensure that the sensor signals line up when using the wrap-around tape style of sensor and that the sensor sites on any device are clean.

After Test: Clients with burns or prolonged use should have the sensor device removed after readings or sites rotated frequently when continuously monitoring.

Contraindications: Prolonged probe-skin contact for the client who is hypothermic or hypovolemic is to be avoided to prevent burns; carbon monoxide poisoning; methemoglobinemia

Interfering Factors: Incorrect placement of sensor; movement of site to which sensor is attached; poor circulation; recent radiogragphy with contrast media; anemia; dirty sensor

Nursing Considerations:

Pediatric: Use the right infant/pediatric size of probe or use wrap-around tapes if digit is very small.

Listing of Related Tests: Arterial blood gas; arterial blood oximetry

---

WEBLINKS

http://RespiratoryCare.medscape.com

Plethysmography
(*PLETH*-iz-*MAHG*-ruh-fee)
(impedance plethysmography; maximal venous outflow test; pulse cuff recording; PCR; venous cuff examination)

30 min.

Type of Test: Manometric

Body Systems and Functions: Cardiovascular system

Normal Findings: Normal arterial or venous wave patterns; ankle/brachial index (ABI) 0.90–1.0

Test Results Time Frame: Within 24 hr

PHYSICAL EXAMINATION, MANOMETRIC, SENSATION, BREATH

Test Description: Plethysmography is a noninvasive diagnostic tool to calculate changes in the size of blood vessels by measuring changes in the volume of blood passing through them. Arterial or venous vessels of the upper or lower extremities can be tested to diagnose peripheral vascular disease, arterial occlusive disease, or deep venous thrombosis. Recorded wave forms depict the varying degrees of occlusion. The most useful data are the segmental limb systolic blood pressures and the ABI, which is diagnostic < 0.90 for arterial occlusive disease. Plethysmography is usually performed instead of or after Doppler vascular studies.

Consent Form: Required

List of Equipment: Pressure cuffs; electrodes and gel; plethysmography machine

Test Procedure:
1. Place client in a supine position.
2. Plethysmography cuffs are put on the extremity to be measured, and the client lies quietly while the machine takes measurements. *Anxiety or tension alters results.*

Clinical Implications and Indications:
1. Diagnoses peripheral vascular disease, arterial occlusive disease, arterial embolus, small-vessel diabetic changes, arterial trauma, and Raynaud's disease
2. Diagnoses venous thrombosis and thrombophlebitis

Nursing Care:
Before Test: Explain the test procedure and the purpose of the test. Assess the client's knowledge of the test. Instruct client to refrain from alcohol, smoking, or caffeine for at least 2 hr before test. Explain that there is no pain during the test.
During Test: Adhere to standard precautions. Instruct client to refrain from talking or moving during the test.

Interfering Factors: Anxiety; environmental temperature; talking; inability to remain still; ingestion of stimulants; depressants; vasoconstrictive substances; shock; low cardiac output; low blood pressure; false positives can occur in people with CHF or arterial insufficiency; false negatives can occur with collateral circulation.

Nursing Considerations:
Pregnancy: Compression of pelvic veins by the fetus during pregnancy may alter results.
Pediatric: Infants and children will need assistance in remaining still during the procedure and age-appropriate comfort measures following the test.
Gerontology: The older person may find it difficult to maintain positions when required to do so for lengthy periods of time during the plethysmography.

Listing of Related Tests: Doppler testing; ultrasound duplex scanning

WEBLINKS

http://americanheart.org

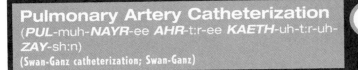

Pulmonary Artery Catheterization
(*PUL*-muh-*NAYR*-ee *AHR*-t:r-ee *KAETH*-uh-t:r-uh-ZAY-sh:n)
(Swan-Ganz catheterization; Swan-Ganz)

30 min.

Type of Test: Manometric

Body Systems and Functions: Cardiovascular system

Normal Findings:

Right atrial pressure (RAP)	3–11 mm Hg
Central venous pressure (CVP)	2.7–12 cm H_2O
Right ventricular systolic pressure	20–30 mm Hg
Right ventricular end-diastolic pressure	<5 mm Hg
Pulmonary artery end-diastolic pressure	8–15 mm Hg
Pulmonary artery pressure (PAP)	20 mm Hg
Pulmonary artery wedge pressure (PAWP or PAOP*)	6–12 mm Hg
Cardiac output (CO)	4–12 mm Hg
Cardiac index	5–8 L/min

*New term for PAWP is pulmonary artery occlusive pressure (PAOP)

Test Results Time Frame: Immediately

Test Description: Pulmonary artery catheterization measures the pumping ability of the heart and can detect early ventricular failure by measuring the pulmonary artery wedge pressure (PAWP or PAOP), which most closely reflects the pressures in the left ventricle, cardiac output, and cardiac index. Preload pressures and fluid volume status on the right side of the heart are obtained from CVP and RAP readings. In addition, oxygenation can be evaluated with intracardiac and mixed venous blood (SVO_2) samples. Right-ventricular pressures are diagnostic for pulmonary hypertension and pulmonary edema. A Swan-Ganz catheter is introduced into the internal jugular, subclavian, or brachial vein and threaded into the superior vena cava, right atrium and ventricle, and the left pulmonary artery. The catheter has four to five ports; when the catheter is fully inserted, the proximal port opens to the right atrium and is used to instill injectate for cardiac output data. The ventricular port opens to the right ventricle and can be used for blood sampling or to instill fluids. The distal port terminates at the end of the catheter and is attached to the flush solution. The balloon inflation port terminates in the pulmonary artery 1 cm from the tip of the catheter. When the balloon is briefly inflated, circulation through the artery is stopped and the PAWP can be measured. Wave patterns are reflected on an oscilloscope. The fourth or fifth lumen has a thermistor to measure core temperature and to calculate cardiac output. The catheter insertion procedure is done in the intensive care unit or in a laboratory with fluoroscopy; the client is continuously monitored in the intensive care unit for cardiac arrhythmias, and other signs/symptoms of complications for the duration the catheter is in the body. The typical length of time that a client needs the catheter is 2–5 days.

PHYSICAL EXAMINATION, MANOMETRIC, SENSATION, BREATH

> **CLINICAL ALERT:**
> Emergency resuscitative equipment and personnel must always be readily available in the event of cardiac arrhythmias when inserting the pulmonary artery catheter.

Consent Form: Required

List of Equipment: Swan-Ganz catheter kit; local anesthetic; IV insertion equipment; emergency equipment

Test Procedure:
1. The Swan-Ganz catheter insertion is performed by a physician in the intensive care unit or in a laboratory, such as the cardiac catheter laboratory, where fluoroscopy and emergency equipment and trained personnel are available for cardiac emergencies.
2. Place the client in the supine position with the entry site exposed, usually the internal jugular, the subclavian, or the brachial vein at the antecubital site. *Ensures correct placement of catheter.*
3. An IV line and fluid are initiated. *Supports emergency medications, if needed.*
4. The entry site is cleansed, a sterile field created, and a local anesthetic given.
5. A vein cut-down is performed to visualize the vein. The catheter is threaded gently through the vasculature into the right atrium. Waveform and pressure readings at this point confirm the position of the catheter if fluoroscopy is not used.
6. The balloon is slightly inflated to help float it through the tricuspid valve, the right ventricle, and the pulmonary artery until it is located in a smaller, more distal pulmonary artery. The balloon is briefly fully inflated to take the PAWP reading, then deflated until it is time for further readings.
7. An x-ray confirms the correct placement of the catheter, the catheter is sutured to the skin, and an occlusive dressing is applied to the site.
8. Readings using the pulmonary artery catheter are performed approximately every 4 hr during its usage (refer to procedure manual for specifics of obtaining the individual hemodynamic readings).

Clinical Implications and Indications:
1. Diagnoses right- or left-ventricular failure. The PAP and PAWP are particularly sensitive to signs of early failure.
2. Diagnoses pulmonary hypertension and other problems such as pulmonary edema or embolus.
3. Determines atrial or ventricular septal defects.
4. Diagnoses pericardial involvement.
5. Determines arterial oxygen content and evaluates tissue oxygen, especially when client is on mechanical ventilation.
6. Measures cardiac contractility after myocardial infarction through evaluation of the cardiac output.
7. Evaluates definitive fluid status after cardiac surgery.
8. Evaluates effect of inotropic medications, fluid infusion, and respiratory treatments.

Nursing Care:

Before Test: Explain the test procedure and the purpose of the test. Assess the client's knowledge of the test. Explain that the client will feel pressure but not pain during the insertion procedure and that the catheter typically is needed for

2–5 days during which the client will be in the intensive care unit for continuous monitoring.

During Test: Adhere to standard precautions. Instruct the client to lie still during the insertion of the catheter. Monitor the client's cardiac and respiratory status continuously.

After Test: Continuous cardiac monitoring (telemetry) for cardiac arrhythmias for the duration the catheter is inserted. Assess the client's cardiac and respiratory status frequently. Assess site for signs/symptoms of bleeding or infection.

Potential Complications: Cardiac arrhythmias; arterial occlusion or embolism; air embolus; perforation of pulmonary artery or myocardium; pneumothorax (if subclavian vein used) during insertion; infection and sepsis; valve damage; catheter knotting

Contraindications: Procedure is performed only in critically ill clients where the risks are outweighed by the benefits of life-saving data.

Interfering Factors: Incorrect placement of catheter; faulty technique in taking pressure measurements

Nursing Considerations:

Pediatric: Infants and children will need assistance in remaining still during the procedure and age-appropriate comfort measures following the test (note: the pulmonary artery catheter is not frequently used in this age range).

Gerontology: In the elderly, there is a decrease of cardiac stroke volume and increased arterial: stiffness resulting in decreased cardiac output and index and in slightly increased right- and left-ventricular pressures.

Listing of Related Tests: Arterial blood gases (ABGs)

WEBLINKS	▤ ▨

www.americanheart.org

Pulmonary Function
(*PUL*-muh-*NAYR*-ee *FUHNGK*-sh:n)
(PFT)
20-60 min.

Type of Test: Breath

Body Systems and Functions: Pulmonary system

Normal Findings: Data are compared with normal reference values using age, height, weight, and gender of client (adult, 70-kg man; 20%–25% lower in women)

TV	500 mL at rest
RV	1,200 mL (approximate)
IRV	3,000 mL (approximate)
ERV	1,200 mL (approximate)
VC	4,800 mL (approximate)

TLC	6,000 mL (approximate)
FRC	3,000–5,000 mL (approximate)
FEV_1	81%–83%
MMEF	25%–75%
FIF	25%–75%
MVV	25%–35% or 170 L/min
PIFR	300 L/min
PEFR	450 L/min

Test Results Time Frame: Within 24 hr

Test Description: Pulmonary function tests provide data on the lung volumes, pattern, and air flow rates involved in respiratory function. The most common pulmonary function test is spirometry, which measures lung volumes, lung capacities, and flow rates. Given the results of spirometry, further testing may be done using gas exchange and diffusion capacity tests, body plethysmography, flow volume loops, and exercise testing. Spirometry can be adapted for testing at the bedside or in an outpatient setting. Spirometry may also be done before and after the bronchoinhaler medications are administered to compare changes in lung function.

Components of spirometry testing

Tidal volume (TV)	Total volume of air inhaled and exhaled in one breath
Residual volume (RV)	Amount of air remaining in lungs after maximal expiratory effort. Cannot be measured but is calculated from FRC – ERV.
Inspired residual volume (IRV)	Maximum amount of air inhaled at point of maximum expiration
Expired residual volume (ERV)	Maximum amount of air exhaled slowly at point of maximum inspiration
Vital capacity (VC)	Maximum amount of air exhaled at the point of maximum inspiration
Total lung capacity (TLC)	Total amount of air that the lungs can hold after maximal inspiration
Inspiratory capacity (IC)	Maximum amount of air inspired after normal expiration
Functional residual capacity (FRC)	Volume of air that remains in the lungs after normal expiration
Forced volume capacity (FVC)	Maximum amount of air that can be forcefully exhaled after full inspiration
Forced expired volume (FEV_1)	Amount of air exhaled in first second of forced vital capacity (FVC)
Maximal midexpiratory flow (MMEF)	Maximal rate of air flow during a forced expiration

Forced inspiratory flow rate (FIF)	Volume inspired from the residual volume (RV) at a point of measurement; expressed in a percent to identify the volume pressure and inspired volume
Peak inspiratory flow rate (PIFR)	Maximum flow of air during a forced maximal inspiration
Peak expiratory flow rate (PEFR)	Maximum flow of air expired during forced vital capacity (FVC)

CLINICAL ALERT:
A bronchodilator should be on hand in the event of bronchospasm with some of the pulmonary function testing (e.g., bronchial provocation test, histamine challenge).

Consent Form: Not required

List of Equipment: Test is performed in a pulmonary function laboratory with special equipment.

Test Procedure:
1. Have client sit in chair next to respiratory equipment.
2. Place soft nose clip on nose. *Enables breathing through the mouth.*
3. Instruct client to breathe through mouthpiece and to follow instructions when to inhale and exhale. Allow some practice breaths, especially for forced timed exhalations. *Ensures accurate results.*
4. The technician will give specific breathing instructions for each measurement.
5. If gas diffusing capacity tests are ordered, the client will inhale gas mixtures of helium and carbon monoxide, hold 1 min, then exhale into a machine that analyzes the concentrations.
6. For the bronchial provocation test, the client inhales methacholine; then a repeat FVC is done after 5 min. A histamine challenge may also be given if there is no change in the FVC. A bronchodilator should be on hand. *For treatment of bronchospasms.*
7. An exercise pulmonary function study may also be done with a variety of spirometry and gas exchange testing done after the client exercises on a treadmill.

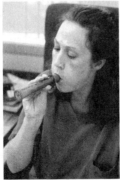

Pulmonary Function Test

PHYSICAL EXAMINATION, MANOMETRIC, SENSATION, BREATH

Clinical Implications and Indications:

1. Diagnoses and differentiates between pulmonary obstructive and restrictive disease or combination of both.
2. Diagnoses chronic obstructive pulmonary disease (COPD) that affects lower airways and function (asthma, bronchitis, emphysema) and upper airways (tumors, infections, or foreign body in pharynx, larynx, or trachea).
3. Diagnoses effect on lung function of disease that affects the chest wall (kyphosis, scoliosis, neuromuscular), interstial tissue (fibrosis), and other conditions such as cysts or ascites.
4. Determines effectiveness of bronchodilator therapy on respiratory function.
5. Evaluates the ability of the client's respiratory system to tolerate surgery and other procedures.
6. Screens high-risk populations, such as workers exposed to potential airway irritants.
7. Evaluates pulmonary function following pneumonectomy or lobectomy surgery.
8. Determines allergic respiratory airway reactive disease.
9. Determines diffusing capacity of lungs in those with congestive heart failure, adult respiratory distress syndrome, and collagen disorders.

Nursing Care:

Before Test: Explain the test procedure and the purpose of the test. Assess the client's knowledge of the test. Check with clinician to see if medications that affect respiratory function should be held before testing. Caution client to refrain from smoking or eating a heavy meal within 4 hr of the test.
During Test: Adhere to standard precautions. Encourage client to follow instructions carefully. Monitor for excessive shortness of breath and fatigue.
After Test: Resume normal diet and any respiratory medications that were held.

Contraindications: Cardiac insufficiency; recent myocardial infarction; chest pain; upper respiratory infection; acute asthma attack

Interfering Factors: Inability of client to cooperate due to confusion or severe shortness of breath; medications that affect respiratory functioning will alter results; improper placement of nose clips or mouthpiece allowing leakage of air

Nursing Considerations:

Pregnancy: Late pregnancy may alter results due to uterine pressure on the diaphram, which limits lung expansion.
Pediatric: Testing can be done on young child as soon as child is capable of following directions on inhaling and exhaling.
Gerontology: In the elderly elasticity of the lungs and vital capacity decrease and compliance is 70% of baseline value by the time a person is 80 years old. Residual volume increases nearly 50% and maximal airflow rates decrease.
Rural: Advisable to arrange for transportation home after recovering from procedure.

Listing of Related Tests: Arterial blood gases (ABGs); pulse oximetry

WEBLINKS

www.nlm.nih.gov

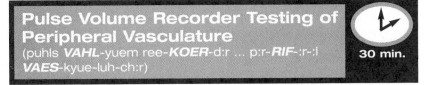

Pulse Volume Recorder Testing of Peripheral Vasculature
(puhls **VAHL**-yuem ree-**KOER**-d:r ... p:r-**RIF**-:r-:l **VAES**-kyue-luh-ch:r)

30 min.

Type of Test: Manometric

Body Systems and Functions: Cardiovascular system

Normal Findings: Normal wave pattern has rapid upstroke, a sharp peak, sharp decline, and a clearly discernable diastolic wave.

Test Results Time Frame: Immediately

Test Description: A pulse volume recorder measures pressure changes in arterial vessels. While inflating and deflating sets of blood pressure cuffs at the distal, middle, and proximal sites of each limb, pressure changes are recorded as wave forms by a transducer. Pulse volume recordings supplement segmental limb pressure studies. Arterial narrowing produces a loss of the diastolic wave, a rounding of the sharp peak, and a decreased slope of wave (flattening and lengthening). The pressure volume recordings are a sensitive indicator to arterial occlusive disease, especially in the feet and toes.

Consent Form: Not required

List of Equipment: The test is done in a laboratory setting with special equipment.

Test Procedure:
1. Remove clothing from each extremity. *Constrictive clothing alters the results.*
2. Place in prone position and tell client to remain still. *Tension or movement alters the results.*
3. Blood pressure cuffs especially measured to fit the client's size are placed at 2.5 cm above the antecubital crease in the arms, above the wrist, as high as possible on the thighs, below the knee, and above the malleolus of the ankle. *Cuffs must meet specific circumference and width specifications to give reliable results.*
4. The recording equipment is attached and the cuffs are inflated and deflated with the pulse volume readings taken at the brachial, radial, ulnar, femoral, popliteal, dorsalis pedis, and posterior tibial levels of the limbs.

Clinical Implications and Indications:
1. Diagnoses and monitors arterial vascular narrowing and occlusions.
2. The test is sensitive to vascular occlusions, which cannot be measured by a Doppler probe.

Nursing Care:
Before Test: Explain the test procedure and purpose of the test. Assess client's knowledge of the test. Instruct client they will experience no discomfort. Inform client to remain still during procedure.
During Test: Adhere to standard precautions.

PHYSICAL EXAMINATION, MANOMETRIC; SENSATION, BREATH

Interfering Factors: Improper size, application, or inflation of cuffs; false negatives occur in upper thigh measurements in situations where a large collateral circulation has developed; inability to remain still

Nursing Considerations:
Gerontology: The older person may find it difficult to maintain positions when required to do so for lengthy periods of time during the procedure.
Rural: Advisable to arrange for transportation home after recovering from procedure (particularly if client is elderly)

Listing of Related Tests: Segmental limb pressure studies

WEBLINKS

www.americanheart.org

Raynaud's Cold Stimulation
(ray-*NOEZ* koeld *STIM*-yue-*LAY*-sh:n)

30-40 min.

Type of Test: Sensation

Body Systems and Functions: Cardiovascular system

Normal Findings: Normal temperature, blood pressure, and skin color of fingers and toes after exposure to cold

Test Results Time Frame: Immediately

Test Description: Raynaud's cold stimulation test measures temperature changes in the fingers after exposure to cold and the time it takes for finger temperature to return to normal after the cold stimulation has been removed. In normal fingers, recovery to baseline temperature occurs in about 10 min. In Raynaud's disease, recovery takes more than 20 min. The test is done after chronic arterial occlusive disease has been ruled out. In Raynaud's disease, intense vasospasm occurs in small arteries and arterioles of the fingers and in some cases the toes are affected. Vasospasm causes ischemia, which in turn causes symptoms, which include severe pain, tingling, and numbness. After the ischemia, hyperemia occurs. In primary Raynaud's symptoms occur under extreme stress or exposure to cold. In secondary Raynaud's symptoms occur in association with other diseases, such as scleroderma and lupus.

Consent Form: Not required

List of Equipment: The test is performed in a laboratory with special equipment.

Test Procedure:
1. Place the client in a sitting position with a thermistor attached to each finger above the nail bed. Wires attach the thermistors to a machine, which records the temperature changes.
2. After baseline temperatures are recorded, immerse the hands in ice water for 20 sec. *Ensures accurate results.*

PHYSICAL EXAMINATION, MANOMETRIC, SENSATION, BREATH

3. After the hands are removed, record temperatures again and every 5 min until baseline is attained.

Clinical Implications and Indications:
1. Evaluates and monitors Raynaud's disease

Nursing Care:
Before Test: Explain the test procedure and the purpose of the test. Assess the client's knowledge of the test. Explain the test will be done by a technician and requires 30–40 min. Instruct the client that there may be slight discomfort while the hands are in the ice water. Have client void before the procedure.
During Test: Adhere to standard precautions.

Contraindications: Infections or gangrene of the digits

Nursing Considerations:
Home Care: Clients with Raynaud's disease should be advised to wear slippers and gloves to insulate their extremities during exposure to cold weather.

WEBLINKS

www.nlm.nih.gov

Rectal Motility
(*REK*-t:l moe-*TIL*-uh-tee)
(anorectal manometry; rectal manometry; rectal sphincteric manometry)

30 min.

Type of Test: Manometric

Body Systems and Functions: Gastrointestinal system

Normal Findings: 40–120 mm Hg. Distention of rectum should cause relaxation of internal sphincter and tightening of external sphincter.

Test Results Time Frame: Within 24 hr

Test Description: The rectal motility manometric test measures pressures within the rectum and evaluates the strength and function of the internal and external sphincters, rectal anal reflexes, and rectal sensation. Using a multisensor catheter with a balloon that is inflated to produce rectal distention, the amount of air required for the client to feel resistance is measured at eight different points along approximately 10 cm of the anorectal canal. During a series of maneuvers by the client, impaired rectal sensation, low basal tone, impaired squeeze pressure, and impaired sphincter function can be evaluated. In normal function, distention of the rectum causes the internal sphincter to relax and the external sphincter to tighten.

Consent Form: Not required

List of Equipment: The procedure is done in a laboratory or office examination room with special equipment.

PHYSICAL EXAMINATION, MANOMETRIC, SENSATION, BREATH

Test Procedure:
1. Instruct client to disrobe from the waist down.
2. Place client in left lateral position with the knees flexed; cover with a drape. *Ensures privacy.*
3. The catheter is inserted into the rectum 8–10 cm.
4. The balloon is inflated distending the rectum for 8–12 sec until resistance is demonstrated. The amount of air is recorded (normal is 30–50 mL).
5. Air is withdrawn in small increments until resistance is no longer felt. This is the threshold of rectal sensation and usually causes relaxation of the internal sphincter with 15 mL air.
6. Instruct the client to squeeze the external sphincter tightly for 2 sec and relax.
7. Pressures are measured at eight points along the catheter with each voluntary squeeze and relaxation.

Clinical Implications and Indications:
1. Diagnoses colonic dilatation, anal alchalasia, intrinsic ganglionic innervations, Hirschsprung's disease, and rectal incontinence
2. Analyzes external sphincter disorders related to other diseases, such as muscular dystrophy, myasthenia gravis, and multiple sclerosis

Nursing Care:
Before Test: Explain the test procedure and the purpose of the test. Assess the client's knowledge of the test. A sodium phosphate enema may be ordered 1–2 hr prior to the procedure. Explain that the procedure is not painful but may be uncomfortable when the balloon is inflated and the rectum is distended. Instruct the client to cooperate with the technician's instructions and communicate when resistance is felt.
During Test: Adhere to standard precautions. Encourage client to follow instructions.
After Test: Caution client to notify health care provider if any rectal bleeding or discharge.

Interfering Factors: Stool in rectum; inability of client to cooperate with instructions; improper placement of catheter and balloon

Nursing Considerations:
Pediatric: Test is not reliable in newborns; young children may need to be sedated.

Listing of Related Tests: Colonic transit time; evacuation protography

WEBLINKS

http://chorus.rad.mcw.edu

Refraction
(ree-**FRAEK**-sh:n)   •
(refraction vision test)

20-30 min.

Type of Test: Physical examination

Body Systems and Functions: Sensory system

Normal Findings:

No refractive error

Overall refractive power for the eye	58 diopters
Refractive power for cornea/aqueous humor	44 diopters
Refractive power for lens	10–14 diopters

Test Results Time Frame: Immediately

Test Description: Refraction is a test performed to determine visual acuity, refractive abnormalities, and strength and curvature of corrective lens powers, which will correct the client's visual acuity. Refraction is the process by which rays of light entering the eye are bent by the different densities of the lens and aqueous humor. The more the eye bends the light rays, the greater is its refractive power, which is measured in diopters. The point at which the rays meet within the eye is called the point of focus. If the rays meet at a point in front of or behind the retina, vision is blurred. The rays must meet exactly on the retina for visual acuity (emmetropia). Corrective lenses change the bend of the light ray so that its point of focus is on the retina. Hyperopia is farsightedness with the rays meeting behind the retina. Myopia is near sightedness with the point of focus in front of the retina. In astigmatism refraction is spread over a diffuse area within the eye due to differing curvatures in the cornea and lens of the eye. After the pupil is dilated by mydriatic eyedrops, an examination of the retina is done with the retinoscope to look for abnormalities. Then different lenses are tried for each eye with the client reading the lines of the Snellen chart to determine the best lens for visual acuity. A prescription is written for the strength/curvature of corrective lens needed for each eye.

Consent Form: Not required

List of Equipment: Test is performed in examination room with special equipment; mydriatic eyedrops (per prescription order)

Test Procedure:

1. Seat the client comfortably in the examining chair. Have the client remove any corrective lens.
2. Administer mydriatic eyedrops per order to both eyes.
3. Repeat eyedrops in 5–15 min.
4. Dim lights and examine retina using the retinoscope light through the dilated pupil. Check for vascular abnormalities, size, shape, and presence of the red reflex.
5. Test different lenses until visual acuity is achieved in both eyes. *Allows determination of correct prescription for corrective lenses.*

PHYSICAL EXAMINATION, MANOMETRIC, SENSATION, BREATH

Clinical Implications and Indications:
1. Diagnoses refractive errors, such as hyperopia, myopia, and astigmatism
2. Determines what lens gives best refractive correction for each eye

Nursing Care:
Before Test: Explain the test procedure and the purpose of the test. Assess the client's knowledge of the test. Inform the client that the test will take 20–30 min in a darkened room, the importance of following the technician's instruction, and to let someone know if there is itching, burning, shortness of breath, tightness in chest or throat, or other abnormal symptoms.

During Test: Adhere to standard precautions. Monitor for allergic reaction to mydriatic eyedrops.

After Test: Instruct client not to drive or operate machinery until distance vision returns; it is normal to have some blurring of vision for up to 2 hr after the eye test; sunglasses should be worn outside until the medicine has lost its effect and the pupils can constrict again.

Potential Complications: Allergic reaction to eyedrops, such as rash, itching, hives, shortness of breath, tightness in throat, bronchospasm, or anaphylactic shock

Contraindications: Narrow-angle glaucoma; allergy to mydriatics used for pupil dilation

Interfering Factors: Inability of client to remain still and to cooperate during test; improper administration of eyedrops to achieve pupil dilation

---

WEBLINKS ▤ ☒

http://www.mic.ki.se/Diseases/c10.html

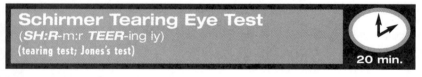

Schirmer Tearing Eye Test
(*SH:R*-m:r *TEER*-ing iy)
(tearing test; Jones's test)

20 min.

Type of Test: Physical examination

Body Systems and Functions: Sensory system

Normal Findings: 10–30 mm of moisture from each eye after 5 min

CRITICAL VALUES:
8 mm is diagnostic of a hyposecretion condition.

Test Results Time Frame: Immediately

Test Description: The Schirmer tearing test measures the amount of tears produced by the lacrimal glands in a specified time period. When no anesthesia is used, the test measures all tears produced and does not differentiate between the basic and reflexive tear production (Schirmer I). Basic (nonreflex) secretions are measured by using topical anesthesia and the filter paper (Jones's test). Reflex secretions are measured when topical anesthesia is used and the nasal mucosa is stimulated for 2 min (Schirmer II). The Schirmer testing is accomplished by holding filter paper against the conjunctiva of both eyes and evaluating the quantity of moisture (tears) that accumulates on the paper. The lacrimal apparatus consists of the lacrimal glands and ducts. They are located above and on the temporal side of each eye. The lacrimal apparatus is responsible for the production of tears, which lubricate the eye. Most often these tests are used to confirm the diagnosis of hyposecretion associated with conditions such as Sjögren's syndrome, an autoimmune disorder that affects the moisture-producing (exocrine) glands of the body. Two types of Sjögren's syndrome exist: primary and secondary Sjögren's syndromes, which occur in the absence of other autoimmune diseases (note: dry eyes, mouth, and other mucous membranes are common complaints).

Consent Form: Required

List of Equipment: Standardized strip of filter paper; timer; cotton applicators/swabs; measuring device in millimeters; topical anesthetic

Test Procedure:
1. Instruct the client to sit comfortably in a room with dim light, maintaining a straight gaze.
2. Blot the interior fornix of the lower eyelid with a cotton applicator. Both eyes are usually tested simultaneously. *Removes tears that are in the eye at the start of the examination.*
3. Fold one end of the filter paper over 5 mm and place in the lower eyelid one-third of the eye-length away from the temporal corner of the eye. *Allows the filter paper to stay in place.*
4. Allow the filter paper to remain in place for 5 min, remove, and measure the distance the tears have traveled.
5. Proceed with the Jones test and place one drop of topical anesthetic in each eye. Repeat steps 1–4. *Allows the filter paper to stay in place without causing a reflexive stimulation of tears.*
6. Proceed with the Schirmer II test by anesthetizing the eyes and placing the filter paper in the lower eyelid, as above. Introduce a cotton applicator into the middle of the nasal cavity to stimulate the nasal mucosa. Assess the amount of tears after 2 min of nasal stimulation. *Tests reflects tearing capacity.*

Clinical Implications and Indications:
1. Diagnoses Sjögren's syndrome, which is more common among women by a ratio of 9:1
2. Evaluates lupus erythematosus, rheumatoid arthritis, and scleroderma
3. Predicts the outcome for some eye surgeries, such as for Stevens-Johnson syndrome
4. Diagnoses keratoconjunctivitis sicca (dry eyes), which often occurs in menopausal and postmenopausal women

Nursing Care:
Before Test: Explain the test procedure and the purpose of the test. Assess the client's knowledge of the test.
During Test: Adhere to standard precautions.
After Test: Assess for corneal abrasions caused from rubbing eyes before anesthetic eye drop medication has worn off.

PHYSICAL EXAMINATION, MANOMETRIC, SENSATION, BREATH

Potential Complications: Corneal abrasions

Interfering Factors: Rubbing eyes increases tearing.

Nursing Considerations:
Pregnancy: *Women with Sjögren's syndrome have a greater chance of bearing children with a serious heart condition.*
Gerontology: *Hormonal replacement therapy tends to decrease the complaints of hyposecretion (keratoconjunctivitis sicca) in postmenopausal women.*

Listing of Related Tests: Slit lamp biomicroscopy

WEBLINKS

www.sjogrens.com; http://www.orthop.washington.edu

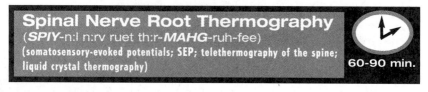

Spinal Nerve Root Thermography
(*SPIY*-n:l n:rv ruet th:r-*MAHG*-ruh-fee)
(somatosensory-evoked potentials; SEP; telethermography of the spine; liquid crystal thermography)

60-90 min.

Type of Test: Sensation

Body Systems and Functions: Neurological system

Normal Findings: Normal distribution of heat patterns of the lumbar, thoracic, and cervical spinal nerve areas; an absence of nerve irritation or soft tissue trauma

Test Results Time Frame: Within 24 hr

Test Description: Spinal nerve root thermography is a noninvasive test that measures the heat emitted from the surface of the skin at two adjacent areas of the spinal column. This test is performed to detect the sensory nerve irritation that is caused when distinct heat patterns at skin sites indicate nerve root injury. Spinal nerve root thermography may be used in combination with several other nervous system tests [e.g., myelography (EMG)]. The spinal nerves are made of two roots: (1) the dorsal root, which carries afferent neuron axons into the CNS, and (2) the ventral root, which carries the axons of the afferent neurons into the periphery. When either of these two roots are irritated, there are abnormal heat productions that the spinal nerve root thermography detects.

Consent Form: Not required

List of Equipment: Infrared thermogram machine; ice water

Test Procedure:
1. Place client in prone position with the area to be scanned left exposed.
2. Skin sites are cooled with water or with alcohol and are blown dry. *Allows for good conduction and even temperatures of the areas to be scanned.*
3. Thermography measuring device is placed on two adjacent skin surfaces and scanning is performed.

Clinical Implications and Indications:

1. Diagnoses herniated disks (extreme change or asymmetric distribution of temperature can indicate the presence of disc protrusion).
2. Changes in temperature may indicate decreased blood flow to an area along the dermatome. Asymmetries of thermal patterns can indicate nerve irritation from herniation of the disc.
3. Assesses condition of nerve roots in lower back region injuries.
4. Diagnoses chronic or acute back pain as related to nerve root involvement.

Nursing Care:

Before Test: Explain the test procedure and the purpose of the test. Assess the client's knowledge of the test. Gather historical data regarding clinical manifestations of musculoskeletal conditions. Instruct client to not smoke 4–6 hr prior to test. Do not allow lotions or powders to be applied before study. Inform client that there is no discomfort associated with this procedure. Instruct client to void before procedure.

During Test: Adhere to standard precautions. Support client during procedure, particularly if they have a history of back pain.

After Test: Give analgesics per protocol.

Interfering Factors: Changes in room temperature; smoking before the test; varicose veins; inability to remain still

Nursing Considerations:

Pediatric: Infants and children will need assistance in remaining still during the procedure and age-appropriate comfort measures following the test (note: somewhat unusual for this age to require this test).

Gerontology: The older person may find it difficult to maintain positions when required to do so for lengthy periods of time.

Listing of Related Tests: EMG; myelography; CAT scan

WEBLINKS

http://adam.excite.com

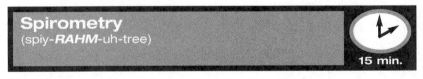

Spirometry
(spiy-***RAHM***-uh-tree)

15 min.

Type of Test: Breath

Body Systems and Functions: Pulmonary system

Normal Findings: Selected lung function measurements (forced expiratory volumes, forced vital capacity, peak expiratory flow rates) are within normal limits.

Test Results Time Frame: Within 24 hr

Test Description: Spirometry measures lung capacity, volume, and flow rates of the respiratory system. The spirometer is an instrument that consists of a bell that is suspended in a container of water. The bell rises and falls as the client breathes into the device. The movement of the bell is then recorded and specific lung measurements are obtained. Various dynamics of ventilation are assessed by this relatively noninvasive procedure, and the effects of pathological diseases (e.g., asthma, COPD, bronchitis) can be evaluated as to their progress and deteriorating effects on the lungs.

CLINICAL ALERT:
Observe client closely for clinical manifestations of syncope during procedure.

Consent Form: Not required

List of Equipment: Spirometer; kymograph or electrical potentiometer

Test Procedure:
1. Assist client into sitting and upright position. *Enhances breathing and full lung expansion.*
2. Place mouthpiece of spirometer in client's mouth; put clip over nose. *Allows only breathing through the mouth.*
3. Instruct client to take maximum inhalation, hold it, and exhale forcibly. Then rest, and repeat activity two to three times.
4. Record measurements.

Clinical Implications and Indications:
1. The severity of asthma is evaluated using spirometry before and after a bronchodilator is administered.
2. Reduced expiratory flow rate is typical in COPD.
3. Assesses damage from smoking.
4. Diagnoses and monitors asthma, COPD, bronchitis, emphysema, and myasthenia gravis.

Nursing Care:
Before Test: Explain the test procedure and the purpose of the test. Assess the client's knowledge of the test. Take baseline vital signs. Withhold bronchodilator medications for 5 hr prior to test.
During Test: Adhere to standard precautions. Provide assurance and support while client is instructed to inhale and exhale during test. Caution client to stop if they feel faint.
After Test: Assess vital signs and compare to baseline. Instruct client to resume medications per protocol.

Contraindications: Angina or recent myocardial infarction

Interfering Factors: Inability to take in deep breaths or follow instructions; sedatives, analgesics, bronchodilators; metabolic acidosis or alkalosis

Nursing Considerations:
Pediatric: Child may need assistance and support while being instructed in the methods of breathing required by the test. Normal care provider may need to assist during the test (note: evaluate this on individual basis).

Gerontology: Elderly clients with history of lung disorders may find this test difficult and need continual assessment for their potential clinical manifestations of deoxygenation (e.g., feeling faint, skin pallor, tachycardia).

Listing of Related Tests: Pulmonary function tests (PFTs); bronchial challenge test; seated and supine spirometry; body plethysmography; pulse oximetry; capnography; arterial blood gases; ventilation-perfusion studies

WEBLINKS

http://www.healthgate.com

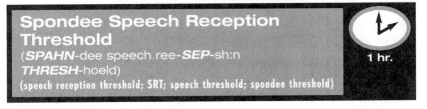

Spondee Speech Reception Threshold
(*SPAHN*-dee speech ree-*SEP*-sh:n *THRESH*-hoeld)

1 hr.

(speech reception threshold; SRT; speech threshold; spondee threshold)

Type of Test: Physical examination

Body Systems and Functions: Sensory system

Normal Findings: 0 decibels (dB) for both right and left ears

CRITICAL VALUES:
12 dB or greater

Test Results Time Frame: Immediately after the test

Test Description: Spondee speech reception threshold tests the ability of the client to understand speech at the lowest threshold. Spondees are two-syllable words presented to the listener as recorded words that are played through the audiometer. The listener is asked to repeat what is heard. This test measures the amount of hearing loss and is often performed as a follow-up to audiometry testing.

Consent Form: Not required

List of Equipment: Electronic audiometer with earphones, voltage unit, prerecorded spondee lists; monitored live voice (MLV) may be used in place of the electronic audiometer.

Test Procedure:
1. The client is seated in a quiet room and listens to the spondees (two-syllable words that receive equal stress on each syllable) and is asked to repeat what he hears.
2. The words are played at about 40 dB above the normal speech threshold. The volume is decreased in 10-dB increments until the listener is unable to correctly repeat the played word. *Assesses the hearing ability of the listener.*

PHYSICAL EXAMINATION, MANOMETRIC, SENSATION, BREATH

Clinical Implications and Indications:

1. Validity of the test depends on the client's familiarity with the words utilized and the accuracy/reliability of the client.
2. Evaluates the ability of the listener to comprehend and respond to everyday speech.

Nursing Care:

Before Test: Explain the test procedure and the purpose of the test. Assess the client's knowledge of the test. Prior to taking the spondee speech test, the client should be examined by a health care professional. Impacted cerumen and otitis media, for example, should be addressed and treated before testing. Hearing aids should be brought to the examination. All medications may be taken before the test.

During Test: Adhere to standard precautions. Provide support as needed.

Interfering Factors: Underlying ear infections; cerumen impaction

Nursing Considerations:

Pediatric: Very young children may have difficulty following directions in the performance of this test.

International: Success with the evaluation is dependent on the client understanding the words used. Clients with English as a second language should be identified ahead of time.

Listing of Related Tests: Pure tone audiometry

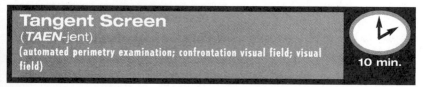

WEBLINKS

http://www.healthgate.com

Tangent Screen
(*TAEN*-jent)
(automated perimetry examination; confrontation visual field; visual field)

10 min.

Type of Test: Physical examination

Body Systems and Functions: Sensory system

Normal Findings: Visual field is normal in size: 90° temporally, 60° nasally, 50° superiorly, and 70° inferiorly.

Test Results Time Frame: Immediate

Test Description: Tangent screen test is a measurement of the full visual field. One eye is occluded while the opposite eye is tested by moving an object throughout the entire visual field. The tested eye is then occluded and the other eye is tested.

Consent Form: Not required

List of Equipment: Tangent screen; hand-held eye occluder; test object

Test Procedure:

1. Position client in a sitting position 3½ feet from the tangent screen (or examiner). *Distance allows for standard evaluation of visual field.*
2. Have client occlude one eye. *Each eye is tested separately to assist in determining disparity between eyes.*
3. While having the client focus on the tangent screen (or spot on the wall), the examiner moves an object (usually a pen) throughout the different fields of vision, noting how wide the visual field is. *When the client is unable to see the object, the end of the visual field is reached.*
4. Have client switch eye occluder to other eye and repeat examination with the new eye. *Each eye's visual field needs to be tested separately.*
5. Record visual field for each eye. *Documentation allows for comparison over time.*

Clinical Implications and Indications:

1. Decreased visual fields can occur with cerebrovascular accidents, retinitis pigmentosa, retinal detachment, aneurysms of the circle of Willis, meningiomas, pituitary tumors, and bitemporal hemianopsia.
2. Evaluates and monitors glaucoma and opthalmic eye vessel damage.

Nursing Care:

Before Test: Explain the test procedure and the purpose of the test. Assess the client's knowledge of the test. Perform visual acuity test prior to visual field test. Perform practice visual field test prior to actual testing.
During Test: Adhere to standard precautions. Move items slowly within the visual field.
After Test: Record results of visual field test.

Interfering Factors: Poor visual acuity

Nursing Considerations:

Pediatric: Children need to be cooperative. Use of toys or other distraction methods may enhance cooperation. Also, children with visual disturbances may perform poorly in school or have problems focusing and thus require early detection of the vision problem.

Listing of Related Tests: Visual acuity

|WEBLINKS|

www.readersdigesthealth.com

Tensilon Test
(*TEN*-suh-lahn)

15 min.

Type of Test: Physical examination

Body Systems and Functions: Neurological system

Normal Findings: No change in muscle strength upon administration of Tensilon

Test Results Time Frame: Immediate

Test Description: Tensilon, an anticholinesterase drug, is injected intra-venously to test for myasthenia gravis. Upon injection of the Tensilon, the person with myasthenia gravis will have marked improvement in muscle strength for about 5 min. If there is no change in muscle strength, the person does not have myasthenia gravis. This test evaluates the ability of nerve impulses to get to muscle fibers for contraction. Myasthenia gravis is a degenerative neurological disease that causes generalized muscle fatigue, respiratory complications usually due to a compromised diaphragm, altered speech tone, and upper extremity weakness.

CLINICAL ALERT:
Client may have anticholingeric crisis after receiving Tensilon medication.

Consent Form: Not required

List of Equipment: Intravenous equipment; Tensilon; needle and syringe; alcohol swab

Test Procedure:
1. Initiate an IV or saline lock if there is not one in place. *Tensilon is given IV so IV access is needed.*
2. Inject Tensilon. *Tensilon is an anticholinesterase that temporarily counters the effects of the myasthenia gravis.*
3. Observe client for up to 5 min. *Response to Tensilon will occur within and last for 5 min.*

Clinical Implications and Indications:
1. No change in muscle strength indicates not having myasthenia gravis.
2. Marked improvement in muscle strength indicates the presence of myasthenia gravis.

Nursing Care:
Before Test: Explain the test procedure and the purpose of the test. Assess client's knowledge of the test. Instruct client to not take any medications 4 hr before the test. Explain that effects of the Tensilon will wear off rapidly.
During Test: Adhere to standard precautions. Observe client for response to Tensilon.
After Test: Encourage client to verbalize fears if test results are positive for myasthenia gravis.

Potential Complications: Anticholinergic crisis

Interfering Factors: Dose of Tensilon

WEBLINKS

http://webmd.lycos.com

Thermography
(th:r-*MAHG*-ruh-fee)

15-30 min.

Type of Test: Physical examination (photodiagnostic)

Body Systems and Functions: Integumentary system

Normal Findings: Relative consistency of temperature of body area and gradual changes in temperature from one area to another

Test Results Time Frame: Within 24 hr

Test Description: Thermography is the use of an infrared device that records temperature in areas of the body. Relatively hot and cold spots are revealed as the area lacks the ability to adapt to changes in temperature. This is most commonly used to study blood flow to the limbs and in detecting breast cancer.

CLINICAL ALERT:
Client should also have a mammogram when having thermography.

Consent Form: Required

List of Equipment: Infrared thermogram machine; ice water

Test Procedure:
1. Client is placed in cold examination room (18°C–22°C). *Cold room allows for detection of pathological changes on the thermogram.*
2. Client disrobes above the waist and infrared images are taken of the breasts (or limb if that is the problem area). *Infrared images can identify hot and cold spots in tissue.*
3. Client's hand is placed in ice water to observe thermodynamic changes. *This elicits a spinal cord reflex to change body temperature.*
4. Infrared images are repeated. *To observe for changes in temperature as reflected in thermogram.*

Clinical Implications and Indications:
1. Extreme change in temperature can indicate the presence of breast cancer.
2. Changes in temperature may indicate decreased blood flow to an extremity.

Nursing Care:
Before Test: Explain the test procedure and the purpose of the test. Assess the client's knowledge of the test.
During Test: Adhere to standard precautions. Provide emotional support. Ensure that no air conditioning or heat vents are directed toward the client.
After Test: Instruct client on follow-up visits.

WEBLINKS

http://www.breastthermography.org/

PHYSICAL EXAMINATION, MANOMETRIC, SENSATION, BREATH

Tilt Table Test
(tilt *TAY*-b:l)
(head uptilt table test)

30-90 min.

Type of Test: Physical examination

Body Systems and Functions: Cardiovascular system

Normal Findings: Client maintains normal to high blood pressure and heart rate with normal state of consciousness.

Test Results Time Frame: Immediate (note: written results within 24 hr)

Test Description: The tilt test is performed to determine the cause of syncope in a client. It is most effective in diagnosing neurally related syncope. The client is monitored while lying on a table, and then the table is tilted to an 80° angle. The health care worker assesses changes in vital signs and client's verbalization of feeling dizzy, lightheaded, or any other clinical manifestations of deoxygenation.

> **CLINICAL ALERT:**
> Careful monitoring of the client's cardiovascular system (e.g., blood pressure, heart rate) during the test is necessary to avoid complications. Clinical manifestations of angina or dyspnea need to be assessed for, and the management is to discontinue the test in the presence of alterations.

Consent Form: Required

List of Equipment: Tilt table; EKG machine; blood pressure cuff; IV equipment; Isuprel

Test Procedure:
1. Connect client to EKG machine and blood pressure monitor and obtain baseline vital signs. *Allows for continuous evaluation of vital signs throughout the test.*
2. Place client in supine position on the tilt table and secure to the table with straps. *Provides for client safety.*
3. The table moves the client to an upright angle of 80°. *Simulates going from flat to upright position.*
4. If there are no abnormal changes, the table is returned to the flat position. *Prepares client for the next stage of testing.*
5. Administer IV isoproternol. *This simulates sympathetic nervous system response.*
6. The tilt table is returned to an 80° position. *Simulates going from flat to upright position.*
7. If an abnormal result is not seen, the table is lowered to flat position, the medication increased, and the tilt table raised again. *Attempts to simulate situation that causes syncope at home.*
8. If client's heart rate and blood pressure drop and there is a resulting loss of consciousness, the medication is stopped and the table is returned to flat position. *Allows client to physiologically return to stable condition.*

9. Observe client for 20 min with periodic vital signs and assessment. *Assures client's return to stable condition.*

Clinical Implications and Indications:

1. A positive tilt table test is when the heart rate and blood pressure drop suddenly and the client gets dizzy and loses consciousness. This is indicative of neurally mediated syncope (treatment may be medications to prevent further episodes of the syncopal episodes).

Nursing Care:

Before Test: Explain the test procedure and the purpose of the test. Assess the client's knowledge of the test. Take baseline vital signs. Instruct client to be NPO after midnight the day of the test. Secure patient on the tilt table with straps across legs and chest.

During Test: Provide reassurance and emotional support to the client throughout the test.

After Test: Assure clients are steady on their feet before leaving and vital signs have returned to normal.

Potential Complications: Chest discomfort

Contraindications: Angina

Interfering Factors: Autonomic nervous system medications

Nursing Considerations:

Gerontology: Use particular caution during test (e.g., monitoring vital signs, assessing potential oxygenation changes) when administering to the elderly, due to the potential respiratory or cardiovascular complications.

WEBLINKS

www.heartsite.com

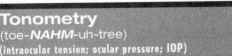

Tonometry
(toe-*NAHM*-uh-tree)
(intraocular tension; ocular pressure; IOP)

5 min.

Type of Test: Manometric

Body Systems and Functions: Sensory system (eyes)

Normal Findings: 20 mm Hg or lower

Test Results Time Frame: Immediate

Test Description: This is the use of a machine to measure intraocular pressure. Clients with glaucoma have higher intraocular pressure. This is a screening test, and further testing needs to be done to confirm glaucoma. The machine measures intraocular pressure either directly when positioned on the cornea or indirectly through a puff of air on the cornea.

PHYSICAL EXAMINATION, MANOMETRIC, SENSATION, BREATH

CLINICAL ALERT:
Usually done in an opthalmologist's or optometrist's office

Consent Form: Not required

List of Equipment: Tonometer

Test Procedure:
1. Place client in upright position in front of tonometer. *Allows easy access to the eye.*
2. Apply topical anesthetic to the eye. *Allows tonometer to be in contact with the eye.*
3. The tonometer is placed against the cornea. *Tonometer measures intraocular pressure.*
4. In noncontact tonometry, a puff of air is used and there is no contact of the tonometer with the eye. *Intraocular pressure is measured indirectly.*

Clinical Implications and Indications:
1. Pressure greater than 20 mm Hg indicates the need for further testing for glaucoma.

Nursing Care:
Before Test: Explain the test procedure and the purpose of the test. Assess the client's knowledge of the test.
During Test: Adhere to standard precautions.
After Test: Provide tissue if tearing occurs. Instruct client to avoid rubbing eyes for at least 30 min after the test.

Potential Complications: Corneal abrasions from contact tonometry

Contraindications: Sensitivity to topical anesthetics

Interfering Factors: Irregular corneas

Nursing Considerations:
Pediatric: Infants and children will need assistance in remaining still during the procedure (e.g., distraction techniques) and age-appropriate comfort measures following the test.

WEBLINKS

HTTP://webmd.lycos.com; www.healthgate.com

Tourniquet Test
(*T:RN*-uh-ket)
(capillary fragility test; negative pressure test; Rumpel-Leede capillary fragility test)

5 min.

Type of Test: Physical examination

Body Systems and Functions: Hematological system

Normal Findings: No petechiae is normal. One to two petechiae is negative.

Test Results Time Frame: Immediate

Test Description: A tourniquet test measures the coagulability of the blood. A tourniquet (e.g., sphygmomanometer) is placed on a client's extremity and positive or negative pressure is applied to various areas of the body to observe for the amount of petechiae produced. The number of petechiae is a reflection of capillary fragility, which can be indicative of various bleeding disorders (note: the normal tourniquet must be applied securely enough to constrict arterial pressure).

CLINICAL ALERT:
Do not repeat test on the same arm. In addition, a tourniquet should never be left in place too long. Ordinarily, it should be removed 12–18 min after application.

Consent Form: Not required

List of Equipment: Sphygmomanometer or suction cup 2 cm in diameter and lubrication

Test Procedure:
Positive pressure test:
1. Place sphygmomanometer on the upper arm. *Upper arm is used so capillaries below the upper arm can be most easily assessed.*
2. Inflate to midway between systolic and diastolic blood pressure (usually between 70 and 90 mm Hg). *Midway between systolic and diastolic pressure allows for continued blood flow but creates enough pressure to assess capillary fragility.*
3. Keep sphygmomanometer inflated for 5 min. *Five minutes is necessary to create enough positive pressure in capillaries below the sphygmomanometer.*
4. Inspect forearm, wrists, hands, and fingers for petechiae. *In positive pressure tests, capillaries below the sphygmomanometer will be affected.*

Negative pressure test:
1. Lubricate suction cup. *Lubrication allows for better seal with skin.*
2. Apply suction cup to upper arm. *Suction cup creates negative pressure on the skin.*
3. Keep negative pressure for 1 min. *Negative pressure requires less time than positive pressure to create enough pressure to demonstrate capillary fragility.*
4. After 5 min, inspect skin under the suction cup for petechiae. *Five minutes is necessary for petechiae to become visible.*

Clinical Implications and Indications:
1. Increased petechiae can be indicative of thrombocytopenia, disseminated intravascular coagulation, vitamin K deficiency, polycythemia vera, purpura senilis, or von Willebrand's disease.
2. The larger and more numerous the petechiae, the greater the bleeding tendency.
3. The scale used for petechiae is: 0–10, 1+; 10–20, 2+; 20–50, 3+; 50 or more, 4+.

PHYSICAL EXAMINATION, MANOMETRIC, SENSATION, BREATH

Nursing Care:

Before Test: Explain the test procedure and the purpose of the test. Assess the client's knowledge of the test. Assess the client's arm for any petechiae, ecchymoses, or infections. Inform client that the test may be uncomfortable but should not be painful.

During Test: Adhere to standard precautions. Provide emotional support during the test.

After Test: Document test outcomes. Observe for bleeding tendencies. Test may need to be repeated on the opposite arm.

Contraindications: An arm with a fistula or arteriovenous shunt; the arm of affected side of postmastectomy

Interfering Factors: Age (postmenopausal women have greater petechiae); individual skin differences in terms of texture, thickness, and termperature; menstruation; presence of measles or influenza; steroid use

Nursing Considerations:

Pediatric: Infants and children will need assistance in remaining still during the venipuncture and age-appropriate comfort measures following the test.
Gerontology: Greater false-positive results in older women.

Listing of Related Tests: Platelet count; partial thromboplastin time

WEBLINKS

www.mdadvice.com

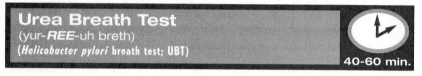

Urea Breath Test
(yur-*REE*-uh breth)
(*Helicobacter pylori* breath test; UBT)

40-60 min.

Type of Test: Breath

Body Systems and Functions: Gastrointestinal system

Normal Findings: Negative for *H. pylori*

Test Results Time Frame: Within 24–48 hr

Test Description: Urea breath test is a noninvasive method to evaluate the presence of *H. pylori. Helicobacter pylori* is a bacteria that invades the stomach or small intestine mucosa producing an enzyme called urease, which can cause ulcers. This disease has become increasingly prevalent in the United States, infecting nearly one-third of the population. It goes on to produce ulcers about 30% of the time. Treating *H. pylori* is especially important in the event that the client needs to be treated with NSAIDs. In the presence of dyspepsia the urea breath test is used since it is the least invasive of tests. If positive, then treatment is recommended. If symptoms persist, an endoscopy is recommended with biopsy.

CLINICAL ALERT:
Ask the female client if she is pregnant or has any allergies. Assess for the presence of heart or lung disease, as they could be contraindicated for this test.

Consent Form: Not required

List of Equipment: Special bag for collecting breath, pudding, and Pranactin

Test Procedure:
1. Provide the client with a cup of pudding to eat and then ask the client to breathe into the collecting bag. *Provides the baseline sample for comparison.*
2. Give the client an oral suspension of Pranactin to drink and wait 30 min. *Detects the presence of H. pylori.*
3. Instruct the client to breathe into the bag again. This air is then sent to the laboratory to be tested for the presence of urease. *The H. pylori bacteria produces urease.*

Clinical Implications and Indications:
1. Evaluates infection with *H. pylori*

Nursing Care:
Before Test: Explain the test procedure and the purpose of the test. Assess the client's knowledge of the test. Instruct client to fast for 4 hr prior to the test. Determine the completion date of antibiotic treatment, if performed.
During Test: Adhere to standard precautions.
After Test: Return to normal activities.

Interfering Factors: False-positives result if the test is performed close to antibiotic treatment, since the test evaluates active infection

Listing of Related Tests: Upper endoscopy

WEBLINKS

http://adam.excite.com

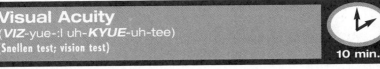

Visual Acuity
(*VIZ*-yue-:l uh-*KYUE*-uh-tee)
(Snellen test; vision test)

10 min.

Type of Test: Physical examination

Body Systems and Functions: Sensory system

Normal Findings: For distance 20/20 (the ability to see a 6-cm letter at 20 ft). For near vision 14/14 (the ability to read what the average person can read at a distance at 14 in.)

Test Results Time Frame: Immediate

PHYSICAL EXAMINATION, MANOMETRIC, SENSATION, BREATH

Test Description: A visual acuity test measures near and far vision, determining the degree of nearsightedness or farsightedness. This test is part of a broader ophthalmologic examination and is often performed in school settings and in health screening programs. The visual acuity test involves testing a client's ability to read a standard Snellen chart. This chart has a variety of symbols located a specific distance from the client (usually 20 ft). The client is asked to describe the type of symbols that can be seen at each "line" of the chart. Overall, the test may be part of a general vision screening time or it may be focused for clients that are suspected of having vision problems. The client may be asked to not wear their corrective devices (glasses, contacts) or the devices may be left in place.

Consent Form: Not required

List of Equipment: Snellen chart (standardized vision chart); E chart for children and illiterate; Jaeger card for near vision; hand-held vision occluder; space with distance of 20 ft.

Test Procedure:
Distance acuity:
1. Place the client in a seated or standing position 20 ft from the chart and have the client cover one eye.
2. The smallest line that the client can read is then indicated and is reported as a fraction. *20/20 indicates that the client can see the same as the average person can at 20 ft.*
3. This test is performed with both eyes with and without glasses. *Determines the vision before and after correction.*

Near acuity:
1. Cover one eye with the occluder and have the client read the Jaeger chart at a distance of 14 in. *This is the normal viewing distance for reading.*
2. Instruct the client to read the smallest line visible. *This will be the nearsight mearsurement.*
3. Perform the test again with the other eye. This is done with and without glasses.
4. This measurement is recorded.

Clinical Implications and Indications:
1. Assesses overall visual acuity in either farsightedness or nearsightedness
2. Assesses nystagmus, distance vision, strabismus, stereopsis, color vision, and peripheral vision

Nursing Care:
Before Test: Explain the test procedure and the purpose of the test. Assess the client's knowledge of the test.
During Test: Adhere to standard precautions.

Interfering Factors: Failure to bring glasses to the examination; old or outdated glasses; inability to follow directions

Nursing Considerations:
Pediatric: For young children or infants, the Snellen chart may be replaced by checking for nystagmus, distance vision, strabismus, stereopsis, color vision, and peripheral vision. School-age children need basic eye examinations in the event of

PHYSICAL EXAMINATION, MANOMETRIC, SENSATION, BREATH

the need for eyeglasses or contacts. Educators need to be informed of signs to look for that indicate this condition (e.g., inability to remain still while the teacher is writing on a white board or chalk board, frequent headaches).

Gerontology: *The elderly naturally develop rapid visual changes as related to the aging process. Consequently, they need to be educated as to the need for annual eye examinations.*

Home Care: *Health care providers need to be aware of common symptoms indicative of potential vision impairments (e.g., frequent falls, inability to dress themselves easily, failure to be able to read simple instructions) and the need for referral of their clients for eye examinations.*

WEBLINKS

http://adam.excite.com

Visual Evoked Response
(*VIZ*-yue-:l ee-voekt)
(VER)

1 hr.

Type of Test: Physical examination

Body Systems and Functions: Neurological system

Normal Findings: Normal symmetric patterns of electrical activity in the range of 8–11 cycles per second

Test Results Time Frame: Within 24–48 hr

Test Description: A visual evoked response is a test that uses the normal EEG techniques with variation specific to identification of lesions in the visual pathways. Lesions in the optic nerves and tracts and multiple sclerosis can be identified with this test. Visual stimulation causes impulses to pass through the optic pathways. This stimulus produces electrical activity, which can be measured in the occipital region. Electrodes placed in this region can measure this electrical activity.

Consent Form: Not required

List of Equipment: Electrodes; electroencephelograph; transducer; water-soluble gel

Test Procedure:
1. Instruct the client to remain still during the procedure. *Moving and talking will affect the accuracy of the test.*
2. The client is generally supine. Seventeen to 21 electrodes are attached to the scalp. Exact placement varies depending on the physician and machine used. Conductive gel ensures a better reading. Unlike the standard EEG, during this test the client will receive a visual stimulus.
3. Recordings are made of the electrical activity of the brain.

PHYSICAL EXAMINATION, MANOMETRIC, SENSATION, BREATH

Clinical Implications and Indications:

1. Evaluates lesions that involve the optic nerves and tracts, multiple sclerosis, and other related brain and nervous system disorders. *Abnormal patterns can indicate seizure disorders.*
2. A visual stimulus creates electrical activity in the occipital region. Abnormal activity in this region can be assessed during this test.
3. Mulitple sclerosis slows VER.
4. Lesions of the optic nerve and optic tract delay the stimulus and the wave response of the VER.
5. EEG has similarities in its clinical implications.

Nursing Care:

Before Test: Explain the test procedure and the purpose of the test. Assess the client's knowledge of the test. Food may be given, but no coffee, tea, or caffeinated beverages are to be given 12 hr prior to the procedure. Hair should be washed and rinsed thoroughly the evening before the procedure. This will allow the EEG electrodes to attach to the scalp.

During Test: Adhere to standard precautions. Instruct client to remain still and quiet.

After Test: Wash or rinse the hair and scalp as necessary to remove the conductive jelly from the electrodes. Reddened areas may appear after removal of the electrodes, which will diminish quickly.

Interfering Factors: Medications that alter results are sedatives, stimulants, and hypoglycemics; oily hair interferes with good conduction; eye and body movement

Nursing Considerations:

Pediatric: Infants and children will need assistance in remaining still during the preocedure and age-appropriate comfort measures following the test.

Listing of Related Tests: Electroencephalography

WEBLINKS

www.healthgate.com

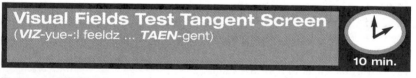

Visual Fields Test Tangent Screen
(*VIZ*-yue-:l feeldz ... *TAEN*-gent)

10 min.

Type of Test: Physical examination

Body Systems and Functions: Sensory system

Normal Findings: Object should remain visualized throughout all vision fields.

CRITICAL VALUES:
Unable to visualize object in one or more fields

Test Results Time Frame: Immediate

Test Description: The visual fields test tangent screen examination is a physical examination of the eyes, which evaluates the condition of the visual fields of a client. The examiner uses objects flashed throughout the visual fields and assesses the inability to visualize objects in all normal fields of vision.

Consent Form: Not required

List of Equipment: Tangent screen; markers (may use black-tipped straight pins); hand-held eye occluder; test objects; visual field chart

Test Procedure:
1. Place client in a sitting, upright position facing a tangent screen, which is placed 3.5 ft in front of them.
2. Ask the client to focus on a central point on the screen, while the examiner momentarily displays objects throughout the normal visual fields.
3. Ask the client to indicate when the objects appear. *Evaluates the visual fields.*

Clinical Implications and Indications:
1. Loss of vision in one or more visual fields may indicate progression or loss of vision in visual field.
2. Inability to visualize objects may indicate meningiomas, pituitary tumors, stroke, clots in the ophthalmic eye vessels, glaucoma, retinitis pigmentosa, retinal detachment or aneurysms or the circle of Willis, and craniopharyngiomas.

Nursing Care:
Before Test: Explain the test procedure and the purpose of the test. Assess the client's knowledge of the test. Instruct the client to fix their eyes on a central point throughout the test and that it will require cooperation and concentration. Have the client wear their normal corrective glasses or contact lens during the test.
During Test: Adhere to standard precautions. Reduce distractions during the test to encourage concentration. Record negative and positive responses during the test.
After Test: Results are determined by the examiner's observations and may indicate the need for further testing.

Interfering Factors: Failure to bring glasses to the examination; old or outdated prescription of eyewear; lack of cooperation or concentration of client

Nursing Considerations:
Pediatric: Children may need special distraction and attention to enable them to follow directions appropriately during the examination.
Gerontology: A higher percentage of the elderly wear corrective lens/contacts and therefore must be considered when examining their visual fields.

Listing of Related Tests: Visual field test

| WEBLINKS |

http://www.med.harvard.edu/AANLIB/hms1.html

PHYSICAL EXAMINATION, MANOMETRIC, SENSATION, BREATH

12

Nuclear Medicine Studies

EXAMINATION BY NUCLEAR MEDICINE

Nuclear medicine tests are studies of the function or physiology of any organ or body system. These tests are different from imaging studies that look at the anatomy of the body, such as magnetic imaging studies, computerized axial tomography studies, or x-rays. To perform nuclear medicine tests, a radioactive substance is introduced into the body and visualized by a camera. The camera visualizes radioactive particles as they are transported within the organ or system of interest. A computer interprets the camera image. A common example of nuclear medicine testing is positron-emission tomography (PET) scans.

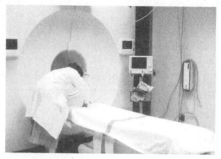

Positron-emission tomography scanner

METHODS OF PERFORMING NUCLEAR MEDICINE STUDIES

The radioactive substance is given orally, by intravenous injection, or occasionally by intramuscular, intracatheter, or intraperitoneal routes, depending on the type of test. Sometimes radioactive testing is combined with laboratory testing, in which case blood or urine specimens are taken after a prescribed amount of time to check for the presence of the radioactive substance. Many facilities have staff that has been specifically educated as to the care management techniques for nuclear medicine testing.

CLIENT CARE IN NUCLEAR MEDICINE TESTING

Client Preparation for a Nuclear Medicine Test

Clients may be understandably uneasy about having a radioactive substance placed into their body. Reassure the client that the amount of radioactivity is low. In general, a person is exposed to less radioactivity from a nuclear medicine test than he would be from an x-ray. The radioactivity will be excreted from the body within hours to days, during which time some simple precautions are maintained. The health care provider should assess the client for:

1. Allergies. Some procedures use a radioactive isotope of substances that are common allergens. Occasionally, clients with a history of allergy to iodine, eggs, or shellfish have allergic responses to nuclear medicine studies. In addition, clients should be assessed for whether they have had allergic responses to previous nuclear medicine testing.
2. Pregnancy. Although the amount of radioactivity is small, it might pose a danger to a developing fetus. Therefore, both clients and health care providers who are pregnant are contraindicated for nuclear medicine testing.
3. Lactation. A woman may be advised to stop breast-feeding for a time after the administration of a radioactive isotope.
4. The presence of any prostheses. They may interfere with the radiation. In addition, any jewelry or metal objects need to be removed before the nuclear medicine testing.
5. Age and current weight. They will be used to calculate the appropriate dosage of radioactive material.

NUCLEAR MEDICINE

Handling of Body Fluids After Testing

Standard precautions for body fluids are required after testing. Careful washing of the hands for both clients and care providers after voiding or bowel movements is necessary. The rationale is that the radioactive isotopes are excreted in the urine and feces. In addition, the client should be encouraged to drink fluids after the nuclear medicine tests to flush the isotopes from the body. There are also specifically marked radioactive waste containers available for IV equipment and syringes used in administering nuclear medicine testing.

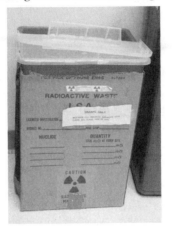

Radioactive waste container for
IV equipment and syringes.

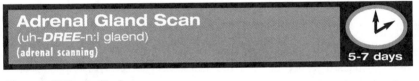

Adrenal Gland Scan
(uh-**DREE**-n:l glaend)
(adrenal scanning)

5-7 days

NUCLEAR MEDICINE

Type of Test: Nuclear scan

Body Systems and Functions: Endocrine system

Normal Findings: Normal adrenal glands without masses and with normal uptake and secretion

Test Results Time Frame: Within 48 hr

Test Description: The adrenal glands are symmetrical endocrine glands that are located on top of each kidney. They synthesize, store, and release a number of hormones that control blood pressure, water balance, and carbohydrate metabolism, among other functions. The adrenal glands mediate the body's response to stress. Since these hormones affect most of the body's systems, either over- or underproduction has major effects on well-being. The scan helps to localize the position of a tumor by noting uptake and storage within the glands.

CLINICAL ALERT:
Have emergency equipment readily available in the event of an anaphylactic reaction to the dye. Pregnant health care workers should avoid caring for clients who have had a nuclear scan for 24 hr postscan.

Consent Form: Required

Test Procedure:
1. Intravenous access is obtained. *Allows access to radionuclide.*
2. Trained personnel administer the intravenous radionuclide. *Helps to minimize risk of exposure to radioactive material.*
3. The client is generally scheduled to return in 24 hr for the first scan.
4. A scan of the renal area and abdomen is done on the second, third, and fourth days following injection. Occasionally a fifth and sixth scan will be necessary.
5. Client is placed in a prone position on the examination table and asked to remain very still for approximately 30 min while the scan is performed. *Ensures accuracy of results.*

Clinical Implications and Indications:
1. Diagnoses pheochromocytomas, carcinomas, and neuroblastomas
2. Monitors the interventions used in treating disease

Nursing Care:
Before Test: Explain the test procedure and the purpose of the test. Assess the client's knowledge of the test. Educate client on need to remain still during scan. Reassure client no pain will be experienced during the test. Instruct client to void before the procedure. Assess if client is pregnant or nursing. Have client remove all jewelry or metal objects. Administer sedatives as ordered. Assess for potential allergies to contrast medium. Inform client that during injection of contrast medium, a burning sensation may be felt for a few seconds behind the eyes or in the jaw, teeth, tongue, or lips. Assess for anxiety and provide sedation as ordered. Administer preoperative medication usually 30 min before procedure. Obtain baseline vital signs and neurological assessment. Instruct client to take Lugol's solution for 2 weeks, starting 2 days before the radioactive iodine is injected. Teach the client that the Lugol's solution will prevent uptake of radioactive iodine by the thyroid.
During Test: Adhere to standard precautions. Assess for allergic reactions to contrast medium. Encourage client to remain still.
After Test: Instruct client and caregivers to wash hands after voiding or bowel movements because the radionuclide is excreted in urine and feces. Encourage client to drink fluids to assist in flushing isotopes from the body. Assess for allergic reactions to contrast medium.

Potential Complications: Anaphylaxis due to allergic reaction to iodinated contrast material

Contraindications: Pregnancy; lactation; previous history of allergy to iodine, eggs, or shellfish; any known allergy to radionuclides; when administering radionuclide, confirm the IV is patent, because leakage at the site may be interpreted as a false positive.

Interfering Factors: Inability to remain still

Nursing Considerations:

Pregnancy: *Radiation and intravenous contrast should be avoided in pregnant women if possible (note: appropriate lead shielding is done to protect the fetus if it is determined this test is necessary). During lactation, the mother must dispose of milk until radioisotope is cleared from the milk.*

Pediatric: *Radionuclide may be harmful to the fetus, and therefore this test is only performed if absolutely necessary. Young children may require sedation.*

Gerontology: *Confused elders may need sedation; a friend or spouse may stay with the client.*

WEBLINKS

http://www.ncbi.nlm.nih.gov

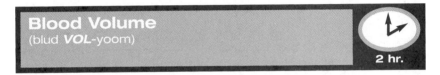

Blood Volume
(blud *VOL*-yoom)

2 hr.

Type of Test: Nuclear scan

Body Systems and Functions: Hematological system

Normal Findings: Total volume:

Adults	55–80 mL/kg
Red cell:	
Men	25–35 mL/kg
Women	20–30 mL/kg
Plasma:	
Adult males/females	30–46 mL/kg

Test Results Time Frame: Within 24 hr

Test Description: Blood volume is a nuclear study that determines the amount of circulating blood volume. It is a combination test for plasma volume and RBC volume by tagging cells and plasma with radioactive material. The results are estimated in milliliters per kilogram.

CLINICAL ALERT:
Pregnant health care workers should avoid caring for clients who have had a nuclear scan for 24 hr postscan. Have emergency equipment readily available in the event of an anaphylactic reaction to the radionuclide.

Consent Form: Not required

List of Equipment: Green-top serum tubes; alcohol swab; needle and five syringes; centrifuge bag; radionuclide

NUCLEAR MEDICINE

Test Procedure:

Nuclear scan general procedures:

1. Intravenous access is obtained. *Allows access for radionuclide.*
2. Trained personnel administer the IV radionuclide. *Helps to minimize risk of exposure to radioactive material.*
3. Client is to increase fluid intake for the next 1–3 hr. *Facilitates renal clearance of radionuclide.*
4. After the required time has passed for radionuclide to circulate and distribute, client is instructed to ensure bladder is empty. *Different radiopharmaceuticals require different times to be distributed. A full bladder will interfere with the pelvis images.*

Procedures specific to RBC scan:

1. Place client supine for 30 min.
2. Draw 20 mL blood and inject into centrifuge bag with 3 mL Strumia formula solution.
3. Add 50 mL Cr-51 to the bag and agitate for 3 min.
4. Fill the bag with 0.9% saline and centrifuge.
5. Inject 5 mL Cr-51 into vein.
6. Draw blood from opposite area at 10 and 40 min.
7. Blood sample counted to determine concentration of radionuclide and compared to the amount administered.

Procedures specific to plasma scan:

1. Place client supine for 30 minutes.
2. Draw blood to count for standard.
3. Inject 2 ml Cr-51 tagged blood into vein.
4. In 10 minutes draw 5 mL blood and centrifuge.
5. Compare to standard.

Clinical Implications and Indications:

1. Evaluates blood and fluid loss from hemorrhage, burns, surgery, and dehydration
2. Differentiates between stress polycythemia and polycythemia vera
3. Determines replacement therapy
4. Monitors response to replacement therapy
5. Evaluates uterine or GI bleeding

Nursing Care:

Before Test: Explain the test procedure and the purpose of the test. Assess the client's knowledge of the test. Educate client on need to remain still during scan. Reassure client no pain will be experienced during the test. Instruct client to void before the procedure. Assess if client is pregnant or nursing. Have client remove all jewelry or metal objects. Administer sedatives as ordered. Assess for potential allergies to contrast medium. Inform client that during injection of radionuclide, a burning sensation may be felt for a few seconds behind the eyes or in the jaw, teeth, tongue, or lips. Assess for anxiety and provide sedation as ordered. Administer preoperative medication usually 30 min before procedure. Obtain baseline vital signs and neurological assessment.

During Test: Support client, providing a calm atmosphere. Observe for allergic reaction to radionuclide.

After Test: Instruct client and caregivers to wash hands after voiding or bowel movements because the radionuclide is excreted in urine and feces. Encourage client to drink fluids to assist in flushing isotopes from the body. Assess for allergic reactions to radionuclide.

Potential Complications: Allergic reaction to radioactive material; bleeding and bruising at venipuncture site

Contraindications: Pregnancy; lactation; previous history of allergy to iodine, eggs, or shellfish; any known allergy to radionuclides; when administering radionuclide, confirm the IV is patent, because leakage at the site may be interpreted as a false positive.

Interfering Factors: Intravenous administration of fluids or blood replacement prior to study; dehydration, overhydration or excessive blood loss; prolonged time for blood sample collection

Nursing Considerations:
Pregnancy: During lactation, the mother must dispose of milk until radioisotope is cleared from the milk.
Pediatric: Radionuclide may be harmful to the fetus and therefore this test is only performed if absolutely necessary. Young children may require sedation.

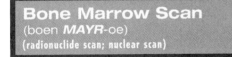

WEBLINKS

www.healthgate.com; www.ncbi.nlm.nih.gov

Bone Marrow Scan
(boen *MAYR*-oe)
(radionuclide scan; nuclear scan)

2 hr.

NUCLEAR MEDICINE

Type of Test: Nuclear scan

Body Systems and Functions: Musculoskeletal system

Normal Findings: Normal uptake, distribution, and excretion of the radionuclide by the bone marrow

Test Results Time Frame: Within 24–48 hr

Test Description: In a bone marrow examination a radionuclide is injected intravenously into the bone marrow. The radioactive material enters the bone marrow and shows the presence of bone marrow abnormalities and identifies sites for bone marrow biopsies.

CLINICAL ALERT:
Pregnant health care workers should avoid caring for clients who have had a nuclear scan for 24 hr postscan.

Consent Form: Required

List of Equipment: Nuclear scanning equipment

Test Procedure:
1. Intravenous access is obtained. *Allows access for radionuclide.*
2. Trained personnel administer the IV radionuclide. *Minimizes risk of exposure to radioactive material.*

3. After the required time, 1 hr for technetium sulfur colloid, 48 hr for indium chlorine, client lies quietly on table during head-to-toe examination. *Allows time for radionuclide to enter bone marrow to vary with type used.*

Clinical Implications and Indications:
1. Identifies presence of hematological malignancy
2. Determines sites for bone marrow biopsy
3. Identifies presence of bone marrow infarct
4. Identifies aplastic anemia
5. Identifies myelofibrosis
6. Diagnoses stages of lymphomas
7. Identifies extreme dullary sites of hematopoiesis

Nursing Care:
Before Test: Explain the test procedure and the purpose of the test. Assess the client's knowledge of the test. Educate client on need to remain still during scan. Reassure client no pain will be experienced during the test. Instruct client to void before the procedure. Assess if client is pregnant or nursing. Have client remove all jewelry or metal objects. Administer sedatives as ordered.
During Test: Adhere to standard precautions.
After Test: Instruct client and caregivers to wash hands after voiding or bowel movements because the radionuclide is excreted in urine and feces. Encourage client to drink fluids to assist in flushing isotopes from the body.

Potential Complications: Allergic reaction to radionuclide

Contraindications: Pregnancy; lactation; previous history of allergy to iodine, eggs, or shellfish; any known allergy to radionuclides; when administering radionuclide, confirm the IV is patent, because leakage at the site may be interpreted as a false positive.

Nursing Considerations:
Pregnancy: During lactation, the mother must dispose of milk until radioisotope is cleared from the milk.
Pediatric: Radionuclide may be harmful to the fetus and therefore this test is only performed if absolutely necessary. Young children may require sedation.

║WEBLINKS▐   ▣▢

www.nmc.dote.hu

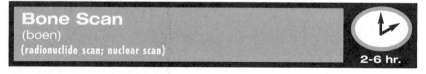

Bone Scan
(boen)
(radionuclide scan; nuclear scan)

2-6 hr.

Type of Test: Nuclear scan

Body Systems and Functions: Musculoskeletal system

Normal Findings: Symmetrical uptake and distribution of the radionuclide and no bone abnormalities

Test Results Time Frame: Within 24–48 hr

Test Description: A bone scan produces high-resolution images of the joints and bones. A radionuclide is injected into the client and a scan is performed. The radionuclide collects at areas of high osteogenesis, hot spots, or areas of absent osteogenesis, cold spots. These hot-spot areas are often detectable months before a radiograph will show abnormalities. The bone scan detects a wide variety of musculoskeletal disorders, as well as evaluating the treatment regimens.

CLINICAL ALERT:
Pregnant health care workers should avoid caring for clients who have had a nuclear scan for 24 hr postscan.

Consent Form: Required

List of Equipment: Nuclear scanning equipment

Test Procedure:
1. Intravenous access is obtained. *Allows access for radionuclide.*
2. Trained personnel administer the IV radionuclide. *Helps to minimize risk of exposure to radioactive material.*
3. Client is to increase fluid intake for the next 1–3 hr. *Facilitates renal clearance of radionuclide.*
4. After the required time has passed for radionuclide to circulate and distribute, client is instructed to ensure bladder is empty. Different radiopharmaceuticals require different times to be distributed. A full bladder will interfere with the pelvic images.
5. Client may need to be placed into different positions during the scan. *Helps to obtain scans of needed areas.*

Clinical Implications and Indications:
1. Evaluates the progression of metastatic bone disease
2. Evaluates bone trauma
3. Monitors degenerative disorders, such as degenerative arthritis, rheumatoid arthritis, and renal osteodystrophy
4. Detects osteomyelitis
5. Identifies areas for potential bone biopsy

Nursing Care:
Before Test: Explain the test procedure and the purpose of the test. Assess the client's knowledge of the test. Educate client on need to remain still during scan. Reassure client no pain will be experienced during the test. Instruct client to void before the procedure. Assess if client is pregnant or nursing. Have client remove all jewelry or metal objects. Administer sedatives as ordered.
During Test: Adhere to standard precautions. Assist client into required positions.
After Test: Instruct client and caregivers to wash hands after voiding or bowel movements because the radionuclide is excreted in urine and feces. Encourage client to drink fluids to assist in flushing isotopes from the body.

Potential Complications: Allergic reaction to radionuclide

Contraindications: Pregnancy; lactation; previous history of allergy to iodine, eggs, or shellfish; any known allergy to radionuclides; when administering radionuclide, confirm the IV is patent, because leakage at the site may be interpreted as a false positive.

NUCLEAR MEDICINE

Nursing Considerations:

Pregnancy: *Radionuclides should be avoided in pregnant women if possible. If performed, the lactating mother must dispose of milk until radioisotope is cleared from the milk.*

Pediatric: *Radionuclide may be harmful to the fetus and therefore this test is only performed if absolutely necessary. Young children may require sedation.*

WEBLINKS 🔖 　　　　　　　　　　　　　　　　　　　　　▣ ☒

www.torrancememorial.org

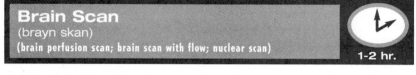

Brain Scan
(brayn skan)
(brain perfusion scan; brain scan with flow; nuclear scan)

1-2 hr.

Type of Test: Nuclear scan

Body Systems and Functions: Neurological system

Normal Findings: Equal and symmetric distribution of brain function and activity with normal uptake and distribution of the radionuclide

Test Results Time Frame: Within 24–48 hr

Test Description: Nuclear brain scans allow the early visualization of physiological functioning of the brain. Brain scans are useful in diagnosing cerebral vascular disease, observing the internal carotid arteries, locating foci seizure activity, and evaluating dementia and Parkinson's disease. Nuclear brain scans combine the use of special radionuclides with gamma cameras and computers to create tomographic images. The gamma camera rotates around the patient's head, thereby creating many thin slices and decreasing the chance of surrounding tissue obscuring the view. The physiological function of the brain can be observed using two different techniques: position emission tomography (PET) and single-photon emission computed tomography (SPECT).

> **CLINICAL ALERT:**
> Pregnant health care workers should avoid caring for clients who have had a nuclear scan for 24 hr postscan.

Consent Form: Required

List of Equipment: Nuclear scanning equipment

Test Procedure:
1. Intravenous access is obtained. *Allows access for radionuclide.*
2. Trained personnel administer the IV radionuclide. *Helps to minimize risk of exposure to radioactive material.*
3. Client is to increase fluid intake for the next 1–3 hr. *Facilitates renal clearance of radionuclide.*
4. Client may need to be placed into different positions during the scan. *Helps to obtain scans of needed areas.*
5. The client lies supine in quiet, dark environment while images are being taken. *Motion during procedure will decrease the quality of images being taken.*

NUCLEAR MEDICINE

Clinical Implications and Indications:

1. Evaluates brain tissue, internal carotid arteries, cerebral vascular disease, or abnormalities
2. Visualizes the function of brain tissue, especially for dementia, organic brain syndrome, Alzheimer's disease, and schizophrenia

Nursing Care:

Before Test: Explain the test procedure and the purpose of the test. Assess the client's knowledge of the test. Educate client on need to remain still during scan. Reassure client no pain will be experienced during the test. Instruct client to void before the procedure. Assess if client is pregnant or nursing. Have client remove all jewelry or metal objects. Administer sedatives as ordered. Advise client to fast for 4 hr prior to examination. Assess for potential allergies to contrast medium. Inform client that during injection of contrast medium, a burning sensation may be felt for a few seconds behind the eyes or in the jaw, teeth, tongue, or lips. Assess for anxiety and provide sedation as ordered. Administer preoperative medication usually 30 min before procedure. Obtain baseline vital signs and neurological assessment.

During Test: Adhere to standard precautions. Assess for allergic reactions to contrast medium. Keep room dark and free of traffic.

After Test: Assess for allergic reactions to contrast medium. Instruct client and caregivers to wash hands after voiding or bowel movements because the radionuclide is excreted in urine and feces. Encourage client to drink fluids to assist in flushing isotopes from the body.

Potential Complications: Anaphylaxis due to allergic reaction to iodinated contrast material

Contraindications: Pregnancy; lactation; previous history of allergy to iodine, eggs, or shellfish; any known allergy to radionuclides; when administering radionuclide, confirm the IV is patent, because leakage at the site may be interpreted as a false positive.

Interfering Factors: Recent nuclear studies

Nursing Considerations:

Pregnancy: Intravenous contrast should be avoided in pregnant women if possible. During lactation, the mother must dispose of milk until radioisotope is cleared from the milk.

Pediatric: Radionuclide may be harmful to the fetus and therefore this test is only performed if absolutely necessary. Young children may require sedation.

NUCLEAR MEDICINE

| WEBLINKS | | ▤▨ |

www.macalstr.edu

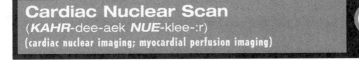

Cardiac Nuclear Scan
(*KAHR*-dee-aek *NUE*-klee-:r)
(cardiac nuclear imaging; myocardial perfusion imaging)

3-4 hr.

Type of Test: Nuclear scan

Body Systems and Functions: Cardiovascular system

Normal Findings: No perfusion defects will be found, as interpreted by the cardiologist.

Test Results Time Frame: Within 30–45 min

Test Description: A cardiac nuclear scan is indicated for the client with chest pain and known or suspected coronary artery disease. Information regarding the location and extent of myocardial ischemia and viability of myocardial tissues is provided. Exercise-induced areas of ischemic cardiac tissue or necrotic cardiac tissue from a previous myocardial infarction reveals decreased radiocompound material uptake known as perfusion defects. Pharmacological stress imaging using adenosine, dipyridamole, or dobutamine may be administered in clients who are unable to exercise. Abnormal results may indicate the need for cardiac catheterization or other studies.

CLINICAL ALERT:
The client is potentially at risk for myocardial ischemia, which could provoke cardiac instability during the testing. Consequently, the care providers must continually assess the client for cardiac abnormalities and have emergency equipment readily available. Pregnant health care workers should avoid caring for clients who have had a nuclear scan for 24 hr postscan.

Consent Form: Required

List of Equipment: Nuclear scanning equipment

Test Procedure:
1. Intravenous access is obtained. *Allows access for radionuclide.*
2. Trained personnel administer the IV radionuclide (e.g., thallium-201, Sestamibi). *Helps to minimize risk of exposure to radioactive material.*
3. Client is to increase fluid intake for the next 1–3 hr. *Facilitates renal clearance of radionuclide.*
4. After the required time has passed for radionuclide to circulate and distribute, client is instructed to ensure bladder is empty. *Different radiopharmaceuticals require different times to be distributed. A full bladder will interfere with the pelvic images.*
5. Client may need to be placed into different positions during the scan and cardiac images are obtained at rest, during exercise or during pharmacological induced stress. *Helps to obtain scans of needed areas during varying circumstances.*
6. A dual-isotope technique protocol employs a rest injection of thallium-201 followed by imaging. Within 1 hr Sestamibi is injected during exercise stress on a treadmill. *Allows for diagnostic evaluation during physical stress.*

Clinical Implications and Indications:
1. Diagnoses coronary artery disease
2. Assesses known coronary stenosis
3. Assesses therapeutic benefits after coronary angioplasty, coronary artery bypass surgery, and medical therapy
4. Risk stratification of stable angina, unstable angina, and post–myocardial infarction

NUCLEAR MEDICINE

Nursing Care:

Before Test: Explain the test procedure and the purpose of the test. Assess the client's knowledge of the test. Educate client on need to remain still during scan. Reassure client no pain will be experienced during the test. Instruct client to void before the procedure. Assess if client is pregnant or nursing. Have client remove all jewelry or metal objects. Administer sedatives as ordered. Instruct client to be NPO for 4–6 hr before the test. Obtain and record resting vital signs, height, and weight (note: radionuclide is based on accurate weight of client). Instruct client to refrain from smoking for 2 hr before the test.

During Test: Monitor and record vital signs, cardiac rhythm, oxygen saturation, and the client's tolerance to stress. Isotopes are injected at designated times during the test. Assess for complications.

After Test: Instruct client and caregivers to wash hands after voiding or bowel movements because the radionuclide is excreted in urine and feces. Encourage client to drink fluids to assist in flushing isotopes from the body. Monitor and record vital signs, cardiac rhythm, oxygen saturation, general physical assessment, and the client's tolerance to stress.

Potential Complications: Nausea and vomiting; headache; dizziness; facial flushing; angina; ST-segment depression or elevation; ventricular arrhythmia

Contraindications: Pregnancy; lactation; previous history of allergy to iodine, eggs, or shellfish; any known allergy to radionuclides; when administering radionuclide, confirm the IV line is patent, because leakage at the site may be interpreted as a false positive; unstable angina; recent myocardial infarction (<48 hr); sick sinus syndrome; second- and third-degree block; hypotension (resting systolic pressure <80 mm Hg); severe aortic stenosis; history of tachyarrhythmias; hypertension (resting systolic pressure >200 mm Hg); poor left ventricular function

Interfering Factors: False-negative scans are caused by inadequate exercise stress, administration of anti-ischemic medications, incorrect interpretation of scans, poor quality images, and a delay in obtaining stress images; causes of false-positive scans include poor technique, cardiomyopathies, coronary vasospasm, and coronary anomalies.

Nursing Considerations:

Pregnancy: During lactation, the mother must dispose of milk until radioisotope is cleared from the milk.

Pediatric: Radionuclide may be harmful to the fetus, and therefore this test is only performed if absolutely necessary. Young children may require sedation.

Listing of Related Tests: Myocardial imaging; radionuclide angiography; multigated acquisition scan

NUCLEAR MEDICINE

| WEBLINKS |

http://www.nhlbi.nih.gov

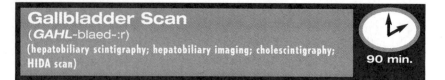

Gallbladder Scan
(***GAHL***-blaed-:r)
(hepatobiliary scintigraphy; hepatobiliary imaging; cholescintigraphy; HIDA scan)

90 min.

Type of Test: Nuclear scan

Body Systems and Functions: Gastrointestinal system

Normal Findings: Normal shape, size, and function of gallbladder; absence of common bile duct (CBD) dilatation; patient cystic; common bile ducts; and absence of stones

Test Results Time Frame: Within 24 hr (unless client has known gallbladder disease and then repeat imaging may be needed at 48 hr)

Test Description: A gallbladder scan is a nuclear medicine test that uses the radionuclide technetium-99m disopropyl. This test obtains images of the hepatobiliary system as an aid to the diagnosis of obstruction within the cystic and common bile ducts and cholecystitis. Gallbladder diease is most common in middle-aged females who are multiparous and obese and have a diet high in fat content. Often clients will experience intolerance of fatty foods, due to the gallbladder's normal function of storing and discharging bile (bile is responsible for the emulsification of fats).

CLINICAL ALERT:
Pregnant health care workers should avoid caring for clients who have had a nuclear scan for 24 hr postscan.

Consent Form: Required

List of Equipment: Nuclear scanning equipment

Test Procedure:
1. Instruct client to fast 4–6 hr before the scan. *Allows for accurate results.*
2. An IV line is established and technetium-99m disopropyl is injected.
3. Images of the right upper abdominal quadrant are taken immediately with the client supine and every 5 min thereafter for 30 min and every 10 min for the next 30 min. Delayed images can be taken at 2, 4, and 24 hr.

Clinical Implications and Indications:
1. Primary diagnostic test for acute cholecystitis.
2. Diagnoses cystic and common bile duct obstruction.
3. Evaluates clients as a follow-up to ultrasonography. It is particulary beneficial when ultrasonography is negative as it is able to detect small stones that are present in the bile ducts.
4. Those clients with known hepatocellular disease will need delayed imaging 6–48 hr after injection.

Nursing Care:
Before Test: Explain the test procedure and the purpose of the test. Assess the client's knowledge of the test. Educate client on need to remain still during scan. Reassure client no pain will be experienced during the test. Instruct client to void before the procedure. Assess if client is pregnant or nursing. Have client

NUCLEAR MEDICINE

remove all jewelry or metal objects. Administer sedatives as ordered. Instruct client to fast for 2–4 hr before test. Take baseline vital signs.
During Test: Adhere to standard precautions.
After Test: Instruct client and caregivers to wash hands after voiding or bowel movements because the radionuclide is excreted in urine and feces. Encourage client to drink fluids to assist in flushing isotopes from the body. Client will be observed and vital signs taken for up to 1 hr after test.

Contraindications: Pregnancy; lactation; previous history of allergy to iodine, eggs, or shellfish; any known allergy to radionuclides; when administering radionuclide, confirm the IV line is patent, because leakage at the site may be interpreted as a false positive.

Interfering Factors: Bilirubin levels >30 mg/dL may decrease hepatic uptake; total parenteral nutrition; alcoholism; barium decreases visualization during the scan.

Nursing Considerations:

Pregnancy: Radionuclides should be avoided in pregnant women if possible. If performed, the lactating mother must dispose of milk until radioisotope is cleared from the milk.
Pediatric: Radionuclide may be harmful to the fetus and therefore this test is only performed if absolutely necessary. Young children may require sedation.
Gerontology: The older person may find it difficult to maintain positions when required to do so for lengthy periods of time during this nuclear scan.
Rural: Advisable to arrange for transportation home after recovering from the nuclear scan.

Listing of Related Tests: Oral cholecystography; CT of the gallbladder; GB ultrasound

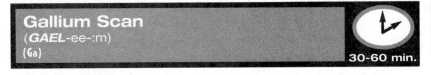

WEBLINKS

http://www.nlm.nih.gov

Gallium Scan
(*GAEL*-ee-:m)
(Ga)

30-60 min.

NUCLEAR MEDICINE

Type of Test: Nuclear scan

Body Systems and Functions: Immunological system

Normal Findings: No localization of gallium citrate in the tissue

Test Results Time Frame: The 1-hr scan may be evaluated within 24 hr (note: repeating the procedure changes the length of time to obtain results).

Test Description: A gallium scan is a nuclear medicine scan that uses the radiopharmaceutical gallium citrate (6–10 mCi). Gallium is a rare metal that has a half-life of 68 min. The gallium is injected intravenously into the client and the tracer follows white blood cells where it localizes in the region of infection or inflammation.

CLINICAL ALERT:
Pregnant health care workers should avoid caring for clients who have had a nuclear scan for 24 hr postscan.

Consent Form: Required

List of Equipment: Nuclear scanning equipment

Test Procedure:
1. Intravenous access is obtained. *Allows access for radionuclide.*
2. Trained personnel administer the IV radionuclide (gallium). *Helps to minimize risk of exposure to radioactive material.*
3. Leave client on an x-ray table in the nuclear medicine department 24, 48, and even 72 hr postinjection for a 1-hr scan.
4. Client may need to be placed into different positions during the scan. *Helps to obtain scans of needed areas.*

Clinical Implications and Indications:
1. Evaluates fevers of unknown origin, osteomyelitis, and abscess
2. Evaluates extent of inflammation and infection
3. Detects metastatic tumors, particularly lymphoma

Nursing Care:
Before Test: Explain the test procedure and the purpose of the test. Assess the client's knowledge of the test. Educate client on need to remain still during scan. Reassure client no pain will be experienced during the test. Instruct client to void before the procedure. Assess if client is pregnant or nursing. Have client remove all jewelry or metal objects. Administer sedatives as ordered. Instruct client to be NPO the morning of the test and the client may be required to have cleansing enemas.
During Test: Adhere to standard precautions.
After Test: Instruct client and caregivers to wash hands after voiding or bowel movements because the radionuclide is excreted in urine and feces. Encourage client to drink fluids to assist in flushing isotopes from the body.

Contraindications: Pregnancy; lactation; previous history of allergy to iodine, eggs, or shellfish; any known allergy to radionuclides; when administering radionuclide, confirm the IV is patent, because leakage at the site may be interpreted as a false positive.

Interfering Factors: Procedure takes hours or days; localization in osteomyelitis may be obscured by overlying acute cellulitis; gallium uptake in the abdomen may be obscured by uptake in the intestines and liver.

Nursing Considerations:
Pregnancy: Radionuclides should be avoided in pregnant women if possible. If performed, the lactating mother must dispose of milk until radioisotope is cleared from the milk.
Pediatric: Radionuclide may be harmful to the fetus and therefore this test is only performed if absolutely necessary. Young children may require sedation.
Gerontology: The older person may find it difficult to maintain positions when required to do so for lengthy periods of time during the nuclear scan.
Rural: Advisable to arrange for transportation home after recovering from the nuclear scan.

Listing of Related Tests: CT; MRI; gallbladder ultrasound

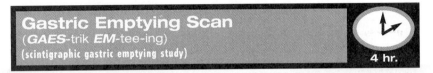

WEBLINKS

http://www.nlm.nih.gov

Gastric Emptying Scan
(*GAES*-trik *EM*-tee-ing)
(scintigraphic gastric emptying study)

4 hr.

Type of Test: Nuclear scan

Body Systems and Functions: Gastrointestinal system

Normal Findings: Liquids usually empty quickly. Solids empty more slowly; gastric emptying tests vary considerably, and individual results should be interpreted cautiously unless the results are unequivocal.

Test Results Time Frame: Within 24 hr

Test Description: The gastric emptying scan involves the ingestion of a test standard meal (typically >200 kcal), labeled with radioactive isotope (technetium-99m for solids and indium-111 for liquids). The test measures the percentage of gastric emptying after 2 and 4 hr. A variety of gastrointestinal abnormalities can be detected with this test.

> **CLINICAL ALERT:**
> Pregnant health care workers should avoid caring for clients who have had a nuclear scan for 24 hr postscan.

Consent Form: Required

List of Equipment: Nuclear scanning equipment

Test Procedure:
1. Intravenous access is obtained. *Allows access for radionuclide.*
2. Trained personnel administer the IV radionuclide. *Helps to minimize risk of exposure to radioactive material.*
3. Client will be in the nuclear medicine department after ingestion of a meal labeled with the radioactive isotope.
4. Scanning will take place 2 and then 4 hr after the meal ingestion.
5. Client may need to be placed into different positions during the scan. *Helps to obtain scans of needed areas.*

Clinical Implications and Indications:
1. Evaluates unexplained nausea and vomiting
2. Diagnoses "motility-like" nonulcer dyspepsia
3. Diagnoses diabetes in clients in whom gastroparesis is suspected (particularly those with poor glycemic control)
4. Evaluates suspected dumping or stasis syndrome post-gastric surgery, refractory gastroesophageal reflux disease, and suspected chronic intestinal pseudo-obstruction
5. Evaluates and monitors a known gastric emptying disturbance where a response to motility-altering drugs is desired

NUCLEAR MEDICINE

Nursing Care:

Before Test: Explain the test procedure and the purpose of the test. Assess the client's knowledge of the test. Educate client on need to remain still during scan. Reassure client no pain will be experienced during the test. Instruct client to void before the procedure. Assess if client is pregnant or nursing. Have client remove all jewelry or metal objects. Administer sedatives as ordered.
During Test: Adhere to standard precautions.
After Test: Instruct client and caregivers to wash hands after voiding or bowel movements because the radionuclide is excreted in urine and feces. Encourage client to drink fluids to assist in flushing isotopes from the body.

Contraindications: Pregnancy; lactation; previous history of allergy to iodine, eggs, or shellfish; any known allergy to radionuclides; when administering radionuclide, confirm the IV line is patent, because leakage at the site may be interpreted as a false positive.

Interfering Factors: Test is not valid if vomiting occurs.

Nursing Considerations:

Pregnancy: During lactation, the mother must dispose of milk until radioisotope is cleared from the milk.
Pediatric: Radionuclide may be harmful to the fetus and therefore this test is only performed if absolutely necessary. Young children may require sedation.

Listing of Related Tests: Upper GI study

WEBLINKS

http://www.imaginis.com

Gastroesophageal Reflux Scan
(*GAES*-troe-uh-*SAHF*-uh-*JEE*-:l *REE*-fluhks)
(GE scintiscan; GER scan)

60 min.

Type of Test: Nuclear scan

Body Systems and Functions: Gastrointestinal system

Normal Findings: A normal scan demonstrates 4% reflux across the esophageal sphincter at any pressure.

Test Results Time Frame: Within 24 hr

Test Description: A gastroesophageal reflux scan is a nuclear medicine test that uses orally administered radioactive contrast (usually technetium-99m sulfur colloid mixed in orange juice) to assess gastric reflux across the esophageal sphincter. Gastric reflux occurs when there is an incompetent esophageal sphincter, as in a hiatal hernia. The client will experience pyrosis (heartburn), indigestion, and a reflux of gastric contents upward into the esophagus. Often the client will self-treat themselves by sitting in an upright position while sleeping and after meals.

CLINICAL ALERT:
Pregnant health care workers should avoid caring for clients who have had a nuclear scan for 24 hr postscan. Have emergency equipment readily available in the event of an anaphylactic reaction to the contrast medium.

Consent Form: Required

List of Equipment: Nuclear scanning equipment

Test Procedure:

1. Place client supine on x-ray table.
2. Intravenous access is obtained. *Allows access for radionuclide.*
3. Trained personnel administer the radionuclide orally (30 mL). *Helps to minimize risk of exposure to radioactive material.*
4. An abdominal binding is applied and gradually tightened to determine the degrees of abdominal pressure. *Increases tendency to have reflux condition.*
5. Nuclear images are obtained and observed at the different pressures (0, 20, 40, 60, 80, and 100 mm Hg) and at 30-sec intervals.

Clinical Implications and Indications:

1. Diagnoses gastroesophageal reflux in clients with nausea, vomiting, and dysphagia of uncertain etiology
2. Assesses gastric reflux across the esophageal sphincter and conditions such as hiatal hernia

Nursing Care:

Before Test: Explain the test procedure and the purpose of the test. Assess the client's knowledge of the test. Educate client on need to remain still during scan. Reassure client no pain will be experienced during the test. Instruct client to void before the procedure. Assess if client is pregnant or nursing. Have client remove all jewelry or metal objects. Administer sedatives as ordered. Assess for potential allergies to contrast medium. Inform client that during injection of contrast medium, a burning sensation may be felt for a few seconds behind the eyes or in the jaw, teeth, tongue, or lips. Assess for anxiety and provide sedation as ordered. Administer preoperative medication usually 30 min before procedure. Obtain baseline vital signs and neurological assessment.

During Test: Adhere to standard precautions. Assess for allergic reactions to contrast medium.

After Test: Instruct client and caregivers to wash hands after voiding or bowel movements because the radionuclide is excreted in urine and feces. Encourage client to drink fluids to assist in flushing isotopes from the body. Assess for allergic reactions to contrast medium.

Potential Complications: Anaphylaxis due to allergic reaction to iodinated contrast material

Contraindications: Previous history of allergy to iodine, eggs, or shellfish; pregnancy; lactation; any known allergy to radionuclides; when administering radionuclide, confirm the IV line is patent, because leakage at the site may be interpreted as a false positive.

Interfering Factors: Results may be affected if recent studies have been done using an opaque dye or contrast medium.

NUCLEAR MEDICINE

Nursing Considerations:

Pregnancy: Contrast materials should be avoided in pregnant women if possible. During lactation, the mother must dispose of milk until radioisotope is cleared from the milk .

Pediatric: Radionuclide may be harmful to the fetus and therefore this test is only performed if absolutely necessary. Young children may require sedation. Assistance may be required to help infant/young child maintain positions required for scanning.

Gerontology: Check serum potassium levels prior to ingestion of the contrast medium in orange juice if client is on potassium replacement or has known renal failure or insufficiency. The older person may find it difficult to maintain positions when required to do so for lengthy periods of time during the scan.

Home Care: Caregivers must wear rubber gloves when discarding the client's urine for 24 hr postprocedure.

Listing of Related Tests: Upper GI series; esophageal manometry; standard acid reflux test

WEBLINKS

http://www.med.harvard.edu

Hepatobiliary Scan
(*HEP*-uh-toe-*BIL*-ee-*AYR*-ee)
(gallbladder scan; HIDA scan; hepatobiliary scintigraphy; hepatobiliary imaging; cholescintigraphy)

90 min.

Type of Test: Nuclear scan

Body Systems and Functions: Hepatobiliary system

Normal Findings: Normal function, size, and shape of gallbladder; absence of obstruction in cystic and common bile ducts

Test Results Time Frame: Within 24 hr

Test Description: Hepatobiliary scan is a radionuclide study that examines the gallbladder, intestines, extrahepatic bile ducts, and hepatic parenchyma. This scan utilizes technetium 99m–labeled derivatives of iminodiacetic acid excreted in the bile. In normal scans, obtained 15–30 min after IV injection, there is a determination of the patency of the bile ducts and the gallbladder and passage of the radionuclide to the common bile duct and small intestine. Clients with hepatocellular disease will need delayed imaging for 6–48 hr after injection.

> **CLINICAL ALERT:**
> Pregnant health care workers should avoid caring for clients who have had a nuclear scan for 24 hr postscan.

Consent Form: Required

List of Equipment: Nuclear scanning equipment; IV line equipment

Test Procedure:
1. Intravenous access is obtained. *Allows access for radionuclide.*

2. Client is placed in the supine position and trained personnel administer the IV radionuclide. *Helps to obtain scans of needed areas and minimizes risk of exposure to radioactive material.*
3. Immediate views of the right upper abdominal quadrant with images taken every 5 min for the first 30 min and every 10 min for the next 30 min. Delayed views may be taken in 2, 4, and 24 hr if the gallbladder cannot be visualized.
4. Client is to increase fluid intake for the next 1–3 hr. *Facilitates renal clearance of radionuclide.*
5. After the required time has passed for radionuclide to circulate and distribute, client is instructed to ensure bladder is empty. *Different radiopharmaceuticals require different times to be distributed. A full bladder will interfere with the pelvis images.*

Clinical Implications and Indications:
1. Diagnoses acute and chronic cholecystitis, biliary obstruction, bile leak, and biliary atresia
2. Assists in the determination of decreased hepatocyte function
3. Diagnoses common duct obstruction caused by tumors or choledocholithiasis

Nursing Care:
Before Test: Explain the test procedure and the purpose of the test. Assess the client's knowledge of the test. Educate client on need to remain still during scan. Reassure client no pain will be experienced during the test. Instruct client to void before the procedure. Assess if client is pregnant or nursing. Have client remove all jewelry or metal objects. Administer sedatives as ordered. Instruct client to be NPO at least 2 hr before the test.

After Test: Instruct client and caregivers to wash hands after voiding or bowel movements because the radionuclide is excreted in urine and feces. Encourage client to drink fluids to assist in flushing isotopes from the body.

Contraindications: Pregnancy; lactation; previous history of allergy to iodine, eggs, or shellfish; any known allergy to radionuclides; when administering radionuclide, confirm the IV line is patent, because leakage at the site may be interpreted as a false positive.

Interfering Factors: A serum bilirubin over 20–30 may interfere with uptake of tracer by the liver; parenchymal liver disease and high bile duct obstruction may lead to failure of imaging of the extrahepatic biliary tree; delayed images would be needed to distinguish acute from chronic cholecystitis.

Nursing Considerations:
Pregnancy: During lactation, the mother must dispose of milk until radioisotope is cleared from the milk.
Pediatric: Radionuclide may be harmful to the fetus, and therefore this test is only performed if absolutely necessary. Young children may require sedation.

Listing of Related Tests: Ultrasound of the gallbladder

NUCLEAR MEDICINE

WEBLINKS

http://webmd.lycos.com

Liver Scan
(*LI*-ver skan)
(liver sonogram; liver echogram; liver ultrasound; liver/spleen scan)

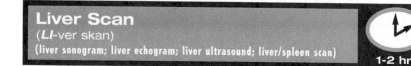

1-2 hr.

Type of Test: Nuclear scan

Body Systems and Functions: Hepatobiliary system

Normal Findings: Normal size, shape, and position of liver and spleen; normal blood flow and cell function; there is normally more uptake of the test substance in the spleen than in the liver.

Test Results Time Frame: Within 24 hr

Test Description: A liver scan is a noninvasive diagnostic technique evaluating the liver and ancillary areas of the gallbladder and diaphragm. It is an ultrasound that passes over the right upper quadrant of the abdomen and provides a three-dimensional picture of the liver. The test determines abnormalities of the liver, including such things as fatty infiltrates, the presence of hepatic fibrosis, and diagnosis of metastatic presence.

CLINICAL ALERT:
Have emergency equipment readily available in the event of an anaphylactic reaction to the radionuclide.

Consent Form: Required

List of Equipment: Intravenous equipment; radioactive substance; rectilinear scanner or gamma camera

Test Procedure:
1. Intravenous access is obtained. *Allows access for radionuclide.*
2. Trained personnel administer the IV radionuclide. *Helps to minimize risk of exposure to radioactive material.*
3. Client may need to be placed into different positions (e.g., supine, lateral, prone) 30 min after injection of the radionuclide. *Helps to obtain scans of needed areas.*

Clinical Implications and Indications:
1. Diagnoses and monitors hepatitis, cirrhosis, liver cancer, cysts, abscesses, tumors, infarctions, granulomas, splenic hematoma, hemangioma, lacerations, portal hypertension, accessory spleen, amyloidosis, and sarcoidosis.
2. Abnormal splenic concentrations reveal unusual splenic size, infarction, ruptured spleen, accessory spleen, tumors, metastatic spread, leukemia, Hodgkin's disease.
3. Areas of absent radioactivity or holes in the spleen are associated with abnormalities that displace or destroy splenic pulp. About 30% of persons with Hodgkin's disease with splenic involvement have a normal spleen scan.

Nursing Care:
Before Test: Explain the test procedure and the purpose of the test. Assess the client's knowledge of the test. Educate client on need to remain still during scan. Reassure client no pain will be experienced during the test. Instruct client to void before the procedure. Assess if client is pregnant or nursing. Have client remove all jewelry or metal objects. Administer sedatives as ordered.

During Test: Adhere to standard precautions.

After Test: Instruct client and caregivers to wash hands after voiding or bowel movements because the radionuclide is excreted in urine and feces. Encourage client to drink fluids to assist in flushing isotopes from the body.

Contraindications: Pregnancy; lactation; previous history of allergy to iodine, eggs, or shellfish; any known allergy to radionuclides; when administering radionuclide, confirm the IV is patent, because leakage at the site may be interpreted as a false positive; not recommended for clients who may not cooperate because of age, mental status, or pain

Interfering Factors: Radioactive substances administered the same day (barium in the intestinal tract can appear as masses); inability to remain still

Nursing Considerations:

Pregnancy: Radionuclides should be avoided in pregnant women if possible. If performed, the lactating mother must dispose of milk until radioisotope is cleared from the milk.

Pediatric: Radionuclide may be harmful to the fetus and therefore this test is only performed if absolutely necessary. Young children may require sedation.

Gerontology: The older person may find it difficult to maintain positions when required to do so for lengthy periods of time during the liver scan.

Home Care: Caregivers must wear rubber gloves when discarding the client's urine for 24 hr postprocedure.

Rural: Advisable to arrange for transportation home after recovering from the liver scan.

WEBLINKS

www.healthgate.com

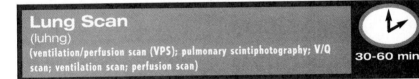

Lung Scan
(luhng)
(ventilation/perfusion scan (VPS); pulmonary scintiphotography; V/Q scan; ventilation scan; perfusion scan)

30–60 min.

NUCLEAR MEDICINE

Type of Test: Nuclear scan

Body Systems and Functions: Pulmonary system

Normal Findings: Even distribution of activity throughout the lungs

Test Results Time Frame: Within 24 hr

Test Description: A lung scan is a nuclear medicine procedure in which the structure and function of the lungs are evaluated. There are three types of lung scans: perfusion scan (the radioactive substance is administered through an IV rather than breathed in), ventilation scan, and inhalation scan. Each of these detects different aspects of the lung's condition.

CLINICAL ALERT:
Have emergency equipment readily available in the event of an anaphylactic reaction to the radionuclide. Pregnant health care workers should avoid caring for clients who have had a nuclear scan for 24 hr postscan.

Consent Form: Required

List of Equipment: Face mask or nebulizer; krypton-85 gas or xenon-133 gas; nuclear scanning equipment

Test Procedure:
1. The client breathes through the mask or nebulizer for about 4 min. A minimal amount of gas is breathed in during this time.
2. Multiple images of the lungs are taken after the inhalation of the radioactive gas or nebulized aerosol.
3. A chest x-ray is also taken either before or immediately after the scan. *Evaluates lung status.*

Clinical Implications and Indications:
1. Diagnoses pulmonary emboli, pulmonary thrombosis, atelectasis, bronchitis, chronic obstructive pulmonary disease, inflammatory fibrosis, lung cancer, and pneumonia
2. Determines the percentage of the lungs that are functioning and an assessment of the pulmonary vasculature

Nursing Care:
Before Test: Explain the test procedure and the purpose of the test. Assess the client's knowledge of the test. Assess for potential allergies to radionuclide. Educate client on need to remain still during scan. Reassure client no pain will be experienced during the test. Instruct client to void before the procedure. Assess if client is pregnant or nursing. Have client remove all jewelry or metal objects. Administer sedatives as ordered. Establish IV line if not already present and if radiology department requests it. Evaluate whether the client is able to cooperate during the test, breathe through a mouthpiece, remain still for 15 min, and hold breath for approximately 10 sec.
During Test: Adhere to standard precautions. Assess for allergic reactions to radionuclide.
After Test: Assess for allergic reactions to radionuclide. Instruct client and caregivers to wash hands after voiding or bowel movements because the radionuclide is excreted in urine and feces. Encourage client to drink fluids to assist in flushing isotopes from the body.

Potential Complications: Anaphylaxis due to allergic reaction to radionuclide

Contraindications: Pregnancy; lactation; previous history of allergy to iodine, eggs, or shellfish; any known allergy to radionuclides; when administering radionuclide, confirm the IV is patent, because leakage at the site may be interpreted as a false positive.

Interfering Factors: False positives may be caused by vasculitis, mitral stenosis, pulmonary hypertension, or an obstruction in the pulmonary artery caused by a tumor.

Nursing Considerations:

Pregnancy: *Radionuclides should be avoided in pregnant women if possible. If performed, the lactating mother must dispose of milk until radioisotope is cleared from the milk.*

Pediatric: *Children must be administered a smaller amount of gas, as there is a greater possibility of airway obstruction. Radionuclide may be harmful to the fetus, and therefore this test is only performed if absolutely necessary. Young children may require sedation.*

Gerontology: *The older person may find it difficult to maintain positions when required to do so for lengthy periods of time during the lung scan.*

Rural: *Advisable to arrange for transportation home after recovering from the lung scan.*

Listing of Related Tests: Lung scan; pulmonary function studies

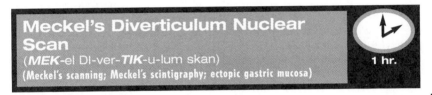

WEBLINKS

www.healthgate.com

Meckel's Diverticulum Nuclear Scan
(*MEK*-el DI-ver-*TIK*-u-lum skan)
(Meckel's scanning; Meckel's scintigraphy; ectopic gastric mucosa)

1 hr.

Type of Test: Nuclear scan

Body Systems and Functions: Gastrointestinal system

Normal Findings: Lack of any focal secreted activity in the abdomen; normal blood distribution and clearance of the radioactive tracer in the duodenum and jejunum

Test Description: Meckel's diverticulum scan assesses a type of diverticulum (outpouching of the gastric mucosa) that is a congenital abnormality of the ileum, usually in the distal third near the ileocecal valve. This diverticulum sometimes continues to the umbilicus with fistula formation. Meckel's diverticulum is estimated to occur in about 2% of the population and is more common in men. It is usually asymptomatic but can become inflamed, especially later in life, and require surgical treatment.

CLINICAL ALERT:
Pregnant health care workers should avoid caring for clients who have had a nuclear scan for 24 hr postscan. A Meckel's diverticulum without functioning gastric mucosa will not visualize.

Consent Form: Required

List of Equipment: Nuclear scanning equipment

Test Procedure:
1. Intravenous access is obtained. *Allows access for radionuclide.*

NUCLEAR MEDICINE

2. Trained personnel administer the IV radionuclide (technetium-99m). *Helps to minimize risk of exposure to radioactive material.*
3. Client is to increase fluid intake for the next 1–3 hr. *Facilitates renal clearance of radionuclide.*
4. After the required time has passed for radionuclide to circulate and distribute, client is instructed to ensure bladder is empty. *Different radiopharmaceuticals require different times to be distributed.*
5. Client may need to be placed into different positions during the scan of the abdomen. *Helps to obtain scans of needed areas.*

Clinical Implications and Indications:
1. Diagnoses and evaluates Meckel's diverticulum.
2. Rectal bleeding is the most common symptom of Meckel's diverticulum.
3. Condition can occur with or without related abdominal symptoms.
4. If Meckel's diverticulum is left untreated, ulceration of the ileum may occur and strangulation may cause intestinal obstruction.

Nursing Care:
Before Test: Explain the test procedure and the purpose of the test. Assess the client's knowledge of the test. Educate client on need to remain still during scan. Reassure client no pain will be experienced during the test. Instruct client to void before the procedure. Assess if client is pregnant or nursing. Have client remove all jewelry or metal objects. Administer sedatives as ordered. Instruct client to fast for up to 12 hr prior to the test (length of time may vary for pediatric clients). Confirm whether client has received a histamine receptor antagonist prior to the procedure (often given for 48 hr prior to scan).
During Test: Adhere to standard precautions.
After Test: Instruct client and caregivers to wash hands after voiding or bowel movements because the radionuclide is excreted in urine and feces. Encourage client to drink fluids to assist in flushing isotopes from the body.

Contraindications: Pregnancy; lactation; previous history of allergy to iodine, eggs, or shellfish; any known allergy to radionuclides; when administering radionuclide, confirm the IV line is patent, because leakage at the site may be interpreted as a false positive.

Interfering Factors: Residual barium in the GI tract from recent x-rays; recent nuclear medicine procedures; false positives may occur with nondiverticular bleeding, intussusception, duplication cysts, or inflammatory bowel disease.

Nursing Considerations:
Pregnancy: Radionuclides should be avoided in pregnant women if possible. If performed, the lactating mother must dispose of milk until radioisotope is cleared from the milk.
Pediatric: Radionuclide may be harmful to the fetus, and therefore this test is only performed if absolutely necessary. Young children may require sedation.

WEBLINKS

http://chorus.rad.mcw.edu/index/4.html

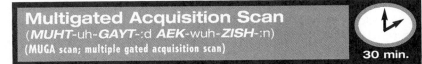

Multigated Acquisition Scan
(*MUHT*-uh-*GAYT*-:d *AEK*-wuh-*ZISH*-:n)
(MUGA scan; multiple gated acquisition scan)

30 min.

Type of Test: Nuclear scan

Body Systems and Functions: Cardiovascular system

Normal Findings: Normal end systolic and diastolic volumes; normal ejection fraction; symmetrical contraction of the left ventricle and normal velocity; no evidence of diminished perfusion, ischemia, or infarction

Test Results Time Frame: Within 24 hr

Test Description: The client receives a radionuclide agent (technetium) intravenously that radiolabels red blood cells. With the use of an electrocardiogram synchronized to computer and gamma scintillator camera, pictures are taken that represent a single cardiac cycle. The results are sequential and can be studied to show left ventricular function, determine ejection fraction, and look for heart wall abnormalities. Exercise-induced areas of ischemic cardiac tissue or necrotic cardiac tissue from a previous myocardial infarction reveal decreased radiocompound material uptake known as perfusion defects. Pharmacological stress imaging using adenosine, dipyridamole, or dobutamine may be administered in clients who are unable to exercise.

CLINICAL ALERT:
Pregnant health care workers should avoid caring for clients who have had a nuclear scan for 24 hr postscan.

Consent Form: Required

List of Equipment: Nuclear scanning equipment

Test Procedure:
1. Insert IV line and attach the client to an ECG.
2. Place client in supine position so that the camera is over the precordium. *Allows for accurate test results.*
3. Trained personnel administer the IV radionuclide. *Helps to minimize risk of exposure to radioactive material.*
4. The scan can begin 1–5 min after the injection and is done with the client at rest and, if desired, repeated during a stress test.

Clinical Implications and Indications:
1. Diagnoses deteriorating cardiovascular function in clients with congestive heart failure or decreasing cardiac ouput
2. Identifies changes in ventricular function following myocardial infarction
3. Determines effectiveness of cardiac medications such as vasodilators on cardiac function
4. Detects developing ventricular aneurysm and valvular regurgitation
5. Diagnoses changing ventricular function causing arrhythmias

Nursing Care:
Before Test: Explain the test procedure and the purpose of the test. Assess the client's knowledge of the test. Educate client on need to remain still during

NUCLEAR MEDICINE

scan. Reassure client no pain will be experienced during the test. Instruct client to void before the procedure. Assess if client is pregnant or nursing. Have client remove all jewelry or metal objects. Administer sedatives as ordered.

During Test: Adhere to standard precautions. Instruct client that they must be in supine position during test (which could last for up to 1 hr).

After Test: Instruct client and caregivers to wash hands after voiding or bowel movements because the radionuclide is excreted in urine and feces. Encourage client to drink fluids to assist in flushing isotopes from the body.

Potential Complications: Allergic reaction to radionuclide

Contraindications: Pregnancy; lactation; previous history of allergy to iodine, eggs, or shellfish; any known allergy to radionuclides; when administering radionuclide, confirm the IV line is patent, because leakage at the site may be interpreted as a false positive; inaccurate ECG; atrial fibrillation

Interfering Factors:
Drug therapy with nitrates; recent nuclear scan; recent barium studies

Nursing Considerations:
Pregnancy: Radiation should be avoided in pregnant women if possible. During lactation, the mother must dispose of milk until radioisotope is cleared from the milk.

Pediatric: Radionuclide may be harmful to the fetus, and therefore this test is only performed if absolutely necessary. Young children may require sedation.

Gerontology: The older person may find it difficult to maintain positions when required to do so for lengthy periods of time (e.g., standing for up to 1 hr during this test).

Rural: Advisable to arrange for transportation home after recovering from procedure.

Listing of Related Tests: Stress test; cardiac flow study; myocardial infarction scan

WEBLINKS

http://www.nhlbi.nih.gov

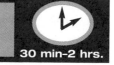

Nuclear Scans
(*NUE*-klee-:r)
(radioisotope scans; radionuclide imaging)

30 min-2 hrs.

Type of Test: Nuclear scan

Body Systems and Functions: Miscellaneous system

Normal Findings: No identified pathology

Test Results Time Frame: Within 24 hr

Test Description: A nuclear scan is taken to examine the physiology or function of any organ system. It may identify the presence of tumors or the presence or progression of disease process upon organ structure. Radionuclides are injected intravenously and once enough time has passed to ensure their distribution in tisse, then a gamma camera is used to identify areas of uptake. A computer stores and processes the information received from the camera.

CLINICAL ALERT:
Pregnant healthcare workers should avoid caring for clients who have had a nuclear scan for 24 hr postscan.

Consent Form: Required

List of Equipment: Nuclear scanning equipment

Test Procedure:
1. Intravenous access is obtained. *Allows access for radionuclide.*
2. Trained personnel administer the intravenous radionuclide. *Helps to minimize risk of exposure to radioactive material.*
3. Client is to increase fluid intake for the next 1–3 hr. *Facilitates renal clearance of radionuclide.*
4. After the required time has passed for radionuclide to circulate and distribute, client is instructed to ensure bladder is empty. *Different radiopharmaceuticals require different times to be distributed. A full bladder will interfere with the pelvis images.*
5. Client may need to be placed into different positions during the scan. *Helps to obtain scans of needed areas.*

Clinical Implications and Indications:
1. Identifies changes in physiology (e.g.,perfusion changes, obstruction, infarction, inflammation).
2. Identifies tumor/cyst presence or growth (e.g., intracranial mass, liver/spleen tumor or cyst, thyroid mass).
3. Scans may be classified by system being studied (e.g., cardiac, endocrine, genitorurinary, gastrointestinal, neurologic, pulmonary, orthopedic), or may be classified as tumor imaging studies (e.g., monoclonal antibody tumor imaging, gallium scans), or as imaging of inflammatory process (e.g., WBC scan).

Nursing Care:
Before Test: Explain the test procedure and the purpose of the test. Assess the client's knowledge of the test. Educate client on need to remain still during scan. Reassure client no pain will be experienced during the test. Instruct client to void before the procedure. Assess if client is pregnant or nursing. Have client remove all jewelry or metal objects. Administer sedatives as ordered. Ensure any specified pre-test requirements have been met (e.g., fasting). Obtain a recent weight for purposes of determining radionuclide dosage.
During Test: Adhere to standard precautions. Unlike X-ray procedures, it is not necessary for the client to be left alone, so a staff or family member may stay with them.
After Test: Instruct client and caregivers to wash hands after voiding or bowel movements because the radionuclide is excreted in urine and feces. Encourage client to drink fluids to assist in flushing isotopes from the body.

Contraindications: Pregnancy; lactation; previous history of allergy to iodine, eggs, or shellfish; any known allergy to radionuclides; when administering radionuclide confirm the IV is patent, because leakage at the site may be interpreted as a false positive.

NUCLEAR MEDICINE

Interfering Factors: More than one administration of radionuclide in one day; inability to remain still; dehydration; drug therapy with antihypertensives; diet or drugs high in iodine (specific to thyroid scan)

Nursing Considerations:

Pregnancy: Radionuclides should be avoided in pregnant women if possible. If performed, the lactating mother must dispose of milk until radioisotope is cleared from the milk.

Pediatric: Radionuclide may be harmful to the fetus and therefore this test is only performed if absolutely necessary. Young children may require sedation.

Gerontology: The older person may find it difficult to maintain positions when required to do so for lengthy periods of time during the nuclear scan.

Rural: Advisable to arrange for transportation home after recovering from the nuclear scan.

Listing of Related Tests: Schilling test; RBC or plasma volumes; positron emission tomography (PET)

WEBLINKS

http://www.entnet.org/score.html

Octreotide Scan
(ahk-*TREE*-uh-tiyd)
(octreoscan, indium octreotide scan, octreotide scintigraphy)

2 hr.

Type of Test: Nuclear scan

Body Systems and Functions: Endocrine system

Normal Findings: No areas of increased uptake

Test Results Time Frame: Within 1–2 weeks

Test Description: Octreotide scanning is used to evaluate neuroendocrine tumors that have a high density of somatostatin receptors. After injection with indium-111 octreotide radiotracer, which targets somatostatin receptors, whole-body scanning is performed several times to identify areas of high uptake. Radionuclides are injected intravenously, and once enough time has passed to ensure their distribution in tissue, a gamma camera is used to identify areas of uptake.

> **CLINICAL ALERT:**
> Pregnant health care workers should avoid caring for clients who have had a nuclear scan for 24 hr postscan.

Consent Form: Required

List of Equipment: Nuclear scanning equipment

Test Procedure:
1. Intravenous access is obtained. *Allows access for radionuclide.*
2. Trained personnel administer the IV radionuclide. *Helps to minimize risk of exposure to radioactive material.*

3. Client may need to be placed in different positions (i.e., supine, lateral, prone) during the scan. *Helps to obtain scans of needed areas.*
4. The client may be given a fatty meal 2 hr after the injection. *Helps clear radioactive drug from gallbladder.*
5. The client is given a strong laxative or enema at 3–4 hours postinjection (note: further laxative may be ordered for the night following the injection. *Helps clear radioactive drug from bowel.*
6. The scan is repeated several times throughout the next 2–5 days. *Ensures accurate results.*

Clinical Implications and Indications:
1. Diagnoses neuroendocrine and carcinoid tumors
2. Identifies areas of granulomatous infections
3. Identifies the staging of clients with Hodgkin's disease

Nursing Care:
Before Test: Explain the test procedure and the purpose of the test. Assess the client's knowledge of the test. Educate client on need to remain still during scan. Reassure client no pain will be experienced during the test. Instruct client to void before the procedure. Assess if client is pregnant or nursing. Have client remove all jewelry or metal objects. Administer sedatives as ordered.
During Test: Adhere to standard precautions.
After Test: Instruct client and caregivers to wash hands after voiding or bowel movements because the radionuclide is excreted in urine and feces. Encourage client to drink fluids to assist in flushing isotopes from the body.

Contraindications: Pregnancy; lactation; previous history of allergy to iodine, eggs, or shellfish; any known allergy to radionuclides; when administering radionuclide, confirm the IV line is patent, because leakage at the site may be interpreted as a false positive; octreotide received as treatment medication within prior 2 weeks

Interfering Factors: Barium in GI tract (mimics masses over liver and spleen)

Nursing Considerations:
Pregnancy: Radionuclides should be avoided in pregnant women if possible. If performed, the lactating mother must dispose of milk until radioisotope is cleared from the milk.
Pediatric: Radionuclide may be harmful to the fetus, and therefore this test is only performed if absolutely necessary. Young children may require sedation.
Gerontology: The older person may experience difficulty with maintaining some positions for lengthy periods of time during the octreotide scan.
Rural: Advisable to arrange for transportation home after recovering from the octreotide scan.

Listing of Related Tests: Single-photon emission computed tomography (SPECT)

NUCLEAR MEDICINE

| WEBLINKS |

http://www.med.harvard.edu

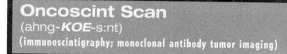

Oncoscint Scan
(ahng-*KOE*-s:nt)
(immunoscintigraphy; monoclonal antibody tumor imaging)

1 hr.

Type of Test: Nuclear scan

Body Systems and Functions: Oncology system

Normal Findings: No areas of the body with increased uptake of radionuclide

Test Results Time Frame: Within 1 week

Test Description: The oncoscint scan is used to detect colon and ovarian cancers through attachment of injected radiolabeled anticarcinoembryonic antigen (CEA) antibodies to the cell surface of these specific cancer cells. A gamma camera is used to obtain whole-body images and thus record any areas of increased radionuclide uptake.

> **CLINICAL ALERT:**
> Pregnant health care workers should avoid caring for clients who have had a nuclear scan for 24 hr postscan.

Consent Form: Required

List of Equipment: Nuclear scanning equipment

Test Procedure:
1. Intravenous access is obtained. *Allows access for radionuclide.*
2. Trained personnel administer the IV radionuclide (monoclonal antibody: radionuclide indium chloride-111). *Helps to minimize risk of exposure to radioactive material.*
3. Images are taken after 48 hr and repeated as requested.
4. Place client supine or prone on an x-ray table. *Positioning related to suspected pathophysiology.*
5. The gamma camera is positioned over the anterior and/or posterior chest, abdomen, and pelvis and each view will take approximately 10–15 min. *Helps to obtain scans of needed areas.*

Clinical Implications and Indications:
1. Diagnoses ovarian and colon cancers

Nursing Care:
Before Test: Explain the test procedure and the purpose of the test. Assess the client's knowledge of the test. Educate client on need to remain still during scan. Reassure client no pain will be experienced during the test. Instruct client to void before the procedure. Assess if client is pregnant or nursing. Have client remove all jewelry or metal objects. Administer sedatives as ordered. Explain that no fasting is required for the test, but some laboratories may request only light meals before scanning. The use of laxatives throughout the scanning period may be recommended to enhance excretion of isotope from the colon, where it tends to accumulate.
During Test: Adhere to standard precautions.

After Test: Instruct client and caregivers to wash hands after voiding or bowel movements because the radionuclide is excreted in urine and feces. Encourage client to drink fluids to assist in flushing isotopes from the body.

Contraindications: Pregnancy; lactation; previous history of allergy to iodine, eggs, or shellfish; any known allergy to radionuclides; when administering radionuclide, confirm the IV line is patent, because leakage at the site may be interpreted as a false positive; recent nuclear medicine studies

Interfering Factors: Movement during imaging; distended bladder could decrease pelvic area visibility.

Nursing Considerations:
Pregnancy: Radionuclides should be avoided in pregnant women if possible. If performed, the lactating mother must dispose of milk until radioisotope is cleared from the milk.
Pediatric: Radionuclide may be harmful to the fetus, and therefore this test is only performed if absolutely necessary. Young children may require sedation.
Gerontology: The older person may find it difficult to maintain positions when required to do so for lengthy periods of time during the nuclear scan.
Rural: Advisable to arrange for transportation home after recovering from procedure.

Listing of Related Tests: CT scan

WEBLINKS

http://www.gretmar.com

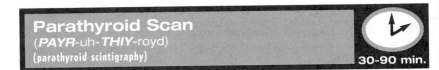

Parathyroid Scan
(*PAYR*-uh-*THIY*-royd)
(parathyroid scintigraphy)

30-90 min.

NUCLEAR MEDICINE

Type of Test: Nuclear scan

Body Systems and Functions: Endocrine system

Normal Findings: No thallium-201 activity above background in computer-subtracted images of thyroid/parathyroid

Test Results Time Frame: Within 1–2 weeks

Test Description: A parathyroid scan involves injecting two radioactive isotopes (technetium-99m and thallium-201) sequentially and intravenously. Then images are taken of the parathyroid. An image subtraction technique that is highly sensitive and specific is used to separate normal thyroid activity from parathyroid abnormalities. The disadvantages of this technique include its being unable to determine the relationship of an identified adenoma to surrounding structures and identify tumors <0.3 g in size accurately.

CLINICAL ALERT:
Pregnant health care workers should avoid caring for clients who have had a nuclear scan for 24 hr postscan.

Consent Form: Required

List of Equipment: Nuclear scanning equipment

Test Procedure:
1. Intravenous access is obtained. *Allows access for radionuclide.*
2. Trained personnel administer the IV radionuclide (thallium-201 chloride and technetium-99m). *Helps to minimize risk of exposure to radioactive material.*
3. Thirty to 60 min after the isotopes are injected the scanner is passed over the neck area and images are recorded.

Clinical Implications and Indications:
1. Detects abnormalities of the parathyroid and surrounding structures
2. Differentiates cysts from solid tumors

Nursing Care:
Before Test: Explain the test procedure and the purpose of the test. Assess the client's knowledge of the test. Educate client on need to remain still during scan. Reassure client no pain will be experienced during the test. Instruct client to void before the procedure. Assess if client is pregnant or nursing. Have client remove all jewelry or metal objects. Administer sedatives as ordered.
During Test: Adhere to standard precautions.
After Test: Instruct client and caregivers to wash hands after voiding or bowel movements because the radionuclide is excreted in urine and feces. Encourage client to drink fluids to assist in flushing isotopes from the body.

Contraindications: Pregnancy; lactation; previous history of allergy to iodine, eggs, or shellfish; any known allergy to radionuclides; when administering radionuclide, confirm the IV line is patent, because leakage at the site may be interpreted as a false positive; recent administration of radionuclides

Interfering Factors: Hypothyroidism; nodular disease; inability to remain still; diffusion of technetium pertechnetate into extracellular tissues

Nursing Considerations:
Pregnancy: Radionuclides should be avoided in pregnant women if possible. If performed, the lactating mother must dispose of milk until radioisotope is cleared from the milk.
Pediatric: Radionuclide may be harmful to the fetus, and therefore this test is only performed if absolutely necessary. Young children may require sedation.
Gerontology: The older person may find it difficult to maintain positions when required to do so for lengthy periods of time during the nuclear scan.
Rural: Advisable to arrange for transportation home after recovering from the parathyroid scan.

Listing of Related Tests: Thyroid scan

WEBLINKS ▯▯

http://www.niddk.nih.gov

Parotid Gland Scan
(puh-*RAHT*-:d glaend)
(salivary gland scan; salivary scintigraphy)

30-90 min.

Type of Test: Nuclear scan

Body Systems and Functions: Gastrointestinal system

Normal Findings: Normal size, shape, and position of parotid and sub-mandibular glands; no duct blockage

Test Results Time Frame: Within 3–5 days

Test Description: A parotid gland scan examines the parotid and sub-mandibular (but not sublingual) salivary glands. These body regions can be imaged with a gamma camera by examining technetium-99 pertechnetate uptake. For investigation of obstructions, repeat imaging is done after discharge of pertechnetate is stimulated with lemon juice.

CLINICAL ALERT:
Pregnant health care workers should avoid caring for clients who have had a nuclear scan for 24 hr postscan.

Consent Form: Required

List of Equipment: Nuclear scanning equipment

Test Procedure:
1. Place the client in supine position with neck extended.
2. Intravenous access is obtained. *Allows access for radionuclide.*
3. Trained personnel administer the IV radionuclide (pertechnetate). *Helps to minimize risk of exposure to radioactive material.*
4. Imaging is started 5 min after injection and views are taken every minute for 30 min. *It takes 5–10 min for pertechnetate to plateau.*
5. Repositioning for anterior, lateral, and oblique views may be necessary and views are taken with the thyroid included in the field. *A normal thyroid acts as a reference.*
6. If testing for obstruction, lemon juice is given to the client to drink or lemon-soaked swabs may be placed between the client's cheeks and gums. *The lemon would normally stimulate discharge of the pertechnetate from the glands within 1–2 min.*

Clinical Implications and Indications:
1. Evaluates symmetry of salivary gland function
2. Monitors gland function after therapeutic head/neck irradiation or surgery
3. Differentiates between types of malignant and benign parotid tumors
4. Diagnoses Sjögren's syndrome, salivary duct obstructions, and parotitis

Nursing Care:
Before Test: Explain the test procedure and the purpose of the test. Assess the client's knowledge of the test. Educate client on need to remain still during scan. Reassure client no pain will be experienced during the test. Instruct client to void before the procedure. Assess if client is pregnant or nursing. Have client remove all jewelry or metal objects. Administer sedatives as ordered.

NUCLEAR MEDICINE

During Test: Adhere to standard precautions.

After Test: Instruct client and caregivers to wash hands after voiding or bowel movements because the radionuclide is excreted in urine and feces. Encourage client to drink fluids to assist in flushing isotopes from the body.

Contraindications: Pregnancy; lactation; previous history of allergy to iodine, eggs, or shellfish; any known allergy to radionuclides; when administering radionuclide, confirm the IV line is patent, because leakage at the site may be interpreted as a false positive.

Interfering Factors: Drug therapy with thyroid-blocking agents or atropine; inability to remain still; nuclear scan within 48 hr prior to test

Nursing Considerations:

Pregnancy: Radionuclides should be avoided in pregnant women if possible. If performed, the lactating mother must dispose of milk until radioisotope is cleared from the milk.

Pediatric: Radionuclide may be harmful to the fetus, and therefore this test is only performed if absolutely necessary. Young children may require sedation.

Gerontology: The older person may find it difficult to maintain positions when required to do so for lengthy periods of time during the parotid gland scan.

Home Care: Caregivers must wear rubber gloves when discarding the client's urine for 24 hr postprocedure if test is performed at home.

Rural: Advisable to arrange for transportation home after recovering from the parotid gland scan.

WEBLINKS

http://chorus.rad.mcw.edu

Positron Emission Tomography
(*PAHZ*-uh-trahn ee-*MISH*-:n tuh-*MAHG*-ruh-fee)
(emission computed tomography; PET)

1-3 hr.

Type of Test: Nuclear scan

Body Systems and Functions: Neurological system

Normal Findings: Normal blood flow and metabolism in organ tissues

Test Results Time Frame: Within 24 hr

Test Description: Positron emission tomography (PET) uses a radionuclide to provide information on the blood flow, O_2 uptake, glucose transport, and metabolic functioning of an organ (see accompanying figure). Neurologically it can detect neurotransmitter receptors. PET can also identify regional lymph node metastasis and evaluate response to therapy. The radionuclide emits positrons (positively charged electrons) as it decays; the positrons combine with electrons in specific tissue cells and emit gamma rays detected by the PET scanner. The information is inputted into a computer, which translates the information into a color-coded image on a screen. PET can only be done in specialized centers because the radionuclides are made in a cyclotron and must be immediately used in the test. The radionuclide is administered either intravenously or by inhalation and has a very short half-life (note: there is no danger from contaminants). PET is most frequently used for neurological diagnosis, but there are numerous other applications, including cardiac, pulmonary, and breast diagnostic studies. Despite the cost, PET scans are being more widely used than previously because of their greater sensitivity and diagnostic value.

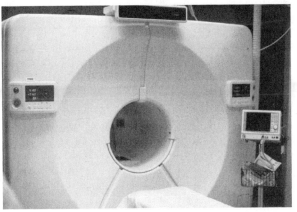

Positron Emission Tomography

CLINICAL ALERT:
Have emergency equipment readily available in the event of an anaphylactic reaction to the dye. Pregnant health care workers should avoid caring for clients who have had a nuclear scan for 24 hr postscan.

Consent Form: Required

List of Equipment: Nuclear scanning equipment

Test Procedure:
1. Intravenous access is obtained. *Allows access for radionuclide.*
2. Trained personnel administer the IV radionuclide. *Helps to minimize risk of exposure to radioactive material.*
3. Depending on what part of the body is being tested, have client in semi-Fowler's position for a brain scan or in supine position for heart, lung, breast, or pelvic study. *Helps to obtain scans of needed areas.*
4. If a brain scan is being done, the head is immobilized. *Ensures accurate results.*
5. Once the test begins, the client must lie perfectly still. *The images will be distorted with any movement.*
6. The client may be asked to speak, read, or repeat material from memory. *Utilizing speech, reading, and memory centers will alter the metabolism and be demonstrated on the screen.*

Clinical Implications and Indications:
1. Diagnoses Alzheimer's, Parkinson's, and Huntington's chorea disease
2. Evaluates brain tumors and response to therapy
3. Diagnoses myocardial infarction, coronary artery disease and the impact on cardiac muscle metabolism, and blockages and aneurysms in cerebral vascular blood flow

4. Diagnoses breast tumors
5. Evaluates brain function and seizure foci of patients with seizure disorders

Nursing Care:

Before Test: Explain the test procedure and the purpose of the test. Assess the client's knowledge of the test. Educate client on need to remain still during scan. Reassure client no pain will be experienced during the test. Instruct client to void before the procedure. Assess if client is pregnant or nursing. Have client remove all jewelry or metal objects. Administer sedatives as ordered. Client must abstain from caffeine, smoking, and alcohol for at least 24 hr before the test. Instruct client to not drink large amounts of fluids within 2 hr of the test unless a Foley catheter will be inserted (performed for pelvic studies). Assess for potential allergies to contrast medium. Inform client that during injection of contrast medium, a burning sensation may be felt for a few seconds behind the eyes or in the jaw, teeth, tongue, or lips. Assess for anxiety and provide sedation as ordered. Administer preoperative medication usually 30 min before procedure. Obtain baseline vital signs and neurological assessment.

During Test: Adhere to standard precautions. Assess for allergic reactions to contrast medium. Instruct client to remain still. Advise client to listen to relaxation tapes or perform mental relaxation exercises during the test.

After Test: Instruct client and caregivers to wash hands after voiding or bowel movements because the radionuclide is excreted in urine and feces. Encourage client to drink fluids to assist in flushing isotopes from the body. Assess for allergic reactions to contrast medium.

Potential Complications: Anaphylaxis due to allergic reaction to iodinated contrast material; phlebitis at injection site

Contraindications: Previous history of allergy to iodine, eggs, or shellfish; pregnancy; lactation; any known allergy to radionuclides; when administering radionuclide, confirm the IV line is patent, because leakage at the site may be interpreted as a false positive.

Interfering Factors: Anxiety, claustrophobia, and movement during the test; hypoglycemia alters the results of metabolic studies.

Nursing Considerations:

Pregnancy: Intravenous contrast should be avoided in pregnant women if possible (note: appropriate lead shielding is done to protect the fetus if it is determined this test is necessary). Radionuclides should be avoided in pregnant women if possible. If performed, the lactating mother must dispose of milk until radioisotope is cleared from the milk.

Pediatric: Radionuclide may be harmful to the fetus, and therefore this test is only performed if absolutely necessary. Young children may require sedation.

Gerontology: The older person may find it difficult to maintain positions when required to do so for lengthy periods of time during the PET.

Listing of Related Tests: CT scans (nonradionuclide); x-ray; magnetic resonance imaging

WEBLINKS

www.cti-pet.com

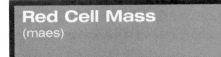

Red Cell Mass
(maes)

30 min.

Type of Test: Nuclear scan

Body Systems and Functions: Hematological system

Normal Findings:

Females	24.24±2.59 mL/kg (standard deviation)
Males	28.27±4.11 mL/kg (standard deviation)

Test Results Time Frame: Within 24 hr

Test Description: Red cell mass is a measurement of the total number of circulating red blood cells expressed in relation to body weight. It reflects the balance between the rate of erythropoiesis by the bone marrow and the rate of red blood cell destruction occurring throughout the body. It is relative to the total quantity of blood in circulation (blood volume) and the quantity of plasma (plasma volume which can change with hydration and natural compensatory mechanisms). Radionuclide testing can also be done for total blood volume and plasma volume, but it can be time consuming and expensive. Normally, the client's history and symptoms are needed to provide the necessary information for this test. A decrease in red cell mass is oligocythemia, which can be caused by an increase in plasma volume, such as pregnancy or overhydration IV fluids or by failure of the bone marrow to produce enough new erythrocytes. An increase in red cell concentration is erythrocytosis, which can be seen in dehydration states, chronic hypoxia, or aberrant erythopoietin production.

CLINICAL ALERT:
Pregnant health care workers should avoid caring for clients who have had a nuclear scan for 24 hr postscan.

Consent Form: Required

List of Equipment: Nuclear scanning equipment; green-top tubes (2) or serum separator tube; needle and syringe or vacutainer; alcohol swab

Test Procedure:
1. Label the specimen tubes. *Correctly identifies the client and the tests to be performed.*
2. Obtain 8-mL blood sample from the extremity that has no IV fluid infusing. *Hemodilution alters the results.*
3. Intravenous access is obtained. *Allows access for radionuclide.*
4. Mix sample with radioactive isotope, and after 15 min, inject intravenously into client.
5. Trained personnel administer the IV radionuclide. *Helps to minimize risk of exposure to radioactive material.*
6. Client is to increase fluid intake for the next 1–3 hr. *Facilitates renal clearance of radionuclide.*
7. After the required time has passed for radionuclide to circulate and distribute, client is instructed to ensure bladder is empty. *Different radiopharmaceuticals require different times to be distributed. A full bladder will interfere with the pelvic images.*

NUCLEAR MEDICINE

8. Client may need to be placed into different positions during the scan. *Helps to obtain scans of needed areas.*
9. Label the specimen tubes. *Correctly identifies the client and the tests to be performed.*
10. Obtain 8-mL blood sample from the extremity that has no IV fluid infusing. *Hemodilution alters the results.*
11. Mix sample with radioactive isotope, and after 15 min, inject intravenously into client.
12. After 15 min draw second 8-mL blood sample, which is prepared for gamma scanning by the technician.

Clinical Implications and Indications:

1. Aids in definitive diagnosis of absolute and relative polycythemia
2. Diagnoses hemolytic anemia and erythrocytosis, including Gaisböck's syndrome

Nursing Care:

Before Test: Explain the test procedure and the purpose of the test. Assess the client's knowledge of the test. Educate client on need to remain still during scan. Reassure client no pain will be experienced during the test. Instruct client to void before the procedure. Assess if client is pregnant or nursing. Have client remove all jewelry or metal objects. Administer sedatives as ordered. Assess for potential allergies to contrast medium. Inform client that during injection of contrast medium, a burning sensation may be felt for a few seconds behind the eyes or in the jaw, teeth, tongue, or lips. Assess for anxiety and provide sedation as ordered. Administer preoperative medication usually 30 min before procedure. Obtain baseline vital signs and neurological assessment. Obtain a recent weight for purposes of determining radionuclide dosage.

During Test: Adhere to standard precautions. Assess for allergic reactions to contrast medium.

After Test: Apply pressure to venipuncture site. Explain that some bruising, discomfort, and swelling may appear at the site and that warm, moist compresses can alleviate this. Monitor for signs of infection. Instruct client and caregivers to wash hands after voiding or bowel movements because the radionuclide is excreted in urine and feces. Encourage client to drink fluids to assist in flushing isotopes from the body. Assess for allergic reactions to contrast medium.

Potential Complications: Anaphylaxis due to allergic reaction to iodinated contrast material; bleeding and bruising at venipuncture site

Contraindications: Pregnancy; lactation; previous history of allergy to iodine, eggs, or shellfish; any known allergy to radionuclides; when administering radionuclide, confirm the IV line is patent, because leakage at the site may be interpreted as a false positive.

Interfering Factors: Active bleeding; edematous upper extremity at site of venipuncture; hemodilution from IV solutions; recent scans with radioisotopes

Nursing Considerations:

Pregnancy: Intravenous contrast should be avoided in pregnant women if possible. Radionuclides should be avoided in pregnant women if possible. If performed, the lactating mother must dispose of milk until radioisotope is cleared from the milk.

NUCLEAR MEDICINE

Pediatric: Radionuclide may be harmful to the fetus, and therefore this test is only performed if absolutely necessary. Young children may require sedation.
Gerontology: The older person may find it difficult to maintain positions when required to do so for lengthy periods of time during the procedure.
Rural: Advisable to arrange for transportation home after recovering from procedure.

Listing of Related Tests: Hematocrit; hemoglobin; plasma volume; reticulocyte count and index; total blood volume

⦿WEBLINKS ☌   ▣▨

www.nlm.nih.gov

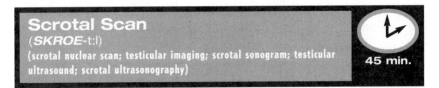

Scrotal Scan
(*SKROE*-t:l)
(scrotal nuclear scan; testicular imaging; scrotal sonogram; testicular ultrasound; scrotal ultrasonography)

45 min.

Type of Test: Nuclear scan

Body Systems and Functions: Reproductive system

Normal Findings: Normal blood flow and structures of the scrotal contents; no tumor, hematoma, torsion, or infection

Test Results Time Frame: Within 24 hr

Test Description: Scrotal scanning is a nuclear test that is performed to evaluate disorders of the testis, epidymis, spermatic cord, and other contents of the scrotal sac. Nuclear scrotal scans combine the use of special radionuclides (e.g., technetium-99, chromium-51) with gamma cameras and computers to create tomographic images. The gamma camera examines the client's scrotal area, thereby creating many thin slices and decreasing the chance of surrounding tissue obscuring the view. The physiological function of the scrotum can be observed through this procedure.

> **CLINICAL ALERT:**
> Pregnant health care workers should avoid caring for clients who have had a nuclear scan for 24 hr postscan.

Consent Form: Not required

List of Equipment: Nuclear scanning equipment

Test Procedure:
1. Intravenous access is obtained. *Allows access for radionuclide.*
2. Trained personnel administer the IV radionuclide. *Helps to minimize risk of exposure to radioactive material.*
3. Client is to increase fluid intake for the next 1–3 hr. *Facilitates renal clearance of radionuclide.*
4. Client may need to be placed into different positions during the scan. *Helps to obtain scans of needed areas.*

NUCLEAR MEDICINE

Clinical Implications and Indications:

1. Evaluates infectious processes and differentiates among such conditions as epididymitis and orchitis
2. Diagnoses hydrocele and varicocele
3. Evaluates the causation for testicular pain and swelling

Nursing Care:

Before Test: Explain the test procedure and the purpose of the test. Assess the client's knowledge of the test. Educate client on need to remain still during scan. Reassure client no pain will be experienced during the test. Instruct client to void before the procedure. Assess if client is pregnant or nursing. Have client remove all jewelry or metal objects. Administer sedatives as ordered.

During Test: Adhere to standard precautions.

After Test: Instruct client and caregivers to wash hands after voiding or bowel movements because the radionuclide is excreted in urine and feces. Encourage client to drink fluids to assist in flushing isotopes from the body.

Contraindications: Pregnancy; lactation; previous history of allergy to iodine, eggs, or shellfish; any known allergy to radionuclides; when administering radionuclide, confirm the IV is patent, because leakage at the site may be interpreted as a false positive.

Nursing Considerations:

Pregnancy: Radionuclides should be avoided in pregnant women if possible. If performed, the lactating mother must dispose of milk until radioisotope is cleared from the milk.

Pediatric: Radionuclide may be harmful to the fetus, and therefore this test is only performed if absolutely necessary. Young children may require sedation.

Gerontology: The older person may find it difficult to maintain positions when required to do so for lengthy periods of time during the scrotal scan.

Rural: Advisable to arrange for transportation home after recovering from scrotal scan.

WEBLINKS	🖵 ☒

http://health.excite.com/

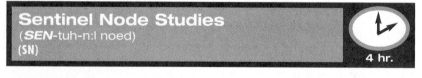

Sentinel Node Studies
(*SEN*-tuh-n:l noed)
(SN)

4 hr.

Type of Test: Nuclear scan

Body Systems and Functions: Oncology system

Normal Findings: No spread of breast cancer or melanoma into the sentinel node(s)

CRITICAL VALUES:
Cancerous cells indicate metastasis of the cancer.

Test Results Time Frame: Within 3–5 days

Test Description: Sentinel node (SN) diagnostics is a method of both treating and evaluating various types of cancerous disorders. Physiologically, the lymph nodes serve as channels and filters of the microcirculation. This is also the first route that cancerous cells will travel if they have left the breast tumor or melanoma site. Previously, removal of the complete lymph node chain was required in order to detect metastasis and help stage the cancer. Removal of this lymph node chain disrupts these filters and can lead to lifelong problems with lymphedema and permanent loss of arm function. Before SN surgery, the client is injected with a radioactive tracer around the tumor site. The nuclear scan locates the diseased areas, then the client is injected with a blue dye, which will be carried by the lymphatic system and will follow the vessels to the SN, where it is deposited. In the operating room, a hand-held gamma probe is placed inside. The probe detects the sentinel node(s), which are removed and sent to the laboratory for testing. If cancer is detected, an axillary dissection must then be performed because cancer has likely spread beyond the SNs into the lymphatic system. However, in the majority of women, no cancer will be found in the SNs and no further surgery is required, eliminating the unnecessary risks and side effects of a full chain removal.

> **CLINICAL ALERT:**
> Pregnant health care workers should avoid caring for clients who have had a nuclear scan for 24 hr postscan.

Consent Form: Required

Test Procedure:
1. Intravenous access is obtained. *Allows access for radionuclide.*
2. Trained personnel administer the IV radionuclide. *Helps to minimize risk of exposure to radioactive material.*
3. Client is to increase fluid intake for the next 1–3 hr. *Facilitates renal clearance of radionuclide.*
4. Client may need to be placed into different positions during the scan and surgical intervention may then be needed. *Helps to obtain scans of needed areas.*

Clinical Implications and Indications:
1. Detects metastasis of breast cancer or melanomas
2. Evaluates the stage of breast cancer and melanomas

Nursing Care:
Before Test: Explain the test procedure and the purpose of the test. Assess the client's knowledge of the test. Instruct client to remain still during scan. Reassure client no pain will be experienced during the test. Instruct client to void before the procedure. Assess if client is pregnant or nursing. Have client remove all jewelry or metal objects. Administer sedatives as ordered.
During Test: Adhere to standard precautions. Assist technician and surgeon throughout the procedures. Provide emotional support to patient. Follow hospital protocol for disposal of radioactive materials from surgery.
After Test: Instruct client and caregivers to wash hands after voiding or bowel movements because the radionuclide is excreted in urine and feces. Encourage client to drink fluids to assist in flushing isotopes from the body. Follow hospital policy for postoperative vital signs. Inform client a blue tint may be present around biopsy site for a few weeks.

NUCLEAR MEDICINE

Potential Complications: Misdiagnosing sentinel node; metastasis of cancer to a nonsentinel node, with a cancer-free sentinel node (2%)

Contraindications: Pregnancy; lactation; previous history of allergy to iodine, eggs, or shellfish; any known allergy to radionuclides; when administering radionuclide, confirm the IV is patent, because leakage at the site may be interpreted as a false positive.

Interfering Factors: Location of the cancer (inner aspect of breast or axilla); history of a lumpectomy; obesity

Nursing Considerations:
Pregnancy: Radionuclides should be avoided in pregnant women if possible. If performed, the lactating mother must dispose of milk until radioisotope is cleared from the milk.
Pediatric: Radionuclide may be harmful to the fetus, and therefore this test is only performed if absolutely necessary. Young children may require sedation.
Gerontology: The older person may find it difficult to maintain positions when required to do so for lengthy periods of time during the sentinel node studies.

WEBLINKS

http://www.obgyn.net

NUCLEAR MEDICINE

Single-Photon Emission Computed Tomography
(*SING*-g:l *FOE*-tahn kuhm-*PYUE*-t:d tuh-*MAHG*-ruh-fee)
(SPECT scan)

30 min.

Type of Test: Nuclear scan

Body Systems and Functions: Neurological system

Normal Findings: Normal organ structures

Test Results Time Frame: Within 24 hr

Test Description: Single-photon emission computed tomography is a nuclear scan that is an imaging test used to scan various organs. A SPECT scan does not require the isotope used in a PET, but it uses the same isotopes as other nuclear scans (technetium-99m). The radionuclide crosses the blood-brain barrier and remains for hours in the body's tissues. During this time, the SPECT camera visualizes images along several planes. This test can detect many types of disorders that the older nuclear scans could not, such as early patterns of dementia.

CLINICAL ALERT:
Pregnant health care workers should avoid caring for clients who have had a nuclear scan for 24 hr postscan. Have emergency equipment readily available in the event of an anaphylactic reaction to the radionuclide.

Consent Form: Required

List of Equipment: Nuclear scanning equipment

Test Procedure:
1. Intravenous access is obtained. *Allows access for radionuclide.*
2. Trained personnel administer the IV radionuclide. *Helps to minimize risk of exposure to radioactive material.*
3. Client is to increase fluid intake for the next 1–3 hr. *Facilitates renal clearance of radionuclide.*
4. After the required time has passed for radionuclide to circulate and distribute, client is instructed to ensure bladder is empty. *Different radiopharmaceuticals require different times to be distributed. A full bladder will interfere with the pelvic images.*
5. Client may need to be placed into different positions during the scan. *Helps to obtain scans of needed areas.*

Clinical Implications and Indications:
1. Evaluates abnormalities of the bone and joints, brain, liver, lungs, heart, and spleen.
2. SPECT scans of the brain evaluate AIDS, Alzheimer's, anoxia, cerebral ischemia, CVA, types of dementias, head trauma, and seizure activity.

Nursing Care:
Before Test: Explain the test procedure and the purpose of the test. Assess the client's knowledge of the test. Educate client on need to remain still during scan. Reassure client no pain will be experienced during the test. Instruct client to void before the procedure. Assess if client is pregnant or nursing. Have client remove all jewelry or metal objects. Administer sedatives as ordered.
During Test: Adhere to standard precautions. Assess for allergic reactions to radionuclide.
After Test: Instruct client and caregivers to wash hands after voiding or bowel movements because the radionuclide is excreted in urine and feces. Encourage client to drink fluids to assist in flushing isotopes from the body. Assess for allergic reactions to contrast medium.

Potential Complications: Anaphylaxis due to allergic reaction to radionuclide

Contraindications: Pregnancy; lactation; previous history of allergy to iodine, eggs, or shellfish; any known allergy to radionuclides; when administering radionuclide, confirm the IV is patent, because leakage at the site may be interpreted as a false positive.

Interfering Factors: Presence of metal objects

Nursing Considerations:
Pregnancy: Radionuclides should be avoided in pregnant women if possible. If performed, the lactating mother must dispose of milk until radioisotope is cleared from the milk.
Pediatric: Radionuclide may be harmful to the fetus, and therefore this test is only performed if absolutely necessary. Young children may require sedation.
Gerontology: The older person may find it difficult to maintain positions when required to do so for lengthy periods of time during the SPECT scan.
Home Care: Home health care providers will need to continue to wash their hands carefully for the first 24 hr after the scan.

NUCLEAR MEDICINE

Rural: *Advisable to arrange for transportation home after recovering from the SPECT scan.*

Listing of Related Tests: Positron emission tomography

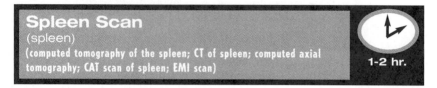

Spleen Scan
(spleen)

(computed tomography of the spleen; CT of spleen; computed axial tomography; CAT scan of spleen; EMI scan)

1-2 hr.

Type of Test: Nuclear scan

Body Systems and Functions: Hepatobiliary system

Normal Findings: A homogenous distribution of the radiolabeled erythrocytes throughout spleen

Test Results Time Frame: Within 24–48 hr

Test Description: Nuclear spleen scans allow the early visualization of physiological functioning of the spleen. Spleen scans are useful in diagnosing the size, shape, and location of the spleen. Nuclear spleen scans combine the use of special radionuclides (e.g., technetium-99, chromium-51) with gamma cameras and computers to create tomographic images. The gamma camera examines the client's upper quadrant of the abdomen, thereby creating many thin slices and decreasing the chance of surrounding tissue obscuring the view. The physiological function of the spleen can be observed because the erythrocytes are sequestered by the spleen and can be identified with the scinticounter.

CLINICAL ALERT:
Pregnant health care workers should avoid caring for clients who have had a nuclear scan for 24 hr postscan. Have emergency equipment readily available in the event of an anaphylactic reaction.

Consent Form: Not required

List of Equipment: Nuclear scanning equipment

Test Procedure:
1. Intravenous access is obtained. *Allows access for radionuclide.*
2. Trained personnel administer the IV radionuclide by adding it to the 5-mL sample of venous blood. *Trained personnel help to minimize risk of exposure to radioactive material.*
3. Client is to increase fluid intake for the next 1– 3 hr. *Facilitates renal clearance of radionuclide.*
4. After the required time has passed for radionuclide to circulate and distribute, client is instructed to ensure bladder is empty. *Different*

radiopharmaceuticals require different times to be distributed. A full bladder will interfere with the pelvic images.

5. Client may need to be placed into different positions during the scan. *Helps to obtain scans of needed areas.*

Clinical Implications and Indications:
1. Determines the size, shape, and location of the spleen.
2. Assists in assessing presence of cancer of the spleen.
3. Serial CT scans of the spleen can be performed at 6-week intervals following blunt trauma to the abdomen to monitor the healing and detect problems. Nonoperative management of the trauma can avoid unnecessary surgery.

Nursing Care:
Before Test: Explain the test procedure and the purpose of the test. Assess the client's knowledge of the test. Educate client on need to remain still during scan. Reassure client no pain will be experienced during the test. Instruct client to void before the procedure. Assess if client is pregnant or nursing. Have client remove all jewelry or metal objects. Administer sedatives as ordered. Ensure any specified pretest requirements have been met (e.g., fasting). Obtain a recent weight for purposes of determining radionuclide dosage.

During Test: Adhere to standard precautions. Instruct client to remain still during procedure.

After Test: Instruct client and caregivers to wash hands after voiding or bowel movements because the radionuclide is excreted in urine and feces. Encourage client to drink fluids to assist in flushing isotopes from the body.

Potential Complications: Bleeding and bruising at venipuncture site

Contraindications: Pregnancy; lactation; previous history of allergy to iodine, eggs, or shellfish; any known allergy to radionuclides; when administering radionuclide, confirm the IV is patent, because leakage at the site may be interpreted as a false positive.

Interfering Factors: Inability to remain still during procedure; amyloidosis, abscess, or tumor may cause filling defects; impaired liver function

Nursing Considerations:
Pregnancy: Radionuclides should be avoided in pregnant women if possible. If performed, the lactating mother must dispose of milk until radioisotope is cleared from the milk.

Pediatric: Instruct client and caregivers to wash hands after voiding or bowel movements because the radionuclide is excreted in urine and feces. Encourage client to drink fluids to assist in flushing isotopes from the body. Radionuclide may be harmful to the fetus, and therefore this test is only performed if absolutely necessary. Young children may require sedation.

Gerontology: The older person may find it difficult to maintain positions when required to do so for lengthy periods of time during the spleen scan.

Listing of Related Tests: Complete blood count (CBC); spleen sonogram

NUCLEAR MEDICINE

WEBLINKS

http://www.vgernet.net

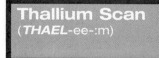

Thallium Scan
(*THAEL*-ee-:m)

5 hr.

Type of Test: Nuclear scan

Body Systems and Functions: Cardiovascular system

Normal Findings: Nonlocalization of thallium in coronary vessels

Test Results Time Frame: Within 24 hr

Test Description: A thallium scan measures cardiac efficiency while the heart is being stressed through exercise using this radioactive imaging agent. This test is used to investigate cardiac perfusion during activity and at rest after activity. It is used to diagnose ischemia. If a client is unable to perform a stress test, dipyridamole may be used to simulate exercise on the heart.

> **CLINICAL ALERT:**
> Pregnant health care workers should avoid caring for clients who have had a nuclear scan for 24 hr postscan.

Consent Form: Required

List of Equipment: Treadmill with ability to increase incline and speed; EKG pads, leads, and EKG monitor; blood pressure cuff; stethescope, IV access, thallium-201 (TI-201).

Test Procedure:

1. Prepare skin and place EKG patches on client's body as for a 12-lead EKG (see description of EKG). *Attach electrodes to EKG monitor. Skin preparation allows for better conduction of electrical signals.*
2. Intravenous access is obtained. *Allows access for radionuclide.*
3. Trained personnel administer the IV radionuclide. *Helps to minimize risk of exposure to radioactive material.*
4. After the required time has passed for radionuclide to circulate and distribute, client is instructed to ensure bladder is empty. *Different radiopharmaceuticals require different times to be distributed. A full bladder will interfere with the pelvic images.*
5. The client begins walking on the treadmill at zero incline and slow pace while the computerized EKG records and monitors heart electroactivity. Then the client progressively walks at greater speeds and greater elevations to increase workload on the heart. *Gradually increasing workload does not overstrain heart.*
6. EKG, heart rate, and blood pressure are continually monitored for signs of abnormality. *Client can be monitored for potential complications during the test.*
7. Inject IV radioactive thallium when the client has reached maximum heart stress. *Thallium allows for visualization of heart structures.*
8. Client lies down on scanning table and scanning begins. *Scan is performed with radiation.* Three static views of cardiac perfusion are taken. *Allows for views of the heart as it returns to rest and at different positions.*

9. A repeat scan is taken 3–4 hr later to evaluate cardiac perfusion at rest. *Resting scan allows for evaluation of the heart's ability to recover from activity.*
10. Client is to increase fluid intake for the next 1–3 hr. *Facilitates renal clearance of radionuclide.*

Clinical Implications and Indications:

1. Normal scan at rest and abnormal during activity indicates ischemia.
2. Abnormal scan at rest and during activity indicates infarction.
3. Specific abnormalities may indicate the need for cardiac catheterization.

Nursing Care:

Before Test: Explain the test procedure and the purpose of the test. Assess the client's knowledge of the test. Educate client on need to remain still during scan. Reassure client no pain will be experienced during the test. Instruct client to void before the procedure. Assess if client is pregnant or nursing. Have client remove all jewelry or metal objects. Administer sedatives as ordered. Instruct client to fast 2 hr prior to the test and throughout the test. Inform client to not smoke 2 hr prior to the test. For dipyridamole test, instruct client to fast for 6 hr with no caffeine intake. Obtain an accurate weight for proper calculation of thallium dose.

During Test: Adhere to standard precautions. Monitor EKG continuously and blood pressure at designated points. Explain to the client to report any chest pain, leg pain, lightheadedness, or extreme shortness of breath immediately during the test.

After Test: Instruct client and caregivers to wash hands after voiding or bowel movements because the radionuclide is excreted in urine and feces. Encourage client to drink fluids to assist in flushing isotopes from the body. Observe client for posttest cardiac symptoms.

Potential Complications: Angina; cardiac dysrhythmias; if dipyridamole is used: nausea, vomiting, headache, and dizziness

Contraindications: Pregnancy; lactation; previous history of allergy to iodine, eggs, or shellfish; any known allergy to radionuclides (e.g., thallium); left and right bundle branch block; left-ventricular hypertrophy; digitalis and quinidine; severe coronary artery disease; angina at rest; dysrhythmias

Interfering Factors: Inadequate or incomplete cardiac stress test; leakage at IV site may be interpreted as a false positive

Nursing Considerations:

Pregnancy: Radionuclides should be avoided in pregnant women if possible. If performed, the lactating mother must dispose of milk until radioisotope is cleared from the milk. Premenopausal women should be advised to use birth control.
Pediatric: Radionuclide may be harmful to the fetus, and therefore this test is only performed if absolutely necessary. Young children may require sedation.

Listing of Related Tests: EKG; stress/exercise test

NUCLEAR MEDICINE

| WEBLINKS |

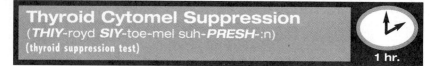

Thyroid Cytomel Suppression
(***THIY**-royd **SIY**-toe-mel suh-**PRESH**-:n)
(thyroid suppression test)

1 hr.

Type of Test: Nuclear scan

Body Systems and Functions: Endocrine system

Normal Findings: Hypothyroid clients with normal uptakes will have a depression of 50% with the second uptake following Cytomel administration.

Test Results Time Frame: Within 24–48 hr

Test Description: The thyroid Cytomel suppression test measures the response of the thyroid metabolic system to the administration of oral triiodothyronine (Cytomel). The uptake of iodine by a normal thyroid gland will decrease following the administration of Cytomel. Abnormal thyroid glands will have sharp suppression of their function to this test. The thyroid is an endocrine gland located in the anterior neck region and partially surrounds the thyroid cartilage and upper rings of the trachea. The primary action of the thyroid gland is to control the basal metabolic rate. The thyroid gland enlarges in hyperthyroidism (goiter), and it may be removed surgically. In addition, a hypothyroid state may exist (e.g., after a thyroidectomy), and the therapy is to administer a synthetic form of thyroid hormones (e.g., synthroid).

> **CLINICAL ALERT:**
> Pregnant health care workers should avoid caring for clients who have had a nuclear scan for 24 hr post scan. This test is rarely done given the availability of TSH assays.

Consent Form: Not required

Test Procedure:

1. Intravenous access is obtained. *Allows access for radionuclide.*
2. Trained personnel administer the IV radionuclide. *Helps to minimize risk of exposure to radioactive material.*
3. A small oral dose of radioactive iodine is given to client. *Radioactive iodine will allow scan to illustrate distribution and structures of the thyroid. Establishes baseline for suppression test.*
4. Radioactivity of the thyroid gland is made at 4–6 hr after ingestion and then again at 24 hr after ingestion. Time is allowed for radioisotope to be distributed.
5. The client is given Cytomel (T3) for 7 days, which suppresses TSH production.
6. Iodine uptake is retaken. *Compares results with baseline.*

Clinical Implications and Indications:

1. If there is no suppression, there is indication of autonomous nodules in the thyroid.

Nursing Care:

Before Test: Explain the test procedure and the purpose of the test. Assess the client's knowledge of the test. Educate client on need to remain still during scan. Reassure client no pain will be experienced during the test. Instruct client to void before the procedure. Assess if client is pregnant or nursing. Have client remove all jewelry or metal objects. Administer sedatives as ordered.

During Test: Adhere to standard precautions.

After Test: Assure the client that the dose of radionuclide used in this test is minute and therefore harmless.

Contraindications: Pregnancy; lactation; previous history of allergy to iodine, eggs, or shellfish; any known allergy to radionuclides; when administering radionuclide, confirm the IV line is patent, because leakage at the site may be interpreted as a false positive.

Nursing Considerations:

Pregnancy: Radionuclides should be avoided in pregnant women if possible. If performed, the lactating mother must dispose of milk until radioisotope is cleared from the milk.

Pediatric: Radionuclide may be harmful to the fetus, and therefore this test is only performed if absolutely necessary. Young children may require sedation.

WEBLINKS	

www.healthgate.com;www.mamc.amedd.army.mil

Thyroid Perchlorate Suppression
(*THIY*-royd p:r-*KLOER*-ayt suh-*PRESH*-:n)
(perchlorate washout test)

3 hr.

NUCLEAR MEDICINE

Type of Test: Nuclear scan

Body Systems and Functions: Endocrine system

Normal Findings: No change in radioactive iodine following administration of perchlorate

Test Results Time Frame: Immediate (note: written results within 24 hr)

Test Description: Test is done in conjunction with thyroid uptake scan. After a thyroid uptake scan is completed, the client ingests 1 g of potassium perchlorate orally. Uptakes are taken hourly for the next 2 hr. This test allows for determination between congenital and acquired thyroid defects.

Consent Form: Required

List of Equipment: Radioactive iodine; scan machine; perchlorate 1 g

Test Procedure:
1. A small oral dose of radioactive iodine is given to client. *Radioactive iodine will allow scan to illustrate distribution and structures of the thyroid.*
2. Radioactivity of the thyroid gland is made at 4–6 hr after ingestion and then again at 24 hr after ingestion. *Time is allowed for radioisotope to be distributed.*

3. Potassium perchlorate 1 g (PO) is administerd to client. *Perchlorate determines trapping or organification of radioactive iodine.*
4. Scan is repeated hourly for 2 hr. *Time is needed to determine amount of organification.*

Clinical Implications and Indications:

1. A decrease of radioisotope uptake <10%–15% after perchlorate administration indicates organic defect which confirms hypothyroidism.

Nursing Care:

Before Test: Explain the test procedure and the purpose of the test. Assess the client's knowledge of the test. Ensure all blood work is drawn prior to administration of radioisotope.

During Test: Adhere to standard precautions. No radiation precautions need to be followed.

After Test: Reassure client that small doses of radioisotopes are injected and no special precautions are required in the home. Encourage client to drink fluids to assist in flushing isotopes from the body.

Listing of Related Tests: Thyroid scan

WEBLINKS

www.healthgate.com; www.mamc.amedd.army.mil

Thyroid Scan
(*THIY*-royd)
(thyroid uptake; nuclear scan; RAUI)

30 hr.

Type of Test: Nuclear scan

Body Systems and Functions: Endocrine system

Normal Findings: Normal distribution of radioactive iodine with absence of nodules; normal size, shape, site, and weight of thyroid

Test Results Time Frame: Immediate (note: written results within 24 hr)

Test Description: Thyroid scans are used to evaluate the size, shape, function, and location of the thyroid gland. This is done through ingestion of radioactive iodine followed by nuclear scanning of the neck. It is most useful in the identification of thyroid nodules, goiter, thyroiditis, and tumors. The thyroid is an endocrine gland located in the anterior neck region and partially surrounds the thyroid cartilage and upper rings of the trachea. The primary action of the thyroid gland is to control the basal metabolic rate. The thyroid gland enlarges in hyperthyroidism (goiter), and it may be removed surgically. In addition, a hypothyroid state may exist (e.g., after a thyroidectomy), and the therapy is to administer a synthetic form of thyroid hormones (e.g., synthroid).

NUCLEAR MEDICINE

CLINICAL ALERT:
Have emergency equipment readily available in the event of an anaphylactic reaction to the dye. Pregnant health care workers should avoid caring for clients who have had a nuclear scan for 24 hr postscan.

Consent Form: Required

List of Equipment: Nuclear scanning equipment

Test Procedure:
1. Administer radioactive iodine in pill or liquid form. *Radioactive iodine collects in the thyroid and is visible upon nuclear scan.*
2. Scan is performed in 4–6 hr. *Allows time for iodine to collect in the thyroid gland.*
3. Instruct client to return for another scan 24 hr later. *Evaluates dissipation of iodine from thyroid.*

Clinical Implications and Indications:
1. Evaluates nodules, enlargement, or other abnormalities of the thyroid gland
2. Identifies whether there is a need for further evaluation of the thyroid gland

Nursing Care:
Before Test: Explain the test procedure and the purpose of the test. Assess the client's knowledge of the test. Assess for potential allergies to contrast medium. Inform client that during injection of contrast medium, a burning sensation may be felt for a few seconds behind the eyes or in the jaw, teeth, tongue, or lips. Assess for anxiety and provide sedation as ordered. Administer preoperative medication usually 30 min before procedure. Obtain baseline vital signs and neurological assessment. Educate client on need to remain still during scan. Reassure client no pain will be experienced during the test. Instruct client to void before the procedure. Assess if client is pregnant or nursing. Have client remove all jewelry or metal objects. Administer sedatives as ordered. Client should be off thyroid medication for 6 weeks prior to the test. Instruct client to fast overnight.
During Test: Adhere to standard precautions. Reassure client during the scan. Assess for allergic reactions to contrast medium.
After Test: Assess for allergic reactions to contrast medium. Instruct client and caregivers to wash hands after voiding or bowel movements because the radionuclide is excreted in urine and feces. Encourage client to drink fluids to assist in flushing isotopes from the body. Resume prescribed thyroid medications.

Potential Complications: Anaphylaxis due to allergic reaction to iodinated contrast material.

Contraindications: Pregnancy; lactation; previous history of allergy to iodine, eggs, or shellfish; any known allergy to radionuclides

Interfering Factors: Iodine-containing foods

NUCLEAR MEDICINE

Nursing Considerations:

Pregnancy: *Radionuclides should be avoided in pregnant women if possible. If performed, the lactating mother must dispose of milk until radioisotope is cleared from the milk. Contrast medium should be avoided in pregnant women if possible.*
Pediatric: *Radionuclide may be harmful to the fetus, and therefore this test is only performed if absolutely necessary. Young children may require sedation.*
Gerontology: *The older person may find it difficult to maintain positions when required to do so for lengthy periods of time during the thyroid scan.*
Rural: *Advisable to arrange for transportation home after recovering from the thyroid scan.*

WEBLINKS

www.healthgate.com

NUCLEAR MEDICINE

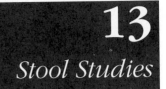

13
Stool Studies

EXAMINATION OF STOOL

Stool tests are performed primarily to confirm the presence of gastrointestinal disorders. These tests are relatively noninvasive in nature and easily implemented. The examination of stool is a common method for evaluating for the presence of gastrointestinal bleeding, normal physiological function, and the abnormal presence of parasites.

PHYSIOLOGY OF STOOL FORMATION

Stool is the end product of digestion, consisting of water, indigestible food material such as cellulose, electrolytes, bile, epithelial cells shed from the intestinal tract, bacteria, inorganic material, and undigested food. The normal brown color of the stool results from the action of bacteria on bile. The average adult excretes 100 to 200 grams of feces daily, which is the end result of 8 to 10 liters of material that enters the intestine daily. The intestines function to digest food, absorb water and electrolytes, and expel wastes in the form of stool from the body.

METHODS OF OBTAINING STOOL SPECIMENS

The stool sample should be sent for analysis while still warm and within one hour. If the stool is to be checked for parasites, immediate transport to the laboratory is imperative. Other tests can be done on a refrigerated specimen if transportation to the laboratory is not immediately possible. Antibiotics and antacids can interfere with bacterial growth while other medications can cause gastrointestinal bleeding.

Stool Specimen Collection Procedure

Stool specimens are collected in either a plastic-hat receptacle placed in the toilet or in a bed pan. The sample should be uncontaminated with either urine or water. Using gloves, a sample is collected from the middle portion of the stool with two clean tongue blades and placed into a specimen container. Any visible anomalies such as blood or pus or organisms should be included in the sample. The sample should be about the size of a walnut. If the stool is unformed, about 15–20 mL are necessary.

Guiac Testing Procedure

A stool smear for analysis of occult blood is collected as above, but a small amount of stool is smeared on a guiac-impregnated paper. A drop of fluid is added to the paper to detect hidden blood. The color blue indicates the presence of blood. The instructions for collection are usually provided directly on the test equipment.

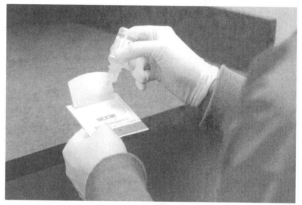

Guiac Testing by Nurse

HANDLING OF STOOL SPECIMENS

STOOL

Stool specimens must be examined in a timely fashion (as described above) to avoid bacterial contamination and for accurate results. In addition, anyone handling the specimen must be careful not to infect himself with the stool products and apply the processes of standard precautions.

Examination of Stool by the Nurse

Nurses observe changes in stool color, odor, consistency, or shape that may indicate a change in health status. In addition, nurses frequently check stools for occult blood as described in the guiac testing procedure. Client education is needed for the test kits that are given for home use. Clients are instructed to mail the sample or deliver the specimen to the laboratory. The clients are advised to follow a meat-free, high-fiber diet (e.g., a diet low in meat or certain vegetables such as turnips) for three days prior to obtaining the stool specimen for testing.

Examination of the Stool by the Laboratory

Laboratory examination of stool provides valuable information about many diseases and bodily systems. Medications must be noted on the laboratory slip to ensure accurate results. The nurse must remember to ask clients about their use of medications and include over-the-counter medications. For example, aspirin is a common cause of gastrointestinal microbleeding and may interfere with test results.

Campylobacter-Like-Organism
(*KAEM*-pi-loe-*BAEK*-t:r liyk *OER*-guh-*NIZ*-:m)
(stool culture for *Campylobacter*)

15 min.

Type of Test: Stool

Body Systems and Functions: Gastrointestinal system

Normal Findings: Normal intestinal flora

Test Results Time Frame: Within 72 hr

Test Description: *Campylobacter* are gram-negative motile rods causing acute gastroenteritis accompanied with diarrhea, abdominal pain, fever, nausea, and vomiting. The bacteria colonize the small and large intestines, causing inflammatory diarrhea with fever. Stools contain leukocytes and blood. The role of toxins in pathogenesis is unclear. For example, *C. jejuni* antigens that cross-react with one or more neural structures may be responsible for triggering the Guillain-Barrè syndrome. Disease incidence peaks in the summer. Domestic and wild animals are the reservoirs for the organisms.

CLINICAL ALERT:
Stool sample must be transported to the laboratory within 1 hr of collection. Three specimens from three consecutive days may be ordered.

Consent Form: Not required

List of Equipment: Clean, dry container to collect stool; tongue depressor; gloves; rectal swab; clean, dry bedpan

Test Procedure:
1. Have client defecate into a clean bedpan, bedside commode, or toilet hat. *Decreases contamination and aids in obtaining stool specimen.*
2. Do not use the stool if it is contaminated with urine or menstrual blood. *Urine and menstrual blood affect stool culture results.*
3. Do not have the client place toilet paper on the stool after defecation. *Toilet paper affects stool culture results.*
4. Use a clean tongue depressor to place 2–3 cm of formed stool or 15 mL of liquid stool in a specimen container. *This amount is necessary for obtaining proper stool culture.*
5. Dispose of remaining stool and tongue depressor. *Decreases chance of spread of pathogen.*

STOOL

6. Include visible mucus, pus, or blood in the specimen. *These may be indicative of disease or contain pathogens.*
7. Label the specimen container and send to laboratory as soon as possible. *Ensures accurate results.*

Clinical Implications and Indications:
1. Evaluates diarrhea of unknown origin
2. Identifies organisms causing gastrointestinal disease and carrier states

Nursing Care:
Before Test: Explain the test procedure and the purpose of the test. Assess the client's knowledge of the test. Assess history of medications, recent travel, dietary changes, and GI disease history.
During Test: Adhere to standard precautions. Assist client if necessary.

Interfering Factors:
Recent use of antimicrobial medications; excessive exposure of sample to air; contamination of stool with urine or blood; failure to transport sample within 1 hr

Nursing Considerations:
Pediatric: Infants and young adults are most often infected.
Rural: Rural settings may predispose to infectious contamination, due to domestic and wild animals being the reservoirs for the organisms. Outbreaks are associated with contaminated animal products or water.
International: Campylobacter jejuni and C. coli infections are endemic worldwide and hyperendemic in developing countries. Infants and young adults are most often infected.

WEBLINKS

www.md.huji.ac.il

Chymex
(*SIY*-meks)
(chymotrypsin)

10 min.

Type of Test: Stool

Body Systems and Functions: Gastrointestinal system

Normal Findings: Positive for small amounts in adults. Greater amounts of chymex are present in children.

Test Results Time Frame: Within 24 hr

Test Description: Chymex is a proteolytic enzyme secreted by the pancreas and found in the small intestine. The chymex test is an indicator of pancreatic function. Three separate specimens indicating abnormal results should be obtained before the diagnosis of pancreatic insufficiency is made. The pancreas is both an exocrine and endocrine organ that is responsible for contributing to the digestive function of the body. A variety of substances is controlled by the pancreas that aid in various metabolic processes (e.g., glucagon, insulin, amylase).

Consent Form: Not required

List of Equipment: Clean, dry container to collect stool; tongue depressor; gloves; rectal swab; clean, dry bedpan

Test Procedure:
1. Have client defecate into a clean bedpan, bedside commode, or toilet hat. *Decreases contamination and aids in obtaining stool specimen.*
2. Do not use the stool if it is contaminated with urine or menstrual blood. *Urine and menstrual blood contaminate stool culture results.*
3. Do not have the client place toilet paper on the stool after defecation. *Toilet paper affects stool culture results.*
4. Use a clean tongue depressor to place 2–3 cm of formed stool or 15 mL of liquid stool in a specimen container. *This amount is necessary for obtaining proper stool culture.*
5. Dispose of remaining stool and tongue depressor. *Decreases chance of spread of pathogen.*
6. Include visible mucus, pus, or blood in the specimen. *These may be indicative of disease or contain pathogens.*
7. Label the specimen container and send to laboratory as soon as possible. *Ensures accurate results.*
8. Collect three separate stool specimens. *Ensures accurate results.*

Clinical Implications and Indications:
1. Decreased levels are found with pancreatic deficiency syndrome, malabsorption disorders, and cystic fibrosis.

Nursing Care:
Before Test: Explain the test procedure and the purpose of the test. Assess the client's knowledge of the test. Ensure the client has not had barium procedures or laxatives for 1 week before the test. A saline or Fleet enema may be administered prior to collecting the specimen.
During Test: Adhere to standard precautions.

Interfering Factors: Bacteria may produce proteolytic enzymes, thus giving false results in the absence of pancreatic enzymes; proteolytic enzymes are destroyed by bacteria within the gastrointestinal tract, thus constipated stool may produce false results; the test is not reliable in adults.

Nursing Considerations:
Pediatric: The chymex test is mainly used in evaluating malabsorption in children under 4 years of age.
Home Care: If home health care provider collects specimen, then rapid transportation to laboratory facilities is required to ensure accurate results.

STOOL

| WEBLINKS |

www.nlm.nih.gov

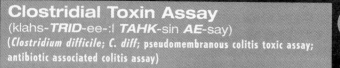

Clostridial Toxin Assay

(klahs-***TRID***-ee-:l ***TAHK***-sin ***AE***-say)

(*Clostridium difficile*; *C. diff*; pseudomembranous colitis toxic assay; antibiotic associated colitis assay)

10 min.

Type of Test: Stool

Body Systems and Functions: Gastrointestinal system

Normal Findings: Negative, no *Clostridium* toxin identified

Test Results Time Frame: Within 24–48 hr

Test Description: Clostridial toxin assay detects *Clostridium difficile*, which is implicated in enteric disease nearly exclusively as a complication of antibiotic therapy (e.g., clindamycin, ampicillin, and the cephalosporins). Antibiotics alter intestinal flora, which provides an environment for conversion of *C. difficile* spores to vegetative forms, with rapid replication and toxin production. Most cases of enteric disease caused by *C. difficile* are manifested by modest diarrhea that resolves when the causative antibiotic is discontinued. Features of *C. difficile*–associated colitis include watery diarrhea (15–30 stools per day), abdominal cramps, lower abdominal tenderness, fever, and leukocytosis. Serious complications include severe dehydration, electrolyte imbalance, hypotension, hypoalbuminemia with anasarca, and toxic megacolon.

CLINICAL ALERT:
Strict enteric isolation precautions must be maintained in clients with *C. difficile*–associated diarrhea.

Consent Form: Not required

List of Equipment: Clean, dry container to collect stool; tongue depressor; gloves; rectal swab; clean, dry bedpan

Test Procedure:
1. Have client defecate into a clean bedpan, bedside commode, or toilet hat. *Decreases contamination and aids in obtaining stool specimen.*
2. Do not use the stool if it is contaminated with urine or menstrual blood. *Urine and menstrual blood affect stool culture results.*
3. Do not have the client place toilet paper on the stool after defecation. *Toilet paper affects stool culture results.*
4. Use a clean tongue depressor to place 2–3 cm of formed stool or 15 mL of liquid stool in a specimen container. *This amount is necessary for obtaining proper stool culture.*
5. Dispose of remaining stool and tongue depressor. *Decreases chance of spread of pathogen.*
6. Include visible mucus, pus, or blood in the specimen. *These may be indicative of disease or contain pathogens.*
7. Label the specimen container and send to laboratory as soon as possible. *Ensures accurate results.*

STOOL

Clinical Implications and Indications:

1. Diagnoses pseudomembranous enterocolitis (often caused by antibiotic therapy)
2. Detects *C. difficile*–associated diarrhea or colitis

Nursing Care:

Before Test: Explain the test procedure and the purpose of the test. Assess the client's knowledge of the test. Instruct client to avoid mixing toilet paper or urine with the stool specimen.
During Test: Adhere to standard and enteric precautions.
After Test: Maintain enteric isolation precautions.

Nursing Considerations:

Pediatric: Studies reveal that infants and children younger than 1 year commonly harbor C. difficile *and its toxin without suffering harmful consequences.*
Gerontology: Aging promotes susceptibility to colonization with C. difficile, *toxin production, and disease.*
Home Care: If home health care provider collects specimen, then rapid transportation to laboratory facilities is required to ensure accurate results.

| WEBLINKS |

www.nlm.nih.gov

Fecal Studies

(*FEE*-k:l)
(fat absorption; fecal fat; quantitative stool fat determination; fecal leukocyte; stool culture; OVA and parasites)

24-72 hr.

Type of Test: Stool

Body Systems and Functions: Gastrointestinal system

Normal Findings: Absence of pathogens and normal amounts of substances found in feces

CRITICAL VALUES:

Clostridium difficile is highly contagious and the client should be placed in contact isolation.

Test Results Time Frame: Within 48 hr of specific test completion

Test Description: Fecal studies are tests that include microscopic, chemical, and microbiological examinations of the feces. Overall, there is less frequency of fecal testing than studies of blood, urine, and other body substances. An obvious rationale for this is that feces cannot be collected on command in the manner of other samples. Nevertheless, fecal analyses are extremely valuable in diagnosing and evaluating a variety of gastrointestinal diseases. Feces are comprised of cellulose and other undigested foods, bacteria, and water. Many other substances are normally found in fecal materials, such as epithelial cells, small amounts of fats, bile pigments, and pancreatic and gastrointestinal secretions.

The average adult eliminates 100–300 g of feces per day. Various tests are performed to evaluate specific substances. Fecal fat is assessed with a quantitative collection of all stools in a 72-hr time period. Fecal leukocyte evaluates the presence of leukocytes in a single stool specimen. Fecal parasites are determined with the microscopic testing of a stool specimen, with the most likely samples being those containing blood and mucus.

CLINICAL ALERT:
A single specimen is often not diagnostic and at least three stool cultures are required for a pathogenic diagnosis.

Consent Form: Not required

List of Equipment: Clean, dry container to collect stool; tongue depressor; gloves; rectal swab; clean, dry bedpan

Test Procedure:
1. Have client defecate into a clean bedpan, bedside commode, or toilet hat. *Decreases chance of contamination and aids in obtaining stool specimen.*
2. Do not use the stool if it is contaminated with urine or menstrual blood. *Affects stool culture results.*
3. Do not have the client place toilet paper on the stool after defecation. *Affects stool culture results.*
4. Have client call nurse as soon as possible after defecation. *Fresh stool is best for stool cultures.*
5. Wear disposable gloves when handling the bedpan and in obtaining the specimen. *Prevents contamination of specimen and protects nurse from pathogens.*
6. Use a clean tongue depressor to place about 2.54 cm of formed stool or 15 mL of liquid stool in a specimen container. *Ensures accurate results.*
7. Dispose of remaining stool and tongue depressor. *Decreases chance of spread of pathogen.*
8. Include visible mucus, pus, or blood in the specimen. *Indicates disease or contain pathogens.*
9. Label the specimen container and send to laboratory as soon as possible.

Clinical Implications and Indications:
1. Detects salmonella, *Shigella*, *Campylobacter jejuni*, enteropathogenic *Escherichia coli*, pure cultures of *Staphylococcus aureus*, *Yersinia enterocolitica*, and various parasites
2. Evaluates leukocytes, epithelial cells, fat (e.g., triglycerides, fatty acids), meat fibers, and parasites
3. Diagnoses inflammatory bowel disorders, pancreatitis, and malabsorption syndrome
4. Evaluates diarrhea of unknown origin

Nursing Care:
Before Test: Explain the test procedure and the purpose of the test. Assess the client's knowledge of the test.
During Test: Adhere to standard precautions. Give client privacy for defecation.
After Test: Ensure client is properly cleaned and dry. Monitor for signs of intestinal infection (e.g., diarrhea).

STOOL

Interfering Factors: Antibiotics, barium, bismuth; toilet paper contamination; diet high in fats; laxatives; urine mixed with the specimen

Nursing Considerations:
Pediatric: Infants and children dehydrate easily during diarrhea and therefore need careful therapeutic management. These ages will need assistance in obtaining an accurate stool specimen.
Gerontology: Elderly clients often have problems with constipation and may have difficulty producing a sample for evaluation.
Home Care: Home health care providers must carefully implement strict standard precautions in clients identified as having parasite infestation.
International: Diarrhea is the leading cause of death worldwide; parasites are frequently found in the gastrointestinal tracts of persons living in third world countries.

Listing of Related Tests: Stool culture; occult blood test

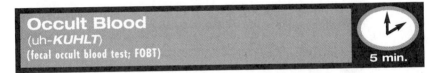

www.cma.ca

Occult Blood
(uh-*KUHLT*)
(fecal occult blood test; FOBT)

5 min.

Type of Test: Stool

Body Systems and Functions: Gastrointestinal system

Normal Findings: Negative for blood

Test Results Time Frame: Immediate if commercial kit used; 2–3 days from laboratory

Test Description: Occult blood tests for the presence of blood in the stool as an indicator of gastrointestinal bleeding. Since smaller amounts of blood are not always visible (e.g., in earlier stages of some GI diseases), a chemical test will confirm its presence and cue further testing and examination for pathophysiology. There are two main methods of tests on the market: those that require direct examination of stool and those that provide testing material that can be thrown into the toilet bowl without direct handling of feces. Caution should be exercised in interpretation of results as the direct stool examination results may be altered by many factors related to diet, medication, and other factors. Urine and emesis should be tested for blood with a dipstick style of testing rather than occult blood kits.

Consent Form: Not required

List of Equipment: *Direct examination of stool:* commercial kit; wooden applicator stick or tongue blade. *Indirect testing:* commercially prepared biodegradable test pad.

STOOL

Test Procedure:
Direct examination of specimen:
1. The client collects a random stool specimen and the feces should be tested from two separate areas. *Blood may be present in isolated areas of sample so testing more than one spot increases chance of capturing target area.*
2. The sample is spread over the identified testing areas of the kit, and the hydrogen peroxide preparation is then applied to the sample spots. *The hydrogen peroxide agent reacts with the pseudoperoxidase activity of any hemoglobin present in sample and oxidizes out as a change in color (usually to blue).*
3. Client reads test and, if positive, informs health care provider. If test is being done in an institution or health care agency, the test can be read on the unit or, if requested, can be sent to the laboratory for testing. Note: Samples should be read within 2 weeks of sampling and should not be refrigerated. *Ensures accurate results.*
4. The test should be repeated for three consecutive stools. *To reduce risk of false negatives/positives and increase chance of identifying presence of blood.*
Indirect testing of specimen:
1. Following a bowel movement, a biodegradable test pad is thrown directly into the toilet bowl.
2. A blue-green color will appear on the test pad if occult blood is present. Again, if the client is doing home testing and gets a positive result, she should inform her health care provider.

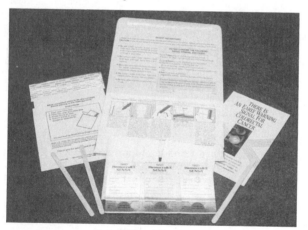

Occult Blood Equipment

Clinical Implications and Indications:
1. Screens for carcinomas (particularly colon) and polyps of GI tract
2. Identifies GI bleeding related to upper GI bleeding (gastric ulcer)
3. Screens for diverticulitis and colitis

Nursing Care:
Before Test: Explain the test procedure and the purpose of the test. Assess the client's knowledge of the test. Instruct client not to eat foods for 2 days that interfere with results. Inform client that one method of collecting the specimen is to place a loose film of plastic wrap across the toilet bowl.

STOOL

During Test: Adhere to standard precautions.

After Test: Instruct client to resume normal diet once testing is complete. Instruct client to report any color changes to their health care provider when using the direct method of testing. Inform client that if positive results are obtained, further testing is likely.

Contraindications: Menstruation; barium enema in last 72 hr

Interfering Factors: Bleeding hemorrhoids; bleeding from constipation; menstruation within 2 days of testing; raw or rare meat, raw broccoli, melons, radishes, cucumbers, horseradish, cauliflower, parsnips, turnips, bananas, apples, and mushrooms; vitamin C–enriched foods or supplements; medications that alter results are rectal medications, aspirin, corticosteroids, nonsteroidal anti-inflammatories, anticoagulants, antimetabolites, and indomethacin.

Nursing Considerations:
Pediatric: Infants and children will need assistance in obtaining stool specimen and age-appropriate comfort measures following the test.
Gerontology: Elderly clients are more at risk for interfering factors associated with constipation and hemorrhoids.
Home Care: If home testing, advise the client to inform the health care provider of positive results. Instruct the client that if sending specimens to laboratory, the sample kits should be closed between sampling and should not be stored in refrigerator or near heat or light.

Listing of Related Tests: Colonoscopy

WEBLINKS

http://chorus.rad.mcw.edu

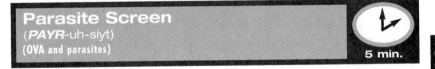

Parasite Screen
(*PAYR*-uh-siyt)
(OVA and parasites)

5 min.

STOOL

Type of Test: Stool

Body Systems and Functions: Gastrointestinal system

Normal Findings: Normal bacteria and microorganisms

Test Results Time Frame: Within 1 week

Test Description: A parasite screen involves the collection of a stool specimen for microscopic examination to rule out the presence of parasites and their eggs. Both a concentrated sample and a stained smear are routinely performed from the collected sample. Some of the more common parasites isolated include protozoa (e.g., *Giardia*), helminths (e.g., roundworm), strongyloides (e.g., threadworm), and *Taenia* (e.g., tapeworm).

Consent Form: Not required

List of Equipment: Clean, dry container to collect stool; tongue depressor; gloves; rectal swab; clean, dry bedpan

Test Procedure:
1. Have client defecate into a clean bedpan, bedside commode, or toilet hat. *Decreases contamination and aids in obtaining stool specimen.*
2. Do not use the stool if it is contaminated with urine or menstrual blood. *Urine and menstrual blood affects stool culture results.*
3. Do not have the client place toilet paper on the stool after defecation. *Toilet paper affects stool culture results.*
4. Use a clean tongue depressor to place 2–3 cm of formed stool or 15 mL of liquid stool in a specimen container. *This amount is necessary for obtaining proper stool culture.*
5. Dispose of remaining stool and tongue depressor. *Decreases chance of spread of pathogen.*
6. Include visible mucus, pus, or blood in the specimen. *These may be indicative of disease or contain pathogens.*
7. Label the specimen container and send to laboratory as soon as possible. *Ensures accurate results.*
8. Usually, three samples on three separate days are submitted. *Increases chance of idenitfying ova and parasites.*
9. Another protocol involves examination of the first sample and follow-up with two samples in high-risk cases, which includes those with chronic or traveller's diarrhea or clients who are immunosuppressed.

Clinical Implications and Indications:
1. Identifies parasitic infestation
2. Investigates prolonged diarrhea or other intestinal symptoms of unknown cause

Nursing Care:
Before Test: Explain the test procedure and the purpose of the test. Assess the client's knowledge of the test.
During Test: Adhere to standard precautions.
After Test: Instruct client to deliver the sample to the laboratory within 2 hr. Emphasize the importance of proper hand washing after each specimen collection.

Interfering Factors: Urine or toilet paper in stool sample; improper storage or delayed delivery time for fresh specimen; medications that alter results are tetracyclines, bismuths (antacids), mineral oil, and castor oil; recent barium studies

Nursing Considerations:
Pediatric: When collecting from the infant or diapered child, the diaper is lined with plastic wrap, and attempts should be made to isolate stool from the urine.
Rural: Rural settings are more likely to have unpurified drinking water, which is a common cause of parasite infestation. Client education should be provided, especially if there is an outbreak of identified parasites in a given area.
International: Obtain information regarding any countries client has visited within the past 3 years. Travellers off the North American continent should be evaluated for a history of drinking unpurified drinking water, which leads to parasitic contamination.

Listing of Related Tests: Stool culture for enteric pathogens; tape-test for pinworms

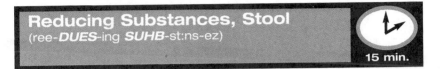

WEBLINKS

www.healthcentral.com

Reducing Substances, Stool
(ree-*DUES*-ing *SUHB*-st:ns-ez)

15 min.

Type of Test: Stool

Body Systems and Functions: Gastrointestinal system

Normal Findings: Negative to trace, <2 mg/g stool

Test Results Time Frame: Within 24 hr

Test Description: Reducing substances is the test that measures the amount of unabsorbed sugars (reducing substances) in the stool sample. Normally, the gastrointestinal border enzymes, primarily sucrase and lactase, aid in rapid absorption of sugar in the upper small intestine. If not absorbed, the sugars remain in the intestine causing osmotic diarrhea by drawing fluids and electrolytes into the intestine. Carbohydrate malabsorption with water diarrhea is a major symptom in short bowel syndrome. It is also present in congenital deficiencies, mucosal injury, and metabolic disorders. As a result of bacterial fermentation, the stools become acidic with a high concentration of lactic acid. The acidity is reflected in the pH of the stool sample.

Consent Form: Not required

List of Equipment: Clean, dry container to collect stool; tongue depressor; gloves; rectal swab; clean, dry bedpan

Test Procedure:
1. Have client defecate into a clean bedpan, bedside commode, or toilet hat. *Decreases contamination and aids in obtaining stool specimen.*
2. Do not use the stool if it is contaminated with urine or menstrual blood. *Urine and menstrual blood affect stool culture results.*
3. Do not have the client place toilet paper on the stool after defecation. *Toilet paper affects stool culture results.*
4. Use a clean tongue depressor to place 2–3 cm of formed stool or 15 mL of liquid stool in a specimen container. *This amount is necessary for obtaining proper stool culture.*
5. Check pH of stool and document results on laboratory requisition and laboratory container. *Acidity of sample is related to sugar content and helpful for interpreting results.*
6. Dispose of remaining stool and tongue depressor. *Decreases chance of spread of pathogen.*
7. Include visible mucus, pus, or blood in the specimen. *These may be indicative of disease or contain pathogens.*

STOOL

8. Label the specimen container and send to laboratory as soon as possible. *Ensures accurate results.*

Clinical Implications and Indications:

1. Diagnoses absence of intestinal enzymes to absorb disaccharides, especially sucrase and lactase, a common problem in short bowel syndrome and congenital deficiency of enzymes.
2. Elevated levels are found with dissacharide deficiency, metabolic disorders, beta-lipoprotein deficiency, celiac disease, cystic fibrosis, and *Giardia* infection.

Nursing Care:

Before Test: Explain the test procedure and the purpose of the test. Assess the client's knowledge of the test.
During Test: Adhere to standard precautions.
After Test: Take pH of stool sample before sending to laboratory.

Interfering Factors: A delay of more than 4 hr between collection and testing invalidates results; medications that decrease levels are colchicines, neomycin, and oral contraceptives; stool coming in contact with paper or cloth during collection alters results.

Nursing Considerations:

Pediatric: Line diaper with plastic wrap to collect specimen because sugar may be absorbed by the fabric or paper of the diaper.

WEBLINKS ⊟ ⊠

www.nlm.nih.gov

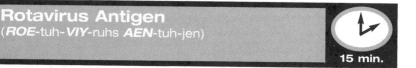

Rotavirus Antigen
(*ROE*-tuh-*VIY*-ruhs *AEN*-tuh-jen)

15 min.

STOOL

Type of Test: Stool

Body Systems and Functions: Gastrointestinal system

Normal Findings: Negative

CRITICAL VALUES:
Positive test

Test Results Time Frame: Within 24 hr

Test Description: Rotavirus is a double-stranded DNA virus and can be detected by enzyme-linked immunosorbent assay (ELISA), enzyme immunoassay (EIA), latex agglutination (LA), and direct electron microscopy. Rotavirus is not routinely cultured.

Consent Form: Not required

List of Equipment: Clean, dry container to collect stool; tongue depressor; gloves; rectal swab; clean, dry bedpan

Test Procedure:
1. Have client defecate into a clean bedpan, bedside commode, or toilet hat. *Decreases contamination and aids in obtaining stool specimen.*
2. Do not use the stool if it is contaminated with urine or menstrual blood. *Urine and menstrual blood affects stool culture results.*
3. Do not have the client place toilet paper on the stool after defecation. *Toilet paper affects stool culture results.*
4. Use a clean tongue depressor to place 2–3 cm of formed stool or 15 mL of liquid stool in a specimen container. *This amount is necessary for obtaining proper stool culture.*
5. Dispose of remaining stool and tongue depressor. *Decreases chance of spread of pathogen.*
6. Include visible mucus, pus, or blood in the specimen. *These may be indicative of disease or contain pathogens.*
7. Label the specimen container and send to laboratory as soon as possible. *Ensures accurate results.*

Clinical Implications and Indications:
1. Rotavirus was identified in 1973 as the cause of "winter vomiting" or "winter diarrhea."
2. It is significant to include a travel history in an interview with the client.
3. Rotavirus disease is spread by the fecal-oral route. It may be contracted from contaminated water sources.

Nursing Care:
Before Test: Explain the test procedure and the purpose of the test. Assess the client's knowledge of the test.
During Test: Adhere to standard precautions.

Nursing Considerations:
Pediatric: Rotavirus is the most common cause of viral gastroenteritis in infants and young children. A vaccine has been developed but has recently been linked to episodes of intussusception and use has been suspended.
Gerontology: Symptoms are more severe in the elderly.
Home Care: Good hand-washing technique should be emphasized.
International: Rotavirus is an international problem often causing endemic acute gastroenteritis in infants and small children. Deaths are usually due to dehydration when unable to be effectively treated in deprived countries.

Listing of Related Tests: Check for blood or neutrophils in the stool

| WEBLINKS |

www.mayohealth.org; http://kidshealth.org

STOOL

Stool Culture
(stuel)
(fecal culture; stool specimen; fecal specimen)

10 min.

Type of Test: Stool

Body Systems and Functions: Gastrointestinal system

Normal Findings: Normal microorganisms found in fecal material include *Candida albicans*, clostidia, enterococci, *Escherichia coli*, *Proteus*, *Pseudomonas*, anaerobic streptococci, staphylococci, and *Helicobacter*. Positive results reported when *Staphylococcus* grows on the culture; no growth in 48 hr indicates negative test.

CRITICAL VALUES:
Clostridium difficile is highly contagious, and the client should be placed in contact isolation.

Test Results Time Frame: Within 48 hr

Test Description: Stool cultures are used to diagnose pathogens, which may be causing abnormal bowel patterns, specifically diarrhea. Stool cultures are most often used to identify parasites, enteric disease pathogens, and viruses. Fecal material is a waste product of the gastrointestinal system. It is normally assessed for its color, odor, and consistency after a rectal examination or after defecation.

CLINICAL ALERT:
A single specimen is not diagnostic; at least three stool cultures are required for a pathogenic diagnosis.

Consent Form: Not required

List of Equipment: Clean bedpan, bedside commode, or toilet hat; specimen container; tongue depressor

Test Procedure:
1. Have client defecate into a clean bedpan, bedside commode, or toilet hat. *Decreases contamination and aids in obtaining stool specimen.*
2. Do not use the stool if it is contaminated with urine or menstrual blood. *Urine and menstrual blood affect stool culture results.*
3. Do not have the client place toilet paper on the stool after defecation. *Toilet paper affects stool culture results.*
4. Use a clean tongue depressor to place 2–3 cm of formed stool or 15 mL of liquid stool in a specimen container. *This amount is necessary for obtaining proper stool culture.*
5. Dispose of remaining stool and tongue depressor. *Decreases chance of spread of pathogen.*
6. Include visible mucus, pus, or blood in the specimen. *These may be indicative of disease or contain pathogens.*
7. Label the specimen container and send to laboratory as soon as possible. *Ensures accurate results.*

STOOL

Clinical Implications and Indications:

1. Diagnoses and monitors *Salmonella, Shigella, Campylobacter jejuni,* enteropathogenic *E. coli, Helicobacter, Clostridium difficile,* and *Yersinia enterocolitica*
2. Evaluates and monitors pure cultures of *S. aureus* and various parasites

Nursing Care:

Before Test: Explain the test procedure and the purpose of the test. Assess the client's knowledge of the test.

During Test: Adhere to standard precautions. Give client privacy for defecation.

After Test: Ensure client is properly cleaned and dry. Monitor for signs of intestinal infection (e.g., diarrhea).

Interfering Factors: Antibiotics; barium; bismuth; urine; menstrual blood; toilet paper contamination

Nursing Considerations:

Pediatric: *Usually only one stool culture ordered. It is not recommended to order stool cultures after 4 days of hospitalization. Infants and children will need assistance in remaining still during the collection of the stool and age-appropriate comfort measures following the test.*

Gerontology: *Precipitating factors leading to decreased bowel elimination in the older adult include lack of bulk in the diet, decreased fluid intake, decreased activity, laxative abuse, and avoidance of the need to defecate. In addition, rectal neurons may degenerate with age, which results in decreased sphincter control and fecal incontinence.*

International: *Diarrhea is the leading cause of death worldwide; parasites are frequently found in the gastrointestinal tracts of persons living in third world countries.*

WEBLINKS

www.amda.ab.ca; www.cma.ca

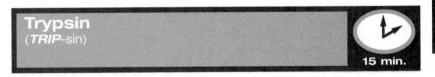

Trypsin
(*TRIP*-sin)

15 min.

STOOL

Type of Test: Stool

Body Systems and Functions: Gastrointestinal system

Normal Findings: Trypsin is found in small amounts in adults and in larger amounts with children.

Test Results Time Frame: Within 24 hr

Test Description: Trypsin is a proteolytic enzyme formed in the intestine from the action of the intestinal juices, which are secreted by the pancreas. Trypsin is used to break down carbohydrates, proteins, and fats. Since intestinal bacteria can destroy trypsin, this test is somewhat unreliable with adults. Testing for trypsin in stool is useful in diagnosing malabsorption in children.

CLINICAL ALERT:
Three separate stool specimens should be tested for positive diagnosis of pancreatic deficiency.

Consent Form: Not required

List of Equipment: Clean, dry container to collect stool; tongue depressor; gloves; rectal swab; clean, dry bedpan

Test Procedure:
1. Have client defecate into a clean bedpan, bedside commode, or toilet hat. *Decreases contamination and aids in obtaining stool specimen.*
2. Do not use the stool if it is contaminated with urine or menstrual blood. *Urine and menstrual blood affects stool culture results.*
3. Do not have the client place toilet paper on the stool after defecation. *Toilet paper affects stool culture results.*
4. Use a clean tongue depressor to place 2–3 cm of formed stool or 15 mL of liquid stool in a specimen container. In addition, obtain three separate stool specimens. *This amount is necessary for obtaining proper stool culture.*
5. Dispose of remaining stool and tongue depressor. *Decreases chance of spread of pathogen.*
6. Include visible mucus, pus, or blood in the specimen. *These may be indicative of disease or contain pathogens.*
7. Label the specimen container and send to laboratory as soon as possible. *Ensures accurate results as the specimen must be tested within 2 hr.*

Clinical Implications and Indications:
1. Elevated levels are normal in children and 95% of adults.
2. Decreased levels are found with pancreatic deficiency, malabsorption, and cystic fibrosis.

Nursing Care:
Before Test: Explain the test procedure and the purpose of the test. Assess the client's knowledge of the test. Older children will need a cathartic prior to obtaining the sample.
During Test: Adhere to standard precautions.

Interfering Factors: Constipation will cause decrease in trypsin (intestinal bacteria destroys trypsin); laxatives and barium; higher levels of intestinal flora in adults destroy trypsin; bacterial proteins can produce a positive result when no trypsin is present.

Nursing Considerations:
Pediatric: Negative amounts in children may indicate lack of trypsin activity and pancreatic deficiency.

WEBLINKS

http://chorus.rad.mcw.edu

14
Ultrasound Studies

EXAMINATION BY ULTRASOUND

Ultrasound studies use soundwaves to produce an image of internal organs, tissues, or fetuses. The soundwaves are very high frequency and inaudible to the human ear, with a frequency of higher than 20,000 cycles/second (normal human hearing is between 16,000–20,000 cycles/second). Pulses of sound are generated by a transducer, which are sent into the client. The ultrasound waves bounce back from the body tissues, producing echoes that the transducer records and displays on a monitor as a picture or into audible sound, which is known as the "Doppler" method. The picture or sound is "real-time" in that it can show motion or hear sounds within the body as they occur. For example, a fetus can be observed moving about, performing musculoskeletal motions as it occurs.

No evidence of any adverse effects has been found for the use of ultrasound. Studies of fetuses exposed to ultrasound waves have not demonstrated any observable risk. Large and continuous doses of ultrasound waves can be used therapeutically to generate heat in tissues for the treatment of low back pain and kidney stones. At diagnostic levels, however, no heat is generated.

History of Ultrasound Procedures

Ultrasound was first used in pregnancy to visualize the developing fetus and to listen to fetal heart tones. Current use includes visualization of many areas of the body, including the heart and blood vessels, and pelvic and abdominal structures. A new Doppler technique translates a color-coded picture of blood flow and can be used to establish the patency of blood vessels. Ultrasound is not useful for studies of bones or air-gas-filled structures in the body, as the soundwaves do not produce a meaningful echo. The use of ultrasound testing has proliferated in routine pregnancy. There is some controversy regarding the cost/benefit ratio for women who are low risk for perinatal complications.

THE ULTRASOUND PROCEDURE

An ultrasound is painless and needs little client preparation. Tests are usually fast and require little time (less than an hour). An informed consent form is usually not required. The procedure includes correct positioning of the client, application of a gel to the skin to assist in the conduction of the sound waves, moving the transducer over the skin above the body part of interest, and recording the images or sounds that are produced.

CLIENT CARE IN ULTRASOUND STUDIES

Ultrasound studies (see Table) are painless, noninvasive, and have very few risks. The two potential complications to share with clients are cavitation, which is the appearance of gas-filled bubbles in a sound field, and the production of heat (as described above). In addition, pregnant clients should be reassured that no evidence has shown any risk to the developing fetus. For some pelvic studies, a full bladder is necessary to use the bladder as an anatomical "marker." Instruct clients to drink at least a quart of water before the test. If the client has an indwelling catheter, it may be necessary to clamp the tubing before the ultrasound is performed. Some abdominal ultrasounds may require that the client be on a special diet or NPO for various lengths of time.

Clients may have interfering factors that affect the ultrasound studies, such as barium contrast, which makes it more beneficial to do barium studies after ultrasound studies; the inability of the client to remain motionless during the ultrasound; and an incorrect placement of the transducer during the procedure.

ULTRASOUND

Abdominal Ultrasound
(ab-*DOM*-in-al *UL*-tra-sound)

30-45 min.

Type of Test: Ultrasound

Body Systems and Functions: Gastrointestinal system

Normal Findings: Normal abdomen and surrounding structures

Test Results Time Frame: Within 24 hr

Test Description: An abdominal ultrasound visualizes all of the upper abdominal organs or the test may be ordered by specific abdominal organ or region. This test is frequently used to detect and monitor abdominal aneurysms. Doppler ultrasonography is a noninvasive test that uses ultrasound waves to identify occlusions of the veins or arteries. Ultrasound waves are transmitted and received from the transducer while it is placed over the circulatory system locations. The returning echoes are amplified and images are recorded on a video and strip recorder.

CLINICAL ALERT:
Sudden onset of abdominal pain or increasing steady abdominal pain, especially with diaphoresis and hypotension, may indicate impending rupture of the abdominal aorta and must be reported immediately. This test may be completed at the client's bedside.

Consent Form: Required

List of Equipment: Ultrasound equipment

Test Procedure:
1. Place client in supine position, expose abdomen, and drape. *Allows privacy.*
2. The technician lubricates the abdominal surface with acoustic gel. *Allows maximum penetration of ultrasound.*
3. The technician positions a transducer over various regions of the abdomen.
4. Images appear on a screen and are saved for analysis.

Clinical Implications and Indications:
1. Diagnoses abdominal aneurysm
2. Monitors small abdominal aneurysms over time
3. Differentiates abdominal aneurysm from a thrombus
4. Diagnoses abdominal problems during pregnancy

Nursing Care:
Before Test: Explain the test procedure and the purpose of the test. Assess the client's knowledge of the test. Instruct the client that there will be no discomfort. Assist client in removing clothing. Provide for privacy. Instruct client not to smoke for 30 min prior to test. Instruct client to fast for 12 hr before the procedure, but encourage fluids. Fasting allows the stomach to be small and empty and allows the gall bladder to be visualized. A full bladder helps to push intestinal contents, especially gas, out of the way. If both ultrasound and x-ray involving barium are to be done, schedule the ultrasound first so that retained barium will not interfere with the ultrasound.
During Test: Adhere to standard precautions. Assist the technician in positioning client. Provide emotional support while the test is performed and evaluate the client for discomfort during the procedure.
After Test: Wipe away the water-soluble gel and reclothe the client when the ultrasound is finished. Encourage client to verbalize fears in terms of test results.

Interfering Factors: Retained barium from a previous upper or lower GI may obscure the results of the ultrasound; inability of client to remain still; obesity or abdominal scars may interfere with the ability of the sound waves to be appropriately deflected from the organ under study; incorrect placement of transducer.

ULTRASOUND

Nursing Considerations:

Pregnancy: *Considered completely safe during pregnancy. The client may inappropriately believe this procedure is radiological in nature. This misconception should be corrected with correct client education.*

Pediatric: *Infants and children will need assistance in remaining still during the procedure and age-appropriate comfort measures following the test.*

Gerontology: *The older person may find it difficult to maintain positions when required to do so for lengthy periods of time.*

Listing of Related Tests: Barium x-rays of the abdomen

WEBLINKS	

http://www.usyd.edu

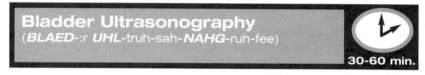

Bladder Ultrasonography
(*BLAED*-:r *UHL*-truh-sah-*NAHG*-ruh-fee)

30-60 min.

Type of Test: Ultrasound

Body Systems and Functions: Renal/urological system

Normal Findings: Normal size, position, and shape of urinary bladder; no urinary residual or masses

Test Results Time Frame: Within 24–48 hr

Test Description: Bladder ultrasonography is a noninvasive test that uses ultrasound waves to examine the bladder's position, shape, and size. Ultrasound waves are transmitted and received from the transducer while it is placed over the bladder location. The returning echoes are amplified and images are recorded on a video and strip recorder.

> **CLINICAL ALERT:**
> This test may be completed at the client's bedside.

Consent Form: Not required

List of Equipment: Ultrasound equipment

Test Procedure:
1. Place client in supine position, expose abdomen, and drape. *Allows privacy.*
2. The technician lubricates the abdominal surface with acoustic gel. *Allows maximum penetration of ultrasound.*
3. The technician positions a transducer over various regions of the abdomen.

Clinical Implications and Indications:
1. Assesses residual urine after voiding for the presence of urinary tract obstruction
2. Diagnoses bladder or pelvis tumors
3. Diagnoses cancer of the bladder

ULTRASOUND

Nursing Care:

Before Test: Explain the test procedure and the purpose of the test. Assess the client's knowledge of the test. Gather history that includes disease or problems with bladder. Encourage fluid intake (e.g., 16 oz) to ensure full bladder or empty bladder immediately before test, if assessing for residual volume. Instruct the client that there will be no discomfort. Assist client in removing clothing from waist down. Provide for privacy.

During Test: Adhere to standard precautions. Assist the technician in positioning of client.

After Test: Provide client opportunity to empty bladder. Remove gel from abdomen.

Contraindications: Third trimester of pregnancy in a transvaginal bladder ultrasound

Interfering Factors: Inability of client to remain still; incorrect placement of transducer; barium or gas in the bowel; residual urine in bladder

Nursing Considerations:

Pediatric: Infants and children will need assistance in remaining still during the procedure and age-appropriate comfort measures following the test.

WEBLINKS

http://adam.excite.com

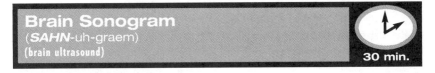

Brain Sonogram
(*SAHN*-uh-graem)
(brain ultrasound)

30 min.

Type of Test: Ultrasound

Body Systems and Functions: Neurological system

Normal Findings: Normal brain tissue, ventricles, and blood flow

Test Results Time Frame: Within 24 hr

Test Description: An ultrasound of the brain is a noninvasive test that uses ultrasound waves to identify occlusions of the veins or arteries. Ultrasound waves are transmitted and received from the transducer while it is placed over the circulatory system locations. The returning echoes are amplified and images are recorded on a video and strip recorder. The test is painless and uses the high-frequency ultrasound waves in varying intensities to observe the brain structure.

CLINICAL ALERT:
This test may be completed at the client's bedside.

Consent Form: Not required

List of Equipment: Ultrasound equipment

ULTRASOUND

Test Procedure:
1. Place client in supine position. *Allows privacy.*
2. The technician lubricates the client's head surface with acoustic gel. *Allows maximum penetration of ultrasound.*
3. The technician positions a transducer over various regions of the skull.
4. The sound waves are received on the machine and recorded. *Allows interpretation at a later time.*

Clinical Implications and Indications:
1. Evaluates and monitors hydrocephalus, abnormal bleeding in the brain, cystic or solid tumors, rubella, cytomegalovirus, and herpes simplex

Nursing Care:
Before Test: Explain the test procedure and the purpose of the test. Assess the client's knowledge of the test. Instruct the client that there will be no discomfort. Assist client in removing clothing. Provide for privacy. Instruct client to not smoke for 30 min prior to test.
During Test: Adhere to standard precautions. Assist the technician in positioning of client and in keeping infant still.
After Test: Encourage client to verbalize fears in terms of test results.

Interfering Factors:
Inability of client to remain still; incorrect placement of transducer; IV access in the scalp area (in an infant)

Nursing Considerations:
Pediatric: Infants and children will need assistance in remaining still during the ultrasound and age-appropriate comfort measures following the test. This procedure can only be performed on infants whose fontanels have not yet closed, since the fontanel allows the passage of ultrasound waves into the brain. Frequently this procedure is completed in the neonatal intensive care unit. Confirm that the client does not have an IV line in the scalp area. Schedule test to be performed after a feeding.
Gerontology: The older person may find it difficult to maintain positions when required to do so for lengthy periods of time during the ultrasound.

WEBLINKS

http://web1.tch.harvard.edu

Breast Sonogram
(brest *SAHN*-uh-graem)
(breast ultrasound; breast ultrasonography)

30 min.

Type of Test: Ultrasound

Body Systems and Functions: Reproductive system

Normal Findings: Normal symmetrical echo pattern of both breasts, which shows no abnormalities or pathological lesions in the subcutaneous, mammary, and retromammary layers

Test Results Time Frame: Within 24–48 hr

Test Description: A breast sonogram is a noninvasive, painless test that uses high-frequency ultrasound waves in varying intensities to record both palpable and nonpalpable masses. Unlike mammography, this test is especially useful in women who have dense breasts or those with silicon implants, because the beam easily penetrates the tissue. Breast sonography can also be performed as an adjunct to mammography or in place of it for those clients who are at risk for mammography (e.g., pregnancy). When ultrasound is used in conjunction with mammography, diagnostic accuracy is improved.

CLINICAL ALERT:
This test may be completed at the client's bedside.

Consent Form: Not required

List of Equipment: Ultrasound equipment

Test Procedure:

Waterless:
1. Position client in supine position on examining table.
2. Expose the chest and drape client. *Provides privacy while allowing access to tissue requiring study.*
3. The technician applies a warmed conductive gel to breast. *Allows maximum penetration of ultrasound.*
4. Client places arms behind head. *Allows access to all breast tissue.*
5. Technician moves transducer over breast tissue and the sound waves are received on the machine and recorded. *Allows interpretation at a later time.*

Water tank:
1. Place client on table in a prone position and immerse each breast in the tank of warm chlorinated water. *Allows waves to be transmitted through the water from a transducer placed at the bottom of the tank.*
2. The technician moves the transducer over the breast tissue and the sound waves are received on the machine and recorded. *Allows interpretation at a later time.*

Clinical Implications and Indications:
1. Verifies the presence of abnormalities found with mammography
2. Differentiates between breast masses, such as cysts, solid tumors, and other lesions in dense breast tissue
3. Detects tumor metastasis to muscle and lymph nodes

Nursing Care:

Before Test: Explain the test procedure and the purpose of the test. Assess the client's knowledge of the test. Instruct the client that there will be no discomfort. Assist client in removing clothing. Provide for privacy. Instruct client to not smoke for 30 min prior to test. Instruct client to not apply any deodorant, powder, or lotions to breast area; obtain history of breast implants, surgeries, and previous or existing abnormalities of the breast.

During Test: Adhere to standard precautions. Assist the technician in positioning of client.

After Test: Encourage client to verbalize fears in terms of test results. Teach client how to perform monthly self-breast exams.

Interfering Factors: Inability of client to remain still; incorrect placement of transducer; use of deodorant, powder, or lotions in breast area; large breasts

ULTRASOUND

Nursing Considerations:

Gerontology: *The older person may find it difficult to maintain positions when required to do so for lengthy periods of time during the ultrasound.*

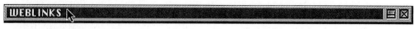

WEBLINKS

www.cancer.org

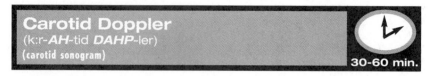

Carotid Doppler
(k:r-*AH*-tid *DAHP*-ler)
(carotid sonogram)

30-60 min.

Type of Test: Ultrasound

Body Systems and Functions: Cardiovascular system

Normal Findings: Normal vascular anatomy and blood flow of the common carotid arteries and internal and external carotids; no evidence of stenosis or occlusion

Test Results Time Frame: Within 24–48 hr

Test Description: A carotid Doppler examination is a noninvasive procedure that examines the arteries supplying the brain. Anatomic and hemodynamic information is provided. During Doppler testing, a signal that represents blood flow can be heard. In general, ultrasonography creates an oscilloscopic image from the echoes of high-frequency sound waves that pass over this system. Various abnormalities of the cardiovascular system are identified with the ultrasound.

Consent Form: Required

List of Equipment: Doppler machine

Test Procedure:
1. Place client in supine position with the neck slightly extended and exposed and drape. *Allows for clear visualization and privacy.*
2. The technician lubricates the neck region with acoustic gel. *Allows maximum penetration of ultrasound.*
3. The technician positions a transducer over various regions of the neck and both carotid vessels are examined.

Clinical Implications and Indications:
1. Evaluates suspected atherosclerotic clinical manifestations (e.g., headache, dizziness, paresthesia, speech difficulties, and visual disturbances).
2. Carotid Doppler testing is usually done in combination with carotid angiography in order to determine the need for carotid endarterectomy. Abnormal images and Doppler signals may indicate plaque, stenosis, occlusion, dissection, aneurysm, and carotid body tumor.

Nursing Care:

Before Test: Explain the test procedure and the purpose of the test. Assess the client's knowledge of the test. Assure client that no pain will be experienced.

During Test: Adhere to standard precautions.

After Test: Encourage client to verbalize fears in terms of test results. Clean site of transducer gel.

Interfering Factors: Obesity; inability to remain still; inadequate gel

Nursing Considerations:

Pediatric: Infants and children will need assistance in remaining still during the procedure and age-appropriate comfort measures following the test.

Gerontology: The older person may find it difficult to maintain positions when required to do so for lengthy periods of time during the Doppler study.

WEBLINKS

http://www.nhlbi.nih.gov

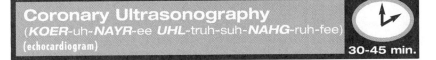

Coronary Ultrasonography
(*KOER*-uh-*NAYR*-ee *UHL*-truh-suh-*NAHG*-ruh-fee)
(echocardiogram)

30-45 min.

Type of Test: Ultrasound

Body Systems and Functions: Cardiovascular system

Normal Findings: Normal position, size, and movement of heart valves and chamber walls

Test Results Time Frame: Within 24–48 hr (note: test results are dependent on the cardiologist's interpretation of results)

Test Description: Coronary ultrasonography is a noninvasive test that uses ultrasound waves to examine the heart's position and size; pericardium and great vessels; valve and chamber movement; and blood flow velocity. Ultrasound waves are transmitted and received by the electrocardiograph and recorded on a video and strip recorder. The two approaches to this test are transthoracic and transesophageal. In the transthoracic approach a transducer is placed on the external chest wall over the precordium. The transesophageal approach involves placing a transesophageal transducer into the client's esophagus. Transesophageal echocardiography provides more specific information at a higher resolution than the precordial approach due to the proximity of the esophagus to the cardiac structures. The various techniques of coronary ultrasonography include M-mode (or motion), two-dimensional, and Doppler. M-mode records detailed motions of cardiac structures and is effective in measuring cardiac chamber dimensions and wall thickness. Two-dimensional coronary ultrasonography provides detailed information about cardiac anatomy and function; it allows for measurement of cardiac dimensions, valvular areas, and chamber volumes. The Doppler technique provides information about coronary blood flow. Note: Stress echocardiography combines exercise or pharmacological stress testing with coronary ultrasonography.

CLINICAL ALERT:
This test may be completed at the client's bedside.

ULTRASOUND

Consent Form: Required

Test Procedure: Transthoracic approach:

Transthoracic approach:
1. Position client in slightly side-lying position.
2. The technician lubricates the chest surface with acoustic gel. *Allows maximum penetration of ultrasound.*
3. The technician positions a transducer over various regions of the chest.

Transesophageal approach:
1. Apply a topical anesthetic to the pharynx. An oral bite block is inserted. *Decreases the risk of damage to the client's teeth, oral structures, and airway.*
2. Place the client in a left lateral decubitus position.
3. The cardiologist inserts the endoscope and performs the test.

Clinical Implications and Indications:
1. Evaluates cardiac performance and hemodynamic parameters
2. Diagnoses mitral/aortic stenosis and regurgitation, tricuspid valve disease, and infective endocarditis
3. Evaluates prosthetic valves, ventricular inlet and outlet abnormalities, and cardiac shunts
4. Detects abnormalities of the great arteries
5. Diagnoses ischemic heart disease, cardiomyopathies, pericardial disease, cardiac tumors, thrombi, and diseases of the aorta
6. Diagnoses myocardial infarctions

Nursing Care:

Before Test: Transthoracic approach: Explain the test procedure and the purpose of the test. Assess the client's knowledge of the test. Instruct the client that there will be no discomfort. Assist client in removing clothing to waist. Provide for privacy. Transesophageal approach: Explain the test procedure and the purpose of the test. Assess the client's knowledge of the test. Ensure client is NPO for 8 hr before procedure. Establish IV access. Remove dentures from client's mouth. Administer preprocedure analgesics and sedatives as ordered. Obtain baseline vital signs and pulse oximetry.

During Test: Transthoracic approach: Adhere to standard precautions. Assist the technician in positioning of client. Transesophageal approach: Adhere to standard precautions. Assist positioning of client. Monitor vital signs, pulse oximetry, and client's tolerance to procedure. Administer IV medications as ordered.

After Test: Monitor vital signs, oxygenation, and level of consciousness. Ensure patent airway. Keep client NPO for a minimum of 1 hr after the procedure. Assess for return of swallowing, coughing, and gag reflexes before allowing food and fluid intake.

Potential Complications: Transesophageal approach: vomiting and aspiration

Contraindications: Transesophageal approach: abnormalities of the esophagus such as esophageal varices and trauma to the esophagus

Interfering Factors: Obesity; trauma to chest wall; pulmonary disease

ULTRASOUND

Nursing Considerations:

Pregnancy: *Fetal echocardiograms are performed through the pregnant woman's abdomen to determine the presence of congenital cardiac defect.*

WEBLINKS

www.acc.org

Doppler Ultrasonography
(*d*AHP-l:r *UHL*-truh-sah-*NAHG*-ruh-fee)
(Doppler studies, vascular; Doppler ultrasound)

30-60 min.

Type of Test: Ultrasound

Body Systems and Functions: Cardiovascular system

Normal Findings: Normal venous system without evidence of occlusion

Test Results Time Frame: Within 24–48 hr

Test Description: Doppler ultrasonography is a noninvasive test that uses ultrasound waves to identify occlusions of the veins or arteries. Ultrasound waves are transmitted and received from the transducer while it is placed over the circulatory system locations. The returning echoes are amplified and images are recorded on a video and strip recorder. Venous patency is determined by the detection of the movement of the RBCs within the veins. The venous system is evaluated due to clinical manifestations that suggest pathology (swelling; painful extremities; presence of edema in the periphery). With single arterial Doppler studies, an evaluation of peripheral arteriosclerosis and occlusive disorders is made with the use of deflating blood pressure cuffs on the calf and ankle. Again, clinical symptomatology provides the impetus for the study (e.g., claudication, pulseless extremity, positive Homans' sign). Double arterial Doppler studies are performed with a pulse Doppler probe to evaluate flow velocities and direction of flow within an artery. The result is a direct visualization and evaluation of stenosis or occluded arteries.

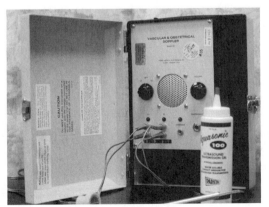

Doppler Ultrasonography Equipment

ULTRASOUND

CLINICAL ALERT:
This test may be completed at the client's bedside.

Consent Form: Not required

List of Equipment: Ultrasound equipment

Test Procedure:
Venous Doppler studies:
1. Position client in supine position, expose skin where testing will occur, and drape. *Allows privacy.*
2. The technician lubricates the skin surface with acoustic gel. *Allows maximum penetration of ultrasound.*
3. The technician positions a transducer over various regions of the abdomen.

Arterial Doppler studies:
1. Position client in supine position, expose skin where testing will occur, and drape. *Allows privacy.*
2. The technician lubricates the skin surface with acoustic gel. *Allows maximum penetration of ultrasound.*
3. Inflate blood pressure cuff above systolic blood pressure, position Doppler immediately distal to cuff, and listen with Doppler as cuff is deflated. *Allows detection of Doppler signal when blood flow sounds are heard.*
4. Repeat testing. *Confirms results.*

Clinical Implications and Indications:
1. Evaluates and detects arterial aneurysms, small or large vessel occlusions, Raynaud's phenomena, embolic arterial occlusive disease, venous occlusions, and varicose veins

Nursing Care:
Before Test: Explain the test procedure and the purpose of the test. Assess the client's knowledge of the test. Instruct the client that there will be no discomfort. Assist client in removing clothing. Provide for privacy. Instruct client to not smoke for 30 min prior to test.
During Test: Adhere to standard precautions. Assist the technician in positioning of client.
After Test: Clean site of transducer gel.

Interfering Factors: Inability of client to remain still; incorrect placement of transducer; occlusions proximal to the site of testing; cigarette smoking due to the nicotine's constriction of peripheral arteries

Nursing Considerations:
Pediatric: Infants and children will need assistance in remaining still during the procedure and age-appropriate comfort measures following the test.
Gerontology: The older person may find it difficult to maintain positions when required to do so for lengthy periods of time during the ultrasonography.
Home Care: Home health care providers should assess clients for clinical manifestations of circulatory occlusions (e.g., painful extremities, edema, pulse changes in extremities) and report to primary care providers.

Listing of Related Tests: Arteriogram studies

WEBLINKS

http://www.entnet.org

Fetal Biophysical Profile
(FEE-t:l *BIY*-oe-'*FIZ*-uh-k:l *PROE*-fiyl)
(biophysical profile; BPP)

30-60 min.

Type of Test: Ultrasound

Body Systems and Functions: Reproductive system

Normal Findings: Score of 8–10 points

CRITICAL VALUES:
Score of less than 4

Test Results Time Frame: Within 24 hr

Test Description: A fetal biophysical profile (BPP) evaluates the fetus during the antepartal period by ultrasonography. This test is comprised of five parameters: fetal heart rate, fetal breathing movement, gross fetal movements, fetal muscle tone, and amniotic fluid volume. The fetal heart rate is measured by the fetal nonstress test, and the other variables are evaluated by ultrasound. These assessment indices are proven as variables that indicate the health of the fetus. Each of the five parameters is scored with either a 2 or a 0, which makes 10 the perfect score and 0 the lowest score. Another parameter that can be observed for is placental grading. Sometimes, repeating the test within 24 hr is encouraged. See table for parameters assessed for in the BPP.

Parameters of fetal biophysical profile

Score of 2	Score of 0
Fetal heart rate (FHR) reactivity over a 20-min time period	FHR of at least 15/min above baseline FHR is nonreactive
Fetal breathing movements	At least 1 normal fetal breathing episode lasting 60 sec within a 30-min time period Absence of breathing episode
Fetal body movements	At least 3 discrete episodes of fetal movements within a 30-min time period 2 or fewer fetal movements in the 30 min
Fetal tone with return to flexion	At least 1 episode of active extension slow extension with a return to only partial extension Measured by flexion/extension movements of arms, legs, trunk, and head
Amniotic fluid volume	At least one pocket of amniotic fluid that measures 1 cm in two perpendicular planes
Fluid is absent in most areas of the uterine cavity	

ULTRASOUND

CLINICAL ALERT:
Be prepared to provide intensive emotional support if test reveals fetal distress.

Consent Form: Not required

List of Equipment: Ultrasound equipment

Test Procedure:
1. Place client in supine position, expose abdomen, and drape. *Allows privacy.*
2. The technician lubricates the abdominal surface with acoustic gel. *Allows maximum penetration of ultrasound.*
3. The technician positions a transducer over various regions of the abdomen.

Clinical Implications and Indications:
1. Evaluates congenital anomalies, intrauterine retardation, and postterm pregnancy
2. Diagnoses and monitors fetal stress, fetal asphyxia, and fetal death

Nursing Care:
Before Test: Explain the test procedure and the purpose of the test. Assess the client's knowledge of the test.
During Test: Adhere to standard precautions.
After Test: If tests reveal fetal distress, provide emotional support.

Interfering Factors: CNS stimulants can increase BPP.

Nursing Considerations:
Pregnancy: Encourage pregnant clients to report abnormalities of fetal movement, as one means of knowing when to perform the BPP. Provide emotional support during this potential time of crisis.
Pediatric: Abnormalities of the fetus may be detected in time to facilitate effective interventions.

Listing of Related Tests: Fetal nonstress test; fetal scalp blood, pH

WEBLINKS ▤▧

http://adam.excite.com

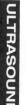

Gallbladder and Biliary System Sonogram
(*GAHL*-blaed-:r *BIL*-ee-*AYR*-ee *SIS*-t:m *SAHN*-uh-graem)

30-60 min.

Type of Test: Ultrasound

Body Systems and Functions: Hepatobiliary system

Normal Findings: Normal hepatobiliary system

Test Results Time Frame: Within 24 hr

Test Description: A gallbladder and biliary system sonogram is an ultrasound that evaluates the hepatobiliary system. Ultrasonography creates an oscilloscopic image from the echoes of high-frequency sound waves that pass over this system. Various abnormalities of the hepatobiliary system are identified with the ultrasound. The hepatobiliary system consists of the liver, gallbladder, and existing duct components. A variety of metabolic processes are influenced and controlled by this system (e.g., glucose metabolism, ammonia conversion, protein metabolism). In addition, bile is produced by the liver and is stored temporarily in the gallbladder, where it stays until needed for digestion. Pathologies of the hepatobiliary system have widespread effects on the human body.

Consent Form: Not required

List of Equipment: Ultrasound equipment

Test Procedure:
1. Position client in supine position, expose abdomen, and drape. *Allows privacy.*
2. The technician lubricates the right upper quadrant of the abdominal surface with acoustic gel. *Allows maximum penetration of ultrasound.*
3. The technician positions a transducer over various regions of the right upper quadrant of the abdomen.
4. Administer sincalide as per protocol if contractility of the gallbladder is to be evaluated.

Clinical Implications and Indications:
1. Diagnoses cholelithiasis and cholecystitis
2. Evaluates the cause of jaundice

Nursing Care:
Before Test: Explain the test procedure and the purpose of the test. Assess the client's knowledge of the test. Instruct client to not eat fats for 24 hr before test and to fast from foods for 8–12 hr before sonogram. Encourage client to drink fluids during this time. Inform client that sincalide may cause nausea, which is aggravated by movement.
During Test: Adhere to standard precautions. Instruct client to remain still during procedure.
After Test: Encourage client to verbalize fears in terms of test results. Clean site of transducer gel.

Contraindications: Administration of sincalide is contraindicated in pregnancy and in children.

Interfering Factors: Inability to remain still; obesity; dehydration

Nursing Considerations:
Pregnancy: Sincalide should not be given in pregnancy.
Pediatric: Sincalide should not be given to children.
Gerontology: The older person may find it difficult to maintain positions when required to do so for lengthy periods of time during the ultrasonography.

ULTRASOUND

WEBLINKS

http://chorus.rad.mcw.edu

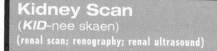

30 min.

Type of Test: Ultrasound

Body Systems and Functions: Renal/urological system

Normal Findings: Normal image indicating normal shape and size of kidneys

Test Results Time Frame: Within 24 hr (immediate evaluation is possible)

Test Description: A renal ultrasound visualizes the parenchyma and associated structures, including renal blood vessels. Doppler ultrasonography is a noninvasive test that uses ultrasound waves over the flank areas to identify occlusions of the veins or arteries. Ultrasound waves are transmitted and received from the transducer while it is placed over the circulatory system locations. The returning echoes are amplified and images are recorded on a video and strip recorder. The kidney is visualized by using the liver or the spleen as comparative structures. The renal ultrasound may be performed with an IVP to define or characterize masses or lesions and can be used in people with iodine allergy.

CLINICAL ALERT:
Renal scans cannot be done over open wounds or dressings. A kidney scan must be performed before radiographic studies involving barium; if not possible, at least 24 hr must elapse between barium procedure and the kidney scan (note: renal biopsy may be done with ultrasound guidance).

Consent Form: May be required

List of Equipment: Ultrasound gel; ultrasound machine

Test Procedure:
1. Position client in supine position, expose flank area, and drape. *Allows privacy.*
2. The technician lubricates the abdominal surface with acoustic gel. *Allows maximum penetration of ultrasound.*
3. Client takes a deep breath and holds it until told to exhale. *Allows upper parts of the kidney to be visualized.*
4. The technician positions a transducer over various regions of the kidney areas.

Clinical Implications and Indications:
1. Detects cysts, solid masses, hydronephrosis, ureteric obstruction, calculi, and abscesses
2. Provides information on size and location of a nonfunctioning kidney
3. Differentiates between bilateral hydronephrosis, polycystic kidneys, and the small, end-stage kidneys of glomerunephritis or polynephritis, solid or cystic lesions

ULTRASOUND

4. Detects the presence of peritoneal fluid
5. Identifies the spread of cancerous conditions from the kidney into the renal vein or inferior vena cava

Nursing Care:

Before Test: Explain the test procedure and the purpose of the test. Assess the client's knowledge of the test. Instruct the client that there will be no discomfort. Assist client in removing clothing. Provide for privacy. Instruct client to not smoke for 30 min prior to test. Instruct client to fast for 12 hr prior to test.
During Test: Adhere to standard precautions. Assist the technician in positioning of client.
After Test: Encourage client to verbalize fears in terms of test results.

Interfering Factors: Inability of client to remain still; incorrect placement of transducer; obesity; retained barium

Nursing Considerations:

Pediatric: Infants and children will need assistance in remaining still during the ultrasound and age-appropriate comfort measures following the test. The kidney scan is often used to monitor renal development in children with hydronephrosis or vesicoureteral reflux (note: a kidney scan is preferable to an IV pyelogram).
Gerontology: The older person may find it difficult to maintain positions when required to do so for lengthy periods of time during the ultrasound.
Rural: Advisable to arrange for transportation home after recovering from kidney scan.

Listing of Related Tests: Renal arteriogram; renal venogram; intravenous pyelogram (IVP)

⟦WEBLINKS ⟧   ▤▨

http://adam.excite.com

Obstetric Sonogram
(ahb-*STET*-rik *SAHN*-uh-graem)
(obstetric ultrasound; ultrasonography)

15-30 min.

Type of Test: Ultrasound

Body Systems and Functions: Reproductive system

Normal Findings: Normal fetal anatomy, position, size, and movement; normal placenta size and position

Test Results Time Frame: Immediate

Test Description: An obstetric sonogram uses high-frequency sound waves that are emitted from a transducer and the ultrasound beams scan the fetus and placenta in thin slices. Ultrasonography creates an oscilloscopic image from the echoes of high-frequency sound waves that passes over this system. The images are reflected back to the same transducer and then are revealed on the monitor screen as a picture. Transabdominal echographic examination of the

ULTRASOUND

pregnant uterus is helpful in determining progress of pregnancy as well as identifying some abnormalities related to the pregnancy. In the first trimester, the scan may be done transvaginally.

CLINICAL ALERT:
If client experiences shortness of breath or drop of blood pressure during the test, it may be necessary to raise the head of the examining table or bed or have client turn onto her side.

Consent Form: Required

List of Equipment: Ultrasonography equipment

Test Procedure:

Transabdominal scan:
1. Place the client on her back with abdomen exposed for transabdominal scan. The client should have a full bladder. *Improves visualization of the uterus and contents.*
2. Apply a gel or lotion to the skin. *Prevents interference of sound and improves scan picture.*
3. The transducer is moved slowly over the abdomen and the picture is visible on the monitor. "Freeze-frames" are produced for the client records. *Ensures continued evaluation of client.*

Transvaginal scan:
1. The perineal area is exposed once insertion of the transducer is imminent. *Allows accurate results.*
2. Apply a gel or lotion to the transducer before it is inserted into the vagina. *Prevents interference of sound and improves scan picture.*
3. Images are obtained of the uterine area. *Ensures continued evaluation of client.*

Clinical Implications and Indications:

1. Confirms pregnancy and abnormal pregnancies (e.g., tubal pregnancy, ectopic pregnancy)
2. Determines the age of the fetus, the rate of fetal growth, and fetal viability
3. Diagnoses congenital fetal abnormalities (18–20 weeks) and the presence of multiple fetus
4. Diagnoses tumors of the female reproductive system and differentiates from normal pregnancy
5. Diagnoses placental abnormalities as well as normal positioning of placenta
6. Identifies pool of amniotic fluid immediately prior to amniocentesis and excessive or decreased amounts of amniotic fluid

Nursing Care:

Before Test: Explain the test procedure and the purpose of the test. Assess the client's knowledge of the test. Inform client that this test does not involve ionizing radiation so both she and her baby will not be exposed as with an x-ray. Ensure that client is suitably attired for procedure after checking on whether a transabdominal or transvaginal scan is to be done. Inform client that transducer gel may be cold. Encourage fluids and discourage voiding prior to transabdominal scan (up to 6 glasses of water in the 2 hr prior to scanning).
During Test: Adhere to standard precautions.

ULTRASOUND

After Test: Remove transducer lubricant from client's abdomen and provide immediate access to bathroom to urinate. In the case of transvaginal scanning, provide opportunity for client to clean excess lubricant from the perineal area.

Contraindications: Latex allergy (for transvaginal scans if transducer cover is made of latex)

Interfering Factors: Inconsistent contact of transducer with skin; inadequate lubricant; posterior positioning of the placenta; empty bladder

Nursing Considerations:
Pregnancy: Emotional support and continued explanations of test procedures are necessary during the obstetric sonogram. Providing objective communication can calm client during this potentially stressful time.
Rural: Advisable to arrange for transportation home after recovering from procedure (note: potentially necessary for the emotional implications after the obstetric sonogram).

Listing of Related Tests: Fetal echocardiograph; pelvic gynecological sonogram; three-dimensional ultrasound

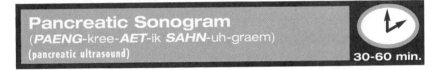

WEBLINKS

www.ob-ultrasound.net

Pancreatic Sonogram
(*PAENG*-kree-*AET*-ik *SAHN*-uh-graem)
(pancreatic ultrasound)

30-60 min.

Type of Test: Ultrasound

Body Systems and Functions: Endocrine/exocrine system

Normal Findings: Normal size and shape of pancreas and surrounding structures

Test Results Time Frame: Within 3 days

Test Description: Pancreatic sonogram is an ultrasound of the pancreas and surrounding anatomy. The pancreas, biliary tree, and gallbladder should all be visible during sonogram. The pancreas is both an exocrine and endocrine organ that is located behind the stomach in front of the first and second lumbar vertebrae. The pancreas is responsible for: secreting glucagon and insulin and the pancreatic juices that contribute to the digestion of all foods in the small intestine. The sonogram can detect abnormalities within the pancreas. Doppler ultrasonography is a noninvasive test that uses ultrasound waves to identify occlusions of the veins or arteries. Ultrasound waves are transmitted and received from the transducer while it is placed over the circulatory system locations. The returning echoes are amplified and images are recorded on a video and strip recorder.

Consent Form: Required

ULTRASOUND

List of Equipment: Ultrasound equipment

Test Procedure:
1. Place client in supine position, expose abdomen, and drape. *Allows privacy.*
2. The technician lubricates the abdominal surface with acoustic gel. *Allows maximum penetration of ultrasound.*
3. The technician positions a hand-held transducer over various regions of the area to image the pancreas and surrounding area. The client may be instructed to hold their breath at certain points during imaging. *Ensures accurate results.*
4. The images are visible on the monitor and recorded on film.
5. Sincalide may be injected and further ultrasound images recorded. *Stimulates gallbladder contraction.*

Clinical Implications and Indications:
1. Evaluates pancreas size and shape
2. Identifies presence of neoplasm, cystic lesions, or pseudocyst
3. Diagnoses and monitors pancreatitis

Nursing Care:
Before Test: Explain the test procedure and the purpose of the test. Assess the client's knowledge of the test. Instruct the client that there will be no discomfort. Assist client in removing clothing. Provide for privacy. Instruct client to not smoke for 30 min prior to test. Ensure client has remained NPO for the requested time (e.g., usually midnight the night before the test or a total of 8–12 hr).
During Test: Adhere to standard precautions. Assist the technician in positioning of client. Inform the client that they may experience discomfort/pressure when the transducer is moved across the abdomen. Instruct client that if sincalide is injected during the procedure, they may experience: abdominal cramping, spasm of the anus or bladder, nausea, dizziness, sweating, and flushing.
After Test: Encourage client to verbalize fears in terms of test results. Instruct client that normal diet can be resumed.

Interfering Factors: Inability of client to remain still; incorrect placement of transducer; barium studies within the last 24–48 hr; open wound or incision overlying ultrasound site; gas in bowel; dehydration; failure to remain NPO for requested time prior to test; obesity

Nursing Considerations:
Pediatric: Infants and children will need assistance in remaining still during the ultrasound and age-appropriate comfort measures following the test.

Listing of Related Tests: CT; cytological evaluation of aspirated fluid from cysts

| WEBLINKS   ▤ ☒ |

http://www.entnet.org

ULTRASOUND

Pelvic Sonogram
(*PEL*-vik *SAHN*-uh-graem)
(lower abdominal ultrasound; pelvis ultrasound; gynecological/
obstetrical sonogram)

30-60 min.

Type of Test: Ultrasound

Body Systems and Functions: Reproductive system

Normal Findings: Normal pelvic organs; normal fetal and placental anatomy, size, and position; normal fetal movement

Test Results Time Frame: Immediate (for obstetrical) if health care provider is present; within 3 days for nonobstetrical

Test Description: A pelvic sonogram, or ultrasound, is generated by bouncing sound waves off internal organs. High-frequency sound waves are emitted from a transducer, and the ultrasound beams scan the area in thin slices that are reflected back to the same transducer. The images then appear in real time on a monitor and freeze-frames can be recorded. The procedure can be performed transabdominally but also may be done transvaginally or transrectally. Frequently used for assessment of obstetrical status and related conditions, this test can also be used for assessment of pelvic abnormalities of both sexes.

CLINICAL ALERT:
Assess for latex allergy in transvaginal or rectal scans if the transducer cover is made of latex.

Consent Form: Required

List of Equipment: Ultrasound equipment

Test Procedure:
1. Instruct the client to drink the required amount of fluid in the 1–2 hr prior to the test. *A full bladder pushes the bowel out of the way of ultrasound waves and also acts as a conductor to reach deeper pelvic organs.*
2. Place client in best position for sonography. *Allows best visualization: supine for transabdominal, lithotomy for transvaginal, and side lying for transrectal.*
3. Expose abdomen, and drape. *Allows privacy.*
4. The technician lubricates the abdominal surface with acoustic gel. *Allows maximum penetration of ultrasound.*
5. The technician positions a transducer over various regions of the abdomen. Then the transducer is moved slowly over the abdomen, and the images are visible on the monitor and can be recorded for future reference. For transvaginal or transrectal sonography, a protective cover is placed over a special probe transducer, lubricated, and inserted. Images are then recorded.

Clinical Implications and Indications:
1. Confirms pregnancy (around 7 weeks) and identifies multiple pregnancies
2. Determines age of fetus, rate of fetal growth, fetal viability, and fetal abnormalities

ULTRASOUND

3. Diagnoses tubal or ectopic pregnancies, placental abnormalities, and placental positioning
4. Identifies excessive or decreased amounts of amniotic fluid as well as location for amniocentesis
5. Diagnoses tumor of female reproductive system; differentiates from normal pregnancy
6. Determines cause of persistent vaginal bleeding, cramping, or lack of menstruation
7. Determines cause of hematuria or difficulty voiding
8. Differentiates between presence of cyst, tumor, or abscess of the pelvic area
9. Diagnoses abnormalities of the prostate gland, vas deferens, or bladder

Nursing Care:

Before Test: Explain the test procedure and the purpose of the test. Assess the client's knowledge of the test. Instruct the client that there will be no discomfort. Assist client in removing clothing. Provide for privacy. Instruct client to not smoke for 30 min prior to test. Remind client that this process does not involve ionizing radiation, and therefore the baby and mother will not be exposed to radiation. For transabdominal, inform client that gel will feel cool and ensure that the appropriate amount of fluid has been taken (up to 6 glasses of water in the 2 hr prior to scanning). Discourage voiding prior to transabdominal sonography.

During Test: Adhere to standard precautions. Assist the technician in positioning of client.

After Test: Encourage client to verbalize fears in terms of test results. Remove transducer lubricant from client's abdomen and provide immediate access for urination and, in the case of transvaginal or rectal sonography, to remove excess lubricant from the perineal area.

Contraindications: Latex allergy (for transvaginal or rectal scans, if transducer cover is made of latex); acute pelvic infection or inflammatory disease (contraindicated due to pain)

Interfering Factors: Inability of client to remain still; incorrect placement of transducer; inadequate lubricant; posterior positioning of the placenta; empty or overdistended bladder; gas or fluid in bowel; barium studies within 2 days prior to sonogram; obesity; pain; metal surgical clips or IUD in place; posthysterectomy changes may mimic recurrent mass.

Nursing Considerations:

Pregnancy: If shortness of breath or a drop in blood pressure is experienced, raise the head of the examining table or have pregnant client turn on side.

Listing of Related Tests: MRI for nonobstetrical purposes; fetal echocardiograph; three-dimensional ultrasound

WEBLINKS

www.radiologyresource.org

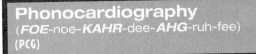

Phonocardiography
(*FOE*-noe-*KAHR*-dee-*AHG*-ruh-fee)
(PCG)

30 min.

Type of Test: Ultrasound

Body Systems and Functions: Cardiovascular system

Normal Findings: Normal heart sounds

Test Results Time Frame: Within 1–2 days

Test Description: Phonocardiography uses one or more microphones that are strapped to the client's chest and records heart sounds externally. Impulses generated from these sounds are recorded on graph paper while ECG tracings are done at the same time. Selective filtering is required to accurately identify heart sounds, clicks, and murmurs. Other external recording techniques such as pulse tracings and echocardiography are usually performed in conjunction with this test. Phonocardiography is now most frequently used as an educational or research measurement tool since its clinical value is limited by the considerable expertise required by the clinician performing and interpreting the test.

Consent Form: May be required

Test Procedure:
1. Place client in supine position, expose thoracic area, and drape. *Allows privacy.*
2. Client lies supine in a quiet room. *Limits noise interference on recording.*
3. The technician lubricates the thoracic surface with acoustic gel. *Allows maximum penetration of ultrasound.*
4. Microphones with selected filters are strapped to the client's chest in the second right intercostal space, at the left lower sternal border, and at the cardiac apex. Four limb ECG leads are applied. *Simultaneous recordings of the ECG and phoncardiograph are taken for comparative purposes.*
5. Other positions may be requested of the client and adjustments made in position of microphones to gather all data for phonocardiography and pulse tracings.
6. Directions will be given to the client to clench fists *(enhances murmurs),* to breathe in and out, or to hold breath.

Clinical Implications and Indications:
1. Locates and times abnormal heart sounds (particularly valvular dysfunctions)
2. Evaluates left-ventricular function
3. Diagnostic instrument often used for educational or research purposes

Nursing Care:
Before Test: Explain the test procedure and the purpose of the test. Assess the client's knowledge of the test. Instruct the client that there will be no discomfort. Assist client in removing clothing. Provide for privacy. Instruct client to not smoke for 30 min prior to test. Explain that the test requires restriction of movement and application of microphones by straps across the chest. Clients with hairy chests may be shaved in areas where microphones will be placed.

ULTRASOUND

During Test: Adhere to standard precautions. Instruct client to remain still in two or more positions. At specific points during the test, instruct client to clench their fists, breathe in and out, and hold their breath. Assist the technician in positioning of client.

After Test: ECG electrodes are removed and skin is cleansed of application gel.

Interfering Factors: Inability to remain still; incorrect placement of transducer; obesity; background noise

Nursing Considerations:

Pediatric: Infants and children will need assistance in remaining still during the ultrasound and age-appropriate comfort measures following the test. While phonocardiography can be a valuable tool in teaching auscultation, the length and restrictions of the test make it impractical for use in teaching infant and child auscultatory sounds.

Listing of Related Tests: ECG; echocardiograph

| WEBLINKS |

www.healthgate.com

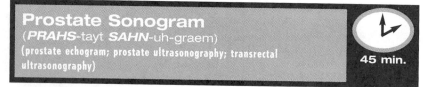

Prostate Sonogram
(*PRAHS*-tayt *SAHN*-uh-graem)
(prostate echogram; prostate ultrasonography; transrectal ultrasonography)

45 min.

Type of Test: Ultrasound

Body Systems and Functions: Reproductive system

Normal Findings: Normal size, shape, and structure of prostate gland with no lumps or narrowing of ureteral passage

Test Results Time Frame: Within 24 hr

Test Description: A prostate sonogram is a test that uses the echo from high-frequency waves as they are reflected off the prostate and surrounding tissues to create an oscilloscope picture. The size and consistency of the prostate tissue can be evaluated as well as a more complete visualization of the tumors. Stricture of the urethra can be detected. The transurethral route is rarely done because the transrectal approach is proven to have far fewer risks but also to be highly accurate. However, a prostate sonogram is not highly accurate in detecting cancers less than 5 mm, those that are well differentiated, and those located in the transition zone. One of the greatest uses for prostate sonography is guiding needle biopsies.

Consent Form: Required

List of Equipment: Transrectal sonogram is done in an examining room with specialized equipment (e.g., ultrasonic gel, sonogram probe).

ULTRASOUND

Test Procedure:

1. Position the client for the transrectal approach on the left side with the knees pulled up toward the chest. *Provides a clear pathway for inserting the sonogram probe.*
2. A digital rectal examination (DRE) is done first. *Provides landmarks and position of nodule or lumps.*
3. The scope is gently introduced into the rectum and a condom covering the end of the scope is enlarged by injecting water into it. *The echo waves move through water with better visualization and less distortion on the screen.*
4. The scope is gently manipulated to get pictures of the prostate.

Clinical Implications and Indications:

1. Diagnoses prostate cancer, prostate abscesses, and perirectal abscesses
2. Identifies the stages of prostate cancer
3. Guides tissue biopsy and radiation seed implantation
4. Evaluates response of tumor to therapy
5. Evaluates the etiology of voiding difficulties

Nursing Care:

Before Test: Explain the test procedure and the purpose of the test. Assess the client's knowledge of the test. There are no food or fluid restrictions. Test should be performed before GI barium studies. A sodium phosphate or biscodyl suppository is usually ordered and can be administered by the client before coming to the procedure. Inform the client that the procedure is uncomfortable because of the pressure of the scope and the enlarged condom.

During Test: Adhere to standard precautions. Assist the technician in positioning of client.

After Test: Encourage client to verbalize fears in terms of test results; provide hygiene cleansing by removing gel from rectum.

Potential Complications: Transurethral route: infection, bleeding. Transrectal route: infection.

Contraindications: Transurethral: bleeding disorder

Interfering Factors: Inability to remain still; incorrect placement of transducer; feces or barium in the rectum

Nursing Considerations:

Pediatric: Infants and children will need assistance in remaining still during the ultrasound and age-appropriate comfort measures following the test.
Gerontology: The older person may find it difficult to maintain positions when required to do so for lengthy periods of time during the ultrasound.
Rural: Advisable to arrange for transportation home after recovering from procedure.

Listing of Related Tests: Prostate biopsy; prostate-specific antigen

ULTRASOUND

| WEBLINKS |

www.cancer.org

Retroperitoneal Ultrasonography
(*RET*-roe-*PAYR*-uh-tuh-*NEE*-:l *UHL*-truh-SAH-*NAHG*-ruh-fee)

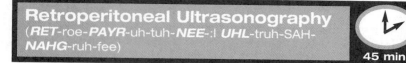

45 min.

Type of Test: Ultrasound

Body Systems and Functions: Lymphatic system

Normal Findings: Retroperitoneal and intrapelvic nodes are not visible or are less than 1.5 cm in diameter.

Test Results Time Frame: 24–48 hr

Test Description: Retroperitoneal ultrasonography is a test to evaluate organ size and pathological states, such as lymhoma and metastatic spread of cancer. Ultrasonography uses high-frequency sound waves transmitted into the abdominal cavity. The waves create echoes that vary with tissue density (solid vs. cystic). The echoes bounce back to a transducer, which gives a pictorial representation of the tissue under study. Retroperitoneal ultrasonography is the preferred method of diagnostics because this area of the body is inaccessible for conventional radiography in the diagnosis of lymphadenopathy. Doppler ultrasound may be used in conjunction to assess organ size, shape, and position. Retroperitoneal ultrasound assesses hepatobiliary, pancreatic, and renal organ size, cysts, tumors, masses, and calculi.

Consent Form: Not required

List of Equipment: Ultrasound equipment

Test Procedure:
1. Position client in supine position.
2. The technician lubricates the chest surface with acoustic gel. *Allows maximum penetration of ultrasound.*
3. The technician positions a transducer over various regions of the areas being visualized.
4. Client takes a deep breath and holds it. *Assists in visualizing organs.*

Clinical Implications and Indications:
1. Detects hydronephrosis
2. Diagnoses and locates renal cysts, tumors, or calculi
3. Evaluates the status following renal transplant
4. Guides antegrade pyelography biopsy, aspiration, or nephrostomy tube insertion
5. Provides an alternative to renal dye imaging tests for clients with allergy response to radiographic dye

Nursing Care:
Before Test: Explain the test procedure and the purpose of the test. Assess the client's knowledge of the test. Instruct the client that there will be no discomfort. Client may need to fast for 8–12 hr prior to the test so that gas in the bowel does not obscure the images.
During Test: Adhere to standard precautions.

ULTRASOUND

After Test: No special posttest instructions; client may resume usual activities and diet.

Interfering Factors: Barium has an adverse effect on quality of abdominal studies so barium studies should be booked after a sonogram; inability of client to remain still during procedure; incorrect placement of the transducer

Nursing Considerations:
Pediatric: Infants and children will need assistance in remaining still during the ultrasound and age-appropriate comfort measures following the test.

‖ⅦEBLINKS ⟍   ▤ ⊠

www.entnet.org

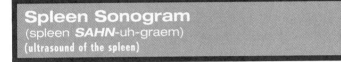

Spleen Sonogram
(spleen *SAHN*-uh-graem)
(ultrasound of the spleen)

30 min.

Type of Test: Ultrasound

Body Systems and Functions: Lymphatic system

Normal Findings: Normal size, structure, and position of the spleen and surrounding organs

Test Results Time Frame: Within 24 hr

Test Description: A spleen sonogram involves an ultrasound probe (transducer) that is moved over the surface of the skin in the vicinity of the spleen. Sound waves are transmitted into the body and echo back from the tissues. These returning sound waves are received by the probe and translated into scans or graphs by a computer. The spleen itself is highly vascular and often damaged in abdominal trauma or as a response to tumors or spleen enlargement from various pathologies.

CLINICAL ALERT:
Trauma to the spleen will make the client hypersensitive to the touch and pressure of the ultrasound equipment.

Consent Form: Not required

List of Equipment: Ultrasound equipment; transducer gel

Test Procedure:
1. Advise client to empty his bladder before the test begins. *Allows for an unobstructed view of the spleen area.*
2. The client is placed on a table in the supine position with the arms extended. *Allows for an unobstructed assessment of the abdomen.*
3. Transducer gel is applied to the area directly over the spleen. *Allows for ultrasound beam to penetrate tissues.*
4. The ultrasound probe is moved methodically over the splenic region. *The spleen is "visualized" by the reflected sound waves from several positions.*

ULTRASOUND

5. The computer records the information, and the size, shape, and some content of the spleen can be identified.

Clinical Implications and Indications:
1. Evaluates tissue abnormalities, such as masses, cysts, and edema (splenomegaly).
2. A splenectomy may be indicated following this examination.
3. Evaluates damage to the spleen from abdominal trauma.

Nursing Care:
Before Test: Explain the test procedure and the purpose of the test. Assess the client's knowledge of the test. Note any acute pain as to its type, location, and severity. Administer analgesics before the procedure to increase comfort during the diagnostic testing.
During Test: Adhere to standard precautions.
After Test: Advise the client that the results will be ready in 1–2 days.

Interfering Factors: Obesity can decrease the sensitivity of the examination; inability of client to remain still during the procedure; incorrect placement of transducer

Nursing Considerations:
Rural: Damage to the spleen in rural settings makes speed a necessity in the transport of the client, due to the potential of hemorrhagic shock and the ensuing crisis.

Listing of Related Tests: CT of spleen; MRI of spleen

WEBLINKS	

http://harvard.edu

Thyroid/Parathyroid Ultrasonography
(*THIY*-royd *PAYR*-uh-*THIY*-royd *UHL*-truh-sah-*NAHG*-ruh-fee)
(thyroid echogram; thyroid sonogram)

30 min.

Type of Test: Ultrasound

Body Systems and Functions: Endocrine system

Normal Findings: Homogeneous structure of thyroid and parathyroid

Test Results Time Frame: Immmediate (note: written report within 24 hr)

Test Description: Thyroid/parathyroid ultrasonography is a noninvasive test that uses ultrasound waves to examine the thyroid/parathyroid position and size. The thyroid/parathyroid ultrasonography helps to determine size of the thyroid and parathyroid glands, detect tumors and cysts, and reveal depth of any thyroid nodules. It is also used to estimate thyroid weight, which is useful in

ULTRASOUND

monitoring treatment for Graves' disease. The thyroid is an endocrine gland located in the anterior neck region and partially surrounds the thyroid cartilage and upper rings of the trachea. The primary action of the thyroid gland is to control the basal metabolic rate. The thyroid gland enlarges in hyperthyroidism (goiter), and it may be removed surgically. In addition, a hypothyroid state may exist (e.g., after a thyroidectomy), and the therapy is to administer a synthetic form of thyroid hormones (e.g., synthroid). The four parathyroid glands are located in pairs on each side of the thyroid gland and among other properties are largely responsible for the balance of calcium and phosphorous metabolism.

Consent Form: Not required

List of Equipment: Ultrasound equipment

Test Procedure:
1. Place client in supine position with neck exposed. *Position enhances ability to obtain accurate ultrasound images.*
2. A pillow may be placed under the client's shoulder. *Allows better contact of ultrasound transducer and enhances client comfort.*
3. The technician lubricates the thyroid surface with acoustic gel. *Allows maximum penetration of ultrasound.*
4. The technician positions a transducer over various regions of the neck.

Clinical Implications and Indications:
1. Evaluates cystic or solid echo patterns.
2. Small nodules (<1 cm) may be nondetectable; lesions larger than 4 cm may give mixed results, making diagnosis difficult.
3. Detects enlarged thyroid or parathyroid glands.

Nursing Care:
Before Test: Explain the test procedure and the purpose of the test. Assess the client's knowledge of the test. Instruct the client that there will be no discomfort. Assist client in removing clothing. Provide for privacy. Instruct client to not smoke for 30 min prior to test.
During Test: Adhere to standard precautions. Assist the technician in positioning of client.
After Test: Encourage client to verbalize fears in terms of test results. Ensure the site is cleaned. Monitor for signs of thyroid disease.

Interfering Factors: Inability of client to remain still; incorrect placement of transducer

Nursing Considerations:
Pediatric: Infants and children will need assistance in remaining still during the ultrasound and age-appropriate comfort measures following the test.
Gerontology: The older person may find it difficult to maintain positions when required to do so for lengthy periods of time during the ultrasound.

ULTRASOUND

WEBLINKS

www.oso.adam.com; http://medline.cos.com

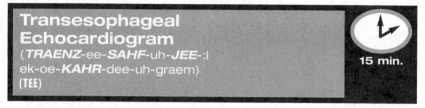

Transesophageal Echocardiogram
(*TRAENZ*-ee-*SAHF*-uh-*JEE*-:l ek-oe-*KAHR*-dee-uh-graem)
(TEE)

15 min.

Type of Test: Ultrasound

Body Systems and Functions: Cardiovascular system

Normal Findings: Normal heart size, wall function, and valve function

Test Results Time Frame: Within 24 hr

Test Description: A transesophageal echocardiogram involves the passage of an ultrasound transducer into the esophagus. The ultrasound produces high-frequency sound waves to induce vibrations to visualize images of heart size, left-ventricular wall motion, valve function, and possible source of emboli. This test is used when posterior heart structures need better visualization than can be supplied by other methods of evaluation.

CLINICAL ALERT:
Confirm resuscitation equipment is present as this procedure may cause respiratory compromise.

Consent Form: Required

List of Equipment: Local anesthetic for throat; sedative; ultrasound transducer; respiratory equipment (for emergencies)

Test Procedure:
1. Confirm correct client and remove dentures. *Correctly identifies the client and the test to be performed and ensures no blockage to the airway.*
2. Place the client in a left lateral decubitus position. *Helps facilitate passage of the scope.*
3. Place client on oxygen if ordered. *Prevents hypoxia during the procedure.*
4. Administer local anesthetic onto the pharynx and tongue and into nose. *Helps facilitate passage of the scope.*
5. Over the next 5–20 min the scope is gently withdrawn and images are viewed/recorded. *Detects structural abnormalities.*

Clinical Implications and Indications:
1. Detects any irregularity in heart size, wall function, and valve function
2. Examines prosthetic heart valves
3. Detects mitral valve regurgitation
4. Diagnoses cardiac tumors and masses
5. Detects congenital heart disorders of the adult
6. Determines aortic dissection site and extent

Nursing Care:
Before Test: Explain the test procedure and the purpose of the test. Assess the client's knowledge of the test. Instruct client to be NPO 6 hr before the proce-

ULTRASOUND

dure. Instruct client that a sedative will be given and the throat will receive a local anesthetic.

During Test: Adhere to standard precautions. Monitor client during procedure (e.g., vital signs, oxygen saturation, and need for suctioning). Reassure client throughout the procedure to reduce anxiety.

After Test: Assess for gag reflex as client will not be able to eat or drink until after the gag reflex returns.

Potential Complications: Aspiration; dysrhythmias; esophageal perforation; hemorrhage; hypoxia

Contraindications: Dysphagia; esophageal disorders; radiation therapy to chest wall

Nursing Considerations:

Pediatric: Sedation or anesthesia is recommended for infants and children. Place the infant or child on a blanket for comfort. After postprocedure monitoring is completed and per health care provider's order, the pediatric client is discharged with an adult who is given instructions.

Gerontology: The older person may find it difficult to maintain positions when required to do so for lengthy periods of time during the transesophageal echocardiogram.

Rural: Advisable to arrange for transportation home after recovering from transesophageal echocardiogram.

WEBLINKS

www.med.umich.edu; www.heartsite.com

ULTRASOUND

15

Urine Studies

EXAMINATION OF URINE

Urine tests are an important and useful diagnostic tool because they are easily obtained and inexpensive. Urine provides important information about a number of physiologic processes, including renal disease, diabetes mellitus, hydration status, and some liver diseases. Most people will have a routine urine examination upon admission to a hospital, and many outpatient settings do routine analyses as well.

PHYSIOLOGY OF URINE FORMATION

Blood is filtered by the kidneys, producing urine to rid the body of wastes and to regulate fluid and electrolyte balance. The normal adult produces between 1.0 to 1.5 liters of urine daily. Enormous amounts of fluids pass through the kidneys every day, as about a thousand liters of blood need to pass through the kidneys to produce one liter of urine.

The nephron is the primary unit of the kidney that produces urine, and each kidney has about one million nephrons. The nephron is composed of the glomerular capsule, the proximal convoluted tubule, the loop of Henle, and the distal convoluted tubule, which empties into a collecting tubule. Every minute about 125 mL of blood is filtered by the glomeruli in an adult male, slightly less in an adult female. The nephrons filter the blood of electrolytes, glucose, water, and small proteins, most of which is reabsorbed in the proximal tubule. Urine in a healthy person contains 96% water and 4% solutes, primarily urea and sodium chloride.

METHODS OF OBTAINING URINE SPECIMENS

Despite the ease of urine collection, many problems in the handling of specimens occur which will provide inaccurate results. Problems can occur with the collection process, the handling of the urine specimen, or with urine testing. Most urine tests require a minimum of 10 cc of urine. Urine is collected through several methods: catheterization, clean-catch, first morning, and pediatric collection.

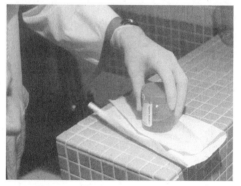

Urine specimen

Catheter Collection Procedure

Catheterized specimens are excellent because they are the least likely to be contaminated by bacteria from the perineum. Their cost and inconvenience, however, make them less useful for routine analysis. When a client is catheterized only to obtain a urine specimen, sterile catherization technique is used and the catheter is removed immediately.

When the client has an indwelling catheter, the specimen is obtained from the specimen port of the catheter tubing. Urine is never collected from the collection bag as it has been sitting at room temperature.

Random Specimen Procedure

Random specimens can be collected when sterile urine is not required, for example, to do an office pregnancy test. The specimen can be collected in any clean container, but should not be contaminated with feces or toilet paper. If the woman has any vaginal bleeding, it should be noted on the collection slip.

Clean-Catch Procedure

Clean-catch urine specimens are collected in a sterile specimen cup or container. Instruct a woman to clean the perineum well before voiding. Tell her to void a small amount into the toilet, then stop. Next start the urine stream again, directing it into the sterile container. Caution her not to place the container onto the perineal skin or to touch the inside of the container with her fingers.

A specimen that contains stool, vaginal discharge, or menstrual blood cannot be used. Men follow the same instructions, but cleanse the outside of the penis before starting the urine stream.

Timed Specimens

Explain to the patient the amount of time that urine will be collected. No urine should be discarded at any time during the collection as it will invalidate the test. Usually the first void is discarded, than all urine is collected into a clean container for the appropriate time, including the last void.

Pediatric Procedure

A number of pediatric collection devices are on the market. Taking urine from a soaked diaper is never an appropriate method of collecting a specimen, since contamination is almost assured.

HANDLING OF URINE SPECIMENS

Urine specimens must be examined within two hours of collection to avoid bacterial contamination. Bacteria that are present within the urine at collection will convert urea to ammonia, giving a false alkaline reading. The alkalinity, in turn, leads to breakdown of casts and proteins. To avoid these problems, urine should be immediately refrigerated if it cannot be analyzed within a two-hour period.

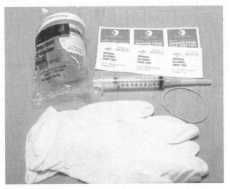

Equipment for obtaining a sterile urine specimen fram an indwelling catheter.

URINE

Examination of Urine by the Nurse

Urine reagent strips (dipsticks)

Reagent strips are used to measure the presence of substances in the urine, including glucose, ketones, proteins, blood, and urea. Instructions are specific to each container, but in general protect strips from light. Timing is crucial for the accurate interpretation of results, and some strips will have several different times at which the strips should be read.

Pregnancy testing

Pregnancy tests vary by manufacture, but most involve adding a few drops of urine to a test strip or stick. Concentrated urine is helpful for detecting early pregnancy, and women are encouraged to use the urine first voided in the morning.

Examination of the Urine by the Laboratory

As the following tests in this chapter demonstrate, laboratory examination of urine provides information about many disease processes and bodily systems. The nurse's role in these studies is to provide appropriate collection and handling of the specimen before it reaches the laboratory.

11-Deoxycortisol
(dee-*AHK*-see-*KOER*-tuh-sahl)
(metyrapone stimulation tests)

72 hr.

Type of Test: Urine; blood

Body Systems and Functions: Metabolic system

Normal Findings: Plasma 11-deoxycortisol elevation <210 mmol/L at 4 hr after the last dose of metyrapone when using 24-hr urine collection; normal response to metyrapone

Test Results Time Frame: Within 5 days

Test Description: 11-Deoxycortisol testing measures deoxycortisol, which is a substance in the development of cortisol. Metyrapone blocks the conversion of II-deoxycortisol to cortisol by 11-beta-hydroxylase, which is the last step in the biosynthetic pathway from cholesterol to cortisol. As a result, cortisol synthesis and secretion fall markedly after metyrapone, and 11-deoxycortisol accumulates in the plasma. 11-Deoxycortisol is essentially devoid of glucocorticoid bioactivity and does not inhibit ACTH secretion. Thus, the lower plasma cortisol concentration in normal individuals leads sequentially to increases in ACTH secretion, adrenal steroidogenesis, and the release of cortisol precursors, especially 11-deoxycortisol, the substrate of 11-beta-hydroxylase. The level of 11-deoxycortisol can be measured either in blood by protein-binding radioassay or radioimmunoassay or in urine as a 17-hydroxycorticosteroid metabolite. The metyrapone test can be performed as an overnight test or as a 2- or 3-day test, which is the standard.

CLINICAL ALERT:
This test reduces cortisol production and as a result should not be performed outside of the hospital in clients suspected of having this disorder.

Consent Form: Not required

List of Equipment: *Blood:* red-top tube or serum separator tube; needle and syringe or vacutainer; alcohol swab. *Urine:* sterile plastic container; ice.

Test Procedure:

Blood:
1. Label the specimen tube and urinary containers. *Correctly identify the client and the tests to be performed.*
2. The 3-day test is begun by obtaining a baseline 24-hr urine collection, usually beginning at 8 AM. Immediately after completing this collection, the client begins taking metyrapone (750 mg every 4 hr for six doses) by mouth with a glass of milk or small snack.
3. Subsequent 24-hr urine specimens (see procedure immediately following) are collected the day of and the day after metyrapone administration for measurement of urine products (17-hydroxycorticosteroids) and creatinine excretion. Plasma 11-deoxycortisol, cortisol, and ACTH can also be measured 4 hr after the last dose of metyrapone.
4. Obtain a 5-mL blood sample.
5. Do not agitate the tube. *Agitation may cause RBC hemolysis.*
6. Send tube and urine collection containers to the laboratory.

24-hr urine:
1. Label the collection container. *Correctly identifies the client and the test to be performed.*
2. Discard the first morning void. Then begin the time of the collection for the next 24 hr, including the void at the end of the 24 hr, and record the last voiding time. *An exact 24-hr count ensures accurate results.*
3. If the client has an indwelling catheter in place, keep the drainage bag on ice and empty the urine into the urine container periodically during the 24-hr period.
4. Keep urine cool during collection. *Higher temperatures alter the results.*
5. If any urine is lost, discard the entire specimen and begin collection again the next day.

Clinical Implications and Indications:
1. Assists in the diagnosis of suspected ACTH deficiency or primary adrenal disease
2. Diagnoses hypercortisolism

Nursing Care:
Before Test: Explain the test procedure and the purpose of the test. Assess the client's knowledge of the test. Instruct client not to discard any urine over the 24-hr time period.
During Test: Adhere to standard precautions. If complications of adrenal insufficiency occur, the client should be infused with physiological saline solution and the test should be discontinued. If any urine is accidentally discarded or contaminated with feces, discard entire specimen and begin test again the following morning.
After Test: Blood: Apply pressure to venipuncture site. Explain that some bruising, discomfort, and swelling may appear at the site and that warm, moist com-

URINE

presses can alleviate this. Monitor for signs of infection. Urine: Document urine quantity, date, and exact hours of collection on requisition.

Potential Complications: Bleeding and bruising at venipuncture site; hypotension, nausea, and vomiting in clients with adrenal insufficiency

Interfering Factors: Oral contraceptives cause false positives; hypothyroidism; hypoglycemia; diabetes mellitus; congestive heart failure; obesity; chronic renal failure; urine contaminated with feces; spillage or inaccurate collection of the 24-hr specimen, including nonrefrigeration or placing on ice; heavy bleeding during menstruation; glucocorticoids

Nursing Considerations:

Pregnancy: Performed only if the benefits outweigh potential complications.
Pediatric: Blood: Infants and children will need assistance in remaining still during the venipuncture and age-appropriate comfort measures following the test. Urine: For collection of 24-hr specimen a collection bag needs to be used for infants and toddlers.

Listing of Related Tests: 17-Hydroxycorticosteroids; plasma ACTH level; hypothalamic and pituitary peptides

WEBLINKS

http://www.niddk.nih.gov

17-Hydroxycorticosteroids
(hiy-*DRAHK*-see-*KOER*-ti-koe-*STER*-oydz)
(17-OHCS)

24 hr.

Type of Test: Urine

Body Systems and Functions: Endocrine system

Normal Findings:

Males	3–10 mg/24 hr
Females	2–6 mg/24 hr
Children to 16 years	2.1–4.1 mg/m^2/24 hr

Test Results Time Frame: Within 24 hr

Test Description: 17-Hydroxycorticosteriods are steroid compounds that are found in urine and are the end product of cortisol secretion by the renal adrenal cortex in response to stress, ACTH, and normal body rhythm. Cortisol is secreted in a diurnal pattern and varies throughout a 24-hr period; therefore, a complete 24-hr urine collection is needed to test cortisol production, adrenocortical function, and pituitary-adrenal activity. Baseline evaluations are done along with a measurement following administration of dexamethasone.

Consent Form: Not required

List of Equipment: Sterile plastic container; ice

Test Procedure:

1. Label the collection container. *Correctly identifies the client and the test to be performed.*

URINE

2. Discard the first morning void. Then begin the time of the collection for the next 24 hr, including the void at the end of the 24 hr, and record the last voiding time. *An exact 24-hr count ensures accurate results.*
3. If the client has an indwelling catheter in place, keep the drainage bag on ice and empty the urine into the urine container periodically during the 24-hr period.
4. Keep urine cool during collection. *Higher temperatures alter the results.*
5. If any urine is lost, discard the entire specimen and begin collection again the next day.

Clinical Implications and Indications:

1. Elevated levels are found with Cushing's disease, Cushing's syndrome, stress, hyperthyroidism, congenital adrenal hyperplasia, and 11-hydroxylase deficiency.
2. Decreased levels are found with Addison's disease, anterior pituitary hypofunction, severe anemia, starvation, congenital adrenal hyperplasia, and 21-hydroxylase deficiency.

Nursing Care:

Before Test: Explain the test procedure and the purpose of the test. Assess the client's knowledge of the test. Instruct client not to discard any urine over the 24-hr time period. Instruct client not to exercise for 24 hr before urine collection.
During Test: Adhere to standard precautions. If any urine is accidentally discarded or contaminated with feces, discard entire specimen and begin test again the following morning.
After Test: Document urine quantity, date, and exact hours of collection on requisition.

Interfering Factors:

Urine contaminated with feces; spillage or inaccurate collection of the 24-hr specimen, including nonrefrigeration or placing on ice; heavy bleeding during menstruation; medications that increase results are ascorbic acid, penicillin, digitalis glycosides, chloralhydrate, corticotropin, diethylstilbestrol, metyrapone, gonadotropin, histamine, betamethasone, chlorthalidone, and cortisone; medications that decrease results are aminoglutethimide, apresoline, medroxyprogesterone, metyrapone, SKF-12185, ethinyl estradiol, norethynodrel, oral contraceptives, printazocine, phenothiazines, chlorpromazine, dexamethasone, levodopa, meperidine, morphine, perphanazine, promazine, propoxyphene, diphenylhydantoin, estrogens, phenobarbital, phenylbutazone, carbon disulfide, MAO inhibitors, salicylates, mitotane, progesterone, and reserpine.

Nursing Considerations:

Pediatric: For collection of 24-hr specimen a collection bag or indwelling catheter needs to be used for infants and toddlers.
Gerontology: Many medications should ideally be withheld for 2 weeks prior to this test, which could have implications for the elderly who regularly take these medications.
Home Care: The home health care provider must be included in the knowledge that the client must not take certain medications for 2 weeks prior to this test.

Listing of Related Tests:

Dexamethasone suppression test; 17-ketogenic steroids; 17-ketosteroids; blood glucose; CBC; serum potassium and sodium; ACTH stimulation test

URINE

WEBLINKS

http://www.niddk.nih.gov

17-Ketosteroids
(*KEE*-toe-*STER*-oydz)
(17-KGS; 17KS)

24 hr.

Type of Test: Urine

Body Systems and Functions: Endocrine system

Normal Findings:

Males:

Under 1 year	<1 mg/day
1–10 years	1 mg/day/year of age
>15 years	9.0–22 mg/day
Adult <70 years	5–23 mg/day
>70 years	3–12 mg/day

Females:

Under 1 year	<1 mg/day
1–10 years	1 mg/day/year of age
>15 years	5.0–15 mg/day
Adult <70 years	3–15 mg/day
>70 years	3–12 mg/day

Test Results Time Frame: Within 24 hr

Test Description: 17-Ketosteroids are a group of metabolites of steroids produced by the adrenal cortex and gonads that appear in the urine. The test is used to detect endocrine disorders, particularly gonadal dysfunction.

Consent Form: Not required

List of Equipment: Sterile plastic container; ice

Test Procedure:

1. Label the collection container. *Correctly identifies the client and the test to be performed.*
2. Discard the first morning void. Then begin the time of the collection for the next 24 hr, including the void at the end of the 24 hr, and record the last voiding time. *An exact 24-hr count ensures accurate results.*
3. If the client has an indwelling catheter in place, keep the drainage bag on ice and empty the urine into the urine container periodically during the 24-hr period.
4. Keep urine cool during collection. *Higher temperatures alter the results.*
5. If any urine is lost, discard the entire specimen and begin collection again the next day.

Clinical Implications and Indications:

1. Elevated levels are found in the early morning and with congenital adrenal hyperplasia, Cushing's disease, Cushing's syndrome, stress, hyperthyroidism, obesity, hirsutism, severe infection, pregnancy, congenital adrenal hyperplasia (note: since the only difference between levels of 17-KGS and 17-OHCS occurs with congenital adrenal hyperplasia, the test can be used to diagnose this disease), and 11-hydroxylase deficiency.

URINE

2. Decreased levels are found with Addison's disease, anterior pituitary hypofunction, severe anemia, starvation, menopause, congenital adrenal hyperplasia, and 21-hydroxylase deficiency.

Nursing Care:

Before Test: Explain the test procedure and the purpose of the test. Assess the client's knowledge of the test. Instruct client not to discard any urine over the 24-hr time period. Levels will rise with stress, so ensure that the client has not undergone significant stress or vigorous physical activity during the collection procedure.

During Test: Adhere to standard precautions. If any urine is accidentally discarded or contaminated with feces, discard entire specimen and begin test again the following morning.

After Test: Document urine quantity, date, and exact hours of collection on requisition.

Interfering Factors: Urine contaminated with feces; spillage or inaccurate collection of the 24-hr specimen including nonrefrigeration or placing on ice; heavy bleeding during menstruation; exercise and stress; pregnancy; medications that alter results are cortisone, metryapone, ampicillin, dexamethasone, and oral contraceptives.

Nursing Considerations:

Pregnancy: Levels rise in the third trimester of pregnancy.
Pediatric: For collection of 24-hr specimen a collection bag or indwelling catheter needs to be used for infants and toddlers.

Listing of Related Tests: 17-Hydroxycorticosteriods; blood glucose; CBC; serum potassium and sodium; ACTH stimulation test; dexamethasone suppression test

WEBLINKS

http://www.ncbi.nlm.nih.gov

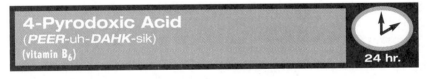

4-Pyrodoxic Acid
(*PEER*-uh-*DAHK*-sik)
(vitamin B$_6$)

24 hr.

Type of Test: Urine

Body Systems and Functions: Miscellaneous system

Normal Findings: 0.5–1.3 mg/day

Test Results Time Frame: Within 24 hr

Test Description: 4-Pyridoxic acid is a major metabolite of vitamin B$_6$. The test is used to measure B$_6$ deficiency. Urine analysis is of limited value in measuring the severity of vitamin B$_6$ deficiency but can give an indication of recent dietary intake.

URINE

Consent Form: Not required

List of Equipment: Sterile plastic container; ice

Test Procedure:
1. Label the collection container. *Correctly identifies the client and the test to be performed.*
2. Discard the first morning void. Then begin the time of the collection for the next 24 hr, including the void at the end of the 24 hr, and record the last voiding time. *An exact 24-hr count ensures accurate results.*
3. If the client has an indwelling catheter in place, keep the drainage bag on ice and empty the urine into the urine container periodically during the 24-hr period.
4. Keep urine cool during collection. *Higher temperatures alter the results.*
5. If any urine is lost, discard the entire specimen and begin collection again the next day.

Clinical Implications and Indications:
1. Decreased levels are found with vitamin B_6 (pyroxidine) deficiency, which can occur with chronic alcoholism, malnutrition, uremia, malabsorption, exposure to hydrazine compounds, normal pregnancies, gestational diabetes, and pellagra.

Nursing Care:
Before Test: Explain the test procedure and the purpose of the test. Assess the client's knowledge of the test. Instruct client not to discard any urine over the 24-hr time period.
During Test: Adhere to standard precautions. If any urine is accidentally discarded or contaminated with feces, discard entire specimen and begin test again the following morning.
After Test: Document urine quantity, date, and exact hours of collection on requisition.

Interfering Factors: Urine contaminated with feces; spillage or inaccurate collection of the 24-hr specimen, including nonrefrigeration or placing on ice; heavy bleeding during menstruation; medications that decrease levels are isoniazid, cycloserine, penicillamine, levodopa, hydralazine, anticonvulsants, and ethanol

Nursing Considerations:
Pediatric: For collection of 24-hr specimen a collection bag or indwelling catheter needs to be used for infants and toddlers.

Listing of Related Tests: Vitamin testing

WEBLINKS

http://alice.ucdavis.edu

URINE

5-Hydroxyindoleacetic Acid
(hiy-*DRAHK*-see-in-*DOEL*-uh-*SEE*-tik)
(5-HIAA)

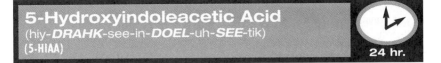

24 hr.

Type of Test: Urine

Body Systems and Functions: Oncology system

Normal Findings: 2–8 mg/24 hr

> **CRITICAL VALUES:**
> Levels of 100 mg/24 hr usually indicate a large carcinoid tumor. Levels could be as high as 1000 mg/24 hr.

Test Results Time Frame: Within 24 hr

Test Description: 5-HIAA is a metabolite of serotonin, which is normally present only in platelets and in argentaffin cells of the intestines. The test is used to detect early carcinoid tumors (argentaffinomas) of the intestines.

Consent Form: Not required

List of Equipment: Sterile plastic container; ice

Test Procedure:
1. Label the collection container. *Correctly identifies the client and the test to be performed.*
2. Discard the first morning void. Then begin the time of the collection for the next 24 hr, including the void at the end of the 24 hr, and record the last voiding time. *An exact 24-hr count ensures accurate results.*
3. If the client has an indwelling catheter in place, keep the drainage bag on ice and empty the urine into the urine container periodically during the 24-hr period.
4. Keep urine cool during collection. *Higher temperatures alter the results.*
5. If any urine is lost, discard the entire specimen and begin collection again the next day.

Clinical Implications and Indications:
1. Elevated levels are found with cancerous argentaffinomas of the intestines. The increase only occurs with 5%–7% of clients with an argentaffinoma.
2. Levels are less elevated with hemorrhage, thrombosis, nontropical sprue, sciatic pain or muscle spasm, oat cell cancer of the bronchus, and bronchial cancerous adenomas.
3. Decreased levels are found with depression, small intestinal resection, mastocytosis, PKU, and Hartnup's disease.

Nursing Care:
Before Test: Explain the test procedure and the purpose of the test. Assess the client's knowledge of the test. Instruct client not to discard any urine over the 24-hr time period. Instruct the client to follow a diet low in serotonin (see Interfering Factors) 4 days before the test and to avoid coffee, tea, and tobacco 3 days before the test.

URINE

During Test: Adhere to standard precautions. If any urine is accidentally discarded or contaminated with feces, discard entire specimen and begin test again the following morning.
After Test: Document urine quantity, date, and exact hours of collection on requisition.

Interfering Factors: Urine contaminated with feces; spillage or inaccurate collection of the 24-hr specimen, including nonrefrigeration or placing on ice; heavy bleeding during menstruation; bananas, plums, pineapples, avocados, eggplants, tomatoes, and walnuts will falsely elevate levels and must be withheld for 4 days before the test; severe gastrointestinal disturbance; diarrhea; medications that increase results are fluorouracil, melphalan, caffeine, nicotine, rauwoldia, reserpine, and phenmetrazine; medications that decrease results are chlorophenylananine, ethanol, imipramine, isocarboxazid, MAO inhibitors, isoniazid, methyldopa, hydrazine derivatives, and streptozotocin.

Nursing Considerations:
Pediatric: For collection of 24-hr specimen a collection bag or indwelling catheter needs to be used for infants and toddlers.
Gerontology: Many medications should ideally be withheld prior to this test, which could have implications for the elderly who regularly take these medications.
Home Care: The home health care provider must be included in the knowledge that the client must not take certain medications and foods prior to this test.

Listing of Related Tests: Vanillylmandelic acid; serotonin

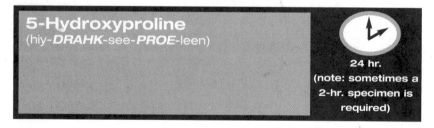

5-Hydroxyproline
(hiy-*DRAHK*-see-*PROE*-leen)

24 hr.
(note: sometimes a 2-hr. specimen is required)

Type of Test: Urine

Body Systems and Functions: Musculoskeletal system

Normal Findings:

2 hr:
Men	0.4–5 mg/2 hr
Women	0.4–2.9 mg/2 hr

24 hr:
Adults (free)	0–2 mg/24 hr
Adults (total)	0.11–0.36 mmol/day

Test Results Time Frame: Within 24 hr

Test Description: 5-Hydroxyproline is an amino acid found in collagen and bone. This test is a reflection of bone reabsorption and an indication of destruction from bone tumors. It is an important measurement for the severity of

Paget's disease but is not primarily the test for the purpose of diagnosis. In adults, hydroxyproline in the urine indicates bone resorption, while alkaline phosphatase in the urine indicates bone formation. Normally, <10% of the hydroxproline is considered free.

CLINICAL ALERT:
Blood samples are preferred for hydroxyproline in the first few months of life.

Consent Form: Not required

List of Equipment: Sterile plastic container; ice

Test Procedure:
1. Label the collection container. *Correctly identifies the client and the test to be performed.*
2. Discard the first morning void. Then begin the time of the collection for the next 24 hr, including the void at the end of the 24 hr, and record the last voiding time. *An exact 24-hr count ensures accurate results.*
3. If the client has an indwelling catheter in place, keep the drainage bag on ice and empty the urine into the urine container periodically during the 24-hr period (note: occasionally, a 2-hr urine specimen is the required amount of urine for this test).
4. Keep urine cool during collection. *Higher temperatures alter the results.*
5. If any urine is lost, discard the entire specimen and begin collection again the next day.

Clinical Implications and Indications:
1. Elevated levels are found with hyperparathyroidism, Paget's disease, Marfan syndrome, Klinefelter's syndrome, osteoporosis, bone tumors, and myeloma.
2. Free hydroxyproline is increased in two hereditary disorders: hydroxyprolinemia and familial iminoglycinuria.

Nursing Care:
Before Test: Explain the test procedure and the purpose of the test. Assess the client's knowledge of the test. Instruct client not to discard any urine over the 24-hr time period. For a 2-hr urine, instruct client to fast from midnight until the collection is done.
During Test: Adhere to standard precautions. If any urine is accidentally discarded or contaminated with feces, discard entire specimen and begin test again the following morning.
After Test: Document urine quantity, date, and exact hours of collection on requisition.

Interfering Factors: Urine contaminated with feces; spillage or inaccurate collection of the 24-hr specimen, including nonrefrigeration or placing on ice; heavy bleeding during menstruation; meat, poultry, fish, and foods containing gelatin falsely elevate levels; medications that increase results are glucocorticoids, aspirin, mithramycin, and calcitonin; ascorbic acid and vitamin D falsely increase levels; skin disorders such as burns and psoriasis may also elevate levels.

Nursing Considerations:
Pediatric: For collection of 24-hr specimen a collection bag or indwelling catheter needs to be used for infants and toddlers.

URINE

Gerontology: *Many foods and some medications should ideally be withheld prior to this test, which could have implications for the elderly who regularly take these medications.*

Home Care: *The home health care provider must be included in the knowledge that their client must not take certain medications and foods prior to this test.*

Listing of Related Tests: Alkaline phosphatase

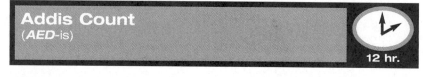

WEBLINKS

http://chorus.rad.mcw.edu

Addis Count
(*AED*-is)

12 hr.

Type of Test: Urine

Body Systems and Functions: Renal/urological system

Normal Findings:

RBCs	<1 million/24 hr
Casts	<100,000/24 hr
WBCs and epithelial cells	<2 million/24 hr

Test Results Time Frame: Within 24 hr

Test Description: The Addis method, or count, for measuring elements in the urine is an older method of quantifying the presence of cells and casts in the urine. Urine is collected for 12 hr, and a numerical count is made of red and white blood cells, epithelial cells, and casts. Laboratory experts believe that the measurement of elements in a single urine sample is as accurate and involves much less time and effort.

Consent Form: Not required

List of Equipment: Sterile plastic container; ice

Test Procedure:

1. Label the collection container. *Correctly identifies the client and the test to be performed.*
2. Discard the first morning void. Then begin the time of the collection for the next 12 hr, including the void at the end of the 12 hr, and record the last voiding time. *An exact 12-hr count ensures accurate results.*
3. If the client has an indwelling catheter in place, keep the drainage bag on ice and empty the urine into the urine container periodically during the 12-hr period.
4. Keep urine cool during collection. *Higher temperatures alter the results.*
5. If any urine is lost, discard the entire specimen and begin collection again the next day.

Clinical Implications and Indications:

1. Cells and casts increase in urine in the presence of renal disease and infection.
2. Evaluates therapeutic interventions for pathology.

URINE

Nursing Care:

Before Test: Explain the test procedure and the purpose of the test. Assess the client's knowledge of the test. Instruct client not to discard any urine over the 12-hr time period.

During Test: Adhere to standard precautions. If any urine is accidentally discarded or contaminated with feces, discard entire specimen and begin test again the following morning.

After Test: Document urine quantity, date, and exact hours of collection on requisition.

Interfering Factors: Urine contaminated with feces; spillage or inaccurate collection of the 12-hr specimen, including nonrefrigeration or placing on ice; heavy bleeding during menstruation; infection

Nursing Considerations:

Pediatric: For collection of 12-hr specimen a collection bag or indwelling catheter needs to be used for infants and toddlers.

WEBLINKS

http://www.creighton.edu

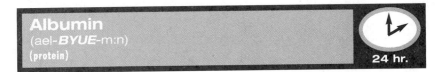

Albumin
(ael-***BYUE***-m:n)
(protein)

24 hr.

Type of Test: Urine

Body Systems and Functions: Renal/urological system

Normal Findings:

Adults	10–140 mg/L in 24 hr
Children	10–100 mg/L in 24 hr

Test Results Time Frame: Within 24 hr

Test Description: Albumin is the smallest protein and the major protein found in blood. The protein, although small, is too large to filter through the renal glomeruli. The presence of albumin in the urine, therefore, is an indicator of renal disease. This test is a quantitative measure of exactly how much albumin is lost in the urine and thereby indicates the extent of kidney damage. Urine albumin can also be used to measure treatment effectiveness for renal damage.

Consent Form: Not required

List of Equipment: Sterile plastic container; ice

Test Procedure:

1. Label the collection container. *Correctly identifies the client and the test to be performed.*
2. Discard the first morning void. Then begin the time of the collection for the next 24 hr, including the void at the end of the 24 hr, and record the last voiding time. *An exact 24-hr count ensures accurate results.*

URINE

3. If the client has an indwelling catheter in place, keep the drainage bag on ice and empty the urine into the urine container periodically during the 24-hr period.
4. Keep urine cool during collection. *Higher temperatures alter the results.*
5. If any urine is lost, discard the entire specimen and begin collection again the next day.

Clinical Implications and Indications:

1. Elevated levels are found with nephritis, glomerulonephritis, polycystic kidneys, kidney tumors, and pyelonephritis.
2. Albumin is a very sensitive indicator of beginning nephropathy for people with diabetes.
3. Nonrenal transient causes of proteinuria are strenuous exercise, fever, CHF, stress, trauma, and seizures.

Nursing Care:

Before Test: Explain the test procedure and the purpose of the test. Assess the client's knowledge of the test. Instruct client not to discard any urine over the 24-hr time period. Teach the client not to undergo strenuous physical activity during the collection procedure. Withhold interfering drugs, if possible, for 48 hr before the test begins.

During Test: Adhere to standard precautions. If any urine is accidentally discarded or contaminated with feces, discard entire specimen and begin test again the following morning.

After Test: Document urine quantity, date, and exact hours of collection on requisition.

Interfering Factors: Urine contaminated with feces; spillage or inaccurate collection of the 24-hr specimen, including nonrefrigeration or placing on ice; heavy bleeding during menstruation; medications that alter results are gallamine, acetaminophen, asparaginase, azathioprine, cyclophosphamide, heroin, niacin, pyrazinamide, thorium dioxide, estrogens, ethinyl estradiol, and dextran.

Nursing Considerations:

Pediatric: For collection of 24-hr specimen a collection bag or indwelling catheter needs to be used for infants and toddlers.

Listing of Related Tests: Urine analysis; total protein

WEBLINKS

http://www.creighton.edu

Aldosterone
(ael-*DAHS*-t:r-oen)

Blood: 5 min.
Urine: 24 hr.

Type of Test: Urine; blood

Body Systems and Functions: Endocrine system

Normal Findings:

Blood:

Women	5–30 ng/dL
Men	6–22 ng/dL

Pediatric:

0–11 months	2–130 ng/dL
1–5 years	2–37 ng/dL
6–9 years	1–24 ng/dL
10–17 years	1–32 ng/dL
Urine	>97–222 mmol/day

Test Results Time Frame: Within 48 hr

Test Description: Aldosterone is the most biologically active of the mineralcorticoids. Aldosterone increases sodium reabsorption and potassium excretion by the kidneys and is therefore involved in the regulation of body water, blood pressure, blood volume, electrolyte balance, and pH.

CLINICAL ALERT:
Diuretics, progestins, estrogens, and licorice should be discontinued at least 2 weeks before the test to obtain accurate results.

Consent Form: Not required

List of Equipment: *Blood:* red-top tube or serum separator tube; needle and syringe or vacutainer; alcohol swab. *Urine:* sterile plastic container; ice.

Test Procedure:

Blood:
1. Label the specimen tube. *Correctly identifies the client and the test to be performed.*
2. Obtain a 5-mL blood sample.
3. Do not agitate the tube. *Agitation may cause RBC hemolysis.*
4. Send tube to the laboratory.

Urine:
1. Label the collection container. *Correctly identifies the client and the test to be performed.*
2. Discard the first morning void. Then begin the time of the collection for the next 24 hr, including the void at the end of the 24 hr, and record the last voiding time. *An exact 24-hr count ensures accurate results.*
3. If the client has an indwelling catheter in place, keep the drainage bag on ice and empty the urine into the urine container periodically during the 24-hr period.
4. Keep urine cool during collection. *Higher temperatures alter the results.*
5. If any urine is lost, discard the entire specimen and begin collection again the next day.

Clinical Implications and Indications:
1. Elevated levels are found in primary aldosteronism, which may be caused by an aldosterone-secreting tumor or by hyperplasia of the adrenal cortex of the kidney.

2. Elevated levels are also found in secondary aldosteronism, when aldosterone excretion is elevated, as in salt depletion, potassium loading, large doses of ACTH, liver cirrhosis, dehydration, and postsurgery.
3. Decreased levels are found with Cushing's syndrome, licorice ingestion, or certain medications.

Nursing Care:

Before Test: Explain the test procedure and the purpose of the test. Assess the client's knowledge of the test. Instruct client not to discard any urine over the 24-hr time period. The client must be upright (sitting or standing) for 4 hr prior to the test and have unrestricted salt intake.

During Test: Adhere to standard precautions. If any urine is accidentally discarded or contaminated with feces, discard entire specimen and begin test again the following morning.

After Test: Apply pressure to venipuncture site. Explain that some bruising, discomfort, and swelling may appear at the site and that warm, moist compresses can alleviate this. Monitor for signs of infection. Document urine quantity, date, and exact hours of collection on requisition.

Potential Complications: Bleeding and bruising at venipuncture site

Interfering Factors: Urine contaminated with feces; spillage or inaccurate collection of the 24-hr specimen, including nonrefrigeration or placing on ice; heavy bleeding during menstruation; levels can be increased in pregnancy and by fetal position.

Nursing Considerations:

Pregnancy: Aldosterone levels are elevated 2–3 times higher during pregnancy.
Pediatric: For collection of 24-hr specimen a collection bag or indwelling catheter needs to be used for infants and toddlers.

Listing of Related Tests: Plasma renin; electrolytes; urine-free cortisol; creatinine

WEBLINKS

http://www.ncbi.nlm.nih.gov

Amino Acids
(uh-*MEE*-noe *AE*-sidz)
(phosphoserine; taurine; aspartic acid; hydroxyproline; threonine; serine; asparagine; glutamic acid; glutamine; proline; glycine; alanine; citrulline; 2-aminobutyric; valine; methionine; isoleucine; leucine; tyrosine; phenylananine; homocystine; tryptophan; ornithine; ysine, 1-methylhistidine; histidine; 3-methylhistidine; arginine)

Blood: 5 min.
Urine: 10 min.

URINE

Type of Test: Urine; blood

Body Systems and Functions: Metabolic system

Normal Findings:

Blood:

Phosphoserine	3–7 μmol/L
Taurine	27–168 μmol/L
Aspartic acid	0–24 μmol/L
Hydroxyproline	0-40 μmol/L
Threonine	79–193 μmol/L
Serine	73–167 μmol/L
Asparagine	14–104 μmol/L
Glutamic acid	0–88 μmol/L
Glutamine	415–694 μmol/L
Proline	102–336 μmol/L
Glycine	120–554 μmol/L
Alanine	210–661 μmol/L
Citrulline	12–55 μmol/L
2-Aminobutyric	3–38 μmol/L
Valine	141–317 μmol/L
Methionine	6–40 μmol/L
Isoleucine	36–98 μmol/L
Leucine	75–175 μmol/L
Tyrosine	21–87 μmol/L
Phenylananine	37–88 μmol/L
Homocystine	0 μmol/L
Tryptophan	20–95 μmol/L
Ornithine	30–106 μmol/L
Lysine	83–238 μmol/L
1-Methylhistidine	0–27 μmol/L
Histidine	31–107 μmol/L
3-Methylhistidine	0–4 μmol/L
Arginine	36–145 μmol/L
Urine	Normal laboratory findings vary among laboratory settings.

Test Results Time Frame: Within 2–5 days

Test Description: Amino acid testing is often an initial screen for congenital abnormalities of metabolism. More than 50 abnormalities of amino acids are recognized. Amino acids are one of a large group of organized compounds that are the building blocks of proteins and are the end products of protein digestion or hydrolysis. They are responsible for human metabolism and growth.

Consent Form: Not required

List of Equipment: *Blood:* green-top tube or plasma separator tube; needle and syringe or vacutainer; alcohol swab. *Urine:* sterile plastic container; ice.

URINE

Test Procedure:
Blood:
1. Label the specimen tube. *Correctly identifies the client and the test to be performed.*
2. Obtain a 5-mL blood sample.
3. Gently invert tube several times, but do not agitate the tube. *Mixes the anticoagulant, but agitation may cause RBC hemolysis.*
4. Send tube to the laboratory immediately. *Plasma must be separated within 30 min of blood draw.*
5. Keep specimen cool. *High temperatures alter the results.*

Urine:
1. Label a sterile urine container. *Correctly identifies the client and the test to be performed.*
2. Obtain a clean-catch specimen of urine (note: first morning voiding preferred, at least 10 mL). *Ensures accurate results.*
3. Keep specimen cool. *High temperatures alter the results.*
4. Send specimen to laboratory. Freeze if the specimen cannot go immediately to the laboratory. Boric acid may also be used. *Both freezing and boric acid prevent protein denaturization.*

Clinical Implications and Indications:
1. Total serum amino acids are increased with diabetic ketoacidosis, malabsorption, fructose intolerance brain damage, Reye's syndrome, renal failure, eclampsia, and specific amino acidopathies.
2. Total urine amino acids are increased with viral hepatitis, multiple myeloma, hyperparathyroidism, rickets, osteomalacia, fructose intolerance, galactosemia, cystinosis, Wilson's disease, and Hartnup disease.
3. Total serum amino acids are decreased with adrenocortical hyperfunction, Huntington's chorea, nephritic syndrome, rheumatoid arthritis, Hartnup disease, fever, and malnutrition.

Nursing Care:
Before Test: Assess the client's knowledge of the test. Explain the test procedure and the purpose of the test.
During Test: Adhere to standard precautions. If any urine is accidentally discarded or contaminated with feces, discard entire specimen and begin test again.
After Test: Blood: Apply pressure to venipuncture site. Explain that some bruising, discomfort, and swelling may appear at the site and that warm, moist compresses can alleviate this. Monitor for signs of infection. Urine: Document urine quantity, date, and exact hours of collection on requisition.

Potential Complications: Bleeding and bruising at venipuncture site

Interfering Factors: Wide variety of medications alter results (note: consult medication text for individual medications); diet can increase or decrease amino acids; urine contaminated with feces; not placing on ice; heavy bleeding during menstruation

Nursing Considerations:
Pediatric: Blood: *Infants and children will need assistance in remaining still during the venipuncture and age-appropriate comfort measures following the test.*
Urine: A collection bag or insertion of a straight catheter is likely needed for infants and toddlers.

URINE

| WEBLINKS |

http://alice.ucdavis.edu

Arylsulfate A
(*AYR*-:l-*SUHL*-fayt)
(ARS A)

24 hr.

Type of Test: Urine

Body Systems and Functions: Immunological system

Normal Findings:

Children	>1 U/L
Men	1.4–19.3 U/L
Women	1.4–11 U/L

Test Results Time Frame: Within 24–48 hr

Test Description: Arylsulfate A is a lysosomal enzyme found in all body cells except mature RBCs. Enzymes are catalysts that enhance reactions without directly participating in them. When the cells and tissues are damaged, enzymes are released. Increased levels of the enzymes are then found in the urine and blood. ARS A is one of the few enzymes that are analyzed in the urine and therefore require a 24-hr urine specimen collection. The main activities of ARS A are found in the liver, pancreas, and kidney.

Consent Form: Not required

List of Equipment: Sterile plastic container; ice

Test Procedure:
1. Label the collection container. *Correctly identifies the client and the test to be performed.*
2. Discard the first morning void. Then begin the time of the collection for the next 24 hr, including the void at the end of the 24 hr, and record the last voiding time. *An exact 24-hr count ensures accurate results.*
3. If the client has an indwelling catheter in place, keep the drainage bag on ice and empty the urine into the urine container periodically during the 24-hr period.
4. Keep urine cool during collection. *Higher temperatures alter the results.*
5. If any urine is lost, discard the entire specimen and begin collection again the next day.

Clinical Implications and Indications:
1. Elevated levels are found with granulocytic leukemia, malignancy of the bladder, colon, or rectum, and a family history of lipid storage diseases.
2. Decreased levels are found with metachromatic leukodystrophy.

Nursing Care:
Before Test: Explain the test procedure and the purpose of the test. Assess the client's knowledge of the test. Instruct client not to discard any urine over the 24-hr time period.
During Test: Adhere to standard precautions. If any urine is accidentally discarded or contaminated with feces, discard entire specimen and begin test again the following morning.
After Test: Document urine quantity, date, and exact hours of collection on requisition.

URINE

Interfering Factors: Urine contaminated with feces; spillage or inaccurate collection of the 24-hr specimen, including nonrefrigeration or placing on ice; abdominal surgery within 1 week of the test, which will falsely elevate levels

Nursing Considerations:
Pediatric: For collection of 24-hr specimen a collection bag needs to be used for infants and toddlers.

Listing of Related Tests: Amylase; lysozyme; leucine aminopeptidase (LAP)

WEBLINKS

http://adam.excite.com

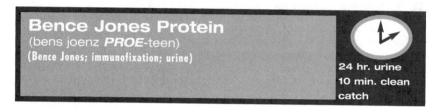

Bence Jones Protein
(bens joenz *PROE*-teen)
(Bence Jones; immunofixation; urine)

24 hr. urine
10 min. clean catch

Type of Test: Urine

Body Systems and Functions: Immunological system

Normal Findings: Negative

CRITICAL VALUES:
>4 g/24 hr

Test Results Time Frame: Within 24 hr

Test Description: Bence Jones is a specific protein associated with multiple myeloma, macroglobulinemia, and malignant lymphoma. It is estimated that 50%–80% of clients with multiple myeloma will have Bence Jones in the urine. Large amounts of Bence Jones proteins cause tubular cells to degenerate due to high levels of protein reabsorption. High levels lead to damaged kidney and are termed myeloma kidney and nephrotic syndrome. In multiple myeloma, large amounts of low-molecular-weight immunoglobulins are synthesized by malignant plasma cells in bone barrow and reabsorbed by the kidney. Excessive amounts cannot be metabolized and spill in to the urine. These proteins have an unusual thermal property that allows them to be identified: They precipitate from urine when heated between 45°C and 60°C and redissolve on boiling. Electrophoresis and immunofixation is the preferred method of testing.

Consent Form: Not required

List of Equipment: Sterile plastic container; ice

Test Procedure:
24-hr urine:
1. Label the collection container. *Correctly identifies the client and the test to be performed.*

URINE

2. Discard the first morning void. Then begin the time of the collection for the next 24 hr, including the void at the end of the 24 hr, and record the last voiding time. *An exact 24-hr count ensures accurate results.*
3. If the client has an indwelling catheter in place, keep the drainage bag on ice and empty the urine into the urine container periodically during the 24-hr period.
4. Keep urine cool during collection. *Higher temperatures alter the results.*
5. If any urine is lost, discard the entire specimen and begin collection again the next day.

Midstream urine specimen:
1. Label a sterile urine container. *Correctly identifies the client and the test to be performed.*
2. Obtain a clean-catch specimen of urine (note: first morning voiding preferred, at least 60 mL). *Ensures accurate results.*
3. Keep specimen cool. *High temperatures alter the results.*
4. Send specimen to laboratory.

Clinical Implications and Indications:
1. Detects multiple myeloma and is used in combination with other testing
2. Diagnoses amyloidosis, Fanconi's syndrome, and Waldenstrom's macroglobulinemia

Nursing Care:
Before Test: Explain the test procedure and the purpose of the test. Assess the client's knowledge of the test. Instruct client in the method of collection that is ordered (clean catch or 24 hr). For 24-hr urine, instruct client not to discard any urine.

During Test: Adhere to standard precautions. If any urine is accidentally discarded or contaminated with feces, discard entire specimen and begin test again the following morning. Collect all urine to specimen container and refrigerate or put on ice.

After Test: Document urine quantity, date, and exact hours of collection on requisition.

Interfering Factors: Urine contaminated with feces; spillage or inaccurate collection of the 24-hr specimen, including nonrefrigeration or placing on ice; severe urinary tract infection; chronic renal insufficiency; specimen contaminated with menstrual blood; medications that alter results are aminosalicylic acid, cephaloridine, penicillin, and sulfisoxazole tolbutamide.

Nursing Considerations:
Pediatric: For 24-hr urine specimen: A collection bag needs to be used for infants and toddlers. For midstream specimen: A collection bag or insertion of a straight catheter is likely needed for infants and toddlers.

WEBLINKS

www.healthcentral.com; www.healthgate.com

URINE

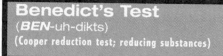

Benedict's Test
(*BEN*-uh-dikts)
(Cooper reduction test; reducing substances)

10 min.

Type of Test: Urine

Body Systems and Functions: Metabolic system

Normal Findings: An absence of homogenetic acids in the urine

> **CRITICAL VALUES:**
> A blue color indicates a negative response on the tablet test (Clinitest).

Test Results Time Frame: Within 24 hr

Test Description: Benedict's test is performed to screen for presence of sugars, reducing substances, and homogenetic acids in the urine. This is primarily used in a genetic condition whereby homogentisic acid is lacking, which causes the client to be unable to metabolize homogentisic acid. Benedict's is a qualitative and quantitative test, which is more sensitive to reducing substances than the single-tablet Cooper reduction test. Benedict's solution is heated and turns orange/red in the presence of ascorbic acid, homogentisic acid, or sugars. If the test is positive, a tablet test (Clinitest) should be performed to differentiate homogenetic acids from glucose.

Consent Form: Not required

List of Equipment: Sterile plastic container; ice

Test Procedure:
1. Label a sterile urine container. *Correctly identifies the client and the test to be performed.*
2. Obtain a clean-catch specimen of urine (note: first morning voiding preferred, at least 60 mL). *Ensures accurate results.*
3. Keep specimen cool. *High temperatures alter the results.*
4. Send specimen to laboratory.

Test results for Benedict's test

Color	Quantitative	Qualitative
Blue	0 mmol/L	Negative
Green	14 mmol/L	Trace
Green + yellow precipitate	28 mmol/L	1+
Yellow-green	56 mmol/L	2+
Brown	83 mmol/L	3+
Orange-red	>110 mmol/L	

URINE

Clinical Implications and Indications:
1. Screens for glucose or amino acid metabolism dysfunction
2. Diagnoses ochronosis
3. Evaluates metabolic disorders

Nursing Care:

Before Test: Explain the test procedure and the purpose of the test. Assess the client's knowledge of the test.

During Test: Adhere to standard precautions. Collect a clean urine sample. Twenty-four-hour urine: If any urine is accidentally discarded or contaminated with feces, discard entire specimen and begin test again.

After Test: Document urine quantity, date, and exact hours of collection on requisition.

Interfering Factors: Low kidney threshold for glucose; urine contaminated with feces; spillage or inaccurate collection of the urine specimen, including nonrefrigeration or placing on ice; medications that alter results are ampicillin, aminosalicylic acid, cephalosporins, chloral hydrate, chloramphenicol, isoniazid, levodopa, nalidixic acid, nitrofurantoin, penicillin G, probenecid, salicylates, streptomycin, and tetracyline.

Nursing Considerations:

Pediatric: A collection bag or insertion of a straight catheter is likely needed for infants and toddlers.

Listing of Related Tests: Clinistix; Clinitest; Diastix; Tes-tape

WEBLINKS

www.acp.edu; www.ncbi.nlm.nih.gov

Cyclic Adenosine Monophosphate
(*SIK*-lik uh-*DEN*-oe-*SEEN MAH*-noe-*FAHS*-fayt)
(cAMP)

4 hr.

Type of Test: Urine

Body Systems and Functions: Endocrine system

Normal Findings: An increase in cyclic adenosine monophosphate (cAMP) diuresis (3.6–4 µmol) is a normal response to injection of parathyroid hormone.

Test Results Time Frame: Within 24 hr

Test Description: cAMP is a nucleotide produced by the kidneys and is involved in many hormonal activities. cAMP acts as a messenger for hormones, transmitting the initial receptor signal to targeted cells. cAMP is the messenger for parathyroid hormone, which increases serum calcium. Urinary cAMP rises after parathyroid administration in clients with hypoparathyroidism and in healthy clients. Clients with pseudohypoparathyroidism (PHP) do not have a rise in urinary cAMP or an increased serum calcium after parathyroid administration. Parathyroid hormone infusion fails to produce renal production of cAMP. Failure of stimulation of cAMP indicates a defect in receptor sites for parathyroid hormone or a problem with cAMP-mediated signal transduction.

URINE

CLINICAL ALERT:

Test results will be inaccurate if any urine specimens are missed within the 4-hr time period.

Consent Form: Required

List of Equipment: Parathyroid hormone; sterile plastic container; ice

Test Procedure:
1. Label the collection container. *Correctly identifies the client and the test to be performed.*
2. Discard the first morning void. Then begin the time of the collection for the next 4 hr, including the void at the end of the 4 hr, and record the last voiding time. *An exact 4-hr count ensures accurate results.*
3. If the client has an indwelling catheter in place, keep the drainage bag on ice and empty the urine into the urine container periodically during the 4-hr period.
4. Keep urine cool during collection. *Higher temperatures alter the results.*
5. If any urine is lost, discard the entire specimen and begin collection again the next day.
6. Infuse the parathyroid hormone via IV line over 15 min. Record the start of the parathyroid hormone at time zero.
7. Ensure that all urine voided for next 4 hr is collected. *Ensures accurate results.*
8. Label the 4-hr urine container with the time the collection is ended.
9. Send specimen to laboratory immediately.

Clinical Implications and Indications:
1. Aids in establishing the diagnosis of parathyroid hormone resistance and pseudohypoparathyroidism

Nursing Care:
Before Test: Explain the test procedure and the purpose of the test. Assess the client's knowledge of the test. Instruct client not to discard any urine over the 4-hr time period.
During Test: Adhere to standard precautions. If any urine is accidentally discarded or contaminated with feces, discard entire specimen and begin test again the following morning.
After Test: Document urine quantity, date, and exact hours of collection on requisition.

Potential Complications: Allergic reaction to parathyroid hormone; hypercalcemia (manifested as lethargy, anorexia, nausea, vomiting, vertigo, and abominal cramps)

Contraindications: High calcium levels; digitalis therapy; sarcoidosis; renal disease; cardiac disease

Interfering Factors: Urine contaminated with feces; spillage or inaccurate collection of the 4-hr specimen, including nonrefrigeration or placing on ice; heavy bleeding during menstruation

Nursing Considerations:
Pediatric: For collection of 4-hr specimen a collection bag or indwelling catheter needs to be used for infants and toddlers.

URINE

WEBLINKS

http://www.niddk.nih.gov

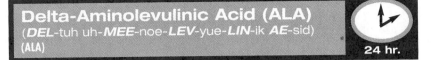

Delta-Aminolevulinic Acid (ALA)
(*DEL*-tuh uh-*MEE*-noe-*LEV*-yue-*LIN*-ik *AE*-sid)
(ALA)

24 hr.

Type of Test: Urine

Body Systems and Functions: Hematological system

Normal Findings: 1.5–7.5 mg/dL/24 hr

Test Results Time Frame: Within 24–48 hr

Test Description: Delta-aminolevulinic acid is a test that uses colorimetric technique (a black light or ultraviolet light test) that screens for the presence of polyphyrins. Polyphyrins are cyclic compounds that are formed from ALA. They play a foundational role in the formation of hemoglobin and other hemoproteins. The test is determined from evaluating the products found in the urine after collecting a 24-hr sample. Normally, very small amounts of the ALA is excreted in the urine, but in certain abnormalities (e.g., lead poisoning, liver cancer) porphyrins are excreted.

CLINICAL ALERT:
Do not expose urine specimen to direct sunlight.

Consent Form: Not required

List of Equipment: Sterile plastic container; ice

Test Procedure:
1. Label the collection container. *Correctly identifies the client and the test to be performed.*
2. Discard the first morning void. Then begin the time of the collection for the next 24 hr, including the void at the end of the 24 hr, and record the last voiding time. *An exact 24-hr count ensures accurate results.*
3. If the client has an indwelling catheter in place, keep the drainage bag on ice and empty the urine into the urine container periodically during the 24-hr period.
4. Keep urine cool during collection. *Higher temperatures alter the results.*
5. If any urine is lost, discard the entire specimen and begin collection again the next day.
6. If a catheter is used, collect urine in a dark-colored plastic bag. *Ensures accurate results.*

Clinical Implications and Indications:
1. Elevated levels are found with lead poisoning, acute porphyria, liver cancer, hereditary coproporphyria, and hepatitis.

Nursing Care:
Before Test: Explain the test procedure and the purpose of the test. Assess the client's knowledge of the test. Instruct client not to discard any urine over the 24-hr time period. Check medications to be sure they do not affect test results.
During Test: Adhere to standard precautions. If any urine is accidentally discarded or contaminated with feces, discard entire specimen and begin test again the following morning.

URINE

After Test: Document urine quantity, date, and exact hours of collection on requisition. Advise client to resume taking any medications that were withheld before the test. Instruct client that urine may appear amber red or burgundy, pale pink, to almost black (note: in the presence of porphyrins).

Interfering Factors: Urine contaminated with feces; spillage or inaccurate collection of the 24-hr specimen, including nonrefrigeration or placing on ice; oral contraceptives; medications that alter results are barbiturates, griseofulvin, and vitamin E (large doses).

Nursing Considerations:
Pediatric: For collection of 24-hr specimen a collection bag needs to be used for infants and toddlers. In addition, increased levels of ALA may be seen in newborns of mothers with porphyria.

WEBLINKS

http://www.entnet.org

Dexamethasone Suppression Test
(*DEK*-suh-*METH*-uh-*SOEN* suh-*PRE*-sh:n)
(cortisol suppression; DST)

24 hr.

Type of Test: Urine; blood

Body Systems and Functions: Endocrine system

Normal Findings: 24-hr urine should be <50% of baseline levels:

Plasma cortisol	<5 mg/dL
Urine-free cortisol	<25 mg/24 hr
Urine for 17-OHCS	4 mg/24 hr

Test Results Time Frame: Within 24–48 hr

Test Description: Dexamethasone suppression testing examines both blood and urine for the presence of cortisol. The test is performed by administering dexamethasone (a synthetic glucocorticoid) to evaluate the production of cortisol. The dexamethasone is given in high or low doses and blood samples are obtained to determine if cortisol is at normal levels in the blood. The low dose is given for screening, and a high-dose test is administered to determine the cause of Cushing's disease (Cushing's disease has no suppression of ACTH).

Consent Form: Not required

List of Equipment: *Blood:* red-top tube or serum separator tube; needle and syringe or vacutainer; alcohol swab. *Urine:* sterile plastic container; ice.

Test Procedure:
Blood:
1. Label the specimen tube. *Correctly identifies the client and the test to be performed.*
2. Obtain a 5-mL blood sample.
3. Do not agitate the tube. *Agitation may cause RBC hemolysis.*

URINE

4. Send tube to the laboratory.
5. For the overnight test, administer 1 mg of dexamethasone orally at 11 AM, followed by a venipuncture for cortisol level the next day at 8 AM.
6. For the high-dose test obtain a baseline of urine-free cortisol by giving oral dexamethasone every 6 hr for 2 days, followed by a 24-hr urine.

24-hr urine:
1. Label the collection container. *Correctly identifies the client and the test to be performed.*
2. Discard the first morning void. Then begin the time of the collection for the next 24 hr, including the void at the end of the 24 hr, and record the last voiding time. *An exact 24-hr count ensures accurate results.*
3. If the client has an indwelling catheter in place, keep the drainage bag on ice and empty the urine into the urine container periodically during the 24-hr period.
4. Keep urine cool during collection. *Higher temperatures alter the results.*
5. If any urine is lost, discard the entire specimen and begin collection again the next day.

Clinical Implications and Indications:
1. Evaluates diurnal suppression of cortisol to confirm Cushing's syndrome.
2. Diagnoses endogenous depression (note: cortisol is depressed in 50% of the cases).
3. Elevated levels of cortisol after dexamethasone administration are found with adrenal hyperplasia, adrenal tumors, and oat cell cancer of the lung.

Nursing Care:
Before Test: Explain the test procedure and the purpose of the test. Assess the client's knowledge of the test. Instruct client not to discard any urine over the 24-hr time period.
During Test: Adhere to standard precautions. If any urine is accidentally discarded or contaminated with feces, discard entire specimen and begin test again the following morning.
After Test: Apply pressure to venipuncture site. Explain that some bruising, discomfort, and swelling may appear at the site and that warm, moist compresses can alleviate this. Monitor for signs of infection. Document urine quantity, date, and exact hours of collection on requisition.

Potential Complications: Bleeding and bruising at venipuncture site

Interfering Factors: Urine contaminated with feces; spillage or inaccurate collection of the 24-hr specimen including nonrefrigeration or placing on ice; heavy bleeding during menstruation; failure to ingest dexamethasone; nuclear scan within previous 24 hr; false positives will occur with alcoholism, anorexia nervosa, severe depression, malnutrition, fever, obesity, pregnancy, and high stress levels; false negatives will occur with Addison's disease and hypopituitarism; medications that increase results are barbiturates, carbamazepine, estrogens, meprobamate, oral contraceptives, phenytoin, reserpine, and spironolactone; medications that decrease results are benzodiazapines, corticosteroids, and cyproheptadine.

URINE

Nursing Considerations:
Pregnancy: Pregnancy causes elevation in test levels.
Pediatric: Infants and children will need assistance in remaining still during the venipuncture and age-appropriate comfort measures following the test. For

collection of 24-hr specimen a collection bag or indwelling catheter needs to be used for infants and toddlers.

Listing of Related Tests: Cortisol stimulation; metyrapone

WEBLINKS

www.ncbi.nlm.nih.gov

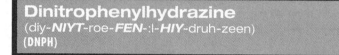

Dinitrophenylhydrazine
(diy-*NIYT*-roe-*FEN*-:l-*HIY*-druh-zeen)
(DNPH)

15 min.

Type of Test: Urine

Body Systems and Functions: Hematological system

Normal Findings: Normal amino acids

Test Results Time Frame: Within 72 hr

Test Description: Dinitrophenylhydrazine is excreted in the urine in metabolic disorders of branched-chain amino acids. Many amino acid abnormalities can be detected in blood and urine fluid analyses. Free amino acids are usually found in urine or acid filtrates of protein containing fluids. Urine testing such as dinitrophenylhydrazine is used in initial screening for genetic metabolic disorders.

> **CLINICAL ALERT:**
> Some of the metabolites involved in this test make the urine smell like maple syrup.

Consent Form: Not required

List of Equipment: Sterile plastic container; ice

Test Procedure:
1. Label a sterile urine container. *Correctly identifies the client and the test to be performed.*
2. Obtain a clean-catch specimen of urine (15 mL). *Ensures accurate results.*
3. Keep specimen cool. *High temperatures alter the results.*
4. Send specimen to laboratory.

Clinical Implications and Indications:
1. Elevated levels are found with cystinuria, Hartnup's homocystinuria, urine disease, PKU, tyrosinosis, lactic acidosis, seizures, and unexplained mental retardation.

Nursing Care:
Before Test: Explain the test procedure and the purpose of the test. Assess the client's knowledge of the test.
During Test: Adhere to standard precautions.
After Test: Keep sample refrigerated or on ice. Document urine quantity, date, and exact hours of collection on requisition.

URINE

Interfering Factors: Urine contaminated with feces; inaccurate collection of the urine specimen, including nonrefrigeration or placing on ice; valproic acid; penicillin derivatives; benzoic acid preservatives; radiopaque dye will increase levels.

Nursing Considerations:
Pediatric: A collection bag or insertion of a straight catheter is likely needed for infants and toddlers.

WEBLINKS

http://adam.excite.com

D-Xylose Absorption
(dee-*ZIY*-loes uhb-*ZOERP*-sh:n)
(xylose tolerance test)

2-4 hr.

Type of Test: Urine; blood

Body Systems and Functions: Hematological system

Normal Findings:
Blood:

		SI units
Adults	25–40 mg/dL	1.67–2.66 mmol/L
Children:		
<10 years	10%–33% of dose ingested	2.01 mmol/L or >30 mg/dL
>10 years	>16% of 25 g dose	

Urine:

	SI units
Adults	4 g of xylose excreted in 5 hr
Children	16%–33% excreted in 5 hr

Test Results Time Frame: Within 24 hr

Test Description: D-xylose absorption test measures d-xylose, which is a sugar that is not metabolized by the body and is normally absorbed by the proximal small intestine and excreted in the urine. D-xylose is used to differentiate malabsorption from maldigestion.

Consent Form: Not required

List of Equipment: Red-top tube or serum separator tube; needle and syringe or vacutainer; alcohol swab

Test Procedure:
1. Instruct client to void at 8 AM and discard the sample. Then begin urine collection.
2. Label all the specimen tubes. *Correctly identifies the client and the test to be performed.*
3. Obtain a 5-mL fasting blood sample.

URINE

4. Administer d-xylose per protocol and follow with 500 mL of water orally.
5. Collect all urine voided for 5 hr after d-xylose.
6. Obtain a 7-mL blood sample at 60 and 120 min after the d-xylose administration. *Allows for d-xylose levels to be determined.*
7. Do not agitate the tubes. *Agitation may cause RBC hemolysis.*
8. Send tubes to the laboratory.

Clinical Implications and Indications:
1. Elevated levels are found with Hodgkin's disease, malabsorption, and scleroderma.
2. Decreased levels are found with amyloidosis, celiac disease, cystic fibrosis, diarrhea, and Wipple's disease.

Nursing Care:
Before Test: Explain the test procedure and the purpose of the test. Assess the client's knowledge of the test. Instruct adults to fast for 8 hr and children for 4 hr before test. Instruct clients not to eat foods containing pentose (sugar). Instruct client not to discard any urine over the 5-hr time period.
During Test: Adhere to standard precautions.
After Test: Apply pressure to venipuncture site. Explain that some bruising, discomfort, and swelling may appear at the site and that warm, moist compresses can alleviate this. Monitor for signs of infection.

Potential Complications: Bleeding and bruising at venipuncture site

Interfering Factors: Vomiting; poor renal function; medications that increase results are aspirin, atropine, and indomethacin.

Nursing Considerations:
Pediatric: Infants and children will need assistance in remaining still during the venipuncture and age-appropriate comfort measures following the test.

WEBLINKS	⊟☒

www.ncbi.nlm.nih.gov

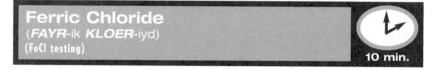

Ferric Chloride
(*FAYR*-ik *KLOER*-iyd)
(FeCl testing)

10 min.

Type of Test: Urine

Body Systems and Functions: Renal/urological system

Normal Findings: Negative

Test Results Time Frame: Within 12 hr

Test Description: Ferric chloride testing is a urine test that measures various color changes when FeCl is added to urine. Specific pathologies react with specific color changes in this testing. Some specific examples are listed below (note: consult with laboratory for more conditions that are tested in this manner):

Condition	Color change
Alcoholism	Red or red-brown
Alkaptonuria	Blue or green
Diabetes	Red or red-brown
Drug ingestion:	
Acetoophenetidines	Red
Aminosalicylic acid	Red-brown
Antipyrines	Red
Cyanates	Red
Phenothiazines	Light purple
Salicylates	Purple
Malnutrition	Red or red-brown
Phenylketonuria	Blue or blue-green

Consent Form: Not required

List of Equipment: Sterile plastic container

Test Procedure:
1. Label a sterile urine container. *Correctly identifies the client and the test to be performed.*
2. Obtain a clean-catch specimen of urine (note: first morning voiding preferred, at least 4 mL). *Ensures accurate results.*
3. Add FeCl (10%) to 1–2 mL of urine. Document color change when FeCl is added if protocol directs in this manner.
4. Keep specimen cool. *High temperatures alter the results.*
5. Send specimen to laboratory if there is no protocol for further evaluation.

Clinical Implications and Indications:
1. Evaluates the various color changes that occur with this test when the following conditions exist: alcoholism, diabetes, drug ingestion, phenylketonuria, starvation, and tyrosinosis

Nursing Care:
Before Test: Explain the test procedure and the purpose of the test. Assess the client's knowledge of the test.
During Test: Adhere to standard precautions.

Interfering Factors: Urine contaminated with feces; phenylalanine; levodopa

Nursing Considerations:
Pediatric: *A collection bag or insertion of a straight catheter is likely needed for infants and toddlers.*

URINE

WEBLINKS

http://adam.excite.com

Glucose, Urine
(*GLUE*-koes)
(urine glucose)

10 min.

Type of Test: Urine

Body Systems and Functions: Endocrine system

Normal Findings: Absent from the urine or negative

Test Results Time Frame: Within 2 min

Test Description: Urine glucose testing uses Clinistix, which are glucose oxidase enzyme paper dipsticks, and Clinitest tablets, which are copper sulfate reduction tablets. Glucose will appear in the urine if the renal tubules are unable to reabsorb all of the glucose back into the blood due to high plasma glucose levels. Glucose is the most important carbohydrate in body metabolism. It is formed during digestion from the hydrolysis of disaccharides and starch. Excess glucose is converted to glycogen in the liver (glycogenesis). Glucose is the primary source of energy within most cells and is oxidized in cell respiration into carbon dioxide and water in the form of adenosine triphosphate (ATP).

CLINICAL ALERT:
Exposure to light or moisture of the Clinitest tablets or strips will degrade them; if darkened, discard.

Consent Form: Not required

List of Equipment: Clinitest tablets; Clinistix reagent strips; dextrose or glucose strips; sterile plastic container

Test Procedure:
1. Have client void and then discard. After drinking 8 oz of fluid, have the client void 30 min later. If client has a Foley catheter, obtain a fresh specimen from the catheter.
2. If using Clinistix, dip reagent strip completely into the urine and hold for 2 sec.
3. Exactly 30 sec after removal from the urine, compare the color of the test pad to colors on the bottle and record results.

Clinical Implications and Indications:
1. Elevated levels are found with diabetes mellitus, gestational diabetes, Cushing's syndrome, hyperthyroidism, uremia, and sepsis.

Nursing Care:
Before Test: Explain the test procedure and the purpose of the test. Assess the client's knowledge of the test. Inform the client that the sample needs to be collected after the first voided specimen.
During Test: Adhere to standard precautions.

Interfering Factors: Discolored tablets with Clinitest or darkened strips with Clinistix will invalidate test results; medications that alter results are ammonium chloride, asparaginase, carbamazepine, corticosteroids, indomethacin, isoniazid, lithium carbonate, nicotinic acid, and thiazide diuretics.

URINE

Nursing Considerations:

Pediatric: *For children suspected of juvenile diabetes, the health care provider must begin assessing the client and family members as to their ability for self-care of this complicated disease process (i.e., diabetes mellitus).*
Gerontology: *Use of the tablets or reading of the strips, depending on method used, may be difficult for those clients with peripheral neuropathy or retinopathy.*
Home Care: *Clients need to check expiration dates.*

Listing of Related Tests: Capillary blood sugars; fasting blood sugars; postprandial glucose

WEBLINKS 🔲🗙

http://www.niddk.nih.gov

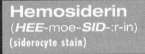

Hemosiderin
(*HEE*-moe-*SID*-:r-in)
(siderocyte stain)

10 min.

Type of Test: Urine

Body Systems and Functions: Metabolic system

Normal Findings: Negative

Test Results Time Frame: Within 24 hr

Test Description: Hemosiderin measures the presence of iron storage granules in urine sediment. This finding is abnormal and is one indication of extensive hemolysis, renal tubular damage, or an iron metabolism disorder. The granules of hemosiderin stain blue when potassium ferrocyanide is added to the sample.

Consent Form: Not required.

List of Equipment: Sterile plastic container; ice

Test Procedure:
1. Label a sterile urine container. *Correctly identifies the client and the test to be performed.*
2. Obtain a clean-catch specimen of urine (note: first morning voiding preferred, at least 50 mL). *Ensures accurate results.*
3. Keep specimen cool. *High temperatures alter the results.*
4. Send specimen to laboratory.

Clinical Implications and Indications:
1. Detects the etiology of RBC hemolysis
2. Evaluates renal tubule dysfunction

Nursing Care:
Before Test: Explain the test procedure and the purpose of the test. Assess the client's knowledge of the test.
During Test: Adhere to standard precautions.
After Test: Document urine quantity, date, and exact hours of collection on requisition.

URINE

Interfering Factors: Urine contaminated with feces; spillage or inaccurate collection of the urine specimen, including nonrefrigeration or placing on ice; heavy bleeding during menstruation; alkaline urine will prevent detection of hemosiderin.

Nursing Considerations:
Pediatric: A collection bag or insertion of a straight catheter is likely needed for infants and toddlers.
Gerontology: Client may need further assessment and intervention if tissue hypoperfusion is assessed related to anemia.

Listing of Related Tests: Total iron; iron saturation; hemoglobin and hematocrit; transbronchial lung biopsy if idiopathic pulmonary hemosiderosis is suspected

WEBLINKS ▣▣

http://www.kumc.edu

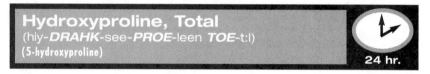

Hydroxyproline, Total
(hiy-**DRAHK**-see-**PROE**-leen **TOE**-t:l)
(5-hydroxyproline)

24 hr.

Type of Test: Urine

Body Systems and Functions: Metabolic system

Normal Findings: 24-hr test (normal laboratory findings vary among laboratory settings):

Adults	10–50 mg/24 hr
Children:	
1–10 years	20–99 mg/24 hr
11–14 years	63–180 mg/24 hr

Test Results Time Frame: Within 5 days

Test Description: Hydroxyproline is an amino acid found in collagen that has increased urinary excretion. The hydroxyproline is increased in various disorders with increased osteoblastic activity, as well as in some diseases involving osteolysis and collagen metabolism. This protein is also increased during periods of rapid growth in children.

Consent Form: Not required

List of Equipment: 3-L metal-free urine collection container with or without preservative depending on laboratory specific directions; ice

Test Procedure:
1. Label the collection container. *Correctly identifies the client and the test to be performed.*
2. Discard the first morning void. Then begin the time of the collection for the next 24 hr, including the void at the end of the 24 hr, and record the last voiding time. *An exact 24-hr count ensures accurate results.*

URINE

3. If the client has an indwelling catheter in place, keep the drainage bag on ice and empty the urine into the urine container periodically during the 24-hr period.
4. Keep urine cool during collection. *Higher temperatures alter the results.*
5. If any urine is lost, discard the entire specimen and begin collection again the next day.

Clinical Implications and Indications:

1. Assists in the detection of tumors having bone metastases
2. Detects disorders associated with increased bone resorption
3. Monitors the treatment of disorders characterized by bone reabsorption, such as Paget's disease

Nursing Care:

Before Test: Explain the test procedure and the purpose of the test. Assess the client's knowledge of the test. Instruct client not to discard any urine over the 24-hr time period.

During Test: Adhere to standard precautions. If any urine is accidentally discarded or contaminated with feces, discard entire specimen and begin test again the following morning.

After Test: Document urine quantity, date, and exact hours of collection on requisition.

Interfering Factors:

Urine contaminated with feces; spillage or inaccurate collection of the 24-hr specimen, including nonrefrigeration or placing on ice; psoriasis or burns can promote collagen turnover and can elevate urine levels; heavy bleeding during menstruation

Nursing Considerations:

Pediatric: For collection of 24-hr specimen a collection bag or indwelling catheter needs to be used for infants and toddlers.

Listing of Related Tests:

Alkaline phosphatase; 2-hr test period/collection for hydroxyproline

WEBLINKS ▯

http://alice.ucdavis.edu

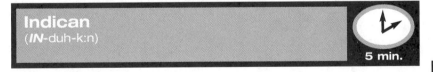

Indican
(*IN*-duh-k:n)

5 min.

URINE

Type of Test: Urine

Body Systems and Functions: Gastrointestinal system

Normal Findings: Small quantities of indoxylsulfate are found in normal urine.

Test Results Time Frame: Within 48 hr

Test Description: Indican is a potassium salt of indoxylsulfate found in sweat and urine and formed when intestinal bacteria convert tryptophan to indole. Indican is excreted in the feces, but also small amounts are excreted in the urine as a result of absorption and detoxification of indole (note: normal urine turns blue when 5 mL of urine is added to 5 mL of ferric chloride reagent). Indican is considered one of the most common intestinal toxins, and its presence in the intestines generally suggests the occurrence of other toxins.

Consent Form: Not required

List of Equipment: Sterile plastic container; ice

Test Procedure:
1. Label a sterile urine container. *Correctly identifies the client and the test to be performed.*
2. Obtain a clean-catch specimen of urine (note: first morning voiding preferred, at least 60 mL). *Ensures accurate results.*
3. Keep specimen cool. *High temperatures alter the results.*
4. Send specimen to laboratory.

Clinical Implications and Indications:
1. Detects indicanemia and indicanuria
2. Assists in the diagnosis of bowel toxemia, which is thought to be implicated in a variety of mental disturbances

Nursing Care:
Before Test: Explain the test procedure and the purpose of the test. Assess the client's knowledge of the test.
During Test: Adhere to standard precautions.
After Test: Document urine quantity, date, and exact hours of collection on requisition.

Interfering Factors: Urine contaminated with feces; spillage or inaccurate collection of the urine specimen, including nonrefrigeration or placing on ice

Nursing Considerations:
Pediatric: A collection bag or insertion of a straight catheter is likely needed for infants and toddlers.

Listing of Related Tests: Ammonia level; indole, phenol; stool cultures

WEBLINKS

www.newfrontier.com

Ketone Bodies
(*KEE*-toen)
(acetone; aceotacetate)

2 min.

Type of Test: Urine

Body Systems and Functions: Endocrine system

Normal Findings: No ketones in urine (quantitative = 0); no deep color on acetone tablet or reagent strip

CRITICAL VALUES:
Abrupt changes in ketone bodies indicate a clinical alert (note: the age of the individual and the test method used by the laboratory produce a range of strongly positive values).

Test Results Time Frame: Less than 2 min with the reagent strip and <1 min with the acetone tablet

Test Description: Ketone bodies measure the ketonuria (an increased amount of ketones in urine), which is indicative of malfunctioning carbohydrate metabolism and of diabetes. A ketone bodies test may aid in the diagnosis of ketoacidosis and diabetic comas. Starvation or diets low in carbohydrates, high in fat, and high in protein also produce ketones.

CLINICAL ALERT:
The presence of ketone bodies in the urine of diabetic or non-diabetic individuals is an alert, but not a crisis. However, in children under 2 years of age ketones may indicate a more serious condition.

Consent Form: Not required

List of Equipment: Ketone reagent strip; acetone tablet; sterile plastic container

Test Procedure:
Dip test:
1. A reagent strip is dipped into a specimen of freshly voided urine. Different reagent strips may vary in activation time; check the manufacturer's information for time specific to the test being used (usually 1 min).
2. Compare the strip with the result information provided by the manufacturer. *Ensures accurate results.*

Tablet test:
1. A fresh drop of urine is placed on an acetone tablet. The tablet must be on a clean surface, such as a clean piece of paper or paper towel. *Ensures accurate test results.*
2. A positive test will result in the tablet becoming purple in appoximately 30 sec.

Clinical Implications and Indications:
1. Fasting elevates ketone levels.
2. A specific diet that contains high amounts of fat and protein and low amounts of carbohydrates may produce ketosis and ketonuria.
3. Ketosis and ketonuria may result from diabetes mellitus, renal glycosuria, glycogen storage disease, anorexia, eclampsia, hypothyroidism, fever, pregnancy, and lactation.
4. Severe illness, heavy stress, and intense excerise may produce increased ketones in the urine of nondiabetic individuals. Other factors that may produce abnormal values are diarrhea, vomiting, postanesthesia, alcoholism, and if phenylketones or levadopa metabolites are present in the urine.

URINE

Nursing Care:
Before Test: Explain the test procedure and the purpose of the test. Assess the client's knowledge of the test.

During Test: Adhere to standard precautions. If any urine is accidentally discarded or contaminated with feces, discard entire specimen and begin test again.

After Test: Document urine quantity, date, and exact hours of collection on requisition.

Potential Complications: The urine specimen must be freshly voided, as false negatives may occur if the ketones are allowed to evaporate.

Interfering Factors: Urine contaminated with feces; heavy bleeding during menstruation; medications that cause false-positive results are aspirin, bromosulfophthalein, captopril, ether, insulin, metformin, penicillamine, phenazopyridine, phenolsulfonphthalein, phenothiazines, salicylates, and sulfobromophthalein.

Nursing Considerations:
Pediatric: A collection bag or insertion of a straight catheter is likely needed for infants and toddlers. Ketonuria and ketosis are more prevalent in pediatric patients.

Listing of Related Tests: Clinitest; Acetest

WEBLINKS

http://www.niddk.nih.gov

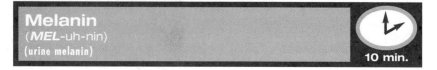

Melanin
(*MEL*-uh-nin)
(urine melanin)

10 min.

Type of Test: Urine

Body Systems and Functions: Oncology system

Normal Findings: No melanin in urine

Test Results Time Frame: Within 24–48 hr

Test Description: Melanin testing is performed to detect the biochemical marker of melanin in the urine. Melanin is the main pigment in the body and is synthesized by the melanocyte in the skin and eyes. Melanin is primarily used as an indicator of melanoma through the process of chromatography.

> **CLINICAL ALERT:**
> Confirmation of cancer may be difficult for the clien to reconcile. Sensitivity toward the client's concerns and fears is very important.

Consent Form: Not required

List of Equipment: Sterile plastic container; ice

URINE

Test Procedure:

1. Label a sterile urine container. *Correctly identifies the client and the test to be performed.*
2. Obtain a freshly voided urine sample. *Ensures accurate results.*
3. Keep specimen cool. *High temperatures alter the results.*
4. Send specimen to laboratory.

Clinical Implications and Indications:

1. Detects a late-stage internal melanoma
2. Evaluates slight increases seen in liver metastasis

Nursing Care:

Before Test: Explain the test procedure and the purpose of the test. Assess the client's knowledge of the test.

During Test: Adhere to standard precautions.

After Test: Document urine quantity, date, and exact hours of collection on requisition.

Interfering Factors: Urine contaminated with feces; spillage or inaccurate collection of the urine specimen, including nonrefrigeration or placing on ice; heavy bleeding during menstruation

Nursing Considerations:

Pediatric: A collection bag or insertion of a straight catheter is likely needed for infants and toddlers.

WEBLINKS	⊟ ⊠

http://www.healthgate.com

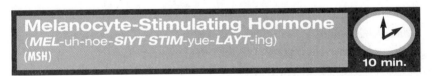

Melanocyte-Stimulating Hormone
(*MEL*-uh-noe-*SIYT STIM*-yue-*LAYT*-ing)
(MSH)

10 min.

Type of Test: Urine

Body Systems and Functions: Endocrine system

Normal Findings: Negative for MSH

Test Results Time Frame: Within 24 hr

Test Description: Melanocyte-stimulating hormone is secreted by the anterior lobe of the pituitary gland. MSH is responsible for affecting pigment metabolism by promoting the synthesis of melanin. The increased level of melanin produces a variation in the normal skin color of a person with Addison's disease.

Consent Form: Not required

List of Equipment: Sterile plastic container; ice

Test Procedure:

1. Label a sterile urine container. *Correctly identifies the client and the test to be performed.*
2. Obtain a freshly voided urine sample. *Ensures accurate results.*

URINE

3. Keep specimen cool. *High temperatures alter the results.*
4. Send specimen to laboratory.

Clinical Implications and Indications:
1. Elevated levels are found with Addison's disease and hyperpituitarism.
2. Evaluates melanoma and metastasis to the liver.

Nursing Care:
Before Test: Explain the test procedure and the purpose of the test. Assess the client's knowledge of the test.
During Test: Adhere to standard precautions. If any urine is accidentally discarded or contaminated with feces, discard specimen and begin test again.
After Test: Document urine quantity, date, and time of collection on requisition.

Interfering Factors: Urine contaminated with feces; spillage or inaccurate collection of the urine specimen, including nonrefrigeration or placing on ice; heavy bleeding during menstruation; cortisol increases MSH.

Nursing Considerations:
Pediatric: A collection bag or insertion of a straight catheter is likely needed for infants and toddlers.

WEBLINKS

www.kumc.edu

Mucopolysaccharides, Qualitative
(*MYUE*-koe-*PAHL*-ee-*SAEK*-:r-iydz *KWAHL*-uh-*TAYT*-iv)
(berry spot test; GAGs; MPS spot; qualitative glycosaminoglycans)

10 min.

Type of Test: Urine

Body Systems and Functions: Metabolic system

Normal Findings: Negative for MPS glycosaminoglycans

Test Results Time Frame: Within 3–7 days

Test Description: Mucopolysaccharide testing screens the urine to identify the presence or absence of mucopolysaccharides. A thin-layer chromatography evaluates the qualitative identification of the type of sulfate(s) being stored (e.g., heparan, keratan, dermatan, chondroitin). Positive results may indicate one of several inherited disorders of connective tissue metabolism. Mucopolysaccharides are a group of polysaccharides that contain hexosamine and proteins that form chemical bonds with water. The mucopolysaccharides are an integral substance of body cells that are found in mucous secretions and synovial fluids.

URINE

CLINICAL ALERT:
Laboratories vary on the timing of the sample. Most laboratories prefer that the sample is not the first void of the morning, which necessitates confirming with the laboratory the appropriate timing of the sample.

Consent Form: Not required

List of Equipment: Sterile plastic container; ice

Test Procedure:
1. Label a sterile urine container. *Correctly identifies the client and the test to be performed.*
2. Obtain a clean-catch specimen of urine (note: first morning voiding is not preferred, at least 5–15 mL). *Ensures accurate results.*
3. Store sample in refrigerator or laboratory may request frozen sample until transport. *Bacterial growth may produce a false-positive result or degrade GAGs, which would result in a false negative.*
4. Send specimen to laboratory.

Clinical Implications and Indications:
1. Increased levels are found with mucopolysaccharidosis and disorders of connective tissue metabolism (e.g., Hunter's, Hurler-Sheie, Morquio, Sanfilippo, Maroteaux/Lamy syndromes).

Nursing Care:
Before Test: Explain the test procedure and the purpose of the test. Assess the client's knowledge of the test.
During Test: Adhere to standard precautions. If urine is accidentally discarded or contaminated with feces, discard entire specimen and begin test with next voiding.
After Test: Document urine quantity, date, and exact hours of collection on requisition.

Interfering Factors: Urine contaminated with feces; spillage or inaccurate collection of the urine specimen, including nonrefrigeration or placing on ice; heavy bleeding during menstruation

Nursing Considerations:
Pediatric: A collection bag or insertion of a straight catheter is likely needed for infants and toddlers.

Listing of Related Tests: Mucopolysaccharide quantitation; creatinine

WEBLINKS

http://www.mic.ki.se/Diseases/c20.html

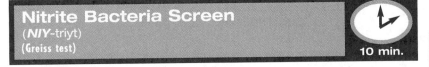

Nitrite Bacteria Screen
(**NIY**-triyt)
(Greiss test)

10 min.

URINE

Type of Test: Urine

Body Systems and Functions: Immunological system

Normal Findings: Negative for bacteria; no appearance of color on dipstick

Test Results Time Frame: Immediately

Test Description: A nitrite bacteria screen examines the first voided urine of the day for bacteriuria. The process is based on the fact that dietary nitrate is converted to nitrite by the enzyme nitrate reductase, which is an enzyme synthesized by gram-negative bacteria. The reagent strips used in this urine test contain reagents that expose this conversion. However, a negative test may not rule out infection since bacteria converts nitrate to nitrite in the bladder after approximately 6 hr. Also, yeasts and some gram-positive bacteria will not result in a positive test since they do not promote a nitrate-to-nitrite conversion.

Consent Form: Not required

List of Equipment: Sterile plastic container; ice; reagent strip; associated color chart

Test Procedure:
1. Label a sterile urine container. *Correctly identifies the client and the test to be performed.*
2. Obtain a clean-catch specimen of urine (note: first morning voiding of at least 15–30 mL preferred to allow enough time for the urine in the bladder to generate a nitrate-to-nitrite conversion). *Ensures accurate results.*
3. Dip reagent strip into urine immediately and compare results against manufacturer's color chart (note: positive results appear in various shades of pink). *Ensures accurate results.*
4. Document response.
5. Send specimen to laboratory.

Clinical Implications and Indications:
1. Diagnoses urinary tract infections
2. Utilized as a self-screening test with a high degree of accuracy (positive response indicates need for follow-up)

Nursing Care:
Before Test: Explain the test procedure and the purpose of the test. Assess the client's knowledge of the test. Instruct client to use the first voided urine sample.
During Test: Adhere to standard precautions. If any urine is accidentally discarded or contaminated with feces, discard entire specimen and begin test again the following morning.
After Test: Document urine quantity, date, and exact hours of collection on requisition. Compare reagent strip against color chart provided. Note any pink color as a positive result. A negative result requires no follow-up unless the client is experiencing signs and symptoms of a urinary tract infection (UTI) (note: indicates a UTI as a result of an organism that does not stimulate a nitrate-to-nitrite conversion).

Interfering Factors: Urine contaminated with feces; spillage or inaccurate collection of the urine specimen, including nonrefrigeration or placing on ice; heavy bleeding during menstruation; random sample (versus overnight) will not have allowed enough time for nitrate to convert to nitrite; diet lacking in green vegetables; medications that alter results are ascorbic acid and antibiotics.

Nursing Considerations:
Pediatric: A collection bag or insertion of a straight catheter is likely needed for infants and toddlers.

URINE

Listing of Related Tests: Urine culture; leukocyte esterase test

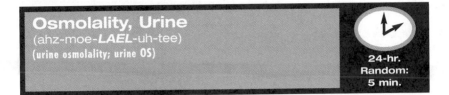

http://www.nlm.nih.gov

Osmolality, Urine
(ahz-moe-*LAEL*-uh-tee)
(urine osmolality; urine OS)

24-hr.
Random:
5 min.

Type of Test: Urine

Body Systems and Functions: Renal/urological system

Normal Findings: 500–800 mOsm/kg; up to 3:1 urine/serum ratio

Test Results Time Frame: Within 24 hr

Test Description: Urine osmolality measures the concentration of numbers of particles of solute in a defined amount of solution. It reflects the kidney's ability to concentrate urine and is directly affected by the hydration status of the subject. The test aids in assessing fluid and electrolyte balance and can be used to determine osmolar gap, which is the difference between the sum of all the expected particles in urine and the actual measurement. Comparisons of urine and serum osmolalities may be useful when investigating fluid and electrolyte balance.

Consent Form: Not required

List of Equipment: Sterile plastic container; ice

Test Procedure:
Random specimen:
1. Label a sterile urine container. *Correctly identifies the client and the test to be performed.*
2. Obtain a clean-catch specimen of urine (note: first morning voiding at 6 AM is discarded and a single sample of at least 10 mL is taken 2 hr later). *Ensures accurate results.*
3. Keep specimen cool. *High temperatures alter the results.*
4. Send specimen to laboratory.
24-hr specimen:
1. Label the collection container. *Correctly identifies the client and the test to be performed.*
2. Discard the first morning void. Then begin the time of the collection for the next 24 hr, including the void at the end of the 24 hr, and record the last voiding time. *An exact 24-hr count ensures accurate results.*
3. If the client has an indwelling catheter in place, keep the drainage bag on ice and empty the urine into the urine container periodically during the 24-hr period.
4. Keep urine cool during collection. *Higher temperatures alter the results.*
5. If any urine is lost, discard the entire specimen and begin collection again the next day.

URINE

Clinical Implications and Indications:

1. Elevated levels are found with (but not limited to) dehydration, hyperglycemia with glycosuria, diarrhea, edema, Addison's disease, SIADH, and uremia.
2. Decreased levels are found with (but not limited to) diabetes insipidus, glomerulonephritis, acute renal failure, hypercalcemia, hypokalemia, hyponatremia, overhydration, sickle cell anemia, multiple myeloma, and urinary tract obstruction.

Nursing Care:

Before Test: Explain the test procedure and the purpose of the test. Assess the client's knowledge of the test. Instruct client not to discard any urine over the 24-hr time period (for 24-hr specimen). Variations exist in pretest dietary restrictions, which the testing facility should clarify. For the fasting sample the client may be requested to eat a high-protein diet for 3 days prior to the test. For all samples the client eats a dry supper the night before and ingests no fluids for the 12 hr prior to testing.

During Test: Adhere to standard precautions. If any urine is accidentally discarded or contaminated with feces, discard entire specimen and begin test again.

After Test: Document urine quantity, date, exact hours of collection on requisition, and random, fasting, or 24-hr specimen. Inform client to return to normal dietary and fluid habits.

Interfering Factors:

Urine contaminated with feces; spillage or inaccurate collection of the 24-hr specimen, including nonrefrigeration or placing on ice; heavy bleeding during menstruation; medications that alter results are antibiotics, diuretics, mannitol, and IV sodium or dextrose; recent use of radiographic contrast agent; high-protein diet

Nursing Considerations:

Pediatric: For collection of 24-hr specimen a collection bag or indwelling catheter needs to be used for infants and toddlers. For random specimen a collection bag or insertion of a straight catheter is likely needed for infants and toddlers.

Listing of Related Tests:

Serum osmolality; specific gravity; BUN; creatinine clearance; IV pyelogram

---

WEBLINKS

http://www.creighton.edu

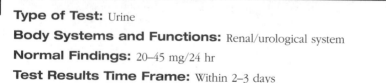

Oxalate
(*AHK*-suh-layt)

24 hr.

Type of Test: Urine

Body Systems and Functions: Renal/urological system

Normal Findings: 20–45 mg/24 hr

Test Results Time Frame: Within 2–3 days

Test Description: Approximately 10% of urinary oxalate is a result of diet, but most of its presence is accounted for as a result of metabolic processes. Since oxalate is not highly soluble, once it is absorbed from the small bowel, it is not metabolized and the amount of absorption in the bowel depends on how much calcium is present. Excretion occurs in the proximal tubule and the amount of oxalate in the urine determines the formation of calcium oxalate calculi (kidney stones). A 24-hr urine is the best average measurement of oxalate as the levels are somewhat higher during the day when the individual is eating.

Consent Form: Not required

List of Equipment: Sterile plastic container; ice

Test Procedure:
1. Label the collection container. *Correctly identifies the client and the test to be performed.*
2. Discard the first morning void. Then begin the time of the collection for the next 24 hr, including the void at the end of the 24 hr, and record the last voiding time. *An exact 24-hr count ensures accurate results.*
3. If the client has an indwelling catheter in place, keep the drainage bag on ice and empty the urine into the urine container periodically during the 24-hr period.
4. Keep urine cool during collection. *Higher temperatures alter the results.*
5. If any urine is lost, discard the entire specimen and begin collection again the next day.

Clinical Implications and Indications:
1. Diagnoses primary hyperoxaluria, which is characterized by excessive amounts of oxalate in tissues in the absence of pyridoxine (vitamin B_{12}) deficiency
2. Diagnoses acquired hyperoxaluria associated with regional ileitis, colitis, Crohn's disease, celiac disease, pancreatic disorders, ethylene glycol intoxication, cirrhosis, and postoperative intestinal bypass or surgical loss of distal small intestine
3. Diagnoses idiopathic hyperoxaluria, which occurs in some individuals who have diets high in vitamin C or oxalate or have a vitamin B_{12} deficiency
4. Decreased levels are found with renal failure or hypercalciuria

Nursing Care:
Before Test: Explain the test procedure and the purpose of the test. Assess the client's knowledge of the test. Ensure client knows there are diet restrictions (listed in Interfering Factors) and not to take vitamin C within 24 hr prior to the test or while the urine is being collected. Instruct client not to discard any urine over the 24-hr time period.
During Test: Adhere to standard precautions. If any urine is accidentally discarded or contaminated with feces, discard entire specimen and begin test again the following morning.
After Test: Document urine quantity, date, and exact hours of collection on requisition.

Interfering Factors: Urine contaminated with feces; spillage or inaccurate collection of the 24-hr specimen, including nonrefrigeration or placing on ice; heavy bleeding during menstruation; calcium and vitamin C ingestion; ingestion of oxalate-containing foods, such as beans, beets, chocolate, cocoa, cola, gelatin, rhubarb, strawberries, tomatoes, and tea

URINE

Nursing Considerations:

Pediatric: *For collection of 24-hr specimen a collection bag or indwelling catheter needs to be used for infants and toddlers.*

Listing of Related Tests: Urine and serum calcium; KUB x-ray; IVP; renal ultrasound

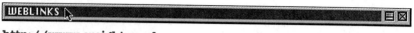

WEBLINKS

http://www.creighton.edu

Phenistix
(fe-***NIS***-tiks)
(urine for PKU)

10 min.

Type of Test: Urine

Body Systems and Functions: Metabolic system

Normal Findings: Negative dipstick (green color does not appear)

Test Results Time Frame: Immediate visualization

Test Description: Phenylketonuria (PKU) is an autosomal, recessive inborn error of metabolism that occurs due to an enzyme deficiency that prevents phenylalanine hydroxylase from being synthesized into tyrosine. Increasing levels of phenylalanine accumulate and are excreted in the urine. Ultimately they may cause irreversible severe mental retardation. Urine screening can be used reliably after the first month and a half of life and once dietary control for PKU has been established. Urine may be tested with a solution of 10% ferric chloride solution or dipped with a test strip that contains a ferric salt. Regular monitoring of actual phenylalanine blood levels is necessary to monitor efficacy of treatment.

CLINICAL ALERT:
False negatives may occur if the test is performed prior to 2 days after birth, since enzyme activity will not have reached normal levels.

Consent Form: Not required

List of Equipment: Phenistix testing strips and associated color chart; alternative is 10% ferric chloride solution

Test Procedure:

1. The newborn must have ingested formula or milk for at least 2 days. *Prior to this the phenylalanine levels would not have normalized.*
2. A Phenistix test strip is pressed into the urine on the infant's diaper. For the older child, the test strip can be dipped directly into a urine sample. The test strip is compared against the color chart that accompanies the product. Ten percent ferric chloride can also be dropped directly on the fresh urine. *Change in color to green is a positive result.*

URINE

3. A positive result requires a follow-up phenylalanine blood level in the previously undiagnosed individual (see Phenylalanine).

Clinical Implications and Indications:
1. Screens for phenylketonuria in the newborn.
2. Infants that are low birth weight as well as individuals with galactosemia or hepatic encephalopathy will also test positive.

Nursing Care:
Before Test: Explain the test procedure and the purpose of the test. Assess the client's knowledge of the test. When an infant is being tested, assess caregiver's understanding of purpose of the test and how it is performed. Review the use of the test strips and how to read them.

During Test: Adhere to standard precautions.

After Test: For adult and child clients, dietary practices and usual testing schedules should be reviewed. Recent research supports both men and women who are PKU positive to maintain the appropriate diet.

Interfering Factors: Sample tested too early from newborn; sample tested from newborn who has not received milk in the first 24–48 hr of life; medications that alter results are antibiotics, salicylates, and chlorpromazine; ketonuria; vomiting/diarrhea; feeding problems; prolonged time period between collection and testing of the urine

Nursing Considerations:
Pregnancy: Women with PKU should be instructed to maintain a low-phenylalanine diet if attempting to conceive and when pregnant.

Pediatric: Review the infant's feeding pattern with the caregiver. Ensure that the caregiver understands that a positive result requires follow-up with a health care provider and a change in the infant's diet.

Listing of Related Tests: Serum phenylalanine level; Guthrie test; serum tyrosine

WEBLINKS 🔲🔀

www.pkunews.org

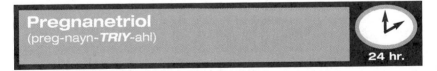

Pregnanetriol
(preg-nayn-*TRIY*-ahl)

24 hr.

URINE

Type of Test: Urine

Body Systems and Functions: Endocrine system

Normal Findings: Normal laboratory findings vary among laboratory settings.

| Adult females | 0.5–2.0 mg/24 hr |
| Adult males | 0.4–2.4 mg/24 hr |

Children:

<6 years	.08<0.1 mg/24 hr
7–16 years	0.3–1.1 mg/24 hr
Males	0.2–0.6 mg/24 hr
Females	0.1–0.6 mg/24 hr

Test Results Time Frame: Within 24 hr

Test Description: Pregnanetriol testing measures the metabolite of 17-hydroxyprogesterone, which is involved in the synthesis of adrenal corticoids. Normally pregnanetriol is excreted in only small amounts in the urine. However, a deficiency of the enzyme that converts 17-hydroxyprogesterone to cortisol causes pregnanetriol to accumulate and be excreted. Because cortisol synthesis is impaired, the adenohypothesis is stimulated to secrete more ACTH. Excessive 17-hydroxyprogesterone may be converted to androgens causing virilization in women and sexual precocity in boys. Pregnanetriol should not be confused with pregnanediol, which is an inactive end product of the metobolism of progesterone and increases during the luteal phase of the menstrual cycle and during pregnancy.

Consent Form: Not required

List of Equipment: Sterile plastic container; ice

Test Procedure:
1. Label the collection container. *Correctly identifies the client and the test to be performed.*
2. Discard the first morning void. Then begin the time of the collection for the next 24 hr, including the void at the end of the 24 hr, and record the last voiding time. *An exact 24-hr count ensures accurate results.*
3. If the client has an indwelling catheter in place, keep the drainage bag on ice and empty the urine into the urine container periodically during the 24-hr period.
4. Keep urine cool during collection. *Higher temperatures alter the results.*
5. If any urine is lost, discard the entire specimen and begin collection again the next day.

Clinical Implications and Indications:
1. Diagnoses adrenogenital syndrome
2. Diagnoses congenital adrenocortical hyperplasia
3. Evaluates causes of hirsutism and virilization
4. Diagnoses Stein-Leventhal syndrome

Nursing Care:
Before Test: Explain the test procedure and the purpose of the test. Assess the client's knowledge of the test. Instruct client not to discard any urine over the 24-hr time period.
During Test: Adhere to standard precautions. If any urine is accidentally discarded or contaminated with feces, discard entire specimen and begin test again the following morning.
After Test: Document urine quantity, date, and exact hours of collection on requisition. Support client if related to potential body image changes.

URINE

Interfering Factors: Urine contaminated with feces; spillage or inaccurate collection of the 24-hr specimen, including nonrefrigeration or placing on ice; heavy bleeding during menstruation; vigorous exercise during the collection period increases androgen release.

Nursing Considerations:
Pediatric: For collection of 24-hr specimen a collection bag or indwelling catheter needs to be used for infants and toddlers.

Listing of Related Tests: Serum 17-hydroxyprogesterone; serum cortisol; urinary 17-ketosteroids

WEBLINKS

www.kumc.edu

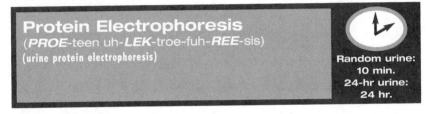

Protein Electrophoresis
(*PROE*-teen uh-*LEK*-troe-fuh-*REE*-sis)
(urine protein electrophoresis)

Random urine:
10 min.
24-hr urine:
24 hr.

Type of Test: Urine

Body Systems and Functions: Renal/urological system

Normal Findings: Total protein:

Albumin	37.9%
Alpha-1 globulin	27.3%
Alpha-2 globulin	19.5%
Beta globulin	8.8%
Gamma globulin	3.3%

Test Results Time Frame: Within 24–48 hr

Test Description: Protein electrophoresis measures the quantitative amount of proteins in the urine. Normally the urine contains very little protein with perhaps a trace of albumin and small amounts of alpha-1 and alpha-2 globulin. Normal renal function allows proteinuria with pregnancy, dehydration, and vigorous exercise. Functional proteinuria occurs in congestive heart failure, fever, and exposure to cold. Electrophoresis separates the proteins in the specimen into band patterns depending on their size, shape, and electrical charge.

Consent Form: Not required

List of Equipment: Sterile plastic container; ice

Test Procedure:
Random specimen:
  1. Label a sterile urine container. *Correctly identifies the client and the test to be performed.*

URINE

2. Obtain a clean-catch specimen of urine (note: first morning voiding preferred, at least 10–29 mL). *Ensures accurate results.*
3. Keep specimen cool. *High temperatures alter the results.*
4. Send specimen to laboratory.

24-hr specimen:
1. Label the collection container. *Correctly identifies the client and the test to be performed.*
2. Discard the first morning void. Then begin the time of the collection for the next 24 hr, including the void at the end of the 24 hr, and record the last voiding time. *An exact 24-hr count ensures accurate results.*
3. If the client has an indwelling catheter in place, keep the drainage bag on ice and empty the urine into the urine container periodically during the 24-hr period.
4. Keep urine cool during collection. *Higher temperatures alter the results.*
5. If any urine is lost, discard the entire specimen and begin collection again the next day.

Clinical Implications and Indications:
1. Diagnoses glomerular and tubular renal disease.
2. Diagnoses effect on the kidney of systemic diseases that cause proteinuria.
3. Detects Bence Jones proteinuria, which is a symptom of monoclonal gammopathies and multiple myeloma.
4. Elevated levels are found with cancer (particularly multiple myeloma), monoclonal gammopathies, crushing injuries and burns, acute infections, and systemic lupus erythematosus.

Nursing Care:
Before Test: Explain the test procedure and the purpose of the test. Assess the client's knowledge of the test. Instruct client not to discard any urine over the 24-hr time period.
During Test: Adhere to standard precautions. If any urine is accidentally discarded or contaminated with feces, discard entire specimen and begin test again the following morning.
After Test: 24-hr urine: Document urine quantity, date, and exact hours of collection on requisition.

Interfering Factors: Urine contaminated with feces; spillage or inaccurate collection of the 24-hr specimen, including nonrefrigeration or placing on ice; heavy bleeding during menstruation; medications that alter results are amphotericin B, amikacin, gentamicin, kanamycin, penicillin, sulfonamides, gold sodium thiomalate, and trimethadione.

Nursing Considerations:
Pregnancy: Normal pregnancy may cause mild proteinuria. Preeclampsia often causes high amounts of proteinuria.
Pediatric: 24-hr urine: For collection of 24-hr specimen a collection bag or indwelling catheter needs to be used for infants and toddlers. Random urine: A collection bag or insertion of a straight catheter is likely needed for infants and toddlers.

Listing of Related Tests: Creatinine clearance; serum protein electrophoresis; serum total protein

URINE

```
WEBLINKS
```
http://webmd.lycos.com

Schilling Test
(**SHIL**-ing)
(vitamin B_{12} absorption test)

24 hr.

Type of Test: Urine

Body Systems and Functions: Hematological system

Normal Findings: Over 10% of vitamin B_{12} is absorbed and >7% of a 1-mg dose of vitamin B_{12} is excreted within the first 24 hr.

Test Results Time Frame: Within 24–48 hr

Test Description: The Schilling test measures the absorption of vitamin B_{12}, which indicates if the client lacks intrinsic factor. Vitamin B_{12} is normally combined with intrinsic factor from the stomach and is then absorbed in the ileum. Any excess vitamin B_{12} is excreted in the urine, which is the rationale for performing this test. A parenteral injection of vitamin B_{12} is administered, and a 24-hr urine sample is collected to determine whether the intrinsic factor is deficient.

CLINICAL ALERT:
Have emergency equipment readily available in the event of an anaphylactic reaction to the dye.

Consent Form: Not required

List of Equipment: Needle and syringe; alcohol swab; vitamin B_{12}; sterile plastic container; ice; cyanocobalamin (0.5 mCi) CO-57

Test Procedure:
1. Administer cyanocobalamin (0.5 mCi) CO-57 in capsule form. Then 2 hr later, give vitamin B_{12} parenterally.
2. Label the urine collection container. *Correctly identifies the client and the test to be performed.*
3. Begin the time of the collection for the next 24 hr, including the void at the end of the 24 hr, and record the last voiding time. *An exact 24-hr count ensures accurate results.*
4. If the client has an indwelling catheter in place, keep the drainage bag on ice and empty the urine into the urine container periodically during the 24-hr period.
5. Keep urine cool during collection. *Higher temperatures alter the results.*
6. If any urine is lost, discard the entire specimen and begin collection again the next day.
7. If excretion is low (<7%), repeat the test.

Clinical Implications and Indications:
1. Diagnoses Crohn's disease, alcoholism, folic acid anemia, gastritis, pernicious anemia, macrocytic anemia, and small intestine malabsorption

Nursing Care:
Before Test: Explain the test procedure and the purpose of the test. Assess the client's knowledge of the test. Instruct client not to discard any urine over the 24-hr time period. Instruct client to fast for 8–12 hr prior to the test. Inform

URINE

client to not take vitamin B or laxatives for 3 days prior to test.
During Test: Adhere to standard precautions. Normal diet is resumed after injection of vitamin B_{12}. Assess for allergic reactions to contrast medium. If any urine is accidentally discarded or contaminated with feces, discard entire specimen and begin test again the following morning.
After Test: Assess for allergic reactions to contrast medium. When urine is handled, use rubber gloves for 24 hr after the specimen is collected. Document urine quantity, date, and exact hours of collection on requisition.

Potential Complications: Anaphylaxis due to allergic reaction to radionuclide material

Contraindications: Pregnancy; breast-feeding

Interfering Factors: Urine contaminated with feces; spillage or inaccurate collection of the 24-hr specimen, including nonrefrigeration or placing on ice; radioactive scan within previous 7 days; diabetes mellitus; kidney disease; hypothyroidism; liver disease; myxedema; pancreatic insufficiency; partial gastrectomy; laxative use

Nursing Considerations:
Pregnancy: Radionuclide should be avoided in pregnant women if possible.
Pediatric: Radionuclide may be harmful to the fetus, and therefore this test is only performed if absolutely necessary. Young children may require sedation. For collection of 24-hr specimen a collection bag or indwelling catheter needs to be used for infants and toddlers.

WEBLINKS	▤ ▨

http://www.methodisthealth.com

Specific Gravity
(spuh-*SIF*-ik *GRAEV*-uh-tee)
(SG; SGU; sp.gr.)

15 min.

Type of Test: Urine

Body Systems and Functions: Renal/urological system

Normal Findings:

		SI units
Adults	1.016–1.030	1.016–1.022
Newborns	1.012	1.012
Infants	1.002–1.006	1.002–1.006

Test Results Time Frame: Immediately to within 24 hr

Test Description: Specific gravity measures the ratio of the density of urine as compared to the density of an equal volume of water (density 1.00). Specific gravity of urine is an indicator of the kidney's ability to reabsorb water and chemicals from the glomerular filtrate. Specific gravity also evaluates

URINE

hydration status and detects problems with antidiuretic hormone levels. Specific gravity is noninvasive, and for a more thorough evaluation of renal concentrating ability, urine osmolality is determined, as well as other concentration tests. There are three ways to obtain the specific gravity. The quickest way to get results is the urine dipstick. This test is available on some nursing units, in home health, and in outpatient clinics. Most laboratories use the refractometer, or total solids (TS) meter. Some machines require only one drop of urine. Other machines need up to 50 mL. The third method involves a urinometer, which is a glass bobber with a weighted bottom, and a calibrated scale is attached to the top. Urine is placed in a graduated cylinder and the urinometer floats in at least 30 mL of urine, and the specific gravity is read from the calibrated scale.

Consent Form: Not required

List of Equipment: Urinometer (hydrometer); sterile plastic container; dipstick

Test Procedure:
1. Label a sterile urine container. *Correctly identifies the client and the test to be performed.*
2. Obtain a clean-catch specimen of 30 mL urine. *Ensures accurate results.*
3. Keep specimen cool. *High temperatures alter the results.*
4. Send specimen to laboratory.
5. If using a urinometer and not sending the urine to the laboratory, place the urine into the urinometer on a level surface.
6. Read the level of the urine as it corresponds to the numerical scale on the glass cylinder.

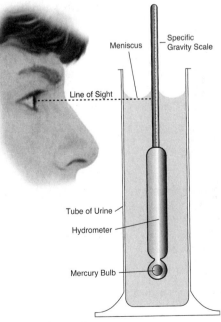

Meniscus

Specific
Gravity Scale

Line of Sight

Tube of Urine

Hydrometer

Mercury Bulb

Urinometer

URINE

Clinical Implications and Indications:

1. Elevated levels are found with congestive heart failure, diarrhea, fever, fluid volume deficit, proteinuria, SIADH, vomiting, and toxemia.
2. Decreased levels are found with diabetes insipidus, chronic renal failure, fluid volume excess, intracranial pressure increases, and malignant hypertension.
3. The specific gravity of urine is dependent on the client's hydration status. This can be very important in sports medicine.
4. Non-insulin-dependent diabetes mellitus can have specific gravity readings from 1.000 to 1.088, depending on the glucose content.

Nursing Care:

Before Test: Explain the test procedure and the purpose of the test. Assess the client's knowledge of the test. Instruct client not to discard any urine over the 24-hr time period.
During Test: Adhere to standard precautions. If any urine is accidentally discarded or contaminated with feces, discard entire specimen and begin test again. Keep urine at room temperature.
After Test: Document specific gravity measurement amount if not done in laboratory.

Interfering Factors:
Urine contaminated with feces; spillage or inaccurate collection of the urine specimen; not keeping urine at room temperature; hydration status

Nursing Considerations:

Pregnancy: Vasopressinase-induced diabetes insipidus may be detected in the last trimester of pregnancy. This condition can resolve spontaneously.
Pediatric: A collection bag or insertion of a straight catheter is likely needed for infants and toddlers.
Home Care: Home health care provider can obtain equipment to perform specific gravity in home setting. Home health providers need to be sure that urine dipsticks are not left in the car where they could be exposed to extreme heat or freezing temperatures.

Listing of Related Tests:
Urinalysis; urine osmolality

WEBLINKS

http://www.rnceus.com/ua/uasg

Thiocyanate
(thiy-oe-*SIY*-uh-nayt)

10 min.

URINE

Type of Test: Urine

Body Systems and Functions: Metabolic system

Normal Findings: Absence of thiocyanate

Test Results Time Frame: Within 6 hr

Test Description: Urine testing for thiocyanate serves as a screening. Thiocyanate is often a metabolite that is found in a variety of chemicals and some medications. Presence in the urine indicates ingestion or exposure to these chemicals and might indicate toxicity. Thiocyanate is a metabolite of cyanide and the vasodilator nitroprusside sodium.

Consent Form: Not required

List of Equipment: Sterile plastic container; ice

Test Procedure:
1. Label a sterile urine container. *Correctly identifies the client and the test to be performed.*
2. Obtain a clean-catch specimen of 10 mL urine. *Ensures accurate results.*
3. Keep specimen cool. *High temperatures alter the results.*
4. Send specimen to laboratory.

Clinical Implications and Indications:
1. Presence of thiocyanate in the urine indicates exposure to toxic chemicals.

Nursing Care:
Before Test: Explain the test procedure and the purpose of the test. Assess the client's knowledge of the test.
During Test: Adhere to standard precautions. If any urine is accidentally discarded or contaminated with feces, discard specimen.
After Test: Document urine quantity, date, and exact hours of collection on requisition. Monitor for signs of drug toxicity and renal failure.

Interfering Factors: Urine contaminated with feces; spillage or inaccurate collection of the urine specimen including nonrefrigeration or placing on ice; heavy bleeding during menstruation

Nursing Considerations:
Pediatric: A collection bag or insertion of a straight catheter is likely needed for infants and toddlers.

WEBLINKS

www.druglibrary.org

Toxicology Screening
(*TAHKS*-uh-*KAHL*-uh-jee)

10 min.

URINE

Type of Test: Urine

Body Systems and Functions: Renal/urological system

Normal Findings: No signs of drugs in urine

Test Results Time Frame: Within 48 hr

Test Description: Toxicology screening that evaluates urine for the presence of drugs is the most common toxicology screening tool. The metabolites of many drugs are excreted in the urine, which allows for their detection. Toxicology screening is becoming increasingly useful as places of employment are requiring drug screening as a condition of employment. Urine testing is relatively easy to teach in its procurement and somewhat inexpensive by comparison to other diagnostic testing methods. Toxicology testing is also used in cases of suspected drug use, victims of motor vehicle accidents, and clients admitted to emergency departments in a comatose state.

CLINICAL ALERT:
There are many ethical and legal implications when toxicology results are positive. Positive test results should be confirmed with equally sensitive tests (e.g., blood tests).

Consent Form: Required

List of Equipment: Sterile plastic container; plastic bag

Test Procedure:
1. A trained individual may observe the urine procurement or privacy is provided and a dye is put in the toilet and temperature strips on urine containers. *Provides assurance that the urine is a fresh specimen from the client.*
2. Obtain a clean-catch specimen of urine and place in plastic bag (note: first morning voiding preferred, at least 50 mL). *Ensures accurate results.*
3. The plastic bag is placed in a sealed sack and marked with tamper-proof tape. *Assures that correct urine sample is tested.*
4. Each person who handles the sample signs a document, which follows the sample. *Assures that correct urine sample is tested.*
5. The specimen is kept for a minimum of 30 days after evaluation of the specimen. *In the event retesting is necessary.*
6. Positive test should be confirmed with a different test method (e.g., blood test). *Urine tests are not 100% accurate.*
7. Results of testing can only be released to authorized personnel. *Protects client confidentiality.*

Clinical Implications and Indications:
1. Any signs of the following drugs are considered positive toxicology tests: amphetamines, barbiturates, benzodiazepines, cannabenoids, cocaine metabolite, codeine, methadone, methaqualone, morphine, phencyclidine, and propoxyphene.
2. It is important to note that many hallucinogens like LSD will not show up in urine testing (note: alcohol is most accurately tested using blood samples).

Nursing Care:
Before Test: Explain the test procedure and the purpose of the test. Assess the client's knowledge of the test. Instruct client as to who will get test results.
During Test: Adhere to standard precautions. If indicated, observe client urine collection.
After Test: Follow procedure for handling specimen. Document urine quantity, date, and exact hours of collection on requisition.

URINE

Interfering Factors: Urine contaminated with feces; inaccurate collection of the urine specimen; heavy bleeding during menstruation; detergents in urine; table salt in urine; low specific gravity of urine; low or high pH of urine

Nursing Considerations:

Pediatric: There could be rare instances where an infant or toddler would need the toxicology screening, and if so, a collection bag or insertion of a straight catheter is likely needed.

Listing of Related Tests: Blood toxicology testing

WEBLINKS

www.recoveryctr.org

Twenty-Four-Hour Urine

(*TWEN*-te for owr *UR*-in)

(24-hr urine; long-term urine specimen)

24 hr.

Type of Test: Urine

Body Systems and Functions: Renal/urological system

Normal Findings: See specific element testing for (note: the 24-hr urine can test for up to 70 different items).

24-hr urine analysis

Test	Preservative
Acid mucopolysaccharides	20 mL toluene
Aldosterone	1 g boric acid/100 mL urine
Amylase	None
Arsenic	None
Cadmium	None
Calcium	None
Catecholamines	20 mL normal acetic acid
Chloride	None
Copper	None
Cortisol (free)	None
Creatinine	None
Creatinine clearance	None
Cyclic AMP	None
Cystine	None
Delta-aminolevulinic acid	1 mL of 33% glacial acetic acid/10 mL urine
Electrolytes Na	None
Estrogens	None
5-HIAA (serotonin)	1 g boric acid
Histamine	None

URINE

Homogentisic acid	None
Hydroxyproline	None
FSH/LH	1 g boric acid
17-Hydroxycorticosteroids	1 g boric acid
17-Ketogenic steroid	1 g boric acid
17-Ketosteroids (total)	1 g boric acid
Magnesium	None
Metanephrine (total)	2 mL acetic acid
Oxalate	None
Phosphorus (inorganic)	None
Pregnanediol	None
Protein (total)	None
Porphobilinogens	None
Potassium	None
Porphyrins	None
Thiocyanate	None
Urea nitrogen	None
Uric acid	None
Vanillylmandelic acid (VMA)	20 mL SN acetic acid before collection

Test Results Time Frame: Within 48 hr

Test Description: A 24-hr urine is collected to more accurately measure the components of urine over time. A single sample is often inaccurate since the kidney excretes substances at different rates and amounts throughout the day; therefore, a 24-hr sample will give a more valid overall evaluation of kidney function. All urine is collected during the 24-hr period. Depending on the elements being examined, various preservatives may be required.

CLINICAL ALERT:
Hospitalized clients using bedpans should be reminded to void before having a bowel movement to prevent contamination of the specimen. Toilet paper should not be placed in the bedpan as it absorbs urine and decreases the amount saved.

Consent Form: Not required

List of Equipment: Sterile plastic container; ice; necessary preservatives

Test Procedure:
1. Label the collection container. *Correctly identifies the client and the test to be performed.*
2. Discard the first morning void. Then begin the time of the collection for the next 24 hr, including the void at the end of the 24 hr, and record the last voiding time. *An exact 24-hr count ensures accurate results.*
3. If the client has an indwelling catheter in place, keep the drainage bag on ice and empty the urine into the urine container periodically during the 24-hr period.
4. Keep urine cool during collection. *Higher temperatures alter the results.*
5. If any urine is lost, discard the entire specimen and begin collection again the next day.

URINE

Clinical Implications and Indications:
1. Evaluates various indications related to renal function and toxicology
2. Monitors the levels of specific substances identified in the urine and the effectiveness of the intervention therapies

Nursing Care:
Before Test: Explain the test procedure and the purpose of the test. Assess the client's knowledge of the test. Explain the consequences of not collecting a voiding to encourage client compliance. If a preservative is added to the container, inform client to take extra precautions to avoid urine spillage. Instruct client not to discard any urine over the 24-hr time period.

During Test: Adhere to standard precautions. If any urine is accidentally discarded or contaminated with feces, discard entire specimen and begin test again the following morning. Continue to keep urine refrigerated if required.

After Test: Document urine quantity, date, and exact hours of collection on requisition.

Interfering Factors: Urine contaminated with feces; spillage or inaccurate collection of the 24-hr specimen, including nonrefrigeration or placing on ice; heavy bleeding during menstruation; improper preservative

Nursing Considerations:
Pediatric: For collection of 24-hr specimen a collection bag or indwelling catheter needs to be used for infants and toddlers.

WEBLINKS ◨◱

http://www.kumc.edu

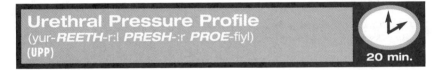

Urethral Pressure Profile
(yur-*REETH*-r:l *PRESH*-:r *PROE*-fiyl)
(UPP)

20 min.

Type of Test: Urine

Body Systems and Functions: Renal/urological system

Normal Findings: Altered pressures of the urethra and sphincter

Test Results Time Frame: Within 24–48 hr

Test Description: Urethral pressure profile involves the placement of a special catheter into the client's bladder. This catheter is attached to a transducer that measures the pressure of the urethra and sphincter. Pressures are recorded at each of the marked areas on the catheter as the catheter is slowly withdrawn from the bladder. The length of the urethra is also recorded. A variety of sphincter and urethral disorders are identified with this test.

Consent Form: Not required

List of Equipment: Urethral pressure catheter; betadine solution; gauze pads; sterile gloves

URINE

Test Procedure:
1. Place client in semi-Fowler's position.
2. Prepare equipment and clean the meatus with betadine or appropriate antimicrobial. *Reduces potential for infection.*
3. Lubricate the catheter tip and slowly insert into the bladder. *Lubrication reduces discomfort.*
4. Slowly withdraw the catheter, recording pressures at each marked area on the catheter. *Differences in pressures indicate stricture or narrowing.*
5. Measure the difference between the start and end of the urethra to determine the length. *The functional length of the urethra is important for diagnosis of the malfunction.*

Clinical Implications and Indications:
1. Low pressures at the sphincter indicate dysfunction.
2. High or variations in pressure along the urethra indicate narrowing or strictures, which may lead to incontinence, bladder infections, and inability to empty the bladder.

Nursing Care:
Before Test: Explain the test procedure and the purpose of the test. Assess the client's knowledge of the test.
During Test: Adhere to standard precautions. Sedation is not used since client participation is required. Instruct client to remain still.
After Test: Encourage the client to increase fluids to dilute the urine. Explain that minor burning, discomfort, and slight bleeding may be noticed during the first urination and that these clinical manifestations are normal.

Potential Complications: A urinary tract infection could occur, especially for individuals with existent inflammation.

Interfering Factors: Inability to remain still

Nursing Considerations:
Pediatric: Provide reading materials or other distractions for children.

Listing of Related Tests: Cystometrogram; rectal electromyogram; cystourethrogram

WEBLINKS

http://www.creighton.edu

Urinalysis
(yur-uh-*NAEL*-uh-sis)
(UA; urine examination; routine urinalysis)

10 min.

URINE

Type of Test: Urine

Body Systems and Functions: Renal/urological system

Normal Findings:

pH	4.5–8; mean 6
Specific gravity	1.010–1.030; usually about 1.015–1.025
Protein	Usually negative
Sugar	Usually negative (may be trace in normal pregnancy)
Ketone	Negative
Nitrites	Negative
Leukocyte esterase	Negative
Microscopic sediment:	
Crystals	Little significance
Casts	Most are pathological (some hyaline casts normal)
WBCs	Few less than 4–5 per high power
RBCs	Occasional less than 2–3 per high power

CRITICAL VALUES:

Color/appearance	Clear/straw
pH	The importance of pH is primarily an indication of acid-base disorders and maintenance of the urine pH for certain urinary conditions.
Specific gravity	1.001–1.010 (low);1.025–1.035 (high)
Protein	Positive
Glucose	Positive
Ketones	Positive
Nitrites	Positive
Leukocyte esterase	Positive
Crystals	Urate crystals may indicate gout. Phosphate and calcium crystals may indicate hyperparathyroidism or malabsorption.
Casts	WBC casts indicate pyelonephritis; RBC casts indicate glomerulonephritis. Hyaline casts indicate proteinuria.
WBCs	>5 indicates urinary tract infection
RBCs	≥5 indicates microscopic hematuria

Test Results Time Frame: Within 24–48 hr

Test Description: A urinalysis provides a wide spectrum of data from which tentative diagnoses can be made. The urinalysis may indicate the need for further studies. Kidney and urinary tract infections can be screened. Diseases unrelated to the kidney can be detected. A small sample of urine is used for a dipstick test. Microscopic examination can be requested if the dipstick reveals pathology.

CLINICAL ALERT:

Report unusual color of urine. Ask the client about recent injury or infections, which may have caused the discoloration. If the pH is 9, suspect that the specimen was old or contaminated, since urine never reaches a pH of 9. Blood in the urine is an indication of renal or urinary tract disease. If repeated tests reveal blood, the client should receive further examination. Protein in urine may be an indication of glomerular disease or

URINE

nephrotic syndrome. Glucose of 4+ is a critical value. Screen the drugs the client is taking to see if they affect glucose results. If a urinalysis tests positive for both leukocyte esterase and nitrites, the urine should be cultured for bacteria.

Consent Form: Not required

List of Equipment: Sterile plastic container; ice; dipsticks

Test Procedure:

1. Label a sterile urine container. *Correctly identifies the client and the test to be performed.*
2. Obtain a clean-catch specimen of urine (note: first morning voiding preferred, at least 15 mL). *Ensures accurate results.*
3. Keep specimen cool. *High temperatures alter the results.*
4. Send specimen to laboratory or dipstick the urine. *The urine needs to be tested fresh for accuracy.*

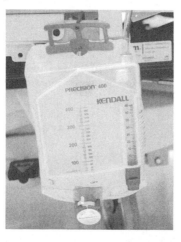

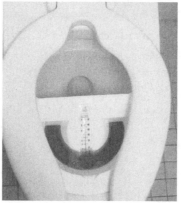

Measuring Urine Output: (A) Foley Drainage Bag; (B) Graduated Container

Clinical Implications and Indications: The following are the variety of components of the urinalysis to be evaluated:

Color/appearance	Blood or pus
Specific gravity	Kidney function test
Hemoglobin	Blood
Glucose	Diabetes
Nitrites	Bacteria in the urine
Ketones	Uncontrolled diabetes, starvation
RBCs	Tumor, calculus, glomerulonephritis
WBCs	Infection
Casts	Kidney disease
Crystals	Calculi

Nursing Care:

Before Test: Explain the test procedure and the purpose of the test. Assess the client's knowledge of the test.

During Test: Adhere to standard precautions. If any urine is accidentally discarded or contaminated with feces, discard entire specimen and begin test again.

After Test: Document urine quantity, date, and exact hours of collection on requisition.

Interfering Factors: Heavy bleeding during menstruation will affect the results; large amounts of vitamin C can give false glucose results; dehydration, contamination with vaginal secretion, and dipstick left in urine too long can all cause false positives for protein; urine contaminated with feces; spillage or inaccurate collection of the specimen, including nonrefrigeration or placing on ice; inadequate cleaning of meatus, excessive time lapse from collection time to testing and contamination can cause false results of the microscopic examination (RBCs, WBCs, casts); certain diets will make the urine more acid or more alkaline; specific gravity will be altered by glucose in the urine and dehydration.

Nursing Considerations:

Pediatric: A collection bag or insertion of a straight catheter is likely needed for infants and toddlers.

Home Care: A urinalysis can be collected by the home health care provider and taken to laboratory, if it is iced and transported immediately after collection. Instruct caregiver to label the sample with date, time, and client name.

Listing of Related Tests: Specific gravity; urine glucose testing

WEBLINKS

http://www.vgernet.net

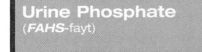

Urine Phosphate
(*FAHS*-fayt)

24 hr.

Type of Test: Urine

Body Systems and Functions: Renal/urological system

Normal Findings: <1,000 mg in 24 hr

Test Results Time Frame: Within 48 hr

Test Description: Urine phosphate is measured with a 24-hr urine, which is collected to more accurately measure the components of urine over time. A single sample is often inaccurate since the kidney excretes substances at different rates and amounts throughout the day; therefore a 24-hr sample will give a more valid overall evaluation of kidney function. All urine is collected to obtain an accurate phosphate level during the 24-hr period.

Consent Form: Not required

List of Equipment: Sterile plastic container; ice

Test Procedure:
1. Label the collection container. *Correctly identifies the client and the test to be performed.*
2. Discard the first morning void. Then begin the time of the collection for the next 24 hr, including the void at the end of the 24 hr, and record the last voiding time. *An exact 24-hr count ensures accurate results.*
3. If the client has an indwelling catheter in place, keep the drainage bag on ice and empty the urine into the urine container periodically during the 24-hr period.
4. Keep urine cool during collection. *Higher temperatures alter the results.*
5. If any urine is lost, discard the entire specimen and begin collection again the next day.

Clinical Implications and Indications:
1. In renal failure the reabsorption of phosphate may be impaired, which decreases the urine phosphate levels.
2. Urine phosphate levels are used primarily as a nutritional indicator since this is a good indication of phosphates in the diet.

Nursing Care:
Before Test: Explain the test procedure and the purpose of the test. Assess the client's knowledge of the test. Instruct client with both verbal and written instructions to ensure compliance. If a preservative is added to the container, tell client to take extra precautions related to spilling the urine. The time is indicated of the first voiding, and this is discarded.
During Test: Adhere to standard precautions. Continue to keep urine refrigerated if required. If any urine is accidentally discarded or contaminated with feces, discard entire specimen and begin test again the following morning.
After Test: The last voiding is included in the collection. Document urine quantity, date, and exact hours of collection on requisition.

Interfering Factors: Utilize the proper preservative; heavy bleeding during menstruation will affect the results; urine contaminated with feces; spillage or inaccurate collection of the 24-hr specimen, including nonrefrigeration or placing on ice

Nursing Considerations:
Pediatric: For collection of 24-hr specimen a collection bag needs to be used for infants and toddlers.

Listing of Related Tests: Urinalysis

```
WEBLINKS
```

http://www.entnet.org

Urobilinogen
(*YUR*-oe-biy-*LIN*-oe-jen)

10 min.

Type of Test: Urine

Body Systems and Functions: Hepatobiliary system

Normal Findings: 0.3–1.0 Ehrlich units in a 2-hr sample

CRITICAL VALUES:
>1.0 Ehrlich units in a 2-hr sample

Test Results Time Frame: Within 48 hr

Test Description: Urobilinogen is a test that assists in evaluating the presence of the substance formed within a complex set of physiological circumstances. Bilirubin is formed from the breakdown of hemoglobin. Bacterial enzymes act on the bilirubin to make urobilinogen in the intestines. Some of the urobilinogen stays in the bowel and is excreted in feces and some enters the bloodstream, where it is further broken down in the liver. There is a smaller amount of urobilinogen that enters the kidneys and is excreted in urine. Unlike bilirubin, urobilinogen is a normal finding in urine. Urobilinogen, however, is colorless. Urine urobilinogen is increased in diseases, which cause an increase in blood breakdown and in liver diseases. Absence of urobilinogen may indicate an obstruction in the bile duct.

CLINICAL ALERT:
Urine urobilinogen breaks done quickly at room temperature and when exposed to light.

Consent Form: Not required

List of Equipment: Sterile plastic container; ice

Test Procedure:
1. Label a sterile urine container. *Correctly identifies the client and the test to be performed.*
2. Obtain a clean-catch specimen of urine (note: the best time for collection is between 1 and 4 PM). *Ensures accurate results and this is the time when excretion rates are highest.*
3. Keep specimen cool. *High temperatures alter the results.*

URINE

4. Protect the specimen from light. *Light causes a breakdown in urobilinogen.*
5. Send specimen to laboratory.

Clinical Implications and Indications:

1. Elevated levels are found with increased destruction of RBCs (e.g., pernicious and hemolytic anemia, malaria) and liver damage (e.g., cirrhosis, acute hepatitis, or biliary disease).
2. Evaluates hemorrhaging into tissues, such as massive bruising or pulmonary injury.

Nursing Care:

Before Test: Explain the test procedure and the purpose of the test. Assess the client's knowledge of the test.
During Test: Adhere to standard precautions. If any urine is accidentally discarded or contaminated with feces, discard entire specimen and begin test again.
After Test: Document urine quantity, date, and exact hours of collection on requisition.

Interfering Factors: Urine contaminated with feces; spillage or inaccurate collection of the urine specimen, including nonrefrigeration or placing on ice; exposure to light; not transporting specimen to laboratory immediately

Nursing Considerations:

Pediatric: A collection bag or insertion of a straight catheter is likely needed for infants and toddlers.

Listing of Related Tests: Urine bilirubin

WEBLINKS

http://www.kumc.edu

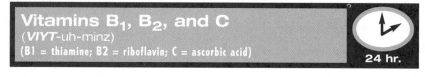

Vitamins B₁, B₂, and C
(*VIYT*-uh-minz)
(B1 = thiamine; B2 = riboflavin; C = ascorbic acid)

24 hr.

Type of Test: Urine

Body Systems and Functions: Gastrointestinal system

Normal Findings:

B1	100–200 µg/24 hr
B2	80–269 mg/g
C	30 µg/24 hr

CRITICAL VALUES:

B1	Measured through transketolase activity, >20%
B2	<30 mg/g
C	<0.2 mg/dL or >2.0 mg/dL

Test Results Time Frame: Within 2 days

URINE

Test Description: Vitamins B1, B2, and C tests for vitamin levels that can detect many abnormalities or conditions. B1, or thiamine, is essential in maintaining a healthy heart and nervous system. Thiamine deficiencies are common in third world countries, producing a disease called beriberi. Thiamin deficiencies in the United States are most frequently seen in alcoholics. Low levels of vitamin C can produce scurvy, which causes hemorrhage and increased need for iron and folic acid. This can lead to various forms of anemia, leukopenia, and thrombocytopenia.

Consent Form: Not required

List of Equipment: Sterile plastic container; ice

Test Procedure:
1. Label the collection container. *Correctly identifies the client and the test to be performed.*
2. Discard the first morning void. Then begin the time of the collection for the next 24 hr, including the void at the end of the 24 hr, and record the last voiding time. *An exact 24-hr count ensures accurate results.*
3. If the client has an indwelling catheter in place, keep the drainage bag on ice and empty the urine into the urine container periodically during the 24-hr period.
4. Keep urine cool during collection. *Higher temperatures alter the results.*
5. If any urine is lost, discard the entire specimen and begin collection again the next day.

Clinical Implications and Indications:
1. B1 deficiency indicates beriberi and Wernicke-Korsakoff syndrome in alcoholics. Branched-chain ketoaciduria may also be caused from thiamine deficiency.
2. B2 deficiency can produce anemia. Riboflavin is necessary for normal RBC function.
3. Lack of vitamin C will produce scurvy, leading to hemorrhage anemia, leukopenia, and sometimes thrombocytopenia. High doses of vitamin C can destroy vitamin B12, leading to B12 deficiency.

Nursing Care:
Before Test: Explain the test procedure and the purpose of the test. Assess the client's knowledge of the test. Instruct client not to discard any urine over the 24-hr time period.
During Test: Adhere to standard precautions. If any urine is accidentally discarded or contaminated with feces, discard entire specimen and begin test again the following morning.
After Test: Document urine quantity, date, and exact hours of collection on requisition.

Interfering Factors: Urine contaminated with feces; spillage or inaccurate collection of the 24-hr specimen, including nonrefrigeration or placing on ice; heavy bleeding during menstruation

Nursing Considerations:
Pregnancy: Vitamins are usually suggested in the prenatal time period as a means of ensuring health in the pregnant woman to both the mother and the fetus.

URINE

Pediatric: For collection of 24-hr specimen a collection bag or indwelling catheter needs to be used for infants and toddlers.
Gerontology: Vitamin deficiencies may exist among the elderly due to their inability to obtain wide varieties of food sources.
International: A variety of vitamin deficiencies may occur in countries with rampant poverty. Consequently, diseases specific to vitamin abnormalities must be assessed by health care providers.

WEBLINKS ▐▌ ▤▨

www.healthgate.com

Water Deprivation
(*WAHT*-:r *DEP*-ruh-*VAY*-sh:n)
(concentration test, urine)

4-20 hr.

Type of Test: Urine

Body Systems and Functions: Renal/urological system

Normal Findings: Specific gravity should be greater than 1.025, or at least 1.020. Below that reflects diabetes insipidus or distal tubular disease with inability to concentrate urine. Osmolality should be greater than 850 mOsm/L. Below that indicates an inability of the body to concentrate urine.

CRITICAL VALUES:
Weight loss >3% of starting weight

Test Results Time Frame: Within 1–2 days

Test Description: The water deprivation test is performed on the client with diabetes insipidus. This disease causes the inability to concentrate urine, and therefore during the water deprivation test the urine will not become concentrated and the serum osmolality will remain high. This is due to the inability of the renal tubules to reabsorb water. Water is withheld for 4–20 hr while the client is closely monitored and the urine tested. During this test antidiuretic hormone (ADH or vasopression) can be given subcutaneously. This hormone stops the massive polyuria and reveals the kidneys effects in the presence of the hormone.

CLINICAL ALERT:
The client with severe diabetes insipidus may become severely dehydrated. The client must be hospitalized and monitored closely during this test. Blood pressure, heart rate, urine osmolality, and urine output should be monitored and recorded every hour. Weigh client every third hour. Report any signs of dizziness, tachycardia, or hypotension. Weight loss greater than 3% of body weight should be reported immediately.

Consent Form: Not required

List of Equipment: Blood pressure cuff; watch; scale; urine cups; urine-measuring device

URINE

Test Procedure:

1. Explain to the client that water will be withheld while vital signs and urine will be monitored.
2. Hold fluids for several hours, documenting the vital signs, urine osmolality, and specific gravity.
3. ADH is injected subcutaneously.
4. Continue to document vital signs, urine amount, specific gravity, and osmolality.
5. One hour after ADH is given, collect urine and blood for osmolality testing.

Clinical Implications and Indications:

1. The client with diabetes insipidus is unable to concentrate urine; therefore during this test the urine will not become concentrated and the serum osmolality with remain high. This is due to the inability of the renal tubules to reabsorb water.
2. Elevated levels with dehydration.
3. Decreased levels are found with congestive heart failure, hypercalcemia, hydronephrosis, polycystic kidneys, pyelonephritis, and sickle cell trait.

Nursing Care:

Before Test: Explain the test procedure and the purpose of the test. Assess the client's knowledge of the test. Provide client with both verbal and written instructions to ensure compliance. Restrict client to 200 mL of fluid with dinner the night before the examination. Explain that they will be very thirsty prior to the test. Instruct client to eat high-protein diet the day before the examination. Ask the client to report any untoward effects of hypotension or tachycardia.
During Test: Adhere to standard precautions. Explain the importance of not drinking during this test.
After Test: Allow client to return to normal diet as tolerated.

Potential Complications: Hypotension; tachycardia; severe dehydration

Contraindications: Subnormal cardiac output

Interfering Factors: Failure to restrict fluids; urine contaminated with feces; spillage or inaccurate collection of the specimen, including nonrefrigeration or placing on ice; not utilizing the proper preservative; heavy bleeding during menstruation; glucosuria

Nursing Considerations:

Pediatric: A collection bag or insertion of a straight catheter is likely needed for infants and toddlers.
Home Care: Clients in home settings often experience dehydration due to their decreased mobility, and therefore this test may be applicable to their condition.

Listing of Related Tests: Specific gravity

URINE

WEBLINKS

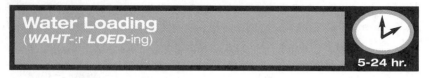

Water Loading
(*WAHT*-:r *LOED*-ing)

5-24 hr.

Type of Test: Urine; blood

Body Systems and Functions: Renal/urological system

Normal Findings:

Serum osmolality	270–290
Urine osmolality, 24 hr	320–920 mOsm/kg H_2O
Random checks	55–1,250 mOsm/kg H_2O

CRITICAL VALUES:
Less than 80% of the water given is excreted in 4–5 hr.

Test Results Time Frame: Within 1–2 days

Test Description: The water loading test is useful in the determination of water and electrolyte disturbances. It can assess hydration, seizures, ADH function, liver disease, and coma. The client is given water to drink over a 30-min period. The urine is measured and osmolarity tested. The serum osmolarity is tested hourly. The urine-to-serum osmolarity ratio and the amount of urine excreted in 4–5 hr can help diagnose a number of conditions.

CLINICAL ALERT:
The urine and serum osmolarities are taken together and compared. When the urine is concentrated, the urine-to-serum osmolarity ratio is high. When the kidneys are unable to concentrate urine, the urine-to-serum osmolality ratio is low. It is always greater than 1.

Consent Form: Not required

List of Equipment: Red-top tube or serum separator tube; needle and syringe or vacutainer; alcohol swab; urine specimen cups; water and urine measuring devices

Test Procedure:
1. Label the collection container. *Correctly identifies the client and the test to be performed.*
2. Discard the first morning void. Then begin the time of the collection for the next 24 hr, including the void at the end of the 24 hr, and record the last voiding time. Three hundred milliliters of water is given to replace fluid lost during the night. *An exact 24-hr count ensures accurate results.* This amount is not counted in the test.
3. The client then drinks 20 mL of water for every kilogram of body weight within 30 min.
4. All urine is measured and tested for hourly serum osmolarity and specific gravity measurements.

5. Greater than 90% of the water given should be excreted within 4–5 hr. The urine osmolality should be less than 100 mOsm/kg and the specific gravity should be less than 1.003.
6. If the client has an indwelling catheter in place, keep the drainage bag on ice and empty the urine into the urine container periodically during the 24-hr period.
7. Keep urine cool during collection. *Higher temperatures alter the results.*
8. If any urine is lost, discard the entire specimen and begin collection again the next day.

Clinical Implications and Indications:
1. If less than 80% of the urine is excreted during the test period, this could be evidence of edema, ascites, obesity, malabsorption syndrome, adrenocortical insufficiency, dehydration, cirrhosis, and CHF.
2. If less than 90% of the urine is secreted yet the urine osmolarity remains above 100 mOsm/kg, this could indicate increased ADH secretion.

Nursing Care:
Before Test: Explain the test procedure and the purpose of the test. Assess the client's knowledge of the test. Instruct client with both verbal and written instructions to ensure compliance. Explain the importance of not drinking water other than that given during the test. Instruct client not to discard any urine over the 24-hr time period. Inform client that they may experience nausea, fullness, fatigue, or the urge to defecate.

During Test: Adhere to standard precautions. Accurate results will not be performed if vomiting occurs. If any urine is accidentally discarded or contaminated with feces, discard entire specimen and begin test again the following morning.

After Test: Allow client to return to normal diet as tolerated. Observe for difficulty breathing, extreme discomfort, or chest pain. Document urine quantity, date, and exact hours of collection on requisition.

Potential Complications: Clients unable to tolerate this test could experience seizures or hyponatremia, which could be fatal.

Interfering Factors: Food, alcohol, or medications before the test; strenuous exercise before the test; urine contaminated with feces; spillage or inaccurate collection of the 24-hr specimen, including nonrefrigeration or placing on ice

Nursing Considerations:
Pediatric: For collection of 24-hr specimen a collection bag or indwelling catheter needs to be used for infants and toddlers.

Listing of Related Tests: Water deprivation test; antidiuretic suppression test

WEBLINKS

URINE

www.healthgate.com

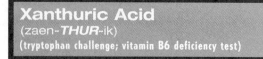

Xanthuric Acid
(zaen-*THUR*-ik)
(tryptophan challenge; vitamin B6 deficiency test)

24 hr.

Type of Test: Urine

Body Systems and Functions: Renal/urological system

Normal Findings: <50 mg/24 hr

CRITICAL VALUES:
>50 mg in 24 hr

Test Results Time Frame: Within 48 hr

Test Description: Xanthuric acid is converted to uric acid by xanthine oxidase and secreted into the urine. Testing is performed by having the client ingest an oral dose of L-tryptophan (xanthuric acid is a major metabolite of the amino acid tryptophan). Test results are measured by the amount of xanthurenic acid in urine after the dosage of tryptophan.

Consent Form: Not required

List of Equipment: Sterile plastic container; ice

Test Procedure:
1. Label the collection container. *Correctly identifies the client and the test to be performed.*
2. Discard the first morning void. Then begin the time of the collection for the next 24 hr, including the void at the end of the 24 hr, and record the last voiding time. *An exact 24-hr count ensures accurate results.*
3. If the client has an indwelling catheter in place, keep the drainage bag on ice and empty the urine into the urine container periodically during the 24-hr period.
4. Keep urine cool during collection. *Higher temperatures alter the results.*
5. If any urine is lost, discard the entire specimen and begin collection again the next day.

Clinical Implications and Indications:
1. Elevated levels are found with poor nutrition, familial xanthurenic acid, and pregnancy.
2. Decreased levels are found with xanthine stones, vitamin B6 deficiency, and xanthinuria.

Nursing Care:
Before Test: Explain the test procedure and the purpose of the test. Assess the client's knowledge of the test. Instruct client not to discard any urine over the 24-hr time period.
During Test: Adhere to standard precautions. If any urine is accidentally discarded or contaminated with feces, discard entire specimen and begin test again the following morning.
After Test: The last voiding is included in the collection. Document urine quantity, date, and exact hours of collection on requisition.

URINE

Interfering Factors: Heavy bleeding during menstruation; urine contaminated with feces; spillage or inaccurate collection of the 24-hr specimen, including nonrefrigeration or placing on ice; increased urine pH; medications that alter results are D-penicillinase, isoniazid, oral contraceptives, and hydralazine.

Nursing Considerations:
Pediatric: For collection of 24-hr specimen a collection bag or indwelling catheter needs to be used for infants and toddlers. In addition, xanthuric crystals are often found in the urine of children with acute lymphocytic leukemia.

WEBLINKS ↳	▤ ⊠

http://www.creighton.edu

URINE

16

Radiologic Studies

EXAMINATION BY RADIOLOGY

Radiologic exams (x-rays) send radiation through the body to form a picture of the internal structures. X-rays turn film black, so areas that allow radiation to pass easily appear dark, while areas that block radiation appear white. Therefore, air-filled lungs appear blackish on an x-ray, while bones appear white. X-rays are used in several basic ways; the most common are standard (plain) films, fluoroscopy, and tomography. In addition, contrast media may be used to enhance visualization.

TYPES OF RADIOLOGIC STUDIES

Plain Films

Plain films are taken without contrast media and detect the presence of gross anomalies. They are relatively easy to administer, and although the client is exposed to radiation from the procedure, the risks are minimal.

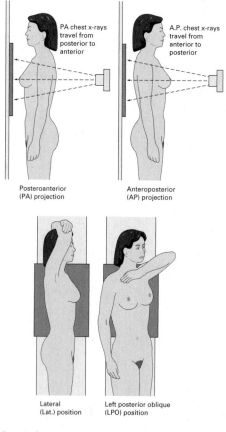

Radiographic projection positions during plain films.

Contrast Films

Contrast films are x-ray studies that involve the administration of a contrast medium. This form of radiologic testing allows for further visualization of the area of focus and is more definitive in its diagnostic ability. In addition, all contrast agents have the potential to induce serious side effects. Some clients receiving a contrast medium with a radiologic study may be at higher risk (see table).

CLIENT PREPARATION FOR RADIOLOGIC STUDIES

Specific Risks of Radiologic Studies

Radiologic studies pose two risks for clients: exposure to radiation and, when contrast agents are used, adverse reactions to the agents. X-rays cause damage to tissue cells and have the potential to induce mutations. Exposure must be kept to minimal levels. Precautionary measures include screening all women for possible pregnancy, as radiation poses a serious risk to a developing fetus. Other screening measures are listed above in the discussion of contrast films. Consent must be given only if the procedure is invasive.

Nursing Considerations during Radiologic Studies

There are a variety of specific considerations for clients having radiologic studies. For example, portable x-ray machines may be brought to the nursing unit if the inpatient client cannot be moved. In addition, clients must be instructed to remain still during the x-ray if they are capable. For many x-rays studies, clients are told to hold in their inhaled breath during the x-ray, with the rationale being to encourage no motion. It also may be necessary to provide sedation to infants and children to ensure good x-ray results. There are usually no dietary restrictions during plain films, but the client is instructed to remove dental prostheses, jewelry, eyeglasses, or any other metal objects like hair clips.

Abdominal Film
(*AB-DO*-min-al film)
(KUB; flat plate of the abdomen; abdominal x-ray)

15 min.

Type of Test: X-ray

Body Systems and Functions: Gastrointestinal system

Normal Findings: Normal abdomen and surrounding structures

Test Results Time Frame: Within 24 hr

Test Description: The abdominal film is taken to aid in the diagnosis of gastrointestinal, biliary system, and urological diseases. It may provide information on the size, shape, and position of the liver, spleen, and kidneys.

> **CLINICAL ALERT:**
> A portable x-ray machine may be brought to the nursing unit if the client cannot be moved.

RADIOLOGIC

Consent Form: Not required

List of Equipment: X-ray machine and related equipment from radiology

Test Procedure:
1. Place client in supine postion on an x-ray table with the arms extended over the head. A protective shield may be placed over the genital region. *Keeps abdomen from being obstructed.*
2. A single film is taken, although if required, another film may be taken in the supine/standing positions.
3. The client is instructed to hold his or her breath when film is taken. *Prevents movement during respiration.*

Clinical Implications and Indications:
1. Evaluates abdominal masses and large tumors (e.g., ovarian or uterine)
2. Diagnoses acute abdominal pain of unknown origin and intestinal obstruction
3. Identifies abnormal air (e.g., bowel perforation/obstruction), fluid (e.g., ascites), or objects in the abdomen
4. Precursor to urological and gastrointestinal tract contrast-mediated studies
5. Detects calcium deposits in blood vessels and lymph nodes, cysts, tumors, and stones
6. Detects abnormal kidney/liver/spleen size, shape, and position
7. Differentiates between gastrointestinal and urological disorders

Nursing Care:
Before Test: Explain the test procedure and the purpose of the test. Assess the client's knowledge of the test. Instruct the client that during the procedure it may be uncomfortable to sit on the hard table or achieve some of the necessary positions; it is important to remain as still as possible during the test; there are no dietary restrictions prior to the test; and it is necessary to remove dental prosthesis, jewelry, eyeglasses, or other metal objects like hair clips before the procedure.
During Test: Adhere to standard precautions. The client is instructed to take a deep breath and hold it or to exhale and not to breathe as the x-ray is taken.
After Test: Monitor bowel sounds in clients who are experiencing abdominal pain (unrelated to the abdominal film procedure).

Contraindications: Abdominal films are not appropriate for some specific conditions, such as hemorrhaging gastrointestinal ulcers, or pregnancy (unless the benefits outweigh the risks to the fetus).

Interfering Factors: Abdominal films should be done after lower GI studies, due to the barium that limits optimal visualization; extreme obesity; ovarian and uterine tumors

Nursing Considerations:
Pregnancy: Radiation should be avoided in pregnant women if possible (note: appropriate lead shielding is done to protect the fetus if it is determined this test is necessary).
Pediatric: Infants and children will need assistance in remaining still during the x-ray and age-appropriate comfort measures following the test.

RADIOLOGIC

Gerontology: *The older person may find it difficult to maintain positions when required to do so for lengthy periods of time.*

Listing of Related Tests: Upper/lower GI studies; abdominal film may be performed prior to an IVP or other renal studies

---

WEBLINKS ⬚⊠

http://adam.excite.com

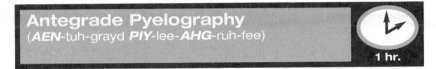

Antegrade Pyelography
(***AEN***-tuh-grayd ***PIY***-lee-***AHG***-ruh-fee)

1 hr.

Type of Test: X-ray

Body Systems and Functions: Renal/urological system

Normal Findings: Normal renal collection system structures; normal renal pressures

Test Results Time Frame: Within 24 hr

Test Description: Antegrade pyelography is percutaneous puncture and injection of contrast dye directly into the renal pelvis. The test provides images of the renal collection system and can be used to check pressure and perfusion of the kidney (Whitaker test). Antegrade pyelography is used to collect direct urine samples, evaluate hydronephrosis, and do calyceal mapping.

> **CLINICAL ALERT:**
> There is the danger of puncture of the kidney and adjacent organs. Therefore health care providers must observe for clinical manifestations of generalized infection (e.g., febrile response, profuse sweating) and symptomatology specific to kidney infection (e.g., flank pain). Have emergency equipment readily available in the event of an anaphylactic reaction to the dye.

Consent Form: Required

List of Equipment: X-ray machine and related equipment from radiology

Test Procedure:
1. Place client in prone position.
2. A 20–22-gauge needle is inserted into the kidney pelvis, guided by ultrasound or fluoroscopy. *Ensures visualization of kidney position.*
3. Urine may be withdrawn. *Allows for either sampling or decompressing the kidney before dye is injected.*
4. Contrast dye is injected into the kidney. *Allows for visualization of structures.*
5. A series of films is taken of the kidney structures.
6. Pressure may be measured via a manometer.

RADIOLOGIC

7. The needle is removed and a sterile dressing is applied. *Prevents contamination and infection of the puncture site.*

Clinical Implications and Indications:

1. Assesses patency and obstruction of the kidney or ureters and the cause of dilitation
2. Evaluates hydrostatic pressures
3. Identifies correct placement of a nephrostomy tube

Nursing Care:

Before Test: Explain the test procedure and the purpose of the test. Assess the client's knowledge of the test. Instruct the client that during the procedure it may be uncomfortable to sit on the hard table or achieve some of the necessary positions; it is important to remain as still as possible during the test; there are no dietary restrictions prior to the test; and it is necessary to remove dental prosthesis, jewelry, eyeglasses, or other metal objects like hair clips before the procedure. Assess for potential allergies to contrast medium. Inform client that during injection of contrast medium, a burning sensation may be felt for a few seconds behind the eyes or in the jaw, teeth, tongue, or lips. Assess for anxiety and provide sedation as ordered. Administer preoperative medication usually 30 min before procedure. Obtain baseline vital signs and neurological assessment.

During Test: Adhere to standard precautions. The client is instructed to take a deep breath and hold it or to exhale and not to breathe as the x-ray is taken and during needle insertion. Instruct client to remain still. Monitor client for signs of intra-abdominal bleeding (e.g., thready pulse, hypotension, abdominal pain, cold, clammy skin). Assess for allergic reactions to contrast medium.

After Test: Assess for allergic reactions to contrast medium. Monitor vital signs until stable, checking for interabdominal bleeding. Monitor intake and output for 24 hr to check for hematuria. Monitor for signs of septicemia (e.g., fever, chills). Have client drink 2–3 L of fluid within 24 hr of the procedure.

Potential Complications: Anaphylaxis due to allergic reaction to iodinated contrast material; perforation; septicemia

Contraindications: Previous history of allergy to iodine, eggs, or shellfish

Nursing Considerations:

Pregnancy: Radiation and intravenous contrast should be avoided in pregnant women if possible (note: appropriate lead shielding is done to protect the fetus if it is determined this test is necessary). There is a potential inability of client to hold still and follow instructions due to the uncomfortable positioning. The obesity from the pregnancy may prevent a needle from reaching the kidney easily and there is a prolonged clotting time due to the pregnancy.

Pediatric: Sedation is recommended for infants and children. Place the infant or child on a blanket for comfort. After postprocedure monitoring is completed and per health care provider's order, the pediatric client is discharged with an adult who is given instructions.

Listing of Related Tests: IVP; renal ultrasound; fluoroscopy

WEBLINKS

http://www.creighton.edu

RADIOLOGIC

Arteriography
(ahr-*TEER*-ee-*AHG*-ruh-fee)
(arteriogram)

**Usually 1–3 hr.
(note: varies
with the site to
be visualized)**

Type of Test: X-ray

Body Systems and Functions: Cardiovascular system

Normal Findings: Normal vessels

Test Results Time Frame: Within 24–48 hr

Test Description: An arteriogram is a radiographic picture of an artery. The picture is taken by injecting a contrast medium into a vessel, usually the femoral or brachial artery, through a catheter. As the medium reaches the area of interest, a series of x-rays are taken to visualize the artery. The arteries are assessed for pathology such as narrowing from atherosclerosis and increased collateral circulation. Common sites of arteriograms are coronary arteries.

CLINICAL ALERT:
Have emergency equipment readily available in the event of an anaphylactic reaction to the dye. Arteriography involves invasive techniques that can place a client at risk. Direct injuries can occur with accidental perforation of a vessel during the test.

Consent Form: Required

List of Equipment: X-ray machine and related equipment from radiology

Test Procedure: (Note: The test procedure varies according to the area to be studied, but the following highlights some common points.)
1. Administer any premedications ordered for the client
2. Place the client on an x-ray table.
3. Initiate an intravenous line. *Allows administration of contrast medium or medications.*
4. A vessel is entered through puncture or cutdown. A catheter may be advanced through the vessel to reach the area to be studied
5. Contrast medium is injected through the catheter
6. Arteriographic films are taken as the contrast medium enters the study area
7. The catheter is removed and pressure applied to the site for 10–15 min. *Prevents hemorrhage.*
8. Bed rest may be required following the procedure.

Clinical Implications and Indications:
1. Arteriograms are done when vessels in the heart or other arteries need to be visualized for abnormalities, obstruction, and hemorrhage.
2. Diagnoses aneurysms.

RADIOLOGIC

Nursing Care:

Before Test: Explain the test procedure and the purpose of the test. Assess the client's knowledge of the test. Assess for potential allergies to contrast medium. Inform client that during injection of contrast medium, a burning sensation may be felt for a few seconds behind the eyes or in the jaw, teeth, tongue, or lips. Assess for anxiety and provide sedation as ordered. Administer preoperative medication usually 30 min before procedure. Obtain baseline vital signs and neurological assessment. Instruct the client that during the procedure it may be uncomfortable to sit on the hard table or achieve some of the necessary positions; it is important to remain as still as possible during the test; there are no dietary restrictions prior to the test; and it is necessary to remove dental prosthesis, jewelry, eyeglasses, or other metal objects like hair clips before the procedure.

During Test: Adhere to strict aseptic technique and standard precautions. Instruct client to lie still and provide reassurance. Monitor vital signs and other vital physical parameters. Assess for allergic reactions to contrast medium. The client is instructed to take a deep breath and hold it or to exhale and not to breathe as the x-ray is taken.

After Test: Monitor vital signs and insertion site. Instruct client to report any signs of infection, fever, or pain at the insertion site. Assess for allergic reactions to contrast medium.

Potential Complications: Nausea/vomiting; cardiac collapse; respiratory arrest; anaphylaxis due to allergic reaction to iodinated contrast material; cerebrovascular accident; renal toxicity

Contraindications: Previous history of allergy to iodine, eggs, or shellfish; anticoagulant therapy; bleeding disorders; dehydration; uncontrolled hypertension

Interfering Factors: Inability to remain still

Nursing Considerations:

Pregnancy: Radiation and intravenous contrast should be avoided in pregnant women if possible (note: appropriate lead shielding is done to protect the fetus if it is determined this test is necessary).

Pediatric: Sedation is recommended for infants and children. Place the infant or child on a blanket for comfort. After postprocedure monitoring is completed and per health care provider's order, the pediatric client is discharged with an adult who is given instructions.

Gerontology: The older person may find it difficult to maintain positions when required to do so for lengthy periods of time during the arteriography.

WEBLINKS 🔲 ☒

http://www.nhlbi.nih.gov

Arthrography
(ahr-*THRAHG*-ruh-fee)

15 min.

Type of Test: X-ray

Body Systems and Functions: Musculoskeletal system

Normal Findings: Intact soft tissue structure of the joint; absence of lesions, fractures, or tears

Test Results Time Frame: Within 24 hr

Test Description: Arthrogaphy is the visualization of a joint by radiographic study, following the injection of radiopaque material into the joint. This test is most commonly performed on the shoulder or knee joint but may also be performed on the hip, ankle, waist, and TMJ. An arthrograph visualizes soft tissue surrounding the joint, including the meniscus, cartilage, ligaments, and joint capsule. Arthrography is useful in identifying both chronic and acute tears of the joint capsule or supporting ligaments. If a tear is present, the contrast medium will leak out of the joint and be visualized on radiograph.

> **CLINICAL ALERT:**
> A portable x-ray machine may be brought to the nursing unit if the client cannot be moved.

Consent Form: Required

List of Equipment: X-ray machine and related equipment from radiology

Test Procedure:
1. Clean the area to be radiographed with an antiseptic solution. *Prevents contamination.*
2. A local anesthetic is administered.
3. A 2-in. needle is inserted into the joint space and the fluid aspirated. With the needle in place, the syringe is removed and replaced with one containing the dye. If fluoroscopic examination shows the needle correctly placed, the dye is injected.
4. After needle removal, the site is rubbed with a sterile sponge. *Prevents air from escaping.*
5. The client is asked to perform range of motion to distribute the dye.
6. A series of films are taken quickly, before the contrast material can be absorbed.

Clinical Implications and Indications:
1. Evaluates persistent unexplained joint pain
2. Identifies abnormalities of synovial membranes, such as synovitis, tumors, or cysts

Nursing Care:
Before Test: Explain the test procedure and the purpose of the test. Assess the client's knowledge of the test. NPO for 8 hr prior to procedure. Assess for potential allergies to contrast medium. Inform client that during injection of contrast medium, a burning sensation may be felt for a few seconds behind the eyes or in

RADIOLOGIC

the jaw, teeth, tongue, or lips. Assess for anxiety and provide sedation as ordered. Administer preoperative medication usually 30 min before procedure. Obtain baseline vital signs and neurological assessment. Instruct the client to remain as still as possible during the procedure, except when instructed to change position. Instruct the client that during the procedure it may be uncomfortable to sit on the hard table or achieve some of the necessary positions; it is important to remain as still as possible during the test; there are no dietary restrictions prior to the test; and it is necessary to remove dental prosthesis, jewelry, eyeglasses, or other metal objects like hair clips before the procedure.

During Test: Adhere to standard precautions. Assess for allergic reactions to contrast medium.

After Test: Assess for allergic reactions to contrast medium. The client is encouraged to rest the joint at least 12 hr. If a knee examination was done, an elastic wrap may be applied. The wrap should remain in place several days. Instruct the client how to rewrap the bandage. Inform the client that he may experience some swelling or discomfort. If this occurs, apply ice and take a mild analgesic. Inform client that crepitant sounds may be heard in the joint, but this will usually disappear in 1–2 days. If symptoms persist, inform client to contact health care provider.

Potential Complications: Anaphylaxis due to allergic reaction to iodinated contrast material

Contraindications: Previous history of allergy to iodine, eggs, or shellfish; pregnancy, unless the benefits outweigh the risks; infectious condition of the joint; exacerbation of arthritis

Interfering Factors: Inability of the client to cooperate during the procedure; incomplete aspiration of the joint, allowing dilution of the contrast material; improper injection of the contrast medium

Nursing Considerations:

Pregnancy: Radiation and intravenous contrast should be avoided in pregnant women if possible (note: appropriate lead shielding is done to protect the fetus if it is determined this test is necessary).

WEBLINKS

http://www.nih.gov

Barium Enema
(*BAYR*-ee-uhm *EN*-uh-muh)
(BE; lower GI)

1 hr.

Type of Test: X-ray

Body Systems and Functions: Gastrointestinal system

Normal Findings: Normal contour, filling, and patency of the colon without distention, overlapping, or torsion

RADIOLOGIC

Test Results Time Frame: Within 24–48 hr

Test Description: A barium enema is a radiological examination of the colon using barium instilled via a rectal tube into the rectum or through an existing colostomy. Fluoroscopy visualizes movement of barium through the large intestine. X-ray is used to spot film various areas of the colon. This test is especially useful in detection of small lesions and polyps. While barium is the agent of choice, a water-soluble solution of iodinated contrast medium may be used. The bowel must be cleaned of fecal materials or prior barium for the test to be a success.

CLINICAL ALERT:
Caution should be used with children, the elderly, or the chronically ill, as the bowel preparation may cause shifts in fluid and electrolyte balance.

Consent Form: Not required

Test Procedure:
1. Place client in supine position for an initial abdominal film.
2. Client is placed in side-lying position and draped. *Provides privacy.*
3. A lubricated rectal tube with a balloon is inserted via the rectum and the balloon is inflated. *Keeps tube in the correct position.*
4. Barium is instilled. (Note: This may cause cramping and a feeling of abdominal fullness with the urge to defecate.)
5. The movement of the barium through the colon to the ileocecal valve is observed by fluoroscopy.
6. The client is assisted with position change to supine, prone, side lying, and erect with films taken in each position. *Ensures accurate results.*
7. When the films are completed, the barium is aspirated and the tube removed.
8. The client is assisted to the bathroom or onto a bedpan. *Expels the remaining barium.*
9. An additional film may be taken following the elimination of the barium.

Clinical Implications and Indications:
1. Determines cause of rectal bleeding, pus, or mucus in the feces
2. Identifies changes in bowel patterns, such as chronic diarrhea, constipation, or diameter of the feces
3. Evaluates unexplained weight loss or anemia
4. Evaluates persistent abdominal pain or distention of unknown etiology
5. Identifies and locates benign or malignant polyps and tumors
6. Evaluates suspected inflammations of the colon or congenital anomalies
7. Evaluates suspected foreign bodies of the colon
8. Evaluates intussusception in children

Nursing Care:
Before Test: Explain the test procedure and the purpose of the test. Assess the client's knowledge of the test. Educate client to dietary regimen and bowel preparation per the institution, which is usually a magnesium citrate liquid, the day prior with administration of suppository or cleansing enemas. In addition, instruct client in the adherence to a low-residue diets for several days prior to the test, with clear liquids the evening prior and NPO the day of the test. Inform the client that bowel preparation may cause cramping and diarrhea.

RADIOLOGIC

During Test: Adhere to standard precautions. Encourage relaxation and controlled breathing. Instruct the client that during the procedure it may be uncomfortable to sit on the hard table or achieve some of the necessary positions; it is important to remain as still as possible during the test; there are no dietary restrictions prior to the test; and it is necessary to remove dental prosthesis, jewelry, eyeglasses, or other metal objects like hair clips before the procedure.
After Test: Encourage an increase in fluid intake. Note and report any signs or symptoms of dehydration, such as decreased urinary output and warm, dry skin. Monitor electrolytes. Note and report any signs or symptoms of bowel perforation, such as severe abdominal pain, nausea and vomiting, or abdominal distention.

Potential Complications: Fluid and electrolyte imbalance; colon perforation

Contraindications: Severe active ulcerative colitis; perforated intestine; tachycardia; toxic megacolon; x-rays, which are usually avoided during pregnancy unless the benefit to the fetus outweighs the potential risk

Interfering Factors: Inability of the client to remain still; inability to assume the proper positions; inability of the client to tolerate or retain barium, air, or other contrast materials in the bowel; excessive feces or residual barium in the bowel; metal objects in the x-ray field

Nursing Considerations:
Pregnancy: Radiation should be avoided in pregnant women if possible (note: appropriate lead shielding is done to protect the fetus if it is determined this test is necessary).
Gerontology: The older person may find it difficult to maintain positions when required to do so for lengthy periods of time during the barium enema.

WEBLINKS

http://chorus.rad.mcw.edu

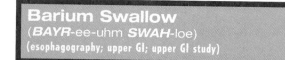

Barium Swallow
(BAYR-ee-uhm SWAH-loe)
(esophagography; upper GI; upper GI study)

30 min.

Type of Test: X-ray

Body Systems and Functions: Gastrointestinal system

Normal Findings: No structural or functional abnormalities

Test Results Time Frame: Within 24 hr

Test Description: A barium swallow is the indirect visualization of the upper gastrointestinal system. A combination of fluoroscopy and a radiological exam is performed to evaluate the anatomical structures and peristalsis of the esophageal lumen, stomach, and small bowel after swallowing barium. This is accomplished by having a mixture of barium sulfate swallowed by the client, and then visualization is made with fluoroscopy.

CLINICAL ALERT:
Have emergency equipment readily available in the event of an anaphylactic reaction to the dye.

Consent Form: Required

List of Equipment: X-ray machine and related equipment from radiology/special studies

Test Procedure:
1. Client is placed supine on the x-ray table or standing in front of an x-ray screen.
2. Baseline films are taken.
3. Client drinks a barium mixture while standing in front of a fluoroscopy screen.
4. Client is then placed on the x-ray table and tilted in various positions. *Ensures accurate results.*
5. Additional barium is then swallowed for a total amount of approximately 400 mL (adult).
6. Final delayed films are taken.

Clinical Implications and Indications:
1. Determines cause of dysphagia, heart burn, or regurgitation
2. Evaluates esophageal motility disorders or esophageal reflux
3. Evaluates suspected strictures, diverticula, tumor, or polyps
4. Evaluates esophageal cancer, hiatal hernia diverticula, ulcers, and achalasia (failure of esophagus to relax)
5. Evaluates stomach disorders, such as gastric cancer, gastric ulcer, gastritis, polyps, and pyloric stenosis
6. Evaluates small-bowel disorders, such as tumor, malabsorption syndrome, and inflammation
7. Diagnoses alcoholic neuropathy, annular pancreas, colitis, cystic fibrosis, Schatzki stricture of lower esophagus ring, ovarian cancer, and primary or idiopathic intestinal pseudo-obstruction

Nursing Care:
Before Test: Explain the test procedure and the purpose of the test. Assess the client's knowledge of the test. Instruct the client to be NPO for 8 hr prior to the test. Assess for allergies if an iodinated contrast is to be used. Inform client that during injection of contrast medium, a burning sensation may be felt for a few seconds behind the eyes or in the jaw, teeth, tongue, or lips. Assess for anxiety and provide sedation as ordered. Administer preoperative medication usually 30 min before procedure. Obtain baseline vital signs and neurological assessment.
During Test: Adhere to standard precautions. Provide reassurance and a calm atmosphere during the procedure. Assess for allergic reactions to contrast medium.
After Test: Instruct client to resume food and increase fluids to facilitate barium elimination, unless contraindicated. Instruct client that stools may be light in color for 3 days. If unable to eliminate barium or stools do not return to normal color, notify physician. Administer a laxative if ordered to prevent constipation. Assess for allergic reactions to contrast medium.

RADIOLOGIC

Potential Complications: Constipation; vasovagal reaction; anaphylaxis due to allergic reaction to iodinated contrast material; aspiration

Contraindications: Intestinal obstruction; upper dysphagia due to possible aspiration; pregnancy; previous history of allergy to iodine, eggs, or shellfish

Interfering Factors: Improper positioning; presence of metallic objects such as jewelry within the x-ray field

Nursing Considerations:
Pregnancy: Intravenous contrast should be avoided in pregnant women if possible (note: appropriate lead shielding is done to protect the fetus if it is determined this test is necessary).

WEBLINKS ⊟☒

http://www.usyd.edu

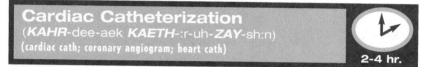

Cardiac Catheterization
(*KAHR*-dee-aek *KAETH*-:r-uh-*ZAY*-sh:n)
(cardiac cath; coronary angiogram; heart cath)

2-4 hr.

Type of Test: X-ray

Body Systems and Functions: Cardiovascular system

Normal Findings: Unblocked coronary arteries; normally functioning heart valves; normal chambers of the heart

Test Results Time Frame: Within 24 hr

Test Description: Cardiac catheterizations are performed in cardiac catheter laboratories by cardiologists. A long, slim hollow catheter is threaded into an artery or vein in the upper groin or arm. This catheter is gently threaded through the vessel to the heart and a radiographic dye is injected (coronary angiogram). This dye outlines the heart, vessels, and pressure gradients across the valves. It also allows the measurement of pressures, oxygen saturation, oxygen content, and cardiac index. A coronary arteriogram involves the placement of the catheter tip at the coronary ostia and injection of radiographic dye into the coronary arteries for visualization. Physicians may perform a left-sided heart catheterization, a right-sided heart catheterization, or both. A left-sided heart catheterization allows the visualization of the left heart chambers, valves, aorta, and coronary arteries and requires arterial access. A right-sided heart catheterization is performed as homodynamic monitoring in special units. A combination heart catheterization enters the right side of the heart allowing the physician to study the right heart chambers and valves as well as the left side.

CLINICAL ALERT:
Have crash cart available in the event of life-threatening arrhythmias during the procedure.

Consent Form: Required

List of Equipment: X-ray machine and related equipment from radiology

Test Procedure:

1. Place client in supine position and confirm correct client and procedure.
2. Intravenous access is obtained. *Allows IV access for medication administration.*
3. Assist physician and technician with medication administration and procedure. *Multifaceted team performs procedure and monitors client.*
4. Monitor client for reaction to radiographic dye. *Potential for allergic reaction.*
5. Accompany client to recovery area and give report. *Facilitates smooth transition of client care.*

Clinical Implications and Indications:

1. Diagnoses coronary artery disease with specific information about atherosclerotic arteries
2. Evaluates coronary occlusions and degree of blockage
3. Evaluates and monitors pulmonary venous return, pulmonary emboli complications, and pulmonary hypertension
4. Detects and evaluates congenital abnormalities, intracardiac tumors, ventricular mural thrombi, septal defects, aneurysms, and valvular defects

Nursing Care:

Before Test: Explain the test procedure and the purpose of the test. Assess the client's knowledge of the test. Instruct the client that during the procedure it may be uncomfortable to sit on the hard table or achieve some of the necessary positions; it is important to remain as still as possible during the test; she is to be NPO prior to the test; and it is necessary to remove dental prosthesis, jewelry, eyeglasses, or other metal objects like hair clips before the procedure. Advise client she may feel warm or taste metallic when dye is injected. Confirm necessary preprocedure tests are complete. Report elevated blood urea nitrogen levels. Hold cardiac prescriptions. Assist client with voiding. Assess for potential allergies to contrast medium. Inform client that during injection of contrast medium, a burning sensation may be felt for a few seconds behind the eyes or in the jaw, teeth, tongue, or lips. Assess for anxiety and provide sedation as ordered. Administer preoperative medication usually 30 min before procedure. Obtain baseline vital signs and neurological assessment.

During Test: Adhere to standard precautions. Assess for allergic reactions to contrast medium. Provide emotional support and continually monitor cardiac status. Assist physician with medication administration. Assist client with positional changes during procedure.

After Test: Assess for allergic reactions to contrast medium. Observe the puncture site for bleeding, and palpate around puncture site to assess for hematoma. If hematoma develops, apply direct pressure with gloved hand for 15 min. Check distal pulses for arterial patency. Monitor vital signs per institution policy. Keep sandbags in place on groin insertion site. Remind client to remain supine for 6 hr with groin insertion site. Assess for angina. Encourage water intake to flush out contrast dye. Report changes in vital signs or cardiac rhythms. At discharge, instruct client not to drive or climb stairs for 24 hr and to avoid heavy lifting, sports, or strenuous housework for 3 days. Advise client to not take baths until

RADIOLOGIC

wound site is healed (note: shower and bandage change are authorized after 24 hr). Inform client to take analgesics and use warm, moist packs for mild discomfort at insertion site and what signs and symptoms to report immediately.

Potential Complications: Anaphylaxis due to allergic reaction to iodinated contrast material; arrhythmias; air embolism; thrombus of catheter; hematoma at insertion site; cardiac tamponade; perforation of heart myocardium; myocardial infarction; congestive heart failure; cerebrovascular accident; infection

Contraindications: Previous history of allergy to iodine, eggs, or shellfish; pregnancy; bleeding tendencies; renal disorders

Interfering Factors: Uncontrolled congestive heart failure; renal insufficiency; electrolyte imbalances; infection; drug toxicity

Nursing Considerations:

Pregnancy: Radiation and IV contrast should be avoided in pregnant women if possible (note: appropriate lead shielding is done to protect the fetus if it is determined this test is necessary).

Pediatric: Sedation is recommended for infants and children. Place the infant or child on a blanket for comfort. After postprocedure monitoring is completed and per health care provider's order, the pediatric client is discharged with an adult who is given instructions (note: cardiac catheterizations are relatively uncommon in younger ages).

Gerontology: The elderly have a greater risk of life-threatening arrhythmias during the procedure. The older person may find it difficult to maintain positions when required to do so for lengthy periods of time during the cardiac catheterization.

Rural: Advisable to arrange for transportation home after recovering from cardiac catheterization.

WEBLINKS

www.voicenet.com

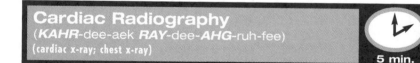

Cardiac Radiography
(*KAHR*-dee-aek *RAY*-dee-*AHG*-ruh-fee)
(cardiac x-ray; chest x-ray)

5 min.

Type of Test: X-ray

Body Systems and Functions: Cardiovascular system

Normal Findings: No abnormalities of the mediastinum, heart, aortic arch, valves, and surrounding structures; normal-appearing heart size and mediastinum width; correctly positioned invasive lines and devices

Test Results Time Frame: Within 30–60 min

Test Description: Cardiac radiography is used to provide important information concerning the status of the heart and surrounding structures. Cardiac radiographic assessment is most often done in conjunction with the routine and

RADIOLOGIC

common chest x-ray. This test is also used to determine correct placement of central lines, pulmonary artery catheters, temporary pacemaker wires, permanent pacemakers, intra-aortic balloon pump catheter, ventricular assist device hoses, and other invasive devices.

CLINICAL ALERT:
A portable x-ray machine may be brought to the nursing unit if an inpatient client cannot be moved.

Consent Form: Not required

List of Equipment: X-ray machine and related equipment from radiology

Test Procedure:
1. Monitoring cables should be positioned out of view of the x-ray (note: client must wear hospital gown that does not have buttons or snaps). *These items may obscure a clear view of the chest.*
2. Place client in standing position to take a cardiac x-ray. If the client cannot stand, an upright position should be maintained. *Ensures accurate results.*
3. Anterior and left lateral views are taken.
4. Instruct client to hold breath when film is taken. *Prevents movement during respiration.*

Clinical Implications and Indications:
1. Cardiomegaly (the heart is enlarged when it occupies space equal to more than one-third of the hemothorax)
2. Diagnoses pericardial effusion
3. Identifies widened mediastinum, which may indicate aortic aneurysm
4. Detects abnormalities in position or size of the large vessels
5. Detects incorrectly placed monitoring devices and invasive lines

Nursing Care:
Before Test: Explain the test procedure and the purpose of the test. Assess the client's knowledge of the test. Instruct the client that the during the procedure it may be uncomfortable to sit on the hard table or achieve some of the necessary positions; it is important to remain as still as possible during the test; there are no dietary restrictions prior to the test; it is necessary to remove dental prosthesis, jewelry, eyeglasses, or other metal objects like hair clips before the procedure. *During Test:* The client is instructed to take a deep breath and hold it or to exhale and not to breathe as the x-ray is taken.

Contraindications: X-rays are usually avoided during pregnancy unless the benefit to the fetus outweighs the potential risk.

Interfering Factors: Obesity; lack of full inspiration; inability to remain still

Nursing Considerations:
Pregnancy: Radiation should be avoided in pregnant women if possible (note: appropriate lead shielding is done to protect the fetus if it is determined this test is necessary).
Pediatric: Sedation is recommended for infants and children. Place the infant or child on a blanket for comfort. After postprocedure monitoring is completed and per health care provider's order, the pediatric client is discharged with an adult who is given instructions.

RADIOLOGIC

Gerontology: The older person may find it difficult to maintain positions when required to do so for lengthy periods of time during the x-ray.

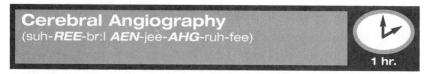

WEBLINKS

http://www.howstuffworks.com

Cerebral Angiography
(suh-*REE*-br:l *AEN*-jee-*AHG*-ruh-fee)

1 hr.

Type of Test: X-ray

Body Systems and Functions: Neurological system

Normal Findings: Absence of pathological conditions in cerebral vasculature and vessels

Test Results Time Frame: Within 24–48 hr

Test Description: Cerebral angiography is a diagnostic procedure that involves the intra-arterial injection of radio-opaque dye into the carotid or vertebral arteries. The femoral, brachial, subclavian, or axillary artery is used as the point of entry. Femoral access is most common. Serial x-ray films are taken in sequence to show arterial and venous phases of cerebral circulation. A radiographic visualization of the cerebral vascular system is then obtained. Cerebral angiography can be performed using local anesthesia or as a component of major surgery while the client is under general anesthesia. For example, cerebral angiography may be done during an aneurysm clipping to verify the clip's position and integrity.

CLINICAL ALERT:
Have emergency equipment readily available in the event of an anaphylactic reaction to the dye.

Consent Form: Required

List of Equipment: Intravenous equipment; x-ray machine and related equipment from radiology or special studies area

Test Procedure:
1. Transport the client to laboratory where cerebral catheterization is done.
2. Place the client in a supine position. Lateral positions may also be necessary. *Ensures optimal visualization of vessels.*
3. Assist with aseptic cleansing of puncture site, administration of local anesthetic, and injection of contrast material.

Clinical Implications and Indications:
1. Diagnoses aneurysms and arteriovenous malformations.
2. The lumen of cerebral blood vessels can be visualized to determine patency, narrowing or stenosis, thrombosis, vasospasm, and displacement of cerebral vessels caused by hematomas, cysts, tumors, and abscesses.

RADIOLOGIC

Nursing Care:

Before Test: Explain the test procedure and the purpose of the test. Assess the client's knowledge of the test. Assess for potential allergies to contrast medium. Inform client that during injection of contrast medium, a burning sensation may be felt for a few seconds behind the eyes or in the jaw, teeth, tongue, or lips. Assess for anxiety and provide sedation as ordered. Administer preoperative medication usually 30 min before procedure. Obtain baseline vital signs and neurological assessment. Educate client on need to remain still during scan. Reassure client no pain will be experienced during the test. Instruct client to void before the procedure. Assess if client is pregnant or nursing. Have client remove all jewelry or metal objects. Administer sedatives as ordered.

During Test: Adhere to standard precautions. Ensure that all health care team members are wearing lead aprons. Position any monitoring devices (e.g., automatic blood pressure, intracranial pressure, and electrocardiogram monitors) in view to allow for continuous observation. Assess for allergic reactions to contrast medium. Instruct client to remain still. Assist with positioning client in supine and lateral positions.

After Test: Maintain the client on complete bedrest for 8 hr. Assess for allergic reactions to contrast medium. Assist with removal of arterial catheter. Ensure that arterial puncture site has achieved complete hemostasis and apply pressure dressing. If the puncture site is the femoral artery, keep the client's leg straight for 8 hr and check pedal pulses and color, sensation, and temperature of affected extremity. Monitor vital signs, assess puncture site for hematoma and bleeding, and do frequent neurological checks. Monitor intake and output. Encourage PO fluids if not contraindicated. Assess for pain at puncture site and provide ordered analgesic medications.

Potential Complications: Anaphylaxis due to allergic reaction to iodinated contrast material; hemorrhage or hematoma at arterial puncture site; seizures; stroke; pulmonary emboli; thrombosis; carotid sinus sensitivity symptoms (hypotension, syncope, and bradycardia); aphasia; visual disturbances

Contraindications: Previous history of allergy to iodine, eggs, or shellfish

Nursing Considerations:

Pregnancy: Radiation and IV contrast should be avoided in pregnant women if possible (note: appropriate lead shielding is done to protect the fetus if it is determined this test is necessary).

Pediatric: Sedation is recommended for infants and children. Place the infant or child on a blanket for comfort. After postprocedure monitoring is completed and per health care provider's order, the pediatric client is discharged with an adult who is given instructions.

Gerontology: The older person may find it difficult to maintain positions when required to do so for lengthy periods of time during the angiography.

Rural: Advisable to arrange for transportation home after recovering from the angiography.

Listing of Related Tests: Digital subtraction angiography

WEBLINKS

www.aann.org

RADIOLOGIC

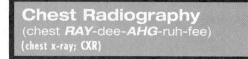

Chest Radiography
(chest *RAY*-dee-*AHG*-ruh-fee)
(chest x-ray; CXR)

5 min.

Type of Test: X-ray

Body Systems and Functions: Pulmonary system

Normal Findings: No abnormalities of lungs, pleura, thorax, soft tissues, mediastinum, heart, and aortic arch; correctly positioned central lines, pulmonary artery catheters, endotracheal tube, nasogastric and nasoenteric tubes, pacemaker wires, and other invasive devices

Test Results Time Frame: Within 30–60 min

Test Description: A chest x-ray is frequently performed in routine adult evaluation during an inpatient hospital admission. It is used in the diagnosis of pulmonary diseases and provides important information concerning the status of the heart, gastrointestinal tract, thyroid gland, bones of the thorax, and diaphragm. It is also used to determine placement of central lines, pulmonary artery catheters, endotracheal tubes, nasogastric and nasoenteric tubes, pacemaker wires, and other invasive devices.

CLINICAL ALERT:
A portable x-ray machine may be brought to the nursing unit if an inpatient client cannot be moved.

Consent Form: Not required

List of Equipment: X-ray machine and related equipment from radiology

Test Procedure:
1. Place client in standing position. If the client cannot stand, an upright position should be maintained. *X-ray films taken in the supine position will not demonstrate fluid levels.*
2. A posteroanterior (PA) position is usually taken first, and then left lateral views are taken. *Ensures accurate results.*
3. The client is instructed to hold his breath when film is taken. *Prevents movement during respiration.*

Clinical Implications and Indications:
1. Abnormal chest x-rays may indicate a wide variety of conditions of the lungs, bony thorax, gastrointestinal tract, heart, diaphragm, and other systems. These conditions include but are not limited to pneumonia, lung abscess, pneumothorax, and pericardial and pleural effusions.
2. Evaluates trauma to bony thorax.
3. Monitors osteoarthritis and cardiac enlargement.
4. Detects incorrectly placed monitoring devices; invasive lines may also be noted.

Nursing Care:
Before Test: Explain the test procedure and the purpose of the test. Assess the client's knowledge of the test. Instruct the client that it may be uncomfortable to

RADIOLOGIC

sit on the hard table or achieve some of the necessary positions; it is important to remain as still as possible during the test; there are no dietary restrictions prior to the test; and it is necessary to remove dental prosthesis, jewelry, eyeglasses, or other metal objects like hair clips before the procedure.

During Test: Adhere to standard precautions. The client is instructed to take a deep breath and hold it or to exhale and not to breathe as the x-ray is taken.

Contraindications: X-rays are usually avoided during pregnancy unless the benefit to the fetus outweighs the potential risk.

Interfering Factors: Obesity; lack of full inspiration; inability to remain still

Nursing Considerations:

Pregnancy: Radiation should be avoided in pregnant women if possible (note: appropriate lead shielding is done to protect the fetus if it is determined this test is necessary).

Pediatric: Sedation is recommended for infants and children. Place the infant or child on a blanket for comfort. After postprocedure monitoring is completed and per health care provider's order, the pediatric client is discharged with an adult who is given instructions.

Gerontology: The older person may find it difficult to maintain positions when required to do so during the chest x-ray.

WEBLINKS ⟋	▤ ⊠

http://RespiratoryCare.medscape.com

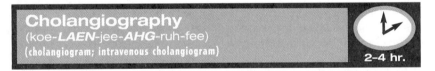

Cholangiography
(koe-*LAEN*-jee-*AHG*-ruh-fee)
(cholangiogram; intravenous cholangiogram)

2–4 hr.

Type of Test: X-ray

Body Systems and Functions: Hepatobiliary system

Normal Findings: No obstructions of the biliary ducts

Test Results Time Frame: Within 24 hr

Test Description: A cholangiography is a radiographic examination of the bile ducts. This test is performed if the gallbladder is not visualized by oral cholecystography or if biliary symptoms are present in a client who has had a previous cholecystectomy. Contrast medium is injected intravenously and films are taken of the upper right abdominal quadrant at 20-min intervals for 1 hr or until the biliary ducts are visualized. Computed tomography is frequently used to allow for better visualization of the ducts. Intravenous cholangiography is being replaced by endoscopic retrograde cholangiopancreatography and percutaneous transhepatic cholangiography in most institutions.

RADIOLOGIC

CLINICAL ALERT:
Have emergency equipment readily available in the event of an anaphylactic reaction to the dye.

Consent Form: Required

List of Equipment: Endoscopic equipment

Test Procedure:
1. Transport client to radiology department.
2. Place client in supine position.
3. Administer IV infusion of iodine dye as ordered while radiographs are taken of region.

Clinical Implications and Indications:
1. Identifies stenosis, obstructions, and calculi of the common bile duct.
2. Cholangiography may be done during laparoscopic cholecystectomy to detect unsuspected common bile duct stones and to confirm the anatomy of the bile ducts.

Nursing Care:
Before Test: Explain the test procedure and purpose of the test. Assess the client's knowledge of the test. Assess for potential allergies to contrast medium. Inform client that during injection of contrast medium, a burning sensation may be felt for a few seconds behind the eyes or in the jaw, teeth, tongue, or lips. Assess for anxiety and provide sedation as ordered. Administer preoperative medication usually 30 min before procedure. Obtain baseline vital signs and neurological assessment. Instruct client to maintain normal diet and remain NPO after midnight the day before the exam. An oral laxative (usually Dulcolax) is administered in the morning on the day before the test. A cleansing enema may be given on the morning of the exam.
During Test: Adhere to standard precautions. Assess for allergic reactions to contrast medium.
After Test: Assess for allergic reactions to contrast medium.

Potential Complications: Anaphylaxis due to allergic reaction to iodinated contrast material; nausea and vomiting

Contraindications: Previous history of allergy to iodine, eggs, or shellfish; bilirubin >3.5 mg/dL

Nursing Considerations:
Pregnancy: Radiation and IV contrast should be avoided in pregnant women if possible (note: appropriate lead shielding is done to protect the fetus if it is determined this test is necessary).
Pediatric: Sedation is recommended for infants and children. Place the infant or child on a blanket for comfort. After postprocedure monitoring is completed and per health care provider's order, the pediatric client is discharged with an adult who is given instructions.
Gerontology: The older person may find it difficult to maintain positions when required to do so for lengthy periods of time during the cholangiography.
Rural: Advisable to arrange for transportation home after recovering from the cholangiography.

Listing of Related Tests: Endoscopic retrograde cholangiopancreatography; percutaneous transhepatic cholangiography

WEBLINKS

http://chorus.rad.mcw.edu

Cholecystography
(*KOE*-lee-sis-*TAHG*-ruh-fee)
(oral cholecystography)

1–3 hr.

Type of Test: X-ray

Body Systems and Functions: Hepatobiliary system

Normal Findings: Normal gallbladder without filling defects and stones

Test Results Time Frame: Within 24–48 hr

Test Description: Cholecystography is an x-ray examination of the gallbladder after oral ingestion of radiopaque dye. The client orally ingests radiopaque, iodinated dye tablets the night before the test. The dye is absorbed by the liver and secreted into the bile, and the bile is concentrated in the gallbladder. X-rays of the right upper quadrant of the abdomen are taken after the client is placed in several different positions. After the initial series of x-rays are taken, the client may be given a high-fat meal or synthetic-fat-containing substance to test the gallbladder's contractility. X-rays are then repeated. A second dose of contrast material may be necessary in up to 25% of clients. Cholecystography is considered a secondary method of identifying stones in the gallbladder. The primary reason for cholecystography is determination of a patent cystic duct before lithotripsy. Sonography of the gallbladder is currently the imaging study of choice due to its ease, rapidity, reliability, and absence of the need for ionizing radiation.

CLINICAL ALERT:
Have emergency equipment readily available in the event of an anaphylactic reaction to the dye.

Consent Form: Required

List of Equipment: X-ray machine and related equipment from radiology

Test Procedure:
1. Place client in sitting, lateral, and supine positions. *Position changes assist the radiologist in differentiating gallstones from air bubbles. Gallstones descend to the bottom of the bile solution, while air bubbles rise to the top.*
2. The client is instructed to hold his breath when film is taken. *Prevents movement during respiration.*
3. Instruct client to remain still during x-ray procedure. *Ensures accurate results.*

RADIOLOGIC

Clinical Implications and Indications:
1. Diagnoses gallbladder disease, such as gallstones, gallbladder polyps, cholestrolosis, and chronic cholecystitis
2. Determines patent cystic duct before lithotripsy

Nursing Care:
Before Test: Explain the test procedure and purpose of the test. Assess the client's knowledge of the test. Assess for potential allergies to contrast medium. Inform client that during injection of contrast medium, a burning sensation may be felt for a few seconds behind the eyes or in the jaw, teeth, tongue, or lips. Assess for anxiety and provide sedation as ordered. Administer preoperative medication usually 30 min before procedure. Obtain baseline vital signs and neurological assessment. Instruct the client to eat a fat-free dinner on the evening before the test and to take the radiopaque iodine tablets by mouth 1–2 hr after dinner. Instruct the client to remain NPO except for water after the radiopaque iodine tablets are taken. Instruct the client to remain completely NPO after bedtime. Instruct the client that during the procedure it may be uncomfortable to sit on the hard table or achieve some of the necessary positions; it is important to remain as still as possible during the test; there are no dietary restrictions prior to the test; and it is necessary to remove dental prosthesis, jewelry, eyeglasses, and other metal objects like hair clips before the procedure.
During Test: Adhere to standard precautions. Assess for allergic reactions to contrast medium. Remind client to remain still. Provide reassurance and a calm atmosphere during the procedure. The client is instructed to take a deep breath and hold it or to exhale and not to breathe as the x-ray is taken.
After Test: Assess for allergic reactions to contrast medium. Instruct client and caregivers to wash hands after voiding or bowel movements because the radionuclide is excreted in urine and feces. Encourage client to drink fluids to assist in flushing radionuclide from the body.

Potential Complications: Anaphylaxis due to allergic reaction to iodinated contrast material

Contraindications: Pregnancy; lactation; previous history of allergy to iodine, eggs, or shellfish; any known allergy to radionuclides; when administering radionuclide, confirm the IV line is patent, because leakage at the site may be interpreted as a false positive; inflammatory condition of abdomen

Interfering Factors: Vomiting or diarrhea will prevent absorption of dye; bilirubin >1.8 mg/dL will prevent adequate visualization of the gallbladder; obstruction of the cystic duct will prevent the dye from entering the gallbladder.

Nursing Considerations:
Pregnancy: Radiation and IV contrast should be avoided in pregnant women if possible (note: appropriate lead shielding is done to protect the fetus if it is determined this test is necessary). Radionuclides should be avoided in pregnant women if possible. If performed, the lactating mother must dispose of milk until radioisotope is cleared from the milk.
Pediatric: Radionuclide may be harmful to the fetus and therefore this test is only performed if absolutely necessary. Young children may require sedation.

RADIOLOGIC

Gerontology: *The older person may find it difficult to maintain positions when required to do so during the cholecystography.*
Rural: *Advisable to arrange for transportation home after recovering from the cholecystography.*

Listing of Related Tests: Cholangiography; percutaneous transhepatic cholangiography; endoscopic retrograde cholangiopancreatography

WEBLINKS

http://catalog.lib.ncsu.edu

Computed Tomography, Abdomen
(kuhm-*PYUE*-t:d tuh-*MAHG*-ruh-fee *AEB*-duh-men)
(CAT scan; CT; computerized axial tomography)

15 min.

Type of Test: X-ray

Body Systems and Functions: Gastrointestinal system

Normal Findings: Interpretation of images determines the absence of pathological conditions and a normal appearing abdomen.

Test Results Time Frame: Within 24 hr

Test Description: Computed tomography images cross sections of tissue structures. A narrow beam of x-rays rotates in a continuous 360° motion around the patient to image the body and provides views of cross-sectional slices of tissue. X-rays only pass through the section of interest. The computer calculates tissue absorption and produces a clear view of tissues. Barium or iodinated contrast agents are routinely used in abdominal CT.

CLINICAL ALERT:
Have emergency equipment readily available in the event of an anaphylactic reaction to the contrast medium.

Consent Form: Required

List of Equipment: Computed tomography scanning equipment

Test Procedure:
1. Computed tomography testing takes place in a designated area of the health care facility where the computed tomography scanner is located.
2. The client is placed in a supine position within the scanner. *Allows for unobstructed view of the desired region being scanned.*
3. Intravenous access is obtained. *Allows access for contrast medium.*
4. Trained personnel administer the intravenous contrast medium. *Helps to provide continuity for administration of contrast medium.*

Clinical Implications and Indications:
1. Evaluates hernias, hematomas, inflammations, infectious processes, ascites, abscesses, abdominal aneurysms, neoplasms, and trauma

RADIOLOGIC

2. Detects abnormalites of the adrenals, GI system, kidney, liver, pancreas, spleen, uterus, and biliary tract

Nursing Care:

Before Test: Explain the test procedure and the purpose of the test. Assess the client's knowledge of the test. Assess for potential allergies to contrast medium. Inform client that during injection of contrast medium, a burning sensation may be felt for a few seconds behind the eyes or in the jaw, teeth, tongue, or lips. Assess for anxiety and provide sedation as ordered. Administer preoperative medication usually 30 min before procedure. Obtain baseline vital signs and neurological assessment. Instruct client to remain still and NPO after midnight, the night before the examination (note: fluids and medications are permitted). Provide instructions concerning body positioning. Start an IV line with infusing solution as ordered. Administer oral and IV contrast medium. Note health care provider's order for specific type of contrast medium to be administered and time of administration. Oral contrast material may be ordered before bed and 1–1.5 hr before the examination.

During Test: Adhere to standard precautions. Position any monitoring devices in view of the control area in order to allow for continuous observation. Assess for allergic reaction to contrast medium. A blanket may be provided for client comfort. Instruct client to lie still and to hold breath when asked.

After Test: Assess for allergic reactions to contrast medium. Encourage client to drink fluids if not contraindicated.

Potential Complications: Anaphylaxis due to allergic reaction to iodinated contrast material

Contraindications: Previous history of allergy to iodine, eggs, or shellfish

Nursing Considerations:

Pregnancy: Intravenous contrast should be avoided in pregnant women if possible.
Pediatric: Sedation is recommended for infants and children under 5 years old. Children greater than 5 years require verbal reassurance. Place the infant or child on a blanket for comfort. If it is necessary to extend the arms over the head, they may be restrained with adhesive tape or Velcro straps. Oral contrast may be mixed with Kool-Aid or fruit juice to mask the unpleasant taste. In neonates and small children, CT scan should be delayed at least 30 sec after all of the IV contrast is administered in order to ensure enhancement of vascular structures. In larger children in whom contrast is given through small-gauge IV catheters (22–24 gauge) with lower flow rates, CT scanning of the abdomen should begin no later than 60 sec after the start of the contrast injection. Adult protocols should be applied to children greater than 45 kg. The pediatric client is discharged with an adult who is given verbal and written instructions.
Gerontology: The older person may find it difficult to maintain positions when required to do so during the computed tomography.

Listing of Related Tests: Upper GI series

WEBLINKS

http://webmd.lycos.com

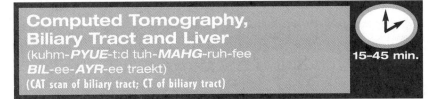

Computed Tomography, Biliary Tract and Liver
(kuhm-**PYUE**-t:d tuh-**MAHG**-ruh-fee **BIL**-ee-**AYR**-ee traekt)
(CAT scan of biliary tract; CT of biliary tract)

15–45 min.

Type of Test: X-ray

Body Systems and Functions: Hepatobiliary system

Normal Findings: Interpretation of images determines the absence of pathological conditions and a normal appearing biliary tract and liver.

Test Results Time Frame: Within 24 hr

Test Description: Computed tomography of the liver and biliary tract is a cross-sectional visualization used to identify tissue characteristics. It is used extensively for evaluating focal and diffuse hepatic disease and biliary obstruction. Computed tomography images cross sections of tissue structures. A narrow beam of x-rays rotates in a continuous 360° motion around the patient to image the body and provides views of cross-sectional slices of tissue. X-rays only pass through the section of interest. The computer calculates tissue absorption and produces a clear view of tissues.

CLINICAL ALERT:
Have emergency equipment readily available in the event of an anaphylactic reaction to the dye.

Consent Form: Required

Test Procedure:
1. Computed tomography testing takes place in a designated area of the health care facility where the computed tomography scanner is located.
2. The client is placed in a supine position within the scanner. *Allows for unobstructed view of the desired region being scanned.*
3. Intravenous access is obtained. *Allows access for contrast medium.*
4. Trained personnel administer the IV contrast medium. *Helps to provide continuity for administration of contrast medium.*

Clinical Implications and Indications:
1. Diagnoses benign and malignant hepatic tumors and abscesses; diffuse diseases such as steatosis, cirrhosis, iron overload, hepatitis, radiation injury; and liver vascular disorders.
2. Confirms the presence of biliary obstruction and determines the level and cause of obstruction and the extent of the disease process.
3. When the contrast agent is administered intravenously, it is quickly redistributed from the vascular to the interstitial space while continuously being excreted by the kidney. In the liver, this process occurs very rapidly, and soon after an IV contrast medium injection has ended, a large amount of hepatic parenchyma is enhanced by contrast.

RADIOLOGIC

Nursing Care:

Before Test: Explain the test procedure and the purpose of the test. Assess the client's knowledge of the test. Assess for potential allergies to contrast medium. Inform client that during injection of contrast medium, a burning sensation may be felt for a few seconds behind the eyes or in the jaw, teeth, tongue, or lips. Assess for anxiety and provide sedation as ordered. Administer preoperative medication usually 30 min before procedure. Obtain baseline vital signs and neurological assessment. Instruct client to be NPO 3–4 hr prior to examination. *During Test:* Assess for allergic reactions to contrast medium. Adhere to standard precautions.
After Test: Assess for allergic reactions to contrast medium.

Potential Complications: Anaphylaxis due to allergic reaction to iodinated contrast material

Contraindications: Previous history of allergy to iodine, eggs, or shellfish

Nursing Considerations:

Pregnancy: Intravenous contrast should be avoided in pregnant women if possible. Pediatric: Sedation is recommended for infants and children. Place the infant or child on a blanket for comfort. After postprocedure monitoring is completed and per health care provider's order, the pediatric client is discharged with an adult who is given instructions.
Gerontology: The older person may find it difficult to maintain positions when required to do so during the CT.

WEBLINKS

http://chorus.rad.mcw.edu

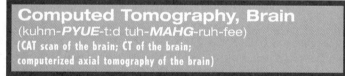

Computed Tomography, Brain
(kuhm-*PYUE*-t:d tuh-*MAHG*-ruh-fee)
(CAT scan of the brain; CT of the brain;
computerized axial tomography of the brain)

15–30 min.

Type of Test: X-ray

Body Systems and Functions: Neurological system

Normal Findings: Interpretation of images determines the absence of pathological conditions and a normal appearing brain.

Test Results Time Frame: Within 24 hr

Test Description: Computed tomography images cross sections of tissue structures of the brain. A narrow beam of x-rays rotates in a continuous 360° motion around the client to image the body and provides views of cross-sectional slices of tissue. X-rays only pass through the section of interest. The computer calculates tissue absorption and produces a clear view of tissues. CT of the brain results in a series of pictures of coronal or horizontal sections. Intravenous injections of iodinated contrast dye may be used. Xenon-enhanced CT of the brain is

RADIOLOGIC

a new technological advancement that provides information about regional alterations in cerebral blood flow. A noncontrasted CT scan is usually performed first and then iodine dye is administered intravenously or xenon/oxygen mix gas is administered via a mask. Intubated clients will have the xenon/oxygen mix given into the endotracheal tube.

CLINICAL ALERT:
Have emergency equipment readily available in the event of an anaphylactic reaction to the dye or the xenon (xenon is an anesthetic agent and may have sedating effects).

Consent Form: Required

List of Equipment: Computed tomography scanning equipment

Test Procedure:
1. Computed tomography testing takes place in a designated area of the health care facility where the computed tomography scanner is located.
2. Place client in a supine position with the client's head securely positioned in a holding device. *Movement during the test may cause artifacts.*
3. Intravenous access is obtained. *Allows access for contrast medium.*
4. Trained personnel administer the IV contrast medium. *Helps to provide continuity for administration of contrast medium.*

Clinical Implications and Indications:
1. Evaluates and monitors intracranial neoplasms, cerebral infarctions, ventricular displacement or enlargement, cortical atrophy, cerebral aneurysms, intracranial hemorrage and hematoma, and arteriovenous malformation.
2. Xenon-enhanced CT of the brain is especially useful in clients being considered for thrombolytic therapy during acute ischemic stroke; assessing subarachnoid hemorrrhage patients for cerebral vasospam; and assessing global cerebral blood flow in traumatic head injury.

Nursing Care:
Before Test: Explain the test procedure and the purpose of the test. Assess the client's knowledge of the test. Assess for potential allergies to contrast medium. Inform client that during injection of contrast medium, a burning sensation may be felt for a few seconds behind the eyes or in the jaw, teeth, tongue, or lips. Assess for anxiety and provide sedation as ordered. Administer preoperative medication usually 30 min before procedure. Obtain baseline vital signs and neurological assessment. Remove hairpins, wigs, and all hair accessories. Instruct client to remain NPO for 4 hr before the examination if iodine dye or xenon gas is to be used. Iodine and xenon may cause nausea and subsequent aspiration. Assure client that the test causes no pain. Provide instructions concerning body positioning. Start an IV line with infusing solution as ordered.

During Test: Adhere to standard precautions. Position any monitoring devices in view of the control area in order to allow for continuous observation. A blanket may be provided for client comfort. Assess for allergic reactions to contrast medium. Assess client for side effects of xenon gas. Instruct client to remain still and not to talk during the test. Sedation may be necessary for clients who are unable to lie still.

RADIOLOGIC

After Test: Assess for allergic reactions to contrast medium and side effects of xenon gas. Encourage client to drink fluids if not contraindicated. If xenon is used, the neurological examination should be delayed 5 min due to the possible sedating effects.

Potential Complications: Anaphylaxis due to allergic reaction to iodinated contrast material; side effects of xenon are mild, temporary lowering of heart rate and blood pressure and sleepiness, which lasts only a few minutes longer than the procedure.

Contraindications: Previous history of allergy to iodine, eggs, or shellfish

Nursing Considerations:
Pregnancy: Intravenous contrast should be avoided in pregnant women if possible.
Pediatric: Sedation is recommended for infants and children. Place the infant or child on a blanket for comfort. Postexamination discharge criteria include alertness, stable vital signs for 1 hr after administration of the sedative, and the ability to tolerate oral fluids. The pediatric client is discharged with an adult who is given verbal and written instructions.
Gerontology: The older person may find it difficult to maintain positions when required to do so during the CT.

⊞WEBLINKS   ⊟☒

www.aann.org

Computed Tomography, Chest
(kuhm-*PYUE*-t:d tuh-*MAHG*-ruh-fee)
(CAT scan of the chest; CT of the chest)

15–45 min.

Type of Test: X-ray

Body Systems and Functions: Pulmonary system

Normal Findings: Interpretation of images determines the absence of pathological conditions and a normal appearing chest.

Test Results Time Frame: Within 24 hr

Test Description: Computed tomography of the chest provides cross-sectional views of the chest and allows for detection of small differences in tissue densities that cannot be seen on conventional radiology. Computed tomography images cross sections of tissue structures. A narrow beam of x-rays rotates in a continuous 360° motion around the patient to image the body and provides views of cross-sectional slices of tissue. X-rays only pass through the section of interest. The computer calculates tissue absorption and produces a clear view of tissues.

CLINICAL ALERT:
Have emergency equipment readily available in the event of an anaphylactic reaction to the contrast medium.

Consent Form: Required

List of Equipment: Computed tomography scanning equipment

Test Procedure:

1. Computed tomography testing takes place in a designated area of the health care facility where the computed tomograpy scanner is located.
2. Place client in a supine, prone, or lateral decubitus position. The arms may be elevated above the head. *Allows for an unobstructed view of the chest region.*
3. Intravenous access is obtained. *Allows access for contrast medium.*
4. Trained personnel administer the IV contrast medium. *Helps to provide continuity for administration of contrast medium.*

Clinical Implications and Indications:

1. Evaluates bronchogenic carcinoma and other neoplasms, such as lymphoma, sarcoma, and potential metastatic disease.
2. Diagnoses chest trauma, enlarged lymph nodes, and pleural effusion.
3. When an IV contrast is administered, evaluation for the presence of an aortic aneurysm can be done.

Nursing Care:

Before Test: Explain the test procedure and the purpose of the test. Assess the client's knowledge of the test. Assess for potential allergies to contrast medium. Inform client that during injection of contrast medium, a burning sensation may be felt for a few seconds behind the eyes or in the jaw, teeth, tongue, or lips. Assess for anxiety and provide sedation as ordered. Administer preoperative medication usually 30 min before procedure. Obtain baseline vital signs and neurological assessment.

During Test: Adhere to standard precautions. Assess for allergic reactions to contrast medium.

After Test: Assess for allergic reactions to contrast medium.

Potential Complications: Anaphylaxis due to allergic reaction to iodinated contrast material

Contraindications: Previous history of allergy to iodine, eggs, or shellfish

Nursing Considerations:

Pregnancy: Intravenous contrast should be avoided in pregnant women if possible.
Pediatric: Chest CT scanning of neonates and small children should be delayed at least 30 sec after 100% of the contrast medium is given in order to ensure enhancement of vascular structures. Sedation is recommended for infants and children. Place the infant or child on a blanket for comfort. After postprocedure monitoring is completed and per health care provider's order, the pediatric client is discharged with an adult who is given instructions.
Gerontology: The older person may find it difficult to maintain positions when required to do so during the CT.

RADIOLOGIC

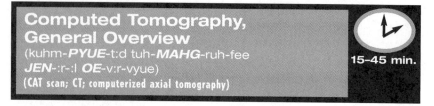

Computed Tomography, General Overview

(kuhm-**PYUE**-t:d tuh-**MAHG**-ruh-fee **JEN**-:r-:l **OE**-v:r-vyue)

(CAT scan; CT; computerized axial tomography)

15–45 min.

Type of Test: X-ray

Body Systems and Functions: Miscellaneous systems

Normal Findings: Interpretation of images determines the absence of pathology.

Test Results Time Frame: Within 24 hr (note: the availability of a radiologist increases the efficiency in obtaining results)

Test Description: Computed tomography images cross sections of tissue structures. A narrow beam of x-rays rotates in a continuous 360°ree; motion around the client to image the body and provide views of cross-sectional slices of tissue. X-rays only pass through the section of interest. The computer calculates tissue absorption and produces a clear view of tissues. A wide variety of abnormalities and pathological condtions can be definitively diagnosed with CT scanning. Computed tomography rooms are often located close to emergency rooms for quick access in a critical client needing immediate diagnostic attention.

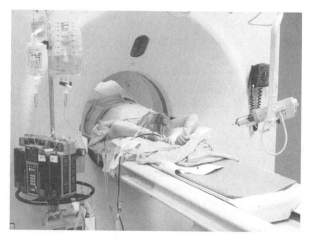

Computed Tomography Testing

CLINICAL ALERT:
Have emergency equipment readily available in the event of an anaphylactic reaction to the contrast medium.

Consent Form: Required

List of Equipment: Computed tomography scanning equipment

RADIOLOGIC

Test Procedure:

1. Computed tomography testing takes place in a designated area of the health care facility where the computed tomography scanner is located.
2. The client is placed in a supine position within the scanner. *Allows for unobstructed view of the desired region being scanned.*
3. Intravenous access is obtained. *Allows access for contrast medium.*
4. Trained personnel administer the IV contrast medium. *Helps to provide continuity for administration of contrast medium.*

Clinical Implications and Indications:

1. CT aids in the diagnosis of an extremely wide range of tumors, infractions, bone displacement, fluid accumulations, and other pathologies specific to the region of the scan.

Nursing Care:

Before Test: Explain the test procedure and the purpose of the test. Assess the client's knowledge of the test. Assess for potential allergies to contrast medium. Inform client that during injection of contrast medium (if prescribed) a burning sensation may be felt for a few seconds behind the eyes or in the jaw, teeth, tongue, or lips. Assess for anxiety and provide sedation as ordered. Administer preoperative medication usually 30 min before procedure. Obtain baseline vital signs and neurological assessment. Provide instruction concerning body positioning. In some tests a barium enema may be required. Instruct client to remain still throughout CT scan. Inform client that closing eyes may assist in not feeling claustrophobic. See specific test for more detailed instructions.

During Test: Adhere to standard precautions. Position any monitoring devices in view of the control area in order to allow for continuous observation. Assess for allergic reaction to contrast medium. A blanket may be provided for client comfort.

After Test: Assess for allergic reactions to contrast medium.

Potential Complications: Anaphylaxis due to allergic reaction to iodinated contrast material

Contraindications: Previous history of allergy to iodine, eggs, or shellfish

Nursing Considerations:

Pregnancy: Intravenous contrast should be avoided in pregnant women if possible. *Pediatric:* Sedation is recommended for infants and children under 5 years old. Children greater than 5 years require verbal reassurance. Place the infant or child on a blanket for comfort. If it is necessary to extend the arms over the head, they may be restrained with adhesive tape or Velcro straps. Oral contrast may be mixed with Kool-Aid or fruit juice to mask the unpleasant taste. Postexamination discharge criteria include alertness, stable vital signs for 1 hr after administration of the sedative, and the ability to tolerate oral fluids. The pediatric client is discharged with an adult who is given verbal and written instructions. *Gerontology:* The older person may find it difficult to maintain positions when required to do so during the CT.

| WEBLINKS

http://www.jeffersonhealth.org

RADIOLOGIC

Computed Tomography, Pancreas

(kuhm-*PYUE*-t:d tuh-*MAHG*-ruh-fee)
(CAT scan of the pancreas; CT of the pancreas; computerized axial tomography of the pancreas)

15–45 min.

Type of Test: X-ray

Body Systems and Functions: Gastrointestinal system

Normal Findings: Interpretation of images determines the absence of pathological conditions and a normal appearing pancreas.

Test Results Time Frame: Within 24 hr

Test Description: Computed tomography images cross sections of the tissue structures of the pancreas. A narrow beam of x-rays rotates in a continuous 360° motion around the client to image the body and provides views of cross-sectional slices of tissue. X-rays only pass through the section of interest. The computer calculates tissue absorption and produces a clear view of tissues. Morphological changes in acute pancreatitis are clearly evident on CT. Acute pancreatitis is defined as an acute inflammatory process of the pancreas with variable involvement of other regional tissues and remote organ systems. The severity of pancreatitis can be assessed on CT by determining the extent of pancreatic inflammation and presence of pancreatic parenchymal necrosis. Oral contrast material is administered to ensure there is no unopacified bowel that could be misinterpreted as pancreatic fluid collection. Intravenous contrast medium is administered if the differentiation between interstitial and necrotizing pancreatitis is necessary.

CLINICAL ALERT:
Have emergency equipment readily available in the event of an anaphylactic reaction to the dye.

Consent Form: Required

List of Equipment: Computed tomography scanning equipment

Test Procedure:
1. Computed tomography testing takes place in a designated area of the health care facility where the computed tomography scanner is located.
2. Place client in a supine position.
3. Intravenous access is obtained. *Allows access for contrast medium.*
4. Trained personnel administer the IV contrast medium. *Helps to provide continuity for administration of contrast medium.*

Clinical Implications and Indications:
1. Evaluates and monitors inflammatory or neoplastic disease
2. Diagnoses acute pancreatitis

Nursing Care:

Before Test: Explain the test procedure and the purpose of the test. Assess the client's knowledge of the test. Assess for potential allergies to contrast medium. Inform client that during injection of contrast medium, a burning sensation may be felt for a few seconds behind the eyes or in the jaw, teeth, tongue, or lips. Assess for anxiety and provide sedation as ordered. Administer preoperative medication usually 30 min before procedure. Obtain baseline vital signs and neurological assessment. Instruct client to remain NPO after midnight before the exam. Provide instructions concerning body positioning. Initiate an IV line for contrast medium.

During Test: Adhere to standard precautions. Assess for allergic reactions to contrast medium. Position any monitoring devices in view of the control area in order to allow for continuous observation. A blanket may be provided for client comfort. Administer oral and IV contrast medium. Note health care provider's order for specific type of contrast medium to be administered and time of administration. Instruct client to hold breath for 24–30 sec while a scan is obtained from the lower chest to the iliac crest.

After Test: Assess for allergic reactions to contrast medium. Encourage client to drink fluids if not contraindicated.

Potential Complications: Anaphylaxis due to allergic reaction to iodinated contrast material

Contraindications: Previous history of allergy to iodine, eggs, or shellfish

Nursing Considerations:

Pregnancy: Intravenous contrast should be avoided in pregnant women if possible (note: the most common cause of pancreatitis during pregnancy is gallstones).

Pediatric: Sedation is recommended for infants and children. Place the infant or child on a blanket for comfort. Postexamination discharge criteria include alertness, stable vital signs for 1 hr after administration of the sedative, and the ability to tolerate oral fluids. The pediatric client is discharged with an adult who is given verbal and written instructions.

Gerontology: The older person may find it difficult to maintain positions when required to do so during the CT.

Listing of Related Tests: Amylase; lipase

```
WEBLINKS
```

http://www.niddk.nih.gov

Computed Tomography, Pelvis
(kuhm-*PYUE*-t:d tuh-*MAHG*-ruh-fee)
(CAT scan of the pelvis; CT of the pelvis;
computerized axial tomography of the pelvis)

15–45 min.

Type of Test: X-ray

Body Systems and Functions: Musculoskeletal system

Normal Findings: Interpretation of images determines the absence of pathological conditions.

Test Results Time Frame: Within 24 hr

RADIOLOGIC

Test Description: Computed tomography images cross sections of tissue structures of the pelvis. A narrow beam of x-rays rotates in a continuous 360° motion around the client to image the body and provides views of cross-sectional slices of tissue. X-rays only pass through the section of interest. The computer calculates tissue absorption and produces a clear view of tissues. CT of the pelvis provides a cross-sectional display of bony and soft tissue pelvic structures. In order to provide for opacification of the rectosigmoid and descending colon, oral contrast is given 6–12 hr before the examination or an enema of contrast material is administered before the examination. In addition, oral contrast is administered at least 1 hr before the examination. During the examination iodine contrast solution is administered intravenously in order to differentiate pelvic arteries and veins from pelvic lymph nodes.

CLINICAL ALERT:
Have emergency equipment readily available in the event of an anaphylactic reaction to the dye.

Consent Form: Required

List of Equipment: Computed tomography scanning equipment

Test Procedure:
1. Computed tomography testing takes place in a designated area of the health care facility where the computed tomography scanner is located.
2. Place client in a supine position.
3. Intravenous access is obtained. *Allows access for contrast medium.*
4. Trained personnel administer the IV contrast medium. *Helps to provide continuity for administration of contrast medium.*

Clinical Implications and Indications:
1. Evaluates and monitors prostatic carcinoma, pelvic neoplasms, carcinoma of the cervix, endometrial neoplasm, ovarian masses, and congenital uterine anomalies
2. Determines the localization of undescended testes

Nursing Care:
Before Test: Explain the test procedure and the purpose of the test. Assess the client's knowledge of the test. Assess for potential allergies to contrast medium. Inform client that during injection of contrast medium, a burning sensation may be felt for a few seconds behind the eyes or in the jaw, teeth, tongue, or lips. Assess for anxiety and provide sedation as ordered. Administer preoperative medication usually 30 min before procedure. Obtain baseline vital signs and neurological assessment. Instruct client to remain NPO after midnight before the examination. Administer contrast material orally or per enema as directed by health care provider. Provide instructions concerning body positioning. Initiate an IV line for contrast medium.

During Test: Adhere to standard precautions. Assess for allergic reactions to contrast medium. Position any monitoring devices in view of the control area in order to allow for continuous observation. A blanket may be provided for client comfort. Administer oral and IV contrast medium. Note health care provider's order for specific type of contrast medium to be administered and time of administration.

RADIOLOGIC

After Test: Assess for allergic reactions to contrast medium. Encourage client to drink fluids if not contraindicated.

Potential Complications: Anaphylaxis due to allergic reaction to iodinated contrast material

Contraindications: Previous history of allergy to iodine, eggs, or shellfish

Nursing Considerations:

Pregnancy: Intravenous contrast should be avoided in pregnant women if possible. Pediatric: Sedation is recommended for infants and children. Place the infant or child on a blanket for comfort. Postexamination discharge criteria include alertness, stable vital signs for 1 hr after administration of the sedative, and the ability to tolerate oral fluids. The pediatric client is discharged with an adult who is given verbal and written instructions.
Gerontology: The older person may find it difficult to maintain positions when required to do so during the CT.

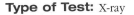
| WEBLINKS |

www.inurse.com

Computed Tomography, Renal
(kuhm-***PYUE***-t:d tuh-***MAHG***-ruh-fee)
(CAT scan of the renal system; CT of the renal system; computerized axial tomography for the renal system)

15–45 min.

Type of Test: X-ray

Body Systems and Functions: Renal/urological system

Normal Findings: The radiologist's interpretation of images determines the absence of pathological conditions.

Test Results Time Frame: Within 24 hr

Test Description: Computed tomography images cross sections of tissue structures of the renal system. A narrow beam of x-rays rotates in a continuous 360° motion around the client to image the body and provide views of cross-sectional slices of tissue. X-rays only pass through the section of interest. The computer calculates tissue absorption and produces a clear view of tissues. Images may be displayed in a two- or three-dimensional mode. Oral and IV contrast materials are used, if not contraindicated, to enhance normal structures and pathological conditions. Pre- and postcontrast images are taken. CT imaging used to demonstrate ureteral calculi in patients with acute renal colic has a high success rate and replaces the traditional IV urogram. Angiomyolipomas' high fat content provides a clear visualization on CT. Hemorrhage is shown as a high-density collection, in contrast to lower density urine, ascites, or old blood. Staging of neoplasms is also accurately achieved by CT imaging, although magnetic resonance imaging may be a slightly better alternative.

RADIOLOGIC

CLINICAL ALERT:
Have emergency equipment readily available in the event of an anaphylactic reaction to the dye.

Consent Form: Required

List of Equipment: Computed tomography scanning equipment

Test Procedure:
1. Computed tomography testing takes place in a designated area of the health care facility where the computed tomography scanner is located.
2. Place client in a supine position.
3. Intravenous access is obtained. *Allows access for contrast medium.*
4. Trained personnel administer the IV contrast medium. *Helps to provide continuity for administration of contrast medium.*

Clinical Implications and Indications:
1. Evaluates and monitors angiomyolipomas, acute or recent hemorrhage in or around the kidneys and the retroperitoneum, renal cell carcinoma and staging of neoplasms of the kidneys, and renal masses and cysts
2. Identifies filling defects in the calyces and renal pelvis
3. Detects calcifications, such as ureteral calculi
4. Diagnoses severe acute pyelonephritis, gas-producing infections, and renal trauma
5. Evaluates benign and malignant diseases of the bladder, prostate, testes, seminal vesicles, and spermatic cords

Nursing Care:
Before Test: Explain the test procedure and the purpose of the test. Assess the client's knowledge of the test. Assess for potential allergies to contrast medium. Inform client that during injection of contrast medium, a burning sensation may be felt for a few seconds behind the eyes or in the jaw, teeth, tongue, or lips. Assess for anxiety and provide sedation as ordered. Administer preoperative medication usually 30 min before procedure. Obtain baseline vital signs and neurological assessment. Instruct client to remain NPO after midnight before the examination. Administer oral contrast agent. Initiate an IV line for contrast medium.

During Test: Adhere to standard precautions. Assess for allergic reactions to contrast medium. Position any monitoring devices in view of the control area in order to allow for continuous observation. A blanket may be provided for client comfort. Administer IV contrast agent as a rapid bolus. Note health care provider's order for specific type of contrast medium to be administered, dose, and time of administration. Instruct client to remain still.

After Test: Assess for allergic reactions to contrast medium. Encourage client to drink fluids if not contraindicated.

Potential Complications: Anaphylaxis due to allergic reaction to iodinated contrast material

Contraindications: Previous history of allergy to iodine, eggs, or shellfish

RADIOLOGIC

Nursing Considerations:

Pregnancy: *Intravenous contrast should be avoided in pregnant women if possible.*
Pediatric: *Sedation is recommended for infants and children. Place the infant or
child on a blanket for comfort. Postexamination discharge criteria include alertness, stable vital signs for 1 hr after administration of the sedative, and the ability
to tolerate oral fluids. The pediatric client is discharged with an adult who is given
verbal and written instructions.*
Gerontology: *The older person may find it difficult to maintain positions when
required to do so during the CT.*

WEBLINKS 🖑

www.nlm.nih.gov

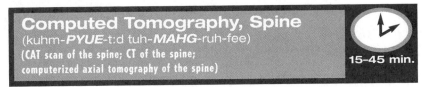

Computed Tomography, Spine
(kuhm-*PYUE*-t:d tuh-*MAHG*-ruh-fee)
(CAT scan of the spine; CT of the spine;
computerized axial tomography of the spine)

15–45 min.

Type of Test: X-ray

Body Systems and Functions: Neurological system

Normal Findings: Interpretation of images determines the absence of
pathological conditions.

Test Results Time Frame: Within 1 hr

Test Description: Computed tomography images cross sections of tissue
structures of the spine. A narrow beam of x-rays rotates in a continuous 360°
motion around the patient to image the body and provides views of cross-sectional slices of tissue. X-rays only pass through the section of interest. The computer calculates tissue absorption and produces a clear view of tissues. A complete spinal cord injury lesion refers to total loss of sensation and voluntary
muscle control below the level of injury due to a complete dissection of the
spinal cord and its neurochemical pathways. An incomplete spinal cord injury
lesion implies preservation of the sensory and/or motor fibers below the lesion.
Incomplete lesions are classified as central, lateral, anterior, or peripheral, indicating the area of damage. Quadriplegia refers to a spinal cord lesion involving
one of the cervical segments of the spinal cord and results in dysfunction of all
extremeties, bowel, and bladder. Paraplegia refers to a lesion involving the thoracic, lumbar, or sacral areas of the spine and results in dysfunction of the lower
extremeties, bowel, or bladder.

CLINICAL ALERT:
Have emergency equipment readily available in the event of an
anaphylactic reaction to the dye. Ensure immobilization and
stabilization of the client's head and neck. Use spinal cord precautions, such as log rolling. The nurse must continuously
remain with the acute trauma, critical client during CT, observing for the client's tolerance to the procedure.

RADIOLOGIC

Consent Form: Required

List of Equipment: Computed tomography scanning equipment

Test Procedure:
1. Computed tomography testing takes place in a designated area of the health care facility where the computed tomography scanner is located.
2. Place client in a supine position.
3. Intravenous access is obtained. *Allows access for contrast medium.*
4. Trained personnel administer the IV contrast medium. *Helps provide continuity for administration of contrast medium.*

Clinical Implications and Indications:
1. Determines the degree and extent of damage to the spinal cord
2. Identifies the presence of blood or bone within the spinal cord
3. Provides a detailed evaluation of cortical bone
4. Diagnoses disc herniation and degenerative spine disease

Nursing Care:
Before Test: Explain the test procedure and the purpose of the test. Assess the client's knowledge of the test. Assess for potential allergies to contrast medium. Inform client that during injection of contrast medium, a burning sensation may be felt for a few seconds behind the eyes or in the jaw, teeth, tongue, or lips. Assess for anxiety and provide sedation as ordered. Administer preoperative medication usually 30 min before procedure. Obtain baseline vital signs and neurological assessment. Radiographic films of the spinal cord are taken and reviewed prior to CT of the spine.
During Test: Adhere to standard precautions. Assess for allergic reactions to contrast medium. Position any monitoring devices in view of the control area in order to allow for continuous observation. A blanket may be provided for patient comfort. Instruct the client to remain still. Closely observe the client who has sustained an acute spinal cord injury for complications and assess vital signs, neurological signs, and intracranial pressure if monitored.

Potential Complications: Anaphylaxis due to allergic reaction to iodinated contrast material. Critical neurological clients may exhibit deterioration during transport for testing.

Contraindications: Previous history of allergy to iodine, eggs, or shellfish

Nursing Considerations:
Pediatric: Sedation is recommended for infants and children. Place the infant or child on a blanket for comfort. Postexamination discharge criteria include alertness, stable vital signs for 1 hr after administration of the sedative, and the ability to tolerate oral fluids. The pediatric client is discharged with an adult who is given verbal and written instructions.

RADIOLOGIC

| WEBLINKS ⬓ | 🖳 🗵 |

www.aann.org

Cystography
(sis-*TAHG*-ruh-*FEE*)
(retrograde cystography)

1 hr.

Type of Test: X-ray

Body Systems and Functions: Renal/urological system

Normal Findings: Normal bladder anatomy and function; absence of abnormalities

Test Results Time Frame: Within 24–48 hr

Test Description: Cystography is a test of the lower urinary tract that provides information concerning the anatomy and integrity of the bladder and urethra. A radiographic contrast agent is instilled into the bladder and radiographic imaging is then performed. Cystography may be performed during a urodynamic study or as a separate test.

CLINICAL ALERT:
A portable x-ray machine may be brought to the nursing unit if the client cannot be moved.

Consent Form: Required

List of Equipment: X-ray machine and related equipment from radiology; urinary catheter equipment

Test Procedure:
1. Place client in supine position.
2. Perform kidney-ureter-bladder (KUB) radiograph.
3. Instill contrast medium into bladder and clamp the catheter.
4. Perform radiographic films with the client in various positions.
5. Unclamp the catheter and allow bladder fluid to drain.
6. Perform postdrainage radiographic film. *Allows evaluation for extravasated contrast material.*

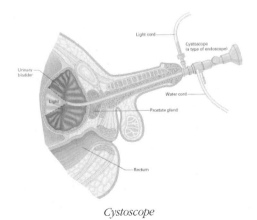

Cystoscope

RADIOLOGIC

Clinical Implications and Indications:

1. Evaluates bladder injury after trauma (including iatrogenic trauma such as after cystoscopic biopsy or resection of a lesion)
2. Detects anastomotic leak after surgery (partial cystectomy, prostatectomy, ureteral reimplantation, renal and pancreatic transplantation)
3. Diagnoses neurogenic bladder, recurrent urinary infections, vesicoureteral reflux, fistulas between the bladder and adjacent organs, and bladder diverticula

Nursing Care:

Before Test: Explain the test procedure and purpose of the test. Assess the client's knowledge of the test. Instruct the client that during the procedure it may be uncomfortable to sit on the hard table or achieve some of the necessary positions; it is important to remain as still as possible during the test; there are no dietary restrictions prior to the test; and it is necessary to remove dental prosthesis, jewelry, eyeglasses or other metal objects like hair clips before the procedure.

During Test: Adhere to standard precautions and sterile technique. The client is instructed to take a deep breath and hold it or to exhale and not to breathe as the x-ray is taken.

After Test: Monitor vital signs every 15 min for 1 hr, every 30 min for 1 hr, and every 2 hr for 24 hr. Record the time of voiding and color and amount of urine. Assess for hematuria, chills, fever, hypotension, elevated pulse and respiratory rate, and other signs of complications.

Potential Complications: Urinary sepsis from urinary tract infection; extravasation of contrast medium into general circulation; bladder rupture or urethral injury during catheterization

Contraindications: X-rays are usually avoided during pregnancy unless the benefit to the fetus outweighs the potential risk.

Interfering Factors: Presence of feces or gas

Nursing Considerations:

Pregnancy: Radiation and IV contrast should be avoided in pregnant women if possible (note: appropriate lead shielding is done to protect the fetus if it is determined this test is necessary).

Pediatric: Sedation is recommended for infants and children. Place the infant or child on a blanket for comfort. After postprocedure monitoring is completed and per health care provider's order, the pediatric client is discharged with an adult who is given instructions. This test is performed in male infants when cystoscopic examination is not possible.

Gerontology: The older person may find it difficult to maintain positions when required to do so during the cystography.

Rural: Advisable to arrange for transportation home after recovering from procedure.

Listing of Related Tests: Cystourethrography

| WEBLINKS |

http://www.creighton.edu

RADIOLOGIC

Fluorescein Angiography
(floer-*ES*-ee-:n *AEN*-jee-*AHG*-ruh-fee)
(FA; eye fundus)

45–60 min.

Type of Test: X-ray

Body Systems and Functions: Sensory system

Normal Findings: Normal retina and choroidal vessels

Test Results Time Frame: Within 24–48 hr

Test Description: Fluorescein angiography (FA) is a radiological examination of the retinal vasculature after the administration of a fluorescein dye. Within 12–15 min, the dye fills the arteries, capillaries, and veins of the retina. Then fluorescein images are taken in sequence and a computer provides views during any of the stages of the filling and emptying of the dye. The retina is the innermost layer of the eye and is responsible for receiving the transmitted images through the eye lens and contains the receptors for vision, the rods, and the cones. FA detects abnormalities in the function of the retina.

CLINICAL ALERT:
Have emergency equipment readily available in the event of an anaphylactic reaction to the dye.

Consent Form: Required

List of Equipment: X-ray machine and related equipment from radiology or special studies; IV equipment (heparin lock)

Test Procedure:
1. Administer mydriatic eye drops 15–30 min before the examination. *Dilates eyes.*
2. Place client in sitting position facing camera.
3. Client is instructed to open eyes wide, close the mouth, and look forward as baseline fundus photographs are taken.
4. Inject fluorescein dye intravenously.
5. Photographs of eye are taken every second for 25–45 sec, with a follow-up photograph taken 30 min later.

Clinical Implications and Indications:
1. Detects vascular disorders affecting visual acuity, tumors, papilledema, and leakage and retinal thickening
2. Evaluates the retina and any circulation abnormalities

Nursing Care:
Before Test: Explain the test procedure and the purpose of the test. Assess the client's knowledge of the test. Instruct client to withhold current eye medications. Inform client that dye can cause skin to be yellow for 1–2 days. Instruct client to void. Assess for potential allergies to contrast medium. Inform client that during injection of contrast medium, a burning sensation may be felt for a few seconds behind the eyes or in the jaw, teeth, tongue, or lips. Assess for

RADIOLOGIC

anxiety and provide sedation as ordered. Administer preoperative medication usually 30 min before procedure. Obtain baseline vital signs and neurological assessment.

During Test: Adhere to standard precautions. Assess for allergic reactions to contrast medium.

After Test: Assess for allergic reactions to contrast medium.

Potential Complications: Anaphylaxis due to allergic reaction to iodinated contrast material

Contraindications: Previous history of allergy to iodine, eggs, or shellfish; allergy to fluorescein

Interfering Factors: Inability of client to keep eyelids open and eyes in a fixed position; cataracts; improper dilation of pupils

Nursing Considerations:

Pediatric: Infants and children will need assistance in remaining still during the procedure and age-appropriate comfort measures following the test.

WEBLINKS ▶	🖿 ⊠

http://health.excite.com

Fluoroscopy
(floer-*AHS*-kuh-pee)

15 min.

Type of Test: X-ray

Body Systems and Functions: Cardiovascular system is common, but body system varies, dependent on site of testing

Normal Findings: Normal pulmonary and diaphragm movement; absence of CAD; normal structures of individual sites where fluoroscopy is performed (e.g., gastrointestinal system, myelography, venography, genitourinary system)

Test Results Time Frame: Within 24 hr

Test Description: Fluoroscopy is an imaging examination in which x-rays are taken through the client to a fluorescent viewing screen. The examiner is able to watch movement in the area being filmed while the study is in progress. A variety of systems are able to be tested (e.g., diaphragm, heart, digestive system). In addition, fluoroscopy is used for needle insertion or biopsy, catheter guidance during placement, or removal of fluid from a body cavity. Fluoroscopy can be used as a single film or videotape and is used in combination with other radiological procedures (e.g., plain films, contrast medium delivery).

Consent Form: Required

RADIOLOGIC

List of Equipment: Fluoroscopy x-ray machine and related equipment from radiology

Test Procedure:
1. Place client in position that allows visualization of selected site. May require client to stand in front of fluoroscopy screen.
2. Administer fluoroscopy x-rays.

Clinical Implications and Indications:
1. Evaluates movement of sites of the body evaluated (e.g., diaphragm, esophagus)
2. Detects variety of structural problems, depending on area of body studied
3. Evaluates and monitors pleural effusion, pleural lesion, pulmonary disease, and lung masses

Nursing Care:
Before Test: Explain the test procedure and the purpose of the test. Assess the client's knowledge of the test. Instruct the client that during the procedure it may be uncomfortable to sit on the hard table or achieve some of the necessary positions; it is important to remain still as possible during the test; there are no dietary restrictions prior to the test; and it is necessary to remove dental prosthesis, jewelry, eyeglasses, or other metal objects like hair clips before the procedure.
During Test: Adhere to standard precautions. Remain still during procedure, except when technician asks client to turn for different projections.

Potential Complications: Radiation exposure (fluoroscopy delivers a much higher dose of radiation than conventional x-rays); infection

Contraindications: X-rays are usually avoided during pregnancy unless the benefit to the fetus outweighs the potential risk; lactation

Interfering Factors: Inability to remain still; uncooperative; metal objects

Nursing Considerations:
Pregnancy: Radiation should be avoided in pregnant women if possible (note: appropriate lead shielding is done to protect the fetus if it is determined this test is necessary).
Pediatric: Sedation is recommended for infants and children. Place the infant or child on a blanket for comfort. After postprocedure monitoring is completed and per health care provider's order, the pediatric client is discharged with an adult who is given instructions.
Gerontology: The older person may find it difficult to maintain positions when required to do so for lengthy periods of time during the fluoroscopy.

Listing of Related Tests: Fluoroscopy of the small intestine; myelogram; venogram

WEBLINKS

http://adam.excite.com

RADIOLOGIC

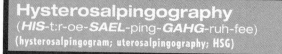

Hysterosalpingography
(*HIS*-t:r-oe-*SAEL*-ping-*GAHG*-ruh-fee)
(hysterosalpingogram; uterosalpingography; HSG)

30 min.

Type of Test: X-ray

Body Systems and Functions: Reproductive system

Normal Findings: No abnormality on fluoroscopic visualization

Test Results Time Frame: Within 24 hr

Test Description: Hysterosalpingography uses fluoroscopic visualization, where a radiopaque iodine-based dye is injected through the cervix, from which it follows the normal anatomical pathway into the uterus, the fallopian tubes, and finally the abdominal cavity. The test allows the exploration of the internal configuration of the uterine cavity. Hysterosalpingography also allows the determination of the patency of the fallopian tubes.

> **CLINICAL ALERT:**
> Have emergency equipment readily available in the event of an anaphylactic reaction to the dye.

Consent Form: Required

List of Equipment: Specialized equipment in special studies areas

Test Procedure:
1. The test should be performed in the first part of the menstrual cycle. *Ensures accurate results.*
2. Client is placed on an x-ray table in a lithotomy position for the initial injection of dye into the cervix.
3. Instruct client to hold breath when film is taken. *Prevents movement during respiration.*
4. Visualization under fluoroscopy is done following the dye through the anatomic pathway.

Clinical Implications and Indications:
1. Investigates uterine abnormalities, including pathology of the internal configuration of the uterine cavity.
2. Assesses patency of the fallopian tubes.
3. Instilling dye into the fallopian tubes may have a beneficial effect on the physiology of the involved organs.
4. The HSG should be scheduled for the interval between cessation of menstrual flow and ovulation to avoid retrograde flow of menstrual tissue into the tubes and the abdominal cavity.

Nursing Care:
Before Test: Explain the test procedure and the purpose of the test. Assess the client's knowledge of the test. Assess for potential allergies to contrast medium. Inform client that during injection of contrast medium, a burning sensation may be felt for a few seconds behind the eyes or in the jaw, teeth, tongue, or lips.

RADIOLOGIC

Assess for anxiety and provide sedation as ordered. Administer preoperative medication usually 30 min before procedure. Obtain baseline vital signs and neurological assessment.

During Test: Adhere to standard precautions. Provide for privacy. Assess for allergic reactions to contrast medium.

After Test: Assess client for possible abdominal discomfort or nausea immediately following the study. Assess for allergic reactions to contrast medium.

Potential Complications: Anaphylaxis due to allergic reaction to iodinated contrast material

Contraindications: Previous history of allergy to iodine, eggs, or shellfish; infections of the vagina or fallopian tubes; uterine bleeding

Interfering Factors: Incorrect timing of study in relation to menstrual cycle; tubal spasms; stricture of the fallopian tubes

Nursing Considerations:
Pregnancy: Radiation and IV contrast should be avoided in pregnant women if possible (note: appropriate lead shielding is done to protect the fetus if it is determined this test is necessary).

Listing of Related Tests: Laparoscopy; hysteroscopy

WEBLINKS

http://biocrs.biomed.brown.edu

Intravenous Pyelography
(*IN*-truh-*VE*-nus *PI*-e-*LOG*-ra-fee)
(excretory urography; IVU; IVP; KUB x-rays)

45 min.

Type of Test: X-ray

Body Systems and Functions: Renal/urological system

Normal Findings: Normal structure and function of the kidneys, ureters, and bladder, as evidenced by the length of time for dye to pass through to the bladder; normal kidney size approximately 3.5 vertebral bodies

> **CRITICAL VALUES:**
> If the blood urea nitrogen (BUN) is over 40 mg/dL, the test may not be performed.

Test Results Time Frame: Immediately after test to 1 day

Test Description: Intravenous pyelography (IVP) is a contrast radiographic study of the kidneys, ureters, and bladder. The IVP is performed by injecting the radiopaque contrast medium to visualize the renal pelvis. Multiple radiographs of the urinary tract are taken while the material is excreted through the normal routes. Any blockage along this tract is readily detected by this examination.

RADIOLOGIC

CLINICAL ALERT:
Have emergency equipment readily available in the event of an anaphylactic reaction to the dye.

Consent Form: Required

List of Equipment: Overhead radiography tube with flat top table (tomographic capabilities are desirable)

Test Procedure:
1. Place client in a supine position on the x-ray table.
2. Following an IV injection of iodine contrast, a series of x-rays are taken at specific time intervals over a 30-min period. *Visualizes the kidney, ureters, and bladder.*
3. The client is then asked to void and a final x-ray is taken (note: tomography studies may also be included during this procedure). *Visualizes bladder emptying.*

Clinical Implications and Indications:
1. Detects renal calculi, acute renal failure, tumors, polycystic kidney disease, hydronephrosis, chronic pyelonephritis, congenital abnormalities, ureteral calculi, urinary retention, and trauma

Nursing Care:
Before Test: Explain the test procedure and the purpose of the test. Assess the client's knowledge of the test. Assess for potential allergies to contrast medium. Inform client that during injection of contrast medium, a burning sensation may be felt for a few seconds behind the eyes or in the jaw, teeth, tongue, or lips. Assess for anxiety and provide sedation as ordered. Administer preoperative medication usually 30 min before procedure. Instruct clients to be NPO for 8–12 hr prior to the test. Clients with renal dysfunction may be given small amounts of water as ordered by their health care provider. Administration of a laxative is usually ordered on the evening before the study and a cleansing enema may be ordered the morning of the study to minimize interference of bowel contents during visualization of the renal and urinary structures. Vital signs, characteristics of the urinary output, urinary patterns, and urinary sensations, the most recent BUN, and other indices of renal function should be noted.
During Test: Adhere to standard precautions. Assess for allergic reactions to contrast medium.
After Test: Assess for allergic reactions to contrast medium. Vital signs should be monitored and documented every 30 min for 1 hr and then resume routine vital signs unless otherwise indicated. Urinary output should be monitored for detection of the renal response to the preprocedural dehydration. Food and fluids should be administered to facilitate rehydration.

Potential Complications: Anaphylaxis due to allergic reaction to iodinated contrast material; hypoglycemia or acidosis may occur in clients who are taking glucophage and receive iodine dye.

Contraindications: Previous history of allergy to iodine, eggs, or shellfish; severe dehydration; pregnancy; renal failure; multiple myeloma

RADIOLOGIC

Interfering Factors: Fecal matter; gas or barium in the bowel obscures visualization; abnormal renal function may prevent adequate visualization.

Nursing Considerations:
Pregnancy: Intravenous contrast should be avoided in pregnant women if possible.
Pediatric: Fasting times should be decreased.
Gerontology: Renal failure in elderly clients who are chronically dehydrated; 12-hr fasting may affect the geriatric client and it may be necessary to encourage activity restrictions if they are weakened by the procedure; the older person may find it difficult to maintain positions when required to do so for lengthy periods of time during the IVP.
Rural: Advisable to arrange for transportation home after recovering from the IVP.

Listing of Related Tests: Kidney scan; renal scan; renal tomography; renal ultrasound

WEBLINKS ⬚	⊟ ⊠

http://www.medexpert.net

Lymphangiography
(lim-*FAEN*-jee-*AHG*-ruh-fee)
(lymphography; lymphangiogram)

3 hr.

Type of Test: X-ray

Body Systems and Functions: Lymphatic system

Normal Findings: Normal filling of the lymphatic vessels and normal size and placement of lymph nodes with regular, uniform opacity

Test Results Time Frame: Within 24–48 hr

Test Description: Lymphangiography is a radiographic study of the lymphatic system following injection of an oil-based contrast medium into a lymphatic vessel. Following location of lymphatic vessels by the intradermal injection of blue contrast medium, a local anesthetic is injected at the catheter insertion site. An incision is made, the vessel is cannulated, and the contrast medium is injected over 1–2 hr. Radiographic films are taken. When adequate visualization of the lymphatic system is accomplished, the catheter is removed, the incision is closed, and a sterile dressing is applied. Radiographic films are repeated in 24 hr for visualization of the lymph nodes. The contrast medium is injected into the lymphatic vessels in the foot for visualization of lymph structures of the leg, inguinal, iliac, retroperitoneum, and thoracic duct. The contrast medium is injected into the hand for visualization of the axillary, supraclavicular, and cervical lymph structures.

> **CLINICAL ALERT:**
> Have emergency equipment readily available in the event of an anaphylactic reaction to the dye.

Consent Form: Required

RADIOLOGIC

List of Equipment: Radiology equipment; contrast dye; antiseptic solutions; local anesthestic; lymphangiography sterile equipment tray

Test Procedure:

1. Place client in supine position on the x-ray table.
2. Blue contrast media is injected intradermally between each of the first three toes. *Stains the lymphatic vessels.*
3. Site is anesthetized and small incision is made on the dorsum of each foot.
4. Lymph vessels are identified and cannulated. *Facilitates low-pressue injection of the iodine contrast media.*
5. When contrast reaches level of third to fourth lumbar vertebrae as seen with fluoroscopy, the injection is stopped.
6. Abdominal pelvic and upper body films are taken. *Demonstrates the lymphatic vessels filling.*
7. Second set of x-rays is taken 12–24 hr later. *Demonstrates filling of the nodes.*

Clinical Implications and Indications:

1. Detects lymphoma metastatic disease and lymphedema

Nursing Care:

Before Test: Explain the test procedure and the purpose of the test. Assess the client's knowledge of the test. Assess for potential allergies to contrast medium. Inform client that during injection of contrast medium, a burning sensation may be felt for a few seconds behind the eyes or in the jaw, teeth, tongue, or lips. Assess for anxiety and provide sedation as ordered. Administer preoperative medication usually 30 min before procedure. Obtain baseline vital signs and neurological assessment. Instruct clients that urine and stool discoloration from the blue dye may last several days. The skin may also have a bluish tinge. Instruct relaxation techniques to clients for remaining still during the prolonged injection of the contrast medium. Instruct client to void before the procedure.

During Test: Adhere to standard precautions. Assess for allergic reactions to contrast medium.

After Test: Assess for allergic reactions to contrast medium. Vital signs should be monitored and recorded every 4 hr for 48 hr. Clients are placed on bed rest for 24 hr with the extremity elevated to minimize peripheral edema. Incision sites may be painful requiring the administration of analgesics; they should be assessed for signs of hematoma formation and infection. Instruct clients in the care of the incision sites (i.e., the sterile dressing should be kept in place for 2 days and the site kept dry and tub baths should not be taken until the sutures are removed in approximately 7 days). Signs of infection should be reported immediately.

Potential Complications: Anaphylaxis due to allergic reaction to iodinated contrast material; lipoid pneumonia

Contraindications: Previous history of allergy to iodine, eggs, or shellfish; multiple myeloma; acute asthma; pregnancy; diabetes; severe pumonary insufficiency; cardiac disease; advanced renal or hepatic disease; sickle cell disease; syphilis; hyperthyroidism; dehydration

RADIOLOGIC

Nursing Considerations:

Pregnancy: *Radiation and IV contrast should be avoided in pregnant women if possible (note: appropriate lead shielding is done to protect the fetus if it is determined this test is necessary).*

Pediatric: *Sedation is recommended for infants and children. Place the infant or child on a blanket for comfort. After postprocedure monitoring is completed and per health care provider's order, the pediatric client is discharged with an adult who is given instructions.*

Gerontology: *The older person may find it difficult to maintain positions when required to do so for lengthy periods of time during the lymphangiography.*

Rural: *Advisable to arrange for transportation home after recovering from lymphangiography.*

| WEBLINKS |

http://adam.excite.com

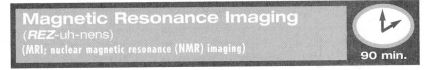

Magnetic Resonance Imaging
(*REZ*-uh-nens)
(MRI; nuclear magnetic resonance (NMR) imaging)

90 min.

Type of Test: X-ray

Body Systems and Functions: Musculoskeletal system

Normal Findings: Normal tissue, blood flow, and structures

Test Results Time Frame: Within 48 hr

Test Description: Magnetic resonance imaging takes take images that are created from the magnetic characteristics of body tissues. Certain atomic nuclei with an odd number of neutrons and protons are subjected to a radiofrequency pulse, which causes them to absorb and release energy. The resulting current passes through a radiofrequency receiver and is then transferred to a cross-sectional image of the body. This testing spares the client from x-ray exposure. Images can be taken at any angle, including sagittal and coronal planes. The MRI is able to provide more detail than some aspects of a computed tomography scan, for example in brain tumors of the posterior fossa. The MRI may also include the use of contrast materials for additional enhancement of its images.

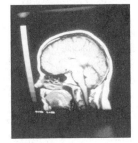

Magnetic Resonance Imaging

RADIOLOGIC

CLINICAL ALERT:
No form of metal is to accompany the client while having the MRI. Clients with claustrophobia may require sedation.

Consent Form: Required

List of Equipment: Radiology equipment

Test Procedure:
1. Place client in supine position on a narrow table with a cylindrical scanner surrounding them as images are taken (note: a loud clicking/banging noise may occur as images are taken).
2. Remove client from MRI device.

Clinical Implications and Indications:
1. The MRI is excellent for showing abnormalities of the brain (e.g., stroke, hemorrhage, tumor, infection, multiple sclerosis, demyelinating disease, dementia), of the head and neck (e.g., carotid artery disease, tumors, sinus disease), of the spine (e.g., herniated disk, spinal stenosis, metastatic disease, spinal cord compression), and heart disease and blood clots.

Nursing Care:
Before Test: Assess the client's knowledge of the test. Explain the test procedure and the purpose of the test. Explain that some clients suffer a feeling of claustrophobia because the magnetic machine has a small-diameter bore for the client's body. Instruct the client to remain still and explain that they cannot move out of the machine, which can cause a feeling of helplessness and claustrophobia. Inform the client that they will hear loud knocking noises emitted from the magnetic coils changing pulse direction. Remove all jewelry, watches, glasses, hairpins, and any other metal objects. Mild sedation may be required to assist client to relax as well as playing music and remaining in verbal contact with the client during the test.

During Test: Adhere to standard precautions. A microphone is available for technicians to communicate with client. Provide positive verbal encouragement during the test to assist client to relax.

Contraindications: The strong magnetic force will affect metal objects and electronic devices; pacemakers; cerebral aneurysms that have been clipped with metal; metal fragments in the eye (e.g., from a working environment)

Interfering Factors: Movement during the test; metal, especially ferrous metal, in the client's body can cause serious injury; metals can also cause artifacts in the images.

Nursing Considerations:
Pediatric: Infants and children will need assistance in remaining still during the magnetic resonance imaging and age-appropriate comfort measures following the test.

RADIOLOGIC

Gerontology: The older person may find it difficult to maintain positions when required to do so for lengthy periods of time during the MRI.

Listing of Related Tests: CT scan

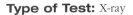

WEBLINKS 🔖

www.medexpert.net

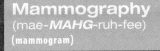

Mammography
(mae-*MAHG*-ruh-fee)
(mammogram)

30 min.

Type of Test: X-ray

Body Systems and Functions: Reproductive system

Normal Findings: Breast tissue within normal limits; normal ducts with gradually narrowing ductal system branches

Test Results Time Frame: Within 24–48 hr

Test Description: Mammography is a radiographic study using a low-dose x-ray technique to examine breast tissue. It is used in conjuction with physical palpation. Mammography is used to screen for pathology in women over 40, and annual mammograms are recommended. Mammography is used to screen for breast cancer or assess for a wide variety of breast tissue anomalies.

CLINICAL ALERT:
Mammograms should be compared with previous mammo-gram testing to provide accurate interpretation.

Consent Form: Not required

List of Equipment: X-ray machine and related equipment from radiology

Test Procedure:
1. The client is placed in a sitting or standing position with her breasts flat-tened in a plastic compressor. *Allows for correct positioning of the breasts.*
2. Instruct client to hold her breath when film is taken. *Prevents movement during respiration.*

Clinical Implications and Indications:
1. Detects breast mass (benign or cancerous), cysts, abcesses, fibrocystic dis-ease, intraductal papilloma of the breasts, occult cancer, supporative mastitis, and Paget's disease of the breasts
2. Evaluates the breasts when clinical manifestations are present
3. Screens for women over 40 and for women at risk for breast cancer
4. Assesses pendulous breasts that are difficult to palpate
5. Provides method of localizing a mass before a biopsy procedure
6. Monitors client after breast biopsy and after cancer management (e.g., sur-gery, radiation, chemotherapy)

RADIOLOGIC

Nursing Care:

Before Test: Explain the test procedure and the purpose of the test. Assess the client's knowledge of the test. Assure client that exposure to radiation is minimal. Respect client's privacy and the sensitive nature of the test, especially if the mammogram is not "routine" but being conducted because of an abnormal breast examination. Instruct the client that during the procedure it may be uncomfortable to sit on the hard table or achieve some of the necessary positions; it is important to remain as still as possible during the test; there are no dietary restrictions prior to the test; and it is necessary to remove dental prosthesis, jewelry, eyeglasses, or other metal objects like hair clips before the procedure.
During Test: Adhere to standard precautions. Provide reassurance and a calm atmosphere during the procedure. The client is instructed to take a deep breath and hold it or to exhale and not to breathe as the x-ray is taken.
After Test: Recommend that client have a routine mammogram every other year over the age of 40 and annually after age 50. Also inform client that women with an increased risk of breast cancer should have a mammogram annually after age 40.

Contraindications: X-rays are usually avoided during pregnancy unless the benefit to the fetus outweighs the potential risk.

Interfering Factors: Inability to remain still; jewelry and clothing; scar tissue from previous surgery; body powders, creams, and deodorants; cystic breasts (common before age 30)

Nursing Considerations:

Pregnancy: Radiation should be avoided in pregnant women if possible (note: appropriate lead shielding is done to protect the fetus if it is determined this test is necessary).
Gerontology: The older person may find it difficult to maintain positions when required to do so for lengthy periods of time during the mammography.

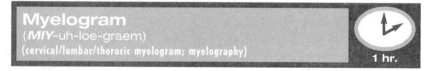

WEBLINKS

http://www.healthgate.com

Myelogram

(*MIY*-uh-loe-graem)
(cervical/lumbar/thoracic myelogram; myelography)

1 hr.

Type of Test: X-ray

Body Systems and Functions: Musculoskeletal system

Normal Findings: Normal outline of subarachnoid space with no visualization of spinal cord abnormalities or obstructions

Test Results Time Frame: Within 24 hr

Test Description: A myelogram is an x-ray of the spine with the subarachnoid space highlighted through augmentation with oil-based or water-based

RADIOLOGIC

agents. In rare instances, air may be used for contrast instead of the injection of liquid medium. The study allows for visualization of spinal cord and nerve roots and assists in identifying abnormalities of the spine, spinal cord, or surrounding structures. MRIs are often used in place of myelograms due to lower associated risk of complications and increasing availability.

CLINICAL ALERT:
Have emergency equipment readily available in the event of an anaphylactic reaction to the dye.

Consent Form:
Required

List of Equipment: X-ray machine and related equipment from radiology; specialized myelography equipment

Test Procedure:
1. Place client in prone or side-lying position, depending on spinal injection site. Secure the client to the table with straps. *Allows for safety during the procedure.*
2. Prepare the puncture site, drape, and administer local anesthetic.
3. Remove a small amount of spinal fluid and inject the contrast agent.
4. As the contrast agent is being injected, the table is tilted and x-rays are taken at various points (note: the table is returned to horizontal and oil-based agent may be removed).
5. Remove the needle and apply a sterile dressing. *Decreases the likelihood of infection.*

Clinical Implications and Indications:
1. Detects injury to spinal nerve roots
2. Identifies herniated or protruding intervertebral disks
3. Identifies meningiomas, neurofibromas, or tumors (primary or metastatic) impinging on spinal cord or within the subarachnoid space

Nursing Care:
Before Test: Explain the test procedure and the purpose of the test. Assess the client's knowledge of the test. Assess for potential allergies to contrast medium. Inform client that during injection of contrast medium, a burning sensation may be felt for a few seconds behind the eyes or in the jaw, teeth, tongue, or lips. Assess for anxiety and provide sedation as ordered. Administer preoperative medication usually 30 min before procedure. Obtain baseline vital signs and neurological assessment. Instruct the client to be NPO 2–4 hr prior to the test. In the case of glucophage, the client should receive instructions regarding injectable insulin. Instruct client to void before procedure.
During Test: Assess for allergic reactions to contrast medium.
After Test: Assess for allergic reactions to contrast medium. Monitor vital signs frequently and instruct client is to lie prone or supine for 8–12 hr. If water-soluble agent is used, the head of the bed sould be elevated to 60°, otherwise 30°–45°. Encourage the client to drink fluids and monitor ouput. Assess for symptoms of headache, fever, stiff neck, and photophobia, which might indicate irritation of meninges or meningitis. Instruct client that phenothiazines or tricyclic antidepressants are usually not restarted for 48 hr.

RADIOLOGIC

Potential Complications: Anaphylaxis due to allergic reaction to iodinated contrast material; headache; seizures; meningitis

Contraindications: Previous history of allergy to iodine, eggs, or shellfish; pregnancy; increased intracranial pressure; multiple sclerosis; bleeding abnomalities; anticoagulants

Interfering Factors: Inability to remain still; medications that alter results are tricyclic antidepressants, phenothiazines, CNS stimulants, and glucophage.

Nursing Considerations:
Pregnancy: Intravenous contrast should be avoided in pregnant women if possible.
Pediatric: Sedation is recommended for infants and children. Place the infant or child on a blanket for comfort. After postprocedure monitoring is completed and per health care provider's order, the pediatric client is discharged with an adult who is given instructions.
Gerontology: The older person may find it difficult to maintain positions when required to do so for lengthy periods of time during the myelogram.
Rural: Client should be told before coming to facility where test is performed that the test may take most of the day. The length of the test is due to additional testing such as CT scan (which is often ordered in conjunction with the myelogram) as well as the minimum 8-hr recovery period.

Listing of Related Tests: CT scan; MRI of spine

WEBLINKS 🔲🗙

www.spineuniverse.com

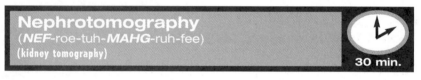

Nephrotomography
(*NEF*-roe-tuh-*MAHG*-ruh-fee)
(kidney tomography)

30 min.

Type of Test: X-ray

Body Systems and Functions: Renal/urological system

Normal Findings:
Normal anatomy of the kidneys, renal pelvis, and ureters

Test Results Time Frame: Within 24 hr

Test Description: Nephrotomography is an x-ray film of the kidney structures that penetrates dense shadows and thereby provides an augmented picture of soft tissue such as that due to masses or normal anatomical structures. An enhanced picture of a plane of an organ is generated that might otherwise have been hidden by surrounding structures. It may be done in isolation or as an adjunct to excretory urography. A contrast medium is added to provide more definitive information about the renal system.

> **CLINICAL ALERT:**
> Have emergency equipment readily available in the event of an anaphylactic reaction to the dye.

RADIOLOGIC

Consent Form: Required

List of Equipment: X-ray machine and related equipment from radiology

Test Procedure:
1. Place the client in supine position on an x-ray table with his arms above his head. *Allows for an unobstructed view of the abdomen.*
2. Place a protective shield over the genital region and take a single film. *To prevent radiation overexposure.*
3. Instruct the client to hold his breath when film is taken. *Prevents movement during respiration.*
4. Radiopaque dye is injected intravenously. *Enhances definition of film information.*
5. A second film (if more than one) is taken.

Clinical Implications and Indications:
1. Provides clearer visualization whenever anatomical information is obscured (e.g., overlying bowel or faint visualization)
2. Provides enhanced anatomical or pathophysiological definition (e.g., changes due to renal failure, presence of mass)

Nursing Care:
Before Test: Explain the test procedure and the purpose of the test. Assess the client's knowledge of the test. Assess for potential allergies to contrast medium. Inform client that during injection of contrast medium, a burning sensation may be felt for a few seconds behind the eyes or in the jaw, teeth, tongue, or lips. Assess for anxiety and provide sedation as ordered. Administer preoperative medication usually 30 min before procedure. Obtain baseline vital signs and neurological assessment. Inform client that if the nephrotomography is being done in combination with other diagnostic test (e.g., IVP), it may require a fasting period. In addition, inform client that bowel preparation may have been ordered to limit feces or gas from obscuring renal system views. Instruct the client that during the procedure it may be uncomfortable to sit on the hard table or achieve some of the necessary positions; it is important to remain as still as possible during the test; and it is necessary to remove dental prosthesis, jewelry, eyeglasses, or other metal objects like hair clips before the procedure.
During Test: Assess for allergic reactions to contrast medium. Instruct client to take a deep breath and hold it or to exhale and not to breathe as the x-ray is taken.
After Test: Assess for allergic reactions to contrast medium. Encourage client to drink fluids to increase excretion of dye.

Potential Complications: Anaphylaxis due to allergic reaction to iodinated contrast material

Contraindications: Previous history of allergy to iodine, eggs, or shellfish; severe cardiovascular disease; multiple myeloma

Interfering Factors: Residual barium

Nursing Considerations:
Pediatric: Sedation is recommended for infants and children. Place the infant or child on a blanket for comfort. After postprocedure monitoring is completed and

per health care provider's order, the pediatric client is discharged with an adult who is given instructions.

Gerontology: *The older person may find it difficult to maintain positions when required to do so for lengthy periods of time during the nephrotomography. In addition, elderly clients should be assessed for weakness and dehydration following test, particularly when this x-ray is combined with other tests that would have required lengthy pretest fasting.*

Rural: *Advisable to arrange for transportation home after recovering from the nephrotomography.*

Listing of Related Tests: Excretory urography

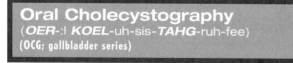

http://www.creighton.edu

Oral Cholecystography
(*OER-*:| *KOEL*-uh-sis-*TAHG*-ruh-fee)
(OCG; gallbladder series)

30–45 min.

Type of Test: X-ray

Body Systems and Functions: Hepatobiliary system

Normal Findings: Normal gallbladder size and structure and no gallstones present

Test Results Time Frame: Within 2 days

Test Description: This x-ray uses augmentation with oral contrast media to identify obstruction of gallbladder or ducts. Ultrasound is often ordered instead of OCG, but some requests are made for OCG since it may provide valuable information regarding gallstone composition (size and number) and cystic duct patency. The gallbladder is an organ located on the underside of the right lobe of the liver. It stores bile, which is received from the liver. Bile is responsible for the emulsification of fats and oils and stimulating peristalsis.

> **CLINICAL ALERT:**
> Have emergency equipment readily available in the event of an anaphylactic reaction to the dye.

Consent Form: Required

List of Equipment: Oral contrast preparation; x-ray equipment

Test Procedure:
1. Contrast medium is ingested by the client prior to the cholecystography.
2. X-rays are taken of the client's right upper quadrant of the abdomen in the prone, left lateral decubitus, and erect positions. Protect the client's genital area with a shield. *Avoids overexposure to radiation.*
3. The client may have to ingest a high-fat meal or synthetic fat agents after the original set of films and then repeat the films 1–2 hr later. *Stimulates the gallbladder and subsequent x-rays will indicate contractility.*

RADIOLOGIC

Clinical Implications and Indications:
1. Diagnoses obstruction or defects of the cystic duct
2. Identifies presence, number, and size of gallstones in the gallbladder
3. Identifies benign or malignant tumor of the gallbladder
4. Diagnoses inflammation of the gallbladder

Nursing Care:

Before Test: Explain the test procedure and the purpose of the test. Assess the client's knowledge of the test. Instruct client to eat high-fat lunch the day prior to the test and ingest a low-fat meal the evening before the test. In addition, instruct client to drink an oral contrast preparation the day before the test (e.g., usually in the evening) and then to fast until the time of the cholecystrography. Instruct the client that during the procedure it may be uncomfortable to sit on the hard table or achieve some of the necessary positions; it is important to remain as still as possible during the test; and to remove dental prosthesis, jewelry, eyeglasses, or other metal objects like hair clips before the procedure. Assess for potential allergies to contrast medium. Inform client that during injection of contrast medium, a burning sensation may be felt for a few seconds behind the eyes or in the jaw, teeth, tongue, or lips. Assess for anxiety and provide sedation as ordered. Administer preoperative medication usually 30 min before procedure. Obtain baseline vital signs and neurological assessment.

During Test: Adhere to standard precautions. The client is instructed to take a deep breath and hold it or to exhale and not to breathe as the x-ray is taken. Assess for allergic reactions to contrast medium.

After Test: Assess for allergic reactions to contrast medium. Instruct client to resume normal diet once the health care provider has determined that no further x-rays will be taken. Changes in diet may be recommended if gallstones are identified on x-ray. Encourage fluid intake, which will enhance excretion of the dye.

Potential Complications: Anaphylaxis due to allergic reaction to iodinated contrast material

Contraindications: Previous history of allergy to iodine, eggs, or shellfish; pregnancy; renal or hepatic disease

Interfering Factors: Barium in bowel; diarrhea; inadequate client preparation; jaundice; liver disease; obstruction of the cystic duct; vomiting

Nursing Considerations:

Pregnancy: Intravenous contrast should be avoided in pregnant women if possible.
Pediatric: Infants and children will need assistance in remaining still during the cholecystography and age-appropriate comfort measures following the test (note: this test is not often performed on this age).
Gerontology: The older person may find it difficult to maintain positions when required to do so for lengthy periods of time during the cholecystography.
Rural: Advisable to arrange for transportation home after recovering from procedure.

Listing of Related Tests: IV cholangiography; ultrasound

WEBLINKS

http://chorus.rad.mcw.edu

RADIOLOGIC

Orbital Films
(*OER*-bit-:l)

15 min.

Type of Test: X-ray

Body Systems and Functions: Musculoskeletal system

Normal Findings: Normal structure, no foreign bodies

Test Results Time Frame: Within 24 hr

Test Description: Orbital x-rays are taken of the bony pyramid-shaped cavity of the skull that contains and protects the eyeball. The orbit is pierced posteriorly by the optic foramen, the optic nerve and ophthalmic artery, the superior and inferior orbital fissures, and several foramina. These x-rays are valuable in the initial evaluation of fractures due to blunt trauma. Intraorbital and intracranial air, sinuses, and lacrimal fossa may also be identified. Hemorrhage may be apparent through presence of an air-fluid level or complete opacification of a sinus, which may be consistent with a fractured orbit.

Consent Form: Not required

List of Equipment: X-ray machine and related equipment from radiology

Test Procedure:
1. The client is seated on the x-ray table with the arms at the side and one ear against the plate so that the client's midsaggital plane is parallel to the plane of the film. *Allows for a lateral projection of the skull and surrounding organs.*
2. A protective shield may be placed over the genital region. *To prevent radiation overexposure.*
3. The client may be asked to reposition during the series of x-rays depending upon required angle. *X-rays are taken of the eye from several angles. Usual angles include oblique coronal view, posterior-anterior plane, and lateral view, but others may be required.*
4. Instruct the client to hold breath when film is taken. *Prevents movement during respiration.*

Clinical Implications and Indications:
1. Identifies bone fractures around the eye
2. Locates foreign bodies in the eyesocket or eye
3. Detects increased bone density associated with Paget's disease or meningioma

Nursing Care:
Before Test: Explain the test procedure and the purpose of the test. Assess the client's knowledge of the test. Instruct the client that during the procedure it may be uncomfortable to sit on the hard table or achieve some of the necessary positions; it is important to remain as still as possible during the test; there are no dietary restrictions prior to the test; and it is necessary to remove dental prosthesis, jewelry, eyeglasses, or other metal objects like hair clips before the procedure.

RADIOLOGIC

During Test: Adhere to standard precautions. Instruct client to reposition head or flex or extend their neck during the x-rays. Instruct the client to take a deep breath and hold it or to exhale and not to breathe as the x-ray is taken.

Contraindications: X-rays are usually avoided during pregnancy unless the benefit to the fetus outweighs the potential risk; suspect or confirmed cranial or cervical injuries

Interfering Factors: Inability to remain still

Nursing Considerations:
Pregnancy: Radiation should be avoided in pregnant women if possible (note: appropriate lead shielding is done to protect the fetus if it is determined this test is necessary).
Pediatric: Sedation may be recommended for infants and children. Place the infant or child on a blanket for comfort. After postprocedure monitoring is completed and per health care provider's order, the pediatric client is discharged with an adult who is given instructions.
Gerontology: The older person may find it difficult to maintain positions when required to do so for lengthy periods of time during the x-ray.

Listing of Related Tests: CT; MRI; angiography

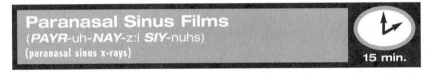

www.healthgate.com

Paranasal Sinus Films
(*PAYR*-uh-*NAY*-z:l *SIY*-nuhs)
(paranasal sinus x-rays)

15 min.

Type of Test: X-ray

Body Systems and Functions: Pulmonary system

Normal Findings: Intact paranasal sinus structures

Test Results Time Frame: Within 24 hr

Test Description: Radiography of the paranasal sinuses is a useful tool in determining the presence of abnormalities in sinus shape and structure. Frequently, abnormalities determined on x-ray will be further examined using CT or MRI to provide more specific detail. Usually a series of four films is taken. The first is the Caldwell projection, which will visualize the frontal and ethmoid sinuses. Next, the Water's projection is taken with the client in both the supine and upright positions to capture the maxillary antra and demonstration of air fluid levels within it. The last projection is lateral to visualize the sphenoid and frontal sinuses.

Consent Form: Not required

List of Equipment: X-ray machine and related equipment from radiology

RADIOLOGIC

Test Procedure:

1. Instruct client to wear a leaded apron. *Minimizes radiation exposure.*
2. Instruct client to maintain different positions of head and body, and a foam-covered head bracket may be applied to the head. *Optimizes visualization of sinuses on film.*
3. Instruct client to hold breath when film is taken. *Prevents movement during respiration.*

Clinical Implications and Indications:

1. Detects unilateral or bilateral abnormalities of the sinuses and surrounding tissue
2. Assists in identifying abnormal growths (benign or malignant tumors, cysts) and determining their size and location (both for initial diagnosis and follow-up to treatment)
3. Diagnoses acute or chronic sinusitis
4. Identifies traumatic damage (bleeding, fracture) to area

Nursing Care:

Before Test: Explain the test procedure and the purpose of the test. Assess the client's knowledge of the test. Instruct the client that during the procedure it may be uncomfortable to sit on the hard table or achieve some of the necessary positions; it is important to remain as still as possible during the test; there are no dietary restrictions prior to the test; and it is necessary to remove dental prosthesis, jewelry, eyeglasses, or other metal objects like hair clips before the procedure. Alert client that a bracket or "vise" may be used to assist in maintaining position but that it is padded and should cause no discomfort.

During Test: Adhere to standard precautions. The client is instructed to take a deep breath and hold it or to exhale and not to breathe as the x-ray is taken.

Contraindications: X-rays are usually avoided during pregnancy unless the benefit to the fetus outweighs the potential risk.

Interfering Factors: Inability to remain still

Nursing Considerations:

Pregnancy: Radiation should be avoided in pregnant women if possible (note: appropriate lead shielding is done to protect the fetus if it is determined this test is necessary).

Pediatric: Sedation is recommended for infants and children. Place the infant or child on a blanket for comfort. After postprocedure monitoring is completed and per health care provider's order, the pediatric client is discharged with an adult who is given instructions. Frontal sinuses are not fully developed until approximately 10 years of age. Sphenoid sinuses develop shortly after the maxillary and ethmoid sinuses, which are present at birth. As a result, a modified Waters and lateral views are all that is needed for evaluation of the young child and infant.

Listing of Related Tests: CT; MRI

WEBLINKS

http://www.rcjournal.com

RADIOLOGIC

Pelvimetry
(pel-**VIM**-uh-tree)
(radiographic pelvimetry; pelvic examination, digital)

15 min.

Type of Test: X-ray

Body Systems and Functions: Reproductive system

Normal Findings: Adequate anteroposterior and transverse diameters of pelvic inlet

Test Results Time Frame: Within 24 hr

Test Description: X-ray pelvimetry is done to estimate cephalopelvic proportions and predict obstetrical outcomes, usually in the last 4 weeks of pregnancy. Although fluoroscopy of the pregnant woman is considered controversial, the introduction of CT pelvimetry has reduced exposure to ionizing radiation and MRI pelvimetry eliminates it. As a result, there has been a resurgence in the use of pelvimetry, but its value continues to be questioned given that many women assessed as having inadequate pelvic proportions go on to deliver vaginally. Research continues to examine the use and value of pelvimetry.

Consent Form: Required

List of Equipment: X-ray machine and related equipment from radiology

Test Procedure:
1. Placed client standing with abdomen against the cassette (lateral erect view). *Allows for anterior-posterior and lateral x-rays to be taken.*
2. Other film angles can be taken: supine with beam above abdomen onto pubis; inlet view with client sitting semireclined; back supported and back arched; and an outlet view taken with the client sitting directly on the cassette, thighs apart and client leaning forward. *Different angles may be requested for viewing the pelvis and surrounding structures.*
3. Instruct client to hold breath when film is taken. *Prevents movement during respiration.*

Clinical Implications and Indications:
1. Obtain a history of previous cesarean sections for cephalic disproportion (note: controversial, as the success rate of vaginal births after cesarean is high despite information that a pelvimetry would provide)
2. Evaluates the need for a cesarean section delivery

Nursing Care:
Before Test: Explain the test procedure and the purpose of the test. Assess the client's knowledge of the test. Instruct the client that during the procedure it may be uncomfortable to sit on the hard table or achieve some of the necessary positions; it is important to remain as still as possible during the test; there are no dietary restrictions prior to the test; and it is necessary to remove dental prosthesis, jewelry, eyeglasses, or other metal objects like hair clips before the procedure.

During Test: Adhere to standard precautions. Client is requested to take a deep breath and hold it or to exhale and not to breathe as x-ray is taken.

RADIOLOGIC

After Test: Client may get dressed after technician or radiologist has confirmed that the x-rays are adequate.

Contraindications: X-rays are usually avoided during pregnancy unless the benefit to the fetus outweighs the potential risk.

Interfering Factors: Superimposition of other anatomical structures over target structures; inability to remain still

Nursing Considerations:
Pregnancy: Radiation should be avoided in pregnant women if possible (note: appropriate lead shielding is done to protect the fetus if it is determined this test is necessary).
Pediatric: Sedation is recommended for infants and children. Place the infant or child on a blanket for comfort. After postprocedure monitoring is completed and per health care provider's order, the pediatric client is discharged with an adult who is given instructions.
International: Adequate pelvic measurements may average differently for different populations.

WEBLINKS   ▤ ☒

www.rcog.org,

Percutaneous Transhepatic Cholangiography
(p:r-kyue-*TAYN*-ee-uhs *TRAENZ*-he-*PAET*-ik koe-*LAEN*-jee-*AHG*-ruh-fee)
(PTC; PTHC)

1 hr.

Type of Test: X-ray

Body Systems and Functions: Hepatobiliary system

Normal Findings: Normal anatomy and filling of cystic, hepatic, and common bile ducts

Test Results Time Frame: Within 24 hr

Test Description: This test is usually performed to determine the site of obstruction in a client with known obstructive jaundice. A 21- or 23-gauge Chiba needle is inserted into the ninth intercostal space in the midaxillary line under fluoroscopy. Dye is injected slowly as the needle is withdrawn until it enters a bile duct and more contrast medium is injected with the aim of completely filling the biliary tree. X-rays are then taken of the anatomy and any obstructions. If an obstruction is confirmed and is extrahepatic, a catheter may be left in place to drain bile externally or a stent may be placed across a stricture internally.

CLINICAL ALERT:
Have emergency equipment readily available in the event of an anaphylactic reaction to the dye.

RADIOLOGIC

Consent Form: Required

List of Equipment: X-ray machine and related equipment from radiology

Test Procedure:
1. Place client is supine position.
2. Local anesthetic is injected into abdominal wall.
3. The needle is advanced through the skin and into the liver (hepatic parenchyma of right lobe) using sonography or fluoroscopy as a guide.
4. Radiographic dye is injected.
5. Instruct client to hold breath when film is taken. *Prevents movement during respiration.*
6. A narrow-diameter catheter may be placed in the biliary tract and left for drainage if obstruction is found or a stent is inserted internally.

Clinical Implications and Indications:
1. Diagnoses site of obstruction in client with known obstructive jandice
2. Confirms presence of obstruction in client with jaundice of unknown origin
3. Identifies type of obstruction (e.g., stone, stricture, tumor)
4. Precursor to radiological, surgical, or endoscopic therapy

Nursing Care:
Before Test: Explain the test procedure and the purpose of the test. Assess the client's knowledge of the test. Instruct the client that during the procedure it may be uncomfortable to sit on the hard table or achieve some of the necessary positions; it is important to remain as still as possible during the test; and it is necessary to remove dental prosthesis, jewelry, eyeglasses, or other metal objects like hair clips before the procedure. Instruct client to eat a fat-free diet for the 24 hr prior to the test. Instruct client to remain NPO from midnight before test. Inform client to take laxatives (if ordered) prior to test. Ensure that the client's type and cross-match were completed and that coagulation studies and other blood work are available. Assess for potential allergies to contrast medium. Inform client that during injection of contrast medium, a burning sensation may be felt for a few seconds behind the eyes or in the jaw, teeth, tongue, or lips. Assess for anxiety and provide sedation as ordered. Administer preoperative medication usually 30 min before procedure. Obtain baseline vital signs and neurological assessment.

During Test: Adhere to standard precautions. The client is instructed to take a deep breath and hold it or to exhale and not to breathe as the x-ray is taken. Assess for allergic reactions to contrast medium.

After Test: Take vital signs per postsurgical protocol and until stable. Inform client that they must maintain bed rest for several hours postprocedure. Observe site for hemorrhage or bile leakage. Maintain NPO status for several hours postprocedure until it is confirmed that client is not going to bleed postoperatively. Maintain a sterile closed drainage system if a stent has been left in place. Inform client that they may have pain for several hours after the test and it may radiate into the right shoulder because of irritation to the diaphragm from leaking bile or blood. Administer pain medication as ordered (note: pain medications may be withheld to avoid masking symptoms of hemorrhage or bile extravasation). Assess for allergic reactions to contrast medium.

RADIOLOGIC

Potential Complications: Anaphylaxis due to allergic reaction to iodinated contrast material; peritonitis; hemorrhage; sepsis

Contraindications: X-rays are usually avoided during pregnancy unless the benefit to the fetus outweighs the potential risk; uncontrolled coagulopathy; uncooperativeness; mild cholangitis (injection of dye can increase biliary pressure and cause bacteremia); previous history of allergy to iodine, eggs, or shellfish

Interfering Factors: Barium studies within 2 days prior to test; client movement during test

Nursing Considerations:
Pregnancy: Radiation and IV contrast should be avoided in pregnant women if possible (note: appropriate lead shielding is done to protect the fetus if it is determined this test is necessary).
Pediatric: Sedation is recommended for infants and children. Place the infant or child on a blanket for comfort. After postprocedure monitoring is completed and per health care provider's order, the pediatric client is discharged with an adult who is given instructions.
Gerontology: The older person may find it difficult to maintain positions when required to do so for lengthy periods of time during the percutaneous transhepatic cholangiography.
Rural: Advisable to arrange for transportation home after recovering from the percutaneous transhepatic cholangiography.

Listing of Related Tests: Endoscopic retrograde cholangiopancreatography (ERCP); liver function studies; CT; sonography

WEBLINKS

www.arup-lab.com

Radiography
(*RAY*-dee-*AHG*-ruh-fee)
(plain film; roentgengram; x-ray)

15–20 min.

Type of Test: X-ray

Body Systems and Functions: Musculoskeletal system

Normal Findings: Negative for bone fracture and tissue masses or abnormalities

Test Results Time Frame: Within 24 hr

Test Description: Radiography is the use of x-rays to visualize bones and soft tissues. X-rays are produced by applying an electron beam to a vacuum tube containing tungsten. The rays produced have a shorter wavelength than those of visible light rays and can penetrate tissues to a varying degree depending on the tissue composition. The x-ray image is a negative image produced on film in special cassettes. Tissue that partially blocks the rays, such as bone, is called radiopaque and produces a white image on the film. Those tissues that

RADIOLOGIC

allow more ray penetration such as the lungs are a grey image on the film. X-rays can be of low energy (1–0.1 AU) used for diagnostic studies to higher energy (0.1–10^{-4} AU) used in radiation therapy for cancer. Radiography can include many uses, including plain x-ray, computed tomography (CT), and radioisotope scans and contrast studies. The plain x-ray, fluoroscopy, CT, and those studies using barium are noninvasive and do not require a signed consent. The plain x-ray is a basic test done for diagnostic screening for many potential problems, which may need additional more expensive or invasive diagnostic tests for further differential diagnosis. Plain film x-ray is the basic diagnostic tool for fractured bones, joint injuries, and pneumonias.

Consent Form: Not required (note: unless test is invasive using iodinated or other types of dyes that are injected intravenously or directly into an organ)

List of Equipment: Tests are done in the medical imaging or x-ray department with trained technicians and specialized equipment.

Test Procedure:
1. Have client remove clothes and all metal or jewelry from the part to be x-rayed. *Metal absorbs all rays so object appears white on film and blocks visualization of tissues behind it.*
2. Have client in gown, and if lying on the x-ray table, place bath blanket over client for warmth and privacy.
3. Splints should not be removed without direction of clinician. If an injury involved, maintain correct positioning of the limb without twisting and with support to all joints.
4. A lead shield is placed over the client's abdomen and genital area to protect the reproductive organs from x-rays.
5. Several x-rays with the camera at different locations and angles are usually taken.

Clinical Implications and Indications: Selected examples of the use of plain film x-rays are:
1. Diagnoses bone fractures
2. Diagnoses presence of foreign body in gastrointestinal tract or in respiratory airways
3. Diagnoses Paget's disease with thickening of bones
4. Diagnoses cardiovascular disorders, such as cardiomyopathy and congestive heart failure
5. Diagnoses pulmonary infections and pleural effusions
6. Diagnoses abnormal tissue mass in thorax, abdomen, or kidneys
7. Diagnoses osteoarthritis in joints or spinal column

Nursing Care:
Before Test: Explain the test procedure and the purpose of the test. Assess the client's knowledge of the test. Instruct the client that during the procedure it may be uncomfortable to sit on the hard table or achieve some of the necessary positions; it is important to remain as still as possible during the test; there are no dietary restrictions prior to the test; and it is necessary to remove dental prosthesis, jewelry, eyeglasses, or other metal objects like hair clips before the procedure.
During Test: The client is instructed to take a deep breath and hold it or to exhale and not to breathe as the x-ray is taken.

RADIOLOGIC

Contraindications: X-rays are usually avoided during pregnancy unless the benefit to the fetus outweighs the potential risk.

Interfering Factors: Inability to remain still; unable to follow instructions

Nursing Considerations:

Pregnancy: X-rays are a known teratogen to fetus and this should be told to the mother.

Pediatric: Sedation is recommended for infants and children. Place the infant or child on a blanket for comfort. After postprocedure monitoring is completed and per health care provider's order, the pediatric client is discharged with an adult who is given instructions.

Gerontology: The older person may find it difficult to maintain positions when required to do so for lengthy periods of time during the x-ray.

WEBLINKS

www.nlm.nih.gov

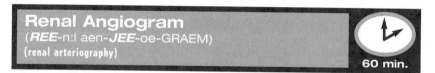

Renal Angiogram
(*REE*-n:l aen-*JEE*-oe-GRAEM)
(renal arteriography)

60 min.

Type of Test: X-ray

Body Systems and Functions: Renal/urological system

Normal Findings: Normal arterial and venous circulation; no abnormal tissues

Test Results Time Frame: Within 24 hr

Test Description: Renal angiography involves injecting contrast dye through a catheter in the renal artery or vein so that the circulation system and tissues of the kidneys can be visualized by x-rays. In the past renal angiography was used more for diagnosis, but it has been largely replaced by noninvasive computerized tomography (CT). The primary uses of renal angiography currently are to evaluate renal stenosis, to detect accessory renal arteries, which are often small but a frequent cause of renal artery hypertension, and as a vehicle for the therapeutic interventions of embolization of accessory blood vessels or aneurysms and for angioplasty of a stenosed renal artery. Venography is rarely done, having been replaced by contrast-enhanced CT.

CLINICAL ALERT:
Have emergency equipment readily available in the event of an anaphylactic reaction to the dye.

Consent Form: Required

List of Equipment: X-ray machine and related equipment from radiology

Test Procedure:
1. Place client in supine position on the x-ray table.
2. Establish an IV line with hydration fluid running. *Hydration is important for the dye to be well excreted through the kidney.*
3. Cleanse femoral entry site with betadine and drape with sterile towels.
4. A local anesthetic is injected under the skin.
5. A catheter is introduced into the femoral artery and threaded through the iliac artery and the aorta into the renal artery. (If a venous image is wanted, the femoral vein is used and the catheter is threaded through the iliac vein and the inferior vena cava and into the renal vein.) Fluoroscopy and a small amount of contrast dye are usually used to determine the catheter location and progression.
6. When the catheter has reached the renal artery or vein, a larger amount of dye is injected through the catheter, and a rapid series of x-rays are taken as the dye moves through the vascular bed.
7. The catheter is removed, a pressure dressing is applied to the groin, and client is monitored closely.

Clinical Implications and Indications:
1. Diagnoses presence of renal tumor and cysts and evaluates extent of vascularity before doing surgery or embolization.
2. Diagnoses presence of renal artery stenosis and evaluates therapeutic angioplasty and treatment of the stinting of renal artery stenosis.
3. Evaluates venovascular hypertension with collection of blood sample for renin evaluation.
4. Evaluates client as a potential kidney donor as well as assessing posttransplant functioning.
5. Diagnoses vascular irregularities, such as aneurysms, emboli, and hematoma.
6. Evaluates renal function in chronic renal failure or hydronephrosis.

Nursing Care:
Before Test: Explain the test procedure and the purpose of the test. Assess the client's knowledge of the test. Assess for potential allergies to contrast medium. Explain that the test will be done by a trained technician in the medical imaging department. Inform client that during injection of contrast medium, a burning sensation may be felt for a few seconds behind the eyes or in the jaw, teeth, tongue, or lips. Assess for anxiety and provide sedation as ordered. Administer preoperative medication usually 30 min before procedure. Obtain baseline vital signs and neurological assessment, instruct client to be NPO for 8 hr prior to the test, and have client void prior to test.

During Test: Adhere to standard precautions. Assess for allergic reactions to contrast medium.

After Test: Instruct client to lie flat with leg on affected side kept straight for 6 hr after the test. Closely monitor vital signs, groin site, and pedal pulses per protocol. Assess for allergic reactions to contrast medium.

Potential Complications: Embolus; hemorrhage; anaphylaxis due to allergic reaction to iodinated contrast material; renal damage from dye

Contraindications: Previous history of allergy to iodine, eggs, or shellfish; anticoagulation or bleeding disorders; end-stage renal disease; pregnancy

RADIOLOGIC

Interfering Factors: Barium or feces can impair image; inability of client to remain still; inability of client to follow diet and medication restrictions

Nursing Considerations:
Pregnancy: Intravenous contrast should be avoided in pregnant women if possible.
Pediatric: Contrast materials may be harmful to fetus. Infants and children will need assistance in remaining still during the procedure and age-appropriate comfort measures following the test.
Gerontology: The older person may find it difficult to maintain positions when required to do so for lengthy periods of time during the renal angiography.
Rural: Advisable to arrange for transportation home after recovering from renal angiography.

Listing of Related Tests: Blood urea nitrogen (BUN); creatinine; renal function tests; renal cystogram; renal scan; renal ultrasound

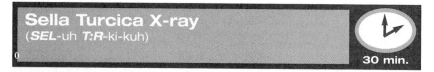

WEBLINKS

http://www.creighton.edu

Sella Turcica X-ray
(*SEL*-uh *T:R*-ki-kuh)

30 min.

Type of Test: X-ray

Body Systems and Functions: Neurological system

Normal Findings: Normal sella turcica and surrounding structures

Test Results Time Frame: Within 24 hr

Test Description: The sella turcica is a deep depression in the superior aspect of the sphenoid bone, located at the base of the cranium. This depression accommodates the pituitary gland (also known as the hypophysis). The auditory canal and organs of hearing are seen on some views of the x-ray.

Consent Form: Not required

List of Equipment: X-ray machine and related equipment from radiology

Test Procedure:
1. The client is seated on the x-ray table with the arms at the side and one ear against the plate so that the client's midsaggital plane is parallel to the plane of the film. *Allows for a lateral projection of the sella turcica and surrounding organs.*
2. Other film angles can be taken in the supine, prone, or sitting position. *Five different angles may be requested for viewing the sella turcica and surrounding structures.*
3. The client is instructed to hold his breath when film is taken. *Prevents movement during respiration.*
4. A head clamp may be used to immobilize the client. *Maintains the appropriate position while the film is taken.*

RADIOLOGIC

Clinical Implications and Indications:

1. Pituitary tumors can present in two ways. First, if the tumor produces a hormone, then hormonal symptoms will be evident, such as Cushing's syndrome or hyperprolactinemic amenorrhea. However, tumors that do not produce abnormally functioning hormones will have an edematous effect on surrounding organs. The client will then present with headache and visual disturbances.
2. MRI is a preferred technique for diagnosing sella turcica problems. Computerized tomography is also used in place of sella turcica films.
3. Often the problem with the sella turcica pituitary is discovered when skull or sinus films are ordered for other situations, such as head trauma or sinus problems.

Nursing Care:

Before Test: Explain the test procedure and the purpose of the test. Assess the client's knowledge of the test. The procedure causes no pain, but it may be uncomfortable to sit on the hard table or achieve some of the necessary positions. There are no dietary restrictions prior to the test. Remove dental prosthesis, jewelry, eyeglasses, or other metal objects like hair clips before the procedure.

During Test: The client is instructed to take a deep breath and hold it or to exhale and not to breathe as the x-ray is taken.

Contraindications:
X-rays are usually avoided during pregnancy unless the benefit to the fetus outweighs the potential risk.

Nursing Considerations:

Pregnancy: Radiation should be avoided in pregnant women if possible (note: appropriate lead shielding is done to protect the fetus if it is determined this test is necessary).

Pediatric: Sedation is recommended for infants and children. Place the infant or child on a blanket for comfort. After postprocedure monitoring is completed and per health care provider's order, the pediatric client is discharged with an adult who is given instructions.

Gerontology: The older person may find it difficult to maintain positions when required to do so for lengthy periods of time during the x-ray.

Listing of Related Tests:
Thyroid testing (T3 and T4); visual fields examination (peripheral vision may be compromised with pituitary tumors); prolactin; testosterone; estradiol

WEBLINKS

http://www.ncbi.nlm.nih.gov

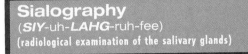

Sialography
(*SIY*-uh-*LAHG*-ruh-fee)
(radiological examination of the salivary glands)

30 min.

RADIOLOGIC

Type of Test: X-ray

Body Systems and Functions: Gastrointestinal system

Normal Findings: Normal salivary glands and surrounding structures

Test Results Time Frame: Within 24 hr

Test Description: Sialography involves injecting a contrast medium into the ducts of the salivary glands, making it possible to distinguish the surrounding tissue and the ductal system. Because the glands and ducts are so close together, only one gland/duct at a time can be examined with the contrast medium. Sialography can identify conditions such as inflammatory lesions, tumors, fistulae, and calculi.

> **CLINICAL ALERT:**
> Have emergency equipment readily available in the event of an anaphylactic reaction to the dye.

Consent Form: Required

List of Equipment: X-ray machine and related equipment from radiology

Test Procedure:
1. Preliminary films are taken without contrast medium. *Establishes the optimum exposure technique.*
2. A secretory stimulant such as a lemon wedge is administered to the client 2–3 min before injecting the contrast medium. *Opens the duct for ready identification of the opening.*
3. Contrast medium is injected via syringe attached to a cannula or catheter and x-rays are taken. *Allows illumination of the salivary glands and ducts.*
4. The client may either be seated or in a recumbent position for some examinations. However, the submaxillary and sublingual glands are best viewed when the client is lying on his back with the torso propped up with several firm pillows and the head fully extended backward. The central ray enters from under the chin.
5. When the x-rays have been completed, the client may suck on lemon wedge. *Stimulates rapid evacuation of the contrast medium.*
6. An x-ray may be taken 10 min after the last lemon wedge is administered. *Verifies the evacuation of the contrast medium.*

Clinical Implications and Indications:
1. Determines the presence and extent of salivary gland and ductal disease due to inflammation, tumors, or fistulae

Nursing Care:
Before Test: Explain the test procedure and the purpose of the test. Assess the client's knowledge of the test. Assess for potential allergies to contrast medium. Inform client that during injection of contrast medium, a burning sensation may be felt for a few seconds behind the eyes or in the jaw, teeth, tongue, or lips. Assess for anxiety and provide sedation as ordered. Administer preoperative medication usually 30 min before procedure. Obtain baseline vital signs and neurological assessment. The procedure may be difficult, and it may be uncomfortable to sit on the hard table or achieve some of the necessary positions. It is important to remain as still as possible during the test. There are no dietary restrictions prior to the test. Remove dental prosthesis, jewelry, eyeglasses, or other metal objects like hair clips before the procedure.

During Test: The client is instructed to take a deep breath and hold it or to exhale and not to breathe as the x-ray is taken. Assess for allergic reactions to contrast medium.

After Test: Assess for allergic reactions to contrast medium. Administer a salivary stimulant such as lemon wedges in order to increase the rate of evacuation of the contrast medium.

Potential Complications: Anaphylaxis due to allergic reaction to iodinated contrast material

Contraindications: Previous history of allergy to iodine, eggs, or shellfish; x-rays are usually avoided during pregnancy unless the benefit to the fetus outweighs the potential risk.

Nursing Considerations:

Pregnancy: Radiation and IV contrast should be avoided in pregnant women if possible (note: appropriate lead shielding is done to protect the fetus if it is determined this test is necessary).

Pediatric: Sedation is recommended for infants and children. Place the infant or child on a blanket for comfort. After postprocedure monitoring is completed and per health care provider's order, the pediatric client is discharged with an adult who is given instructions.

Listing of Related Tests: Prostate-specific antigen (PSA)

⎸ WEBLINKS ⎹ ▨⊠

www.oncolink.upenn.edu

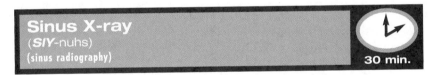

Sinus X-ray
(*SIY*-nuhs)
(sinus radiography)

30 min.

Type of Test: X-ray

Body Systems and Functions: Musculoskeletal system

Normal Findings: Normal sinus and surrounding structures

Test Results Time Frame: Within 24 hr

Test Description: The x-ray of the sinuses is taken to aid in the diagnosis of sinusitis. Opacity without bone destruction is usually seen for diagnosis. Bone destruction could indicate other processes, such as a tumor.

> **CLINICAL ALERT:**
> Potentially, a portable x-ray machine may be brought to the nursing unit if the client cannot be moved. Also, untreated sinus infections are potentially dangerous conditions and therefore necessitate treatment.

Consent Form: Not required

RADIOLOGIC

List of Equipment: X-ray machine and related equipment from radiology

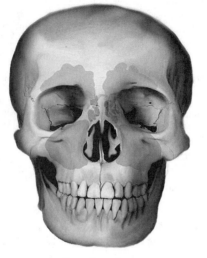

Sinus Locations

Test Procedure:

1. The client is seated on the x-ray table with the arms at the side and one ear against the plate so that the client's midsaggital plane is parallel to the plane of the film. *Allows for a lateral projection of the sinuses and surrounding organs.*
2. Other film angles can be taken in the supine, prone, or sitting position. *Different angles may be requested for viewing the sinuses and surrounding structures.*
3. The client is instructed to hold his breath when film is taken. *Prevents movement during respiration.*
4. A head clamp may be used to immobilize the client. *Maintains the appropriate position while the film is taken.*

Clinical Implications and Indications:

1. Evaluates acute or chronic sinusitis
2. Evaluates obstruction of the nasal sinuses (note: deviation of the nasal septum is common with sinusitis)
3. Detects tumors or abscesses when sinus films are ordered for evaluation of sinus problems

Nursing Care:

Before Test: Explain the test procedure and the purpose of the test. Assess the client's knowledge of the test. Instruct the client that during the procedure it may be uncomfortable to sit on the hard table or achieve some of the necessary positions; it is important to remain as still as possible during the test; there are no dietary restrictions prior to the test; and it is necessary to remove dental prosthesis, jewelry, eyeglasses, or other metal objects like hair clips before the procedure.

RADIOLOGIC

During Test: The client is instructed to take a deep breath and hold it or to exhale and not to breathe as the x-ray is taken.

Contraindications: X-rays are usually avoided during pregnancy unless the benefit to the fetus outweighs the potential risk.

Nursing Considerations:
Pregnancy: Radiation should be avoided in pregnant women if possible (note: appropriate lead shielding is done to protect the fetus if it is determined this test is necessary).
Pediatric: Sedation is recommended for infants and children. Place the infant or child on a blanket for comfort. After postprocedure monitoring is completed and per health care provider's order, the pediatric client is discharged with an adult who is given instructions.
Home Care: Health care provider should be advised that if client has persistent "head cold" symptomatology, with suspected sinus congestion, then further diagnostics may be necessary. Undiagnosed sinus infections are potentially dangerous conditions.

Listing of Related Tests: CT scans; MRI

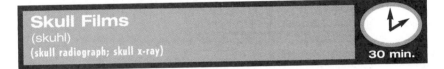

| WEBLINKS |

http://www.sinuses.com; http://health.indiamart.com; http://www.entnet.org

Skull Films
(skuhl)
(skull radiograph; skull x-ray)

30 min.

Type of Test: X-ray

Body Systems and Functions: Musculoskeletal system

Normal Findings: Normal skull and surrounding structures

Test Results Time Frame: Within 24 hr

Test Description: The x-ray of the skull is taken to aid in the diagnosis of skull fracture, head injury, radiopaque tumor, or foreign body. Opacity without bone destruction is usually seen for diagnosis. Bone destruction could indicate other processes, such as a tumor.

CLINICAL ALERT:
Clients who have lost consciousness for over 2 min should be admitted to the hospital for observation. Often head injury is accompanied by neck injury, so the client should continue to be assessed for cord compression. The lack of skull fracture does not eliminate the possibility of severe head injury. In addition, a portable x-ray machine may be brought to the nursing unit if the client cannot be moved.

RADIOLOGIC

Consent Form: Not required

List of Equipment: X-ray machine and related equipment from radiology

Test Procedure:

1. The client is seated on the x-ray table with the arms at the side and one ear against the plate so that the client's midsaggital plane is parallel to the plane of the film. *Allows for a lateral projection of the skull and surrounding organs.*
2. Other film angles can be taken in the supine, prone, or sitting position. *Different angles may be requested for viewing the skull and surrounding structures.*
3. The client is instructed to hold his breath when film is taken. *Prevents movement during respiration.*
4. A head clamp may be used to immobilize the client. *Maintains the appropriate position while the film is taken.*

Clinical Implications and Indications:

1. Evaluates head injury.
2. Tumors may be discovered when skull or sinus films are ordered for other situations, such as head trauma or sinus problems.

Nursing Care:

Before Test: Explain the test procedure and the purpose of the test. Assess the client's knowledge of the test. Instruct the client that during the procedure it may be uncomfortable to sit on the hard table or achieve some of the necessary positions; it is important to remain as still as possible during the test; there are no dietary restrictions prior to the test; and it is necessary to remove dental prosthesis, jewelry, eyeglasses, or other metal objects like hair clips before the procedure.

During Test: The client is instructed to take a deep breath and hold it or to exhale and not to breathe as the x-ray is taken.

Contraindications: X-rays are usually avoided during pregnancy unless the benefit to the fetus outweighs the potential risk.

Nursing Considerations:

Pregnancy: Radiation should be avoided in pregnant women if possible (note: appropriate lead shielding is done to protect the fetus if it is determined this test is necessary).

Pediatric: Sedation is recommended for infants and children. Place the infant or child on a blanket for comfort. After postprocedure monitoring is completed and per health care provider's order, the pediatric client is discharged with an adult who is given instructions. Also, health care provider should be wary of headaches in children and assess the child for symptomatology of potential head injuries.

Home Care: Health care provider should report persistent headache or any falls that potentially produce injury to the skull.

Listing of Related Tests: CT scan; cervical spine radiographs; arteriography; magnetic resonance imaging (MRI)

Small-Bowel Series
(smahl boul)
(SBF; small-bowel enema; small-bowel series; small-intestine radiography and fluoroscopy)

2–6 hr.

Type of Test: X-ray

Body Systems and Functions: Gastrointestinal system

Normal Findings: No abnormalities in the small-bowel shape, position, or motility

Test Results Time Frame: Within 24–48 hr

Test Description: A small-bowel series is a fluoroscopy of the small intestine after the ingestion of barium sulfate. The barium is a contrast material and enters the stomach and empties into the duodenal area, where it continues to be transported through the small bowel.

Consent Form: Required

List of Equipment: X-ray equipment, fluoroscope, barium

Test Procedure:
1. Place client in supine, standing, and lateral positions.
2. Instruct client to drink 16–20 oz of a barium mixture, and the progress of the mixture is monitored using a fluoroscope as the contrast medium passes through the bowel. *Allows for visualization of the areas in question.*
3. The examination table can tilt. *Facilitates the passage of the contrast medium.*
4. If enteroclysis is to be performed, barium is pumped through a small tube that empties into the small bowel. *Provides specific visualization of the small bowel.*
5. The examiner may palpate the abdomen. *Facilitates the movement of barium and to visualize on the fluoroscope the effects of palpation.*
6. If a barium enema is to be done as well, it generally is done first, the colon cleared out, and the rest of the x-rays are done the following morning. *Provides for the maximal visualization of all segments of the small intestine and colon.*

Clinical Implications and Indications:
1. Detects cancer of the esophagus, stomach, and small intestine
2. Diagnoses pyloric stenosis (narrowing of the sphincter of the stomach), ulcers, polyps, Crohn's disease, enteritis, diverticula, and hiatal hernia
3. Evaluates malabsorption syndromes, inflammation, weight loss, diarrhea, and Hodgkin's disease

Nursing Care:
Before Test: Explain the test procedure and the purpose of the test. Assess the client's knowledge of the test. Instruct client to refrain from smoking from midnight prior to the test. Usual bowel preparation includes having a restrictive diet for 2–3 days before the test (clear soup, unsweetened gelatin, black coffee, no milk products, no roughage), being NPO after midnight the night before the

RADIOLOGIC

examination, and to taking no medications, anticholinergics, or narcotics for 24 hr before the test. Arrange for a ride home after the test. On the day before the examination, drink one 8-oz glass of water every hour for 3 consecutive hours. Add magnesium citrate to the next glass of water, and follow by drinking two more 8-oz glasses of water in the next 2 hr. Take four bisacodyl tablets with one 8-oz glass of water, and follow with another glass of water in the next hour. A suppository may also be used the night before the examination. On the day of the examination, remove all jewelry, dentures, and contacts. Diabetics may have small amounts of clear liquids in the morning of the examination if needed. Inform client that the barium is flavored to enhance its ingestion.

During Test: Adhere to standard precautions. Assist client with the different positions required during the test.

After Test: Instruct client to drink 4–6 glasses of water for 2 days to prevent constipation. Administer cathartic if necessary. Inform client that stool will be discolored for up to 72 hr after the test from the barium.

Potential Complications: Aspiration of the contrast material; bowel obstruction; constipation

Contraindications: Perforation of small intestine; obstruction of small bowel; severe cardiovascular disease

Interfering Factors: Narcotic use; inadequate bowel preparation; movement during the test

Nursing Considerations:
Pregnancy: Extreme caution should be exercised during pregnancy.
Pediatric: Restraints are often used to prevent movement during the examination. The quality of the films can be dramatically decreased if there is movement. Play-preparation may be helpful. Children should be NPO for at least 4 hr prior to the test. Age-appropriate comfort measures following the test.
Gerontology: The elderly may need special attention given to the potential problems with constipation.
Home Care: Health care providers can administer cathartics, juices, and water when client returns home to prevent constipation.

Listing of Related Tests: Oral cholecystography

WEBLINKS

http://health.excite.com

Spinal Films
(*SPIY*-n:l)
(spinal x-rays; cervical, thoracic, lumbar, sacral, or coccygeal x-ray studies)

20 min.

Type of Test: X-ray

Body Systems and Functions: Musculoskeletal system

RADIOLOGIC

Normal Findings: Normal vertebral bodies; no abnormal curvatures or fracture of the spine

Test Results Time Frame: Within 24 hr

Test Description: Spinal films examine the cervical, thoracic, and lumbosacral spine areas with radiological techniques. The spinal films can detect fractures and the presence of masses and potentially identify the causative agent for back pain. The procedure is noninvasive and is often the initial diagnostic tool used for spine injuries.

Consent Form: Not required

List of Equipment: X-ray machine and related equipment from radiology

Test Procedure:
1. The client is placed on the x-ray table in a supine position. *Allows for first projection of the spine.*
2. Other film angles can be taken in the side-lying position. *Different angles may be requested for viewing the spine.*
3. The client is instructed to hold his breath when film is taken. *Prevents movement during respiration.*

Clinical Implications and Indications:
1. Diagnoses tumor or destruction of vertebral bodies
2. Assesses back or neck pain for possible arthritis, spondylosis, or spondylolisthesis
3. Evaluates management of scoliosis or lordosis
4. Evaluates congenital spinal cord defects
5. Evaluates potential vertebral fractures or abnormal curvatures

Nursing Care:
Before Test: Explain the test procedure and the purpose of the test. Assess the client's knowledge of the test. Instruct the client that during the procedure it may be uncomfortable to sit on the hard table or achieve some of the necessary positions; it is important to remain as still as possible during the test; there are no dietary restrictions prior to the test; and it is necessary to remove dental prosthesis, jewelry, eyeglasses, or other metal objects like hair clips before the procedure.
During Test: The client is instructed to take a deep breath and hold it or to exhale and not to breathe as the x-ray is taken.

Contraindications: X-rays are usually avoided during pregnancy unless the benefit to the fetus outweighs the potential risk.

Interfering Factors: Positioning difficulties, particularly when fractures are present; inability to remain still; metal objects

Nursing Considerations:
Pregnancy: Radiation should be avoided in pregnant women if possible (note: appropriate lead shielding is done to protect the fetus if it is determined this test is necessary).
Pediatric: Sedation is recommended for infants and children. Place the infant or child on a blanket for comfort. After postprocedure monitoring is completed and

RADIOLOGIC

per health care provider's order, the pediatric client is discharged with an adult who is given instructions.

Gerontology: *The older person may find it difficult to maintain positions when required to do so for lengthy periods of time.*

WEBLINKS ⬛⬛

http://adam.excite.com

Splenoportography
(*SPLEE*-noe-poer-*TAHG*-ruh-fee)
(percutaneous splenoportogram; direct splenoportography)

1 hr.

Type of Test: X-ray

Body Systems and Functions: Hepatobiliary system

Normal Findings: Splenic and portal veins are smooth, having normal caliber and no obstructions or strictures noted.

Test Results Time Frame: Within 24 hr

Test Description: Splenoportography involves radiography of the spleen and portal vein. A radiopaque contrast medium is injected into the spleen and then x-rays are taken to evaluate the function of the spleen.

CLINICAL ALERT:
Have emergency equipment readily available in the event of an anaphylactic reaction to the dye.

Consent Form: Required

List of Equipment: Fluoroscopy, x-ray equipment, and sheathed needle

Test Procedure:
1. Advise client to empty his bladder before the test begins.
2. The client is placed on a table in the supine position with the arms extended. *Allows for an unobstructed access to the abdomen.*
3. The physician introduces a sheathed needle into the splenic pulp. The needle is withdrawn and the sheath remains in place. *Allows for the injection of contrast material.*
4. The contrast material is injected at 5–6 mL/sec for 5–7 sec. X-rays are taken during this time. *The spleen is seen on radiographic examination. The splenic and portal veins drain the contrast material, and this progression is observed by x-ray.*

Clinical Implications and Indications:
1. Evaluates suspected splenic vein or portal vein thrombosis
2. Determines spleen involvement in leukemia, lymphoma, and melanoma
3. Evaluates spleen enlargement

RADIOLOGIC

Nursing Care:

Before Test: Explain the test procedure and the purpose of the test. Assess the client's knowledge of the test. The client should be NPO at least 4 hr prior to the procedure. Assess for potential allergies to contrast medium. Inform client that during injection of contrast medium, a burning sensation may be felt for a few seconds behind the eyes or in the jaw, teeth, tongue, or lips. Assess for anxiety and provide sedation as ordered. Administer preoperative medication usually 30 min before procedure. Obtain baseline vital signs and neurological assessment. Blood typing should be performed in advance. BUN, creatinine, PT, PTT, and platelet count should all be recorded on the chart. If this is done on an outpatient basis, the client should arrange for a ride to and from the facility. *During Test:* Adhere to standard precautions. Assess for allergic reactions to contrast medium. Monitor vital signs every 10 min. *After Test:* The client is on bedrest for about 6 hr following the procedure. Vital signs should be assessed every 15–30 min in the first hour, then every 30 min for 2 hr and every hour after that. Assess for allergic reactions to contrast medium.

Potential Complications: Anaphylaxis due to allergic reaction to iodinated contrast material; internal hemorrhage; shock; splenic rupture

Contraindications: Bleeding abnormalities; low platelet count; ascites; acute renal failure; elevated PT or PTT; previous history of allergy to iodine, eggs, or shellfish

Interfering Factors: Inability of client to remain still

Nursing Considerations:

Pregnancy: Radiation and IV contrast should be avoided in pregnant women if possible (note: appropriate lead shielding is done to protect the fetus if it is determined this test is necessary).
Gerontology: The older person may find it difficult to maintain positions when required to do so for lengthy periods of time during the splenoportography.

Listing of Related Tests: CT of the spleen; MRI of the spleen

| WEBLINKS | | ▣ ☒ |

http://www.healthgate.com

Upper Gastrointestinal Series
(*GAES*-troe-in-*TEST*-in-:l)
(upper GI; barium swallow; UGI)

45 min.

Type of Test: X-ray

Body Systems and Functions: Gastrointestinal system

Normal Findings: No structural or abnormal findings

Test Results Time Frame: Within 24–48 hr

RADIOLOGIC

Test Description: An upper GI series involves swallowing a barium mixture (or dye preparation) that shows up on x-ray. As the client swallows this mixture, x-rays or fluoroscopic pictures are made of the upper GI tract. The form, position, peristaltic action, function, and abnormalities can be visualized of the esophagus, duodenum, and upper portion of the jejunum. The barium passes through the GI tract at a normal rate, and there should not be a reflux (which indicates a hiatal hernia or incompetent cardiac sphincter) or leakage into the abdominal cavity.

Consent Form: Not required

List of Equipment: Barium mixture (or gastrografin); fluoroscope; x-ray machine and related equipment from radiology

Test Procedure:
1. The client drinks the barium as the fluoroscopy machine visualizes the GI tract.
2. X-rays may be taken at the completion of the fluoroscopy.
3. Instruct client to hold breath when film is taken. *Prevents movement during respiration.*

Clinical Implications and Indications:
1. Diagnoses ulcers, hiatal hernia, diverticula, gastritis, enteritis, strictures, varices, pyloric stenosis, and volvulus of the stomach
2. Evaluates and monitors tumors
3. Identifies esophageal reflux
4. Detects foreign bodies

Nursing Care:
Before Test: Explain the test procedure and the purpose of the test. Assess the client's knowledge of the test. Instruct the client that during the procedure it may be uncomfortable to sit on the hard table or achieve some of the necessary positions; it is important to remain as still as possible during the test; and it is necessary to remove dental prosthesis, jewelry, eyeglasses, or other metal objects like hair clips before the procedure. Instruct client to eat a light meal the evening before the test and then fast for 12 hr prior to the procedure. Most medications are held after midnight before the test (particularly those that affect GI motility). Diabetic clients should be scheduled early in the morning.
During Test: Adhere to standard precautions. The barium is often found to have a chalky, unpleasant taste. The client is instructed to take a deep breath and hold it or to exhale and not to breathe as the x-ray is taken.
After Test: Instruct client to take a laxative or enema due to the constipation produced by the barium. Instruct the client to rest after the procedure and explain that stools will be light colored for 24–72 hr.

Potential Complications: Aspiration of contrast material; constipation

Contraindications: X-rays are usually avoided during pregnancy unless the benefit to the fetus outweighs the potential risk; suspected ileus; obstruction; gastrointestinal perforation

Interfering Factors: Retained food or fluids may interfere with visualization during the study; it may be difficult to perform the test on a debilitated client.

RADIOLOGIC

Nursing Considerations:

Pregnancy: *Radiation should be avoided in pregnant women if possible (note: appropriate lead shielding is done to protect the fetus if it is determined this test is necessary).*

Pediatric: *Sedation is recommended for infants and children. Place the infant or child on a blanket for comfort. After postprocedure monitoring is completed and per health care provider's order, the pediatric client is discharged with an adult who is given instructions.*

Gerontology: *The older person may find it difficult to maintain positions when required to do so for lengthy periods of time during the upper GI.*

Rural: *Advisable to arrange for transportation home after recovering from the upper GI.*

Listing of Related Tests: Small-bowel x-ray; radiography; fluoroscopy

WEBLINKS

http://www.entnet.org

Urethrography, Retrograde
(yur-ri-***THRAHG***-ruh-fee ***RET***-roe-grayd)
(x-ray of bladder and urethra)

30–40 min.

Type of Test: X-ray

Body Systems and Functions: Renal/urological system

Normal Findings: No functional or anatomical abnormalities noted

Test Results Time Frame: Within 48 hr

Test Description: Retrograde urethrography involves visualizing the bladder and the urethra with x-ray after a radiographic dye is inserted into the bladder via a urinary catheter. Autourethrography, in which the client instills the contrast medium, has been found, in some cases, to decrease the client's anxiety and enhance the tolerance of the procedure. It also allows the radiologist to not have to remain with the client during the procedure.

CLINICAL ALERT:
Have emergency equipment readily available in the event of an anaphylactic reaction to the dye. Instruct client to increase fluid intake for a few days and to observe for signs and symptoms of urinary infection (e.g., fever, chills, frequency of or odor to urine).

Consent Form: Not required

List of Equipment: X-ray machine and related equipment from radiology; catheter insertion kit (antiseptic solution, gauze, lubricant, sterile gloves); urinary catheter; radiographic dye; penile clamp

RADIOLOGIC

Test Procedure:
1. Place client in supine position.
2. Utilizing aseptic technique, cleanse the opening of the urethra with betadine solution. *Reduces the possibility of urinary tract infection postprocedure.*
3. Lubricate the catheter and insert it into the urethra. *Reduces urethra trauma.*
4. Insert the radiographic dye using a syringe.
5. Remove catheter and apply penis clamp for male clients. *Retains the dye for x-ray.*

Clinical Implications and Indications:
1. Identifies congenital abnormalities of the bladder and urethra.
2. Diagnoses fistulas, calculi, false passages or diverticula of the urethra and bladder, lacerations or tears in the urethra from trauma, and strictures of the urethra.
3. Evaluates and monitors treatment of bladder tumors.
4. Detects incomplete emptying, which is determined by having the client void and repeating the x-ray. *Retained dye will reveal the amount of retained urine for a client unable to empty the bladder.*

Nursing Care:
Before Test: Explain the test procedure and the purpose of the test. Assess the client's knowledge of the test. Explain that some discomfort will be experienced during insertion of the catheter. Instruct the client that during the procedure it may be uncomfortable to sit on the hard table or achieve some of the necessary positions; it is important to remain as still as possible during the test; there are no dietary restrictions prior to the test; and it is necessary to remove dental prosthesis, jewelry, eyeglasses, or other metal objects like hair clips before the procedure. Assess for potential allergies to contrast medium. Inform client that during injection of contrast medium, a burning sensation may be felt for a few seconds behind the eyes or in the jaw, teeth, tongue, or lips. Assess for anxiety and provide sedation as ordered. Administer preoperative medication usually 30 min before procedure. Obtain baseline vital signs and neurological assessment.
During Test: Adhere to standard precautions. Assess for allergic reactions to contrast medium.
After Test: Assess for allergic reactions to contrast medium. No activity restrictions required. Advise the client to increase fluids for a few days and inform the client that he may notice some burning with the first urination. Instruct client to report continued burning or bleeding.

Potential Complications: Anaphylaxis due to allergic reaction to iodinated contrast material; postprocedure urinary tract infection

Contraindications: Previous history of allergy to iodine, eggs, or shellfish

Nursing Considerations:
Pregnancy: Radiation and IV contrast should be avoided in pregnant women if possible (note: appropriate lead shielding is done to protect the fetus if it is determined this test is necessary).
Pediatric: Sedation is recommended for infants and children. Place the infant or child on a blanket for comfort. After postprocedure monitoring is completed and per health care provider's order, the pediatric client is discharged with an adult who is given instructions.

RADIOLOGIC

Gerontology: *The older person may find it difficult to maintain positions when required to do so for lengthy periods of time during the urethrography.*
Rural: *Advisable to arrange for transportation home after recovering from urethrography*

Listing of Related Tests: Retrograde cystography

WEBLINKS

http://www.compsoc.man.ac.uk

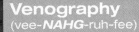

Venography
(vee-*NAHG*-ruh-fee)

1 hr.

Type of Test: X-ray

Body Systems and Functions: Cardiovascular system

Normal Findings: No anatomical or functional abnormalities

Test Results Time Frame: Within 24–48 hr

Test Description: Venography is a test that produces an x-ray of the venous system. The venography is often performed on an extremity to evaluate an obstruction. Dye is injected into the vein of an arm or leg, and x-rays are taken of the flow through the veins. Recorded results specifically identify the structure and flow of the venous system.

CLINICAL ALERT:
Have emergency equipment readily available in the event of an anaphylactic reaction to the dye. If client is diabetic, ensure that metformin/glucophage is discontinued prior to test the day before and for several days after the test. Vital signs and puncture site should be evaluated every 15 min for the first few hours postprocedure. A cold or numb extremity should be reported immediately.

Consent Form: Not required

List of Equipment: Needle and syringe; alcohol swab; x-ray table and equipment; catheters; dye; sedative; three-way stopcock

Test Procedure:
1. Prepare the site to be injected using aseptic techniques. *Reduces infection.*
2. Sedate the client per protocol. *Movement during the procedure affects the test.*
3. Apply a tourniquet above the site to be examined. *Increases venous filling, producing a better image.*
4. Inject dye into the catheter after it is threaded into the appropriate vein.
5. X-rays are taken of the extremity.

RADIOLOGIC

Clinical Implications and Indications:
1. Determines venous obstruction
2. Evaluates venous valvular function
3. Reveals the presence of deep vein thrombosis

Nursing Care:
Before Test: Explain the test procedure and the purpose of the test. Assess the client's knowledge of the test. Provide IV access for sedation and postoperative care. Assess for potential allergies to contrast medium. Inform client that during injection of contrast medium, a burning sensation may be felt for a few seconds behind the eyes or in the jaw, teeth, tongue, or lips. Assess for anxiety and provide sedation as ordered. Administer preoperative medication usually 30 min before procedure. Obtain baseline vital signs and neurological assessment.
During Test: Adhere to standard precautions. Assess client comfort. If uncomfortable, sedate per protocol. Assess for allergic reactions to contrast medium.
After Test: Apply pressure to venipuncture site. Explain that some bruising, discomfort, and swelling may appear at the site and that warm, moist compresses can alleviate this. Monitor for signs of infection. Vital signs, puncture site, and neurological checks are done every 15 min for a few hours postprocedure. Sudden onset of pain, numbness, tingling, or cold sensation should be reported immediately. If bleeding occurs, apply pressure to the site. Assess for allergic reactions to contrast medium.

Potential Complications: Bleeding and bruising at venipuncture site; anaphylaxis due to allergic reaction to iodinated contrast material

Contraindications: Previous history of allergy to iodine, eggs, or shellfish

Interfering Factors: Inability to remain still causes poor picture quality.

Nursing Considerations:
Pregnancy: Radiation and IV contrast should be avoided in pregnant women if possible (note: appropriate lead shielding is done to protect the fetus if it is determined this test is necessary).
Pediatric: Infants and children will need assistance in remaining still during the venipuncture and age-appropriate comfort measures following the test.

Listing of Related Tests: Vascular x-ray; angiography; arteriography

| WEBLINKS |

http://www.entnet.org

List of References

Abeloff, M. D., Armitage, J. O., Lichter, A. S., & Niederhuber, J. E. (2000). *Clinical oncology* (2nd ed.). New York: Churchill Livingstone.

Abrams, C. (2000). ADH-associated pathologies. *Medical Laboratory Observer, 32*(1), 24–36.

Ahmed, T., Kamota, T., Sumazaki, R., Shibasaki, M., Hirano, T., & Takita, H. (1997). Circulating antibodies to common food antigens in Japanese children. *Diabetes care, 20*(1), 74–76.

Allan, C., Kaltsas, G., Perry, L., Lowe, D., Reznek, R., Carmichael, D., & Monson, J. (2000). Concurrent secretion of aldosterone and cortisol from an adrenal adenoma-value of MRI in diagnosis. *Clinical Endocrinology, 53*(6), 749-753.

Allgaier, A., Goethe, R., Wisselink, H., Smith, H., & Valentin-Weigand, P. (2001). Relatedness of streptococcus suis isolates of various serotypes and clinical backgrounds as evaluated by macrorestriction analysis and expression of potential virulence traits. *Journal of Clinical Microbiology, 39* (2), 445-453.

Almass, R., Robertson, B., Linderholm, B., Lundberg, E., Saugstad, O., & Moen, A. (2000). Reversal of meconium inhibition of pulmonary surfactant by ferric chloride, copper chloride, and acetic acid. *American Journal of Respiratory Critical Care Medicine, 162* (5), 1789-1794.

American Diabetes Association. (1999). Clinical Practice Recommendations 1999. *Diabetes Care, 22*(3), 43–46.

American Diabetes Association: Report of the Expert Committee on the Diagnosis and Classification of Diabetes Mellitus. (1999). *Diabetes Care, 22*(2), 23–27.

American Gastroenterological Association Medical Position Statement. (1998). Evaluation of dyspepsia, *Gastroenterology, 114,* 575–579.

Aminoff, M. (2000). Nervous system. In L. M. Tierney, Jr., S. J. McPhee, & M. A. Papadakis (Eds.), *Current medical diagnosis & treatment 2000* (pp. 959–1000). New York: Lange Medical Books/McGraw-Hill.

Anand, S. S., Bates, S., & Ginsberg, J. S., et al (1999). Recurrent venous thrombosis and heparin therapy. *Archives of Internal Medicine, 159*(17), 2029–2031.

Annibale, B., Lahner, E., Bordi, C., Martino, G., Caruana, P., Grossi, C., Negrini, R., & Delle, F. (2000). Role of helicobacter pylori infection in pernicious anemia. *Digestive Liver Disease, 32* (9), 756-762.

Armstrong, D., & Cohen, J. (1999). *Infectious diseases* (Vol. 2). London: Mosby.

Armstrong, P. J. H. (1999). *Your guide to continuing cardiac care.* Medford, OR: Rogue Valley Medical Center.

Augoustides, J., Weiss, S., & Pochettino, A. (2000). Hemodynamic monitoring of the postoperative adult cardiac surgical patient. *Seminar of Thoracic Cardiovascular Surgery, 12*(4), 309–315.

Bakker, A. J. (1999). Detection of microalbuminuria: Receiver operating characteristic curve analysis favors albumin-to-creatinine ratio over albumin concentration. *Diabetes Care, 22*(2), 307–313.

Ballas, S., & Marcolina, M. (2000). Determinants of red cell survival and erythropoietic activity in patients with sickle cell anemia in the steady state. *Hemoglobin, 24* (4), 277-286.

Ballinger, P. W. (1998). *Merrill's atlas of radiographic positions and radiologic procedures* (pp. 252–263). Saint Louis: C. V. Mosby Company.

Behrman, R. E., Kliegman, R. M., and Jenson, H. B. (2000). *Nelson textbook of pediatrics* (16th ed.). Philadelphia: W. B. Saunders.

Berci, G, & Cuschieri, A. (1997). *Bile duct and bile duct stones.* Philadelphia: W. B. Saunders.

Bingley, P. J., Bonifacio, E., Williams, A. J. K., Genovese, S., Bottazzo, G. F., & Gale, E. A. M. (1997). Prediction of IDDM in the general population: Strategies based on combinations of autoantibody markers. *Diabetes, 46*(11), 1701–1710.

Bishop, M. L., Duben-Engelkirk, J. L., & Fodey, E. P. (2000). *Clinical chemistry: Principles, procedures and correlations.* Philadelphia: Lippincott, Williams and Wilkins.

Blaivas, M., Sierzenski, P., & Lambert, M. (2001). Emergency evaluation of patients presenting with acute scrotum using bedside ultrasonography. *Academic Emergency Medicine, 8* (1), 90-3.

Borchardt, K. A., & Noble, M. A. (1997). *Sexually transmitted diseases:* Epidemiology, pathology, diagnosis, and treatment. Boca Raton: CRC Press.

Bouckenooghe, A., & Shandera, W. K. (2000). Infectious diseases: Viral & rickettsial. In L. M Tierney, Jr., S. J. McPhee, & M. A. Papadakis (Eds.), *Current medical diagnosis and treatment 2000* (pp.1313–1315). New York: Lange Medical Books/McGraw-Hill.

Branca, F., & Vatuena, S. (2000). Calcium, physical activity and bone health—building bones for a stronger future. *Public Health Nutrition, 4* (1A), 117-123.

Brant, L. J. (Ed.) (1999). *Clinical practice of gastroenterology* (Vol. 1). Philadelphia: Current Medicine.

Brenner, B. M. (Ed.). (2000). *Brenner and Rector's The kidney* (6th ed., Vol. 2). Philadelphia: W. B. Saunders.

Brenner, H., Bode, G., Adler, G., Hoffmeister, A., Koenig, W., & Rothenbacher, D. (2001). Alcohol as a gastric disinfectant? The complex relationship between alcohol consumption and current Helicobacter pylori infection. *Epidemiology, 12* (2), 209-214.

Bretzel, R. (2000). Current status and perspectives in clinical islet transplantation. *Journal of Hepatobiliary Pancreatic Surgery, 7* (4), 374-379.

Bron, A. J., Daubas, P., Siou-Mermet, R., & Trinquand, C. (1998). Comparison of the efficacy and safety of two eye gels in the treatment of dry eyes: Lacrinorm and Viscotears. *Eye, 12*(5), 839–847.

Brown, K. (2000). *Management guidelines for women's health nurse practitioners.* Philadelphia: F. A. Davis Company.

Bucher, L., & Melander, S. (1999). *Critical care nursing.* Philadelphia: W. B.Saunders.

Burtis, C. A., & Ashwood, E. R. (1999). *Tietz textbook of clinical chemistry* (3rd ed.). Philadelphia: W. B. Saunders.

Bussey, E. (2000). Senate hears testimony on anthrax vaccine shortage, *Reuters Health News,* July 18; Handelman, A. (1999). *S. Biohazard.* New York: Random House; Tucker, J. B. (2000). *Toxic terror: Assessing terrorist use of chemical and biological weapons.* Cambridge, MA: MIT Press.

Calatayud, S., Ramirez, M., Sanz, M., Moreno, L., Hernandez, C., Bosch, J., Pique, J., Esplugues, J. (2001). Gastric mucosal resistance to acute injury in experimental portal hypertension. *British Journal of Pharmacology, 132* (1), 309-317.

Camilleri, M., Hasler, W. L., Parkman, H., et al. (1998). Measurement of gastrointestinal motility in the GI laboratory. *Gastroenterology, 115,* 747.

Carr, D., Smith, K., Parsons, L., Chansky, K., & Shields, L. (2000). Ultrasonography for cervical length measurement: Agreement between transvaginal and translabial techniques. *Obstetrical Gynecology, 96* (4), 554-558.

Carrieri, M., Trevisan, A., Bartolucci, G. (2001). Adjustment to concentration-dilution of spot urine samples: correlation between specific gravity and creatinine. *International Archives of Occupational and Environmental Health, 74* (1), 63-67.

Cavanaugh, G. M. (1999). *Nurses manual of laboratory and diagnostic tests* (3rd ed.). Philadelphia, PA: F. A. Davis.

Cavuoti, D., Baskin, L., & Jialal, I. (1998). Detection of oligoclonal bands in cerebrospinal fluid by immunofixation electrophoresis. *American Journal of Clinical Pathology, 109*(5), 585–588.

CDC Diabetes Cost-Effectiveness Study Group. (1998). The cost-effectiveness of screening for type 2 diabetes. *Journal of the American Medical Association, 22*(1), 121–127.

Centers for Disease Control. (1998e). 1998 Guidelines for treatment of sexually transmitted diseases. *MMWR CDC Surveillance Summaries, 47*(RR-01), 1–102.

Chambers, H. F. (2000). Infectious diseases: Bacterial & chlamydial. In L. M. Tierney, Jr., S. J. McPhee, & M. A. Papadakis (Eds.), *Current medical diagnosis & treatment 2000* (pp. 1364–1365). New York: Lange Medical Books/McGraw-Hill.

Connolly, B., Johnstone, F., Gerlinger, T., & Puttler E. (2000). Methicillin-resistant *Staphylococcus aureus* in a finger felon. *Journal of Hand Surgery — American Volume, 25*(1), 173–175.

Coster, S., Gulliford, M., Seed, P., Powrie, J., & Swaminathan, R. (2000). Self-monitoring in Type 2 diabetes mellitus: a meta-analysis. *Diabetes Medicine, 17* (11), 755-761.

Creasy, R. K., & Resnik, R. (1999). Maternal-fetal medicine (4th ed.). Philadelphia: Lippincott.

Crino, J. (1999). Ultrasound and fetal diagnosis of perinatal infection. *Clinical Obstetrics and Gynecology, 42* (1), 71-80.

Critchley, M. (1997). Octreotide scanning for carcinoid tumours. *Postgraduate Medical Journal, 73*(861), 399–402.

Davidkina, I., Peltolab, H., Leinikkia, P., & Vallea, M. (2000). Duration of rubella immunity induced by two-dose measles, mumps and rubella (MMR) vaccination. *Vaccine, 18* (27), 3106-3112.

Davila, R. M., Miranda, C. M., & Smith, M. E. (1998). Role of cytopathology in the diagnosis of ocular malignancies. *Acta Cytologica, 42*(2), 362–366.

Demoly, P., Michel, F-B, & Bousquet, J. (1998). In vivo methods for study of allergy skin tests, techniques, and interpretation. In E. Middleton Jr., E. F. Ellis, J. W. Yuninger, C. E. Reed, N. F. Adkinson, & W. W. Busse (Eds.), *Allergy principles and Practice* (5th ed.). St. Louis, MO: Mosby.

DeNoon, D. J. (1999, November 1). U.S. military unprotected as adenovirus attacks. *Antiviral Weekly,* p. 20.

D'Epiro, N. W. (2000). Deciphering autoimmune disease in women. *Patient Care, 34*(7), 49–52.

Desch, L. (2001). Longitudinal stability of visual evoked potentials in children and adolescents with hydrocephalus. *Developmental Medicine and Child Neurology, 43* (2), 113-117.

DeVita, V. T., Helman S., & Rosenberg, S. A. (1997). *Cancer: principles and practice of oncology.* Philadelphia: Lippincott-Raven.

Diaz, J. D. (1999). Voluntary ingestion of organophosphate insecticide by a young farmer. *Journal of Emergency Nursing, 25*(4), 266–268.

DiBiase, A., Petrone, G., Conte, M., Seganti, L., Ammendolia, M., Tinari, A., Iosi, F., Marchetti, M., & Superti, F. (2000). Infection of human enterocyte-like cells with rotavirus enhances invasiveness of Yersinia enterocolitica and Y. pseudotuberculosis. *Journal of Medical Microbiology, 49* (10), 897-904.

DiSaia, P. J., & Creasman W. T. (1997). *Clinical gynecologic oncology* (5th ed.). St. Louis: Mosby.

Doldi, N., Papaleo, E., De Santis, L., & Ferrari, A. (2000). Treatment versus no treatment of transient hyperprolactinemia in patients undergoing introcytoplasmic sperm injection programs. *Gynecological Endocrinology, 14* (6), 437-441.

Early, P., & Sodee, D. B. (1995). *Principles and practice of nuclear medicine* (2nd ed.). St. Louis: Mosby

Eastwood, G. L., & Avunduk, C. (1998). *Manual of gastroenterology.* Boston: Little, Brown and Company.

Ellet, M. (2000). Hepatitis C, E, F, G, and non-A-G. *Gastroenterological Nursing, 23*(2), 67–72.

Elsheikh, A., Keramopoulos, A., Lazaris, D., Ambela, C., & Louvrou, N. (2000). Breast tumors during adolescence. *European Journal of Gynecological Oncology, 21*(4), 408–410.

Engstrom, M., Jonsson, L., Grindlund, M., & Stalberg, E. (2000). Electroneurographic facial muscle pattern in Bell's palsy. *Otolaryngeal Head and Neck Surgery, 122* (2), 290-297.

Eschenbach, D., Patton, D., Meier, A., Thwinn, S., Aura, J., Stapleton, A., & Hooton, T. (2000). Effects of oral contraceptive pill use on vaginal flora and vaginal epithelium. *Contraception, 62* (3), 107-112.

Estes, M. E. Z. (1998). *Health assessment and physical examination.* Albany: Delmar.

EUCLID Study Group. (1997). Randomised placebo-controlled trial of lisinopril in normotensive patients with insulin-dependent diabetes and normoalbuminuria or microalbuminuria. *Lancet, 349*(9068), 1787–1793.

Evans-Stoner, N. (1997). Nutrition assessment: A practical approach. *Nursing Clinics of North America, 32*(4), 637–650.

Fair, J., & Fletcher B. J. (Eds). (2000). Abnormal blood lipids. *Journal of Cardiovascular Nursing, 14*(2), 1–103.

Fall, P. J. (2000). A stepwise approach to acid-base disorders: Practical patient evaluation for metabolic acidosis and other conditions. *Postgraduate Medicine,107*(3), 249–250, 253–254, 257–258.

Fauci, S. F., Braunwald, E., Isselbacher, K. J., Wilson, J., Martin, J. B., Kasper, D. L., Hauser, S. L., & Longo, D. L. (1998). *Harrison's principles of internal medicine* (14th ed.). New York: McGraw-Hill.

Feldman, M., Scharschmidt, B. F., & Sleisenger, M. H. (1998). *Sleisenger & Fordtran's*

gastrointestinal and liver disease (6th ed.). Philadelphia: W. B. Saunders.

Ferguson, G. T. (1998). Screening and early intervention for COPD. *Hospital practices, 33*(67), 34-39.

Filteau, S. M., et al. (2000). Use of retinol binding protein: Transthyretin ratio for assessment of vitamin A status during the acute phase response. *British Journal of Nutrition, 83*(5), 513–520.

Fishman, A., et al. (1997). *Fishman's pulmonary diseases and disorders.* New York: McGraw-Hill.

Fitzgerald, P. A. (2000). Endocrinology. In L. M. Tierney, Jr., S. J. McPhee, & M. A. Papadakis (Eds.), *Current medical diagnosis and treatment 2000* (pp. 1086–1087). New York: Lange Medical Books/McGraw-Hill.

Fowler, S. (1999). Duplex scans aids in determining need for carotid endarterectomy. *Journal of Neuroscience Nursing, 31*(6), 369.

Fraser, R. S., Muller, N. L., Coleman, N., & Pare, P. D. (1999). *Fraser and Pare's diagnosis of diseases of the chest* (4th ed., Vol. 1). Philadelphia: W. B. Saunders.

Frumiento, C., Sartorelli, K., & Vane, D. (2000). Complications of splenic injuries: Expansion of the nonoperative theorem. *Journal of Pediatric Surgery, 35*(5), 788–791.

Fuhrman, M., Herrmann, V., Masidonski, P., & Eby, C. (2000). Pancytopenia after removal of copper from total parenteral nutrition. *Journal of Parenteral Enteral Nutrition, 24*(6), 361–366.

Futterman, L., & Lemberg, L. (2001). Lp(a) lipoprotein: an independent risk factor for coronary heart disease after menopause. *American Journal of Critical Care, 10* (1), 63-67.

Gant, R. H., Henkin, R., & Gonce-Morton, P. (1999). ECGs and pacemakers. *Critical Care Nurse, 19*(5), 61–68.

Garcia-Criado, A., Gilabert, R., Real, I., Arguis, P., Bianchi, L., Vilana, R., Salmeron, J., Valdecasas, J., & Bru, C. Early detection of hepatic artery thrombosis after liver transplantation by Doppler ultrasonography: Prognostic implications. *Journal of Ultrasound Medicine, 20* (1), 51-58.

Gawlinski, A. (1997). *American Association of Critical Care Nurses protocols for practice: Hemodynamic monitoring series.* Aliso Viejo, CA: AACN Critical Care Publication.

Geleijnse, M., Elhendy, A., Fioretti, P., Roelandt, J. (2000). Dobutamine stress myocardial perfusion imaging. *Journal of the American College of Cardiology, 36* (7), 2017-2027.

Giustina, A., & Beldhuis, J. D. (1998). Pathophysiology of the neuroregulation of growth hormone secretion in experimental animals and the human. *Endocrine Review, 19,* 713–717.

Goldfrank, L. R., et al. (1998). *Goldfrank's toxicology emergencies* (6th ed.). New Haven, CT: Appelton & Lange.

Gordon, R., Slamovits, T., Rosenbaum, P., & Bello, J. (1999). Calcified scleral plaques imaged on orbital computed tomography. *American Journal of Ophthalmology, 127* (4), 461-463.

Gorevic, P. D. (1997). Drug allergy. In A. P. Kaplan (Ed.), *Allergy* (pp. 626–631). Philadelphia: W. B. Saunders.

Gosbell, I., Sullivan, E., & Maidment, C. (1999). An unexpected result in an evaluation of a serological test to detect syphilis. *Pathology, 31* (4), 398-402.

Gray, M. (1997). *Genitourinary disorders* (2nd ed.). St. Louis, MO: Mosby.

Greenbaum, L., Simckes, A., McKenney, D., Kainer, G., Nagaraj, S., Trachtman, H., & Alon, U. (2000). Pediatric biopsy of a single native kidney. *Pediatric Nephrology, 15* (1), 66-69.

Groenwald, S., Frogge, M. H., Goodman, M., & Yarbro, C. H. (1997). *Cancer nursing: Principles and practice* (4th ed.). Boston: Jones and Bartlett Publishers.

Guermandi,E., Vegetti, W., Bianchi, M., Uglietti, A., Ragni, G., & Crosignani, P. (2001). Reliability of ovulation tests in infertile women. *Obstetrical Gynecology, 97* (1), 92-96.

Guzman, C., Walsh, M., Reddy, V., Donthrieddy, V., Mahmood, F., Bode, A., Turner, J., Jacobs, J., & Sowers, J. (2001). *Altered myosin light-chain phosphorylation in resting platelets from premenopausal women with diabetes, 50* (2), 151-156.

Gyawali, P., & Rangedara, D. C. (1999). Iatrogenically revealed myasthenia gravis. *International Journal of Clinical Practice, 53*(8), 645.

Haas, M., Reinacher, D., Pun, K., Wong, N., & Mooradian, A. (2000). Induction of the apolipoprotein AI gene by fasting: A relationship with ketosis but not with ketone bodies. *Metabolism, 49* (12), 1572-1578.

Haga, H. J., Hulten, B., Bolstad, A. I., Ulvestad, E., & Jonsson, R. (1999). Reliability and sensitivity of diagnostic tests for primary Sjogren's syndrome. *Journal of Rheumatology, 26*(3), 604–608.

Hanly, P., & Pierratos, A. (2001). Improvement of sleep apnea in patients with chronic renal failure who undergo nocturnal hemodialysis. *New England Journal of Medicine, 344* (2), 102-107.

Harris, T., Borsanyi, S., Messari, S., Stanford, K., & Brown, G. (2000). Morning cortisol as a risk factor for subsequent major depressive disorder in adult women. *British Journal of Psychiatry, 177*(6), 505–510.

Hellman, D. B., & Stone, J. H. (2000). Arthritis and musculoskeletal disorders. In L. M Tierney, Jr., S. J. McPhee, & M. A. Papadakis (Eds.), *Current medical diagnosis and treatment 2000* (pp. 836–838). New York: Lange Medical Books/McGraw-Hill.

Heslin, J. M. (1997). Peptic ulcer disease: Making a case against the prime suspect. *Nursing '97, 27*(1), 34–39.

Hickey, J. V. (1997). *The clinical practice of neurological and neurosurgical nursing* (4th ed.). Philadelphia: Lippincott.

Hochberg, M. C. (1996). Sjogren's syndrome. In J. C. Bennett & F. Plum (Eds.), *Cecil textbook of medicine* (20th ed., pp. 1488–1490). Philadelphia: Saunders.

Holmes, K. K., Mardh, P., Sparling, P. F., Lemon, S. P., Stamm, W. E., Piot, P., & Wasserheit, J. N. (1999). *Sexually transmitted diseases* (3rd ed.). New York: McGraw-Hill.

Holmquist, M., Chabelewski, F., Blount, T., Edwards, C., McBride, V., & Petroski, R. (1999). A critical pathway: Guiding care for organ donors. *Critical Care Nurse, 19*(2), 84–98.

Horner, M. (1998). Continuing education forum: Diagnosis and management of acute pancreatitis. *Journal of American Academy of Nurse Practitioners, 10*(10), 471–477.

Howden, C., & Hunt, R. (1998). Guidelines for management of H pylori infection. *Journal of Gastroenterology, 93*(12), 2330–2338.

Hudak, C. M., Gallo, B. M., & Morton, P. G. (1998). *Critical care nursing* (7th ed.). Philadelphia: Lippincott.

Hunter, M., Angelicheva, D., Levy, H., Pueschel, S., & Kalaydjieva, L. (2001). Novel mutations in the GALK I gene in patients with galactokinase deficiency. *Human Mutations, 17* (1), 77-78.

Huonker, M., Schumacher, Y., Ochs, A., et al. (1999). Cardiac function and hemodynamics in alcoholic cirrhosis and effects of transjugular intrahepatic portosystemic stent shunt. *Gut, 44*(5), 743–748.

Hurwitz, R., & Kaptein, J. (2001). How well does contralateral testis hypertrophy predict the absence of the nonpalpable testis. *Journal of Urology, 165* (2), 588-592.

Husseini, A., Abdul-Rahim, H., Awartani, F., Giacaman, R., & Jervell, J. (2000). Type 2 diabetes mellitus, impaired glucose tolerance and associated factors in a rural Palestinian village. *Diabetic Medicine, 17*(10), 746–748.

Jackler, R., & Kaplan, M. J. (2000). Ear, nose and throat. In L. M. Tierney, Jr., S. J. McPhee, & M. A. Papadakis (Eds.), *Current medical diagnosis and treatment 2000* (pp. 223–263). New York: Lange Medical Books/McGraw-Hill.

Jacobson, A., Shapiro, C., Abbeele, A., & Kaplan, W. (2001). Prognostic significance of the number of bone scan abnormalities at the time initial bone metastatic recurrence in breast carcinoma. *Cancer, 91* (1), 17-24.

Jenni, R., & Berger-Bachi, B. (1998). Teichoic acid content in different lineages of *Staphylococcus aureus. Archives of Microbiology, 170*(3), 171–178.

Johnson, G. A. (1997). Paracentesis. In M. S. Jastremski & M. Dumas (Eds.), *Emergency procedures* (2nd ed., pp. 167–172). Philadelphia: W. B. Saunders Company.

Johnson, R. J., & Feehally, J. (2000). *Comprehensive clinical nephrology*. London: Mosby.

Kanski, J. (1999). *Clinical ophthalmology: A systematic approach.* Oxford: Butterworth Heinemann.

Khan, R., Laster R., & Bertorini, T. (2000). Rapid growth of a basilar aneurysm. *American Journal of Medical Science, 320*(4), 281–285.

Khastgir, G., Studd, J., Holland, N., Alaghband-Zadeh, J., Fox, S., & Chow, J. (2001). Anabolic effect of estrogen replacement on bone in postmenopausal women with osteoporosis: histomorphometric evidence in a longitudinal study. *Journal of Clinical Endocrinology and Metabolism, 86* (1), 289-295.

King, B. (1997). Preserving renal function. *RN, 60*(98), 34–49.

King, K. S. (1999). Oral androstenedione and adaptations to resistance training in young men. *JAMA, 22*(1), 2020–2028.

Kirby, R. B. (1999). Maternal phenylketonuria: A new cause for concern. *Journal of Obstetric, Gynecologic, and Neonatal Nursing, 28*(3), 227–233.

Kirk, J. M. (2000). Inconsistencies in sweat testing in UK laboratories. *Archives of Disease in Childhood, 82*(5), 425–427.

Klein, R., & Klein, B. (1998). Relation of glycemic control to diabetic complications and health outcomes. *Diabetes Care, 21*(Suppl. 3), 39–43.

Knight-Madden, J., & Serjeant, G. (2001). Invasive pneumococcal disease in homozygous sickle cell disease: Jamaican experience 1973-1997. *Journal of Pediatrics, 138* (1), 65-70.

Knox, T., Spiegelman, D., Skinner, S., & Gorbach, S. (2000). Diarrhea and abnormalities of gastrointestinal function in a cohort of men and women with HIV infection. *American Journal of Gastroenterology, 95* (12), 3482-3489.

Kobayashi, T. K., Kaneko, C., Sugishima, S., Kusukawa, J., & Kameyama, T. (1999). Scrape cytology of oral pemphigus: Report of a case with immunocytochemistry and light, scanning electron and transmission electron microscopy. *Acta Cytologica, 43*(2), 289–294.

Kontoyiannia, D. P., Ruoff, K., & Hooper, D. C. (1998). *Nocardia* bacteremia: Report of 4 cases and review of the literature. *Medicine, 77*(4), 255–268.

Korinko, A., & Urick, A. (1997). Maintaining skin integrity during radiation therapy. *American Journal of Nursing, 97*(2), 40–44.

Koutroumanidis, M., et al. (2000). Significance of interictal bilateral temporal hypometabolism in temperal lobe epilepsy. *Neurology, 54*(9), 1811–1821.

Kronborg, O. (2000). Screening for early colorectal cancer. *World Journal of Surgery, 24*(9), 1069–1074

Kuhn, S., Davies, H. D., Katzko, G., Jadavji ,T., & Church, D. L. (1999). Evaluation of the Strep A OIA assay versus culture methods: Ability to detect different quantities of group A *Streptococcus. Diagnostic Microbiology and Infectious Disease, 34*(4), 275–280.

Kulke, M. H. (1999). Carcinoid tumors. *New England Journal of Medicine, 340,* 858.

Kunin, C. M. (1997). *Urinary tract infections: Detection, prevention and management.* Baltimore: William & Wilkins.

Kuper, B. C., & Failla, S. (2000). Systemic lupus erythematosus: A multisystem autoimmune disorder. *Nursing Clinics of North America, 35*(1), 253–265.

Kuritzky, L. (2000). Oral androstenedione administration and serum testosterone concentrations in young men. *Internal Medicine Alert, 22*(8), 64.

Latham, P., & Dullye, K. (2001). Complications of thoracoscopy. *Anesthesiology Clinics of North America, 19* (1), 187-200.

Lavie, C. J., Milani, R. V., & Mehra, M. R. (2000). Choosing a stress test. *Patient Care, 34*(3), 81–82, 91–92, 94.

Lee, G. R., Foerster, J., Lukens, J., Paraskevas, F., Greer, J. P., & Rodgers, G. M. (1999). *Wintrobe's clinical hematology* (10th ed., Vol. 1). Baltimore: Williams & Wilkins.

Levy, M., & Cernacek, P. (1996). *Clinical and Investigative Medicine, 19*(6), 435–443.

Liberman, L., Dershaw, D. D., Glassman, J. R., Abramson, A. F., Morris, E. A., LaTrenta, L. R., & Rosen, P. P. (1997). Analysis of cancers not diagnosed at stereotactic core breast biopsy. *Radiology, 203*(1), 151–157.

Lim, S., Ali, A., Law, H., Ng, I., Chung, M., & Lee, S. (2001). An anemic patient with pheotypical beta-thalassemic trait has elevated levels of structurally normal beta-globin mRNA in reticulocytes. *American Journal of Hematology, 65* (3), 243-250.

Lindau, T. (2001). Wrist arthroscopy in distal radial fractures using a modified horizontal technique. *Arthroscopy, 17*(1), 5–9.

LoBuono, C. (2000). Serum ACE activity assay identifies nonadherent patients. *Patient Care, 34*(3), 228.

Lynch, J. (1997). Bacterial pneumonia. In M. G. Khan & J. P. Lynch (Eds.), *Pulmonary disease diagnosis and therapy: A practical approach* (pp. 306–307). Baltimore: Williams & Wilkins.

Maes, M., Verkerk, R., Delmeire, L., Van Gastel, A., & Van Hunsel, F. (2000). Serotonergic markers and lowered plasma branched-chain-amino acid concentrations in fibromyalgia. *Psychiatry Research, 97*(1), 11–20.

Marchigiano, G. (1999). Calcium intake in midlife women: One step in preventing osteoporosis. *Orthopedic Nursing, 18*(5), 11–18.

Marshall, N., Chapple, C., & Kotre, C. (2000). Diagnostic reference levels in interventional radiology. *Physics in Medicine and Biology, 45* (12), 3833-3846.

Massaro, L. M. (1998). Xenon-enhanced CT: Clinical applications. *Journal of Cardiovascular Nursing, 13*(1), 45–56.

Mattioli, A., Vandelli, R., & Mattioli, G. (2000). Doppler echocardiographic evaluation of right ventricular function in patients with right ventricular infarction. *Journal of Ultrasound Medicine, 19* (12), 831-836.

McNeely, M. D., & Brigden, M. L. (2000). Laboratory diagnosis of erythroid disorders. In R. C. Tilton, A. Balows, D. C. Hohnadel, & R. Reiss (Eds.), *Clinical laboratory medicine* (pp. 402–409). Saint Louis: Mosby.

Mehta, J. L., Saldeen, T. G., & Rand, K. (1998). Interactive role of infection, inflammation and traditional risk factors in atherosclerosis and coronary artery disease. *Journal of the American College of Cardiology, 31*(6), 1217–1225.

Merrick, M. V. (1998). *Essentials of nuclear medicine.* London: Springer.

Molzahn, A. E., Northcott, H. C., & Dossetor, J. B. (1997). Quality of life of individuals with end-stage renal disease: Perceptions of patients, nurses, and physicians. *ANNA Journal, 24*(3), 325–333.

Monteiro, L., Mascarel, A., Sarasqueta, A., Bergey, B., Barberis, C., Talby, P., Roux, D., Shouler, L., Goldfain, D., Lamouliatte, H., & Megraud, F. (2001). Diagnosis of helicobacter pylori infection: Noninvasive methods compared to invasive methods and evaluation of two new tests. *American Journal of Gastroenterology, 96* (2), 353-358.

Moorthy, R., & Narsing, A. R. (1997). Approach to the uveitis patient. In K. W. Wright (Ed.), *Ophthalmology* (pp. 481–483). Baltimore: Williams & Wilkins.

Morrison, J. J., Sinnatamby, R., Hackett, G. A., & Tudor, J. (1995). Obstetric pelvimetry in the UK: An appraisal of current practice. *British Journal of Obstetrical Gynecology, 102,* 748–750.

Mullen, D., Eisen, R., Newman, R., Perrone, P., & Wilsey, J. (2001). The use of carbon marking after stereotactic large-core needle breast biopsy. *Radiology, 218* (1), 255-260.

Muniz, A., & Evans, T. (2000). Chronic paronychia, osteomyelitis, and paravertebral abscess in a child with blastomycosis. *Journal of Emergency Medicine, 19* (3), 245-248.

Murray, H. W., Pepin, J., Nutman, T. B., Hoffman, S. L., & Mahmoud, A. A. F. (2000). Tropical medicine. *British Medical Review, 320*(7233), 490–494.

Nicholas, H. (1998). Sexually transmitted diseases. Gonorrhoea: Symptoms and treatment. *Nursing Times, 94*(8), 52–54.

Nicol, N. (2000). Managing atopic dermatitis in children and adults. *Nurse Practitioner, 25*(4), 58–76.

Niederman, M., Skerrett, S., & Yamauchi, T. (1998). Antibiotics or not? Managing patients with respiratory infections. *Patient Care, 32*(1), 60–64, 67.

Noor, M., & Beutler, E. (1998). Acquired sulfhemoglobinemia. An underreported diagnosis? *Western Journal of Medicine, 169*(6), 386–389.

Odom, R., James, W., & Berger, T. G. (2000). *Andrews' diseases of the skin: Clinical dermatology* (9th ed.). Philadelphia: W. B. Saunders.

Oertel, L. B. (1999). Monitoring warfarin therapy. *Nursing, 29*(11) 41–45.

Offidani, A., Amerio, P., Bernaredini, M., Feliciani, C., & Bossi, G. (2000). Role of cytomegalovirus replication in alopecia areata pathogenesis. *Journal of Cutaneous Medical Surgery, 4* (2), 63-65.

Ogino, S., & Redline, R. (2000). Villous capillary lesions of the placenta: Distinctions between chorangioma, chorangiomatosis, and choriangiosis. *Human Pathology, 31* (8), 945-954.

O'Hanlon-Nichols, T. (1998). Basic assessment series: A review of the adult musculoskeletal system. *American Journal of Nursing, 98*(6), 48–52.

O'Neil, B., & Ross, M. (2001). Cardiac markers protocols in a chest pain observation unit. *Emergency Medicine Clinics of North America, 19* (1), 67-86.

Ousehal, A., Abdelouafi, A., Belaabidia, B., Essodegui, F., Kadiri, B., & Kadiri, R. (2001). Malignant stromal tumors of the small bowel: Report of 9 cases. *Journal of Radiology, 82* (1), 35-40.

Ovington, L. G. (1998). The well-dressed wound: An overview of dressing types. *Wounds, 10*(suppl. A), 1A–11A.

Papia, G., Louie, M., Tralla, A., Johnson, C., Collins, V., & Simor, A. E. (1999). Screening high-risk patients for methicillin-resistant *Staphylococcus aureus* on admission to the hospital: Is it cost effective? *Infection Control and Hospital Epidemiology, 20*(7), 473–477.

Pereira-Lima, J., Jakobs, R., Busnello, J., Benz, C., Blaya, C., Riemann, J. (2000). The role of serum liver enzymes in the diagnosis of choledocholithiasis. *Hepatogastroenterology, 47* (36), 1522-1525.

Pillitteri, A. (1999). *Maternal and child health nursing* (3rd ed.). Philadelphia: Lippincott.

Poole, G. V., Thomae, K. R., & Hauser, C. J. (1996). Laparoscopy in trauma. *Surgical Clinics of North America, 76*(3), 547–555.

Porth, C. M. (1998). *Pathophysiology concepts of altered health states* (3rd ed.). San Francisco: J. B. Lippincott Co.

Probert, J., Mills, R., Persad, R., & Sethia, K. (2000). Imaging assessment of uncomplicated bladder outflow obstruction. *International Journal of Clinical Practice, 54*(1), 22–24.

Reust, C. (2001). Does the increased sensitivity of the new Papanicolaou (Pap) tests improve the cost-effectiveness of screening for cervical cancer? *Journal of Family Practice, 50* (2), 175.

Reyes, Romero, M. (2001). The physiological role of estriol during fetal development is to act as antioxidant at lipophilic milieus of the central nervous system. *Medical Hypotheses, 56* (1), 107-109.

Rifai, A., Bazarbashi, S., & Kandil, A. (2000). Positron emission tomography in Hodgkin's disease: Correlation with computed tomography and gallium 67 citrate imaging. *Clinical Positron Imaging, 3* (4), 179.

Ristikankare, M., Hartikainen, J., Heikkinen, M., Janatuinen, E., & Julkunen, R. (2001). The effects of gender and age on the colonoscopic examination. *Journal of Clinical Gastroenterology, 32* (1), 69-75.

Rodriguez, D., & Lewis, S. L. (1997). Nutritional management of patients with acute renal failure. *ANNA Journal, 24*(2), 232–236.

Rodriguez, I., Kilborn, M., Liu, X., Pezzullo, J., & Woosley, R. (2001). Drug-induced QT prolongation in women during the menstrual cycle. *JAMA, 285* (10), 1322-1326.

Rose, D., & King, B. (1997). Preserving renal function. *RN, 60*(98), 34–49.

Ross, J., & Cohen, M. (2001). Biomarkers for the detection of bladder cancer. *Advances in Anatomic Pathology, 8* (1), 37-45.

Rostaing, L, Izopet, J., Sandres, K., Cisterne, J., Puel, J., & Durand, D. (2000). Changes in hepatitis C virus RNA viremia concentrations in long-term renal transplant patients after introduction of mycophenolate mofetil. *Transplantation, 69* (5), 991-994.

Rutherford, R. B. (2000). *Vascular surgery* (5th ed., Vol.1). Philadelphia: W. B. Saunders Company.

Sabol, V. K., & Friedenberg, F. K. (1997). *Diarrhea. AACN Clinical Issues, 8*(3), 425–436.

Sanders, R. C. (1997). *Clinical sonography: A practical guide* (2nd ed.). Boston: Little, Brown and Company.

Sanford, J. (1998). *Guide to antimicrobial therapy.* Dallas: Antimicrobial Therapy.

Santiago, J., Nolledo, M., Kinzler, W., Santiago, T. (2001). Sleep and sleep disorders in pregnancy. *Annals of Internal Medicine, 134* (5), 396-408.

Schmidt, W., Wahnschaffe, U., Schafer, M., Zippel, T., Arvand, M., Meyerhans, A., Rjecken, E., & Ullrich, R. (2001). Rapid increase of mucosal CD4 T cells followed by clearance of intestinal crytosporidiosis in an AIDS patient receiving highly active antiretrovira therapy. *Gastroenterology, 120* (4), 984-987.

Schwab, J., Schmidt, H., Coch, M., Bernhoeft, F., Waas, W., Raedle-Hurst, H., & Waldecker, B. (2001). Results and significance of holter monitoring after direct percutaneous transluminal coronary angioplasty for acute myocardial infarction. *American Journal of Cardiology, 87* (4), 466-469.

Sergides, I. G., Austin, R. C. T., & Winslet, M. C. (1999). Radioimmunodetection: Technical problems and methods of improvement. *European Journal of Surgical Oncology, 25,* 529-539.

Seto, E., Segall, G., & Terris, M. (2000). Positron emission tomography detection of osseous metastases of renal cell carcinoma not identified on bone scan. *Urology, 55* (2), 286.

Shields, H., Weiner, M., Henry, D., Lloyd, J., Ransil, B., Lamphier, D., Gallagher, D., Antonioli, D., & Rosner, B. (2001). Factors that influence the decision to do an adequate evaluation of a patient with a positive stool for occult blood. *American Journal of Gastroenterology, 96* (1), 196-203.

Sinha, P., Krumm, R., & Mozley, P. (2001). Gallbladder stone shown on a hepatobiliary scan. *Clinical Nuclear Medicine, 26* (1), 80-81.

Smith, A., & Hughes, P. L. (1998). The estrogen dilemma. *American Journal of Nursing, 98*(4), 17–20.

Smith, A., Justin, T., Michaeli, D., & Watson, S. (2000). Phase I/II study of G17-DT, an anti-gastrin immunogen, in advanced colorectal cancer. *Clinical Cancer Research, 6* (12), 4719-4724.

Smith, S. D., Wheeler, M. A., & Weiss, R. M. (1998). Detection of urinary tract infections by reduction of nitroblue tetrazolium. *Kidney International, 54,* 1331–1336.

Somach, S., & Morgan, M. (2001). Benign keratosis with a spectrum of follicular differentiation: A case series and an investigation of a potential role of human papilloma virus. *Journal of Cutaneous Pathology, 28* (3), 156-159.

Somers, J., Das, V., Dell'Osso, L., & Leigh, R. (2000). Saccades to sounds: Effects of tracking illusory visual stimuli. *Journal of Neurophysiology, 84* (1), 96-101.

Speroff, L., Glass, R. H., & Kase, N. (1999). *Clinical gynecologic endocrinology and infertility* (6th ed.). Philadelphia: Lippincott Williams & Wilkins.

Sra, J., Bhatia, A., Krum, D., & Akhtar, M. (2000). Endocardial noncontact activation mapping of idiopathic left ventricular tachycardia. *Journal of Cardiovascular Electrophysiology, 11* (12), 1409-1412.

Stirling, C., Simpson, K., & Boulton-Jones, M. (2000). Serum creatinine can predict adequacy of peritoneal dialysis—Preliminary report. *Clinical Nephrology, 54*(5), 400–403.

Stone, J. E. (1998). Urine analysis in the diagnosis of mucopolysaccharide disorders. *Annals of Clinical Biochemistry, 35*(2), 207–225.

Stone, R. (1998). Differential diagnosis. Acute abdominal pain. *Lippincott's primary care practice, 2*(4), 341–357.

Sullivan, J. (2001). Misconceptions in the debate on the iron hypothesis. *Journal of Nutritional Biochemistry, 12* (1), 33-37.

Tanaka, K., Aimyam, T., Imai, J., Morishita, Y., Fukatsu, T., & Kakukma, S. (1995). Serum cryoglobulin and chronic hepatitis C virus disease among Japanese patients. *American Journal of Gastroenterology, 90*(10), 1847–1852.

Testoni, P., & Bagnolo, F. (2001). Pain at 24 hours associated with amylase levels greater than 5 times the upper normal limit as the most reliable indicator of post-ERCP pancreatitis. *Gastrointestinal Endoscopy, 53* (1), 33-39.

Theraiult, M., Dort, J., Sutherland, G., & Zochodne, D. W. (1997). A prospective quantitative study of sensory deficits after whole sural nerve biopsies in diabetic and nondiabetic patients. *Neurology, 50,* 480–484.

Thisyakorn, U., Pancharoen, C., & Wilde, H. (2001). Immunologic and virologic evaluation of HIV-1 infected children after rabies vaccination. *Vaccine, 19* (11), 1534-1537.

Thomas, D. P. (1997). Hypercoagulability in venous and arterial thrombosis. *Annals of Internal Medicine, 126*(8) 638–644.

Tsutsumi, S., Hosouchi, Y., Shimura, T., Asao, T., & Kojima, T. (2000). Double cystic duct detected by endoscopic retrograde cholangiopancreatography and confirmed by intraoperative cholangiography in laparoscopic cholecystectomy: A case report. *Hepatogastroenterology, 47*(35), 1266–1268.

Turner, J., Bui, T., Lerner, R., & Barbas, C. (2000). An efficient benchtop system for multigram-scale kinetic resolutions using aldolase antibodies. *Chemistry, 6*(15), 2772–2774.

Tutschek, B., Reinhard, J., Kogler, G., Wernet, P., & Niederacher, D. (2000). Clonal culture of fetal cells from maternal blood. *Lancet, 18*(9243), 1736–1737.

Udey, M. C., & Stanley, J. R. (1999). Pemphigus-diseases of antidesmosomal autoimmunity. *Journal of the American Medical Association, 282*(6), 572–576.

Uslu, R., Sanli, U., Sezgin, C., Karabulut, B., Terzioglu, E., Omay, S., & Goker, E. (2000). Arsenic trioxide-mediated cytotocity an apoptosis in prostate and ovarian carcinoma cell lines. *Clinical Cancer Research, 6*(12), 4957–4964.

Vaccaro, J., & Brody, J. (2000). CT cystography in the evaluation of major bladder trauma. *Radiographics, 20*(5), 1373–1381.

Van Langevelde, P., Van Dissel, J. T., Ravensbergen, E., Appelmelk, B. J., Schrijver, I. A., & Groeneveld, P. H. (1998). Antibiotic-induced release of lipoteichoic acid and peptidoglycan from *Staphylococcus aureus*: Quantitative measurements and biological reactivities. *Antimicrobial Agents and Chemotherapy, 42*(12), 3073–3078.

VanElsacker-Niele, A. M., & Kroes, A. C. (1999). Human parvovirus B19: Relevance in internal medicine. *Netherlands Journal of Medicine, 54*(6), 221–230.

Walling, A. D. (1998). Evaluating the risk of fetal loss following amniocentesis. *American Family Physician, 58*(8), 1851–1852.

Wallman, C. M. (1998). Newborn genetic screening. *Neonatal Network, 17*(3), 55–60.

Walsh, P. C., Retick, A. B., Vaughan, E. D. Jr., & Wein, A. J. (1998). *Campbell's urology* (7th ed.). Philadelphia: W.B. Saunders.

Wang, S. H., & Robinson, L. R. (1998). Considerations in reference values for nerve conduction studies. *Physical Medicine and Rehabilitation Clinics of North America, 9*(4), 907–923.

Weber, M., Neutel, J., & Smith, D. (2001). Contrasting clinical properties and exercise responses in obese and lean hypertensive patients. *J. Am. Coll. Cardiol., 37* (1), 169-174.

Weiskopg, R. B., Viele, M. K., & Feiner, J. (1998). Human cardiovascular and metabolic response to acute, severe isovolemic anemia. *Journal of the American Medical Association, 279,* 212–217.

Willows, N., Dewailly, E., & Gray, K. (2000). Anemia and iron status in Inuit infants from northern Quebec. *Canadian Journal of Public Health, 91* (6), 407-410.

Wilson, J. D., Foster, D. W., Kronenberg H. M., & Larsen, P. R. (1998). *Williams textbook of endocrinology* (9th ed.). Philadelphia: W.B. Saunders.

Wolf, Y., Johnson, B., Hill, B., Rubin, G., & Fogarty T. (2000). Duplex ultrasound scanning versus computed tomographic angiography for postoperative evaluation of endovascular abdominal aortic aneurysm repair. *Journal of Vascular Surgery, 32*(6), 1142–1148.

Wong, A., & Sharpe, J. (2000). A comparison of tangent screen, Goldmann, and Humphrey perimetry in the detection and localization of occipital lesions. *Ophthalmology, 107* (3), 527-544.

Wroblewski, B. M., Stefanovic, C. R., et. al. (1997). The challenges of idiopathic pulmonary hemosiderosis and lung transplantation. *Critical Care Nurse, 17,* 35–39.

Wu, X., Yeh, Sj., Jeng, T. W., & Khalil, O. S. (2000). Noninvasive determination of hemoglobin and hematocrit using a temperature-controlled localized reflectance tissue photometer. *Annals of Biochemistry, 287*(2), 284–293.

Yaney, G., Civelek, V., Richard, A., Dillon, J., Deeney, J., Hamilton, J., Korchak, H., Tornheim, K., Corkey, B., & Boyd, A. (2001). Glucagon-like peptide 1 stimulates lipolysis in clonal pancreatic beta-cells. *Diabetes, 50* (1), 56-62.

Yang, J., Tao, Q., Flinn, I., Murray, P., & Post, L. (2000). Characterization of Epstein-Barr virus-infected B cells in patients with posttransplantation lymphoproliferative disease: Disappearance after rituximab therapy does not predict clinical response. *Blood, 96*(13), 4055–4063.

Young, W. F. Jr. (1999). Primary aldosteronism: A common and curable form of hypertension. *Cardiology Review, 7*(4), 207–214.

Zoccali, C., Benedeto, F., Mallamaci, F., Tripepi, G., Candela, V., Labate, C., & Tassone, F. (2001). Left ventricular hypertrophy and nocturnal hypoxemia in hemodialysis patients. *Journal of Hypertension, 19* (2), 287-293.

Appendix A
Abbreviation List

2,3-DPG	2,3-diphosphoglycerate
ABG	arterial blood gas
Acetyl-Coa	acetyl coenzyme A
ACTH	adrenocorticotropic hormone
ADH	antidiuretic hormone
ADL	activities of daily living
ADP	adenosine diphosphate
ADR	adverse drug reaction
AGF	angiogenesis factor
AIDS	acquired immunodeficiency syndrome
ALT	alanine transferase
ANA	antinuclear antibodies
ANS	autonomic nervous system
APTT	activated partial thromboplastin time
ARC	AIDS-related complex
ASA	aminosalysilic acid
AST	aspartate aminotransferase
AT	axillary temperature
ATP	adenosine triphosphate
AV	atrioventricular
BCR	bulbocavernosus reflex
BMI	body mass index
BMR	basal metabolic rate
BP	blood pressure
BSE	breast self-examination
BUN	blood urea nitrogen
CAD	coronary artery disease
CAT	computerized axial tomography
CBC	complete blood count
CDC	Centers for Disease Control and Prevention
CHD	coronary heart disease
CHF	congestive heart failure
CNS	central nervous system
COPD	chronic obstructive pulmonary disease
CPK	creatine phosphokinase
CPM	continuous passive motion
CPN	central parenteral nutrition
CPR	cardiopulmonary resuscitation
CPT	chest physiotherapy
CSF	cerebrospinal fluid
CST	computerized simulation testing

CT	computerized tomography
CVA	cerebrovascular accident
DIC	disseminated intravascular coagulation
DNA	deoxyribonucleic acid
DNR	do not resuscitate
DUS	Doppler ultrasound stethoscope
DVT	deep vein thrombosis
ECG	electrocardiogram (also known as EKG)
EDTA	ethylenediaminetetraacetic acid
EEG	electroencephalogram
EN	enteral nutrition
ESR	erythrocyte sedimentation rate
ET	ear canal temperature
FAS	fetal alcohol syndrome
FHR	fetal heart rate
FiO_2	fraction of inspired oxygen
FSH	follicle-stimulating hormone
GAS	general adaptation syndrome
GCS	Glasgow Coma Scale
GFR	glomerular filtration rate
GI	gastrointestinal
GPT	glutamic pyruvic acid
Gtt	drop
GTT	glucose tolerance test
HBD	alpha-hydroxybutyrate dehydrogenase
HBV	hepatitis B virus
Hct	hematocrit
HDL	high-density lipoprotein
HEPA	high-efficiency particulate air
Hgb	hemoglobin
HIV	human immunodeficiency virus
HPN	home parenteral nutrition
HSV	herpes simplex virus
ICU	intensive care unit
IFA	immunofluorescent antibody
Ig	immunoglobulin
IM	intramuscular
I&O	intake and output
IPPB	intermittent positive-pressure breathing
IV	intravenous
IVP	intravenous pyelogram
KUB	kidney-ureter-bladder
LDH	lactate dehydrogenase
LDL	low-density lipoprotein
LH	luteinizing hormone
LLQ	left lower quadrant
LOC	level of consciousness

LUQ	left upper quadrant
MAC	mid-upper-arm-circumference
MAO	monoamine oxidase
MDR	multidrug resistant
MG	myasthenia gravis
MH	malignant hyperthermia
MI	myocardial infarction
mm Hg	millimeters of mercury
MRI	magnetic resonance imaging
MRSA	methicillin-resistant *Staphylococcus aureus*
NG	nasogastric
NPO	(*non per os*) nothing by mouth (to eat or drink)
NS	nutrition support
OSHA	Occupational Safety and Health Administration
OT	oral temperature
OTC	over the counter
P	pulse
PA	pulmonary artery; posteroanterior
PaO$_2$	partial pressure of oxygen dissolved in arterial blood plasma (also known as PAO$_2$)
Pap	Papanicolaou test
PAT	pulmonary artery temperature
PCA	patient-controlled analgesia
PCO$_2$	partial pressure of carbon dioxide dissolved in arterial blood plasma
PEG	percutaneous endoscopic gastrostomy
PERRLA	pupils equal, round, reactive to light, and accommodation
PET	positron emission tomography
pH	hydrogen ion concentration of a solution
PID	pelvic inflammatory disease
PIE	problem, intervention, evaluation
PIEE	pulsed irrigation enhanced evacuation
PKU	phenylketonuria
PMR	progressive muscle relaxation
PMS	premenstrual syndrome
PN	parenteral nutrition
PNI	psychoneuroimmunology
PNS	peripheral nervous system
PO	(*per os*) by mouth
PO$_2$	partial pressure of oxygen in a mixture of gases or in solution
PPN	peripheral parenteral nutrition
PRN	(*pro re nata*) as needed
PT	prothrombin time
PTT	partial thromboplastin time
PURT	prompted urge response toileting
q.d.	every day
q.i.d.	four times a day

R	respiration
RAS	reticular activating system
RBC	red blood cell
RDA	recommended dietary allowances
RDDA	recommended daily dietary allowances
RLQ	right lower quadrant
RNA	ribonucleic acid
ROM	range of motion
RT	rectal temperature
RUQ	right upper quadrant
SaO$_2$	percent saturation of arterial blood (hemoglobin) with oxygen
SA	sinoatrial
SAECG	signal-averaged electrocardiography percent saturation of arterial blood (hemoglobin) with oxygen
SGPT	serum glutamic pyruvic acid
SI	International System of Units
SIADH	syndrome of inappropriate antidiuretic hormone
SL	sublingual
SLE	systemic lupus erythematosus
SLT	social learning theory
SMI	sustained maximum inspiration
SO$_2$	percent saturation of blood (hemoglobin) with oxygen
SPECT	single-photon emission computed tomography
STD	sexually transmitted disease
SUI	stress urinary incontinence
T	temperature
TB	tuberculosis
TENS	transcutaneous electrical nerve stimulation
TMJ	temporomandibular joint
TNA	total nutrient admixture
TPN	total parenteral nutrition
TQM	total quality management
TSE	testicular self-examination
TSH	thyroid-stimulating hormone
UTI	urinary tract infection
VLDL	very low density lipoprotein
VMA	vanillymandelic acid
V/Q	ventilation/perfusion (mismatch)
VRE	vancomycin-resistant enterococci
WB	Western blot
WBC	white blood cell
WNL	within normal limits

Units of Measurement Conversion Table

Metric System
Mass

Unit of Measurement		Grams		Grains
1 kilogram	=	1000.0	=	15,432.35
1 hectogram	=	100.0	=	1,543.23
1 decagram	=	10.0	=	154.323
1 gram	=	1.0	=	15.432
1 decigram	=	0.1	=	1.5432
1 centigram	=	0.01	=	0.15432
1 milligram	=	0.001	=	0.01543

Weights and Measures
Volume

Milliliters (mL)	Fluid Drams (fl oz)	Cubic Inches (in.^{3})	Fluid Ounces (fl oz)	Fluid Quarts (qt)	Liters (L)
1.0	0.2705	0.061	0.03381	0.00106	0.001
3.679	1.0	0.226	0.125	0.00391	0.00369
16.3866	4.4329	1.0	0.5541	0.0173	0.01639
29.573	8.0	1.8047	1.0	0.03125	0.02957
949.332	256.0	57.75	32.0	1.0	0.9463
1000.0	270.52	61.025	33.815	1.0567	1.0

Weight

Grains (gr)	Grams (g)	Apothecaries' Ounces (oz)	Avoirdupois Pounds (lb)	Kilograms (kg)
1.0	0.0648	0.00208	0.0001429	0.000065
15.432	1.0	0.03215	0.002205	0.0001
480.0	31.1	1.0	0.06855	0.0311
7000.0	453.5924	14.583	1.0	0.45354
15,432.358	1000.0	32.15	2.2046	1.0

Household Measures and Weights

1 teaspoon = ⅛ fl oz = 1 dram
3 teaspoons = 1 tablespoon
1 tablespoon = ½ fl oz = 4 drams
1 tumbler or glass = 8 fl oz = 1 pint
16 teaspoons (liquid) = 1 cup
12 tablespoons (dry) = 1 cup
1 cup = 8 fl oz
Approximate equivalents: 60 gtts = 1 teaspoon = 5 ml = 60 minims = 60 grains =
1 dram = ⅛ ounce

Appendix B
Venipuncture and Skin Puncture Procedures

Procedure 1 Venipuncture

Equipment

◊ Sterile packages of 70% isopropanol (antiseptic) and povidone-iodine (topical anti-infectant)
◊ Sterile needle and syringe or vacutainer system (20- or 21-gauge needle for cubital vein puncture on an adult)

◊ Sterile 2 × 2 cotton gauze
◊ Tourniquet
◊ Nonsterile gloves
◊ Bandage or sterile adhesive bandage
◊ Collecting tubes

Action	Rationale
1. Check identification band.	1. Ensures correct client.
2. Wash hands.	2. Decreases transmission of microorganisms.
3. Explain procedure to client.	3. Reduces anxiety; promotes cooperation.
4. Place client in a sitting or supine position; lower side rail.	4. Promotes client comfort; provides access to the site.
5. Prepare supplies: • Open sterile packages. • Label specimen tubes with the client's data.	5. Promotes efficiency; ensures accuracy of specimen collection regarding the client's identifying data and date and time of collection.
6. Position arm straight. If possible, place extremity in dependent position.	6. Provides access to vein. Increases venous dilation and visibility.
7. Apply the tourniquet 6–10 cm above the elbow. Tourniquet should only obstruct venous blood flow, not arterial. Check for a distal pulse.	7. Restricted arterial blood flow prevents venous filling.
8. Select a dilated vein. If a vein is not visible, instruct client to open and close a fist; or stroke extremity from proximal to distal, tap lightly over a vein, and apply warmth.	8. Commonly used veins are the basilic or median cubital. Alternate sites are lower arm veins (cephalic or median antebrachial) and hand veins (basilic). Methods to increase venous dilation.

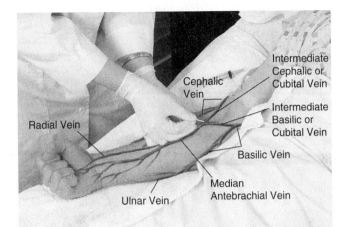

Cephalic Vein

Intermediate Cephalic or Cubital Vein

Intermediate Basilic or Cubital Vein

Radial Vein

Basilic Vein

Median Antebrachial Vein

Ulnar Vein

Nurse selects site for venipuncture and holds skin taut over site with needle held at 30° angle.

Action	Rationale
9. Palpate the vein for size and pliancy; be sure it is well seated.	9. Locates a well-dilated vein; vein does not roll.
10. Release the tourniquet.	10. Prevents hemoconcentration.
11. Cleanse puncture site with isopropanol, let dry and cleanse with povidone-iodine, let dry or wipe with sterile gauze, and do not touch site after cleansing. If the client is allergic to iodine, only use isopropanol and cleanse skin for 30 sec.	11. Povidone-iodine reduces bacteria on the skin's surface; it must be dry to be effective.
12. Place equipment in easy reach and position yourself to access the puncture site.	12. Promotes efficiency.
13. Reapply the tourniquet (time should not exceed 3 min).	13. Restricts blood flow; distends vein.
14. Don gloves.	14. Decreases exposure to blood-borne organisms.
15. Perform venipuncture:	15.
• Remove cap from 20- or 21-gauge needle.	• Large-bore needle prevents hemolysis.
• With nondominant hand, stabilize the vein by holding the skin taut over the puncture site (apply downward tension on the forearm with your thumb).	• Prevents the vein from rolling when the needle is pushed against the outer wall of the vein.

Procedure 1 Venipuncture (*continued*)

Action	Rationale
• With dominant hand, hold the needle.	• Provides for a downward movement toward vein.
• Puncture the skin into the straightest part of vein with a steady, moderately fast movement. (When the vein is entered, you will feel a slight give and can see blood at the needle's hub.)	• Decreases risk of going through the vein; decreases discomfort.
• Apply moderate negative pressure by puncturing the vacuum tube or by gently retracting the syringe plunger. (When first performing a venipuncture, use a syringe. It takes greater dexterity to puncture the vacuum tube with a two-sided needle; if you apply too much pressure, you will go through the vein.)	• When first performing a venipuncture, use a syringe. It takes greater dexterity to puncture the vacuum tube with a two-sided needle; if you apply too much pressure, you will go through the vein.
16. Remove the tourniquet once blood is flowing into the tube or syringe; collect the specimen(s).	16. Prevents hemolysis.
17. Remove the needle and immediately apply pressure to site for 2–3 min or 5–10 min if client is taking anticoagulant medication. Keep the arm straight.	17. Decreases bleeding. Bending the arm can reopen the puncture site.
18. Have the client maintain pressure on the puncture site.	18. Facilitates clotting.
• *Note:* Green stoppers contain sodium heparin (anticoagulant); they must be mixed promptly after collection.	• Prevents coagulation of blood in test tube.
19. Apply a sterile bandage or adhesive bandage to puncture site.	19. Facilitates clotting.
20. If using a needle and syringe, transfer the blood into test tube under moderate pressure.	20. Prevents hemolysis.
21. Dispose the needle or needle/syringe into a sharps container.	21. Prevents needle stick.
22. Remove gloves; wash hands.	22. Decreases transmission of microorganisms.

NURSING PROCESS HIGHLIGHT

Intervention

Clients with a depressed white blood cell count are susceptible to infection. Whenever you have to puncture the skin of a client with a depressed white blood cell count, cleanse the puncture site for 2–3 min.

Arterial Puncture

Assessment of arterial blood gases (ABGs) reveals the ability of the lungs to exchange gases by measuring the partial pressures of oxygen (PO_2) and carbon dioxide (PCO_2) and evaluates the pH of arterial blood. Blood gases are ordered to evaluate:

- Oxygenation
- Ventilation and the effectiveness of respiratory therapy
- Acid-base level of the blood

Procedure 2   Skin Puncture

Equipment

◊ Antiseptic—70% isopropanol or povidone-iodine
◊ Sterile 2 × 2 gauze
◊ Sterile lancet

◊ Hand towel or absorbent pad
◊ Microhematocrit tubes or micropipette (collection tubes)
◊ Nonsterile gloves

Action	Rationale
1. Wash hands.	1. Decreases transmission of microorganisms.
2. Check client's identification band.	2. Ensures correct client.
3. Explain procedure to client.	3. Allays anxiety and encourages cooperation.
4. Prepare supplies: • Open sterile packages. • Label specimen collection tubes. • Place in easy reach.	4. Ensures efficiency.
5. Don gloves.	5. Decreases the health care provider's exposure to blood-borne organisms.
6. Select site: • Lateral aspect of the fingertips in adults/children.	6. Avoids damage to nerve endings and calloused areas of the skin.

Procedure 2   Skin Puncture (*continued*)

Action	Rationale
7. Place the hand or heel in a dependent position; apply warm compresses if fingers or heel is cool to touch.	7. Increases the blood supply to the puncture site.
8. Place hand towel or absorbent pad under the extremity.	8. Prevents soiling the bed linen.
9. Cleanse puncture site with an antiseptic and allow to dry; use 70% isopropanol if client is allergic to iodine.	9. Reduces skin surface bacteria; povidone-iodine must dry to be effective.
10. With nondominant hand apply light pressure by gently squeezing the area above/around the puncture site. Do not touch puncture site.	10. Increases blood supply to puncture site; maintains asepsis.
11. With the sterile lancet at a 90° angle to the skin, use a quick stab to puncture the skin (about 2 mm deep).	11. Provides a blood sample with minimal discomfort to the client.

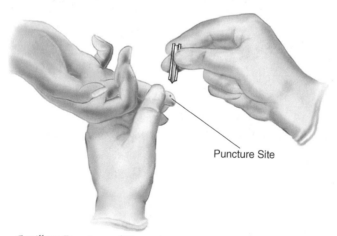

Puncture Site

Capillary Puncture of Fingertip.

12. Wipe off the first drop of blood with a sterile 2 × 2 gauze; allow the blood to flow freely.	12. Pressure at the puncture site can cause hemolysis.
13. Collect the blood into the tube(s). If a platelet count is to be collected, obtain this specimen first.	13. Allows blood collection; avoids aggregation of platelets at the puncture site.

Action	**Rationale**
14. Apply pressure to the puncture site with a sterile 2 × 2 gauze.	14. Controls bleeding.
15. Place contaminated articles into a sharps container.	15. Reduces risk for needle stick.
16. Remove gloves; wash hands.	16. Reduces transmission of microorganisms.
17. Position client for comfort with call light in reach.	17. Provides for comfort and communication.

Appendix C
Cancer Tumor Markers and Laboratory Tests Used in the Diagnosis and Monitoring of Malignant Tumors

Laboratory Test	Reference Value	Elevations in Specific Type of Cancer
Acid phosphatase (ACP)	0.0–0.8 U/L	Prostate; breast; bone; multiple myeloma
Alpha-fetoprotein (AFP)	< 10 ng/ml	Lung; testicular; colon; stomach
Aspartate aminotransferase (AST)	5–40 U/mL	Liver
Beta-2 microglobulin	< 2 µg/mL	Multiple myeloma; lymphoma
CA-15-3	< 22 U/ml	Breast; lung; ovarian benign disease
CA-19-9	< 37 AU/mL	Pancreas; colon; gastric
CA-50	< 17 U/mL	Colorectal; digestive tract; pancreas
CA-125	< 35 U/mL	Ovary; pancreas; breast; colon
Calcitonin	< 100 pg/mL	Thyroid; small-cell lung; breast
Carcinoembryonic antigen (CEA)	0–2.5 ng/mL nonsmokers, < 3.0 ng/mL smokers	Colorectal; breast; lung; stomach; pancreas; prostate
Estrogen receptors	Negative, < 10 fmol/mg	Breast
Human chorionic gonadotropin (HCG)	0–5 IU/L	Choriocarcinoma; gonadal germ cell; lung; liver; stomach; pancreas; endometrium
Progesterone receptor assay	Negative, < 10 fmol/mg	Breast
Prostatic acid phosphatase (PAP)	0.26–0.83 U/L	Adenocarcinoma of prostate
Prostate-specific antigen (PSA)	0–4 ng/mL	Prostate cancer; prostatitis; nodular prostatic hyperplasia
Protein electrophoresis	Negative	Myeloma; lymphoma (note: elevated in connective tissue disorders; chronic renal failure; benign monoclonal gammopathy)
Tissue polypeptide antigen (TPA)	80–100 U/L	Breast; colon; lung; pancreas

Bibliography

Nicholl, I., & Dunlop, M. (1999). Molecular markers of prognosis in colorectal cancer. *Journal of the National Cancer Institute, 91*(16), 1267.

Potosky, A., Harlan, L., Stanford, J., Gilliland, F., Hamilton, A., Albertsen, P., Eley, J., Liff, J., Deapen, D., Stephenson, R., Legler, J., Ferrans, C., Talcott, J., & Litwin, M. (1999). Prostate cancer practice patterns and quality of life: The prostate cancer outcomes study. *Journal of the National Cancer Institute, 91*(20), 1719–1724.

Ryan, D. (2000). A lab primer. *RN, 63*(1), 27–30.

Smeltzer, S., & Bare, B. (2000). *Brunner & Suddarth's textbook of medical-surgical nursing* (9th ed.). Philadelphia: Lippincott.

Welch, D., & Rinker-Shaeffer, C. (1999). What defines a useful marker of metastasis in human cancer? *Journal of National Cancer Institute, 91*(16), 1351–1353.

Appendix D
Consent Form Sample

TULANE MEDICAL CENTER
Hospital and Clinic
1415 Tulane Avenue
New Orleans, Louisiana 70112

Consent for medical procedure and acknowledgement
of receipt of information

Date_____

In keeping with the Louisiana State Law, you are being asked to sign a confirmation that we have discussed your contemplated operation or medical procedure. We have already discussed with you the common problems or risks. We wish to inform you as completely as possible. Please read the form carefully. Ask about anything that you do not understand and we will be pleased to explain it.

1.] I hereby authorize and direct Dr._____, with associates or assistants of his choice, to perform

upon_____, the following surgical, diagnostic, or medical procedure
_____
_____

including any necessary or advisable anesthesia.

2.] In general terms, the nature and purpose of this operation or medical procedure is:
_____
_____
_____

3.] This procedure has been explained to me. Alternate methods have also been explained to me, as have the advantages and disadvantages. I am advised that though good results are expected, the possibility and nature of complications cannot be accurately anticipated and that, therefore, there can be no guarantee as expressed or implied either as to the result of surgery or as to cure. The possible risks include death, brain damage, quadriplegia, paraplegia, loss of organ, loss of an arm or leg, or disfiguring scars.

4.] I authorize the administration of a blood transfusion and such additional transfusion as may be deemed advisable in judgement of the attending physician, or his associates or assistants.
It has been fully explained that blood transfusions are not always successful in producing a desirable result and that there is a possibility of ill effects, such as the transmission of infectious hepatitis or other diseases or blood impairments. Also, it has been explained that emergencies may arise when it may not be possible to make adequate cross-matching tests, and that immediate need may make it necessary to use existing stocks of blood which may not include compatible blood types.

5.] I further authorize the doctors to perform any other procedure that in their judgement is advisable for my well being. I hereby authorize and direct the above named physician and associates or assistants to provide such additional services as they may deem reasonable and necessary including, but not limited to, the administration of any anesthetic agent, or the services of the X-ray department or laboratories, and I hereby consent thereto.

6.] I hereby state that I have read and understand this consent, all questions about the procedure or procedures have been answered in a satisfactory manner, and that all blanks were filled in prior to my signature.

Witness_____ Signature_____
(patient or person authorized to consent)

Witness_____ Relationship_____
(required only for telephone consent or consents signed with an X)

I certify that all blanks in this form were filled in prior to signature and that I explained them to the patient or his representative before requesting the patient or his representative to sign it.

Signature_____
(above named physician to sign)

CONSENT FOR MEDICAL PROCEDURE AND ACKNOWLEDGEMENT
OF RECEIPT OF INFORMATION

Order by priority when consenting to medical/surgical procedure (except for care and treatment of mentally ill)
1. Any competent adult, age 18 or older, for himself.
2. Any parent, whether an adult or minor, for his minor child.
3. Any married person, whether an adult or minor, for his/her spouse if spouse is unable to consent.
4. Any person temporarily standing in place of a parent whether formally served or not for the minor under his care and any guardian for his ward.
5. Any female regardless of age or marital status, for herself when given in connection with pregnancy or childbirth.
6. In the absence of a parent, any adult, for his minor brother or sister.
7. In the absence of a parent, any grandparent for his minor grandchild.

(Courtesy Tulane University Hospital and Clinic, New Orleans, LA).

Appendix E
Therapeutic Blood Levels of Selected Drugs

Drug	Therapeutic Level	Toxic Level
Alcohols		
Ethanol	0.1 g/dL	100 mg/dL
Methanol	—	20 mg/dL
Antibiotics		
Amikacin	20–25 µg/mL	35 µg/mL
SI units	34–43 µmol/L	60 µmol/L
Gentamicin	4–8 µg/mL	12 µg/mL
SI units	8.4–16.8 µmol/L	25.1 µmol/L
Kanamycin	20–25 µg/mL	35 µg/mL
SI units	42–52 µmol/L	73 µmol/L
Streptomycin	25–30 µg/mL	> 30 µg/mL
SI units	—	—
Tobramycin	2–8 µg/mL	12 µg/mL
SI units	4–17 µmol/L	25 µmol/L
Anticonvulsants		
Barbiturates		
Amobarbital	7 µg/mL	30 µg/mL
SI units	30 µmol/L	132 µmol/L
Pentobarbital	4 µg/mL	15 µg/mL
SI units	18 µmol/L	66 µmol/L
Phenobarbital	10 µg/mL	> 55 µg/mL
SI units	43 µmol/L	> 230 µmol/L
Primidone	1 µg/mL	> 10 µg/mL
SI units	4 µmol/L	> 45 µmol/L
Benzodiazepines		
Clonazepam	5–70 ng/mL	> 70 ng/mL
SI units	55–222 µmol/L	> 222 µmol/L
Diazepam (Valium)	5–70 ng/mL	> 70 ng/mL
SI units	0.01–0.25 µmol/L	> 0.25 µmol/L
Hydantoins		
Phenytoin (Dilantin)	10–20 µg/mL	> 20 µg/mL
SI units	40–80 µmol/L	> 80 µmol/L
Succinimides		
Euthosuximide (Zarontin)	40–80 µg/mL	100 µg/mL
SI units	283–566 µmol/L	708 µmol/L

Drug	Therapeutic Level	Toxic Level
Other		
Carbamazepine (Tegretol)	2–10 µg/mL	12 µg/mL
SI units	8–42 µmol/L	50 µmol/L
Valproic acid (Depakene)	50–100 µg/mL	> 100 µg/mL
SI units	350–700 µmol/L	> 700 µmol/L
Bronchodilators		
Aminophylline/theophylline	10–18 µg/mL	20 µg/mL
Cardiac Drugs		
Disopyramide (Norpace)	2–4.5 µg/mL	> 9 µg/mL
SI units	5.9 µmol/L	26 µmol/L
Quinidine	2.4–5 µg/mL	> 6 µg/mL
SI units	7–15 µmol/L	> 18 µmol/L
Procainamide (Pronestyl)	7–15 µg/mL	> 12 µg/mL
SI units	17–35 µmol/L	> 50 µmol/L
Lidocaine	2–6 µg/mL	> 9 µg/mL
SI units	8–25 µmol/L	> 38 µmol/L
Bretylium	5–10 mg/kg	30 mg/kg
Verapamil	5–10 mg/kg	> 15 mg/kg
Diltiazem	50–200 ng/mL	> 200 ng/mL
Nifedipine	5–10 mg/kg	90 mg/kg
Digitoxin	10–25 ng/mL	30 ng/mL
SI units	13–33 nmol/L	39 nmol/L
Digoxin	0.5–2 ng/mL	> 2.5 ng/mL
SI units	0.6–2.5 nmol/L	> 3.0 nmol/L
Phenytoin (Dilantin)	10–18 µg/mL	> 20 µg/mL
SI units	40–71 µmol/L	> 80 µmol/L
Quinidine	2.3–5 µg/mL	> 5 µg/mL
SI units	7–15 µmol/L	> 15 µmol/L
Narcotics		
Codeine		> 0.005 mg/dL
SI units		> 17 nmol/dL
Hydromorphone (Dilaudid)		> .1 mg/dL
SI units		> 350 nmol/L
Methadone		> 0.2 mg/dL
SI units		6.46 µmol/L
Meperidine (Demerol)		0.5 mg/dL
SI units		20 µmol/L
Morphine		0.005 mg/dL
Psychiatrics		
Amitriptyline (Elavil)	100–250 ng/mL	> 300 ng/mL
SI units	361–902 nmol/L	> 1083 nmol/L

Drug	**Therapeutic Level**	**Toxic Level**
Imiprimine (Tofranil)	100–250 ng/mL	> 300 ng/mL
SI units	357–898 nmol/L	> 1071 nmol/L
Lithium (Lithonate)	0.8–1.4 mEq/L	1.5 mEq/L
SI units	0.8–1.4 μmol/L	1.5 μmol/L
Salicylates		
Aspirin	2–20 mg/dL	> 30 mg/dL
SI units	0.1–1.4 mmol/L	> 2.1 mmol/L
Other		
Acetaminophen	0–25 μg/mL	> 150 μg/mL
SI units	0–170 μmol/L	> 1000 μmol/L
Bromides	75–150 mg/dL	> 150 mg/dL
SI units	7–15 mmol/L	> 15 mmol/L
Prochlorperazine	0.5 μg/mL	1.0 μg/mL

Appendix F
Blood Sample for Central Line

- Gather equipment (the sizes of the needle and syringe to obtain the blood sample are determined by the amount of blood needed for the test and the type and size of central line catheter).

- Check the client's identification band.

- Wash hands and don gloves to prevent exposure to blood-borne organisms.

- Select a port that is not used routinely for an infusion.

- Cleanse the port of the lumen with an antiseptic.

- Insert the needle into the port and aspirate the discard volume according to agency protocol; dispose of the syringe containing the discarded blood into a sharps container.

- Access the port and withdraw the blood sample.

- Apply the same principles used in venipuncture to prevent the hemoconcentration and hemolysis of blood when withdrawing the sample.

- Transfer the sample into the correct collection tubes and discard the contaminated needle and syringe into the sharps container.

- Instill the required heparin solution to prevent the lumen from clotting.

- Transport specimen to the laboratory.

- Remove gloves; wash hands.

Appendix G
Reference Laboratory Values

Reference Values for Hematology

Laboratory Tests	Conventional Units	SI Units
Acid hemolysis	No hemolysis	No hemolysis
Alkaline phosphatase	14–100	14–100
Cell counts		
Erythrocytes		
Male	4.6–6.2 million/mm³	4.6–6.2 × 10¹²/L
Female	4.2–5.4 million/mm³	4.2–5.4 × 10¹²/L
Children (varies with age)	4.5–5.1 million/mm³	4.5–5.1 × 10¹²/L
Leukocytes, total	4,500–11,000 million/mm³	4.5–11.0 × 10⁹/L
Leukocytes, differential counts		
Myelocytes	0%	0/L
Band neutrophils	3–5%	150–400 × 10⁶/L
Segmented neutrophils	54–62%	3,000–5,800 × 10⁶/L
Lymphocytes	25–33%	1,500–3,000 × 10⁶/L
Monocytes	3–7%	300–500 × 10⁶/L
Eosinophils	1–3%	50–250 × 10⁶/L
Basophils	0–1%	15–50 × 10⁶/L
Platelets	150,000–400,000/mm³	150–400 × 10⁹/L
Reticulocytes	25,000–75,000/mm³	25–75 × 10⁹/L
Coagulation tests		
Bleeding time	2.75–8.0 min	2.75–8.0 min
Coagulation time	5–15 min	5–15 min
D-dimer	< 0.5 µg/mL	< 0.5 mg/L
Factor VIII and other coagulation factors	50–150% of normal	0.5–1.5 of normal
Fibrin split products	< 10 µg/mL	< 10 mg/L
Fibrinogen	200–400 mg/dL	2.0–4.0 g/L
Partial thromboplastin time (PTT)	20–35 sec	20–35 sec
Prothrombin time (PT)	12.0–14.0 sec	12.0–14.0 sec
Coombs' test		
Direct	Negative	
Indirect	Negative	
Corpuscular values of erythrocytes		
Mean corpuscular hemoglobin	26–34 pg/cell	26–34 pg/cell
Mean corpuscular volume	80–96 µm³	80–96 fL
Mean corpuscular hemoglobin concentration (MCHC)	32–36 g/dL	320–360 g/L
Haptoglobin	20–165 mg/dL	0.20–1.65 g/L
Hematocrit		
Male	40–54 mL/dL	0.40–0.54

Laboratory Tests	Conventional Units	SI Units
Female	37–47 mL/dL	0.37–0.47
Newborn	49–54 mL/dL	0.49–0.54
Children (varies with age)	35–49 mL/dL	0.35–0.49
Hemoglobin		
Male	13.0–18.0 g/dL	8.1–11.2 mmol/L
Female	12.0–16.0 g/dL	7.4–9.9 mmol/L
Newborn	16.5–19.5 g/dL	10.2–12.1 mmol/L
Children (varies with age)	11.2–16.5 g/dL	7.0–10.2 mmol/L
Hemoglobin, fetal	< 1.0% of total	< 0.01 of total
Hemoglobin A1C	3–5% of total	0.03–0.05 of total
Hemoglobin A2	1.5–3.0% of total	0.015–0.03 of total
Hemoglobin, plasma	0.0–5.0 mg/dL	0.0–3.2 µmol/L
Methemoglobin	30–130 mg/dL	19–80 µmol/L
Erythrocyte sedimentation rate (ESR)		
Wintrobe		
Male	0–5 mm/hr	0–5 mm/h
Female	0–15 mm/hr	0–15 mm/h
Westergren		
Male	0–15 mm/hr	0–15 mm/h
Female	0–20 mm/hr	0–20 mm/h

Appendix H
Routine Serum Electrolytes

ELECTROLYTE/NORMAL RANGE

CLINICAL SIGNIFICANCE

Sodium
135–148 mEq/L, adult
138–144 mEq/L, children
133–144 mEq/L, newborns

Increased: excessive intake of sodium without water; salt water drowning; high solute concentration (tube feeding, IV, hyperalimentation) without fluid correction; diarrhea; diabetes insipidus; primary aldosteronism; renal failure. *Decreased:* excessive intake of water without sodium (oral, IV therapy, tap water enemas); heart failure; cirrhosis; nephrosis and massive diuretic therapy.

Potassium (serum)
3.5–5.0 mEq/L, adult
3.4–4.7 mEq/L, children
3.7–5.9 mEq/L, newborns

Increased: high potassium intake (oral, IV therapy, rapid infusion of aged blood); renal disease; drugs (adrenal steroids, potassium-conserving diuretics, potassium penicillin, chemotherapeutic agents); Addison's disease; burns and other massive tissue trauma; metabolic and respiratory acidosis. *Decreased:* drugs (diuretics, diuretics and digitalis); metabolic alkalosis; primary aldosteronism; Cushing's disease; vomiting and gastric suction.

Calcium
Total: 8.4–10.5 mg/dL
Ionized: 1.13–1.32 mmol/L

Increased: hyperparathyroidism; bone catabolism (multiple myeloma, leukemia, bone tumors); immobility. *Decreased:* renal failure; sprue; pancreatitis; Crohn's disease; hyperphosphatemia; drugs (aminoglycosides, antacids containing aluminum, caffeine, cisplatin, corticosteriods, loop diuretics, mithracin, phosphate).

ELECTROLYTE/NORMAL RANGE*	CLINICAL SIGNIFICANCE
Chloride 96–109 mEq/L, adult 98–105 mEq/L, children 94–112 mEq/L, newborn	*Increased:* hyperparathyroidism; drug (ammonium chloride, ion exchange resin, phenylbutazone); metabolic acidosis; respiratory acidosis; dehydration. *Decreased:* prolonged vomiting and gastric suction; diarrhea; diuretics (ethacrynic acid and furosemide).
Magnesium 1.3–2.0 mEq/L, adult 1.6–2.6 mEq/L, children 1.4–2.9 mEq/L, newborn	*Increased:* chronic renal failure, drugs (magnesium sulfate, antacids, enemas containing magnesium, sedatives); acute adrenalcortical insufficiency. *Decreased:* chronic diarrhea and alcoholism, nontropical sprue, steatorrhea, hereditary malabsorption, starvation, bowel resection, diuretics (mannitol, urea, glucose); hypoparathyroidism.
Phosphate 2.7–4.5 mg/dL, adult 4.5–5.5 mg/dL, children 4.5–6.7 mg/dL, newborn	*Increased:* renal insufficiency; intake, IV solutions and enemas; blood transfusion; muscle necrosis; hypoparathyroidism. *Decreased:* alcohol withdrawal; hyperventilation; diabetic ketoacidosis; phosphate-binding antacids.

List of tests by body system and function

Neurological system

Brain Scan	748
Brain Sonogram	815
Caloric Study	691
Cerebral Angiography	936
Cerebrospinal Fluid Examination	501
Computed Tomography, Brain	946
Computed Tomography, Spine	957
Electroencephalography	586
Nerve Biopsy	533
Nerve Conduction Studies	599
Poliomyelitis 1, 2, 3 Titer	343
Positron Emission Tomography	774
Pseudocholinesterase	362
Sella Turcica X-ray	988
Single-Photon Emission Computed Tomography	782
Soluble Amyloid Beta-Protein Precursor	677
Spinal Nerve Root Thermography	720
St. Louis Encephalitis	416
Striational Antibody	420
Tensilon Test	725
Visual Evoked Response	735

Oncology system

5-Hydroxyindoleacetic Acid	853
Acid Phosphatase	54
Carcinoembryonic Antigen	133
Cathepsin-D	500
Cytologic Examination	513
DNA Ploidy	514
HER–2 NEU Oncogene	517
Lipid-Associated Sialic Acid	280
Mediastinoscopy	629
Melanin	882
Oncoscint Scan	770
Progesterone Receptor Assay	547
Sentinel Node Studies	780

Pulmonary system

Acid-Fast Bacterial Culture and Stain, Sputum	642
Adenovirus Antibody Titer	57
Anthrax	77
Bordetella pertussis	497
Bronchoscopy	612
Chest Radiography	938
Computed Tomography, Chest	948
Cytology, Sputum	654
Hypersensitivity Pneumonitis Serology	242
Laryngoscopy	628
Lung Biopsy	526
Lung Scan	761
Mantoux Skin Test	527
Methacholine Challenge	697
Mycoplasma Titer	310
Oximetry	703
Paranasal Sinus Films	979
pH	326
Pleural Biopsy	544
Pneumocystis IFA	342
Pulmonary Function	709
Respiratory Syncytial Virus, Antibodies IgG and IgM	384
Sleep Studies	604
Spirometry	721
Sputum Examination	678
Thoracentesis	683
Thoracoscopy Scan	637

Renal/urological system

Addis Count	856
Albumin	857
Antegrade Pyelography	923
Bladder Ultrasonography	814
Blood Urea Nitrogen	121
Cadmium	124
Catecholamines	136
Chloride	139
Computed Tomography, Renal	955
Creatinine	163
Cystography	959
Cystometry	693
Ferric Chloride	874
Glomerular Basement Membrane Antibody	210
Intravenous Pyelography	965
Inulin Clearance	262
Kidney Biopsy	521
Kidney Scan	826
Kidney Stone Analysis	523
Nephrotomography	974
Osmolality, Urine	887
Oxalate	888
Pelvic Floor Sphincter Electromyography	601
pH	326
Protein Electrophoresis	893
Renal Angiogram	986
Renin Assay	379
Specific Gravity	896
Toxicology Screening	899
Twenty-Four-Hour Urine	901

List of tests by type

General Index